CW01497833

Thoracic Tumours

WHO Classification of Tumours Editorial Board

International Agency for Research on Cancer

World Health
Organization

Suggested citation

WHO Classification of Tumours Editorial Board. Thoracic tumours.
Lyon (France): International Agency for Research on Cancer; 2021.
(WHO classification of tumours series, 5th ed.; vol. 5).
https://publications.iarc.fr/595.

Sales, rights, and permissions

Print copies are distributed by WHO Press, World Health Organization, 20 Avenue Appia, 1211 Geneva 27, Switzerland
Tel.: +41 22 791 3264; Fax: +41 22 791 4857; email: bookorders@who.int; website: https://whobluebooks.iarc.fr

To purchase IARC publications in electronic format, see the IARC Publications website (https://publications.iarc.fr).

Requests for permission to reproduce or translate IARC publications – whether for sale or for non-commercial distribution – should be submitted through the IARC Publications website (https://publications.iarc.fr/Rights-And-Permissions).

Third-party materials

If you wish to reuse material from this work that is attributed to a third party, such as figures, tables, or boxes, it is your responsibility to determine whether permission is needed for that reuse and to obtain permission from the copyright holder. See *Sources*, pages 491–498. The risk of claims resulting from infringement of any third-party-owned component in the work rests solely with the user.

General disclaimers

The designations employed and the presentation of the material in this publication do not imply the expression of any opinion whatsoever on the part of WHO or contributing agencies concerning the legal status of any country, territory, city, or area, or of its authorities, or concerning the delimitation of its frontiers or boundaries. Dotted and dashed lines on maps represent approximate border lines for which there may not yet be full agreement.

The mention of specific companies or of certain manufacturers' products does not imply that they are endorsed or recommended by WHO or contributing agencies in preference to others of a similar nature that are not mentioned. Errors and omissions excepted, the names of proprietary products are distinguished by initial capital letters.

All reasonable precautions have been taken by WHO to verify the information contained in this publication. However, the published material is being distributed without warranty of any kind, either expressed or implied. The responsibility for the interpretation and use of the material lies with the reader. In no event shall WHO or contributing agencies be liable for damages arising from its use.

First print run (10 000 copies)

Updated corrigenda can be found at https://publications.iarc.fr

IARC Library Cataloguing-in-Publication Data

Names: WHO Classification of Tumours Editorial Board.
Title: Thoracic tumours / edited by WHO Classification of Tumours Editorial Board.
Description: Fifth edition. | Lyon: International Agency for Research on Cancer, 2021. | Series: World Health Organization classification of tumours. | Includes bibliographical references and index.
Identifiers: ISBN 9789283245063 (pbk.) | ISBN 9789283245070 (ebook)
Subjects: MESH: Thoracic Neoplasms.
Classification: NLM WJ 160

This volume was produced in collaboration with

The International Association for the Study of Lung Cancer (IASLC)

The International Thymic Malignancy Interest Group (ITMIG)

The International Mesothelioma Panel (IMP)

The WHO classification of thoracic tumours presented in this book reflects the views of the WHO Classification of Tumours Editorial Board that convened via video conference 16–18 March 2020.

The WHO Classification of Tumours Editorial Board

For the complete list of all contributors and their affiliations, see pages 480–486.

For the complete list of all contributors and their affiliations, see pages 480–486.

WHO Classification of Tumours
Thoracic Tumours

Edited by	The WHO Classification of Tumours Editorial Board
IARC Editors	Dilani Lokuhetty
	Valerie A. White
	Ian A. Cree
Epidemiology	Ariana Znaor
Project Assistant	Asiedua Asante
Assistants	Anne-Sophie Hameau
	Laura Brispot
Technical Editor	Jessica Cox
Principal Information Assistant	Alberto Machado
Layout	Meaghan Fortune
	Catarina Marques
Printed by	Omnibook
	74370 Argonay, France
Publisher	International Agency for Research on Cancer (IARC)
	150 Cours Albert Thomas
	69372 Lyon Cedex 08, France

Contents

List of abbreviations

2D	two-dimensional
3D	three-dimensional
AFB	autofluorescence bronchoscopy
AMP	Association for Molecular Pathology
ATS	American Thoracic Society
bp	base pair(s)
CAP	College of American Pathologists
CNS	central nervous system
COG	Children's Oncology Group
CT	computed tomography
D_{LCO}	diffusing capacity of the lung for carbon monoxide
DNA	deoxyribonucleic acid
EBV	Epstein–Barr virus
EPD	extended pleurectomy/decortication
EPP	extrapleural pneumonectomy
ER	estrogen receptor
ERS	European Respiratory Society
ETP	early T-cell precursor
FDC	follicular dendritic cell
FDG	18F-fluorodeoxyglucose
FISH	fluorescence in situ hybridization
FNA	fine-needle aspiration
H&E	haematoxylin and eosin
H/RS cell	Hodgkin/Reed–Sternberg cell
HCV	hepatitis C virus
HIV	human immunodeficiency virus
HPF	high-power field(s)
HPV	human papillomavirus
IARC	International Agency for Research on Cancer
IASLC	International Association for the Study of Lung Cancer
ICD-11	International Classification of Diseases, 11th revision
ICD-O	International Classification of Diseases for Oncology
ICD-O-3	International Classification of Diseases for Oncology, 3rd edition
Ig	immunoglobulin
INRG	International Neuroblastoma Risk Group
ITMIG	International Thymic Malignancy Interest Group
kb	kilobase(s)
M:F ratio	male-to-female ratio
MALT	mucosa-associated lymphoid tissue
MIM number	Mendelian Inheritance in Man number
MITF	melanogenesis-associated transcription factor
MRI	magnetic resonance imaging
mRNA	messenger ribonucleic acid
N:C ratio	nuclear-to-cytoplasmic ratio
NCI	United States National Cancer Institute
NMDAR	N-methyl-D-aspartate receptor
NOS	not otherwise specified
NSE	neuron-specific enolase
PAS	periodic acid–Schiff
PASD	periodic acid–Schiff with diastase
PCR	polymerase chain reaction
PET	positron emission tomography
PR	progesterone receptor
RNA	ribonucleic acid
RT-PCR	reverse transcriptase polymerase chain reaction
SEER Program	Surveillance, Epidemiology, and End Results Program
STAS	spread through airspaces
TCGA	The Cancer Genome Atlas
TNM	tumour, node, metastasis
UICC	Union for International Cancer Control
UV	ultraviolet
WLB	white-light reflectance bronchoscopy

Foreword

The WHO Classification of Tumours, published as a series of books (also known as the WHO Blue Books) and now as a website (https://tumourclassification.iarc.who.int), is an essential tool for standardizing diagnostic practice worldwide. It also serves as a vehicle for the translation of cancer research into practice. The diagnostic criteria and standards that make up the classification are underpinned by evidence evaluated and debated by experts in the field. About 200 authors and editors participate in the production of each book, and they give their time freely to this task. I am very grateful for their help; it is a remarkable team effort.

This fifth volume of the fifth edition of the WHO Blue Books has, like the preceding four, been led by the WHO Classification of Tumours Editorial Board, composed of standing and expert members. The standing members, who have been nominated by pathology organizations, are the equivalent of the series editors of previous editions. The expert members for each volume, equivalent to the volume editors of previous editions, are selected on the basis of informed bibliometric analysis and advice from the standing members. The diagnostic process is increasingly multidisciplinary, and we are delighted that several radiology and clinical experts have joined us to address specific needs.

The most conspicuous change to the format of the books in the fifth edition is that tumour types common to multiple systems are dealt with together – so there are separate chapters on mesenchymal tumours, germ cell tumours, haematolymphoid tumours, and ectopic tumours of thyroid and parathyroid origin. There is also a chapter on genetic tumour syndromes. Genetic disorders are of increasing importance to diagnosis in individual patients, and the study of these disorders has undoubtedly informed our understanding of tumour biology and behaviour over the past decade.

We have attempted to take a more systematic approach to the multifaceted nature of tumour classification; each tumour type is described on the basis of its localization, clinical features, epidemiology, etiology, pathogenesis, histopathology, diagnostic molecular pathology, staging, and prognosis and prediction. We have also included information on macroscopic appearance and cytology, as well as essential and desirable diagnostic criteria. This standardized, modular approach makes it easier for the books to be accessible online, but it also enables us to call attention to areas in which there is little information, and where serious gaps in our knowledge remain to be addressed.

Table A Approximate number of fields per 1 mm² based on the field diameter and its corresponding area

Field diameter (mm)	Field area (mm²)	Approximate number of fields per 1 mm²
0.40	0.126	8
0.41	0.132	8
0.42	0.138	7
0.43	0.145	7
0.44	0.152	7
0.45	0.159	6
0.46	0.166	6
0.47	0.173	6
0.48	0.181	6
0.49	0.188	5
0.50	0.196	5
0.51	0.204	5
0.52	0.212	5
0.53	0.221	5
0.54	0.229	4
0.55	0.237	4
0.56	0.246	4
0.57	0.255	4
0.58	0.264	4
0.59	0.273	4
0.60	0.283	4
0.61	0.292	3
0.62	0.302	3
0.63	0.312	3
0.64	0.322	3
0.65	0.332	3
0.66	0.342	3
0.67	0.352	3
0.68	0.363	3
0.69	0.374	3

The organization of the WHO Blue Books content now follows the normal progression from benign to malignant – a break with the fourth edition, but one we hope will be welcome.

The volumes are still organized by anatomical site (digestive system, breast, soft tissue and bone, etc.), and each tumour type is listed within a taxonomic classification that follows the format below, which helps to structure the books in a systematic manner:

- Site; e.g. lung
- Category; e.g. epithelial tumours
- Family (class); e.g. papillomas
- Type; e.g. bronchial papillomas
- Subtype; e.g. glandular papilloma

The issue of whether a given tumour type represents a distinct entity rather than a subtype continues to exercise pathologists, and it is the topic of many publications in the literature. We continue to deal with this issue on a case-by-case basis, but we believe there are inherent rules that can be applied. For example, tumours in which multiple histological patterns contain shared truncal mutations are clearly of the same type, despite the differences in their appearance. Equally, genetic heterogeneity within the same tumour type may have implications for treatment. A small shift in terminology in the fifth edition is that the term "variant" in reference to a specific kind of tumour has been wholly superseded by "subtype", in an effort to more clearly differentiate this meaning from that of "variant" in reference to a genetic alteration.

Another important change in this edition of the WHO Classification of Tumours series is the conversion of mitotic count from the traditional denominator of 10 HPF to a defined area expressed in mm^2. This serves to standardize the true area over which mitoses are enumerated, because different microscopes have high-power fields of different sizes. This change will also be helpful for anyone reporting using digital systems. The approximate number of fields per 1 mm^2 based on the field diameter and its corresponding area is presented in Table A.

We are continually working to improve the consistency and standards within the classification. In addition to having moved to the International System of Units (SI) for all mitotic counts, we have standardized genomic nomenclature by using Human Genome Variation Society (HGVS) notation. In this volume, we have also further standardized our use of units of length, adopting the convention used by the International Collaboration on Cancer Reporting (http://www.iccr-cancer.org) and the UK Royal College of Pathologists (https://www.rcpath.org/), so that the size of tumours is now given exclusively in millimetres (mm) rather than centimetres (cm). This is clearer, in our view, and avoids the use of decimal points – a common source of medical errors.

The WHO Blue Books are much appreciated by pathologists and of increasing importance to practitioners of other clinical disciplines involved in cancer management, as well as to researchers. The editorial board and I certainly hope that the series will continue to meet the need for standards in diagnosis and to facilitate the translation of diagnostic research into practice worldwide. It is particularly important that cancers continue to be classified and diagnosed according to the same standards internationally so that patients can benefit from multicentre clinical trials, as well as from the results of local trials conducted on different continents.

Dr Ian A. Cree

Head, WHO Classification of Tumours Group
International Agency for Research on Cancer

March 2021

ICD-O topographical coding of thoracic tumours

The ICD-O topography codes for the main anatomical sites covered in this volume are as follows {872}:

C33 Trachea
    C33.9 Trachea

C34 Bronchus and lung
    C34.0 Main bronchus
    C34.1 Upper lobe, lung
    C34.2 Middle lobe, lung
    C34.3 Lower lobe, lung
    C34.8 Overlapping lesion of lung
    C34.9 Lung NOS

C37 Thymus
    C37.9 Thymus

C38 Heart, mediastinum, and pleura
    C38.0 Heart
    C38.1 Anterior mediastinum
    C38.2 Posterior mediastinum
    C38.3 Mediastinum NOS
    C38.4 Pleura NOS
    C38.8 Overlapping lesion of heart, mediastinum, and pleura

C39 Other and ill-defined sites within respiratory system and intrathoracic organs
    C39.0 Upper respiratory tract NOS
    C39.8 Overlapping lesion of respiratory system and intrathoracic organs
    C39.9 Ill-defined sites within respiratory system

C76 Other and ill-defined sites
    C76.1 Thorax NOS

C77 Lymph nodes
    C77.1 Intrathoracic lymph nodes

ICD-O morphological coding: Introduction

The ICD-O coding system uses a topography (T) code and a morphology (M) code together, but these are presented in separate lists for ease of use. Behaviour is coded /0 for benign tumours; /1 for unspecified, borderline, or uncertain behaviour; /2 for carcinoma in situ and grade III intraepithelial neoplasia; /3 for malignant tumours, primary site; and /6 for malignant tumours, metastatic site. Behaviour code /6 is not generally used by cancer registries. For various reasons, the ICD-O morphology terms may not always be identical to the entity names used in the WHO classification, but they should be sufficiently similar to avoid confusion. The designation "NOS" ("not otherwise specified") is provided to make coding possible when subtypes exist but exact classification may not be possible in small biopsies or certain other scenarios. Therefore, it is usual to have "NOS" even when a more specific alternative term is listed in ICD-O.

ICD-O coding of tumours of the lung

Epithelial tumours
Papillomas
8052/0   Squamous cell papilloma, NOS
8053/0   Squamous cell papilloma, inverted
8260/0   Glandular papilloma
8560/0   Mixed squamous cell and glandular papilloma

Adenomas
8832/0   Sclerosing pneumocytoma
8251/0   Alveolar adenoma
8260/0   Papillary adenoma
8140/0   Bronchiolar adenoma / ciliated muconodular papillary
        tumour[†]
8470/0   Mucinous cystadenoma
8480/0   Mucous gland adenoma

Precursor glandular lesions
8250/0   Atypical adenomatous hyperplasia
    Adenocarcinoma in situ
8250/2   Adenocarcinoma in situ, non-mucinous
8253/2   Adenocarcinoma in situ, mucinous

Adenocarcinomas
    Minimally invasive adenocarcinoma
8256/3   Minimally invasive adenocarcinoma, non-mucinous
8257/3   Minimally invasive adenocarcinoma, mucinous
    Invasive non-mucinous adenocarcinoma
8250/3   Lepidic adenocarcinoma
8551/3   Acinar adenocarcinoma
8260/3   Papillary adenocarcinoma
8265/3   Micropapillary adenocarcinoma
8230/3   Solid adenocarcinoma
8253/3   Invasive mucinous adenocarcinoma
8254/3   Mixed invasive mucinous and non-mucinous
        adenocarcinoma
8480/3   Colloid adenocarcinoma
8333/3   Fetal adenocarcinoma
8144/3   Adenocarcinoma, enteric-type
8140/3   Adenocarcinoma, NOS

Squamous precursor lesions
8070/2   Squamous cell carcinoma in situ
8077/0   Mild squamous dysplasia
8077/2   Moderate squamous dysplasia
8077/2   Severe squamous dysplasia

Squamous cell carcinomas
8070/3   Squamous cell carcinoma, NOS
8071/3   Squamous cell carcinoma, keratinizing
8072/3   Squamous cell carcinoma, non-keratinizing
8083/3   Basaloid squamous cell carcinoma
8082/3   Lymphoepithelial carcinoma

Large cell carcinomas
8012/3   Large cell carcinoma

Adenosquamous carcinomas
8560/3   Adenosquamous carcinoma

Sarcomatoid carcinomas
8022/3   Pleomorphic carcinoma
8031/3   Giant cell carcinoma
8032/3   Spindle cell carcinoma
8972/3   Pulmonary blastoma
8980/3   Carcinosarcoma

Other epithelial tumours
8023/3   NUT carcinoma
8044/3   Thoracic SMARCA4-deficient undifferentiated tumour[†]

Salivary gland–type tumours
8940/0   Pleomorphic adenoma
8200/3   Adenoid cystic carcinoma
8562/3   Epithelial-myoepithelial carcinoma
8430/3   Mucoepidermoid carcinoma
8310/3   Hyalinizing clear cell carcinoma[†]
8982/0   Myoepithelioma
8982/3   Myoepithelial carcinoma

Lung neuroendocrine neoplasms
Precursor lesion
8040/0   Diffuse idiopathic neuroendocrine cell hyperplasia

Neuroendocrine tumours
8240/3   Carcinoid tumour, NOS / neuroendocrine tumour, NOS
8240/3   Typical carcinoid / neuroendocrine tumour, grade 1
8249/3   Atypical carcinoid / neuroendocrine tumour, grade 2

Neuroendocrine carcinomas
8041/3   Small cell carcinoma
8045/3   Combined small cell carcinoma
8013/3   Large cell neuroendocrine carcinoma
8013/3   Combined large cell neuroendocrine carcinoma

Tumours of ectopic tissues
8720/3   Melanoma
9530/0   Meningioma

Mesenchymal tumours specific to the lung
8992/0   Pulmonary hamartoma
9220/0   Chondroma
9170/3   Diffuse lymphangiomatosis[†]
8973/3   Pleuropulmonary blastoma
9137/3   Intimal sarcoma
8827/1   Congenital peribronchial myofibroblastic tumour
8842/3   Pulmonary myxoid sarcoma with *EWSR1-CREB1* fusion

PEComatous tumours
9174/3*   Lymphangioleiomyomatosis
8714/0   PEComa, benign
8714/3   PEComa, malignant

Haematolymphoid tumours

9699/3	MALT lymphoma
9680/3	Diffuse large B-cell lymphoma, NOS
9766/1	Lymphomatoid granulomatosis, NOS
9766/1	Lymphomatoid granulomatosis, grade 1
9766/1	Lymphomatoid granulomatosis, grade 2
9766/3	Lymphomatoid granulomatosis, grade 3
9712/3	Intravascular large B-cell lymphoma
9751/1	Langerhans cell histiocytosis
9749/3	Erdheim–Chester disease

―――――――

These morphology codes are from the International Classification of Diseases for Oncology, third edition, second revision (ICD-O-3.2) {1256}. Behaviour is coded /0 for benign tumours; /1 for unspecified, borderline, or uncertain behaviour; /2 for carcinoma in situ and grade III intraepithelial neoplasia; /3 for malignant tumours, primary site; and /6 for malignant tumours, metastatic site. Behaviour code /6 is not generally used by cancer registries.

This classification is modified from the previous WHO classification, taking into account changes in our understanding of these lesions.

Subtype labels are indented.

* Codes marked with an asterisk were approved by the IARC/WHO Committee for ICD-O at its meeting in October 2020.

† Labels marked with a dagger constitute a change in terminology of a previous code.

ICD-O coding of tumours of the pleura and pericardium

Mesothelial tumours
Benign and preinvasive mesothelial tumours
9054/0   Adenomatoid tumour
9052/1   Well-differentiated papillary mesothelial tumour[†]
9050/2* Mesothelioma in situ

Mesothelioma
9050/3   Localized mesothelioma[†]
9050/3   Diffuse mesothelioma, NOS[†]
9051/3   Sarcomatoid mesothelioma
9052/3   Epithelioid mesothelioma
9053/3   Mesothelioma, biphasic

Haematolymphoid tumours
9678/3   Primary effusion lymphoma
9680/3   Diffuse large B-cell lymphoma associated with chronic inflammation

---

These morphology codes are from the International Classification of Diseases for Oncology, third edition, second revision (ICD-O-3.2) {1256}. Behaviour is coded /0 for benign tumours; /1 for unspecified, borderline, or uncertain behaviour; /2 for carcinoma in situ and grade III intraepithelial neoplasia; /3 for malignant tumours, primary site; and /6 for malignant tumours, metastatic site. Behaviour code /6 is not generally used by cancer registries.

This classification is modified from the previous WHO classification, taking into account changes in our understanding of these lesions.

Subtype labels are indented.

* Codes marked with an asterisk were approved by the IARC/WHO Committee for ICD-O at its meeting in October 2020.

[†] Labels marked with a dagger constitute a change in terminology of a previous code.

ICD-O coding of tumours of the heart

Benign tumours

8820/0	Papillary fibroelastoma[†]
8840/0	Myxoma, NOS
8810/0	Fibroma, NOS
8900/0	Rhabdomyoma, NOS
8904/0	Adult cellular rhabdomyoma
8850/0	Lipoma, NOS
	Lipomatous hamartoma of atrioventricular valve
	Hamartoma of mature cardiac myocytes
	Mesenchymal cardiac hamartoma
9120/0	Haemangioma, NOS
9122/0	Venous haemangioma
9131/0	Capillary haemangioma
9123/0	Arteriovenous haemangioma
9121/0	Cavernous haemangioma
	Conduction system hamartoma
8454/0	Cystic tumour of atrioventricular node

Malignant tumours

9120/3	Angiosarcoma
8890/3	Leiomyosarcoma, NOS
8802/3	Pleomorphic sarcoma

Haematolymphoid tumours

9680/3	Diffuse large B-cell lymphoma, NOS
9680/3	Fibrin-associated diffuse large B-cell lymphoma[†]

These morphology codes are from the International Classification of Diseases for Oncology, third edition, second revision (ICD-O-3.2) {1256}. Behaviour is coded /0 for benign tumours; /1 for unspecified, borderline, or uncertain behaviour; /2 for carcinoma in situ and grade III intraepithelial neoplasia; /3 for malignant tumours, primary site; and /6 for malignant tumours, metastatic site. Behaviour code /6 is not generally used by cancer registries.

This classification is modified from the previous WHO classification, taking into account changes in our understanding of these lesions.

Subtype labels are indented.

[†] Labels marked with a dagger constitute a change in terminology of a previous code.

ICD-O coding of mesenchymal tumours of the thorax

Adipocytic tumours
8850/0   Lipoma, NOS
8850/0   Thymolipoma
8850/3   Liposarcoma, NOS
8851/3   Liposarcoma, well differentiated
8852/3   Myxoid liposarcoma
8854/3   Pleomorphic liposarcoma
8858/3   Dedifferentiated liposarcoma

Fibroblastic and myofibroblastic tumours
8821/1   Desmoid-type fibromatosis
8815/1   Solitary fibrous tumour, NOS
8817/0   Calcifying fibrous tumour
8825/1   Inflammatory myofibroblastic tumour
8811/3   Myxofibrosarcoma

Vascular tumours
9120/0   Haemangioma, NOS
9121/0   Cavernous haemangioma
9122/0   Venous haemangioma
9132/0   Intramuscular haemangioma
9123/0   Arteriovenous haemangioma
9170/0   Lymphangioma, NOS
9173/0   Cystic lymphangioma
9133/3   Epithelioid haemangioendothelioma
9120/3   Angiosarcoma

Skeletal muscle tumours
8900/3   Rhabdomyosarcoma, NOS
8910/3   Embryonal rhabdomyosarcoma
8912/3   Spindle cell rhabdomyosarcoma
8920/3   Alveolar rhabdomyosarcoma
8901/3   Pleomorphic rhabdomyosarcoma

Peripheral nerve sheath and neural tumours
8693/3   Extra-adrenal paraganglioma
9580/0   Granular cell tumour
9580/3   Granular cell tumour, malignant
9560/0   Schwannoma
9540/3   Malignant peripheral nerve sheath tumour
9490/0   Ganglioneuroma
9490/3   Ganglioneuroblastoma
9500/3   Neuroblastoma

Tumours of uncertain differentiation
9040/3   Synovial sarcoma, NOS
9041/3   Synovial sarcoma, spindle cell
9042/3   Synovial sarcoma, epithelioid cell
9043/3   Synovial sarcoma, biphasic
9364/3   Ewing sarcoma
9367/3*   *CIC*-rearranged sarcoma
9368/3*   Sarcoma with *BCOR* genetic alterations
9366/3*   Round cell sarcoma with *EWSR1*–non-ETS fusions

These morphology codes are from the International Classification of Diseases for Oncology, third edition, second revision (ICD-O-3.2) {1256}. Behaviour is coded /0 for benign tumours; /1 for unspecified, borderline, or uncertain behaviour; /2 for carcinoma in situ and grade III intraepithelial neoplasia; /3 for malignant tumours, primary site; and /6 for malignant tumours, metastatic site. Behaviour code /6 is not generally used by cancer registries.

This classification is modified from the previous WHO classification, taking into account changes in our understanding of these lesions.

Subtype labels are indented.

* Codes marked with an asterisk were approved by the IARC/WHO Committee for ICD-O at its meeting in October 2020.

ICD-O coding of tumours of the thymus

Epithelial tumours
Thymomas
8580/3   Thymoma, NOS
8581/3   Thymoma, type A
8582/3   Thymoma, type AB
8583/3   Thymoma, type B1
8584/3   Thymoma, type B2
8585/3   Thymoma, type B3
8580/1   Micronodular thymoma with lymphoid stroma
8580/3   Metaplastic thymoma
9010/0   Lipofibroadenoma

Squamous carcinomas
8070/3   Squamous cell carcinoma, NOS
8123/3   Basaloid carcinoma
8082/3   Lymphoepithelial carcinoma

Adenocarcinomas
8140/3   Adenocarcinoma, NOS
8260/3   Low-grade papillary adenocarcinoma[†]
8200/3   Thymic carcinoma with adenoid cystic carcinoma–like
             features
8144/3   Adenocarcinoma, enteric-type

Adenosquamous carcinomas
8560/3   Adenosquamous carcinoma

NUT carcinomas
8023/3   NUT carcinoma

Salivary gland–like carcinomas
8430/3   Mucoepidermoid carcinoma
8310/3   Clear cell carcinoma
8033/3   Sarcomatoid carcinoma
8980/3   Carcinosarcoma

Undifferentiated carcinomas
8020/3   Carcinoma, undifferentiated, NOS

Thymic carcinomas
8586/3   Thymic carcinoma, NOS

Thymic neuroendocrine neoplasms
Neuroendocrine tumours
8240/3   Carcinoid tumour, NOS / neuroendocrine tumour, NOS
8240/3   Typical carcinoid / neuroendocrine tumour, grade 1
8249/3   Atypical carcinoid / neuroendocrine tumour, grade 2

Neuroendocrine carcinomas
8041/3   Small cell carcinoma
8045/3   Combined small cell carcinoma
8013/3   Large cell neuroendocrine carcinoma

These morphology codes are from the International Classification of Diseases for Oncology, third edition, second revision (ICD-O-3.2) {1256}. Behaviour is coded /0 for benign tumours; /1 for unspecified, borderline, or uncertain behaviour; /2 for carcinoma in situ and grade III intraepithelial neoplasia; /3 for malignant tumours, primary site; and /6 for malignant tumours, metastatic site. Behaviour code /6 is not generally used by cancer registries.

This classification is modified from the previous WHO classification, taking into account changes in our understanding of these lesions.

Subtype labels are indented.

[†] Labels marked with a dagger constitute a change in terminology of a previous code.

ICD-O coding of germ cell tumours of the mediastinum

9061/3	Seminoma
9070/3	Embryonal carcinoma
9071/3	Yolk sac tumour
9100/3	Choriocarcinoma
9080/0	Mature teratoma
9080/1	Immature teratoma of the thymus
9085/3	Mixed germ cell tumour
9084/3	Teratoma with somatic-type malignancies
9086/3	Germ cell tumour with associated haematological malignancy

These morphology codes are from the International Classification of Diseases for Oncology, third edition, second revision (ICD-O-3.2) {1256}. Behaviour is coded /0 for benign tumours; /1 for unspecified, borderline, or uncertain behaviour; /2 for carcinoma in situ and grade III intraepithelial neoplasia; /3 for malignant tumours, primary site; and /6 for malignant tumours, metastatic site. Behaviour code /6 is not generally used by cancer registries.

This classification is modified from the previous WHO classification, taking into account changes in our understanding of these lesions.

Subtype labels are indented.

ICD-O coding of haematolymphoid tumours of the mediastinum

9679/3	Mediastinal large B-cell lymphoma
9699/3	MALT lymphoma
9837/3	T-lymphoblastic leukaemia/lymphoma
9650/3	Classic Hodgkin lymphoma, NOS[†]
9663/3	Classic Hodgkin lymphoma, nodular sclerosis
9652/3	Classic Hodgkin lymphoma, mixed cellularity
9651/3	Classic Hodgkin lymphoma, lymphocyte-rich
9653/3	Classic Hodgkin lymphoma, lymphocyte depletion
9596/3	Grey zone lymphoma[†]
9758/3	Follicular dendritic cell sarcoma
9930/3	Myeloid sarcoma

These morphology codes are from the International Classification of Diseases for Oncology, third edition, second revision (ICD-O-3.2) {1256}. Behaviour is coded /0 for benign tumours; /1 for unspecified, borderline, or uncertain behaviour; /2 for carcinoma in situ and grade III intraepithelial neoplasia; /3 for malignant tumours, primary site; and /6 for malignant tumours, metastatic site. Behaviour code /6 is not generally used by cancer registries.

This classification is modified from the previous WHO classification, taking into account changes in our understanding of these lesions.

Subtype labels are indented.

[†] Labels marked with a dagger constitute a change in terminology of a previous code.

ICD-O coding of ectopic tumours of thyroid and parathyroid origin

Thyroid neoplasms
8260/3   Papillary carcinoma of thyroid
8330/0   Follicular adenoma
8330/3   Follicular carcinoma
8345/3   Medullary thyroid carcinoma

Parathyroid neoplasms
8140/0   Parathyroid adenoma
8140/3   Parathyroid carcinoma

These morphology codes are from the International Classification of Diseases for Oncology, third edition, second revision (ICD-O-3.2) {1256}. Behaviour is coded /0 for benign tumours; /1 for unspecified, borderline, or uncertain behaviour; /2 for carcinoma in situ and grade III intraepithelial neoplasia; /3 for malignant tumours, primary site; and /6 for malignant tumours, metastatic site. Behaviour code /6 is not generally used by cancer registries.

This classification is modified from the previous WHO classification, taking into account changes in our understanding of these lesions.

Subtype labels are indented.

TNM staging of lung, pleural, and thymic tumours

Lung, Pleural, and Thymic Tumours

Introductory Notes

The classifications apply to carcinomas of the lung including non-small cell and small cell carcinomas, bronchopulmonary carcinoid tumours, malignant mesothelioma of pleura, and thymic tumours.

Each site is described under the following headings:
- Rules for classification with the procedures for assessing T, N, and M categories; additional methods may be used when they enhance the accuracy of appraisal before treatment
- Anatomical subsites where appropriate
- Definition of the regional lymph nodes
- TNM clinical classification
- pTNM pathological classification
- Stage

Regional Lymph Nodes

The regional lymph nodes extend from the supraclavicular region to the diaphragm. Direct extension of the primary tumour into lymph nodes is classified as lymph node metastasis.

TNM staging of carcinomas of the lung

Lung
(ICD-O-3 C34)

Rules for Classification
The classification applies to carcinomas of the lung including non-small cell carcinomas, small cell carcinomas, and bronchopulmonary carcinoid tumours. It does not apply to sarcomas and other rare tumours.

Changes in this edition from the seventh edition are based upon recommendations from the International Association for the Study of Lung Cancer (IASLC) Staging Project (see references).[1–6]

There should be histological confirmation of the disease and division of cases by histological type.

The following are the procedures for assessing T, N, and M categories:

T categories	Physical examination, imaging, endoscopy, and/or surgical exploration
N categories	Physical examination, imaging, endoscopy, and/or surgical exploration
M categories	Physical examination, imaging, and/or surgical exploration

Anatomical Subsites
1. Main bronchus (C34.0)
2. Upper lobe (C34.1)
3. Middle lobe (C34.2)
4. Lower lobe (C34.3)

Regional Lymph Nodes
The regional lymph nodes are the intrathoracic nodes (mediastinal, hilar, lobar, interlobar, segmental, and subsegmental), scalene, and supraclavicular lymph nodes.

TNM Clinical Classification
T – Primary Tumour
TX	Primary tumour cannot be assessed, *or* tumour proven by the presence of malignant cells in sputum or bronchial washings but not visualized by imaging or bronchoscopy
T0	No evidence of primary tumour
Tis	Carcinoma in situ[a]

T1 Tumour 3 cm or less in greatest dimension, surrounded by lung or visceral pleura, without bronchoscopic evidence of invasion more proximal than the lobar bronchus (i.e., not in the main bronchus)[b]
- T1mi Minimally invasive adenocarcinoma[c]
- T1a Tumour 1 cm or less in greatest dimension[b]
- T1b Tumour more than 1 cm but not more than 2 cm in greatest dimension[b]
- T1c Tumour more than 2 cm but not more than 3 cm in greatest dimension[b]

T2 Tumour more than 3 cm but not more than 5 cm; or tumour with *any* of the following features[d]
- Involves main bronchus regardless of distance to the carina, but without involvement of the carina
- Invades visceral pleura
- Associated with atelectasis or obstructive pneumonitis that extends to the hilar region either involving part of or the entire lung
  - T2a Tumour more than 3 cm but not more than 4 cm in greatest dimension
  - T2b Tumour more than 4 cm but not more than 5 cm in greatest dimension

T3 Tumour more than 5 cm but not more than 7 cm in greatest dimension or one that directly invades any of the following: parietal pleura, chest wall (including superior sulcus tumours) phrenic nerve, parietal pericardium; or separate tumour nodule(s) in the same lobe as the primary

T4 Tumour more than 7 cm or of any size that invades any of the following: diaphragm, mediastinum, heart, great vessels, trachea, recurrent laryngeal nerve, oesophagus, vertebral body, carina; separate tumour nodule(s) in a different ipsilateral lobe to that of the primary

N – Regional Lymph Nodes
NX	Regional lymph nodes cannot be assessed
N0	No regional lymph node metastasis
N1	Metastasis in ipsilateral peribronchial and/or ipsilateral hilar lymph nodes and intrapulmonary nodes, including involvement by direct extension
N2	Metastasis in ipsilateral mediastinal and/or subcarinal lymph node(s)
N3	Metastasis in contralateral mediastinal, contralateral hilar, ipsilateral or contralateral scalene, or supraclavicular lymph node(s)

M – Distant Metastasis

M0 No distant metastasis
M1 Distant metastasis

M1a	Separate tumour nodule(s) in a contralateral lobe; tumour with pleural or pericardial nodules or malignant pleural or pericardial effusion[e]
M1b	Single extrathoracic metastasis in a single organ[f]
M1c	Multiple extrathoracic metastasis in a single or multiple organs

Notes

[a] Tis includes adenocarcinoma in situ and squamous carcinoma in situ.

[b] The uncommon superficial spreading tumour of any size with its invasive component limited to the bronchial wall, which may extend proximal to the main bronchus, is also classified as T1a.

[c] Solitary adenocarcinoma (not more than 3 cm in greatest dimension), with a predominantly lepidic pattern and not more than 5 mm invasion in greatest dimension in any one focus.

[d] T2 tumours with these features are classified T2a if 4 cm or less, or if size cannot be determined, and T2b if greater than 4 cm but not larger than 5 cm.

[e] Most pleural (pericardial) effusions with lung cancer are due to tumour. In a few patients, however, multiple microscopic examinations of pleural (pericardial) fluid are negative for tumour, and the fluid is non-bloody and is not an exudate. Where these elements and clinical judgment dictate that the effusion is not related to the tumour, the effusion should be excluded as a staging descriptor.

[f] This includes involvement of a single non-regional node.

pTNM Pathological Classification

The pT and pN categories correspond to the T and N categories.

pN0 Histological examination of hilar and mediastinal lymphadenectomy specimen(s) will ordinarily include 6 or more lymph nodes/stations. Three of these nodes/stations should be mediastinal, including the subcarinal nodes, and three from N1 nodes/stations. Labelling according to the IASLC chart and table of definitions given in the TNM Supplement {3331} is desirable. If all the lymph nodes examined are negative, but the number ordinarily examined is not met, classify as pN0.

pM – Distant Metastasis*

pM1 Distant metastasis microscopically confirmed

Note

* pM0 and pMX are not valid categories.

Stage

Occult carcinoma	TX	N0	M0
Stage 0	Tis	N0	M0
Stage IA	T1	N0	M0
Stage IA1	T1mi	N0	M0
	T1a	N0	M0
Stage IA2	T1b	N0	M0
Stage IA3	T1c	N0	M0
Stage IB	T2a	N0	M0
Stage IIA	T2b	N0	M0
Stage IIB	T1a–c,T2a,b	N1	M0
	T3	N0	M0
Stage IIIA	T1a–c,T2a,b	N2	M0
	T3	N1	M0
	T4	N0,N1	M0
Stage IIIB	T1a–c,T2a,b	N3	M0
	T3,T4	N2	M0
Stage IIIC	T3,T4	N3	M0
Stage IV	Any T	Any N	M1
Stage IVA	Any T	Any N	M1a,b
Stage IVB	Any T	Any N	M1c

References

1 Rami-Porta R, Bolejack V, Giroux DJ, et al. The IASLC Lung Cancer Staging Project: the new database to inform the 8th edition of the TNM classification of lung cancer. *J Thorac Oncol* 2014; 9: 1618–1624.

2 Rami-Porta R, Bolejack V, Crowley J, et al. The IASLC Lung Cancer Staging Project: proposals for the revisions of the T descriptors in the forthcoming 8th edition of the TNM classification for lung cancer. *J Thorac Oncol* 2015; 10: 990–1003.

3 Asamura H, Chansky K, Crowley J, et al. The IASLC Lung Cancer Staging Project: proposals for the revisions of the N descriptors in the forthcoming 8th edition of the TNM classification for lung cancer. *J Thorac Oncol* 2015; 10: 1675–1684.

4 Eberhardt WEE, Mitchell A, Crowley J, et al. The IASLC Lung Cancer Staging Project: proposals for the revisions of the M descriptors in the forthcoming 8th edition of the TNM classification for lung cancer. *J Thorac Oncol* 2015; 10: 1515–1522.

5 Goldstraw P et al. The IASLC Lung Cancer Staging Project: proposals for the revision of the TNM stage grouping in the forthcoming (eighth) edition of the TNM classification for lung cancer. *J Thorac Oncol* 2016; 11: 39–51.

6 Nicholson AG, Chansky K, Crowley J, et al. The IASLC Lung Cancer Staging Project: proposals for the revision of the clinical and pathological staging of small cell lung cancer in the forthcoming eighth edition of the TNM classification for lung cancer. *J Thorac Oncol* 2016; 11: 300–311.

TNM staging of pleural mesothelioma

Pleural Mesothelioma
(ICD-O-3 C38.4)

Rules for Classification
The classification applies only to malignant mesothelioma of the pleura.

There should be histological confirmation of the disease.

Changes in this edition from the seventh edition are based upon recommendations from the International Association for the Study of Lung Cancer (IASLC) Staging Project.

The following are the procedures for assessing T, N, and M categories:

T categories	Physical examination, imaging, endoscopy, and/or surgical exploration
N categories	Physical examination, imaging, endoscopy, and/or surgical exploration
M categories	Physical examination, imaging, and/or surgical exploration

Regional Lymph Nodes
The regional lymph nodes are the intrathoracic, internal mammary, scalene, and supraclavicular nodes.

TNM Clinical Classification
T – Primary Tumour
TX Primary tumour cannot be assessed
T0 No evidence of primary tumour
T1 Tumour involves ipsilateral parietal pleura, with or without involvement of visceral, mediastinal or diaphragmatic pleura.
T2 Tumour involves the ipsilateral pleura (parietal or visceral pleura), with at least one of the following:
- invasion of diaphragmatic muscle
- invasion of lung parenchyma

T3 Tumour involves ipsilateral pleura (parietal or visceral pleura), with at least one of the following:
- invasion of endothoracic fascia
- invasion into mediastinal fat
- solitary focus of tumour invading soft tissues of the chest wall
- non-transmural involvement of the pericardium

T4 Tumour involves ipsilateral pleura (parietal or visceral pleura), with at least one of the following:
- chest wall, with or without associated rib destruction (diffuse or multifocal)
- peritoneum (via direct transdiaphragmatic extension)
- contralateral pleura
- mediastinal organs (oesophagus, trachea, heart, great vessels)
- vertebra, neuroforamen, spinal cord
- internal surface of the pericardium (transmural invasion with or without a pericardial effusion)

N – Regional Lymph Nodes
NX Regional lymph nodes cannot be assessed
N0 No regional lymph node metastasis
N1 Metastases to ipsilateral intrathoracic lymph nodes (includes ipsilateral bronchopulmonary, hilar, subcarinal, paratracheal, aortopulmonary, paraesophageal, peridiaphragmatic, pericardial fat pad, intercostal and internal mammary nodes)
N2 Metastases to contralateral intrathoracic lymph nodes. Metastases to ipsilateral or contralateral supraclavicular lymph nodes

M – Distant Metastasis
M0 No distant metastasis
M1 Distant metastasis

pTNM Pathological Classification
The pT and pN categories correspond to the T and N categories.

pM – Distant Metastasis*
pM1 Distant metastasis microscopically confirmed

Note
* pM0 and pMX are not valid categories.

Stage – Pleural Mesothelioma
Stage IA	T1	N0	M0
Stage IB	T2,T3	N0	M0
Stage II	T1,T2	N1	M0
Stage IIIA	T3	N1	M0
Stage IIIB	T1,T2,T3	N2	M0
	T4	Any N	M0
Stage IV	Any T	Any N	M1

TNM staging of epithelial tumours of the thymus

Thymic Tumours
(ICD-O-3 C37.9)

Rules for Classification
The classification applies to epithelial tumours of the thymus, including thymomas, thymic carcinomas and neuroendocrine tumours of the thymus. It does not apply to sarcomas, lymphomas and other rare tumours.

This classification is new to the 8th edition and is based upon recommendations from the International Association for the Study of Lung Cancer (IASLC) Staging Project and the International Thymic Malignancies Interest Group (ITMIG) (see references).[1–3]

There should be histological confirmation of the disease and division of cases by histological type.

The following are the procedures for assessing T, N, and M categories:

T categories	Physical examination, imaging, endoscopy, and/or surgical exploration
N categories	Physical examination, imaging, endoscopy, and/or surgical exploration
M categories	Physical examination, imaging, and/or surgical exploration

Regional Lymph Nodes
The regional lymph nodes are the anterior (perithymic) lymph nodes, the deep intrathoracic lymph nodes and the cervical lymph nodes.

TNM Clinical Classification
T – Primary Tumour

TX	Primary tumour cannot be assessed
T0	No evidence of primary tumour
T1	Tumour encapsulated or extending into the mediastinal fat, may involve the mediastinal pleura.
T1a	No mediastinal pleural involvement
T1b	Direct invasion of the mediastinal pleura
T2	Tumour with direct involvement of the pericardium (partial or full thickness).
T3	Tumour with direct invasion into any of the following: lung, brachiocephalic vein, superior vena cava, phrenic nerve, chest wall, or extrapericardial pulmonary artery or vein.
T4	Tumour with direct invasion into any of the following: aorta (ascending, arch or descending), arch vessels, intrapericardial pulmonary artery, myocardium, trachea, or oesophagus

N – Regional Lymph Nodes

NX	Regional lymph nodes cannot be assessed
N0	No regional lymph node metastasis
N1	Metastasis in anterior (perithymic) lymph nodes
N2	Metastasis in deep intrathoracic or cervical lymph nodes

M – Distant Metastasis

M0	No pleural, pericardial or distant metastasis
M1	Distant metastasis
M1a	Separate pleural or pericardial nodule(s)
M1b	Distant metastasis beyond the pleura or pericardium

pTNM Pathological Classification
The pT and pN categories correspond to the T and N categories.

pM – Distant Metastasis*

pM1   Distant metastasis microscopically confirmed

Note
* pM0 and pMX are not valid categories.

Stage – Thymus Tumours

Stage I	T1	N0	M0
Stage II	T2	N0	M0
Stage IIIA	T3	N0	M0
Stage IIIB	T4	N0	M0
Stage IVA	Any T	N1	M0
	Any T	N0,N1	M1a
Stage IVB	Any T	N2	M0,M1a
	Any T	Any N	M1b

References
1   Nicholson AG, Detterbeck FC, Marino M, et al. The IASLC/ITMIG thymic epithelial tumors staging project: proposals for the T component for the forthcoming (8th) edition of the TNM classification of malignant tumors. *J Thorac Oncol* 2014; 9: s73–s80.
2   Kondo K, Van Schil P, Detterbeck FC, et al. The IASLC/ITMIG thymic epithelial tumors staging project: proposals for the N and M components for the forthcoming (8th) edition of the TNM classification of malignant tumors. *J Thorac Oncol* 2014; 9: s81–s87.
3   Detterbeck FC, Stratton K, Giroux D, et al. The IASLC/ITMIG thymic epithelial tumors staging project: proposal for an evidence-based stage classification system for the forthcoming (8th) edition of the TNM classification of malignant tumors. *J Thorac Oncol* 2014; 9: s65–s72.

TNM staging of tumours of soft tissues

Soft Tissues
(ICD-O-3 C38.1, 2, 3, C47-49)

Rules for Classification
There should be histological confirmation of the disease and division of cases by histological type and grade.

The following are the procedures for assessing T, N, and M categories:

T categories   Physical examination and imaging
N categories   Physical examination and imaging
M categories   Physical examination and imaging

Anatomical Sites
1. Connective, subcutaneous, and other soft tissues (C49), peripheral nerves (C47)
2. Retroperitoneum (C48.0)
3. Mediastinum: anterior (C38.1); posterior (C38.2); mediastinum, NOS (C38.3)

Histological Types of Tumour
The following histological types are not included:
- Kaposi sarcoma
- Dermatofibrosarcoma (protuberans)
- Fibromatosis (desmoid tumour)
- Sarcoma arising from the dura mater and brain
- Angiosarcoma, an aggressive sarcoma, is excluded because its natural history is not consistent with the classification.

Note
Cystosarcoma phyllodes is staged as a soft tissue sarcoma of the superficial trunk.

Regional Lymph Nodes
The regional lymph nodes are those appropriate to the site of the primary tumour. Regional node involvement is rare and cases in which nodal status is not assessed either clinically or pathologically could be considered N0 instead of NX or pNX.

TNM Clinical Classification
T – Primary Tumour
TX   Primary tumour cannot be assessed
T0   No evidence of primary tumour

Extremity and Superficial Trunk
T1   Tumour 5 cm or less in greatest dimension
T2   Tumour more than 5 cm but no more than 10 cm in greatest dimension
T3   Tumour more than 10 cm but no more than 15 cm in greatest dimension
T4   Tumour more than 15 cm in greatest dimension

Retroperitoneum
T1   Tumour 5 cm or less in greatest dimension
T2   Tumour more than 5 cm but no more than 10 cm in greatest dimension
T3   Tumour more than 10 cm but no more than 15 cm in greatest dimension
T4   Tumour more than 15 cm in greatest dimension

Head and Neck
T1   Tumour 2 cm or less in greatest dimension
T2   Tumour more than 2 cm but no more than 4 cm in greatest dimension
T3   Tumour more than 4 cm in greatest dimension
T4a Tumour invades the orbit, skull base or dura, central compartment viscera, facial skeleton, and/or pterygoid muscles
T4b Tumour invades the brain parenchyma, encases the carotid artery, invades prevertebral muscle or involves the central nervous system by perineural spread

Thoracic and Abdominal Viscera
T1   Tumour confined to a single organ
T2a Tumour invades serosa or visceral peritoneum
T2b Tumour with microscopic extension beyond the serosa
T3   Tumour invades another organ or macroscopic extension beyond the serosa
T4a Multifocal tumour involving no more than two sites in one organ
T4b Multifocal tumour involving more than two sites but not more than 5 sites
T4c Multifocal tumour involving more than five sites

N – Regional Lymph Nodes
NX   Regional lymph nodes cannot be assessed
N0   No regional lymph node metastasis
N1   Regional lymph node metastasis

M – Distant Metastasis
M0   No distant metastasis
M1   Distant metastasis

pTNM Pathological Classification
The pT and pN categories correspond to the T and N categories.

pM – Distant Metastasis*
pM1 Distant metastasis microscopically confirmed

Note
* pM0 and pMX are not valid categories

Stage – Extremity and Superficial Trunk and Retroperitoneum

Stage IA	T1	N0	M0	G1,GX Low Grade
Stage IB	T2,T3,T4	N0	M0	G1,GX Low Grade
Stage II	T1	N0	M0	G2,G3 High Grade
Stage IIIA	T2	N0	M0	G2,G3 High Grade
Stage IIIB	T3,T4	N0	M0	G2,G3 High Grade
	Any T	N1*	M0	Any G
Stage IV	Any T	Any N	M1	Any G

Note
* AJCC classifies N1 as stage IV for extremity and superficial trunk.

Stage – Head and Neck and Thoracic and Abdominal Viscera

There is no stage for soft tissue sarcoma of the head and neck and thoracic and abdominal viscera.

Staging of Hodgkin and non-Hodgkin lymphomas

Hodgkin Lymphoma

Introductory Notes

The current staging classification for Hodgkin Lymphoma is a modification of the Ann Arbor classification first adopted in 1971. Over the past 45 years the practice has changed, making the previously used staging laparotomy and the resulting pathological staging classification obsolete. The recent consensus conference that took place in 2012 in Lugano suggested even more simplified system putting together stage I and II as Limited Stage and stage III and IV as Advanced Stage lymphoma. The Lugano Classification, a modification of the Ann Arbor classification, has been published and accepted by the UICC.[1]

Clinical Staging (cS)

It is determined by history, clinical examination, imaging, blood analysis, and the initial biopsy report. Bone marrow biopsy must be taken from a clinically or radiologically non-involved area of bone.

Liver Involvement
Clinical evidence of liver involvement must include either enlargement of the liver and at least an abnormal serum alkaline phosphatase level and two different liver function test abnormalities, or an abnormal liver demonstrated by imaging and one abnormal liver function test.

Spleen Involvement
Clinical evidence of spleen involvement is accepted if there is palpable enlargement of the spleen confirmed by imaging.

Lymphatic and Extralymphatic Disease
The lymphatic structures are as follows:
- Lymph nodes
- Waldeyer ring
- Spleen
- Appendix
- Thymus
- Peyer patches

The lymph nodes are grouped into regions and one or more (2, 3, etc.) may be involved. The spleen is designated S and extralymphatic organs or sites E.

Lung Involvement
Lung involvement limited to one lobe, or perihilar extension associated with ipsilateral lymphadenopathy, or unilateral pleural effusion with or without lung involvement but with hilar lymphade-nopathy is considered as **localized** extralymphatic disease.

Liver Involvement
Liver involvement is always considered as **diffuse** extralymphatic disease.

Clinical Stages (cS)
Limited Stage
Stage I
Involvement of a single lymph node region (I), or localized involvement of a single extralymphatic organ or site (IE).

Stage II
Involvement of two or more lymph node regions on the same side of the diaphragm (II), or localized involvement of a single extralymphatic organ or site and its regional lymph node(s) with or without involvement of other contiguous lymph node regions on the same side of the diaphragm (IIE).

Bulky Stage II
Stage II disease with a single nodal mass greater than 10 cm in maximum dimension or greater than a third of the thoracic diameter as assessed on CT.

Advanced Stage
Stage III
Involvement of lymph node regions on both sides of the diaphragm (III), which may also be accompanied by involvement of the spleen (IIIS).

Stage IV
Disseminated (multifocal) involvement of one or more extralymphatic organs, with or without associated lymph node involvement; or non-contiguous extralymphatic organ involvement with involvement of lymph node regions on the same or both sides of the diaphragm.

A and B Classification (Symptoms)
Each stage should be divided into A and B according to the absence or presence of defined general symptoms. These are:
1. Unexplained weight loss of more than 10% of the usual body weight in the 6 months prior to first attendance
2. Unexplained fever with temperature above 38 °C
3. Night sweats

Note
Pruritus alone does not qualify for B classification nor does a short, febrile illness associated with a known infection.

Reference
1   Cheson BD, Fisher RI, Barrington SF, et al. Recommendations for initial evaluation, staging, and response assessment of Hodgkin and non-Hodgkin lymphoma: the Lugano classification. *J Clin Oncol* 2014; 32: 3059–3068.

Non-Hodgkin Lymphomas

The Lugano classification, a modification of the Ann Arbor classification, is recommended as for Hodgkin lymphoma with the exception of the elimination of the A or B classification of symptoms (see above).

In Stage II disease, bulk is defined as larger than 6 cm in greatest dimension in follicular lymphoma, and 10 cm in largest dimension has been recommended for diffuse large cell lymphoma.

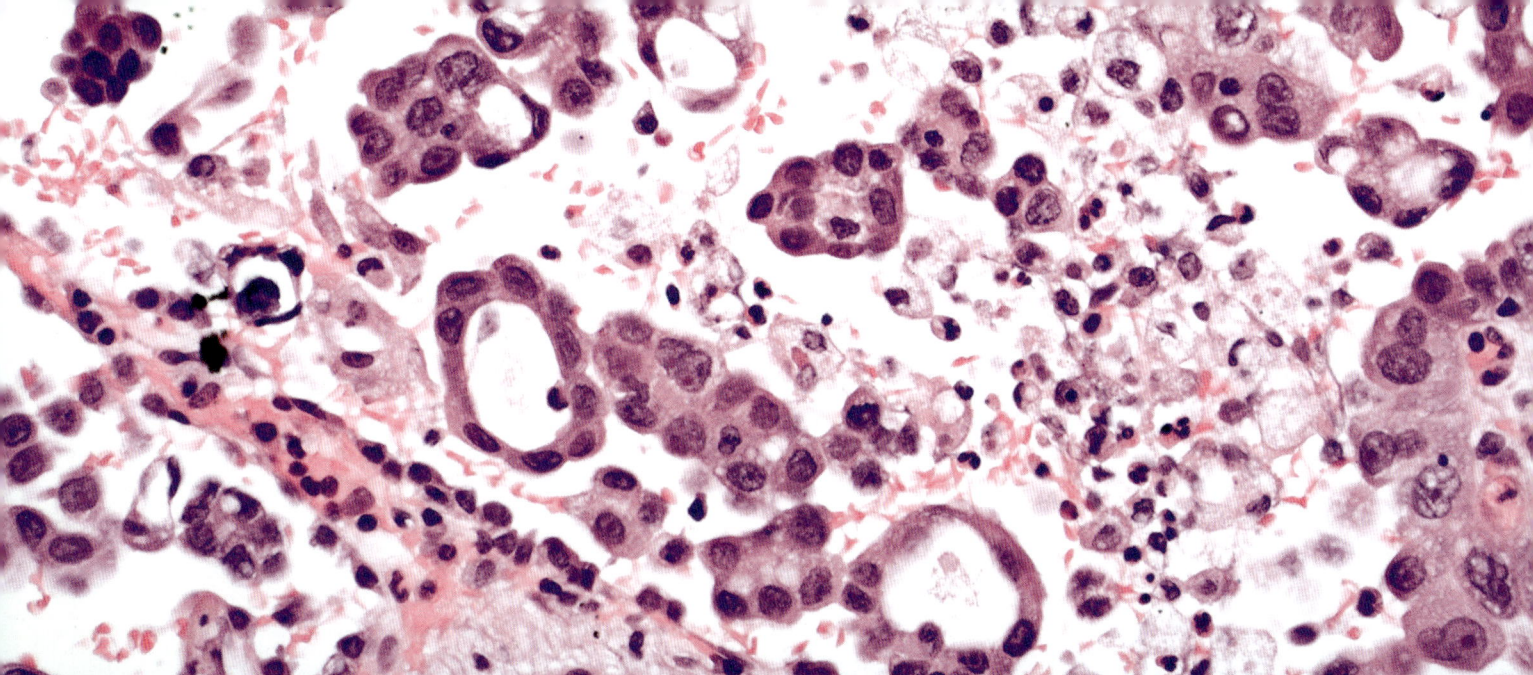

1

Tumours of the lung

Edited by: Borczuk AC, Chan JKC, Cooper WA, Dacic S, Kerr KM, Lantuejoul S, Marx A, Nicholson AG, Scagliotti GV, Thompson LDR, Travis WD, Tsao MS, Yatabe Y

Papillomas
Adenomas
Precursor glandular lesions
Adenocarcinomas
Squamous precursor lesions
Squamous cell carcinomas
Large cell carcinomas
Adenosquamous carcinoma
Sarcomatoid carcinomas
Other epithelial tumours
Salivary gland–type tumours
Lung neuroendocrine neoplasms
Tumours of ectopic tissues
Mesenchymal tumours specific to the lung
Haematolymphoid tumours

Tumours of the lung: Introduction

Tsao MS
Asamura H
Borczuk AC
Dacic S
Devesa SS
Kerr KM
MacMahon H

Rusch VW
Samet JM
Scagliotti GV
Travis WD
Van Schil PEY
Yatabe Y
Znaor A

During the past 15 years, the world has witnessed accelerating advances in the treatment of lung cancer patients, translating into significant improvements in patient survival. These improvements have largely been propelled by rapid advances in our knowledge of molecular aberrations occurring in this disease, technological advances in how we interrogate these aberrations, and development of new therapeutics to overcome them. Nevertheless, histological classification of the tumours remains the backbone of lung cancer diagnosis and patient management. This fifth edition of the WHO classification of thoracic tumours represents the current state of science in lung cancer classification, based primarily on histopathological features and patterns, but closely integrated with immunohistochemistry and genetic features of the tumours.

Epidemiology and etiology
Tobacco smoking
Lung cancer is the most common cause of cancer death worldwide, reflecting the global epidemic characteristics of the cause of most cases: tobacco smoking {1743}. Mortality and incidence rates have generally been highest in high-income countries, in particular the USA and European countries, but are now declining progressively, particularly in younger males and females. Lung cancer has long been more common in men than in women, but in many high-income countries (e.g. the USA, Denmark, and Sweden), incidence rates in men and women have begun converging {1738}. Lung cancer remains the leading cause of cancer incidence and mortality, with more than 2 million new cases and 1.7 million deaths estimated globally in 2018 {309}. Around the world, the current spatial and temporal patterns of lung cancer occurrence largely reflects historical patterns of cigarette smoking; rates are low in much of Africa, while the highest rates are observed in Europe, Asia, and North America. Rates are consistently lower among women, with the highest M:F ratio (of ~5) reported from northern Africa and western Asia, and the lowest (1.2) from Oceania {309,1931}.

Through decades of research, many causal risk factors for lung cancer have been identified, including smoking combustible tobacco products, radon exposure in indoor environments and mines, other occupational agents (e.g. asbestos), and outdoor air pollution {48}. Cigarette smoking is the leading cause of lung cancer, with 1.19 million lung cancer deaths attributable to smoking worldwide in 2017 {928}. The risks in smokers increase with the duration of smoking and the number of cigarettes smoked daily, and they progressively decline after smoking cessation (although never to the level among never-smokers). Lung cancer does occur among never-smokers, at estimated rates as low as 5–10 cases per 100 000 population annually, but at higher rates in some populations according to data from cohort studies {3035}; by contrast, the rates in smokers are as much as 20–30 times as high. However, in the USA,

it is estimated there are 17 000–26 000 annual deaths from lung cancer in never-smokers – as a separate entity this would be the seventh leading cause of cancer mortality {2497}. Possible etiological factors for lung cancer among never-smokers include exposure to secondhand tobacco smoke, radon, various occupational agents, outdoor air pollution, and airborne particles specifically, as well as emissions from indoor coal burning; but in most cases, a specific cause cannot be identified, and the patterns and types of mutations differ from those seen in typical smoking-associated lung cancers {714,370}.

Histological types
Almost all lung cancers are carcinomas. The predominant histological types are adenocarcinoma, squamous cell carcinoma (SCC), small cell lung carcinoma (SCLC), and large cell carcinoma (LCC). Preinvasive lesions, benign epithelial tumours, lymphoproliferative tumours, and other miscellaneous tumours also occur, but they are relatively rare. The International Agency for Research on Cancer (IARC) has collected cancer incidence data from population-based registries around the world and published *Cancer Incidence in Five Continents: Volume XI* in 2017 {308}. Table 1.01 presents the numbers of cases diagnosed during 2008–2012 and incidence rates per 100 000 person-years, age-adjusted to the "World" standard, for lung and bronchus cancers (ICD-O topographical code: C34) overall and for microscopically verified carcinomas, by sex and histological type, for selected registries, which had to have ≥ 80% of their reported cases with microscopic verification of the diagnosis and ≥ 100 cases in each sex in order to be included. The percentage of cases that were microscopically verified ranged from 98% in Sétif (Algeria) to 81% in Mumbai (India). The proportion of carcinomas that were classified as "other and unspecified" (O&U) ranged from > 24% in British Columbia (Canada) to < 1% in Sétif.

With few exceptions, specific risk factors have not been linked to particular histological types of lung cancer. Over the now-lengthy course of the tobacco epidemic, there has been a notable shift in the histological types of lung cancer occurring within the population, as well as in the associations of the various histological types with cigarette smoking. Smoking is associated with all common carcinoma types, but the strongest associations are with SCC and SCLC. When the strong association of cigarette smoking with lung cancer was first characterized in the 1950s, SCC was the predominant histological type in smokers, while adenocarcinoma was the most frequent type in never-smokers. For non-adenocarcinomas, the relative risk associated with smoking was about 10 in studies carried out in the 1950s and 1960s, while smoking was associated with an approximate doubling of risk for adenocarcinoma. In the 1960s, a shift began in the major histological types of lung cancer in high-income countries; the relative frequency of adenocarcinoma increased,

Table 1.01 Age-standardized (World) incidence rates per 100 000 person-years of total and microscopically verified lung (ICD-O topographical code: C34) carcinoma cases in selected populations by histological type and sex, 2008–2012

Population	Males								Females								M:F carcinoma incidence rate ratios					
	Lung cancer		Microscopically verified carcinoma rates						Lung cancer		Microscopically verified carcinoma rates											
	Cases[a]	Rate[b]	Total	SCC	AC	SCLC	LCC	O&U	Cases[a]	Rate[b]	Total	SCC	AC	SCLC	LCC	O&U	Total	SCC	AC	SCLC	LCC	O&U
Algeria, Sétif	412	19.8	17.8	7.2	5.0	0.3	5.2	0.0	104	4.6	3.6	0.8	1.4	0.0	1.3	0.0	4.9	8.7	3.5	7.5	4.0	NE
Brazil, Goiânia	539	21.1	15.7	5.2	5.4	1.6	2.4	1.1	425	12.1	8.6	2.3	3.5	0.8	1.1	0.8	1.8	2.2	1.6	1.9	2.1	1.5
Canada, British Columbia	7 452	34.1	29.2	6.7	10.7	3.8	0.8	7.2	7 078	30.1	26.4	3.6	12.4	3.4	0.7	6.3	1.1	1.9	0.9	1.1	1.1	1.2
USA: White	481 135	45.5	40.2	11.1	14.9	5.9	1.6	6.7	426 869	34.9	31.4	5.7	14.0	5.4	1.0	5.2	1.3	2.0	1.1	1.1	1.5	1.3
USA: Black	62 206	57.3	50.4	14.3	20.0	4.9	2.3	8.9	47 908	32.1	29.3	5.8	13.8	3.5	1.1	5.1	1.7	2.5	1.4	1.4	2.1	1.7
China, Hong Kong SAR	13 856	44.5	37.6	7.0	18.6	3.9	0.8	7.3	7 473	20.9	18.3	1.0	13.9	0.5	0.2	2.7	2.1	7.0	1.3	8.3	3.7	2.8
India, Mumbai	2 578	9.8	7.6	1.3	3.1	1.2	0.9	1.1	1 097	4.1	3.1	0.3	1.7	0.4	0.3	0.4	2.5	4.5	1.8	3.1	2.7	2.7
Japan, Hiroshima	8 543	45.7	40.3	9.6	20.5	4.2	3.0	3.1	4 230	18.6	17.1	1.1	13.7	0.9	0.7	0.8	2.4	8.7	1.5	4.9	4.3	4.1
Republic of Korea	73 653	46.7	39.5	14.4	13.9	5.9	0.8	4.6	31 092	14.7	12.3	1.1	9.0	0.8	0.2	1.2	3.2	13.4	1.5	7.0	4.6	3.8
Turkey, İzmir	9 097	82.6	72.0	26.4	17.7	12.4	2.3	13.2	1 285	10.2	8.5	1.3	3.7	1.5	0.3	1.6	8.5	20.0	4.8	8.1	7.7	8.4
Slovakia	5 855	54.0	44.8	21.6	11.2	7.2	3.0	1.7	1 948	13.1	10.8	2.8	5.0	1.6	0.7	0.7	4.1	7.7	2.2	4.5	4.6	2.4
Denmark	11 483	42.5	37.8	10.0	14.9	6.2	1.7	5.1	10 733	36.7	33.0	4.5	17.3	5.4	1.3	4.5	1.1	2.2	0.9	1.1	1.3	1.1
France, Lille	1 729	70.7	62.3	18.1	26.4	7.0	5.1	5.8	484	15.4	13.9	1.9	7.7	2.1	0.9	1.3	4.5	9.5	3.4	3.4	5.7	4.3
Italy, Turin	5 775	42.7	36.7	7.8	11.4	2.9	9.5	5.2	2 084	13.7	12.0	1.9	4.9	0.8	2.8	1.7	3.1	4.1	2.3	3.5	3.5	3.0
Ireland	6 355	38.9	33.2	11.1	11.2	4.7	1.3	4.9	4 666	25.4	22.1	5.0	9.1	4.0	0.7	3.3	1.5	2.2	1.2	1.2	1.8	1.5
Australia	31 597	33.1	28.1	6.4	10.7	3.5	3.0	4.6	21 429	21.0	18.4	2.3	8.8	2.4	1.7	3.2	1.5	2.8	1.2	1.5	1.8	1.4
New Zealand: Maori	818	71.9	56.5	21.8	13.7	10.6	1.8	8.6	1 090	83.4	66.2	18.6	21.2	14.5	2.1	9.8	0.9	1.2	0.6	0.7	0.8	0.9

AC, adenocarcinoma; LCC, large cell carcinoma; NE, not estimable; O&U, other types of carcinoma and carcinoma unspecified; SCC, squamous cell carcinoma; SCLC, small cell lung carcinoma.
[a]Cases: number of cases 2008–2012. [b]Rates: age-standardized (World) incidence rates per 100 000 person-years.
Note: The four rate values based on < 10 cases (in Algeria, Sétif) are indicated with italics.

Estimated age-standardized incidence rates (World) in 2018, lung, males, all ages

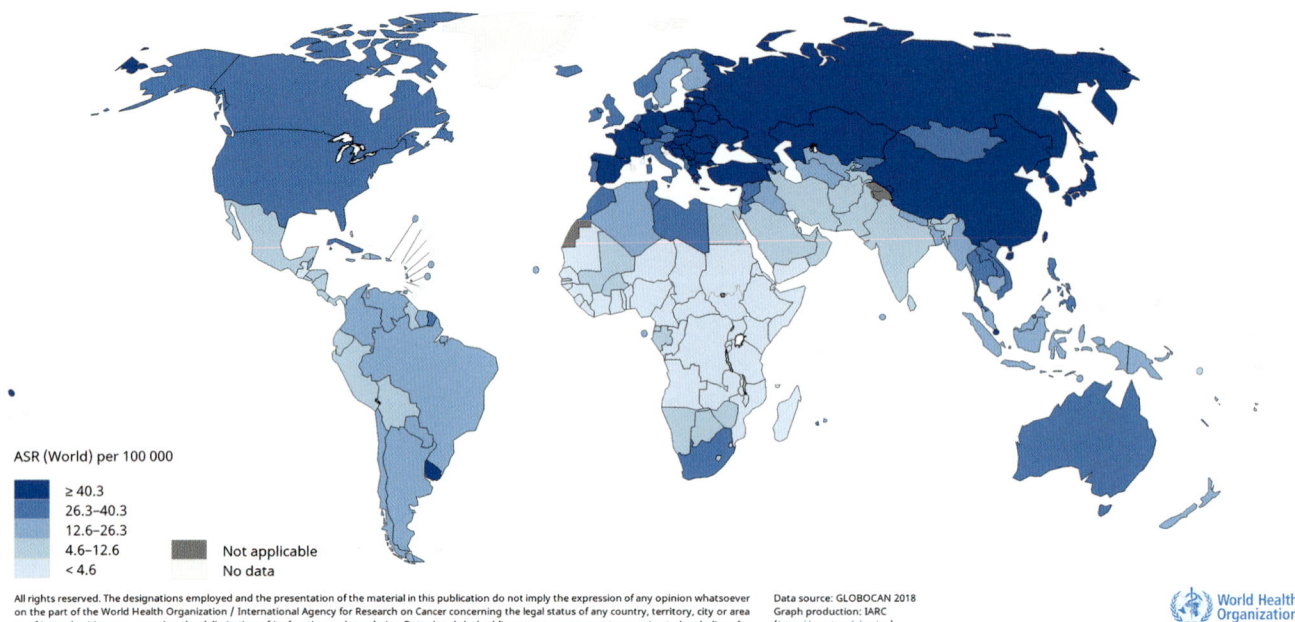

ASR (World) per 100 000

- ≥ 40.3
- 26.3–40.3
- 12.6–26.3
- 4.6–12.6
- < 4.6
- Not applicable
- No data

Data source: GLOBOCAN 2018
Graph production: IARC
(http://gco.iarc.fr/today)
World Health Organization

World Health Organization
© International Agency for Research on Cancer 2018

A

Estimated age-standardized incidence rates (World) in 2018, lung, females, all ages

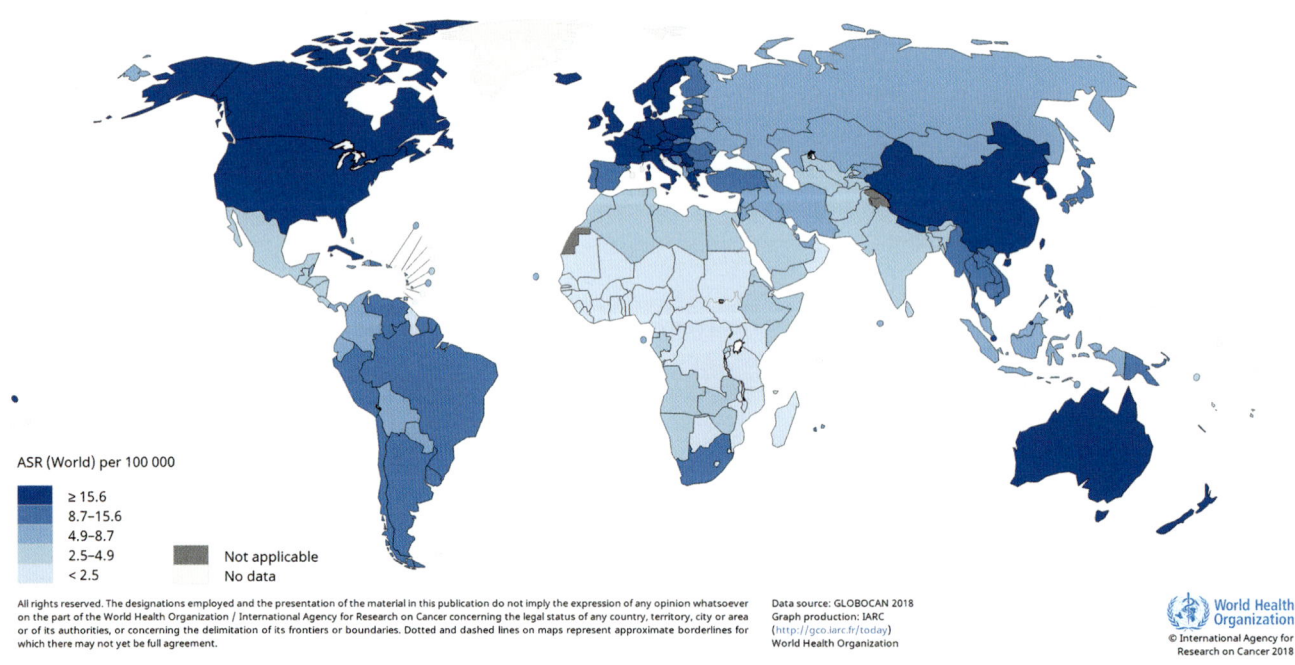

ASR (World) per 100 000

- ≥ 15.6
- 8.7–15.6
- 4.9–8.7
- 2.5–4.9
- < 2.5
- Not applicable
- No data

Data source: GLOBOCAN 2018
Graph production: IARC
(http://gco.iarc.fr/today)
World Health Organization

World Health Organization
© International Agency for Research on Cancer 2018

B

Fig. 1.01 Lung cancer map. Estimated age-standardized global incidence rates (ASRs; World), per 100 000 person-years, of lung cancer in 2018 among males (**A**) and females (**B**).

while SCC and SCLC declined. These trends were first noted in cancer registry data in the USA and have also been documented in other countries {368B}. Illustrative data for the USA are based on the nine registries in the US National Cancer Institute (NCI)'s Surveillance, Epidemiology, and End Results (SEER) Program, which have contributed data since the mid-1970s. During 1977–2016, a total of 609 225 cancers of the lung or bronchus were diagnosed in the populations covered by these registries, of which 89.8% were microscopically confirmed {2910}. After exclusion of cases specified as non-carcinomas or likely to be metastatic carcinoma, 546 061 cases were available for analysis. These were grouped into six major categories: SCC, SCLC, adenocarcinoma, LCC, other specified carcinomas, and unspecified carcinoma {1660}. The unspecified category is composed of carcinoma NOS, non-small cell carcinoma (a new code introduced in ICD-O-3), and malignant neoplasm NOS.

The relative proportions of the histological types have varied considerably over the years. During the earliest period (1977–1981), SCC accounted for 32% of cases in the USA; but by 2012–2016, the proportion had declined to 22%. Adenocarcinoma accounted for < 30% of cases during the earliest years, but the proportion increased to > 50% by 2012–2016. The SCLC proportion decreased from 17% to 13%, and the LCC proportion from 8% to 1%. The proportion that were other specified carcinomas rose from 2% to 5%. The proportion that were unspecified carcinoma rose from 12% to 23% during 2002–2006, and then dropped to 8%. These recent trends reflect improvements in the determination of histological type over the past decade (especially for LCC and adenocarcinoma), such as the introduction of immunohistochemical staining with TTF1 and squamous markers {3074}. This is one likely explanation for the marked decrease in the proportion with LCC. There is now an increased emphasis on the accurate determination of histological type, because of treatment and outcome implications.

Lung cancer incidence

The overall lung cancer incidence rate in the USA for both sexes (per 100 000 person-years, age-adjusted using the World standard) increased from 38.4 during 1977–1981 to peak at 43.5 during 1987–1991, and then decreased to 28.8 during 2012–2016, notably lower than it had been 35 years prior, probably related to declines in the prevalence of cigarette smoking. The rates of the various histological types peaked at slightly different times in the USA. SCC peaked earliest, in 1982–1986; SCLCs and LCCs peaked during 1987–1991; and adenocarcinoma peaked during 1992–1996. The rates of unspecified carcinoma and other specified carcinomas did not peak until 2002–2006 and 2007–2011, respectively. The differences in the timing of the rate peaks among the histological types in the USA probably reflect changes in the construction of cigarettes, the composition of the tobacco, and inhalation patterns.

Lung cancer incidence trends have differed by sex, with overall rates decreasing among males in the USA since the mid-1980s and increasing among females through the late 1990s {1660}. Among males, SCC peaked in the late 1970s, SCLCs and LCCs in the mid-1980s, adenocarcinoma around 1990, and other specified carcinomas in the mid-1990s. Among females, the peaks were later: in the late 1980s for SCCs, SCLCs, and LCCs; in the late 1990s for adenocarcinoma; and in the late 2000s for other specified carcinomas. The M:F incidence rate

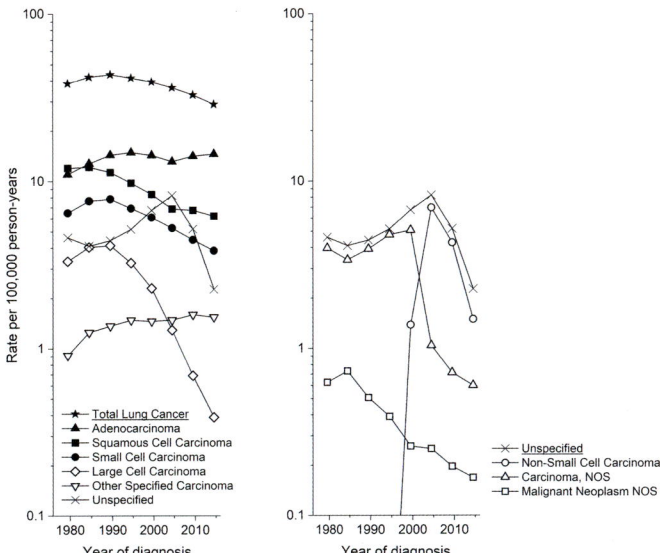

Fig. 1.02 Lung cancer. Trends in lung cancer incidence rates (age-adjusted using the World standard) from 1977–1981 to 2012–2016 in nine registries of the US National Cancer Institute (NCI)'s SEER Program, by histological type.

ratio for lung cancer overall decreased from 2.8 to 1.2 over the study period, reflecting much higher smoking rates among males in the past and more-rapid declines in the prevalence of smoking among males than females. The ratio was highest for SCC, dropping from 5.0 to 1.9, followed by that for LCC, which decreased from 2.7 to 1.4. The M:F incidence rate ratio of SCLC decreased from 2.4 to 1.2, that of adenocarcinoma from 1.9 to 1.1, and that of other specified carcinomas from 1.8 to 0.9 – with these last two findings reflecting the disappearance of the male excess in risk. In recent years, overall US lung cancer incidence rates among adults aged 30–49 years have been higher among women than men {1301}. Among both males and females, the rate of unspecified carcinoma decreased substantially since the mid-2000s, in concert with increasing rates of adenocarcinoma and stabilizing rates of SCC and other specified carcinomas. These trends reflect improving determination of the non-small cell carcinoma cell types as medical technology advanced with

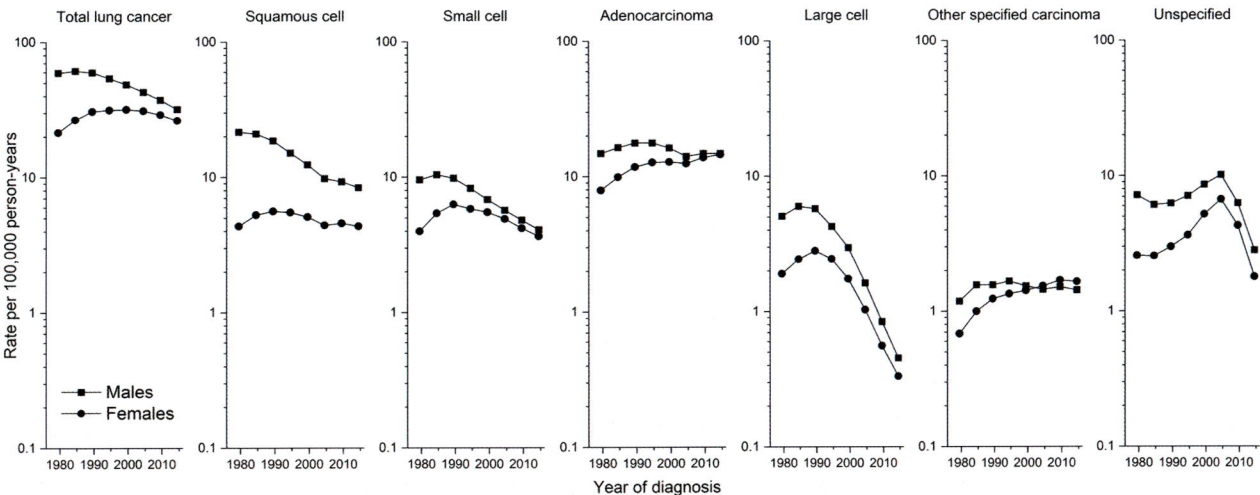

Fig. 1.03 Lung cancer. Trends in lung cancer incidence rates (age-adjusted using the World standard) from 1977–1981 to 2012–2016 in nine registries of the US National Cancer Institute (NCI)'s SEER Program, by histological type and sex.

Table 1.02 Occupational agents and exposure circumstances classified by the IARC Monographs Programme (https://monographs.iarc.fr/) that have *sufficient evidence of human carcinogenicity* for the lung and other thoracic sites

Site	Agent, mixture, or exposure circumstances
Lung	
	Acheson process, occupational exposures associated with
	Aluminium production
	Arsenic and inorganic arsenic compounds
	Asbestos (all forms)
	Beryllium and beryllium compounds
	Bis(chloromethyl) ether; chloromethyl methyl ether (technical grade)
	Cadmium and cadmium compounds
	Chromium (VI) compounds
	Coal, indoor emissions from household combustion
	Coal gasification
	Coal-tar pitch
	Coke production
	Dioxin (2,3,7,8-tetrachlorodibenzo-*para*-dioxin)
	Engine exhaust, diesel
	Hematite mining (underground)
	Iron and steel founding
	MOPP (vincristine-prednisone-nitrogen mustard-procarbazine mixture)
	Nickel compounds
	Opium (consumption of)
	Outdoor air pollution
	Painting (occupational exposure)
	Particulate matter in outdoor air pollution
	Plutonium
	Radon-222 and its decay products
	Rubber production industry
	Silica dust, crystalline
	Soot
	Sulfur mustard
	Tobacco smoke, secondhand
	Tobacco smoking
	Welding fumes
	X-radiation, γ-radiation
Mesothelium (pleura and peritoneum)	
	Asbestos (all forms)
	Erionite
	Fluoro-edenite
	Painting

however, overall lung cancer incidence trends indicate continuing increases among women {1931}.

The explanations for these time trends in lung cancer histology relate to changes in the design and characteristics of manufactured cigarettes – the globally dominant cause of lung cancer. Over the course of the decade before this shift began, and continuing during the subsequent decades, cigarettes were changed by the addition of filters, ventilation holes, and other modifications that were intended to reduce the dose of tar and nicotine, as measured by a machine. But as a result of these changes, puff volume may have increased, causing a shift from more central deposition of tobacco smoke to more peripheral deposition. SCCs and SCLCs generally arise in the more proximal airways, whereas adenocarcinomas mostly originate in the peripheral airways. Thus, more peripheral deposition probably increases the risk for adenocarcinoma. The levels of tobacco-specific nitrosamines in cigarette smoke have also increased as a result of design changes. In animal models, these nitrosamines cause adenocarcinomas specifically.

The evidence on shifting trends in lung cancer histological types was comprehensively reviewed in the US Surgeon General's 2014 report {3114}. The report includes four important conclusions related to the changing patterns of lung cancer:

The evidence is sufficient to conclude that the risk of developing adenocarcinoma of the lung from cigarette smoking has increased since the 1960s.

The evidence is sufficient to conclude that the increased risk of adenocarcinoma of the lung in smokers results from changes in the design and composition of cigarettes since the 1950s.

The evidence is not sufficient to specify which design changes are responsible for the increased risk of adenocarcinoma, but there is suggestive evidence that ventilated filters and increased levels of tobacco-specific nitrosamines have played a role.

The evidence shows that the decline of SCC follows the trend of declining smoking prevalence.

Occupational exposure and other factors

Smoking is the most important risk factor for lung cancer development – for adenocarcinoma as well as for both SCLC and SCC – but many other agents and exposure circumstances are causally linked to lung cancer risk (see Table 1.02). Lung adenocarcinomas can also develop in never-smokers, among whom they are the most frequent histological subtype. In addition to smoking, other reported causal factors include exposure to secondhand tobacco smoke, radon, and other ionizing radiation, asbestos, and indoor air pollution, as well as underlying chronic lung disease (e.g. pulmonary fibrosis, chronic obstructive pulmonary disease, α1-antitrypsin deficiency, and tuberculosis) and family history. For some of these factors (e.g. radon and asbestos exposure), there is evidence that smoking acts synergistically to increase risk. There have been rare reports of families with an inherited genetic predisposition to lung cancer associated with germline *EGFR* {198,925,2226,3142} or *ERBB2* {3361} mutation. Genome-wide association studies have indicated some genetic links to lung cancer risk in smokers {284}.

Clinical features
Presenting signs and symptoms
The vast majority (80–90%) of patients with lung cancer are symptomatic at the time of initial diagnosis. Symptoms, signs,

therapeutic implications. In European countries, adenocarcinoma trends are stabilizing in men but still increasing in women {1739}. Long-term good-quality data by histological type are not available from most low- and middle-income countries;

Table 1.03 Lung cancer presenting symptoms {677,2345}

Category	Symptom	Pathogenesis
Primary tumour		
	Cough	Airway obstruction, atelectasis, infection, airway inflammation
	Haemoptysis	Airway inflammation or necrosis, tumour necrosis and cavitation
	Dyspnoea	Airway compression, lymphangitic spread, pleural effusion, thromboembolism, pericardial effusion
	Pain from invasion of chest wall or brachial plexus, hoarseness from impingement of the recurrent laryngeal nerve, superior vena cava syndrome, Horner syndrome (ptosis, miosis, anhidrosis) from invasion of the sympathetic chain and stellate ganglion, pericardial tamponade	Direct extension
Metastases		
	Headache, bony pain, weight loss, anorexia, fatigue	Sites: brain, bone, liver, adrenal gland, and lung
Paraneoplastic syndromes		
	Hyponatraemia	Syndrome of inappropriate antidiuretic hormone secretion
	Hypercalcaemia	PTHrP
	Cushing syndrome (SCLC, carcinoid)	Ectopic corticotropin
	Hypertrophic pulmonary osteoarthropathy	
	Lambert–Eaton myasthenic syndrome (SCLC)	
	Encephalomyelitis–subacute sensory neuropathy (SCLC)	

SCLC, small cell lung carcinoma.

and abnormalities in laboratory test results relating to the lung cancer can be classified as follows: (1) those related to the primary lesion, (2) those related to intrathoracic spread, (3) those related to distant metastasis, and (4) those related to paraneoplastic syndromes. The growth in the lung of the primary tumour may be divided into central and peripheral patterns, and those two types of presentation can be associated with different symptoms. Some of the more common symptoms include progressive shortness of breath, cough, chest pain/pressure, hoarseness or loss of voice, and haemoptysis. Symptoms related to disseminated disease include weight loss; abdominal pain due to secondary involvement of the liver, adrenals, and other organs; and pain due to bone metastases. Cerebrospinal metastases or meningeal seeding may cause neurological symptoms. Patients with SCLC are more likely than patients with non-small cell lung carcinoma (NSCLC) to present with symptoms referable to distant metastases. At presentation, brain metastases are identified in many patients with lung cancer, and during the course of illness, ≥ 20% of patients with lung cancer develop CNS metastases {3068}. The presenting symptoms of lung cancer are summarized in Table 1.03.

Presenting signs and symptoms often depend on the extent of disease and the sites of metastases. Most patients present with locally advanced or metastatic lung cancer. In the USA, of patients whose stage is known, just 16% present with disease confined to the primary site, another 23% have disease involving regional nodes, and > 60% have evidence of distant metastatic disease at the time of diagnosis {2911}.

The presenting findings and stage distribution of lung cancer may change with local implementation of CT screening for lung cancer among high-risk groups. Patients who are diagnosed with lung cancer as part of a programme of low-dose CT screening are less likely to be diagnosed with stage IV disease and more likely to have an adenocarcinoma identified {2081, 631}. In the US National Lung Screening Trial study, 50% of the screen-detected cancers were diagnosed at stage I {2081}.

Paraneoplastic symptoms

Paraneoplastic syndromes, which occur in as many as 10% of patients with lung cancer, are a group of clinical disorders associated with malignant diseases that are not directly related to the physical effects of primary or metastatic tumour. These syndromes may be due to the production of biologically active substances or due to other, presently unclear, mechanisms. Paraneoplastic symptoms are unrelated to the size of the primary tumour, in some cases can precede the diagnosis of malignant disease, and at other times may occur late in the illness or herald the first sign of recurrence {186}.

Paraneoplastic symptoms are common in lung cancer. Endocrine and paraneoplastic syndromes are less common in adenocarcinoma than in other histological types of lung cancer. SCLC is characterized by neuroendocrine activity, and some of the peptides secreted by the tumour mimic the activity of pituitary hormones {2221,2820}. Neurological symptoms may also be a paraneoplastic phenomenon, which might include sensory, sensorimotor, and autoimmune neuropathies and encephalomyelitis. The symptoms may precede the primary diagnosis by many months, and they may be the presenting complaint. They may also be the initial sign of relapse from remission. Hypercalcaemia is rare in SCLC and almost pathognomonic for SCC.

Initial evaluation of a patient with a possible diagnosis of lung cancer routinely involves imaging and surgical procedures to define the extent of disease; these can include CT, PET, MRI, bronchoscopy, transthoracic needle biopsy, FNA, mediastinoscopy, and endobronchial ultrasound–guided needle aspiration. These procedures should be tailored to allow accurate staging (i.e. detecting sites of nodal metastases and distant disease) and to procure sufficient material to obtain all required information for treatment (including histological and molecular analysis).

Imaging

Primary lung cancer usually occurs as a nodule or mass, although more-complex patterns frequently occur. Lung cancer is often detected initially by chest radiography, and increasingly by CT, either as an incidental finding or in the context of a lung cancer screening programme. Lung cancer is most common in the periphery of the lungs and in the upper lobes.

For lung cancer detection, CT is approximately 4 times as sensitive as chest radiography, which has relatively poor sensitivity and specificity for nodules < 20 mm in diameter, particularly when the nodule is partially obscured by overlapping anatomy {627}. Newer radiographic detectors and image processing provide superior lesion conspicuity, and thus improved detection of lung nodules compared with older computed radiography or screen/film imaging, although accuracy is still operator-dependent to a substantial degree {627}. CT provides superior detail in terms of tumour size, margination, location, and morphology. Contiguous thin-section CT reconstruction allows improved distinction between ground-glass, part-solid, and solid tumours, as well as better detection accuracy for small amounts of calcium or fat. Thin sections (~1 mm) also provide better characterization of tumour margins and more-accurate comparison of nodules over time to determine interval growth. Reconstruction and archiving of contiguous transverse thin sections are therefore now recommended for all adult thoracic CTs, regardless of the clinical indication {1758}. For screening CT and surveillance of suspect nodules, low-dose technique without iodinated contrast is appropriate {1758}, but a diagnostic scan with intravascular contrast allows more-accurate evaluation of hilar, mediastinal, and abdominal disease.

Visual detection of nodules is best performed on thicker CT sections and is facilitated by use of postprocessing techniques such as maximum intensity projection reconstructions, and increasingly by automated nodule detection using artificial intelligence (AI), for which thin-section data are generally required.

Lung cancer tumours typically start as more or less spherical, and they show margins that range from smooth to lobulated, irregular, or spiculated. Although correlation between imaging findings and cell type is approximate at best, adenocarcinoma most commonly occurs as a peripheral nodule or mass, whereas about two thirds of squamous cell tumours occur in the central part of the lung, with resulting obstructive atelectasis or pneumonia. However, peripheral SCCs are becoming more common, and when arising as a peripheral nodule, squamous carcinoma often cavitates. Calcium can be seen on CT in approximately 10% of lung cancers, due to either tumour dystrophic calcification or incorporation of pre-existing benign calcium deposits. Calcification tends to occur in large, central tumours, but it does not predict histological subtype {1008}.

PET with FDG plays an important role in lung cancer staging, and when combined with CT is far superior to CT alone for identification of both locoregional disease and distant metastases. Several studies have shown that PET-CT results in modification of stage and clinical management in 10–33% of lung cancer cases {85}. Sensitivity and specificity are in the range of 95% and 80%, respectively, with lower accuracy for lesions < 10 mm in size and for subsolid nodules with a small or absent solid component. False negative results may also be seen in neuroendocrine tumours (NETs) and in mucinous adenocarcinoma. False positive results can occur in nodules and enlarged lymph nodes caused by infection. Newer tracers, such as 68Ga-DOTATATE, have proved superior to FDG in evaluation of NETs {1412}.

Histopathology and staging

Since the 2015 publication of the fourth-edition volume *WHO Classification of Tumours of the Lung, Pleura, Thymus and Heart* {3068}, the histopathological classification remains intact, except for a few newly described entities. The fourth edition witnessed for the first time the introduction of immunohistochemistry markers as basis for more-precise histological classification of poorly differentiated non-small cell carcinomas and a new classification of lung cancer based on small biopsies and cytology. This fifth-edition volume includes the new SMARCA4-deficient undifferentiated tumour as a highly aggressive poorly differentiated lung cancer subtype, strongly associated with smoking in most cases, that requires immunohistochemistry and/or genetic markers as diagnostic criteria (see *Thoracic SMARCA4-deficient undifferentiated tumour*, p. 111). Bronchiolar adenoma / ciliated muconodular papillary tumour is now recognized as a new adenoma subtype on the basis of its characteristic histopathological appearance and the frequent presence of mutations – especially in *BRAF, EGFR, KRAS, HRAS, AKT1*, and *ALK* (see *Bronchiolar adenoma / ciliated muconodular papillary tumour*, p. 48). In addition, because of the lack of complete correlation between lymphoepithelioma-like histology and EBV-encoded small RNA 1 (EBER1) in situ hybridization positivity, the nomenclature for lymphoepithelioma-like carcinoma has been changed to "lymphoepithelial carcinoma", which includes EBV-positive and EBV-negative subtypes. The term "enteric adenocarcinoma" has been changed to "enteric-type adenocarcinoma" throughout the classification. This new term recognizes that primary lung and thymic adenocarcinomas can have enteric-type morphology and differentiation.

The subclassification of non-mucinous lung adenocarcinoma has largely been accepted by the pathology community, but some issues related to clinical utility remain unresolved. A large number of publications have supported the favourable prognosis for lepidic-predominant adenocarcinomas, adenocarcinoma in situ, and minimally invasive adenocarcinoma, as well as the poor prognostic association of the predominant micropapillary and solid subtypes {2398,1941}. In the setting of adjuvant therapy, there are two studies (one of which includes a pivotal adjuvant chemotherapy trial patient cohort) that demonstrated that high-grade solid/micropapillary histological subtyping correlated with survival benefit with adjuvant chemotherapy {3092, 2709A}. These results provide strong evidence that future adjuvant trials should incorporate adenocarcinoma subtypes as a stratification factor.

In January 2017, the eighth edition of the Union for International Cancer Control (UICC) tumour, node, metastasis (TNM) staging classification system for lung cancer replaced the seventh edition {985,2422,113,748,2099}. The new staging system was developed based on the survival outcome of 94 708 patients collected internationally, with an external validation using the database of the NCI's SEER Program {2423,451,681}. Major revisions involve the T and M staging, with N staging largely unchanged. The new edition introduced Tis (adenocarcinoma in situ) and T1mi for minimally invasive adenocarcinoma. Based on significant differences in overall survival, the T stage is subdivided (T1a–c; T2a–b) by every 10 mm for tumours measuring 10–50 mm, and tumours > 50 mm but ≤ 70 mm are now staged as T3, while those > 70 mm are staged as T4. The T2 classification is now used for tumours that involve the main bronchus, invade the visceral pleura, or are associated with atelectasis or obstructive pneumonitis that extends to the hilar region involving either part of or the whole lung. Involvement of the diaphragm has a T4 prognosis. Invasion of the mediastinal pleura was seldom used and has been discontinued {2422,2105}. A major change involves the recommendation to use only the invasive tumour component for pathological T size of subsolid nodules with non-mucinous adenocarcinoma with a lepidic component {3067}. In this context, there is currently an effort by the Pathology Committee of the International Association for the Study of Lung Cancer (IASLC) to devise clearer histological criteria to define the invasive tumour component, because previous studies have demonstrated a lack of consistent reproducibility in diagnosing invasion {3036}. Other data have shown good agreement in the diagnosis of adenocarcinoma in situ versus minimally invasive adenocarcinoma and excellent reliability in measuring invasion {262}. The eighth edition also provides guidelines on how to stage lung cancers with multiple tumour nodules, in relation to the distinction between separate primary tumours and intrapulmonary metastases, although the actual staging criteria remain essentially the same {682,680,684,683}. Using comprehensive histological assessment allows good reproducibility between pathologists {2104}. For M stage, the criteria for the M1a category remain unchanged from the seventh edition, while single metastatic lesions in a single distant organ are newly designated as M1b, and multiple lesions in a single organ or multiple lesions in multiple organs are reclassified as M1c {748}.

Molecular pathology and biomarker testing

In the fourth edition of the WHO classification, descriptions of genomic aberrations in various lung cancer types, including adenocarcinoma, SCC, carcinoid, and large cell neuroendocrine carcinoma (LCNEC), were included. The complexity may be explained by the histological composition of the lung. Anatomically, lung epithelial cells are divided into two compartments that are associated with differing lung functions (see Fig. 1.04).

In 2015, *EGFR* mutations and *ALK* fusions were the only driver mutations that required routine clinical testing for non-squamous NSCLCs {1693}. Since then, more driver genes with available drugs have been identified (see *Invasive non-mucinous adenocarcinoma of the lung*, p. 64), as targeted therapies for patients harbouring driver mutations in these genes have become available {2817,821}. These new developments have led to an update of the CAP/IASLC/AMP guideline on molecular testing in lung cancer {1692}. In addition, testing for PDL1 is now recommended for advanced-stage non-neuroendocrine carcinomas, because patients with a PDL1 tumour proportional

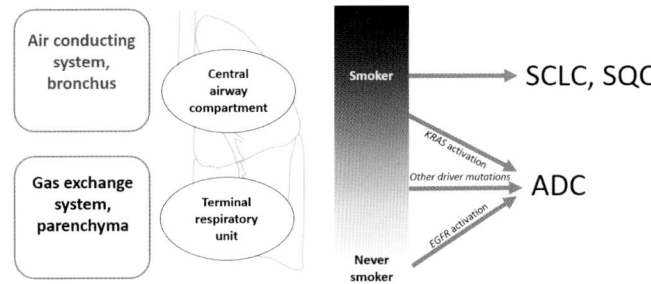

Fig. 1.04 Lung cancer molecular pathogenesis. The concept of the two-compartment model in the putative molecular pathogenesis of lung cancer. The central airway compartment's main function is air conduction, while respiratory exchange occurs in the terminal respiratory unit of the peripheral compartment. In these compartments, different stem cell niches have been identified, and accordingly, different types of lung cancer develop in the two compartments. Carcinogens from tobacco smoke appear to target both central and peripheral airways, although predominantly affecting the central compartment. In contrast, unidentified factors, which appear to specifically target the terminal respiratory unit, are associated with lung cancers in never-smokers. *EGFR* mutations are associated with never-smokers, whereas *KRAS* mutations are more frequently seen in smokers. Other driver mutations also exist. This model illustrates only the major pathways, and other (minor) pathways may also exist.

score ≥ 50% are eligible for first-line treatment with the anti-PD1 therapy pembrolizumab {1596}.

The classification and our understanding of the molecular aberrations in pulmonary NETs were unchanged for decades, but since 2015, new genome sequencing data have emerged for carcinoid as well as high-grade neuroendocrine carcinomas (NECs) {816,937}. On the basis of mutation and gene expression profiles, carcinoid tumours appear to be composed of multiple molecular subgroups (see *Carcinoid/neuroendocrine tumour of the lung*, p. 133). Whole-genome sequencing analysis of SCLCs revealed that loss of tumour suppressor genes *TP53* and *RB1*, sometimes by complex genomic rearrangements, is obligatory in these high-grade NETs {937}. There is currently great hope of translating this scientific progress into novel therapies {2367}.

Therapy and outcome

In the past 20 years, the decision-making process of the entire thoracic oncology community has been transformed by several breakthrough discoveries that have profoundly modified our diagnostic and therapeutic strategies.

Historically, the simple distinction between NSCLC and SCLC together with the assessment of the extent of the disease were the critical steps to drive treatment decisions. After the initial implementation in the clinic of targeted therapies and antifolate agents, it became evident that the safety and efficacy of some therapeutic agents vary by tumour histology. Bevacizumab, an antibody to VEGF, is contraindicated in patients with SCC because clinical trials have demonstrated a higher risk of fatal or life-threatening haemoptysis {1321A}. Histological classification is also relevant with the use of pemetrexed, which is a cytotoxic chemotherapy commonly used in patients with adenocarcinomas {2703A}. The combination of pemetrexed and cisplatin compared with gemcitabine and cisplatin led to poorer overall survival in patients with squamous cell NSCLC versus adenocarcinoma or other NSCLCs {2703A,2648A}.

Another radical change was driven by the full sequencing of the human genome, with a rapid expansion of knowledge about human DNA and genetic variation. However, sequencing technologies remained relatively expensive and time-consuming, and clinical applications in subsequent years were mostly limited to the evaluation of rare monogenic Mendelian disorders. The development of massively parallel sequencing (also called next-generation sequencing) has accelerated the implementation of genomic sequencing in clinical practice, with applications such as exome sequencing and multigene panels ordered regularly in clinical practice and innovative applications steadily emerging. The rapid pace of adoption has created challenges for all stakeholders in clinical genomic sequencing, from standardizing varying interpretation approaches in clinical molecular laboratories to ensuring that clinicians are prepared for new types of clinical information {1537}.

The advent of a wide array of targeted therapies further generated a dramatic change in the way we diagnose and treat patients with NSCLC. Over the past 15 years, cancer treatment has seen increased focus on personalized medicine, leading to stratification of patient management on the basis of biomarker status. Major cancer types (lung, breast, colorectal, melanoma) have become increasingly segmented, with each segment now being recognized as having specific treatment options and outcomes. In many cases, cancer is no longer a single tumour type diagnosis but is defined by a combination of factors, including histology and biomarker status. Identification of newer biomarker niches is likely to fragment the patient populations within these cancers further. Currently, in lung adenocarcinoma, predictive testing for *EGFR* mutations and *ALK*, *ROS1*, and NTRK fusions, as well as for *BRAF* mutations, regardless of sex, race, smoking history, or other risk factors, is prioritized over other molecular predictive tests {1691}. This paradigm for targeted therapies in oncology allows the right patients to receive the most active therapy, while those who are unlikely to benefit can be spared the cost and potential morbidity associated with ineffective therapeutic interventions.

Newer treatment options, biomarker-based patient segmentation, and availability of biomarker-based treatment approaches have added to the treatment complexity over the years. In parallel, innovative clinical-trial designs such as umbrella and basket studies or master protocols – today central components of drug development – are highlighting the need to better appraise tumour biology, drug efficacy, and the potential benefits for patients. Emerging drug-development paradigms are driving new ways of working collaboratively to accelerate progress. The Lung Cancer Mutation Consortium, from 2009 through 2012, which comprised 14 sites in the USA, enrolled patients with metastatic lung adenocarcinomas and tested their tumours for 10 drivers. Actionable drivers were detected in 64% of lung adenocarcinomas, and the study showed that multiplex testing aided physicians in selecting therapies {1539}. Although individuals with drivers who received a matched targeted agent lived longer {2759}, randomized trials are still required to determine whether targeting therapy based on oncogenic drivers improves survival {2583}. However, by generating truly patient-centric clinical trials, oncologists have taken important early steps into the evolving era of precision medicine.

More recently, the therapeutic opportunities in thoracic malignancies have been dramatically changed, by multiple phase III studies of immune checkpoint inhibitors. These studies have completely changed the approach taken to treatment of advanced-stage lung cancer. There is now evidence in the first-line setting of the superiority of immunotherapy over cytotoxic chemotherapy, at least in a subset of patients, as well as the possibility to combine immunotherapy and chemotherapy {720}. Today, cancer immunotherapy is rapidly advancing and can now be considered to be the "fifth pillar" of cancer therapy, joining the ranks of surgery, cytotoxic chemotherapy, targeted therapy, and radiation.

The challenges ahead are to discover why immunotherapy treatments work so dramatically well in some cancers and in some patients while not at all in others, and how tumours that are initially sensitive to treatment can acquire resistance. For cancer immunotherapy to be effective, we must find ways to manipulate the immune system in the patients who show little or no immune response to their tumours, even to the point where the tumour microenvironment is an "immune desert" with no tumour-infiltrating T cells {905}. The next directions for immune therapy include mechanisms to increase innate activation of anti-tumour T cells, altering the tumour microenvironment that will confer immunogenicity to the tumour, engineering an anti-tumour immune response through adoptive T-cell therapy, or inhibiting tumour-mediated immune suppression.

Future perspective

Beyond the initial genome profiling of lung SCC and adenocarcinoma {369,370}, more-recent comprehensive genome sequencing studies involving resected non-small cell carcinomas have provided new insights into intratumoural and intertumoural genomic and immunogenetic heterogeneity of lung cancers {626,1290,1861,2534,1329}, as well as clonal evolution during various stages of lung cancer progression {236,467}. These data have partly contributed to our understanding of heterogeneity in tumour response to therapies, development of drug resistance mechanisms, and clonal differences between primary and metastatic tumour nodules {1680,2478,407}. These advances will probably lead to more-intense characterization of the tumour cellular heterogeneity and immune microenvironment, using multiplex immunohistochemistry and deep or machine learning technologies {2845,2276,3216}. Furthermore, as neoadjuvant treatment using novel therapies in early-stage lung cancer patients is being explored for both clinical research and therapeutic purposes, recommendations have been proposed on how to process and examine neoadjuvant-treated lung cancer specimens {3077}. It is hoped that these new developments will help to further refine the accuracy of lung cancer classification and its clinical implementation and value.

Small diagnostic samples

Travis WD
Al-Dayel FH
Bubendorf L
Chung JH
Rekhtman N
Scagliotti GV

Rationale for classification in small biopsy and cytology specimens

Pathological diagnosis is key to the management of lung cancer, in addition to careful consideration of risk factors and signs and symptoms, assessment of the extent of the disease (locally and outside the thoracic boundaries), and – in the case of resectable disease – evaluation of the cardiopulmonary and metabolic status of the patient. For the 70% of lung cancer patients who present with advanced-stage, unresectable disease, diagnosis must be based primarily on small biopsy and cytology specimens {3074}.

Precise histological classification (and in many cases molecular and/or biomarker testing) of lung cancer is essential because of the clinical need for tailoring systemic therapies according to histological type as well as molecular/biomarker profiles {3068,3071,2760,1161}. However, achieving this goal can be

Box 1.01 Guidelines for good practice of small biopsies and cytological preparations {3073,3074}

1. For small biopsies and cytology, non-small cell carcinoma should be further classified into a more specific type, such as adenocarcinoma or squamous cell carcinoma, whenever possible.

2. The term "non-small cell lung carcinoma NOS" should be used as little as possible, and only when a more specific diagnosis is not possible.

3. When a diagnosis is made in a small biopsy or cytology specimen in conjunction with special studies, it should be clarified whether the diagnosis was established on the basis of light microscopy alone or whether special stains were required.

4. The term "non-squamous cell carcinoma" should not be used by pathologists in diagnostic reports. This categorization is used by clinicians to define groups of patients whose tumours comprise several histological types and who can be treated in a similar manner; in small biopsies and cytology, pathologists should classify non-small cell lung carcinoma as adenocarcinoma, squamous cell carcinoma, non-small cell lung carcinoma NOS, or other terms (see Table 1.04, p. 30).

5. The above classification of adenocarcinoma vs other histologies and the terminology in Table 1.04 (p. 30) and Table 1.05 (p. 31) should be used in routine diagnosis, future research, and clinical trials, to ensure a uniform classification of disease cohorts in relation to tumour subtypes, stratified according to diagnoses made by light microscopy alone vs diagnoses requiring special stains.

6. When paired cytology and biopsy specimens exist, they should be reviewed together to achieve the most specific and concordant diagnosis.

7. The terms "adenocarcinoma in situ" and "minimally invasive adenocarcinoma" should not be used for diagnosis of small biopsies or cytology specimens. If a non-invasive pattern is present in a small biopsy, it should be referred to as a lepidic growth pattern. Similarly, if a cytology specimen has the attributes of adenocarcinoma in situ, the tumour should be diagnosed as an adenocarcinoma, possibly with a comment that this may represent, at least in part, adenocarcinoma in situ.

8. The term "large cell carcinoma" should not be used for diagnosis in small biopsy or cytology specimens and should be restricted to resection specimens where the tumour is thoroughly sampled to exclude a differentiated component.

9. In biopsies of tumours that show sarcomatoid features (marked nuclear pleomorphism, malignant giant cells, or spindle cell morphology), these should be initially classified as above in relation to adenocarcinoma; non-small cell carcinoma, favour adenocarcinoma; squamous cell carcinoma; or non-small cell carcinoma, favour squamous cell carcinoma, because this is apt to influence management, with an additional statement that giant and/or spindle cell features (depending on what feature) are present. If such features are not present, the term "non-small cell carcinoma NOS" should be used, again with a comment on the sarcomatoid features.

10. Staining for neuroendocrine immunohistochemical markers should be performed only in cases where there is suspected neuroendocrine morphology.

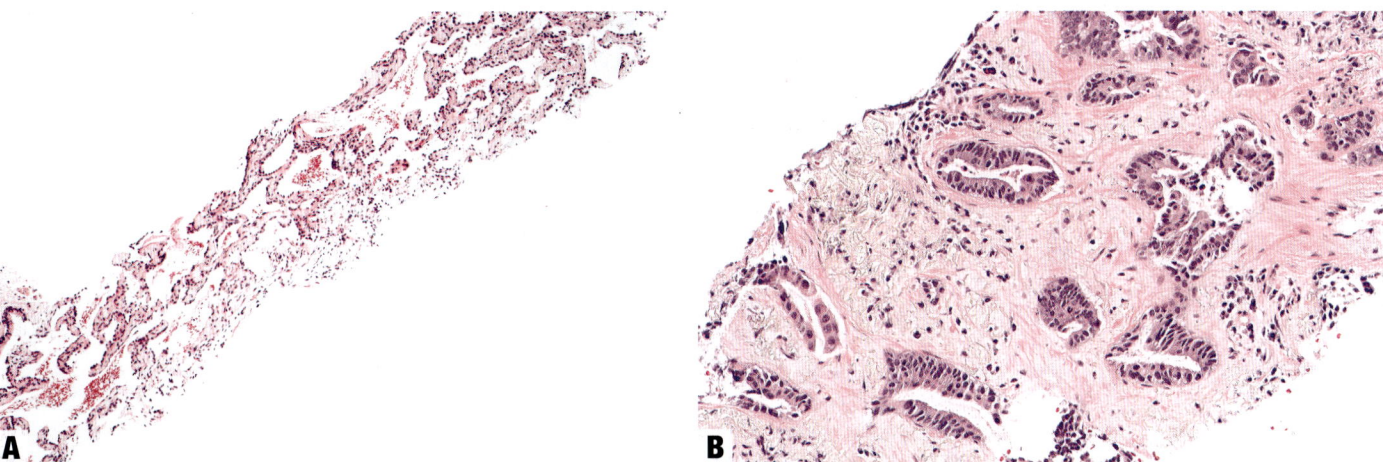

Fig. 1.05 Adenocarcinoma. **A** Lepidic pattern in core biopsy. This tumour shows preservation of alveolar architecture with uniform proliferation of crowded atypical pneumocytes. There is mild fibrotic thickening of alveolar walls. **B** Acinar pattern in core biopsy. This tumour consists of an acinar arrangement of glands with epithelial cells lining luminal spaces.

Table 1.04 Terminology in small biopsy and cytology versus resection specimens for adenocarcinoma and squamous cell carcinoma {3074,3068,3081}

Morphology/stains	Terminology for small biopsies and cytology specimens	Terminology for resection specimens
Morphological squamous cell patterns clearly present	Squamous cell carcinoma	Squamous cell carcinoma
Morphological adenocarcinoma patterns clearly present		
	Adenocarcinoma (list the patterns in the diagnosis)	Adenocarcinoma Predominant pattern: • Lepidic • Acinar • Papillary • Solid • Micropapillary
	Adenocarcinoma with lepidic pattern (if pure, list the differential diagnosis on the right and add a comment that an invasive component cannot be excluded)	Minimally invasive adenocarcinoma, adenocarcinoma in situ, or an invasive adenocarcinoma with a lepidic component
	Invasive mucinous adenocarcinoma (list the patterns; use the term "mucinous adenocarcinoma with lepidic pattern" if pure lepidic pattern and mention the differential diagnosis listed on the right)	Invasive mucinous adenocarcinoma Minimally invasive adenocarcinoma or adenocarcinoma in situ, mucinous type
	Adenocarcinoma with colloid features	Colloid adenocarcinoma
	Adenocarcinoma with fetal features	Fetal adenocarcinoma
	Adenocarcinoma with enteric features[a]	Enteric adenocarcinoma
Morphological squamous cell patterns not present, but supported by stains (i.e. p40+)	Non-small cell carcinoma, favour squamous cell carcinoma[b]	Squamous cell carcinoma (non-keratinizing pattern may be a component of the tumour)[b]
Morphological adenocarcinoma patterns not present, but supported by special stains (i.e. TTF1+)	Non-small cell carcinoma, favour adenocarcinoma[b]	Adenocarcinoma (solid pattern may be just one component of the tumour)[b]
No clear adenocarcinoma, squamous, or neuroendocrine morphology or staining pattern	Non-small cell carcinoma NOS[a,c]	Large cell carcinoma

[a]Metastatic carcinomas should be carefully excluded with clinical and appropriate but judicious immunohistochemical examination.

[b]The categories do not always correspond to solid-predominant adenocarcinoma or non-keratinizing squamous cell carcinoma, respectively. Poorly differentiated components in adenocarcinoma or squamous cell carcinoma may be sampled.

[c]The non-small cell carcinoma NOS pattern can be seen not only in large cell carcinomas but also when the solid, poorly differentiated component of adenocarcinomas or squamous cell carcinomas is sampled but does not express immunohistochemical markers or mucin.

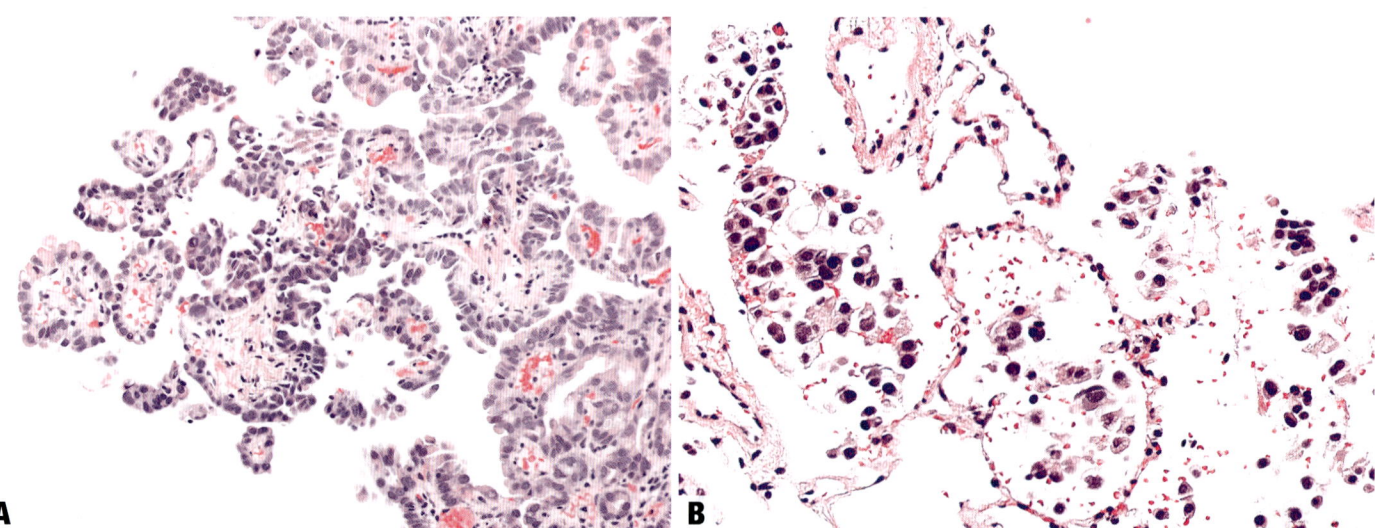

Fig. 1.06 Adenocarcinoma. **A** Papillary pattern in core biopsy. This tumour shows papillary architecture with fibrovascular cores surrounded by several layers of pseudostratified atypical epithelial cells. In addition, there are some smaller glandular structures that resemble micropapillary because they do not show fibrovascular cores, but in this small specimen and in the presence of the prominent papillary growth, it is not possible to exclude the possibility that these might be tangential cuts of true papillary structures. **B** Micropapillary pattern in core biopsy. This tumour shows small nests of malignant epithelial cells arranged in small papillae that lack fibrovascular cores. The nests of tumour cells are mostly within alveolar spaces.

Table 1.05 Terminology for small biopsies and cytology versus resection specimens for small cell carcinoma, large cell neuroendocrine carcinoma, adenosquamous carcinoma, and pleomorphic carcinoma {3074,3068,3081}

Terminology for small biopsies and cytology specimens	Terminology for resection specimens
Small cell carcinoma	Small cell carcinoma
Non-small cell carcinoma with neuroendocrine morphology and positive neuroendocrine markers, possible large cell neuroendocrine carcinoma	Large cell neuroendocrine carcinoma
Morphological squamous cell and adenocarcinoma patterns both present: non-small cell carcinoma NOS	Adenosquamous carcinoma (if both components ≥ 10%)
Comment that adenocarcinoma and squamous components are present, and that this could represent adenosquamous carcinoma	
Morphological squamous cell or adenocarcinoma patterns not present, but immunohistochemical stains favour separate squamous and adenocarcinoma components: non-small cell carcinoma NOS	Adenocarcinoma, squamous cell carcinoma, adenosquamous carcinoma, or large cell carcinoma with unclear immunohistochemical features
Specify the results of the immunohistochemical stains and the interpretation, and comment that this could represent adenosquamous carcinoma, but that diagnosis requires a resection specimen	
Non-small cell carcinoma with spindle cell and/or giant cell carcinoma	Pleomorphic, spindle cell, and/or giant cell carcinoma
Mention if adenocarcinoma or squamous carcinoma is present. Comment that this could represent a pleomorphic carcinoma; however, that diagnosis requires a resection specimen.	

challenging in small tumour samples of primary or metastatic lung tumours obtained through FNA or tiny bronchoscopy biopsies, in which the precise tumour classification may be hampered by scant viable cells and/or poor tumour differentiation. Therefore, a multidisciplinary strategy to obtain adequate biopsy not only for diagnosis but also for molecular and biomarker testing is important. A limited panel of immunohistochemical markers has been shown to reliably distinguish histological types of most non-small cell lung carcinomas (NSCLCs), allowing for preservation of tissue for molecular testing.

Tissue remains the main issue in the era of targeted therapies and immunotherapy because of the clear need to identify subsets of patients who benefit most from these tailored approaches. Histological heterogeneity and biological heterogeneity are well-known phenomena, which might significantly affect our capability to detect specific molecular targets, as well as prediction of sensitivity to specific molecular targeted agents. The heterogeneity of response and outcome associated with specific molecular features is probably a reflection of biological heterogeneity, which might not be captured in small biopsies or cytology specimens.

Over the past 15 years, outstanding breakthrough therapeutic successes have included EGFR tyrosine kinase inhibitors for tumours with *EGFR* sensitizing mutations; ALK, ROS1, BRAF, RET, and NTRK inhibitors; and the recent addition of immune checkpoint pathway inhibitors, in either the second or the front-line treatment of NSCLC {2364,2363,2445}. Of note, these immunotherapy approaches require matching known antigens or pathways with specific antibodies. Consequently, coupling diagnostics and therapeutics is also a major feature of immunotherapy.

Biopsy approaches

There are many different approaches to obtaining small biopsies and cytology specimens for lung cancer diagnosis. These include FNA and exfoliative specimens such as sputum, bronchial washings and secretions, bronchial brushings, and bronchoalveolar lavages. FNA of mass lesions can be guided by endobronchial ultrasound or CT. Confirmation of specimen adequacy at the time of the procedure can be aided by rapid on-site evaluation, including telepathology methods {2664,334, 2457,290,1299}. Molecular testing including next-generation sequencing can show high diagnostic yield in cytology samples with cell blocks or ethanol-fixed smears or liquid-based preparations {2457,3109,2361}. Obtaining multiple biopsy samples that can be used separately for immunohistochemical staining versus molecular testing is helpful. The optimal approach varies from one institution to another depending on the local expertise of the physicians (pulmonologists, radiologists, surgeons, cytopathologists) obtaining the specimens.

Another recent advance is the use of cell-free DNA from plasma as a source of tumour-derived DNA for molecular testing. This has proved to be a useful method for non-invasive detection of driver mutations (*EGFR* mutations and *ALK* fusions), particularly in the setting of resistance to tyrosine kinase inhibitor therapy {109,733,1507,1949,3097,1734}. Although this is a specific test in most circumstances, it suffers from low sensitivity.

Diagnostic terminology and criteria for lung cancer in small biopsy and cytology specimens

A classification for lung cancer diagnosis in non-resection specimens (mostly small biopsies and cytology) initially proposed in the 2011 IASLC/ATS/ERS lung adenocarcinoma classification was also recommended in the 2015 WHO classification – see Box 1.01 (p. 29), Table 1.04, and Table 1.05 {3074,3068}. This provided a workflow for managing small biopsy and cytology samples, emphasizing the need for making an accurate diagnosis including specific histological typing of non-squamous cell carcinomas, which may represent primary or metastatic adenocarcinoma, using ancillary techniques such as immunohistochemistry, as well as highlighting the need for molecular testing {3074,3068}. To spare as much tissue as possible for molecular testing, it is recommended to use only a limited panel of immunohistochemical markers and/or mucin stains to diagnose and subtype NSCLC {3068}.

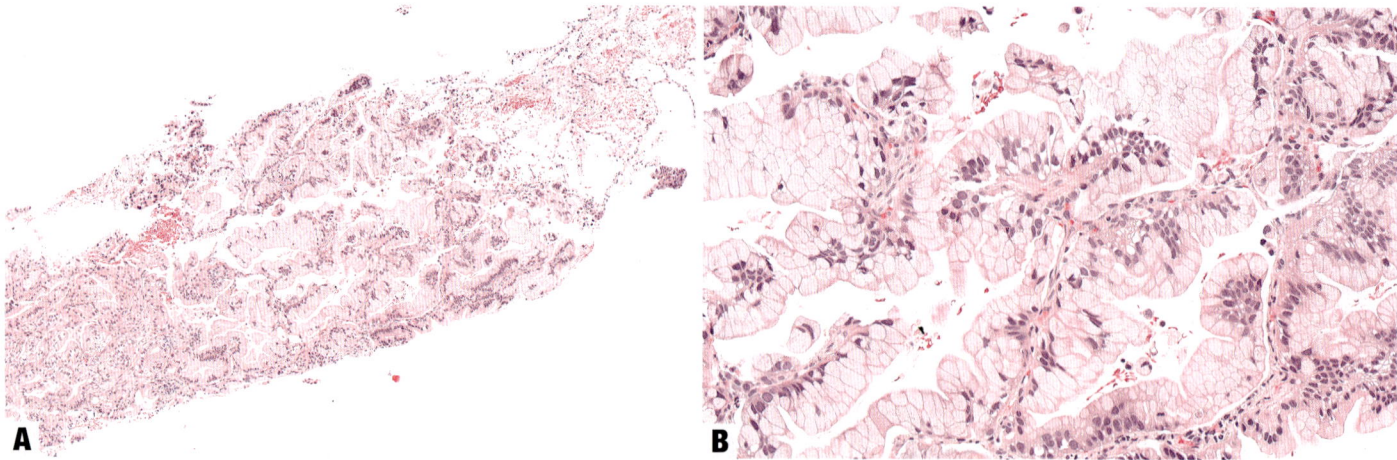

Fig. 1.07 Invasive mucinous adenocarcinoma in core biopsy. **A** This tumour shows acinar and papillary arrangements of mucinous tumour cells. **B** This higher power of the same tumour highlights the cytological features of the tumour cells with abundant apical mucinous cytoplasm and small mostly basally oriented nuclei.

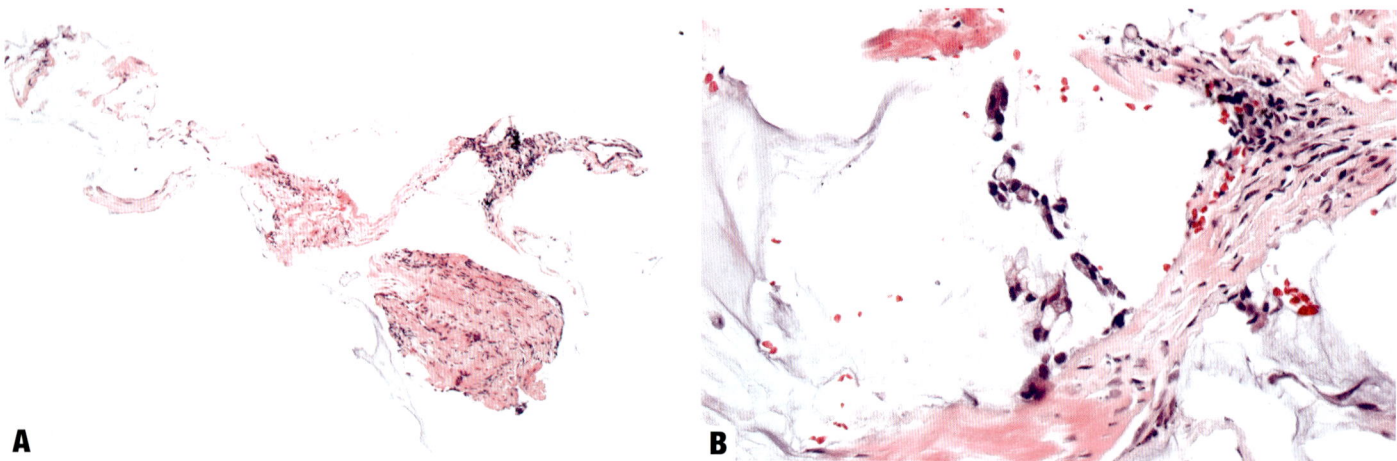

Fig. 1.08 Colloid adenocarcinoma in core biopsy. **A** This tumour consists mostly of abundant pools of mucin expanding airspaces. **B** On closer examination, there are cytologically bland tumour cells floating within the mucin pools that show prominent intracytoplasmic mucin.

If clear glandular morphology or keratinization is present in small biopsies or cytology specimens, the diagnosis of adenocarcinoma or squamous cell carcinoma (SCC), respectively, can be made without a need for special stains, unless TTF1

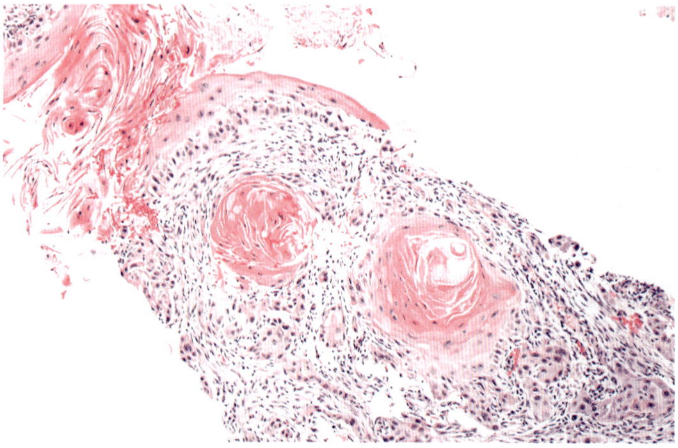

Fig. 1.09 Squamous cell carcinoma, core biopsy. This tumour shows nests of malignant cells with focal keratinization. There is nuclear enlargement, hyperchromatic nuclear chromatin, and prominent nucleoli.

staining is desired to confirm lung origin (see Box 1.01, p. 29) {3074,1608,3068}.

Adenocarcinoma

The patterns that indicate adenocarcinoma differentiation include lepidic, acinar, papillary, micropapillary, solid, fetal, and enteric patterns. In addition, invasive mucinous adenocarcinoma and colloid adenocarcinoma are distinctive patterns of adenocarcinoma.

The cytological aspects of adenocarcinoma are summarized in more detail in the sections specifically about adenocarcinomas of the lung (beginning on p. 60). Briefly, features in cytology specimens that favour adenocarcinomas include papillary or pseudopapillary formations, acinar gland-like structures, 3D balls of cells, and a picket-fence or drunken-honeycomb appearance in mucinous tumours {1608,2511,932}.

It can be helpful to record the adenocarcinoma patterns present in small biopsies or cytology specimens, although unlike for resection specimens, documenting relative percentages of the patterns is not recommended {3074,3068}. In some clinical circumstances, such as stereotactic body radiation therapy or thermal ablation therapy, the presence of a solid and/

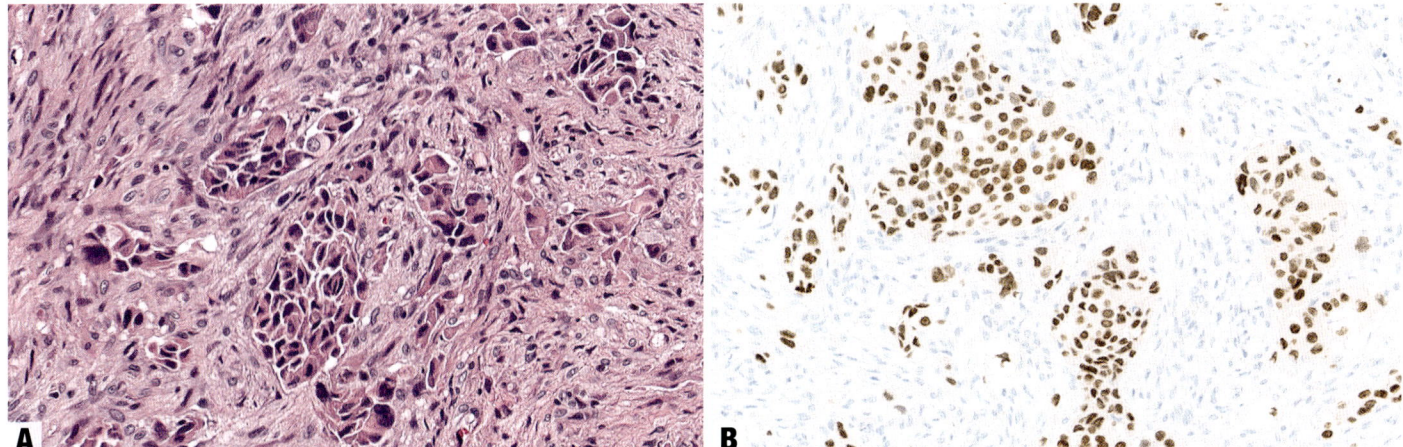

Fig. 1.10 Non-small cell carcinoma, favour adenocarcinoma, in core biopsy of thoracic spine metastases. **A** This tumour consists of a pure solid pattern of malignant cells lacking any glandular or squamous morphology. **B** There is diffuse strong staining for TTF1.

or micropapillary pattern in core biopsies from lung adenocarcinoma patients is associated with poor outcomes {1648,907}.

Squamous cell carcinoma

Squamous cell differentiation can be demonstrated morphologically by the presence of keratinization, squamous pearls, and intercellular bridges {2457,932}. Cytology of SCC is dealt with in more detail in *Squamous cell carcinoma of the lung* (p. 89), but on Pap stains the tumour cell cytoplasm appears orange, bright yellow, or red.

NSCC, favour adenocarcinoma

In poorly differentiated carcinomas with a solid pattern where TTF1 and/or mucin stains are positive but p40 is negative, the diagnosis is "non-small cell carcinoma (NSCC), favour adenocarcinoma" (see Table 1.04, p. 30). In cases where both TTF1 and p40 are negative, the diagnosis of adenocarcinoma can be supported if mucin stains are positive. It is also possible to identify features of adenocarcinoma on cytology specimens to allow for this diagnosis even if the biopsy shows a solid NSCC that is negative for TTF1, p40, and mucin stains. So, in poorly differentiated tumours, correlation between biopsy and cytology findings is useful.

In order to make more accurate diagnoses in poorly differentiated NSCCs that lack morphological glandular or squamous differentiation, it is essential to perform immunohistochemistry or mucin staining to make a specific diagnosis. Solid adenocarcinomas can exhibit prominent eosinophilic cytoplasm suggesting keratinization or SCC, making it impossible to distinguish adenocarcinoma from SCC in this setting.

Although immunohistochemistry is required for NSCC with solid patterns, the number of special stains should be minimized in order to maximize the tissue available for molecular testing. In most tumours, staining for only TTF1 and p40 will allow for a precise diagnosis of adenocarcinoma or SCC.

NSCC, favour SCC

In poorly differentiated carcinomas with a solid pattern, if the tumour is p40-positive but TTF1-negative, the diagnosis should be "NSCC, favour SCC" (see Table 1.04, p. 30). p40 is the preferred squamous marker, because p63 can stain 20–30% of lung adenocarcinomas. Therefore, if a tumour expresses both p63 and TTF1 in the same tumour cells, it should be classified as "favour adenocarcinoma". Furthermore, because as many as 20% of adenocarcinomas are negative for TTF1, a tumour expressing p63 could be misclassified as SCC {239}. Therefore,

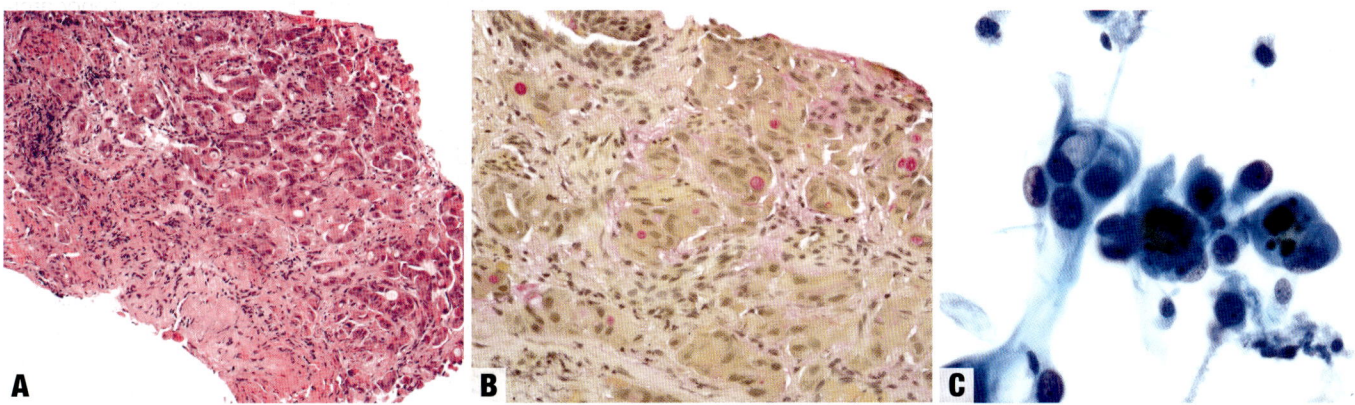

Fig. 1.11 Non-small cell carcinoma, favour adenocarcinoma, in core biopsy. **A** This tumour consists of a pure solid pattern of malignant cells lacking any glandular or squamous morphology. **B** The tumour cells show focal positive staining for intracytoplasmic mucin with the mucicarmine stain. **C** This cytology shows a cluster of tumour cells arranged around a small lumen with focal intracytoplasmic mucin.

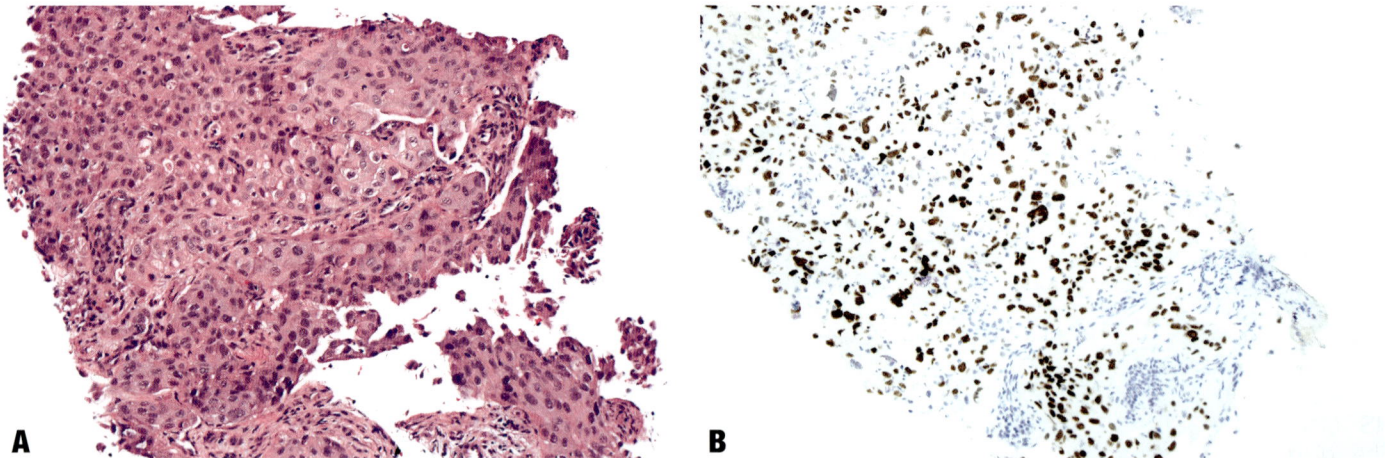

Fig. 1.12 Non-small cell carcinoma, favour adenocarcinoma. Solid adenocarcinoma with pseudosquamous morphology in core biopsy. **A** This adenocarcinoma shows a pure solid pattern, with abundant eosinophilic cytoplasm and sharp intracytoplasmic borders, that is reminiscent of squamous morphology. **B** However, the tumour is diffusely positive for TTF1, and it was negative for p40 (not shown).

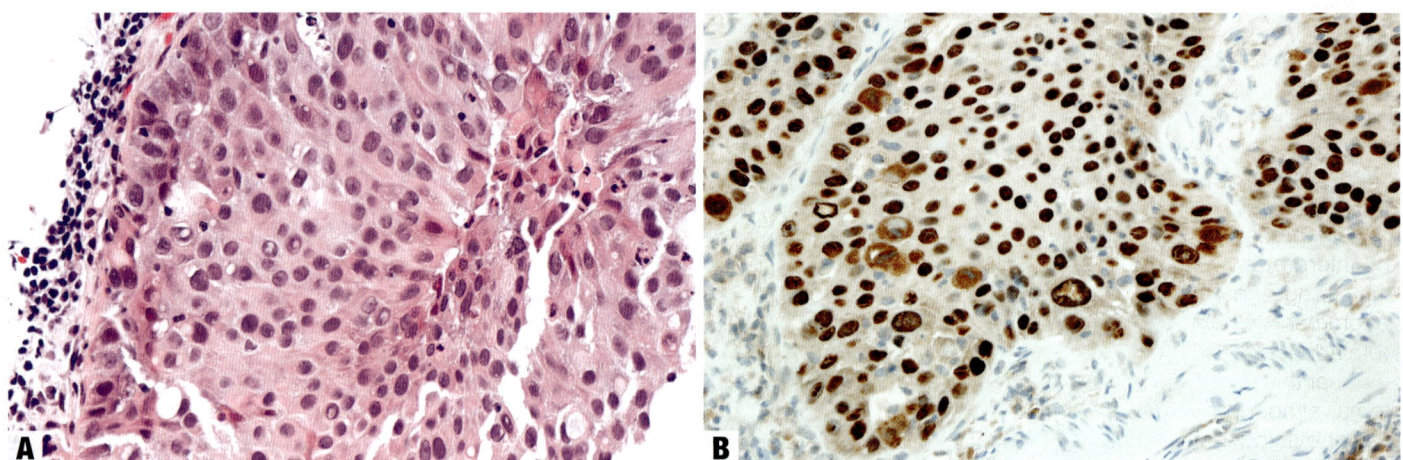

Fig. 1.13 Non-small cell carcinoma, favour squamous cell carcinoma. **A** In core biopsy. This tumour consists of a pure solid pattern of malignant cells lacking any glandular or squamous morphology. **B** This tumour shows diffuse positive staining for p40.

diffuse positive staining for p40 favours SCC, and p63 should be avoided if possible.

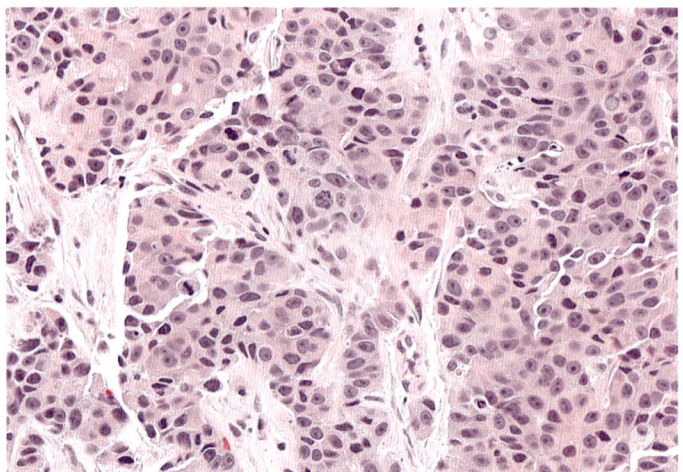

Fig. 1.14 Non-small cell carcinoma NOS in supraclavicular lymph node metastases. This tumour consists of a pure solid pattern of malignant cells lacking any glandular or squamous morphology. Immunohistochemistry for TTF1 and p40 was negative.

NSCC not otherwise specified

The term "NSCC not otherwise specified (NOS)" is appropriate for poorly differentiated carcinomas that, by morphology, mucin staining, and immunohistochemistry (negative TTF1 and p40), lack adenocarcinoma or SCC differentiation, or if the immuno-histochemical staining pattern is indeterminate (see Table 1.04, p. 30). It is important in such cases to perform an additional limited immunohistochemical workup to confirm that the tumour is a carcinoma and to exclude several common possible meta-static tumour types if this can be done without compromising molecular testing (see Chapter 9: *Metastases*). The choice of which stains to perform is dependent upon H&E morphology and clinical circumstances.

If the diagnosis of carcinoma is confirmed and a metastatic tumour appears to be excluded, the diagnosis of NSCC-NOS can be made. It is useful to mention in the report that although these findings are consistent with a primary carcinoma of the lung, they are not specific.

The term "NSCC-NOS" should be used as infrequently as possible and only after a more specific subtyping cannot be made by morphology or special staining. In some cases, when poorly differentiated carcinomas are encountered without any block or unstained slides to pursue a further workup, the diagnosis of NSCC-NOS can be made; however, it should be clearly stated that this is being done only because material is not available for further workup {3074,3068}.

The term "large cell carcinoma" should not be applied in small biopsy or cytology specimens because this is a diagnosis that can be made only in lung cancer resection specimens. In addition, the term "non-squamous cell carcinoma" should be avoided by pathologists in diagnostic reports. It is a term used by clinicians to lump categories of patients whose tumours comprise several histological types, such as adenocarcinoma and NSCC-NOS, who can be treated in a similar manner (see Table 1.04, p. 30, and Table 1.05, p. 31).

NSCC with adenocarcinoma and squamous differentiation

The diagnosis of adenosquamous carcinomas cannot be made on the basis of small biopsy and/or cytology specimens, because it requires a resection specimen with ≥ 10% of each component. However, tumours demonstrating two populations of tumour cells can occasionally be recognized in small biopsy or cytology samples (see Table 1.05, p. 31). It is most straightforward when both components are present morphologically, the adenocarcinoma shows glandular (lepidic, acinar, papillary, micropapillary) morphology, and the SCC is keratinizing. Adenosquamous carcinoma can also be seen in small specimens when one or both tumour components are undifferentiated, requiring TTF1 or p40 staining to recognize them. Although TTF1 expression is usually compelling, caution is advised in the interpretation of p40 (or especially p63) expression unless it is strong and diffuse in the relevant area. In such cases, the recommended diagnosis is NSCC-NOS, with a comment that both adenocarcinoma and squamous differentiation are present and that this raises the consideration of adenosquamous carcinoma, although that diagnosis cannot be made in small biopsies or cytology.

NSCC with spindle and/or giant cell features

Pleomorphic carcinoma cannot be diagnosed on the basis of small biopsy or cytology specimens, because it requires a resection specimen showing ≥ 10% of spindle and/or giant cell components (see Table 1.05, p. 31). However, if small biopsies or cytology specimens show NSCC with spindle and/or giant cell carcinoma patterns, a comment should be made that their presence raises the possibility of a pleomorphic carcinoma {3068}. The presence of TTF1 expression, even if focal, may favour adenocarcinoma differentiation and also support a lung primary. The diagnosis of pulmonary blastoma or carcinosarcoma is very challenging on small biopsy or cytology specimens. However, if both the glandular and sarcomatous components, with the appropriate morphology, are obtained in the specimen, these diagnoses can be made (see *Pulmonary blastoma*, p. 106, and *Carcinosarcoma of the lung*, p. 109).

Adenocarcinoma with lepidic pattern

If a pure lepidic pattern is seen in a small biopsy, the differential diagnosis includes adenocarcinoma in situ, minimally invasive adenocarcinoma, or invasive adenocarcinoma with a lepidic component. This differential diagnosis should be mentioned in a comment; however, each of these diagnoses requires a resection specimen and cannot be made on the basis of small

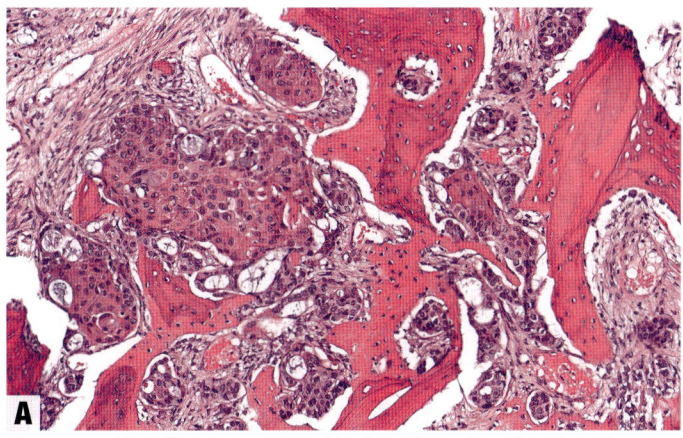

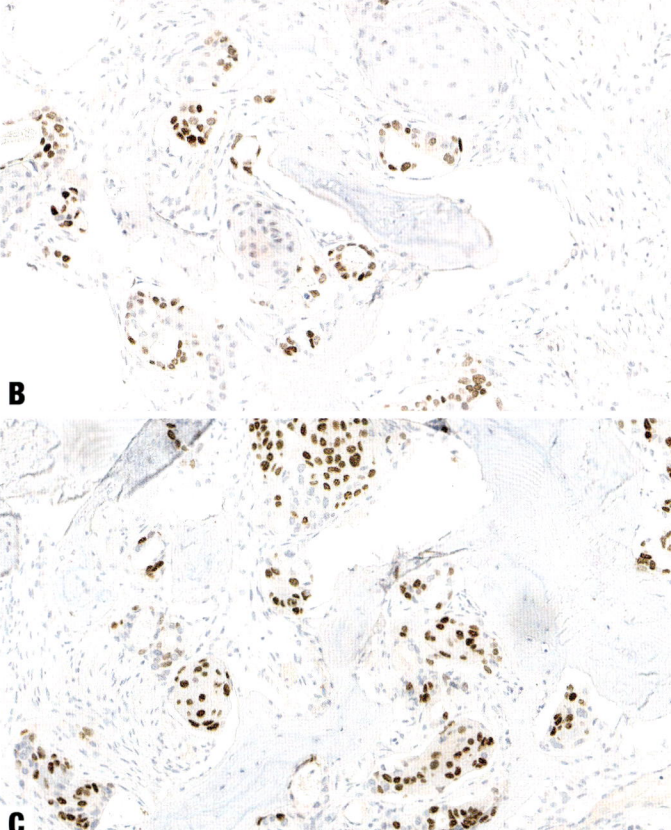

Fig. 1.15 Non-small cell carcinoma NOS with adenocarcinoma and squamous cell carcinoma differentiation in metastases to bone. **A** The tumour shows two components: acinar adenocarcinoma and keratinizing squamous cell carcinoma. **B** The adenocarcinoma component stains positively for TTF. **C** The squamous cell carcinoma component stains positively for p40.

biopsies or cytology specimens. Correlation with CT findings may help narrow the differential diagnosis, depending on the size of the total tumour and/or the size of the ground-glass or solid components {3081}.

Neuroendocrine tumours (NETs)
Carcinoid tumour NOS
The term "carcinoid tumour / NET NOS" is introduced to be used in three settings where the distinction between typical carcinoid (TC) and atypical carcinoid (AC) may not be possible or

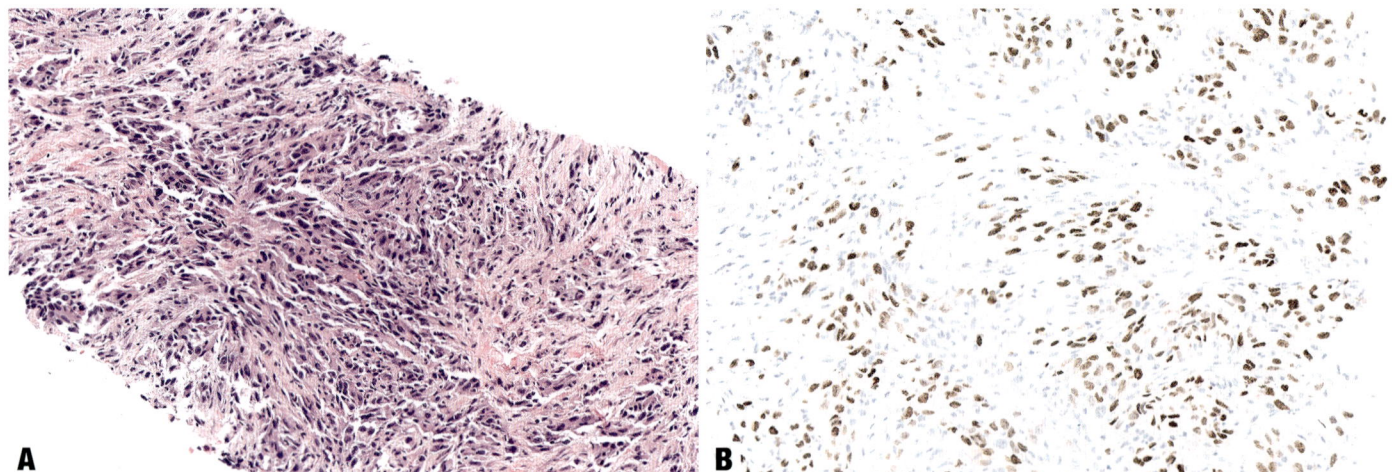

Fig. 1.16 Non-small cell carcinoma, favour adenocarcinoma with spindle cell features, in core biopsy. **A** The tumour in this small specimen consists purely of malignant spindle cells. **B** The tumour stains positively for TTF1.

appropriate. In such cases, rather than specifying TC or AC, it is suggested to record the mitotic count, the presence or absence of necrosis, and (if available) the Ki-67 index {2458}. First, in small biopsies or cytology, the distinction between TC and AC is not possible in most cases because of the limited sampling of tumour or a poor-quality specimen. Second, this term should be used for metastatic carcinoids. The diagnostic criteria for distinguishing TC from AC were established on lung resection specimens {3079,3084} and not on specimens from metastatic sites {2458}. Metastatic pulmonary carcinoid patients are often treated by medical oncologists who also manage gastrointestinal/pancreatic NETs, where Ki-67 is used to stratify patients for therapeutic decisions {2712,173,1368}. So documenting Ki-67 may be useful in the metastatic setting, although mitotic counts and necrosis remain the main diagnostic criteria in resected pulmonary carcinoids. In metastatic pulmonary carcinoids, further study is needed to determine the role of Ki-67 in classification, prognostication, and therapeutic management {2712,2500, 173,1368,1807,379,2458}. This topic is addressed in more detail in *Carcinoid/neuroendocrine tumour of the lung* (p. 133). Third, in some cases, only representative slides of a resected carcinoid tumour are provided for review, rather than the entire set of tumour slides. In such cases, it is not possible to exclude the presence of an increased mitotic count or necrosis on slides not provided, to fully address the differential diagnosis of TC versus AC. See *Lung neuroendocrine neoplasms: Introduction* (p. 127) and *Carcinoid/neuroendocrine tumour of the lung* (p. 133) for more explanation regarding use of the term "carcinoid tumour NOS".

Small cell lung carcinoma (SCLC)

The diagnosis of SCLC is readily established based on small biopsies and cytology specimens. There is a high degree of reproducibility for the diagnosis of SCLC versus NSCLC on H&E sections {3179A,1159A,368A,856A}, but the distinction from large cell neuroendocrine carcinoma (LCNEC) may be more challenging {3077A,659A}. The rate of agreement in SCLC diagnosis can be improved by the use of immunohistochemistry {3038,3390}. With regard to other NETs, Ki-67 is most helpful in the separation of SCLC from carcinoids in crushed biopsies. When biopsies are difficult to interpret, it can be useful to compare with concurrent cytology specimens, which may show material that is more diagnostic. More details regarding SCLC and LCNEC diagnosis are addressed in *Small cell lung carcinoma* (p. 139) and *Large cell neuroendocrine carcinoma of the lung* (p. 144) {3038}.

NSCC with features of LCNEC

LCNEC is challenging to diagnose in small biopsies and/or cytology, particularly because of the need to meet the criteria of neuroendocrine morphology, which can be difficult to identify in small tissue samples. However, because core biopsies are being obtained more often, in order to acquire larger amounts of tissue for molecular testing, neuroendocrine morphological features including peripheral palisading, organoid nesting patterns, or rosette-like structures are more readily recognized than in the past when smaller biopsies were obtained (see *Large cell neuroendocrine carcinoma of the lung*, p. 144) {3068}. In the absence of neuroendocrine morphology, it is not recommended to perform staining for neuroendocrine markers in NSCC-NOS {3070}. The diagnosis of LCNEC, even in small biopsies, requires both neuroendocrine morphology and positive immunohistochemical markers (see Table 1.05, p. 31). A recently proposed scoring system incorporates both neuroendocrine morphology and immunohistochemical markers, but this requires further validation {145}. In tumours that lack neuroendocrine morphology, the clinical significance of positive neuroendocrine immunohistochemical markers is not known {3068}.

Pathology reports for lung cancer diagnoses in small biopsy and cytology specimens

Reports of lung cancer diagnoses based on small biopsies and cytologies need to include the following: (1) a pathological or cytopathological diagnosis according to the 2021 WHO classification, (2) results of immunohistochemical and/or mucin stains, (3) a comment about the differential diagnosis (when appropriate), and (4) a statement of whether any material has been submitted for molecular testing (and the results if available). It can be useful to specify which block was used. Depending on the institutional workflow, the percentage of viable tumour cells in the specimen should be documented by either the surgical pathologist or the molecular team.

Bronchial papillomas

Flieder DB
Agaimy A

Definition

Squamous cell papilloma is a papillary tumour consisting of delicate connective tissue fronds lined with squamous epithelium; it can be solitary or multiple, and exophytic or inverted. Glandular papilloma is a benign papillary tumour lined by non-ciliated columnar cells, with varying numbers of cuboidal and goblet cells. Mixed squamous and glandular papilloma is an endobronchial papillary tumour showing an admixture of squamous and glandular epithelium; each epithelial type should constitute at least one third of the epithelium.

ICD-O coding

8052/0 Squamous cell papilloma, NOS
8053/0 Squamous cell papilloma, inverted
8260/0 Glandular papilloma
8560/0 Mixed squamous cell and glandular papilloma

ICD-11 coding

2F0Y & XH50T2 Benign neoplasms of other specified respiratory and intrathoracic organs & Squamous cell papilloma, NOS
2F0Y & XH3BK2 Benign neoplasms of other specified respiratory and intrathoracic organs & Glandular papilloma
2F0Y & XH1TX5 Benign neoplasms of other specified respiratory and intrathoracic organs & Mixed squamous cell and glandular papilloma

Related terminology

Acceptable: squamous papilloma; columnar cell papilloma; mixed papilloma.

Subtype(s)

Squamous cell papilloma, exophytic; squamous cell papilloma, inverted; glandular papilloma; mixed squamous cell and glandular papilloma

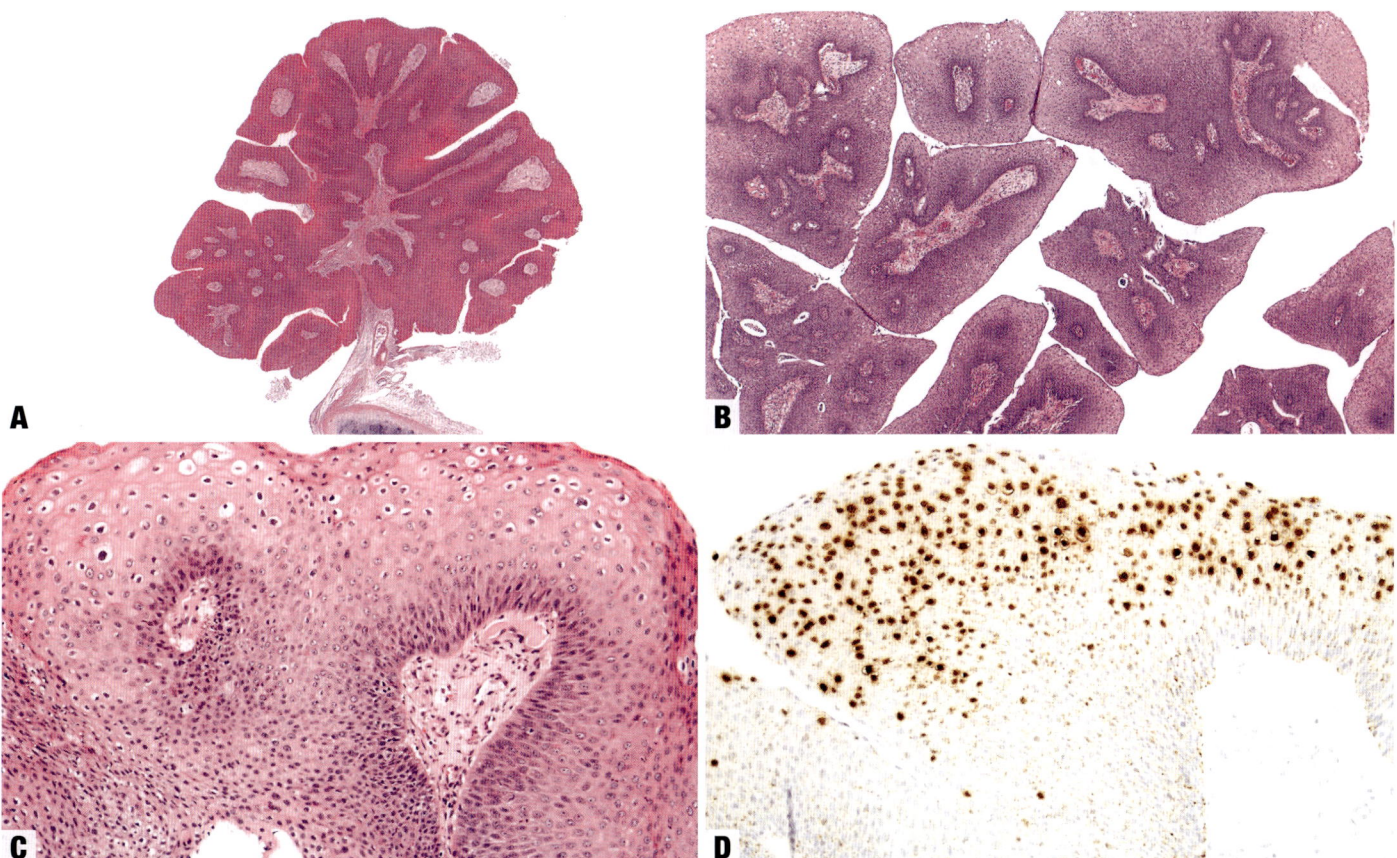

Fig. 1.17 Exophytic squamous cell papilloma. **A** This endobronchial tumour features papillary fronds lined by mature squamous epithelium. **B** This bronchoscopic sample demonstrates the papillary nature of the tumour and the vascular nature of the stroma. The epithelium is acanthotic. **C** Koilocytosis is apparent in the upper epithelial layers. **D** In situ hybridization staining for HPV subtypes 6 and 11.

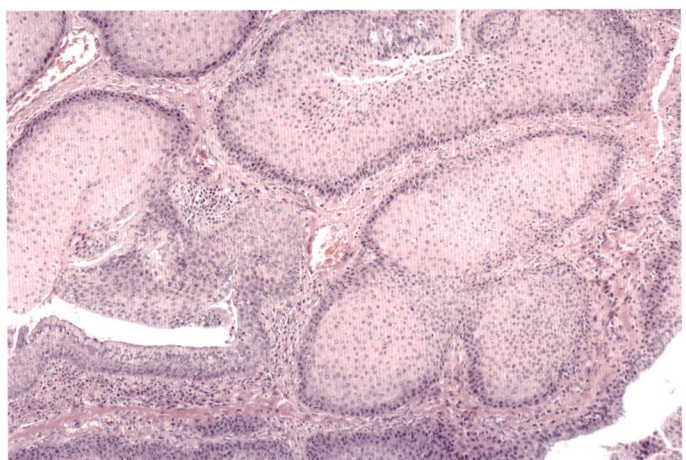

Fig. 1.18 Inverted squamous cell papilloma. Mature squamous epithelium grows into the stromal component of this endobronchial tumour.

Localization

Solitary papillomas are usually central and endobronchial, and rarely peripheral and endobronchiolar. Lung manifestation of squamous laryngotracheal papillomatosis may involve the bronchial tree and/or lung parenchyma with multifocal papillomas {853,1599}.

Clinical features

Most patients present with obstructive symptoms or haemoptysis, but as many as 25% may be asymptomatic, presenting with incidental radiographic detection {1583,844}. High-resolution CT findings demonstrate endobronchial plaques, nodules, or airway thickening in addition to air trapping, atelectasis, consolidation, and bronchiectasis {1488,2049}. PET avidity is reported in several studied glandular and mixed papillomas {2985,1828}. Lung involvement by squamous papillomatosis demonstrates diffuse, poorly defined, non-calcified parenchymal centrilobular opacities, as well as cavitated thick-walled nodules {2559}.

Epidemiology

Solitary squamous cell papillomas are exceedingly rare, accounting for < 1% of all lung neoplasms, but they are far more common than either glandular or mixed papillomas {3090,844}. Squamous cell and mixed papillomas are 3 times as common

in men as in women, while glandular papillomas have an equal sex distribution. Patients are usually in their sixth decade of life {3090}. Squamous papillomatosis involving the bronchial tree or lung parenchyma is related to laryngotracheal papillomatosis {1068}.

Etiology

HPV plays a pathogenetic role in less than half of solitary squamous cell papillomas but in virtually all papillomatosis lesions {1068,844,1599}. Serotypes 6 and 11 are reported in simple and multiple squamous papillomas, while subtypes 16, 18, and 31/33/35 may play a role in malignant transformation {2376, 2377}. HPV has not been identified in non-squamous papillomas. The majority of patients with solitary papillomas are tobacco smokers, but an etiological role has not been established {3090,844}.

Pathogenesis

In HPV-infected lesions, the double-stranded circular DNA virus infects the basal epithelial layer. Viral genome integration into host DNA genome increases expression of the E6 and E7 oncoproteins, which inactivate tumour-suppressor proteins p53 and RB1, in addition to other actions, all leading to cellular proliferation {939}.

Macroscopic appearance

Solitary papillomas arise from the wall of mainstem, secondary, or tertiary bronchi. They range from 7 to > 90 mm, with a median size of 15 mm {844}. Almost all form exophytic, polypoid, tan-white, and friable lesions, protruding into airway lumina. Distal and sometimes proximal airways may be bronchiectatic. The distal lung may show secondary obstructive effects such as atelectasis, consolidation, or honeycomb change {763}. Multiple lesions may impart a velvety appearance to the bronchial mucosa. Involved lung is bronchiectatic, with cavities filled with white-tan friable papillary fronds {664}.

Histopathology

Squamous cell papilloma

Squamous cell papillomas feature arborizing loose fibrovascular cores covered by stratified squamous epithelium. Exophytic tumours have orderly epithelial maturation and often keratinized surface cells. Acanthosis, parakeratosis, and intraepithelial

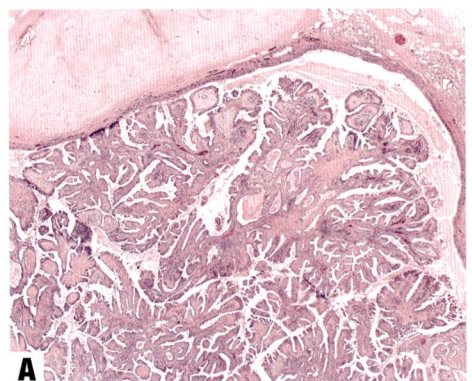
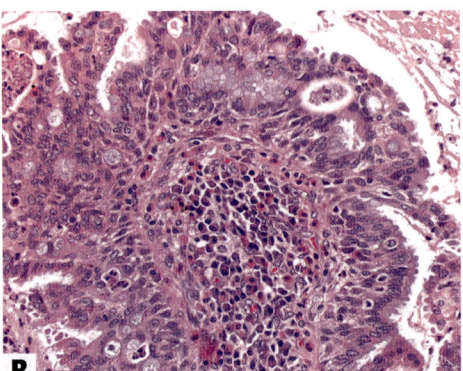
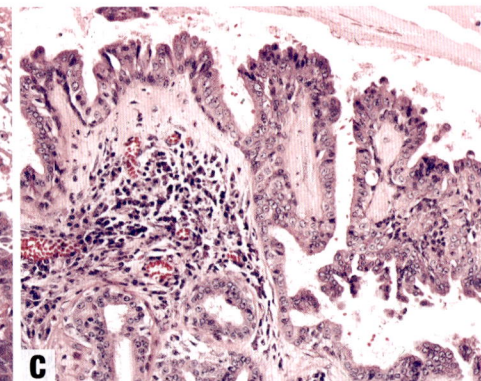

Fig. 1.19 Glandular papilloma. **A** Papillary endobronchial lesion with cytologically bland glandular epithelial cells proliferating along fibrovascular cores. **B** Uniform cytologically bland columnar cells admixed with occasional mucous cells line inflamed stromal cores. **C** Higher power of papillary endobronchial lesion with cytologically bland glandular epithelial cells proliferating along fibrovascular cores.

neutrophils are common {844,1867}. Less than 25% of solitary papillomas feature typical HPV viral cytopathic effect, including binucleate forms, wrinkled nuclei, and perinuclear haloes. Occasional dyskeratotic cells, large atypical cells, and mitotic figures above the basal layer can be seen. Dysplasia is graded according to the current WHO classification (see *Squamous dysplasia and carcinoma in situ of the lung*, p. 85).

Inverted papillomas are also exophytic, but they have squamous epithelial invaginations. Cells may extend into seromucinous glands, but basal lamina invests the endophytic nests. Cells are usually non-keratinizing and demonstrate orderly maturation {844}.

Squamous cell papillomas may occasionally infiltrate beyond the bronchial wall, with parenchymal involvement featuring either solid intra-alveolar nests of cytologically bland non-keratinizing cells or large cysts lined by similar cells. Reactive type II pneumocytes lining alveolar walls may be prominent. Surrounding lung may be inflamed or fibrotic. Viral cytopathic effect is usually seen in instances of pulmonary laryngotracheal papillomatosis. Immunohistochemical or in situ DNA hybridization studies correlate with the morphological finding of koilocytosis.

The differential diagnosis includes inflammatory polyp and squamous cell carcinoma (SCC). Endobronchial inflammatory polyps show conspicuous inflammation and, despite focal squamous metaplasia, they lack true papillary architecture, stromal cores, and proliferative epithelium. SCCs, which can be endobronchial and papillary, feature malignant cytological features even when stromal invasion and desmoplasia are not apparent. Inverted papillomas can be indistinguishable from invasive SCC; however, parenchymal destruction and overt cytological atypia favour a diagnosis of malignancy. The recognition of even focal carcinoma within a papilloma warrants a diagnosis of carcinoma; therefore, small biopsy samples showing mature papillary squamous epithelium may not exclude the diagnosis of SCC.

Glandular papilloma

Glandular papillomas feature broad epithelial-lined fronds with vascular or hyalinized stromal cores. Stratified or pseudostratified columnar epithelium may form micropapillary tufts. Uniform non-ciliated columnar cells have eosinophilic cytoplasm and round regular nuclei, and interspersed mucinous cells may be seen. The cytoplasm can be clear, but nuclear atypia, mitoses, and necrosis are absent. Stromal cores often contain sheets of plasma cells {763}.

The differential diagnosis includes primary and metastatic adenocarcinomas and other adenomas. Complete excision is necessary for definitive diagnosis. In superficial endoscopic biopsies, the term "papillary glandular neoplasm" may be appropriate, because invasive adenocarcinoma cannot be excluded without thorough histological sampling of the lesion. Carcinomas feature epithelial crowding and malignant cytological features yet lack basal, ciliated, and mucinous cells. Bronchiolar adenomas arise in peripheral small airways, not proximal bronchi. They can be papillary and feature a spectrum of cuboidal to ciliated cells with a continuous layer of basal cells {444}. *BRAF* mutations are reported in almost 30% of these tumours (see *Bronchiolar adenoma / ciliated muconodular papillary tumour*, p. 48). The presence of ciliated cells should raise concern to exclude bronchiolar adenoma. Indeed, some peripheral

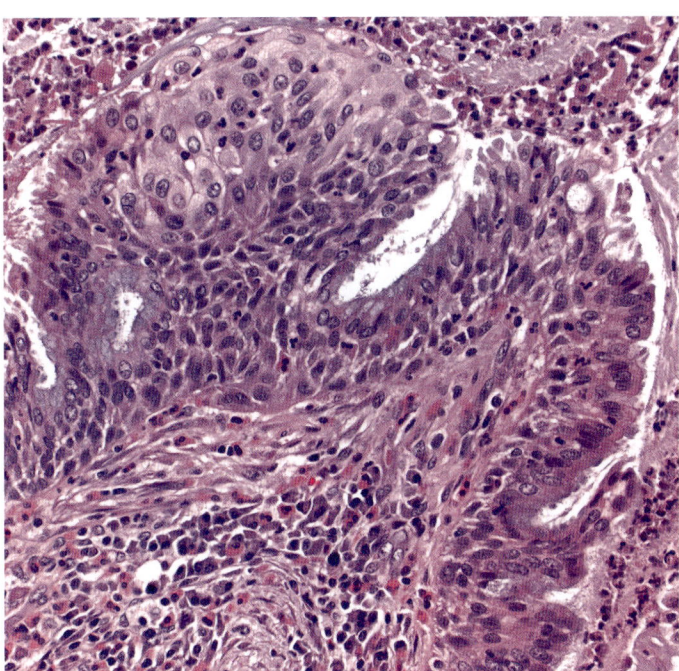

Fig. 1.20 Mixed squamous cell and glandular papilloma. The papillary frond is lined with discrete foci of glandular and squamous epithelium.

papillary tumours with ciliated cells previously thought to be glandular papillomas were probably bronchiolar adenomas. Mucus gland adenoma (see *Mucous gland adenoma of the lung*, p. 53) occurs in proximal bronchi and is composed of mucus-filled cysts and tubules, the latter of which are absent in glandular papillomas. Glandular papillomas also differ from papillary adenomas (see *Papillary adenoma of the lung*, p. 46), which are peripheral parenchymal tumours without an attachment to an airway, composed of a single layer of tumour cells with pneumocytic differentiation.

Mixed squamous and glandular papillomas

Histology mirrors the findings in pure squamous cell and glandular papillomas; however, most of the epithelium lining fibrovascular cores is glandular, with interspersed squamous islands. Each epithelial type should constitute at least one third of the epithelium. The pseudostratified ciliated and non-ciliated cuboidal to columnar cells with scattered mucin-filled cells are distinct from the acanthotic and focally keratinizing squamous epithelium {1245,2629,1665}. Glandular atypia and necrosis are not seen, but squamous atypia ranges from mild to severe. Viral cytopathic effect is not present. A definitive diagnosis can be rendered only on a completely resected tumour.

The differential diagnosis mirrors that of pure squamous cell and glandular papillomas, with the addition of mucoepidermoid carcinoma and adenosquamous carcinoma. The former is primarily composed of mucous glands with intermediate and/or squamoid cells, rather than keratinizing squamous epithelium, and the latter is a high-grade carcinoma.

Cytology

Exfoliated samples from squamous cell papillomas demonstrate sheets and single squamous cells with sharp cellular borders and dense, glassy cytoplasm. Cells may be multinucleated, and

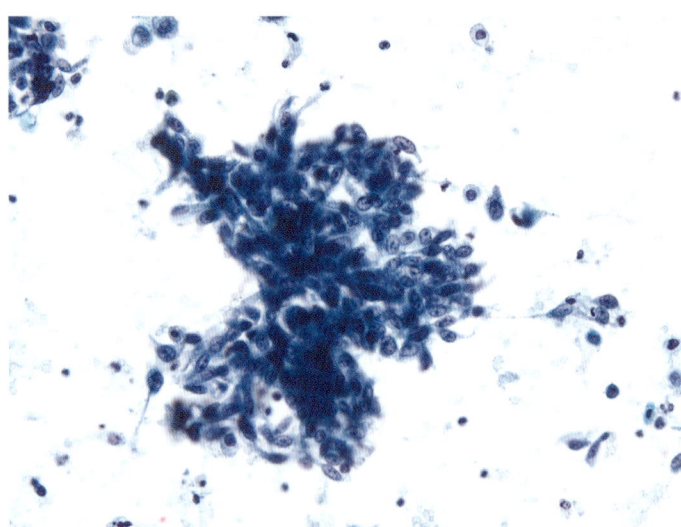

Fig. 1.21 Laryngotracheal papillomatosis involving the lung. This cluster of squamous cells with well-defined cytoplasmic borders and dense cytoplasm also has a suggestion of perinuclear haloes (PAP stain).

nuclei vary from small and pyknotic to large with uneven chromatin. Perinuclear haloes and degenerative vacuoles may be seen. Smaller basal cells featuring scant basophilic cytoplasm and round regular nuclei mix with neutrophils in the background. FNA samples feature well-developed 3D branching papillae lined by crowded non-keratinized round to oval cells with scant, dense cytoplasm. Single cells are also seen. Irregular nuclear contours, enlarged nuclei, anisonucleosis, and/or prominent nucleoli may be seen, but keratinization, mitoses, karyorrhexis, and necrosis are absent {2277,1593}.

Bronchial brushings from mixed papillomas demonstrate that squamous cells outnumber glandular cells. Squamous cells are both keratinized and non-keratinized, feature mild nuclear atypia, and lack koilocytic change. Scattered single columnar cells are ciliated and non-ciliated with granular nuclei without atypia {2629,1338}. Intraoperative imprint cytology additionally showed cohesive clusters of columnar cells.

Diagnostic molecular pathology
Not relevant

Essential and desirable diagnostic criteria
Essential:
- Squamous cell papilloma: papillary fronds with delicate connective tissue fibrovascular cores lined by mature squamous epithelium
- Glandular papilloma: papillary tumour lined by non-ciliated columnar, cuboidal, and/or goblet cells
- Mixed squamous and glandular papilloma: papillary tumour lined by mixed squamous and glandular epithelium – each type should constitute at least one third of the epithelium

Desirable:
- Usually in an endobronchial location
- Complete excision with thorough histological evaluation to exclude carcinoma

Staging
Not relevant

Prognosis and prediction
Surgically resected solitary squamous cell papillomas do not recur, but as many as 20% of patients treated with endoscopic removal have local tumour recurrences {844,1867}. Transformation into SCC is uncertain, and most reported cases represent inadequately sampled or misdiagnosed carcinoma; however, HPV-associated papillomas in the setting of papillomatosis (particularly associated with subtypes 16, 18, and 31/33/35) are recognized as having malignant potential {2376,2377}. Laryngotracheal papillomatosis can spread into the lower respiratory tract in as many as 5% of patients, and into the alveolar parenchyma in < 5% of juvenile cases {853,1396,935}. Bronchial and pulmonary involvement may be related to prior treatments or reflux disease. These lesions may develop into abscesses and eventually bronchiectasis. Malignant transformation does not exceed 2% {973}. This disease is incurable, although antiviral and immunomodulatory therapies, as well as HPV vaccines, are promising {61,220,1274}.

Glandular papillomas are benign tumours that may recur if not completely removed {844}. Malignant transformation has not been reported.

Surgical resection appears curative for mixed squamous and glandular papillomas {1245,844,1526}. SCC arising in a mixed squamous and glandular papilloma has been reported {1583}.

Sclerosing pneumocytoma

Beasley MB
Chou TY
Soares FA
Wang EH

Definition

Sclerosing pneumocytoma is a tumour of pneumocytic origin composed of a dual population of surface cells resembling type II pneumocytes and round cells. The tumour demonstrates varying amounts of solid, papillary, sclerotic, and haemorrhagic patterns.

ICD-O coding

8832/0 Sclerosing pneumocytoma

ICD-11 coding

2F0Z & XH7436 Benign neoplasms of respiratory and intrathoracic organs, unspecified & Sclerosing pneumocytoma

Related terminology

Not recommended: sclerosing haemangioma (obsolete).

Subtype(s)

None

Localization

Sclerosing pneumocytoma is typically solitary and peripheral. Rarely, tumours are multiple; occur as an endobronchial mass; or are situated in the hilum, visceral pleura, or mediastinum {688,1428}.

Clinical features

Patients are typically asymptomatic, with the tumour often discovered incidentally. Radiographs show a solitary circumscribed mass, which may rarely be calcified or cystic {2069, 2401,2602,3213,2753}.

Epidemiology

Sclerosing pneumocytoma occurs in a wide age range (11–80 years), with female predominance. The incidence is higher in eastern Asian populations and rare among individuals of European descent {468,689,1355,1554,1742}.

Etiology

The tumour is thought to derive from primitive respiratory epithelium {468,689,1355,438,3199}.

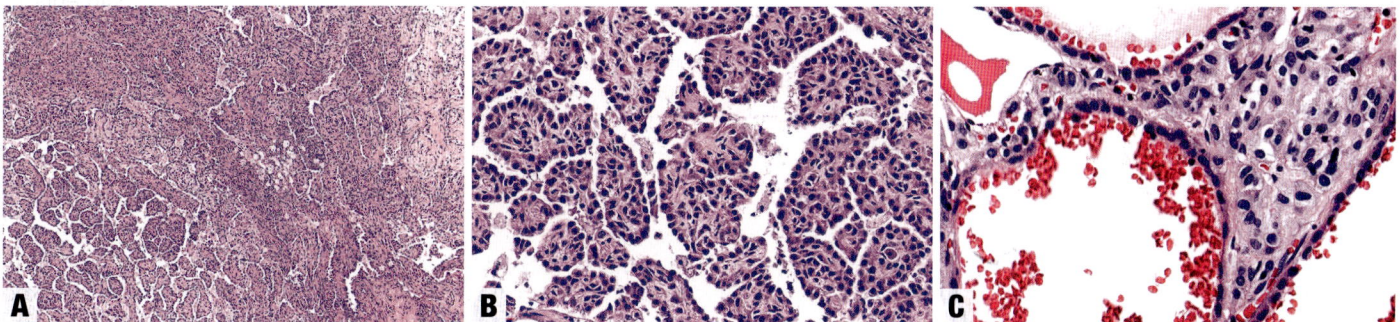

Fig. 1.22 Sclerosing pneumocytoma. **A** Low power showing a mixture of papillary, solid, and sclerotic patterns. **B** Papillary structures are covered by surface cells overlying stromal round cells. **C** Blood-filled spaces are lined by surface cells.

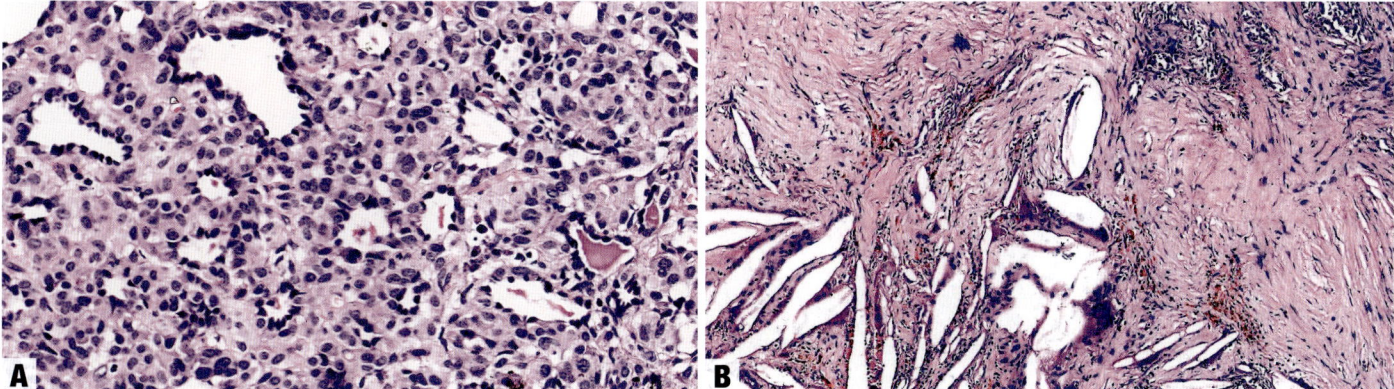

Fig. 1.23 Sclerosing pneumocytoma. **A** The solid region consists of round cells with small tubules lined by surface cells. **B** Inflammatory cells and cholesterol clefts in the sclerotic region. The tumour shows a sclerosing fibrous stroma.

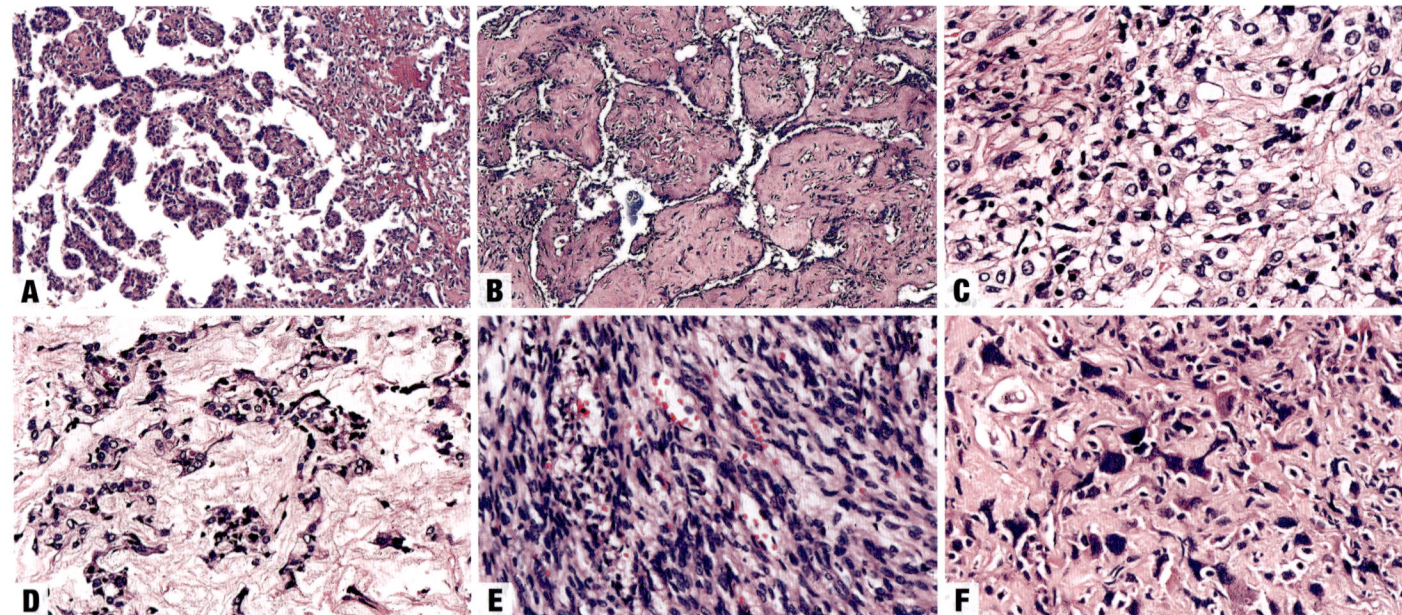

Fig. 1.24 Sclerosing pneumocytoma. **A** Delicate papillary structures mimicking true papillae. **B** Formation of sclerotic papillae. **C** Signet-ring morphology occurring in round cells. **D** Cords of round cells in a background stroma with myxoid change. **E** Stromal cells show spindle morphology, positive for TTF1 (not shown). **F** Multinucleated giant cells composed of fused surface cells.

Pathogenesis

Although sclerosing pneumocytoma is presumably derived from primitive pulmonary epithelium, the pathogenesis is unknown. However, molecular data have demonstrated the same monoclonal pattern in both the round and surface cells, consistent with a true neoplasm {3199}. *AKT1* internal tandem duplications (ITDs), point mutations, and short indels have been identified in nearly all sclerosing pneumocytomas. These mutations are mutually exclusive and occur in the Pleckstrin homology domain, a critical component in the activation of the AKT1 protein {1332,3397}. A *BRAF* p.V600E mutation has been reported in one case {1309}.

Macroscopic appearance

The tumours are well-circumscribed masses that are solid and show a variegated grey-tan to yellow on cut section, with foci of haemorrhage. Cystic degeneration and calcification may be evident.

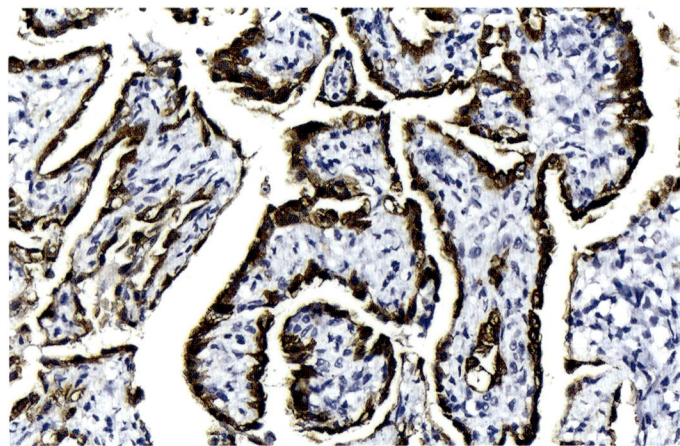

Fig. 1.25 Sclerosing pneumocytoma. Surface cells are positive for pancytokeratin while round cells are negative.

Histopathology

The key feature of sclerosing pneumocytoma is the presence of two cell types: cuboidal surface cells and round stromal cells, both of which are considered neoplastic. The surface cells are cuboidal and morphologically similar to type II pneumocytes. The round cells are small, with well-defined borders and central bland nuclei with fine chromatin and scant small nucleoli. The tumours typically have a combination of growth patterns: papillary, sclerotic, solid, and haemorrhagic. In the papillary pattern, complex papillary structures are covered by surface cells overlying a core of round cells as opposed to true fibrovascular cores. The sclerotic area is composed of fibrosis with hyalinized collagen, in which variable inflammatory cells, haemosiderin deposition, cholesterol clefts, calcification, and ossification may be seen. The solid pattern is composed of sheets of round cells, in which there may be tubular or incomplete adenoid structures surrounded by surface cells. In the haemorrhagic pattern, large blood-filled spaces may be present, lined by cuboidal epithelial cells {468,689,1554}. Fusion of surface cells into multinucleated giant cells, formation of sclerotic papillae due to the replacement of round cells by collagen, delicate papillary structures mimicking true papillae with fibrovascular cores, a spindle or signet-ring morphology of the round cells, and myxoid matrix surrounding round cell cords may be present as diagnostic pitfalls {1689,1713}.

Immunohistochemistry

Both surface and round cells are positive for EMA and TTF1. Pancytokeratin, CAM5.2, CK7, and napsin A stain the surface cells diffusely, but the round cells are usually negative or weakly positive. Neuroendocrine markers are negative. ER and PR staining has also been reported in some cases in the round cells {689,1355,438,1239,2538,2640,2663,3370,3198}.

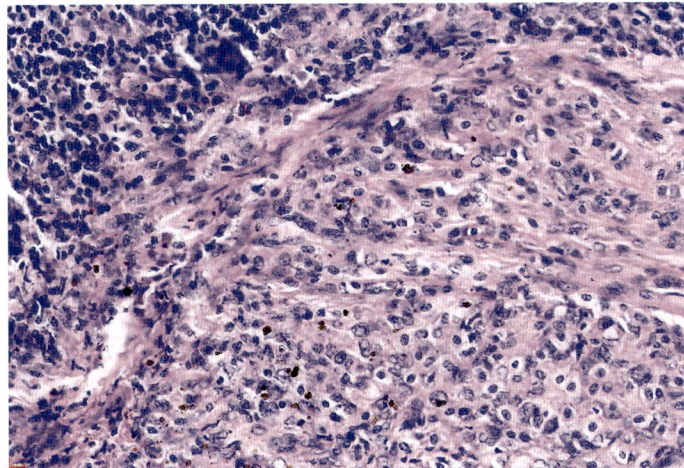

Fig. 1.26 Sclerosing pneumocytoma. Only round cells are evident in the involved lymph node.

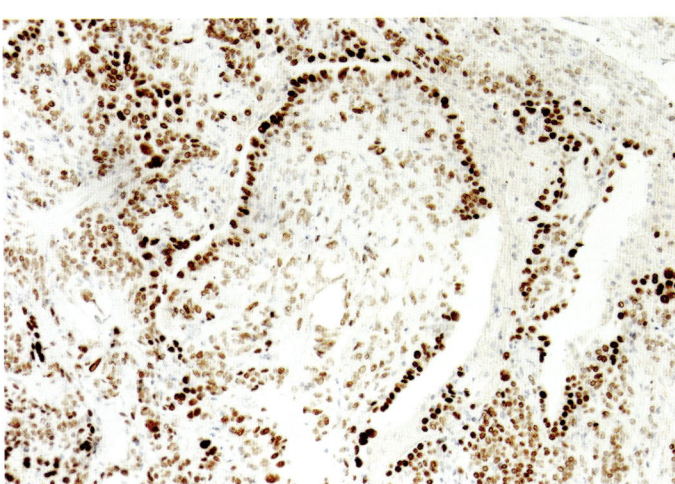

Fig. 1.27 Sclerosing pneumocytoma. This TTF1 stain highlights not only the surface tumour cells but also the underlying solid nests of round cells.

Differential diagnosis

The differential diagnosis consists primarily of carcinoid tumours and papillary adenocarcinoma. Rarely, either may coexist with sclerosing pneumocytoma {1713,3224,509}. In general, the multiple growth patterns, presence of bland cytological features, a dual cell population, and the characteristic immunostaining profile discriminate sclerosing pneumocytoma from other entities. However, accurate diagnosis on small biopsy, cytology, or frozen section may be difficult {437,1769,2590,3378,3339}.

Cytology

FNA may show a dual cell population, as well as hyalinized stromal fragments. The round cells are small, round to spindle-shaped, and arranged in cohesive papillary clusters or flat sheets. Nuclear pleomorphism, overlap, grooves, and inclusions may be seen. Prominent nucleoli and hyperchromasia may be present {1773,242,1165,1564}.

Diagnostic molecular pathology

Molecular data have demonstrated the same monoclonal pattern in both the round and surface cells, consistent with a true neoplasm {3199}. *AKT1* alterations are present in nearly all sclerosing pneumocytomas and may be useful for diagnosis in selected cases.

Essential and desirable diagnostic criteria

Essential:
- Well-circumscribed lesion composed of a dual population of surface and round cells
- A mixture of papillary, sclerotic, solid, and haemorrhagic growth patterns is usually present

Desirable:
- Distinctive immunostaining profile: TTF1 and EMA being positive in surface and round cells and cytokeratin staining being positive in the surface cells but weak or absent in the round cells

Staging

Not relevant

Prognosis and prediction

Most sclerosing pneumocytomas behave in a benign fashion. However, although cases with lymph node metastases and distant organ metastases have occasionally been reported, these findings do not appear to adversely affect prognosis {1939A}.

Alveolar adenoma

Beasley MB
Sauter JL

Definition
Alveolar adenoma is a well-circumscribed tumour consisting of cystic spaces lined by a single layer of type II pneumocytes overlying a spindle-rich stroma.

ICD-O coding
8251/0 Alveolar adenoma

ICD-11 coding
2F00.Y & XH9356 Other specified benign neoplasm of middle ear or respiratory system & Alveolar adenoma

Related terminology
None

Subtype(s)
None

Localization
Tumours are typically solitary and peripheral. Rare hilar tumours have been reported {3442,348,2595}.

Clinical features
Tumours are usually incidental findings in asymptomatic patients. Radiologically, the tumours are well circumscribed, homogeneous, and non-calcified. Cystic spaces may be seen on CT or MRI, and low-level PET positivity has been reported {348,879,2141}.

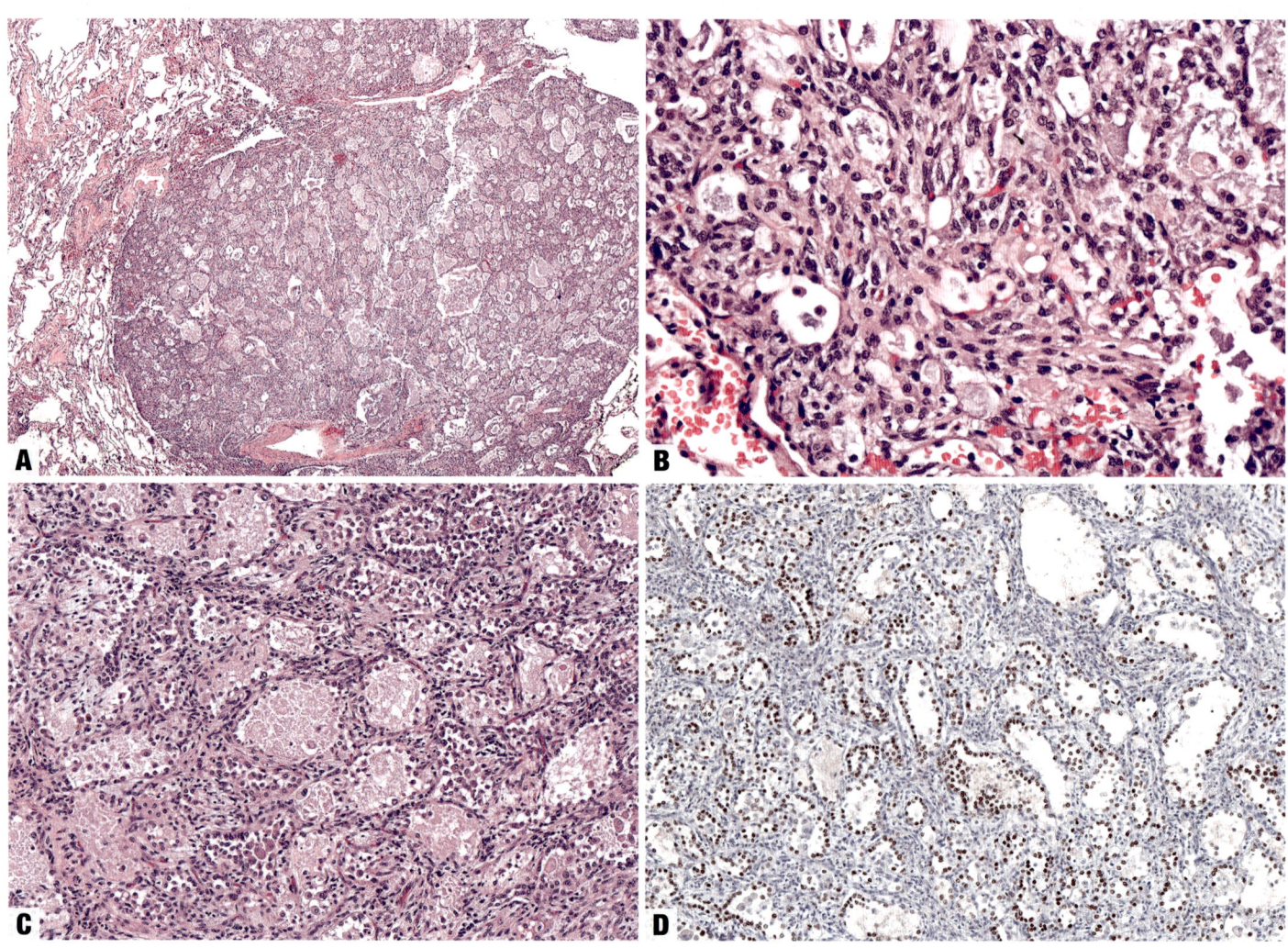

Fig. 1.28 Alveolar adenoma. **A** A well-circumscribed (but not encapsulated) tumour comprising multiple cystic spaces lined by thin walls of alveolar tissue. **B** Multiple small cysts resembling alveolar tissue with hyperplastic pneumocytes and alveolar macrophages within lumina. **C** Alveolar spaces in the tumour are filled with proteinaceous material. **D** TTF1 is positive in cuboidal cyst lining cells.

Epidemiology

Alveolar adenoma is very rare, has a slight female predominance, and has a reported age range of 39–74 years {3442,348,2595}.

Etiology

The etiology of alveolar adenoma is controversial. Chromosomal aberrations support a neoplastic origin, but it is unclear whether both epithelial and mesenchymal components are neoplastic {410}.

Pathogenesis

Alveolar adenoma appears to represent a combined proliferation of alveolar pneumocytes and septal mesenchyme, but the pathogenesis is unknown. No characteristic molecular profile has been identified. Microsatellite abnormalities have been demonstrated in the epithelial component but not the mesenchymal component {410}. Diploid DNA pattern has been reported {2595}. A non-balanced translocation t(10;16) has been reported in some cases {2525}.

Macroscopic appearance

Tumours measure 7–60 mm and are well demarcated, with smooth, lobulated, multicystic pale-yellow to tan cut surfaces {3442,348,2595}.

Histopathology

Alveolar adenomas are well circumscribed; composed of multiple cystic spaces frequently resembling alveolar spaces that are filled with eosinophilic granular material; and lined by cytologically bland, flattened to cuboidal epithelial cells, which correspond to type II pneumocytes by immunohistochemical and electron microscopic evaluation {348,2189}. Associated stroma may be myxoid or collagenous, containing cytologically bland spindle cells {348,3442}.

Cyst lining cells are positive for cytokeratin, TTF1, napsin A, and surfactant protein. Stromal cells are negative for these markers and may show focal staining for SMA and MSA and rare staining for S100 and CD34 {348,639}. Cytokeratin and TTF1 staining of the pneumocytes differentiates alveolar adenoma from lymphangioma, where the endothelial cells are keratin-negative. Lack of staining for TTF1 in stromal cells, along with the absence of a spectrum of solid papillary, sclerotic, and haemorrhagic patterns, helps differentiate alveolar adenoma from sclerosing pneumocytoma, which typically lacks cystic structures and shows TTF1-positive stromal cells.

Cytology

Cytological features of alveolar adenoma are poorly described.

Diagnostic molecular pathology

Not clinically relevant

Essential and desirable diagnostic criteria

Essential:
- Well-circumscribed tumour composed of cystic spaces frequently resembling alveolar spaces, lined by a single layer of type II pneumocytes overlying a mesenchymal, sometimes myxoid, stroma of variable thickness

Desirable:
- The pneumocytes are characteristically positive for TTF1

Staging

Not relevant

Prognosis and prediction

Alveolar adenomas are benign and surgical excision is curative {348}.

Papillary adenoma of the lung

Beasley MB
Sauter JL

Definition
Papillary adenoma is a circumscribed papillary neoplasm composed of cytologically bland, cuboidal to columnar cells lining fibrovascular cores.

ICD-O coding
8260/0 Papillary adenoma

ICD-11 coding
2F0Z & XH09B0 Benign neoplasms of respiratory and intrathoracic organs, unspecified & Papillary adenoma, NOS

Related terminology
None

Subtype(s)
None

Localization
Papillary adenoma of the lung is a peripheral solitary neoplasm with no lobar predilection {2830,575,676}.

Clinical features
There is typically an incidental radiological finding of a well-defined nodule.

Epidemiology
Tumours are rare (< 30 reported) with a male predominance and an age range of 2 months to 70 years (median: 34 years) {2830,575}.

Etiology
Unknown

Pathogenesis
Ultrastructural findings suggest derivation from a combination of type II pneumocytes and club cells, suggesting possible derivation from stem cells with bidirectional differentiation {799, 676,575,887}. One case has been reported with FGFR2-IIIb overexpression {1827}.

Macroscopic appearance
There are well-circumscribed, unencapsulated nodules/masses (reported sizes: 2–60 mm) with white-tan or yellow cut surfaces lacking gross papillae or necrosis {575,1110}.

Histopathology
Papillary adenomas are circumscribed nodules composed of papillary structures with fibrovascular cores lined by a single layer of cuboidal epithelium without nuclear atypia or mitoses and with a low Ki-67 proliferation index {2830,1110,1569,2125, 2262}.

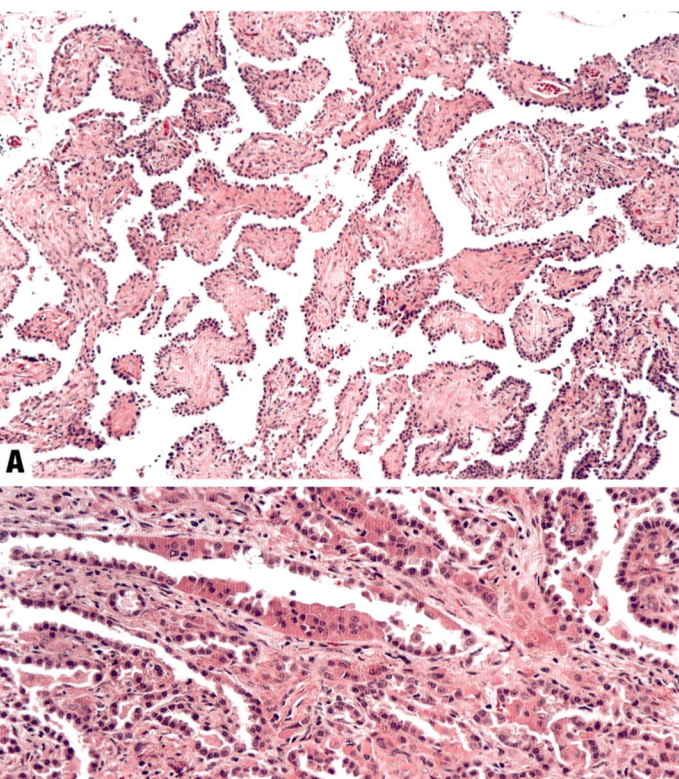

Fig. 1.29 Papillary adenoma. **A** A neoplasm composed of papillae with true fibrovascular cores. **B** At higher power, bland cuboidal cells line the surface of fibrovascular cores.

Immunohistochemistry
Surface epithelial cells, but not stromal cells, are positive for TTF1, CK7, pancytokeratin, surfactant protein, and EMA {575, 1110,2125,2727,3363}.

Differential diagnosis
Sclerosing pneumocytoma is composed of two cell types, with papillary structures containing a TTF1-positive cellular rather than a fibrovascular core and more-varied growth patterns, including papillary, sclerotic, haemorrhagic, and solid growth {575,2101}.

Alveolar adenomas are usually encapsulated and comprise multiple cysts lined by type II pneumocytes with characteristic spindle/inflammatory stroma and without papillary morphology {348,2595}.

Papillary adenocarcinomas generally show a greater degree of cellular proliferation, nuclear atypia, complex branching architecture, and infiltrative growth. Mitotic activity and necrosis may be present.

Cytology

Cytological features include cohesive papillary clusters with bland-appearing medium-sized epithelial cells with no nuclear atypia, prominent nucleoli, or pleomorphism {871}. Papillary adenoma can be difficult to distinguish from papillary adeno-carcinoma cytologically {1929}.

Diagnostic molecular pathology

Diagnostic molecular pathology is not clinically required {575, 2059}.

Essential and desirable diagnostic criteria

Essential:
- Unencapsulated circumscribed peripheral papillary glandular neoplasm with a single layer of cytologically bland cuboidal to columnar cells lining fibrovascular cores
- No nuclear atypia, minimal to no mitoses, no necrosis, no complex branching architecture, and absence of invasion

Desirable:
- Expression of TTF1

Staging

Not relevant

Prognosis and prediction

Behaviour is benign and resection is curative {575,2125,676, 199,3218,1688}.

Bronchiolar adenoma / ciliated muconodular papillary tumour

Chang JC
Beasley MB
Ishikawa Y
Rekhtman N
Yoshida A

Definition

Bronchiolar adenoma / ciliated muconodular papillary tumour (BA/CMPT) is a benign peripheral lung tumour composed of bilayered bronchiolar-type epithelium containing a continuous basal cell layer.

ICD-O coding

8140/0 Bronchiolar adenoma / ciliated muconodular papillary tumour

ICD-11 coding

2F0Y & XH6VL9 Benign neoplasms of other specified respiratory and intrathoracic organs & Atypical adenoma

Related terminology

Not recommended: peripheral papilloma; solitary peripheral ciliated glandular papilloma.

Subtype(s)

None

Localization

BA/CMPTs are located in the peripheral lung in a peribronchiolar location, and they are not associated with proximal bronchi.

Clinical features

These tumours are typically incidental findings. They may appear as solid or ground-glass nodules on CT, with some showing cavitation {1360,1264,444}.

Epidemiology

BA/CMPTs affect middle-aged to elderly patients, with a median age of 72 years. There is no sex predilection.

Etiology

Unknown

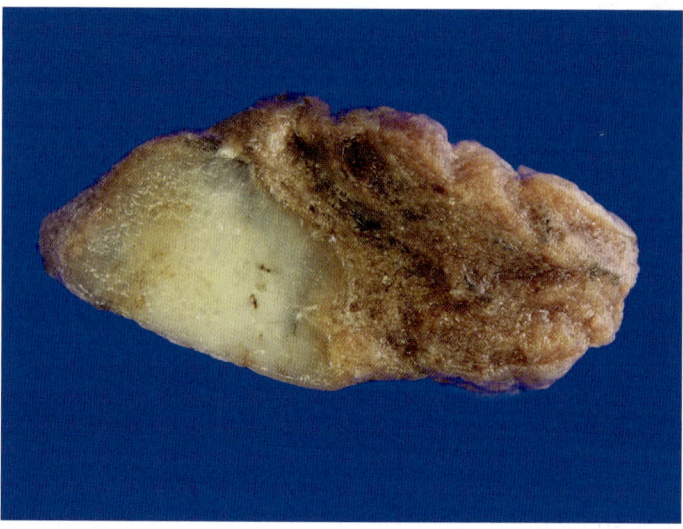

Fig. 1.30 Bronchiolar adenoma / ciliated muconodular papillary tumour. This 20 mm circumscribed subpleural nodule has a white to tan smooth cut surface.

Pathogenesis

BRAF driver mutation is the most common, with other mutually exclusive driver alterations, including in *EGFR*, *KRAS*, *HRAS*, and *ALK*, having been reported in both BAs and CMPTs, supporting their nosological relationship {2947,3116,1359,444}.

Macroscopic appearance

BA/CMPTs are well-circumscribed tan-white to grey nodules with a firm, cystic, or mucoid cut surface. They measure 2–45 mm, most commonly 5–15 mm.

Histopathology

BA/CMPTs are nodular proliferations involving peribronchiolar lung parenchyma. The tumours show papillary and/or flat (glandular) architecture and are composed of bilayered

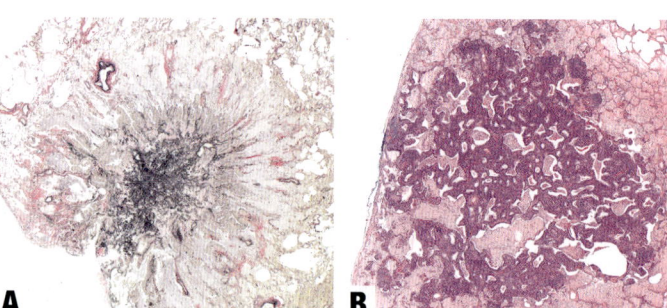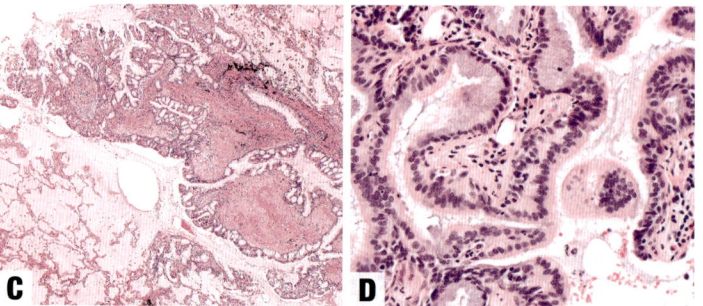

Fig. 1.31 Bronchiolar adenoma / ciliated muconodular papillary tumour. **A** Bronchiolar adenomas sometimes show a central scar as seen at the left, which should not be mistaken for evidence of malignancy. **B** This peripheral subpleural bronchiolar adenoma forms a nodular proliferation of bronchiolar-type epithelial cells overlying thickened alveolar walls, with a moderate lymphoid infiltrate. Airspaces are filled with mucin but the tumour shows mostly flat rather than papillary surfaces. **C** A peribronchiolar papillary tumour surrounded by abundant mucus. **D** Proximal-type bronchiolar adenoma / ciliated muconodular papillary tumour shows abundant ciliated and mucinous cells overlying a continuous layer of basal cells.

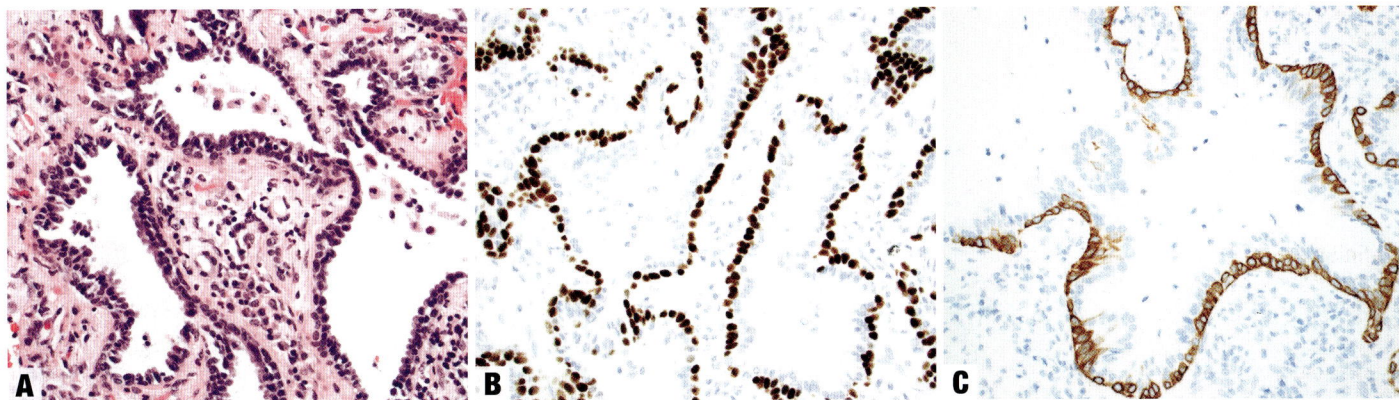

Fig. 1.32 Bronchiolar adenoma / ciliated muconodular papillary tumour. **A** Distal-type bronchiolar adenoma resembling distal bronchiolar epithelium. This tumour is composed of bland luminal cuboidal epithelial cells overlying a continuous basal cell layer. **B** A p40 immunostain highlights the presence of a continuous basal cell layer. **C** A CK5/6 immunostain highlights the presence of a continuous basal cell layer.

cellular elements with luminal epithelial cells and subjacent basal cells. The luminal cells may consist of mucous cells and ciliated cells (referred to by some as proximal-type BA or classic CMPT), whereas cells resembling type II pneumocytes and club cells (formerly known as Clara cells) may predominate (referred to by some as distal-type BA or non-classic CMPT) {1360,444,3510,2945}. Micropapillary tufts of ciliated cells and a minor degree of discontinuous spread are common and should not be regarded as features of malignancy. Some cases have overlapping features between distal and proximal types. Nuclear atypia is absent and mitoses are rare. The diagnosis is difficult to make on a small biopsy, although it may be suspected.

Although there is a spectrum of varying morphological and immunohistochemical features ranging from proximal (papillary or flat, mainly mucinous and ciliated cells, TTF1– or rarely weakly +) to distal (flat, mainly cuboidal type II pneumocytes and club cells, TTF1+) tumours, there may be overlapping features. The main reason for appreciating this spectrum is to aid in diagnosis rather than to categorize each tumour into a specific proximal or distal pattern.

Immunohistochemistry
The continuous basal cell layer is highlighted by p40 or CK5/6. The luminal epithelial cells tend to be diffusely positive for TTF1 in distal-type BA, while only focally positive or negative in proximal-type BA (classic CMPT).

Differential diagnosis
The continuous basal cell layer, ciliated cells, and the lack of nuclear atypia are features that may be useful in distinguishing this tumour from adenocarcinoma (including adenocarcinoma in situ). This distinction can be very difficult on frozen section or small biopsies {2756A}. The bilayered cellular elements with luminal epithelial cells and subjacent basal cells are the most useful criteria to favour BA over adenocarcinoma in situ. Both mucinous and non-mucinous adenocarcinomas in situ also lack cytological atypia, similar to BA, and some distal BAs lack ciliated cells, show tumour cells growing along alveolar wall surfaces (resembling lepidic growth), and may resemble mucinous adenocarcinoma in situ. p40 and/or CK5/6 may be very helpful in such cases. Papillomas are characteristically central

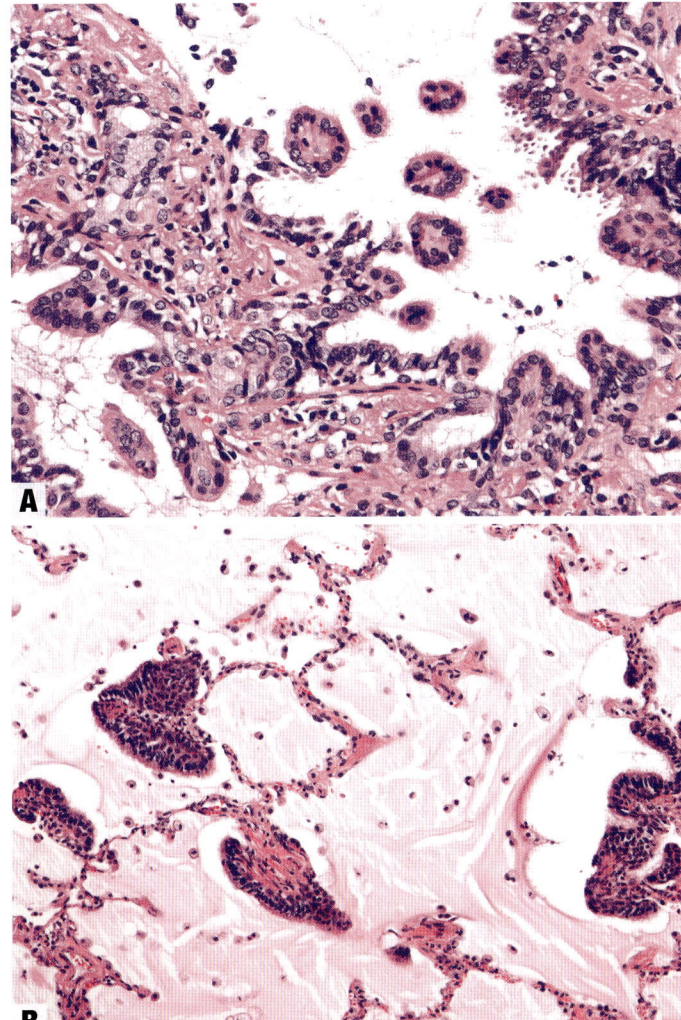

Fig. 1.33 Bronchiolar adenoma. Micropapillary tufts (**A**) and skipping growth (**B**) are common and should not be mistaken for malignant features.

and endobronchial, unlike BA/CMPTs, which are peripheral and bronchiolocentric; the histological findings can be otherwise indistinguishable, although glandular papillomas should lack ciliated cells (see *Bronchial papillomas*, p. 37). Peribronchiolar metaplasia tends to show ill-defined borders and is usually a multifocal process, often in the setting of interstitial lung disease or small airway injury. Foci are generally small and consistently demonstrate ciliated cells. BA/CMPT is unrelated to atypical adenomatous hyperplasia, previously referred to as bronchioloalveolar adenoma {1924,444}.

Cytology
Cytological smears show ciliated columnar cells and mucous cells without atypia, as well as abundant extracellular mucin {1918}.

Diagnostic molecular pathology
Detection of driver alterations is not necessary for diagnosis.

Essential and desirable diagnostic criteria
Essential:
- Circumscribed peribronchiolar lung nodule of papillary and/or flat glandular epithelium
- A bilayered cellular proliferation of luminal epithelial cells and subjacent basal cells
- Luminal cells consisting of mainly mucous cells and ciliated cells in proximal-type areas, but mainly type II pneumocytes and club cells in distal-type areas
- Lack of nuclear atypia and inconspicuous or absent mitoses

Desirable:
- p40 and CK5/6 expression in basal layer
- TTF1-positive luminal cells with more-diffuse staining in distal-type areas and either focal or negative staining in proximal-type areas
- positive BRAF immunohistochemistry or *BRAF* mutation may be confirmatory in the appropriate morphological context

Staging
Not relevant

Prognosis and prediction
BA/CMPT is benign. All patients reported to date remain free of recurrence and metastasis after surgical resections {1360, 444,3510}.

Mucinous cystadenoma of the lung

Yoshida A
Beasley MB

Definition

Mucinous cystadenoma is a localized cystic mass filled with mucin and surrounded by columnar mucinous epithelium without significant atypia or invasive growth.

ICD-O coding

8470/0 Mucinous cystadenoma

ICD-11 coding

2F0Z & XH6H73 Benign neoplasms of respiratory and intrathoracic organs, unspecified & Mucinous cystadenoma, NOS

Related terminology

None

Subtype(s)

None

Localization

Mucinous cystadenomas involve the periphery of the lung.

Clinical features

The lesions are usually found incidentally in asymptomatic patients.

Epidemiology

Mucinous cystadenoma is exceedingly rare. There is mild female predominance, and most patients are in their sixth or seventh decade of life.

Etiology

No predisposing factors are known.

Pathogenesis

Unknown

Macroscopic appearance

The lesion consists of a localized mucin-filled cyst not associated with an airway. The tumour size ranges from < 10 to 70 mm. The cyst wall is thin and lacks mural nodules.

Histopathology

The tumour consists of a localized cyst filled with mucin, which may be surrounded by a fibrous wall {909}. The lining of the cyst wall consists of a discontinuous single layer of low-cuboidal to tall columnar mucin-secreting epithelium. Nuclear atypia is absent or at most mild, and mitoses are absent or rare {1527, 1084}. Mild papillary folding may be present {1527,2555}, but micropapillary fronds, necrosis, overt cytological atypia, or invasive growth is absent. Extravasated acellular mucin may be associated with foreign body giant cell reaction and chronic inflammation {1025,1527}.

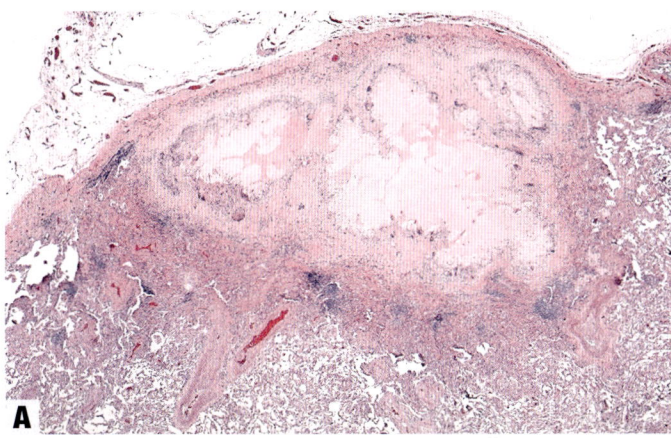

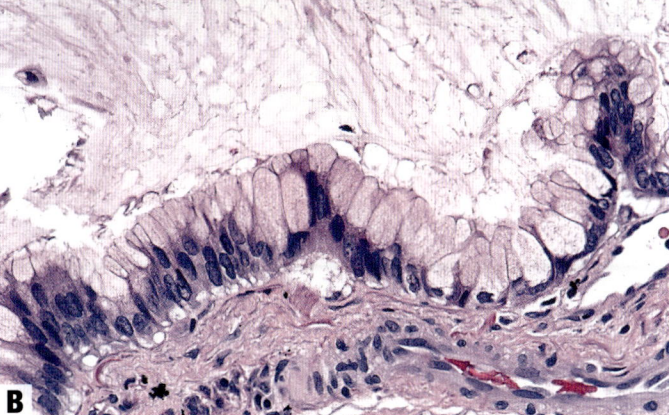

Fig. 1.34 Mucinous cystadenoma. **A** A subpleural cystic tumour is surrounded by a fibrous wall and contains abundant mucus. **B** Columnar epithelial cells line the wall of the cyst. Most of the nuclei are basally oriented, but there is focal nuclear pseudostratification. The apical cytoplasm is filled with abundant mucin.

Immunohistochemistry

The lining cells are positive for pancytokeratin and are rarely positive for CEA {1527}. TTF1 and surfactant protein are usually negative {1084,1527}.

Differential diagnosis

The primary entity in the differential diagnosis is colloid carcinoma of the lung, which includes what was previously known as mucinous cystadenocarcinoma. The spread of the tumour beyond the wall of the cyst in either a lepidic or an invasive fashion, significant cytological atypia, and necrosis are indicators of malignancy {3062,2555,909}. Thorough sampling is necessary, because malignant histology may be only focally present within a tumour that otherwise appears benign {909}. Metastatic carcinoma from the gastrointestinal tract or ovary should be excluded by extensive workup. Developmental and postinfectious bronchogenic cysts may also be a consideration. They usually show coexistent ciliated cells, in contrast to mucinous cystadenoma. A subset of mucinous cystic neoplasms harbouring borderline histology with regard to nuclear and architectural atypia has been described, although there is no consensus on diagnostic criteria, and cases have been reported to behave in a benign fashion {1001,909}.

Cytology
FNA specimens may contain mucin and/or goblet cells, but a diagnosis requires surgical excision.

Diagnostic molecular pathology
Genetic abnormalities have not been reported.

Essential and desirable diagnostic criteria
Essential:
- Circumscribed mucin-filled lung cyst surrounded by mucinous cells
- Overt cytological atypia and invasion are absent

Staging
Not relevant

Prognosis and prediction
Mucinous cystadenoma is benign, and surgical excision is curative.

Mucous gland adenoma of the lung

Yoshida A
Beasley MB

Definition
Mucous gland adenoma is a benign, predominantly exophytic tumour of the bronchus, resembling seromucinous bronchial glands.

ICD-O coding
8480/0 Mucous gland adenoma

ICD-11 coding
2F00.Y & XH5RX2 Other specified benign neoplasm of middle ear or respiratory system & Mucous gland adenoma

Related terminology
None

Subtype(s)
None

Localization
Mucous gland adenoma arises in the proximal airways, most commonly in the lobar or segmental bronchi. A few tumours with a similar histology have been reported in the lung periphery {1389}.

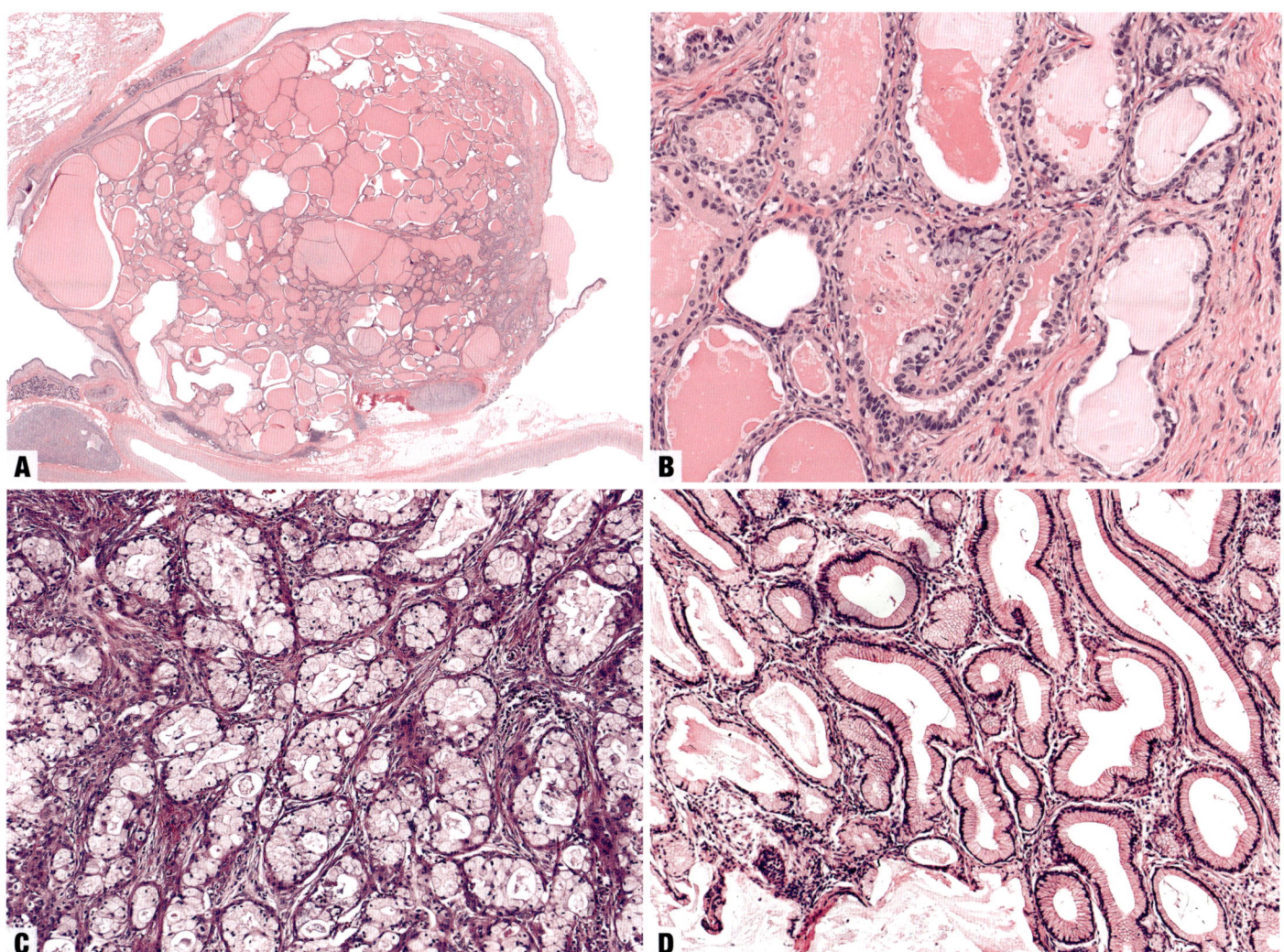

Fig. 1.35 Mucous gland adenoma. **A** This polypoid endobronchial tumour shows numerous dilated cystic glands, many of which contain mucin. **B** These glands are surrounded by a spectrum of cells ranging from flat epithelial cells with scant cytoplasm to intermediate-sized cuboidal cells and other large cells with abundant apical cytoplasmic mucin and small basally oriented nuclei. **C** This tumour consists of tumour cells growing in solid nests and small glands with abundant intracytoplasmic mucin and small basally oriented nuclei. **D** These large and medium-sized glands are lined by columnar epithelial cells with abundant apical cytoplasmic mucin and small basally oriented nuclei.

Clinical features

Patients typically present with symptoms of obstruction, including cough, haemoptysis, dyspnoea, and recurrent pneumonia {771}. Imaging shows a well-defined mass {1573}.

Epidemiology

Mucous gland adenoma is extremely rare. It has no sex predilection and has a wide age range (25–67 years) {771}.

Etiology

Unknown

Pathogenesis

Unknown

Macroscopic appearance

Mucous gland adenomas are well-circumscribed, predominantly exophytic endobronchial nodules confined above the cartilaginous plates. The cut surface is tan to pink, may be solid or cystic, and is often mucoid. The size range is 8–68 mm {771}.

Histopathology

Mucous gland adenomas are well circumscribed and comprise numerous mucin-filled cystic spaces, and they may include non-dilated microacinar, glandular, or tubular structures. Papillary architecture is less common. The tumour cells are cytologically bland columnar, cuboidal, or flattened mucus-secreting cells. Oncocytic cells, clear cells, or ciliated cells may be present. Hyperchromasia, pleomorphism, and mitoses are generally absent. A usually minor component of spindle cell stroma may be hyalinized or contain inflammatory cells.

Immunohistochemistry

The epithelial cells are positive for EMA, keratin, and CEA, whereas they are negative for TTF1. The stromal cells may show occasional expression of keratins, SMA, and S100, indicating a myoepithelial component {1106,771,2191}.

Differential diagnosis

The lack of intermediate cells discriminates mucous gland adenoma from low-grade mucoepidermoid carcinoma. Cellular composition and location are different from endobronchial papillomas and other adenomas. Endobronchial metastasis from extraneous sites should be excluded by clinical history and cellular atypia. Invasive mucinous adenocarcinomas involve the alveolar parenchyma rather than showing exclusive endobronchial growth.

Cytology

Not clinically relevant

Diagnostic molecular pathology

Not clinically relevant

Essential and desirable diagnostic criteria

Essential:

- Well-circumscribed endobronchial tumour
- Acini / tubules / papillary growth of mucous cells with no atypia
- At least focal resemblance to normal seromucinous glands

Staging

Not relevant

Prognosis and prediction

Mucous gland adenomas are benign and cured by resection.

Atypical adenomatous hyperplasia of the lung

Matsubara D
MacMahon H
Mino-Kenudson M
Mitsudomi T

Definition

Atypical adenomatous hyperplasia (AAH) is a small (usually ≤ 5 mm), localized proliferation of mildly to moderately atypical type II pneumocytes and/or club cells lining alveolar walls and sometimes respiratory bronchioles. Within the category of preinvasive lesions, AAH is a putative precursor of adenocarcinoma in situ (AIS).

ICD-O coding

8250/0 Atypical adenomatous hyperplasia

ICD-11 coding

2F0Z & XH5QL3 Benign neoplasms of respiratory and intrathoracic organs, unspecified & Atypical adenomatous hyperplasia

Related terminology

Not recommended (obsolete): atypical alveolar hyperplasia; bronchial adenoma; atypical bronchioloalveolar hyperplasia; atypical alveolar epithelial hyperplasia; atypical alveolar cell hyperplasia.

Subtype(s)

None

Localization

AAH occurs in the peripheral, parenchymal lung, often close to the pleura {2056,2126}.

Clinical features

AAH is usually undetectable by imaging techniques, but larger lesions may be visible as faint, non-solid, focal nodules of a few millimetres, sometimes retrospectively noted, on high-resolution CT. The lesions are typically incidentally found during examination of surgical specimens, most of which bear lung cancer, especially adenocarcinoma. In rare autopsy studies, precursor lesions have been reported in 2–4% of patients not bearing cancer {2860,3406}. The rate is higher in surgical specimens from patients with lung cancer (as high as 19% for women and 9.3% for men), particularly in cases of pulmonary adenocarcinoma (as high as 30.2% for women and 18.8% for men) {453}. When the lesions are completely resected, the disease-free survival rate is 100% – see below {3143,1345}. AAH is not included in TNM staging.

Epidemiology

See *Invasive non-mucinous adenocarcinoma of the lung* (p. 64); *CYP19A1* polymorphisms have been shown to be associated with lung adenocarcinoma with AAH, and this may play a role by causing differences in estrogen levels {1501}.

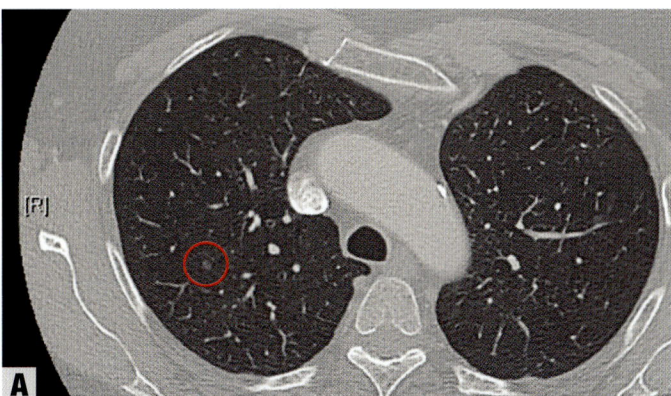

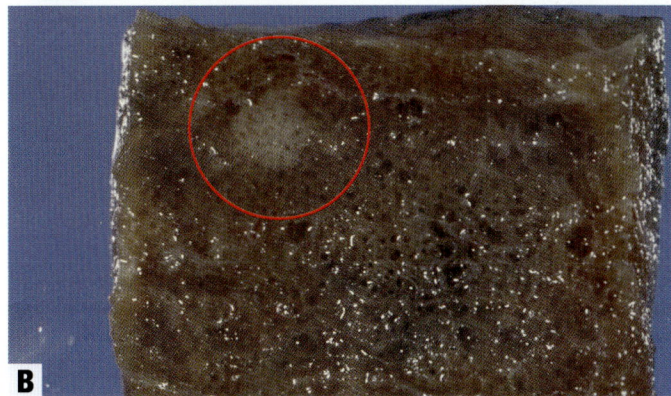

Fig. 1.36 Atypical adenomatous hyperplasia. **A** A 5 mm ground-glass nodule (circle) consistent with atypical adenomatous hyperplasia. **B** This 4 mm circumscribed subpleural tan nodule (circle) represents atypical adenomatous hyperplasia.

Etiology

The etiology is unknown; see *Tumours of the lung: Introduction* (p. 20).

Pathogenesis

Ploidy and clonality studies have shown a clonal/neoplastic nature for AAH {2067}. Loss of heterozygosity on 3p, 9p, 16p, 17q, and 17p has been detected {2785,2958,3328}. The frequency of somatic copy-number aberrations and clonal mutations is lower in AAH than in AIS {1195}.

AAH has been reported to harbour driver mutations such as in *KRAS*, *EGFR*, and *BRAF*, in as many as 33%, 35%, and 29% of cases, respectively, supporting the concept that AAH is a precursor lesion of lung adenocarcinoma and an early event of peripheral lung adenocarcinogenesis {2270,2601,2784,2803, 2958,3427}.

See *Tumours of the lung: Introduction* (p. 20) and *Invasive non-mucinous adenocarcinoma of the lung* (p. 64) for further information.

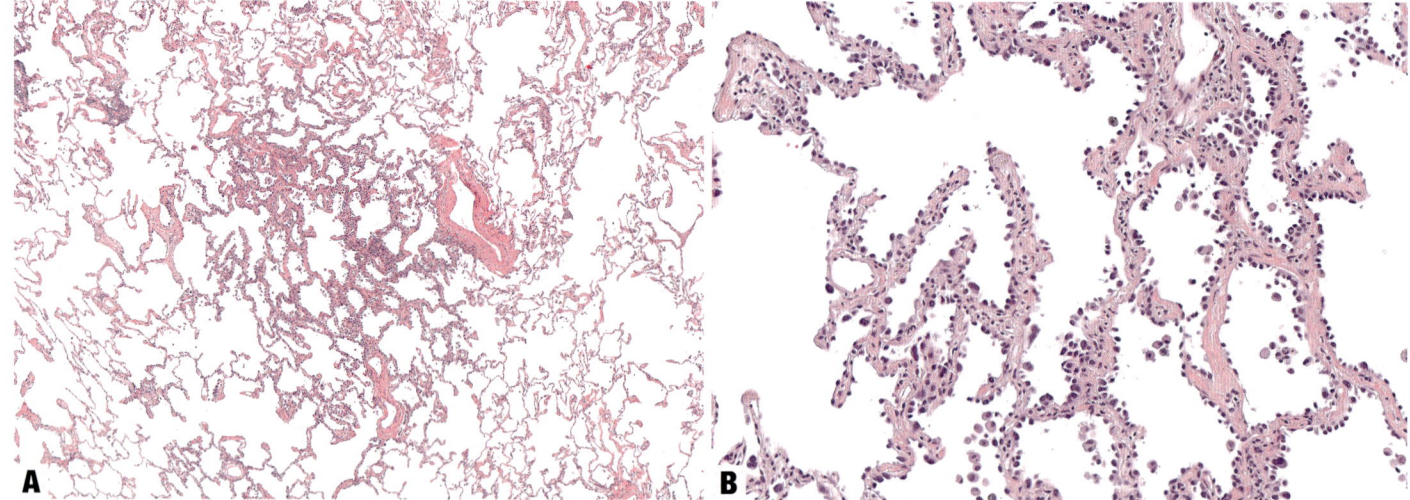

Fig. 1.37 Atypical adenomatous hyperplasia. **A** This ~2 mm nodular atypical pneumocyte proliferation shows preservation of alveolar walls lined by cuboidal pneumocytes, many of which show gaps between them. **B** These preserved alveolar walls are lined by atypical cuboidal pneumocytes, many of which show gaps between them.

Macroscopic appearance

AAH is most often an incidental microscopic finding, but when seen grossly, it is a millimetre-sized, poorly defined, greyish or tan-yellow nodule.

Histopathology

AAH is a small localized lesion (usually ≤ 5 mm) often arising in the centriacinar region, close to respiratory bronchioles. Mildly to moderately atypical type II pneumocytes and/or club cells proliferate along alveolar walls. Inconspicuous pseudo-papillae may also be present {1929,3072,3074}. Club cells are recognized as columnar, with cytoplasmic snouts and pale eosinophilic cytoplasm. Type II pneumocytes are cuboidal or dome-shaped, with fine cytoplasmic vacuoles or clear to foamy cytoplasm. Intranuclear eosinophilic inclusions may be present. The lining of rounded, cuboidal, low columnar cells with round to oval nuclei shows gaps between cells located on the alveolar wall basement membrane. Double nuclei are common, but mitoses are extremely rare. There is a continuum of morphological changes between AAH and AIS {1471,3072,3074,1994}. A spectrum of cellularity and atypia occurs in AAH. Although AAH has sometimes been classified into low-grade and high-grade types {1499,2057}, such grading is not recommended {3074}. AAH expresses TTF1 {1472}.

Differential diagnosis

Distinction between cellular and cytologically anomalous AAH and non-mucinous AIS can be difficult. AIS is usually larger (> 5 mm), but the size is not an absolute criterion; thus, multiple characteristics in addition to size, including architectural and cytological features, are needed to make this distinction. AIS typically exhibits a more cellular, crowded, homogeneous, cuboidal or columnar cell population. There is usually a less graded, more abrupt transition to the adjacent non-neoplastic alveolar lining cells in AIS. Columnar cells are taller in AIS, and overlapping and mild stratification of cells may be seen – features not seen in AAH. AAH also needs to be distinguished from reactive pneumocyte hyperplasia secondary to parenchymal inflammation or fibrosis in which the alveolar lining cells are not the dominant feature and are more diffusely distributed. In addition, in reactive conditions, the inflammatory changes are usually more widely distributed than the reactive alveolar lining cells. AAH also needs to be distinguished from micronodular pneumocyte hyperplasia, which shows less cytological atypia and characteristically occurs in women with lymphangioleiomyomatosis and/or tuberous sclerosis.

Cytology

Not relevant

Diagnostic molecular pathology

Not clinically relevant (in most cases)

Essential and desirable diagnostic criteria

Essential:
- Increased numbers of type II pneumocytes and club cells lining alveoli in a discontinuous monolayer
- Mild atypia
- Small localized lesion, usually ≤ 5 mm, discrete from surrounding alveolar parenchyma
- Surrounding parenchyma devoid of inflammation or fibrosis

Staging

Not clinically relevant

Prognosis and prediction

Patients with resected AAH are cured upon resection. Because the diagnosis of AAH cannot be established without removal of the lesion, there are no data demonstrating its in vivo progression to AIS, minimally invasive adenocarcinoma, or invasive adenocarcinoma. However, because the lesions are frequently found in non-neoplastic lung adjacent to resected lung cancers, and most frequently in patients with multiple adenocarcinomas, it is well accepted that this progression probably occurs in a subset of lung adenocarcinomas {1279,2933}. Further, the prognosis of lung adenocarcinomas with AAH has not been shown to be different from that of those without AAH {2931}.

Adenocarcinoma in situ of the lung

Kadota K
MacMahon H
Matsubara D
Mino-Kenudson M
Mitsudomi T

Definition

Adenocarcinoma in situ (AIS) is a small (≤ 30 mm), localized adenocarcinoma with growth restricted to neoplastic cells along pre-existing alveolar structures (pure lepidic growth with no invasive features). The diagnosis of AIS requires a resection specimen where the lesion has been completely sampled, and it cannot be made based on small biopsy or cytology specimens.

ICD-O coding

8250/2 Adenocarcinoma in situ, non-mucinous
8253/2 Adenocarcinoma in situ, mucinous

ICD-11 coding

2E62.2 & XH1FR9 Carcinoma in situ of bronchus or lung & Non-mucinous adenocarcinoma in situ of the lung
2E62.2 & XH6BU6 Carcinoma in situ of bronchus or lung & Mucinous adenocarcinoma in situ of the lung

Related terminology

Not recommended: bronchioloalveolar carcinoma (obsolete).

Subtype(s)

Adenocarcinoma in situ of the lung, non-mucinous; adenocarcinoma in situ of the lung, mucinous

Localization

AIS occurs in the peripheral lung – often close to the pleura {2126}.

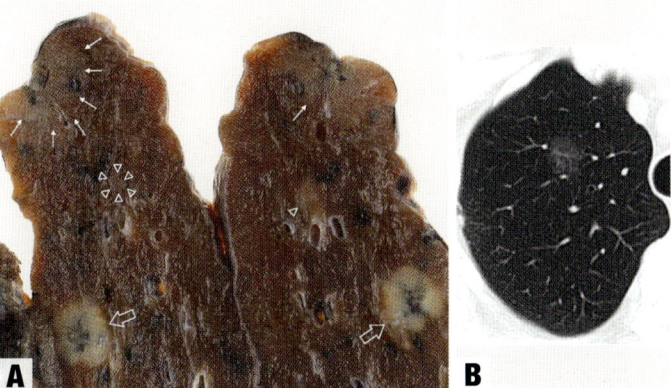

Fig. 1.38 A Macroscopic comparison of atypical adenomatous hyperplasia, adenocarcinoma in situ, and invasive adenocarcinoma in one lung. The two cut surfaces are arranged as a mirror image. From top to bottom: adenocarcinoma in situ (thin arrows), atypical adenomatous hyperplasia (arrowheads), and invasive adenocarcinoma (thick arrows) are seen. **B** Non-mucinous adenocarcinoma in situ. CT shows a circumscribed ground-glass nodule lacking any solid component.

Clinical features

AIS is usually an incidental finding on CT performed for other medical reasons, including screening. The tumours are usually ≤ 20 mm but can be as large as 30 mm. By CT they are characteristically non-solid, but they may be part-solid or even solid, especially in mucinous AIS. AIS may have a so-called bubble-like appearance on CT {128}. Preinvasive lesions are locally slow-growing tumours without lymphatic or vascular invasion or distant metastases.

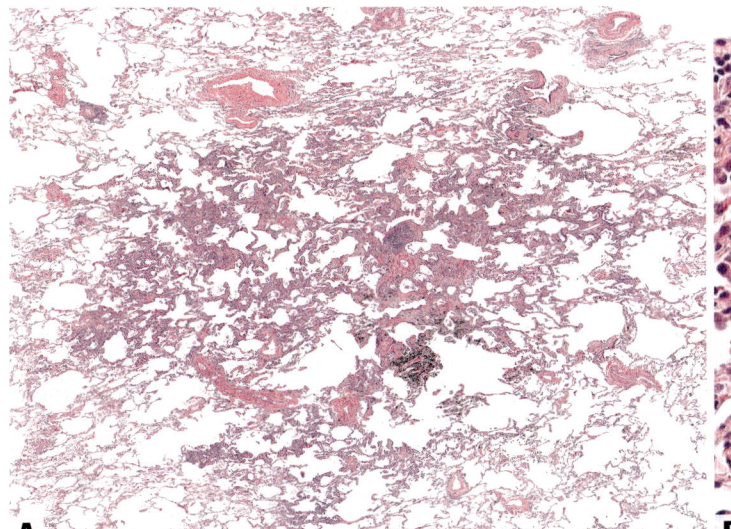
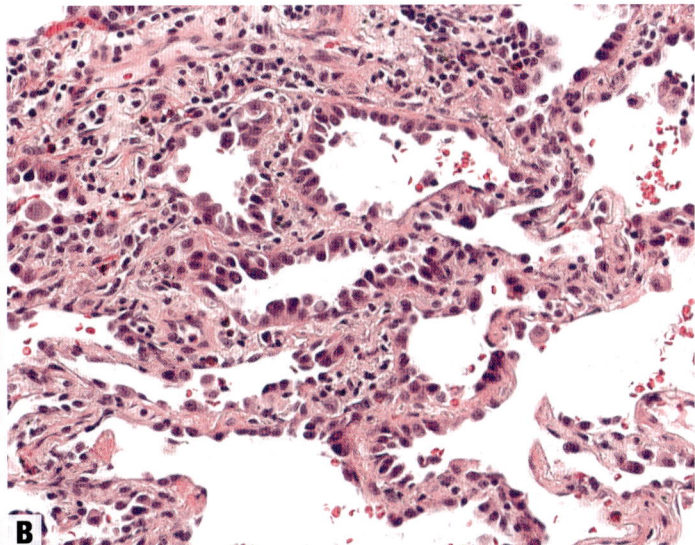

Fig. 1.39 Adenocarcinoma in situ, non-mucinous. **A** This adenocarcinoma in situ is a circumscribed nodular atypical pneumocyte proliferation without invasive growth. **B** The atypical cuboidal pneumocytes line the intact alveolar walls in a crowded manner. No invasion is seen.

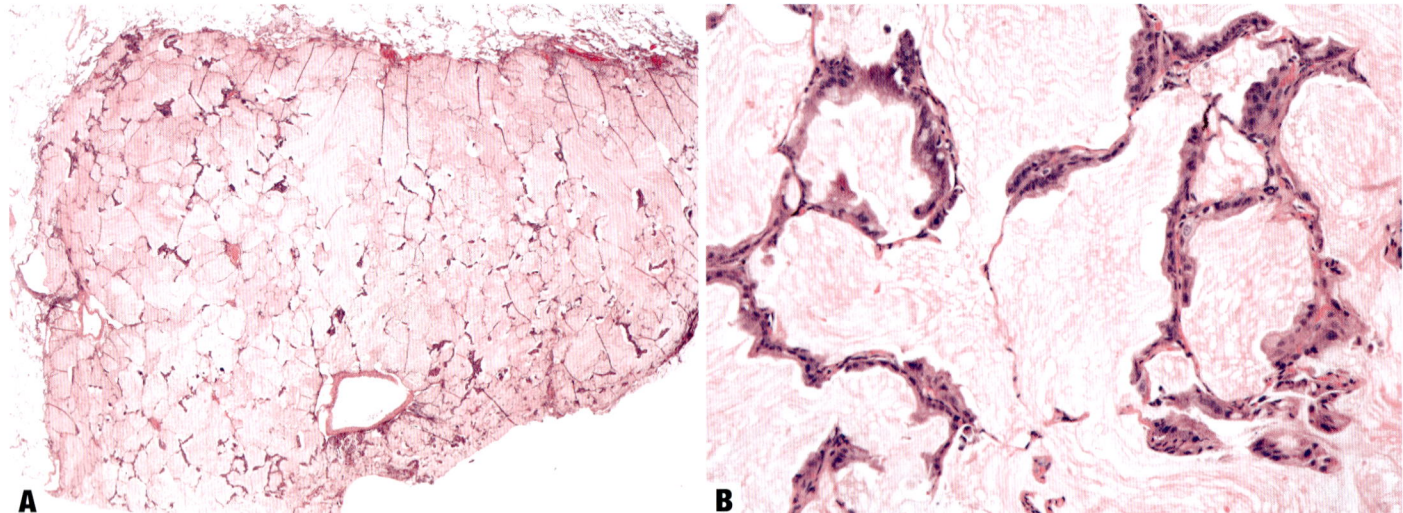

Fig. 1.40 Adenocarcinoma in situ, mucinous. **A** This circumscribed tumour consists of mucinous tumour cells growing in a lepidic pattern along the surface of alveolar walls. No invasive growth within the tumour and no spread beyond the edge of the tumour is seen. There is abundant intra-alveolar mucin. **B** The tumour consists of cuboidal to columnar-shaped tumour cells with apical mucin and small basally oriented nuclei growing in a lepidic manner along the surface of alveolar walls. The alveolar spaces are filled with abundant mucin. No invasive growth is seen.

Epidemiology
See *Tumours of the lung: Introduction* (p. 20).

Etiology
See *Tumours of the lung: Introduction* (p. 20).

Pathogenesis
In the multistep progression model, AIS is an intermediate step between precursor lesion, atypical adenomatous hyperplasia (AAH), and minimally invasive adenocarcinoma (MIA). Because driver mutations are involved in early lung cancer development, driver mutations similar to those seen in early invasive adenocarcinoma may be seen in AIS. Studies from Asian countries show mutation rates of 40–86% for *EGFR* and 0–4% for *KRAS* mutations {3102,3434}, whereas studies from North America show a lower *EGFR* mutation rate of 24% and a higher *KRAS* mutation rate of 10% {2400}. In terms of progression-associated genes, the molecular pathogenesis of the progression from AAH to AIS remains unclear. However, although *EGFR* mutation was found in one third of AAH cases, it was present in almost half of AIS cases, and in two thirds of MIAs {1494}. This increasing incidence of driver gene mutations suggests progression from AAH to AIS, and further to MIA {1494}.

Macroscopic appearance
AIS is a poorly defined nodule measuring up to 30 mm in size, with a tan or pale cut surface. The lesions lack a solid appearance unless markedly compressed or collapsed, and tiny airspaces can often be seen on the cut surface. The tumour should be completely sampled and microscopically examined to confirm that there is no invasive component.

Histopathology
AIS is a localized, small (≤ 30 mm) adenocarcinoma with growth restricted to neoplastic cells along pre-existing alveolar structures (lepidic growth), lacking stromal, vascular, alveolar space or pleural invasion or necrosis {3074,3068}. Tumour cells are arranged in continuous monolayers, sometimes with evidence

of cell overlap or mild stratification. Papillary or micropapillary patterns are absent, similar to in AAH, although minor cellular tufting may be seen. Intra-alveolar tumour cells, either within the tumour or spread in airspaces in the surrounding parenchyma, are absent. AIS is subdivided into non-mucinous and mucinous subtypes. Virtually all cases of AIS are non-mucinous, typically showing type II pneumocyte and/or club cell differentiation.

Box 1.02 Adenocarcinoma in situ – diagnostic criteria {3074,3072,3068}

- A small localized tumour (≤ 30 mm)
- Pure lepidic growth
- No stromal, vascular, or pleural invasion
- No pattern of invasive adenocarcinoma (e.g. acinar, papillary, micropapillary, solid, colloid, enteric, fetal, or invasive mucinous adenocarcinoma)
- No spread through airspaces
- Cell type mostly non-mucinous (type II pneumocytes or club cells) but very rarely may be mucinous (tall columnar cells with basal nuclei and abundant cytoplasmic mucin, sometimes resembling goblet cells)
- Nuclear atypia is inconspicuous
- Septal widening with sclerosis/elastosis is common, particularly in non-mucinous adenocarcinoma in situ

Box 1.03 Adenocarcinoma in situ – good practice points {3074,3072,3068,3081}

- The tumour should be completely sampled. If desired, a small piece may be snap frozen for research if there is no solid component on CT or gross examination and there are no worrisome areas for invasion. If possible and required, this tissue may need to be examined by frozen section if invasion is suspected.
- Size may be underestimated on gross examination, so correlation with CT findings may be necessary to determine tumour size.
- If a solid component is present on CT or gross examination, the lesion should be evaluated very carefully, because this often correlates with an invasive component.
- For adenocarcinoma in situ, particularly mucinous adenocarcinoma in situ, great care must be taken to be sure the lesion is solitary and sharply circumscribed, without miliary spread in adjacent lung parenchyma.
- The criteria for adenocarcinoma in situ can be applied in the setting of multiple tumours only if the other tumours are regarded as synchronous primaries rather than intrapulmonary metastases.

However, there is no recognized clinical significance to the distinction between type II pneumocytes and club cells, so this morphological distinction is not recommended. The exceptionally rare cases of mucinous AIS that occur as a solitary nodule (≤ 30 mm) consist of tall columnar cells with basal nuclei and abundant cytoplasmic mucin; sometimes these cells resemble goblet cells. Nuclear atypia is usually minimal and low-grade in non-mucinous AIS, but it is virtually absent in mucinous AIS. Alveolar septal widening with sclerosis/elastosis is common in AIS, particularly the non-mucinous subtype. The criteria for AIS can be applied in the setting of multiple tumours only if the other tumours are regarded as synchronous primaries rather than intrapulmonary metastases. In the setting of multiple non-mucinous adenocarcinomas, irrespective of the clonality of the other tumours, a lesion that is morphologically qualified as AIS should be classified as AIS – see below. AIS expresses TTF1 and napsin A.

The diagnosis of AIS requires a resection specimen where the lesion has been completely sampled, and it cannot be made based on small biopsy or cytology specimens.

Differential diagnosis

Non-mucinous AIS must be distinguished from MIA, lepidic-predominant adenocarcinoma, and AAH. The lepidic pattern should be distinguished from the acinar or the papillary pattern in the setting of parenchymal collapse and/or emphysema {3036,2741}. The distinction between mucinous AIS and MIA is similar, in that invasive foci should be identified in the latter. Mucinous AIS also needs to be differentiated from bronchiolar adenoma based on the absence of the continuous basal layer in the former. Clinical correlation is needed to exclude a metastatic mucinous adenocarcinoma from sites such as the pancreas. Solitary lesions of small size (≤ 30 mm) and a discrete circumscribed border support AIS, whereas larger, irregular lesions are more likely to be invasive. Where growth shows a pattern of lobar consolidation, particularly for mucinous lesions, invasive disease is more likely. AIS can appear as multiple (often subtly different) synchronous primary lesions, and it is important to distinguish this scenario from airspace spread of invasive disease, in the context of either invasive mucinous adenocarcinoma or, even more rarely, multifocal, monotonously similar, non-mucinous adenocarcinoma. There is insufficient evidence that a 100% disease-free survival rate can occur with tumours that morphologically fit the criteria for AIS but measure > 30 mm. These tumours should be classified as lepidic-predominant adenocarcinoma (and staged as T1a), with a comment that they may represent AIS.

Cytology

The typical cytological features of non-mucinous AIS include relatively low-grade (i.e. bland, small, and monomorphous) nuclei, fine chromatin, inconspicuous pinpoint nucleoli, nuclear grooves, nuclear pseudoinclusions, and cell arrangement in orderly strips and small flat monolayers {127,2164,3162,3083}. Overall, the cytological features can closely resemble those of papillary thyroid carcinoma. Tumour cells are often admixed with alveolar macrophages. As with small biopsies, specific diagnosis of AIS cannot be made in cytological specimens, because the presence of an unsampled higher-grade invasive component cannot be excluded. Low-grade adenocarcinomas with other patterns, particularly the papillary pattern, can also have overlapping cytological features. Because of the bland cytology, the distinction of AIS from benign cellular elements (including reactive pneumocytes and mesothelial cells) is a challenging diagnostic issue {3468}. Mucinous AIS is extremely rare, but it would be expected to show features similar to those of invasive mucinous adenocarcinoma (see *Invasive non-mucinous adenocarcinoma of the lung*, p. 64).

Diagnostic molecular pathology
Not clinically relevant (in most cases)

Essential and desirable diagnostic criteria
See Box 1.02 and Box 1.03.

Essential:
- A small (≤ 30 mm diameter) localized lesion comprising pure lepidic growth
- Stromal, vascular, or pleural invasion, as well as spread through airspaces and invasive adenocarcinoma patterns, all absent
- Adenocarcinoma cells line alveolar walls in a continuous layer; tufting and overlapping may be present
- A completely resected tumour that is entirely sampled and evaluated histologically

Desirable:
- Nuclear atypia and alveolar septal thickening are variable

Staging
In the eighth edition of the TNM classification, AIS is classified as Tis (AIS), and TisN0M0 is defined as stage 0 {3067}.

Prognosis and prediction
Patients with AIS should have 100% disease-free and recurrence-free survival rates if the lesion is completely resected {3102,3074,1263,2126,1345}. These non-invasive lesions can be carefully observed when detected on chest CT as pure ground-glass opacities < 10 mm {1758}. However, if the size or density increases, surgical resection should be considered. Approximately half of resected AIS lesions show tumour growth during the preoperative observation period, with a median volume-doubling time of 811 days {1349}. Factors associated with growth of ground-glass nodules include initial tumour diameter, smoking history, and presence of *EGFR* mutation {1492}. Although results of randomized trials are not yet available, sublobar resections (i.e. anatomical segmentectomy or wide wedge excision) may be valid oncological procedures, assuming that complete resection is achieved {3143}. In the prospective Japan Clinical Oncology Group 0201 study, radiological non-invasive peripheral lung adenocarcinoma could be defined as an adenocarcinoma of < 20 mm with ≤ 25% of the tumour diameter showing consolidation (solid appearance) {2932}.

Minimally invasive adenocarcinoma of the lung

Matsubara D
Kadota K
MacMahon H
Yokose T

Definition

Minimally invasive adenocarcinoma (MIA) is a small (≤ 30 mm), solitary adenocarcinoma with a predominantly lepidic pattern and ≤ 5 mm invasion. The diagnosis of MIA requires a resection specimen where the lesion has been completely sampled and evaluated histologically. This diagnosis cannot be made on the basis of small biopsy or cytology specimens.

ICD-O coding

8256/3 Minimally invasive adenocarcinoma, non-mucinous
8257/3 Minimally invasive adenocarcinoma, mucinous

ICD-11 coding

2C25.Z & XH2098 Malignant neoplasms of bronchus or lung, unspecified & Minimally invasive adenocarcinoma, mucinous
2C25.Z & XH3QM0 Malignant neoplasms of bronchus or lung, unspecified & Minimally invasive adenocarcinoma, non-mucinous

Related terminology

Not recommended: microinvasive adenocarcinoma; bronchioloalveolar carcinoma (obsolete).

Subtype(s)

Minimally invasive adenocarcinoma, non-mucinous; minimally invasive adenocarcinoma, mucinous; minimally invasive adenocarcinoma, mixed non-mucinous and mucinous

Localization

MIA occurs in the lung periphery {3480,3494,1263}.

Clinical features

MIAs are usually discovered by CT screening or as an incidental finding on CT performed for other medical reasons.

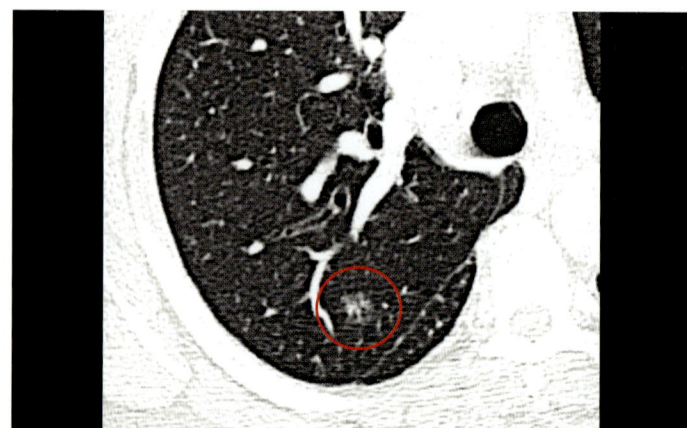

Fig. 1.41 Minimally invasive adenocarcinoma. CT appearance. This part-solid nodule (circle) is mostly ground-glass, with a small solid component measuring < 5 mm.

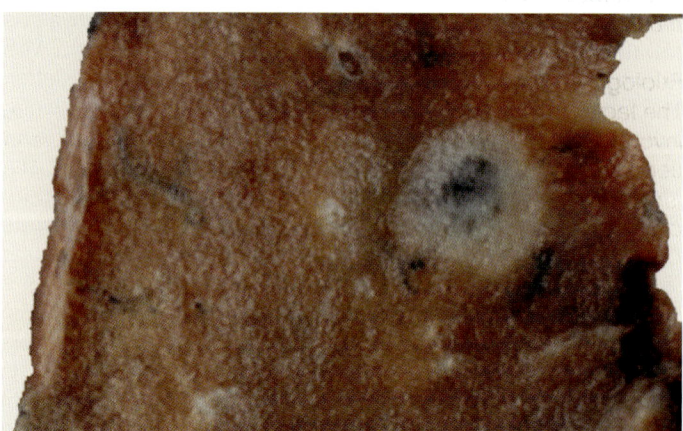

Fig. 1.42 Macroscopy of a minimally invasive non-mucinous adenocarcinoma. This tumour has a small central solid component (< 5 mm) corresponding to the invasive component, surrounded by a poorly defined area that represents the lepidic component.

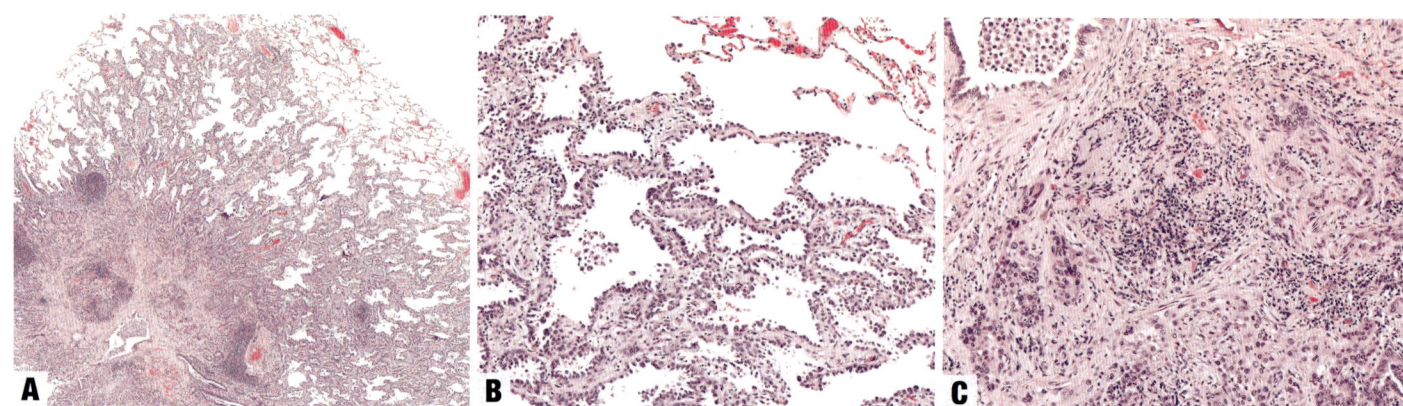

Fig. 1.43 Minimally invasive adenocarcinoma. **A** This lepidic-predominant tumour with a total size of 26 mm had an invasive area measuring 4 mm. The tumour mostly shows a lepidic pattern of growth (top and right), but there is a nodule of invasive adenocarcinoma (bottom left). **B** The lepidic component shows crowded atypical pneumocytes lining alveolar walls with preserved architecture. **C** This invasive area of the tumour shows a solid and acinar pattern surrounded by desmoplastic stroma.

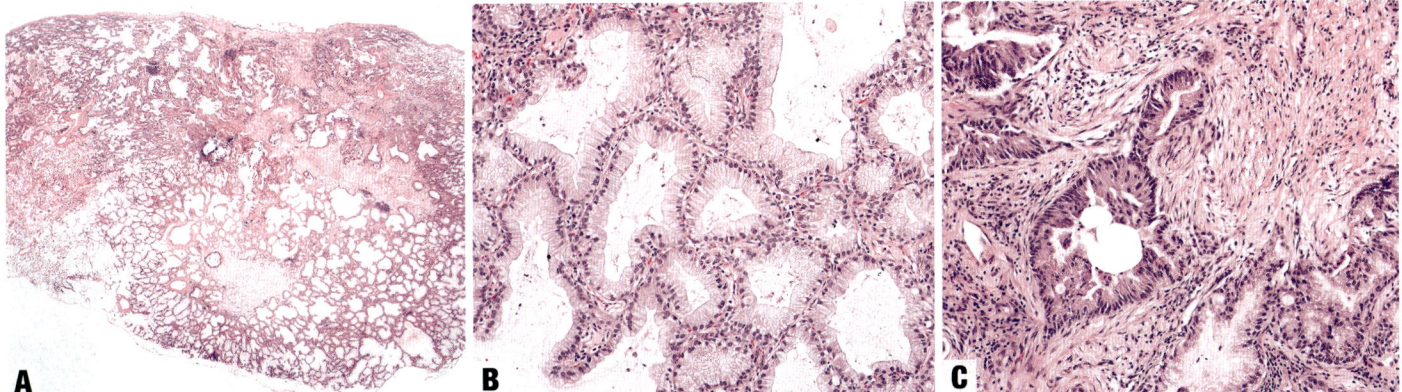

Fig. 1.44 Minimally invasive adenocarcinoma, mucinous. **A** This mucinous minimally invasive adenocarcinoma shows a lepidic-predominant pattern, with several foci of invasion associated with fibrous stroma. **B** This area shows lepidic growth, which was the predominant pattern of this tumour. There are columnar cells with abundant apical cytoplasmic mucin and small basally oriented nuclei growing along the surface of preserved alveolar walls. **C** This area of the tumour shows an invasive pattern of mucinous adenocarcinoma with desmoplastic stroma surrounding infiltrative glands lined by tumour cells with abundant intracytoplasmic mucin.

MIA is variable in its CT presentations, but when the tumour is non-mucinous, most often it shows a part-solid nodule, with a ≤ 5 mm solid component {3480,3494,1263}. In contrast, mucinous MIA usually shows a solid-dominant nodule by CT {1263}.

Epidemiology

See *Tumours of the lung: Introduction* (p. 20) and *Invasive non-mucinous adenocarcinoma of the lung* (p. 64).

Etiology

The factors implicated in the etiology of MIA are similar to those involved in the etiology of adenocarcinoma in situ (AIS) and conventional invasive adenocarcinoma. See *Tumours of the lung: Introduction* (p. 20) and *Invasive non-mucinous adenocarcinoma of the lung* (p. 64).

Pathogenesis

See *Tumours of the lung: Introduction* (p. 20) and *Invasive non-mucinous adenocarcinoma of the lung* (p. 64).

A multistep progression of lung adenocarcinoma is presumed with some lung adenocarcinomas, in which atypical adenomatous hyperplasia progresses to AIS, followed by invasive adenocarcinoma. This presumption is supported by the findings of recent studies by next-generation sequencing {1195,2400}. Because MIA is an early invasive adenocarcinoma, its genetic alterations may reveal early molecular events related to invasion. In addition to repression of *TGFBR2* and amplification of *PDCD6* and *TERT* {129,274}, *EGFR* amplification in association with *EGFR* mutation is involved in the transition from AIS to MIA {2762,2803,3393}. In the progression from AIS/MIA to invasive adenocarcinoma, mutations in *TP53*, *KRAS*, and *NF1*; arm-level

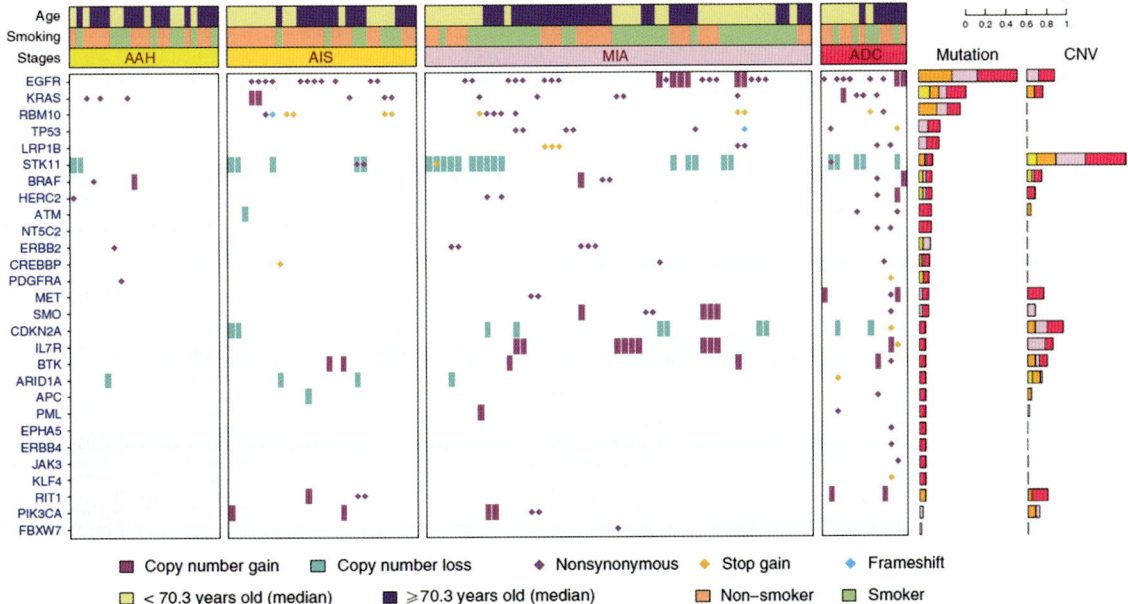

Fig. 1.45 Cancer gene mutations and copy-number aberrations in atypical adenomatous hyperplasia (AAH), adenocarcinoma in situ (AIS), minimally invasive adenocarcinoma (MIA), and invasive adenocarcinoma (ADC) {1195}. Cancer gene mutations were defined as non-synonymous mutations in known cancer genes identical to those previously reported and frameshift indels or truncating mutations in tumour suppressor genes. Cancer genes located in chromosomal segments with copy-number gains (red) or losses (green) are shown. A threshold of $\log_2$ ratio (indeterminate pulmonary nodule vs germline DNA) of > 2 or ≤ 2 was used to screen for chromosomal gains or losses, respectively. CNV, copy-number variation.

Box 1.04 Minimally invasive adenocarcinoma – diagnostic criteria {3074,3072,3068,3081}

- A small tumour (≤ 30 mm)
- A solitary adenocarcinoma
- Predominantly lepidic growth
- ≤ 5 mm invasive component in greatest dimension
- Invasive component to be measured includes
  - Any histological subtype other than a lepidic pattern (e.g. acinar, papillary, micropapillary, solid, colloid, fetal, or invasive mucinous adenocarcinoma)
  - Tumour cells infiltrating myofibroblastic stroma
- Minimally invasive adenocarcinoma diagnosis is excluded if the tumour
  - Invades lymphatics, blood vessels, or pleura
  - Contains tumour necrosis
  - Spreads through airspaces
- Cell type mostly non-mucinous (type II pneumocytes or club cells) but rarely may be mucinous (tall columnar cells with basal nuclei and abundant cytoplasmic mucin, sometimes resembling goblet cells)

Box 1.05 Minimally invasive adenocarcinoma – good practice points {3074,3072, 3068,3081}

- Same list of good practice points from Box 1.03 (p. 58) in the section *Adenocarcinoma in situ of the lung*
- If a single focus of invasion is present on one slide of tumour, it can be measured with a ruler and it should be ≤ 5 mm.
- If the manner of histological sectioning of the tumour makes it impossible to measure the size of invasion, an estimate of invasive size can be made by multiplying the total percentage of the invasive (non-lepidic) components by the total tumour size.
- Because most of the literature on the topic of adenocarcinoma in situ and minimally invasive adenocarcinoma deals with tumours ≤ 20 or 30 mm, there is insufficient evidence to support that 100% disease-free survival can occur in such tumours > 30 mm. These tumours should be classified as lepidic-predominant adenocarcinoma, suspect adenocarcinoma in situ or minimally invasive adenocarcinoma.

copy-number alterations; and HLA loss of heterozygosity have been reported to be involved {473,2400,3484}. Multiregion exome sequencing has also shown progressive genomic evolution at the single nucleotide level and demarcated evolution at the chromosomal level {1195}.

Macroscopic appearance

Most MIAs are peripheral nodules, showing a small (≤ 5 mm), central, solid area surrounded by frequently collapsed peripheral lung tissue. Anthracotic pigmentation and pleural puckering may also be observed. Tumour size may be underestimated on gross examination, so correlation with high-resolution CT findings may be helpful for accurate size determination. The entire tumour needs to be examined histologically to make the diagnosis of MIA {3074,3068}.

Histopathology

MIA is a small, solitary adenocarcinoma (≤ 30 mm), with a predominantly lepidic pattern and ≤ 5 mm invasion {3072,3074}. If the invasive area is in a single focus on one slide, the size of the invasive area should be measured in the largest dimension with a ruler {1345,3072}. If (1) there are multiple foci of invasion, (2) the invasive areas are on more than one slide, or (3) invasive size is difficult to measure, the invasive size can be estimated by multiplying the total size of the tumour by the total percentage of the non-lepidic or invasive components {1345}. If the estimated invasive size is ≤ 5 mm, a diagnosis of MIA is

warranted. Additional issues regarding the distinction between lepidic versus invasive patterns are discussed in *Invasive non-mucinous adenocarcinoma of the lung* (p. 64).

MIA is usually non-mucinous but rarely may be mucinous or mixed {275,1761,3400,3433}. Non-mucinous MIA typically shows type II pneumocyte and/or club cell differentiation. Mucinous MIA shows columnar cells with abundant apical mucin and small, often basally oriented nuclei, and it may show goblet cell morphology. By definition, MIA is solitary and discrete. The invasive component to be measured in MIA is defined as histological subtypes other than a lepidic pattern (i.e. acinar, papillary, micropapillary, or solid, or less often colloid, enteric, fetal, and/or invasive mucinous adenocarcinoma) or tumour cells infiltrating the myofibroblastic stroma. MIA is excluded if the tumour invades lymphatics, blood vessels, or pleura; contains tumour necrosis; or spreads through airspaces (outside the tumour). Tangential sectioning or collapse of lung tissue in lepidic adenocarcinoma can be difficult to distinguish from papillary or acinar patterns. Issues of differential diagnosis between lepidic, acinar, and papillary patterns, as well as reproducibility, are addressed in *Invasive non-mucinous adenocarcinoma of the lung* (p. 64).

Immunohistochemistry

Non-mucinous MIA is positive for pneumocyte markers, including TTF1 and napsin A. Mucinous MIA is usually negative for pneumocyte markers, whereas CK20 and HNF4α are often positive {1835}.

Cytology

The diagnosis of MIA cannot be made by cytology. Features typical of adenocarcinoma are seen (see *Invasive non-mucinous adenocarcinoma of the lung*, p. 64) {2511,1608}. However, one study found that the presence of large or 3D tumour cell clusters and especially irregular nuclear contours favour invasive adenocarcinoma rather than MIA {1837}. Features such as nuclear pleomorphism, prominent nucleoli, or intranuclear cytoplasmic inclusions are not useful for distinguishing invasive adenocarcinoma from MIA {1837}.

Diagnostic molecular pathology

Molecular testing is not required for the diagnosis. Whether to perform molecular testing on MIAs is best determined by each institution {1692}.

Essential and desirable diagnostic criteria

See Box 1.04 and Box 1.05.

Essential:

- A small (≤ 30 mm) lepidic-predominant adenocarcinoma with an invasive component ≤ 5 mm
- Invasive component to be measured includes any histological subtype other than a lepidic pattern (e.g. acinar, papillary, micropapillary, or solid, or less often colloid, enteric, fetal, or invasive mucinous adenocarcinoma) and tumour cells infiltrating myofibroblastic stroma
- The following should be absent: invasion of lymphatics, blood vessels, or pleura, as well as tumour necrosis or spread through airspaces
- A completely resected tumour that is entirely sampled and evaluated histologically

Desirable:

- The percentage of each of the invasive components should be recorded
- The tumour can be non-mucinous (type II pneumocytes or club cells) and rarely can be mucinous or mixed mucinous and non-mucinous
- If a tumour with pure lepidic growth has only been partly sampled, the diagnosis of lepidic adenocarcinoma should be rendered with a comment that the diagnosis of AIS or MIA cannot be made without complete histological sampling

Staging

MIA is staged as T1mi {3067,315}. The criteria for MIA can be applied in the setting of multiple tumours only if the other tumours are regarded as separate primaries rather than intrapulmonary metastases. In the setting of multiple non-mucinous adenocarcinomas, irrespective of clonality of the other tumours, a lesion that is morphologically qualified by the criteria described herein should be classified and staged as MIA.

Prognosis and prediction

Patients with tumours that meet the criteria for MIA should have 100% disease-free and recurrence-free survival if the tumour is completely resected. Multiple studies have found that patients with these tumours had 100% disease-free survival {1345,1761, 3072,3102,1263}. It remains to be determined whether patients with MIA still have 100% disease-free survival if the area of invasion shows a poorly differentiated component (e.g. solid or micropapillary adenocarcinoma) or if there is a giant cell and spindle cell component that does not meet the criteria for pleomorphic carcinoma.

Invasive non-mucinous adenocarcinoma of the lung

Cooper WA
Bubendorf L
Kadota K
Ladanyi M
MacMahon H
Matsubara D
Russell PA
Scagliotti GV
Sholl LM
Van Schil PEY
Warth A
Yoshizawa A

Definition
Invasive non-mucinous adenocarcinoma is a non-small cell lung carcinoma (NSCLC) with morphological or immunohistochemical evidence of glandular differentiation.

ICD-O coding
8140/3 Invasive non-mucinous adenocarcinoma
8250/3 Lepidic adenocarcinoma
8551/3 Acinar adenocarcinoma
8260/3 Papillary adenocarcinoma
8265/3 Micropapillary adenocarcinoma
8230/3 Solid adenocarcinoma

ICD-11 coding
2C25.0 Adenocarcinoma of bronchus or lung

Related terminology
Not recommended: bronchioloalveolar/bronchoalveolar carcinoma (obsolete).

Subtype(s)
Lepidic adenocarcinoma; acinar adenocarcinoma; papillary adenocarcinoma; micropapillary adenocarcinoma; solid adenocarcinoma

Localization
Adenocarcinomas are more likely to be peripherally located in the lung than other types of NSCLC, but tumours may also occur in a central location.

Clinical features
In general, clinical manifestations of lung cancer relate to local growth of the primary lesion, locoregional extension into neighbouring structures or lymph nodes, distant spread, or paraneoplastic syndromes. Clinically, adenocarcinomas are not different from other types of lung cancers, although para-neoplastic symptoms (see *Tumours of the lung: Introduction,* p. 20) are less common than in squamous cell or small cell carcinoma. Most patients present with locoregionally advanced or metastatic disease, apart from those identified through screening programmes. Commonly occurring symptoms are cough, dyspnoea, haemoptysis, or symptoms related to distant spread, such as central neurological symptoms due to brain metastases or peripheral pain due to bone metastases (see also *Tumours of the lung: Introduction,* p. 20).

Imaging
Non-mucinous adenocarcinoma often appears initially on CT as a small pure ground-glass nodule, which evolves over several years into a part-solid and eventually completely solid tumour {1123}. In other cases, it first becomes visible as a completely solid nodule. The histological correlate for the solid component

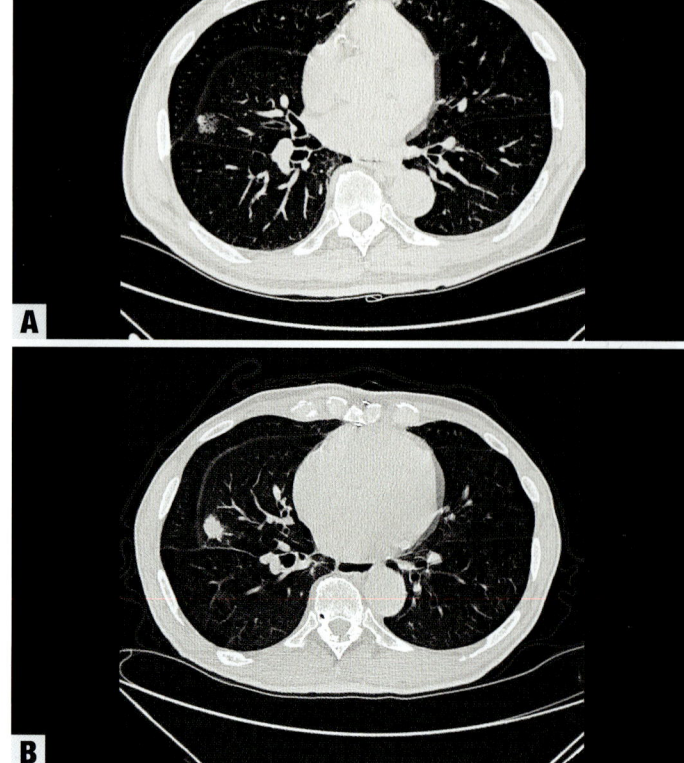

Fig. 1.46 Adenocarcinoma. **A** A ground-glass nodule with a typical appearance of lepidic adenocarcinoma with a small solid component at its anterolateral margin, probably minimally invasive at this time. **B** CT 4 years later shows that the nodule has become completely solid, consistent with invasive adenocarcinoma. This reflects indolent progression from a part-solid lepidic carcinoma to a solid invasive adenocarcinoma.

is typically invasive adenocarcinoma, while the non-solid component corresponds to a lepidic growth pattern {3075}. When adenocarcinoma contains both solid and non-solid components radiologically, the prognosis correlates more closely with size of the solid component than with size of the non-solid component {2054}. Focal calcification can be seen in a small proportion of all lung cancer cell types, including adenocarcinoma, due to dystrophic calcification or incorporation of pre-existing postinfectious calcium deposits {1766,1444}. Multiple primary lung cancers, usually adenocarcinomas, are increasingly recognized and must be distinguished from metastatic disease {112}. FDG PET is important for detecting sites of local and distant metastatic disease. The standardized uptake value for the tracer in the tumour also has prognostic implications. MRI may be useful in selected cases for assessing direct invasion of the chest wall (e.g. for superior sulcus tumours) {1754,397,2895,3054,327}.

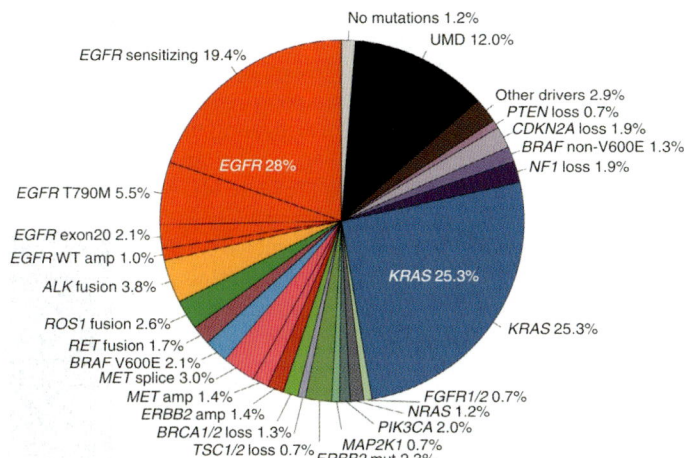

Fig. 1.47 Spectrum of oncogenic drivers assigned to 860 patients with lung adenocarcinoma identified by the MSK-IMPACT assay {1325A}. amp, amplification; mut, mutation; UMD, unknown mitogenic driver; WT, wildtype.

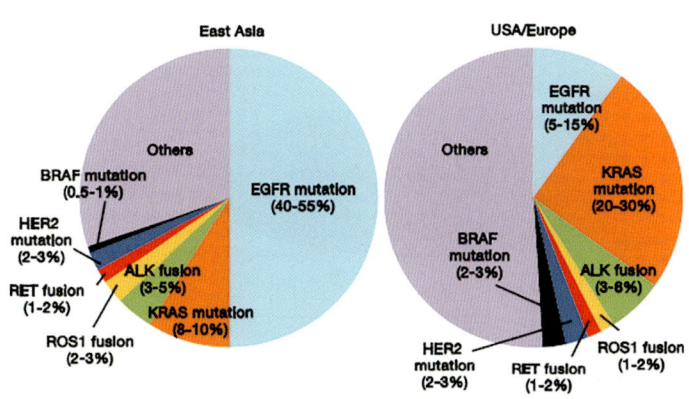

Fig. 1.48 Adenocarcinoma, invasive non-mucinous. Pie charts showing the proportion of various oncogenic driver mutations found in adenocarcinomas from eastern Asia and USA/Europe {1501A}.

Epidemiology

See *Tumours of the lung: Introduction* (p. 20).

Etiology

In Europe, smoking accounts for approximately 90% of lung cancers in men and 60% in women {2776}, with the strongest relationship observed in squamous cell carcinoma and small cell lung carcinoma, followed by lung adenocarcinoma {1431}. Heavy smokers have a 30-fold increased risk of dying of lung cancer by the age of 65 years compared with non-smokers {1847}. Lung adenocarcinoma, unlike other types of lung cancer, is also associated with non-smokers – especially female non-smokers {3184}. More-modern filtered cigarettes that contain lower tar and nicotine are thought to have contributed to the increased incidence of lung adenocarcinoma compared with other histological types of lung cancer due to their association with deeper inhalation and subsequent delivery of carcinogens to the peripheral lung {1004}. Other tobacco smoking products, such as cigars, cigarillos, and pipes, are also associated with a greater risk of lung cancer {252}, although to date no clear association has been identified with vaping products. Although no single environmental or genetic factor is known to account for lung cancer in non-smokers, exposure to environmental tobacco smoke (from a spouse or workplace exposure) is a known risk factor for lung adenocarcinoma in non-smokers {1439,2844}. Among non-smokers, indoor air pollution from wood fire, the burning of other solid fuels, and high-temperature cooking is also associated with lung cancer {1700,1221}.

Other factors that contribute to lung cancer development include occupational exposures to silica, asbestos, heavy metals, polycyclic aromatic hydrocarbons, and welding fumes {404, 2267,1778}; residential and occupational radiation exposure {1531}; air pollution {1732,1700}; pulmonary tuberculosis {770}; HIV infection {1468}; and a family history of lung cancer {143, 1736}. Genome-wide association studies have shown genetic alterations at 15q25 (*CHRNA5*, *CHRNA3*, and *CHRNB4*) {2903}, of the *TERT* gene on 5p15 {3459}, and at 6q23-q25 {143} are associated with increased genetic susceptibility to lung cancer {3089}. Germline mutations in *TP53* (Li–Fraumeni syndrome; see *Li–Fraumeni syndrome*, p. 474), *EGFR* p.T790M

mutations, and some *ERBB2* mutations are also associated with development of lung adenocarcinoma {390,198,925,415,2169, 2391,3361}.

Pathogenesis

The mechanisms by which cigarette smoking leads to lung cancer are well defined. More than 80 carcinogens have been identified in cigarette smoke {2791}, which has a proinflammatory and mutagenic effect in the lung and airways. Carcinogens in cigarette smoke produce DNA adducts that can lead to mutations crucial to the initiation and progression of lung adenocarcinomas {1107}. Molecular alterations are thought to accumulate in a stepwise manner in the development of lung adenocarcinomas {1471}, with early alterations identified in preneoplastic lesions (atypical adenomatous hyperplasia and adenocarcinoma in situ), including *KRAS* {3290} and *EGFR*

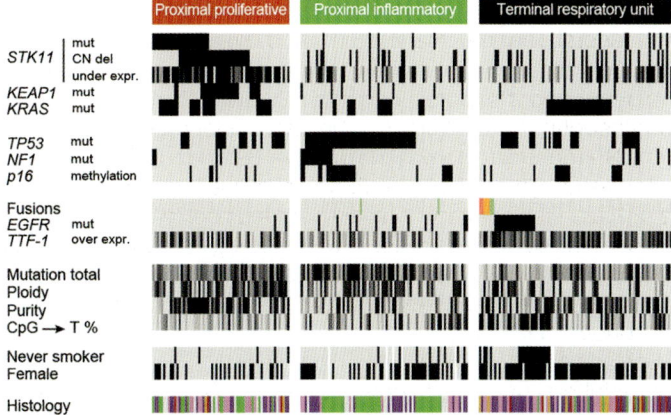

Fig. 1.49 Gene expression subtypes in lung adenocarcinoma. Gene expression subtypes integrated with genomic alterations and clinical and pathological features {370}. To coordinate the naming of the transcriptional subtypes with the histopathological, anatomical, and mutation classifications of lung adenocarcinoma, an updated nomenclature has been proposed: the terminal respiratory unit (formerly "bronchioid"), the proximal inflammatory (formerly "squamoid"), and the proximal proliferative (formerly "magnoid") transcriptional subtypes. CN del, copy-number deletion; expr., expression; mut, mutation.

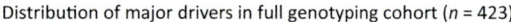

Distribution of major drivers in full genotyping cohort (*n* = 423)

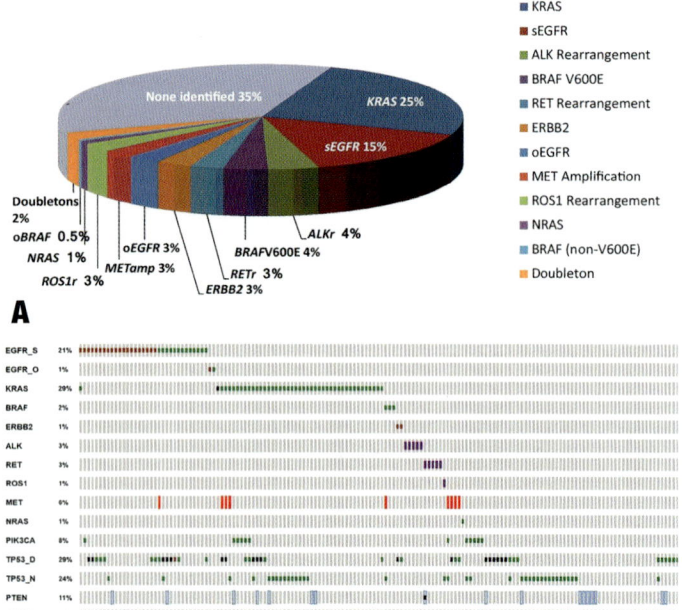

Legend:
- ■ KRAS
- ■ sEGFR
- ■ ALK Rearrangement
- ■ BRAF V600E
- ■ RET Rearrangement
- ■ ERBB2
- □ oEGFR
- ■ MET Amplification
- ■ ROS1 Rearrangement
- ■ NRAS
- ■ BRAF (non-V600E)
- ■ Doubleton

Labels on pie: None identified 35%, KRAS 25%, sEGFR 15%, ALKr 4%, BRAFV600E 4%, RETr 3%, ERBB2 3%, METamp 3%, oEGFR 3%, ROS1r 3%, NRAS 1%, oBRAF 0.5%, Doubletons 2%

A

Co-mutation plot rows (percentages):
EGFR_S 21%, EGFR_O 1%, KRAS 29%, BRAF 2%, ERBB2 1%, ALK 3%, RET 3%, ROS1 1%, MET 6%, NRAS 1%, PIK3CA 8%, TP53_D 29%, TP53_N 24%, PTEN 11%, STK11 11%

Genetic alteration: Amplification | Fusion | Truncating mutation | Inframe mutation | Missense mutation

Protein alteration: Loss of expression

B

Fig. 1.50 Distribution of major drivers and co-mutation plot in lung adenocarcinomas. Mutations and co-mutation plot in the Lung Cancer Mutation Consortium (LCMC2). **A** Distribution of oncogenic drivers in full genotyping cohort. The relative proportion of the various driver mutations is shown for the 423 subjects with complete testing for 12 genes. No *AKT1* or *MAP2K1* mutations were detected in this set. *sEGFR*, sensitizing *EGFR* mutation; *oEGFR*, other *EGFR* mutations; *ALKr*, *RETr*, and *ROS1r* denote rearrangements in the respective genes; *METamp* denotes amplification of *MET*; *oBRAF* denotes a mutation other than V600E; and "doubletons" denotes samples with two or more of the oncogenic drivers shown here. **B** Co-mutation plot. Genetic and expression alterations in the 14 core genes plus key tumour suppressor genes in 154 lung adenocarcinomas with complete analysis. No *AKT1* or *MAP2K1* mutations were detected in this set. EGFR_S, sensitizing *EGFR* mutations; EGFR_O, other *EGFR* mutations; TP53_D, disruptive alterations; TP53_N, non-disruptive alterations.

{3393} mutations, as well as loss of heterozygosity involving multiple tumour suppressor genes {2958,1337}. Growth signalling pathways that are frequently involved in the pathogenesis of lung adenocarcinomas include the EGFR (HER1)/RAS/PI3K pathway and the p53/RB1/p14/STK11 growth inhibitory pathway {302}. Inactivating mutations of the tumour suppressor gene *TP53* occur in approximately 45% of lung adenocarcinomas {1614,708} and are commonly smoking-related, with G>T and C>A transversions {852A,2146A}. Activating mutations in *KRAS* occur in approximately 20% of lung adenocarcinomas and are strongly associated with smoking {2562,1614}. Activating mutations involving *EGFR* occur more commonly in females, never-smokers, and Asians (70% in never-smokers from eastern Asia, 40% in never-smokers of European descent vs 11% in smokers of European descent) {3498A} (see Box 1.06). A small subset of adenocarcinomas are driven by genetic rearrangements such as *ALK* fusions. Patients with these tumours are younger than those with ALK-negative tumours, with no clear ethnic differences {1873,3497} (see Box 1.07). Other factors involved in the pathogenesis of lung adenocarcinoma include inhibition of apoptosis, telomerase activation, and evasion of host immunity.

Macroscopic appearance

Most invasive adenocarcinomas appear as grey-white nodules with central scarring fibrosis associated with anthracotic pigmentation and pleural puckering {3102}. The peripheral lepidic component may result in a poorly defined border, and individual preserved alveolar spaces may be visible. In fresh unfixed specimens, lepidic tumour components may be difficult to discern.

Histopathology

Non-mucinous lung adenocarcinomas usually consist of a complex admixture of architectural patterns (lepidic, acinar, papillary, micropapillary, and solid) and are classified into subtypes according to the predominant architectural pattern using comprehensive histological subtyping {3074}. In resection specimens, each pattern should be estimated in a semiquantitative manner and recorded in 5–10% increments totalling 100%. Using 5% increments allows for greater flexibility in choosing a predominant pattern when tumours have two patterns of relatively similar percentages. Although it is possible to have equal percentages of two prominent components, a single predominant component should be chosen. In such cases, recording all percentages in the report will makes it clear that the tumour had a relatively even mixture of several patterns {3068}. Using 5% increments also avoids the need to use 10% for small amounts of components, such as micropapillary or solid patterns, where

Box 1.06 Characteristics of *EGFR* mutations in lung adenocarcinoma

- The mutations occur in the kinase domain of the receptor tyrosine kinase, and they lead to constitutive activation of downstream signalling without ligand binding.
- Although females and never-smokers are preferentially affected, the biological basis for these associations is not well understood. However, every new case of advanced adenocarcinoma should be tested for the presence of *EGFR* mutations.
- The two most common mutations – the point mutation at codon 858 (p.L858R) and the in-frame deletions in exon 19 – account for > 90% of cases, although many other mutations (e.g. mutations at codon G719 and in-frame insertions in exon 20) are reported in the literature.
- These *EGFR* mutations are highly suggestive of lung adenocarcinoma. Among adenocarcinomas, *EGFR* mutations are frequently detected in cases with lepidic and papillary growth, and they are associated with TTF1 positivity.
- Genetic alterations of other major lung cancer driver genes, such as *KRAS*, *ALK*, *ROS1*, *BRAF*, *RET*, and *ERBB2*, are mutually exclusive with *EGFR* mutations, presumably because these all converge on the same intracellular signalling pathways, and a single impairment in these pathways is sufficient to drive tumour formation.
- Rare families with germline *EGFR* mutations (p.R776G, p.R776H, p.T790M, p.V843I, and p.P848L) have higher risk of lung adenocarcinoma, which can be multifocal, particularly in the case of germline *EGFR* p.T790M mutations.
- *EGFR* mutations in lung adenocarcinoma show ethnic differences, with prevalence ranges of 10–15% in people of European descent and 30–40% in Asians.
- *EGFR* mutation is a prognostic factor as well as a factor predictive of response to EGFR tyrosine kinase inhibitor treatment.
- *EGFR* mutations in exon 20, in-frame insertions, and (rarely) p.T790M mutations are associated with primary resistance to first- and second-generation EGFR tyrosine kinase inhibitors, and acquisition of an additional p.T790M mutation is the most common cause of secondary resistance to EGFR tyrosine kinase inhibitors.

even small amounts of 5% have consistently been shown to correlate with poor prognosis {3373,3509,2634,424,2120,3094, 2953}.

Lepidic

This pattern consists of bland pneumocytic cells (type II pneumocytes or club cells) growing along the surface of alveolar walls. In lepidic-predominant adenocarcinoma, there is also an invasive component measuring > 5 mm in greatest dimension. The invasive component is defined as a histological pattern other than a lepidic pattern (i.e. acinar; papillary; micropapillary; solid; or less commonly, colloid, fetal, enteric, and/or invasive mucinous adenocarcinoma [IMA]) and/or myofibroblastic stroma associated with invasive tumour cells. Diagnostic features that help distinguish minimally invasive adenocarcinoma (MIA) from lepidic-predominant adenocarcinoma are presented in Table 1.06. A diagnosis of lepidic adenocarcinoma rather than MIA should be made if the cancer (1) invades the lymphatic system, blood vessels, or pleura; (2) exhibits tumour necrosis; (3) contains an invasive component > 5 mm; or (4) shows spread through airspaces (STAS). If the invasive area is in a single focus on one slide, the size of the invasive area should be measured in the largest dimension microscopically {1345,3072}. If (1) there are multiple foci of invasion, (2) the invasive areas are on more than one slide, or (3) invasive size is difficult to measure, the invasive size can be estimated by multiplying the total size of the tumour by the total percentage of the non-lepidic or invasive components {1345,1361,3067,3068}. Alveolar wall collapse can result in thickening of alveolar walls, with increased interstitial connective tissue raising the consideration of the acinar pattern; however, clear invasive growth is lacking. Some lepidic tumours have prominent hyperplastic lymphoid stroma. It is understood that lepidic growth can occur in metastatic tumours to the lung as well as in IMAs. However, the specific term "lepidic adenocarcinoma" refers to a non-mucinous adenocarcinoma showing lepidic growth as its predominant component, distinguishing these tumours from IMAs. Lepidic growth may also be composed of neoplastic cells with more-marked nuclear atypia resembling that of the adjacent invasive patterns. Diagnostic features that help distinguish lepidic / in situ growth of adenocarcinoma from invasive adenocarcinoma are presented in Table 1.07 (p. 68). Compared with tumours with lepidic components resembling type II pneumocytes or club cells ("precursor lepidic"), those with marked nuclear atypia ("outgrowth lepidic") show increased Ki-67 proliferation index and p53 immunohistochemistry alterations {1965}. Despite evidence that these forms

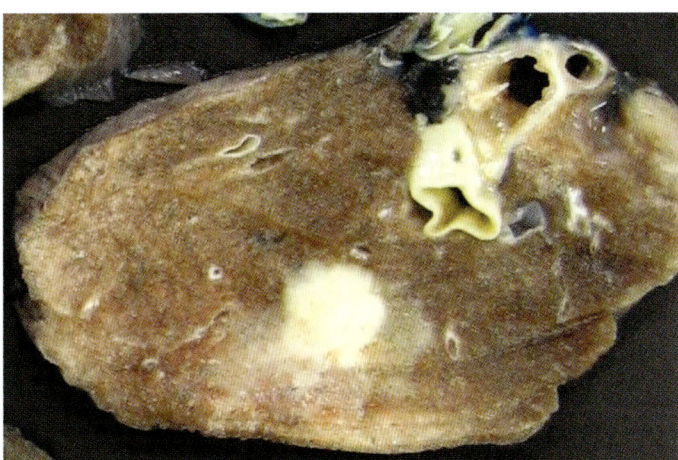

Fig. 1.51 Non-mucinous lung adenocarcinoma. Gross image shows a solid white component that corresponds to invasive adenocarcinoma microscopically and an adjacent paler poorly defined spongy area that corresponds to lepidic adenocarcinoma.

Box 1.07 Characteristics of *ALK* gene fusions in lung cancer

- *ALK* fusions are detected in various tumours of the lung, thyroid, oesophagus, soft tissue, kidney, colorectum, and bladder, and the fusion partner genes vary among the tumour types. *EML4-ALK* fusion is most frequently and almost exclusively found in carcinomas of the lung.
- *ALK* rearrangement in lung cancer is strongly associated with adenocarcinoma histology, in particular with acinar and/or solid growth pattern, or with cellular features of signet-ring cell carcinoma.
- *EML4-ALK* fusion accounts for > 90% of *ALK* rearrangements in lung adenocarcinomas. Other (less common) *ALK* fusion partners include *KIF5B*, *KLC1*, *TFG*, and others.
- Like *EGFR* mutations, *ALK* rearrangement is frequent in never-smokers, but it is less associated with female sex.
- The median age of patients with ALK-positive lung cancer is about 10 years younger than that of patients with ALK-negative cancer.
- ALK-positive lung adenocarcinoma constitutes 4–5% of non-small cell lung carcinomas, and ethnic differences have not been reported, unlike with *EGFR* mutations.
- *ALK* rearrangement is predictive of response to ALK inhibitor treatment, but it is not a prognostic factor.

of lepidic growth are biologically distinct, it is not recommended to make this distinction in clinical practice, because of the lack of sufficient evidence, that adjusts for the impact of the invasive components, to indicate a worse overall survival for the outgrowth versus the precursor cases {1965}.

Table 1.06 Distinction of minimally invasive adenocarcinoma from lepidic-predominant adenocarcinoma

Diagnostic feature	Minimally invasive adenocarcinoma	Lepidic-predominant adenocarcinoma
Size of total tumour	Lepidic-predominant tumour ≤ 30 mm	Lepidic-predominant tumour of any size *or* Tumour that otherwise meets the criteria for minimally invasive adenocarcinoma but is > 30 mm
Size of invasive focus	≤ 5 mm	> 5 mm
Invasion of visceral pleura or blood vessels or lymphatic vessels	Absent	May be present
Tumour necrosis	Absent	May be present
Spread through airspaces	Absent	May be present

Table 1.07 Features to help distinguish lepidic pattern of adenocarcinoma from invasive adenocarcinoma

Diagnostic feature	Lepidic pattern of adenocarcinoma[a]	Invasive adenocarcinoma
Histological pattern	Lepidic	Acinar, papillary, micropapillary, or solid
Myofibroblastic stroma	Absent	May be present
Intra-alveolar macrophages	May be present	Usually absent
Alveolar architecture	Preserved	Lost

[a]This includes non-mucinous adenocarcinoma in situ or lepidic pattern of adenocarcinoma within a minimally invasive adenocarcinoma or an invasive non-mucinous adenocarcinoma.

Acinar

This pattern is characterized by glands that may be round to oval or have a more jagged outline with central luminal spaces surrounded by tumour cells {3072,3074,3068}. The tumour cells and/or glandular spaces may contain mucin. The neoplastic glands invade through myofibroblastic stroma and/or replace the background alveolar architecture of the lung. In contrast, in lepidic adenocarcinoma, the background alveolar architecture is intact. Acinar adenocarcinoma can occasionally be difficult to distinguish from lepidic adenocarcinoma, particularly

when there is lung parenchymal collapse in which the lepidic pattern appears as nests or strands of tumour cells mimicking the neoplastic glands of acinar adenocarcinoma. The presence of alveolar macrophages in residual compressed alveolar spaces, preservation of the underlying alveolar architecture, and absence of myofibroblastic stroma are helpful features in favour of lepidic adenocarcinoma, whereas neoplastic glands invading through myofibroblastic stroma indicate acinar adenocarcinoma. The cribriform pattern is defined by invasive back-to-back fused tumour glands with multiple spaces lacking intervening stroma {1346}. Cribriform arrangements are regarded as a pattern of acinar adenocarcinoma that is associated with poor prognosis {1346,1991,3228,1339,1543,3068}.

Papillary

This pattern is characterized by growth of glandular tumour cells along the surface of fibrovascular cores {3072,3074,3068}. The presence of myofibroblastic stroma, as is seen in acinar adenocarcinoma, is not needed to diagnose this pattern. Accordingly, lepidic adenocarcinoma may mimic papillary adenocarcinoma, particularly in areas of lepidic pattern in which there has been tangential sectioning of alveolar walls or lung parenchymal collapse as can be seen after surgery {3037}. Papillary adenocarcinoma shows a morphological spectrum based on size of papillary structures and nuclear grade, which corresponds to

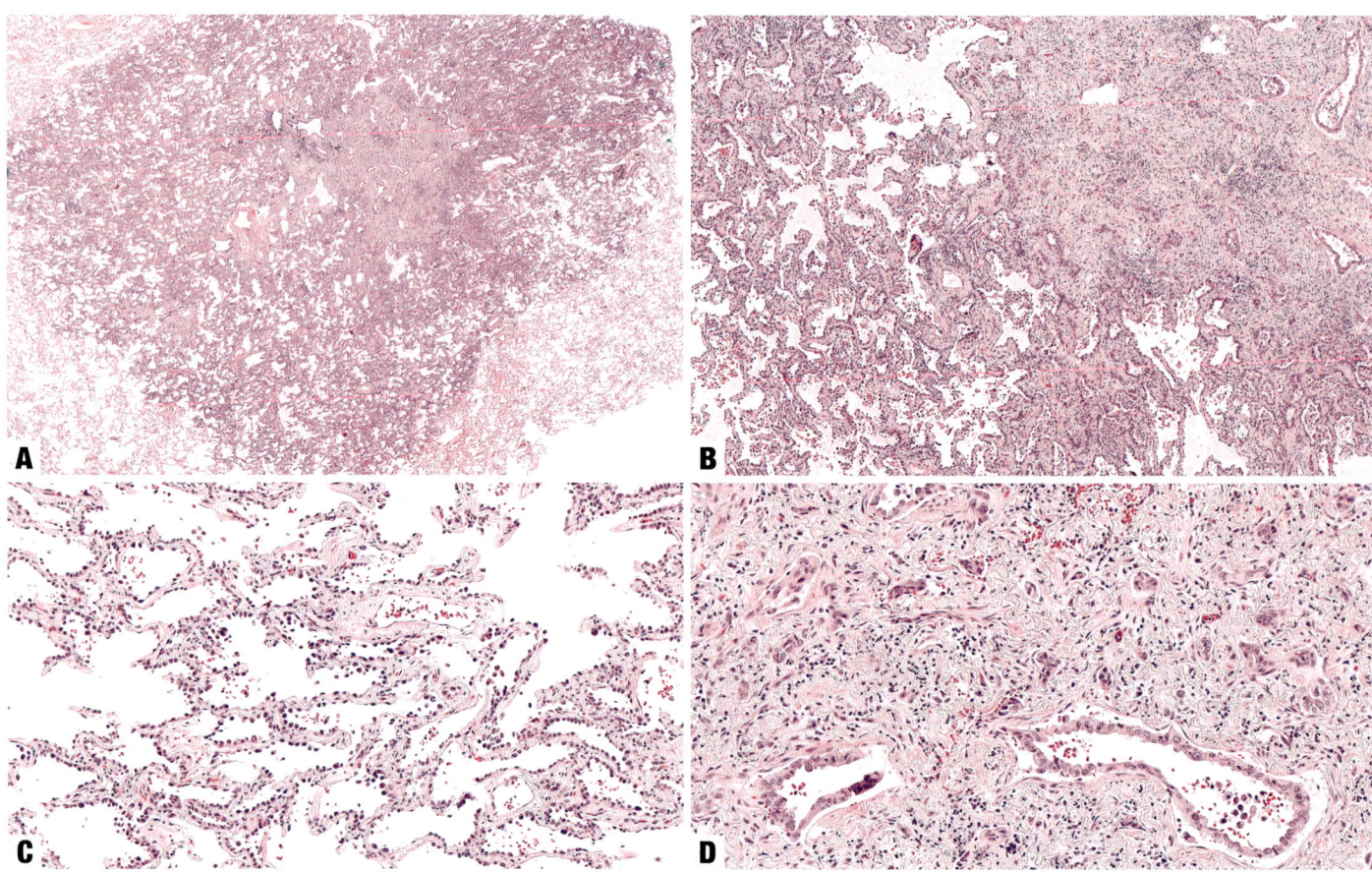

Fig. 1.52 Lepidic-predominant adenocarcinoma. **A** This tumour, measuring a total size of 29 mm, consists of a predominant lepidic component and an invasive component measuring 12 mm. In this image there is a central fibrous scar invaded by an acinar and solid pattern adenocarcinoma. **B** The lepidic component (left) surrounds the invasive area (right) with an acinar and solid pattern invading in a fibrous stroma. **C** This lepidic area shows alveolar walls lined by a marked proliferation of atypical pneumocytes without invasive growth. **D** This area of invasive adenocarcinoma shows an acinar and solid pattern. The solid pattern consists of infiltrating small nests of tumour cells.

prognosis {3226}. If papillary structures are noted filling air-spaces surrounded by acinar or lepidic patterns, the tumour pattern is classified as papillary adenocarcinoma, rather than acinar or lepidic adenocarcinoma.

Solid

This pattern consists of polygonal tumour cells arranged in sheets, lacking recognizable lepidic, acinar (including cribriform), papillary, or micropapillary architecture. To confirm glandular differentiation in solid tumours, immunohistochemical expression of a pneumocyte marker (TTF1 and/or napsin A) with negative p40 {3039} or histochemical demonstration of intracellular mucin (e.g. PASD or mucicarmine stain) in ≥ 5 tumour cells in each of two high-power fields (~0.4 mm²) is required for diagnosis {3074}. TTF1 immunohistochemistry is more sensitive than mucin stains to diagnose solid adenocarcinoma {1907}. Both squamous and large cell carcinomas may show rare tumour cells with intracellular mucin.

Micropapillary

This pattern is composed of tumour cells growing in papillary tufts forming florets that lack fibrovascular cores, which may appear detached from and/or connected to alveolar walls. Ring-like glandular structures may float within alveolar spaces, and psammoma bodies may be seen {3074}. The morphological spectrum of the micropapillary pattern was recently expanded by recognition of a filigree pattern consisting of tumour cells growing in delicate, lace-like, narrow stacks of ≥ 3 cells, without fibrovascular cores {767,3519A}. When airspaces surrounded by lepidic, acinar, or papillary patterns contain micropapillary adenocarcinoma, the pattern should be classified as micropapillary, because of the comparably poorer prognosis of this pattern {767}. Micropapillary adenocarcinoma can also show a stromal invasive pattern {2160}.

Clear cell and signet-ring features

Clear cell and signet-ring changes are cytological features that can be seen in a variety of patterns, including acinar, papillary, solid, and micropapillary patterns {3074}. Therefore, these are not regarded to be specific patterns and are not included in comprehensive histological description. However, it may be useful to record the percentage of tumour cells that show clear cell or signet-ring cytological features for comparison of histological features if these tumours recur or metastasize {3074}.

Invasion

Invasion is defined as (1) histological patterns other than a lepidic pattern (i.e. acinar, papillary, micropapillary, and/or solid, or less commonly invasive mucinous, colloid, fetal, and enteric adenocarcinoma), (2) myofibroblastic stroma associated with invasive tumour cells, (3) vascular or pleural invasion, and (4) STAS.

Reproducibility for major patterns, invasive pattern, and measurement of invasion

Reproducibility studies evaluating the major adenocarcinoma patterns, for the distinction of adenocarcinoma in situ, MIA versus invasive adenocarcinoma, and measurement of invasion have shown variable results depending on whether the analysis focuses on difficult cases or on cohorts representative of

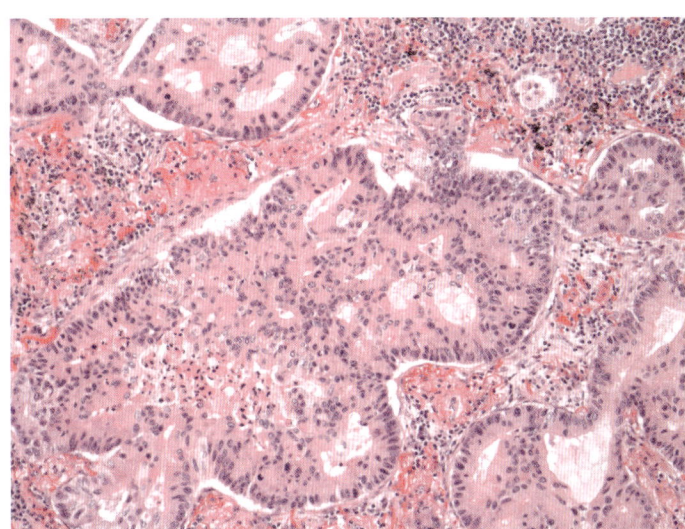

Fig. 1.53 Acinar adenocarcinoma. A cribriform component is associated with a worse prognosis.

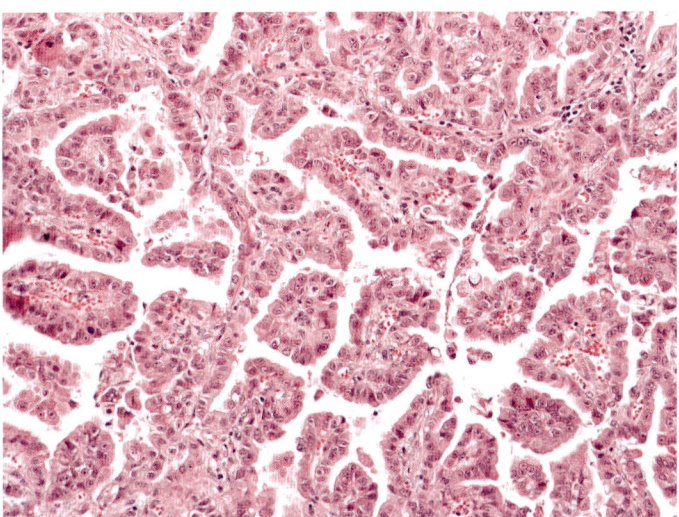

Fig. 1.54 Papillary adenocarcinoma. This tumour consists of neoplastic glandular cells growing along the surface of fibrovascular cores.

routine clinical practice. Understandably the reproducibility is lower for analyses focusing on difficult cases.

Reproducibility was moderate to substantial and fair to moderate in selected typical and difficult cases, respectively {3225, 3036,2741}. After a training session, reproducibility was shown to improve to almost perfect {3225}. When cohorts representative of routine hospital cases were used, the agreements were good for distinction among adenocarcinoma in situ, MIA, and stage IA adenocarcinoma, and in resected adenocarcinomas of all histological patterns, 21% of predominant patterns with different prognostic scores were mismatched, suggesting that the classification scheme captured prognostic differences {262, 266}.

In studies evaluating whether invasion is present or not, for typical cases the reported agreement is moderate to good {3036,266} and for difficult cases it ranges from slight to fair {2741,3036}. Agreement regarding measurement of invasion in typical cases has been reported to be excellent {262}, but for difficult cases it is reported to be slight or poor {3036,2741}.

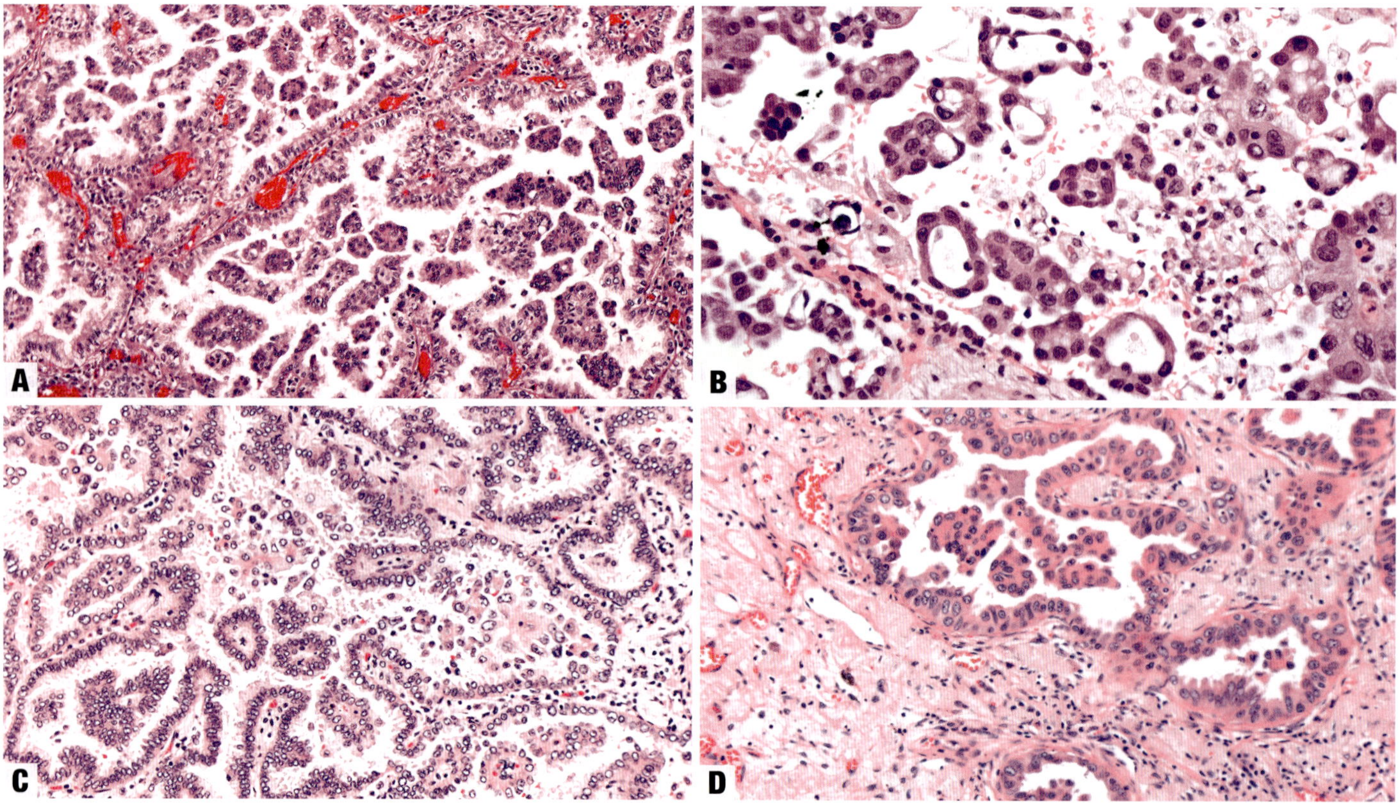

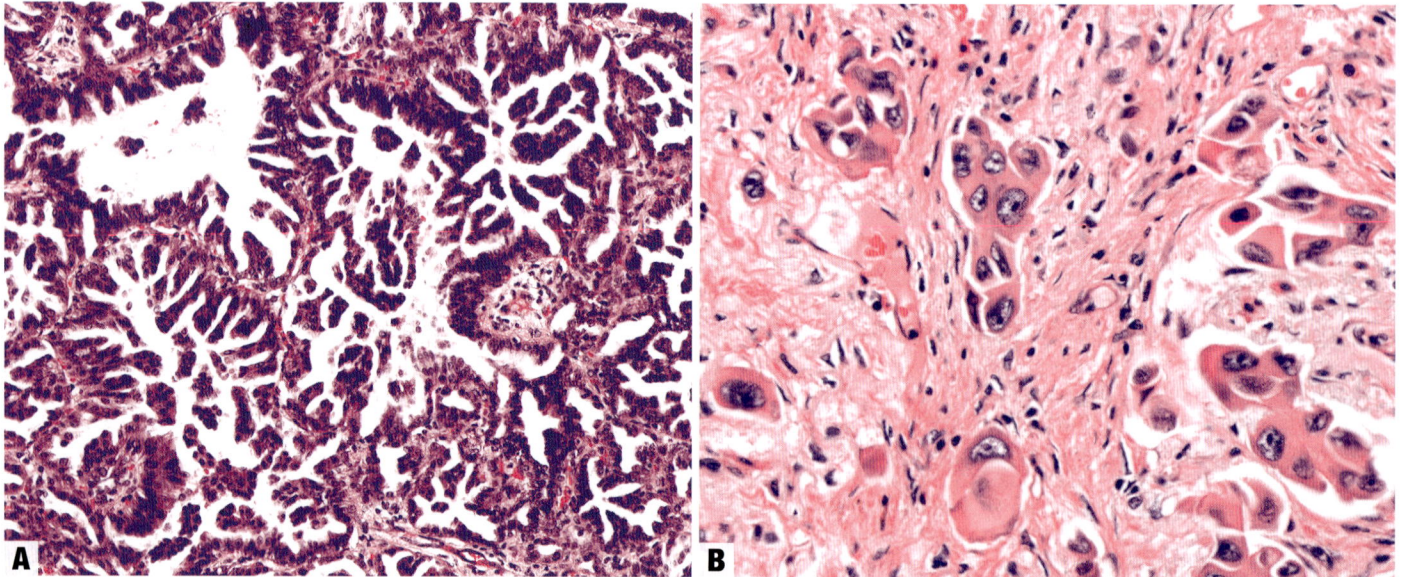

Fig. 1.55 Micropapillary adenocarcinoma. **A** This tumour consists of extensive micropapillary clusters of tumour cells lacking fibrovascular cores. **B** This micropapillary pattern shows numerous ring-like structures. **C** Although this tumour shows a papillary architecture, because there are numerous tumour cells with a micropapillary architecture within the airspaces, this should be classified as micropapillary and not papillary adenocarcinoma. **D** Although there is an acinar adenocarcinoma structure, this should be classified as micropapillary adenocarcinoma due to the airspace pattern of micropapillary tumour cells.

Fig. 1.56 Micropapillary adenocarcinoma. **A** Filigree pattern. This tumour shows extensive stacks of tumour cells with a thickness of ≤ 3 tumour cells, extending from the alveolar walls towards the airspaces, forming a filigree pattern. **B** Stromal pattern. This micropapillary adenocarcinoma shows extensive infiltration of fibrous stroma within lymphatics.

Immune response and microenvironment

Within the tumour microenvironment, there are various non-neoplastic cells including stromal fibroblasts and endothelial cells, as well as immune cells including T cells, B cells, and macrophages, some of which have prognostic relevance {474, 737,895,1033,1271,1407,1411,1464,1834,2126,2655,2736,2838, 2960,3193,3284,3371}, implicating cross-talk between cancer cells and the microenvironment in tumour progression.

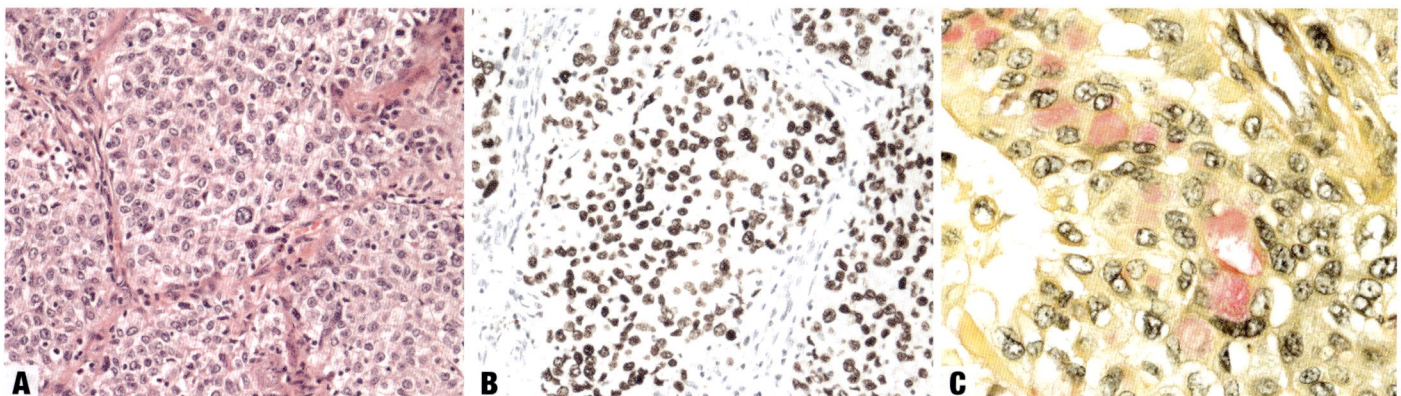

Fig. 1.57 Solid adenocarcinoma. **A** The tumour consists of morphologically undifferentiated solid nests of tumour cells. **B** TTF1 immunohistochemistry shows diffuse nuclear staining, confirming a solid adenocarcinoma (p40 was negative). **C** Adenocarcinoma, solid, with mucin. This mucicarmine stain highlights prominent intracytoplasmic mucin.

Table 1.08 Proposed grading of resected early-stage invasive non-mucinous lung adenocarcinoma

Grade	Differentiation	Patterns
1	Well-differentiated	Lepidic-predominant with no or < 20% high-grade pattern
2	Moderately differentiated	Acinar or papillary-predominant with no or < 20% high-grade pattern
3	Poorly differentiated	Any tumour with ≥ 20% high-grade pattern (solid, micropapillary, cribriform, or complex glandular pattern[a])

[a]Fused glands or single cells infiltrating in a desmoplastic stroma.

Tumour spread through airspaces

Tumour STAS is defined as tumour cells within airspaces in the lung parenchyma beyond the edge of the main tumour {1342, 2193}. This should be distinguished from findings suggesting artefactual spread of tumour cells, such as (1) randomly situated and ragged-edged clusters of tumour cells often at the edge of the tissue section or out of the plane of section of the tissue, (2) lack of continuous spread in airspaces from the tumour edge to the most distant airspace tumour cells, (3) the presence of jagged edges of tumour cell clusters, (4) normal benign pneumocytes or bronchial cells with benign cytological features or presence of cilia, or (5) linear strips of cells that are lifted off alveolar walls {1342}. STAS in adenocarcinoma is composed of three morphological patterns: micropapillary structures, solid nests of tumour cells filling airspaces, and discohesive single cells {1342}. A number of independent studies have shown STAS to be a predictor of worse clinical outcome in resected lung adenocarcinoma as well as all major histological lung cancer types investigated {1342,2193,3229,146,69}. In addition, in patients with STAS, limited resection probably contributes to a significantly higher risk of recurrence than lobectomy {1342, 146}. Because STAS is thought to represent a manifestation of tumour spread, it is not included in the total percentage of patterns or in tumour size for staging.

Immunohistochemistry

Immunohistochemistry can be a useful ancillary technique to confirm a primary lung adenocarcinoma rather than a pulmonary metastasis (see *Metastases*, p. 451) and is also required for the diagnosis of solid-predominant lung adenocarcinoma (unless histochemical staining confirms the presence of intracytoplasmic mucin), or to make a diagnosis of "non-small cell lung carcinoma, favour adenocarcinoma" in a morphologically undifferentiated tumour in small biopsy or cytology specimens (see *Small diagnostic samples*, p. 29). Although there is no immunohistochemical marker with 100% sensitivity or specificity for pulmonary adenocarcinomas, the pneumocyte markers TTF1 and napsin A are positive in the majority of cases (~75–80%) {3227, 2456}, and TTF1 is recommended when a limited panel is used {3390}. The currently available antibody clones for TTF1 have a variable staining performance, with clone 8G7G3/1 being the most specific and SPT24 being more sensitive {3390}. Even focal positivity for TTF1 is sufficient to favour glandular differentiation in the appropriate context {3390}. Double positivity in the same tumour for TTF1 and p40 usually indicates an adenocarcinoma {3390}, although adenosquamous carcinoma should also be considered (see *Adenosquamous carcinoma of the lung*, p. 100). When evaluating tumours, positive immunoreaction for TTF1 in entrapped pneumocytes must be carefully excluded. Tumours other than lung adenocarcinomas also express TTF1 (e.g. neuroendocrine tumours [NETs], thyroid tumours, and some female genital tract carcinomas) {3482,3390} and napsin A (e.g. renal cell carcinomas) {2209}. CK7 is not specific for pulmonary adenocarcinomas {3390}.

Grading

The predominant histological pattern of lung adenocarcinoma is associated with prognosis, with lepidic-predominant tumours having the best prognosis, acinar and papillary-predominant tumours having an intermediate prognosis, and solid-predominant and micropapillary-predominant tumours having the worst prognosis {3074,3433,3102}. Significant efforts have been made to build on these data and develop a robust histological grading scheme for lung adenocarcinoma. In a recent large study undertaken by the International Association for the Study of Lung Cancer (IASLC) Pathology Committee, a combination of predominant histological pattern plus worst pattern (≥ 20% of a high-grade solid, micropapillary, cribriform, or complex

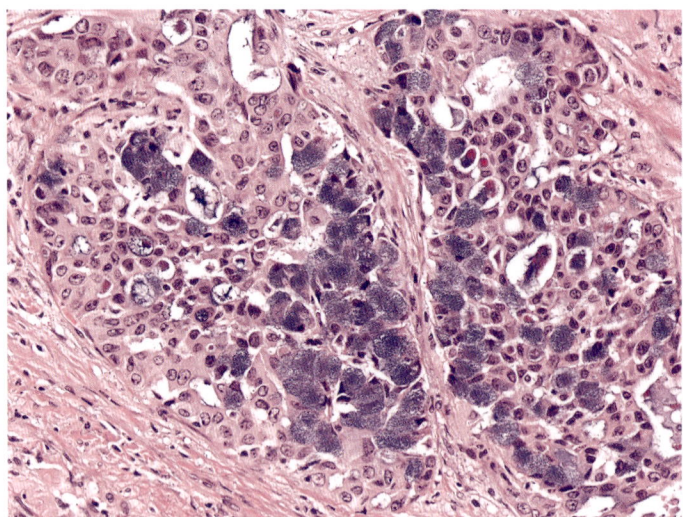

Fig. 1.58 Adenocarcinoma with *ALK* fusion shows signet-ring features. This adenocarcinoma with an *ALK* fusion shows solid, acinar, and mucinous features.

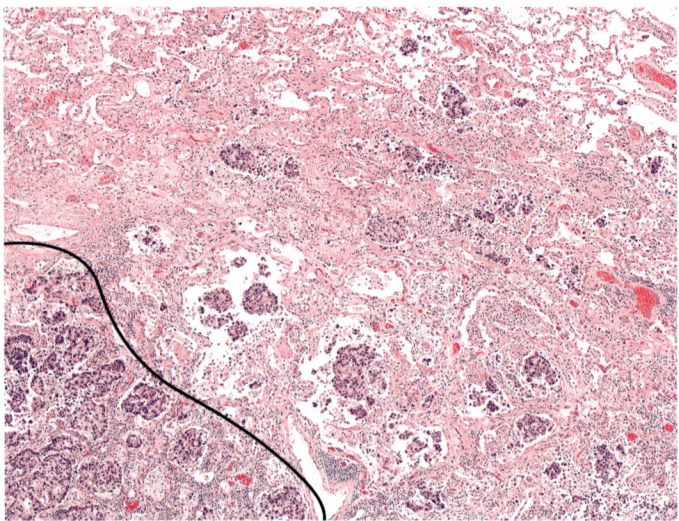

Fig. 1.59 Spread through airspaces in adenocarcinoma. Many airspace clusters of tumour cells spread far beyond the tumour edge (marked by black line) in a continuous manner (lower-left corner), forming the lesion of spread through airspaces.

glandular pattern [fused glands or single cells infiltrating in a desmoplastic stroma]) significantly improved prediction of patient outcome in a training cohort and an independent validation cohort of early-stage resected lung adenocarcinomas, and it was superior to other models incorporating mitotic count, nuclear grade, cytological grade, STAS, or necrosis {1990A}. This has led to the recommendation of a three-tiered grading system for resected early-stage lung adenocarcinoma (see Table 1.08, p. 71).

Differential diagnosis
The differential diagnosis of pulmonary adenocarcinomas involves (1) distinction from other lung cancer types, (2) distinction from mesothelioma, (3) distinction of multiple lung primaries from intrapulmonary metastasis, and (4) distinction from metastases from extrapulmonary sites.

For the distinction from other lung cancers, particularly squamous cell carcinoma or large cell neuroendocrine carcinoma

(LCNEC), close attention to morphological features, as well as appropriate immunohistochemical stains, is usually sufficient.

For multiple lung adenocarcinomas, essential factors include comprehensive histological subtyping considering the predominant and secondary/tertiary growth patterns, the presence/absence of lepidic growth, cytological characteristics (e.g. cell size, clear cell change, nuclear atypia, mitotic count), and stromal features (e.g. degree of desmoplasia and inflammation) {962,2104}. Comparative molecular profiling can also be helpful {963,1788,2902,2270}. A multidisciplinary approach with clinical, radiological, morphological, and molecular correlation may be needed in difficult cases {684}.

Separation of lung adenocarcinomas from metastases from extrapulmonary sites is based on respective clinical and radiological information, along with comparative morphological criteria, immunophenotyping, and/or molecular testing (see *Metastases*, p. 451).

Cytology
Although the diagnosis of adenocarcinoma is readily established based on cytology, histological subtyping can be difficult. Acinar or papillary structures are easier to detect in cell block sections, but ethanol-fixed conventional smears or liquid-based preparations are superior in terms of nuclear and cytoplasmic details. There has generally been a good correlation of morphological NSCLC subtyping between histological and cytological specimens {2772,3466,1608,413}. In addition to the presence of mucin, several morphological features of cell aggregates or individual cells have been shown to be associated with adenocarcinoma. 3D clusters are more common than true acinar or papillary formations. Typical features of individual non-mucinous adenocarcinoma cells are columnar cell shape, delicate or vacuolated cytoplasm, nuclear grooves and/or intranuclear cytoplasmic inclusions, and non-hyperchromatic vesicular nuclei with open chromatin and large nucleoli {1608}. In clinical practice, cytopathologists often use these features to suspect or even diagnose non-mucinous adenocarcinoma {2772,1608,413}. For the time being, there is insufficient published evidence to allow for a definitive diagnosis of non-mucinous adenocarcinoma based on single or combined cytomorphological features other than unequivocal acinar or papillary formations. However, in the presence of typical cytological features, it is reasonable to comment that a non-mucinous adenocarcinoma is likely. Cytology specimens, particularly cell blocks, can be very useful for immunohistochemistry and molecular testing {2457,2517,702}. When specimens like large pleural effusions are obtained, the fluid available beyond what is needed for diagnosis should be processed to prepare cell blocks.

Diagnostic molecular pathology
Several oncogenic driver gene alterations are now known in lung adenocarcinomas, including in *EGFR* {1752,2239,2258}, *KRAS* {3403}, *BRAF* {320,2241}, *ALK* {2797}, *ROS1* {2487}, *RET* {1699,2971,3407}, *NTRK1–3* {3128,2531}, *MET* {2242,130,704, 2678}, *ERBB2* (*HER2*) {97,2856}, *MAP2K1* (*MEK1*) {98}, *NRAS* {2157}, and *NRG1* {817}. Targeted therapies are available for patients whose tumours harbour *EGFR*, *ALK*, *ROS1*, *BRAF*, *MET*, *RET*, and NTRK-family alterations. Clinical trials of targeted agents for *KRAS* p.G12C mutations {1956} are showing

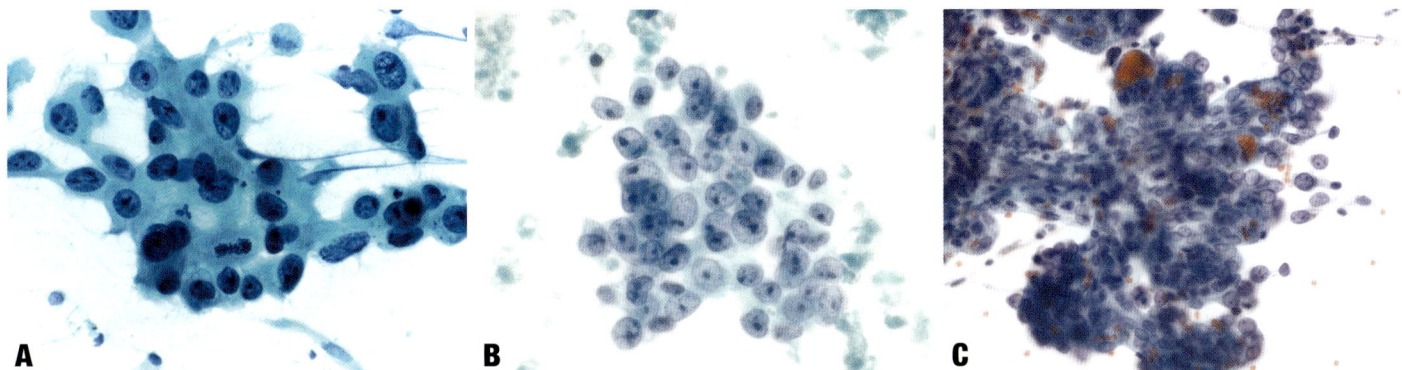

Fig. 1.60 Non-mucinous adenocarcinoma. **A** Cytology smear showing cells with vesicular nuclei, prominent nucleoli, and relatively abundant pale delicate cytoplasm (Pap stain). **B** Tumour cells with large, vesicular nuclei, prominent nucleoli, and delicate translucent cytoplasm. Necrotic debris in the background. **C** Papillary formation with a delicate fibrovascular core (Pap). Tumour cells with vesicular nuclei and delicate cytoplasm. Congested capillaries filled with erythrocytes.

significant promise. Thus, optimal management of patients with lung adenocarcinomas requires comprehensive analysis of a substantial number of oncogenes.

Notably, *EGFR* and *ERBB2* mutations and *ALK*, *ROS1*, *RET*, and NTRK-family fusions are enriched in TTF1-positive adenocarcinomas {2578,460,2789,3422,2253} arising in never smokers {800}, and *EGFR* mutations are uniquely enriched in women and in eastern Asian populations {36,1909}. In contrast, *KRAS*, *NRAS*, and *MAP2K1* (*MEK1*) mutations are highly enriched in smokers, whereas *BRAF* and *MET* mutations (specifically those leading to *MET* exon 14 skipping) are observed in both smokers and never-smokers. About two thirds of lung adenocarcinomas harbour an oncogenic mutation or fusion within one of the aforementioned genes, all of which drive signalling through the RAS/MAPK pathway. Of the remaining "oncogene-negative" tumours, a small subset may contain rare fusion events, enriched in never-smokers; others show a combination of tumour suppressor gene alterations and focal amplifications in members of the RAS/MAPK pathway, enriched in smokers {203,367}. High tumour mutation burden tends to correlate with smoking status; accordingly, smoking mutation signatures are highly enriched in lung tumours, including adenocarcinomas. Other mutation processes implicated in development and progression of adenocarcinoma include DNA cytosine deaminase (APOBEC) activity and, rarely, mismatch repair deficiency {2840}. Hypermutation processes such as APOBEC, as well as acquisition of additional oncogenic mutations in genes such as *PIK3CA* and *NF1*, contribute to tumour clonal heterogeneity and adenocarcinoma progression {1290,2524}.

Unlike the specific genetic alterations seen in other tumours (e.g. sarcomas, lymphomas, and leukaemias), there are no specific histological–molecular correlations in lung cancer {3072,3074}, although statistical associations have been drawn between *KRAS* mutations and IMA and tumours with a predominantly solid pattern {661,2012,3392,2455,2577,3434} and between *EGFR* mutation and lepidic-predominant non-mucinous adenocarcinomas {1312}, as well as between *ALK* and *ROS1* rearrangements and cribriform pattern, signet-ring cell features, and psammomatous calcification {1864,3424,3514,265}.

Essential and desirable diagnostic criteria
Essential:
- Malignant epithelial tumour with glandular differentiation by architecture (lepidic, acinar, papillary, micropapillary, cribriform) or a pure solid pattern with (1) immunohistochemical expression of pneumocyte markers associated with adenocarcinoma (e.g. TTF1 or napsin A) or (2) histochemical demonstration of intracytoplasmic mucin (e.g. PASD) in a solid tumour in ≥ 5 tumour cells in each of two high-power fields (~0.4 mm²)
- The tumour does not fulfil criteria of other types of adenocarcinoma (e.g. IMA), although minor components of other types may be present (up to 5%)
- After comprehensive histological subtyping in 5–10% increments, the tumours are classified according to their predominant pattern

Desirable:
- Record the percentages of each histological pattern in pathology reports to document the predominant histological pattern (subtype) and any components of high-grade patterns to determine the tumour grade (see Table 1.08, p. 71)
- Immunohistochemical and/or molecular characterization of driver mutations

Staging
The eighth edition of the Union for International Cancer Control (UICC) / American Joint Committee on Cancer (AJCC) TNM staging system for NSCLC is used for staging all NSCLCs, including adenocarcinomas, to provide prognostic information that can assist in management decisions. This updated staging schema came into effect in January 2017 and was based on an IASLC database of 94 708 patients from 16 countries, with the majority of cases from Japan {2423}. The most significant change in the new staging classification is the use of the solid or invasive tumour size for the cT or pT factor, respectively {75,3067}. This only applies to non-mucinous lung adenocarcinomas with a lepidic component. Although the IASLC database was unable to address the prognostic value of measuring the invasive tumour component of non-mucinous lung adenocarcinomas rather than total tumour size (due to lack of pre-planned collection of these data elements), this approach is recommended by the UICC {3331} and is supported by several retrospective studies {3433,3230,1762,3104,1217,3105,1361}.

Prognosis and prediction

As is the case for other histological types of lung cancer, TNM classification and performance status significantly influence the choice of treatment and strongly predict survival. Never-smoker status and female sex are favourable prognostic factors, independent from the stage of the disease {1404}. Tumour size ≥ 25 mm and solid and micropapillary patterns {424,2120,2579, 3230,3434} are predictors of poor prognosis. The prognosis for stage I lepidic-predominant adenocarcinoma is excellent {2579, 3102,3230,3433}, and most of the tumours that recur have some high-risk factor, such as a close margin in limited resection and presence of a micropapillary component, or invasion of blood vessels and/or pleura {1345}. In some studies, this prognostic significance is also preserved in more-advanced stages {3230}. The relatively good prognosis of CT screen–detected lung cancer is driven by the predominance of early-stage adenocarcinomas with favourable histological features {843}. STAS has been shown to be associated with poor prognosis in multiple studies, particularly in patients who underwent limited resection {755, 471,146,1706,1340}. The proposed IASLC grading system has demonstrated prognostic significance but needs further validation {1990A}.

Lung tumours frequently harbour driver mutations, which are generally mutually exclusive {900,1463,2257}; among them, *EGFR* mutation, *ALK*/*ROS1*/*RET* rearrangements, *MET* exon 14 skipping alterations, and *BRAF* p.V600E mutation are strongly correlated with the probabilities of response to targeted tyrosine kinase inhibitors {1952,2329,2362,2530,2709,2721,2808,730A, 3333A}.

Immune checkpoint inhibitors such as anti-PD1/PDL1 antibodies improve survival of a subset of advanced lung cancer patients, including patients with adenocarcinomas {278,300, 807,1127,2445,2496}. PDL1 expression {1127,2445} and tumour mutation burden {1115,2446,1745} have been associated with treatment response but are not sufficient to ensure the response {365}.

Invasive mucinous adenocarcinoma of the lung

Cooper WA
Chang JC
Chou TY
MacMahon H
Warth A
Yoshizawa A

Definition

Invasive mucinous adenocarcinoma (IMA) is a primary lung adenocarcinoma with tumour cells showing goblet cell or columnar cell morphology with abundant intracytoplasmic mucin.

ICD-O coding

8253/3 Invasive mucinous adenocarcinoma
8254/3 Mixed invasive mucinous and non-mucinous adenocarcinoma

ICD-11 coding

2C25.0 & XH7GY6 Adenocarcinoma of bronchus or lung & Adenocarcinoma of lung, mucinous

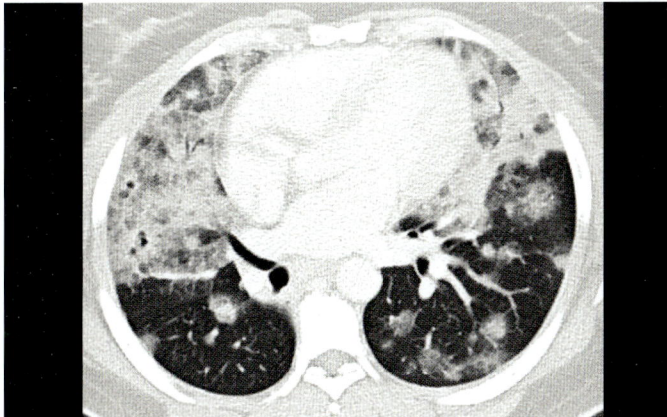

Fig. 1.61 Invasive mucinous adenocarcinoma. CT section through the lower lungs showing diffuse bilateral airspace and ground-glass opacity with nodular components, secondary to invasive mucinous adenocarcinoma.

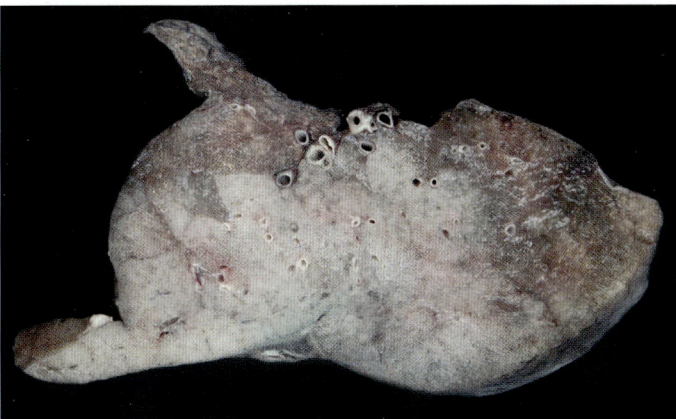

Fig. 1.62 Invasive mucinous adenocarcinoma. Macroscopic image shows a poorly defined tumour with a soft mucoid appearance.

Related terminology

Not recommended: mucinous bronchioloalveolar/bronchoalveolar carcinoma (obsolete).

Subtype(s)

Invasive mucinous adenocarcinoma; mixed invasive mucinous and non-mucinous adenocarcinoma

Localization

IMAs are located peripherally in the lung and have a high frequency of multifocal, multilobar, and bilateral tumours, which may reflect aerogenous spread {541,914,3074}.

Clinical features

Signs and symptoms

See *Tumours of the lung: Introduction* (p. 20). Patients may also present with bronchorrhoea {2961,2374}.

Imaging

A spectrum of radiological findings exist, including solid and part-solid nodules or pneumonic-like patterns {1634,3232}. Air bronchograms are common. Because these tumours produce pulmonary consolidation, they are commonly misdiagnosed as pneumonia at initial presentation. Multilobar and bilateral lung involvement is common, often raising concern for metastases from an extrapulmonary primary.

Epidemiology

IMAs are less common than non-mucinous adenocarcinomas, accounting for 3–10% of lung adenocarcinomas {2579,3102, 3433,361,1093}. Approximately 55% of cases occur in females {3074,1093}, but there may be geographical differences. The demographic features, including smoking rates, are similar to those of non-mucinous lung adenocarcinomas {3325,3074}.

Etiology

IMAs are frequently associated with exposure to tobacco smoke {2743}, and the etiology is similar to that of non-mucinous adenocarcinomas (see *Tumours of the lung: Introduction*, p. 20). Etiology is also covered extensively in *Invasive non-mucinous adenocarcinoma of the lung* (p. 64).

Pathogenesis

IMAs develop through acquisition of genetically distinct driver mutations, most commonly involving the *KRAS* oncogene (~60%) {2743}. Unlike in non-mucinous lung adenocarcinomas, *TP53* mutations are rare and tumour mutation burden is generally low, even in smokers. In those without *KRAS* mutations, oncogenic fusions are frequently found, especially in never-smokers, and most commonly involve *NRG1*, leading to activation of the PI3K/AKT signalling pathway {2059,2743}. *NKX2-1*

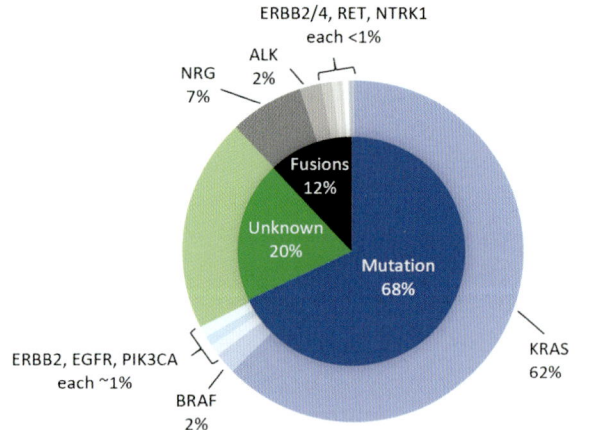

Fig. 1.63 Invasive mucinous adenocarcinoma. Pie chart of molecular alterations in invasive mucinous adenocarcinomas.

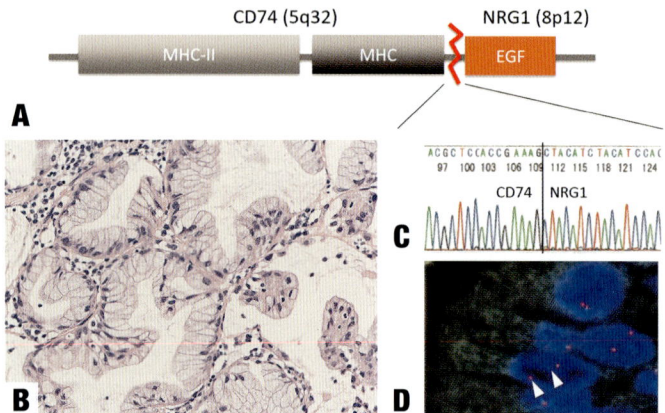

Fig. 1.64 Invasive mucinous adenocarcinoma with *CD74-NRG1* fusion. **A** The fusion leads to expression of the EGF-like domain of NRG1 III-β3, thereby providing the ligand for ERBB2/ERBB3 receptor complexes. **B** The fusion is specific to invasive mucinous adenocarcinoma. **C** A direct sequence of RT-PCR transcript showed the fusion of *CD74* with *NRG1*. **D** Separate signals with *NRG1* break-apart FISH demonstrate *NRG1* rearrangement.

mutations have been identified in 19% of IMAs, leading to loss of expression of its protein product, TTF1 {1216}.

Macroscopic appearance

IMAs usually appear as poorly circumscribed lesions with a soft, gelatinous/mucoid appearance. There may be disseminated nodules or a diffuse pneumonia-like consolidation across large areas or whole lobes.

Histopathology

Tumour cells show a goblet and/or columnar cell morphology with abundant intracytoplasmic mucin and small, basally oriented nuclei. Nuclear atypia is usually inconspicuous or absent. The surrounding alveolar spaces are often mucin-filled. Although IMAs often show lepidic-predominant growth, extensive sampling usually reveals invasive foci, including an acinar, papillary, micropapillary, solid, or cribriform growth pattern {934}. Tumours with a mixture of mucinous and non-mucinous components should be classified as mixed invasive mucinous and non-mucinous adenocarcinoma if there is ≥ 10% of each component. It should be noted that the invasive component of invasive mucinous carcinomas often contains less intracytoplasmic mucin than lepidic components.

Immunohistochemistry

IMAs express CK7 and may show focal coexpression of CK20 and/or CDX2 but are usually negative for TTF1 and napsin A {1216,1534,1603,3101,3341}. HNF4α {2892} and GATA6 {2050} have recently been described in this type of adenocarcinoma, but neither of these markers is specific.

Grading

There is no established grading system for IMAs.

Differential diagnosis

IMAs are separated from mucinous adenocarcinoma in situ and minimally invasive adenocarcinoma on the basis of specified criteria (see *Adenocarcinoma in situ of the lung*, p. 57, and

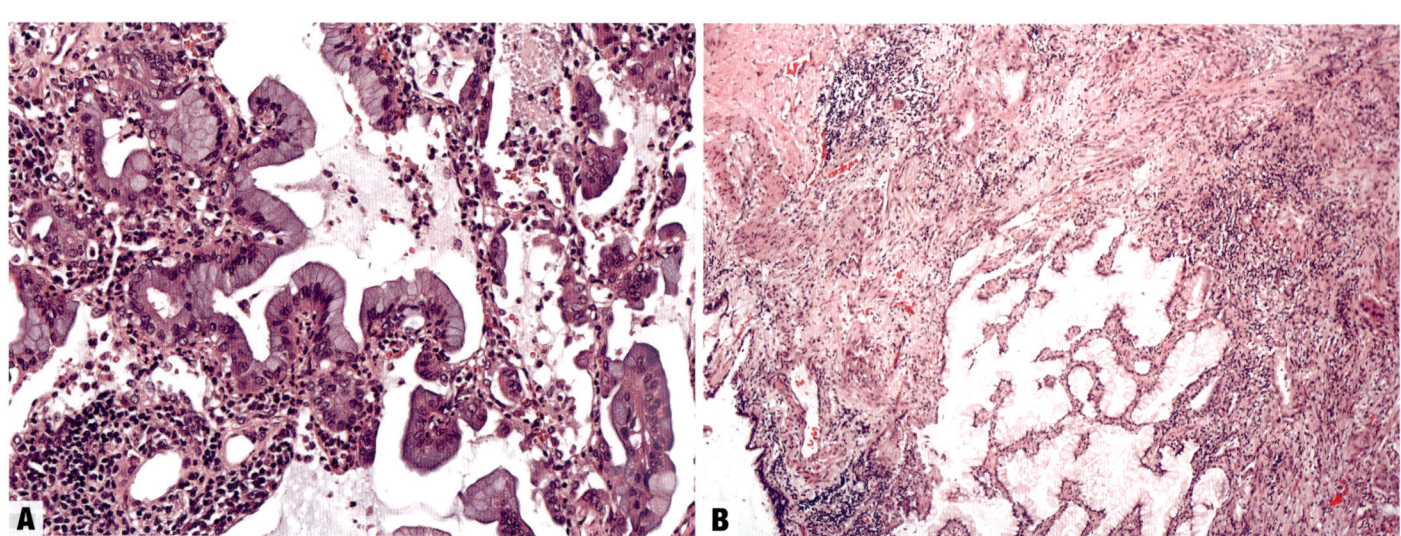

Fig. 1.65 Invasive mucinous adenocarcinoma. **A** Columnar mucinous cells with minimal cytological atypia growing in a lepidic growth pattern. Tumour cells show abundant apical cytoplasmic mucin and small basally oriented nuclei. **B** This area of invasive mucinous adenocarcinoma demonstrates areas with lepidic and acinar patterns; there is also a fibrotic focus, which contains invasive tumour with a desmoplastic stroma.

Table 1.09 Differences between invasive mucinous adenocarcinomas and non-mucinous adenocarcinomas (non-mucinous adenocarcinoma in situ [AIS], minimally invasive adenocarcinoma [MIA], and lepidic-predominant adenocarcinoma [LPA]) {3075,2743}

	Invasive mucinous adenocarcinoma	Non-mucinous lung adenocarcinoma (AIS, MIA, LPA)
Demographics		
Female:male	55:45	70:30
Smokers	~45%	~45%
CT features	Pneumonic-like consolidation, air bronchograms; frequently multifocal/multilobar	Mostly solitary ground-glass attenuation; small solid component may be seen in MIA and LPA
Cell type	Columnar cells with abundant intracytoplasmic mucin and/or goblet cells	Type II pneumocytes and/or club cells
Immunohistochemistry		
CK7	~90%	~90%
CK20	~50%	~5%
TTF1	~40%	~75%
Napsin A	~33%	~75%
Genetic alterations		
KRAS	~60% (mostly p.G12D and p.G12V)	~15% (mostly p.G12C)
EGFR	~1%	45%
Oncogenic fusions	~12% (NRG > *ALK* > *ERBB2/4*, *RET*, NTRK)	~5% (*ALK* > *ROS1* > *RET*, NTRK)

Minimally invasive adenocarcinoma of the lung, p. 60), although such tumours are extremely rare. Due to their similar morphology, IMAs must be specifically separated from metastatic adenocarcinomas from extrapulmonary sites including the pancreatobiliary system, gastrointestinal tract, and ovary. Mucinous breast carcinomas usually express GATA3 and ER {3287}. SATB2 expression and strong CK20 and CDX2 can help in distinction from mucinous colorectal adenocarcinomas, which occasionally also express TTF1 {1534}. Clinical and radiological correlation is important, particularly in difficult cases. Differences between IMAs and non-mucinous adenocarcinoma in situ, minimally invasive adenocarcinoma, and lepidic-predominant adenocarcinoma are presented in Table 1.09.

Cytology

Cytologically, IMAs exhibit cohesive flat sheets of mildly atypical columnar cells in a drunken-honeycomb pattern {1992, 3073}. The cells lack cilia and contain abundant apical intracytoplasmic mucin. Papillary, papilliform, and (less commonly) solid 3D groups of cells may be seen. A mucinous background may be present.

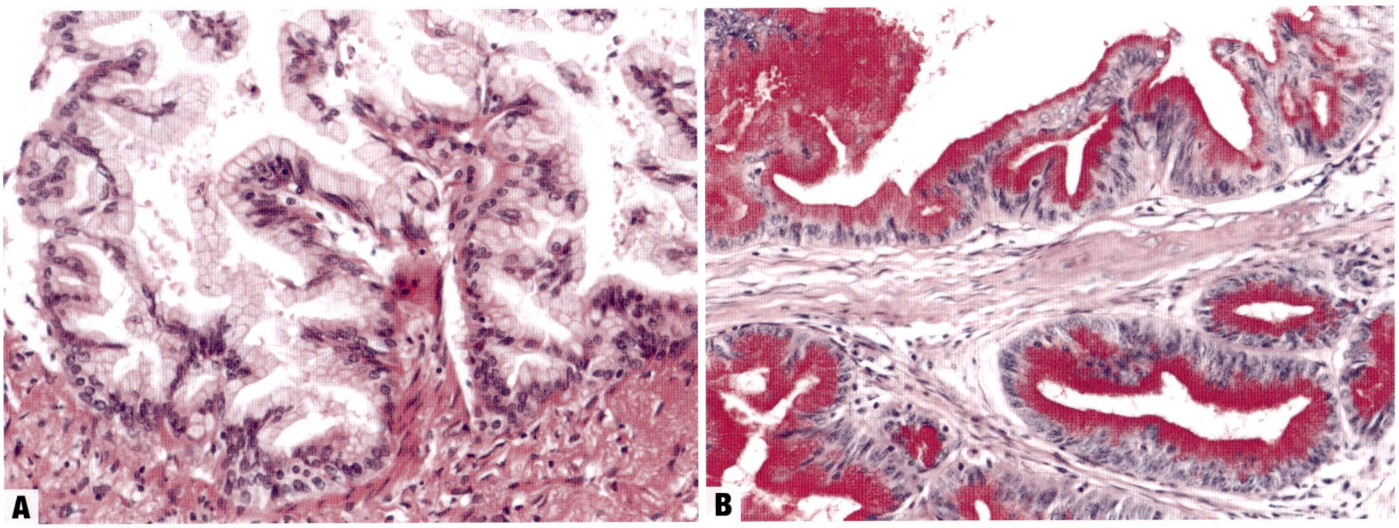

Fig. 1.66 Invasive mucinous adenocarcinoma. **A** Uniform columnar cells forming papillary structures. **B** PASD stain demonstrates abundant intracellular mucin.

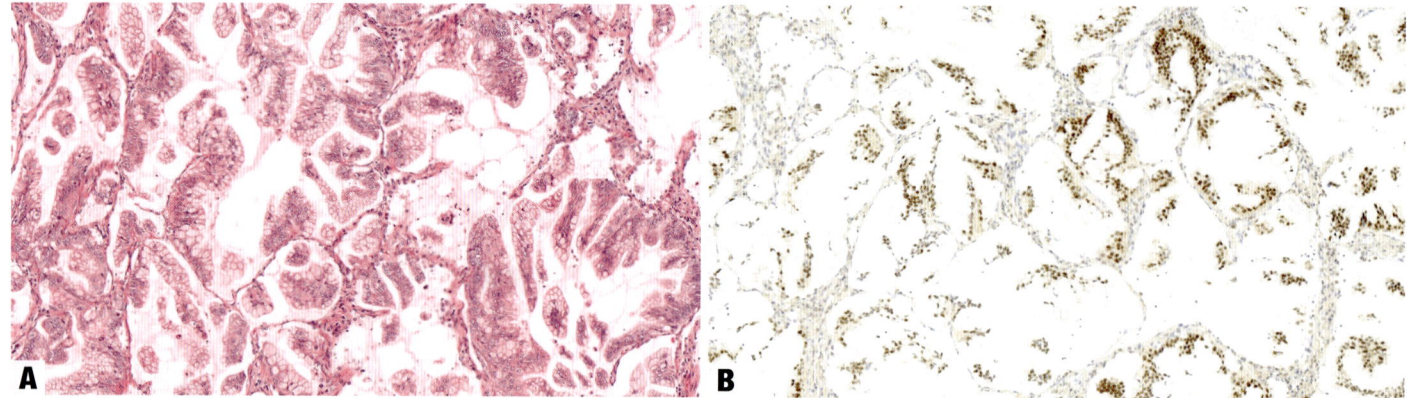

Fig. 1.67 Invasive mucinous adenocarcinoma. **A** Columnar mucinous cells with minimal cytological atypia growing in a lepidic growth pattern. **B** Immunohistochemical stain for HNF4α.

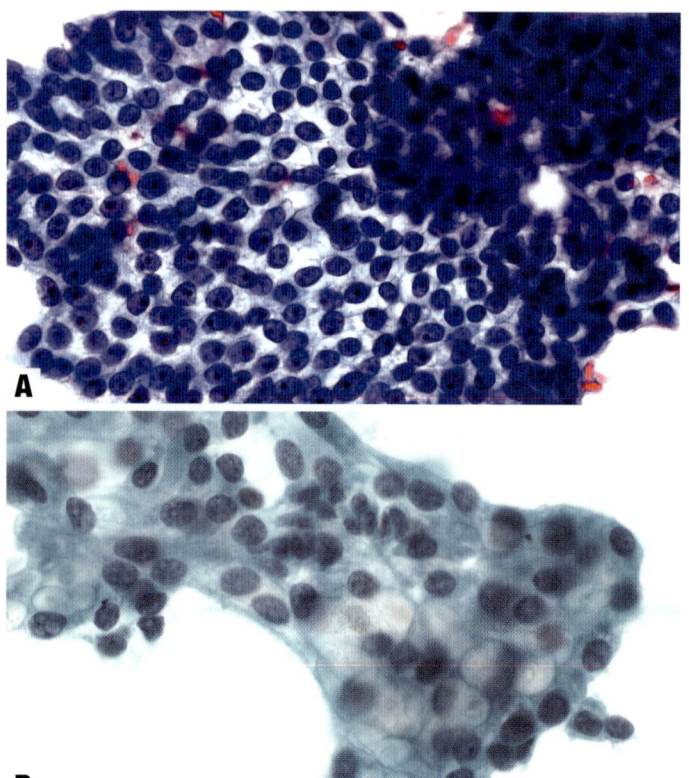

Fig. 1.68 Invasive mucinous adenocarcinoma. **A** A disorderly sheet of fairly uniform epithelial cells in a drunken-honeycomb pattern (Diff-Quik stain). **B** The cells show abundant intracytoplasmic mucin (Pap stain).

Diagnostic molecular pathology

The commonest molecular alterations in IMAs are *KRAS* mutations (~60% of cases), mostly p.G12D and p.G12V, similar to in gastrointestinal carcinomas {2743}. Unlike in non-mucinous adenocarcinomas, *EGFR* mutations are rare (~1% of cases)

{2059,2743,1216}. Oncogenic fusions that are mutually exclusive with *KRAS* mutations occur in about 12% of cases and provide therapeutic (or potentially therapeutic) targets. The commonest fusions involve *NRG1*, followed by *ALK*, *ERBB2*, *ERBB4*, *BRAF*, *RET*, *ROS1*, and *NTRK1* {2743,2059}.

Essential and desirable diagnostic criteria

Essential:
- Adenocarcinoma composed of goblet and/or columnar cells with abundant apical intracytoplasmic mucin frequently with small basally oriented nuclei
- Exclusion of metastatic mucinous adenocarcinoma from other sites
- Does not fulfil criteria for mucinous adenocarcinoma in situ or minimally invasive adenocarcinoma

Desirable:
- Confirmation of intracytoplasmic mucin with a histochemical stain (e.g. PASD)

Staging

The same criteria are used to stage IMAs as for other non-small cell lung carcinomas. For IMAs, the entire tumour size (including lepidic components) is used for the T descriptor, because total tumour size is predictive of survival in this tumour type {3067}. Unlike with non-mucinous adenocarcinomas, there should be no adjustment for invasive size, according to the percentage of lepidic versus invasive components.

Prognosis and prediction

The prognosis of IMA is not as well-characterized as that of non-mucinous adenocarcinoma. Early studies showed an intermediate to poor prognosis compared with that of non-mucinous adenocarcinoma {2579,3433}; however, recent reports have demonstrated similar outcomes {2743,3230,3434,1633,263}, possibly relating to varying growth patterns (pneumonic-type vs solitary-type) {1633,3232}.

Colloid adenocarcinoma of the lung

Jain D
MacMahon H
Pelosi G
Riely G
Rusch VW
Van Schil PEY

Definition
Colloid adenocarcinoma is an invasive adenocarcinoma where extensive pools of extracellular mucin distend alveolar spaces and destroy alveolar walls, up to the complete effacement of underlying lung parenchyma.

ICD-O coding
8480/3 Colloid adenocarcinoma

ICD-11 coding
2C25.Z & XH7GY6 Malignant neoplasms of bronchus or lung, unspecified & Adenocarcinoma of lung, mucinous

Related terminology
Not recommended: mucinous cystadenocarcinoma; mucinous cystic tumour of borderline malignancy.

Subtype(s)
None

Localization
Most tumours occur in the peripheral lung parenchyma {2545}.

Clinical features
These are commonly incidentally detected localized masses on imaging {1821}.

Epidemiology
The epidemiology is similar to that of other adenocarcinomas.

Etiology
The etiology is similar to that of other adenocarcinomas.

Pathogenesis
Because gastrointestinal differentiation would be responsible for pathogenesis of mucinous tumours of the lung, its pathogenesis may overlap with that of mucinous/colloid gastrointestinal

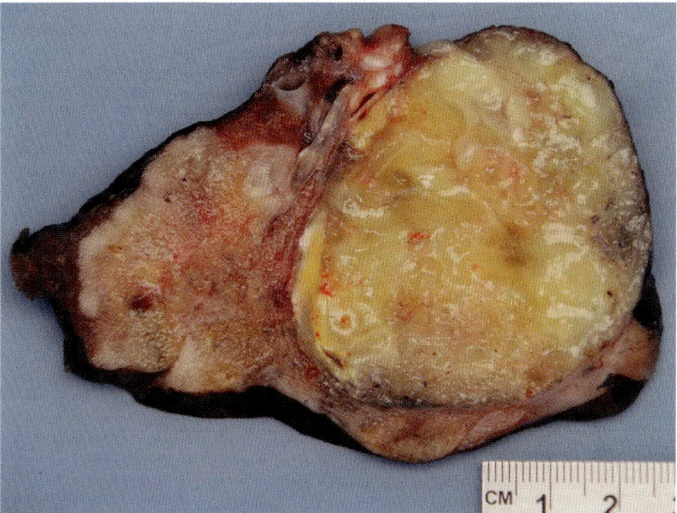

Fig. 1.69 Colloid adenocarcinoma. This circumscribed tumour shows a yellow gelatinous cut surface.

adenocarcinoma where most mucin is extracellularly accumulated.

Macroscopic appearance
Tumours are variably circumscribed, unencapsulated, solitary, soft, gelatinous nodules, which are mucoid in appearance and bulging on cut surface. Tumour size ranges from 5 to 100 mm {1966,3476}. Uncommonly, these tumours may appear markedly cystic.

Histopathology
Colloid adenocarcinoma shows abundant extracellular mucin in pools, which distend alveolar spaces and destroy their walls, showing an overtly invasive growth pattern into the alveolar spaces. Mucin deposits enlarge and dissect through the lung parenchyma, creating pools of mucin-rich matrix. The tumour cells are mucin-laden cuboidal to tall columnar cells, sometimes

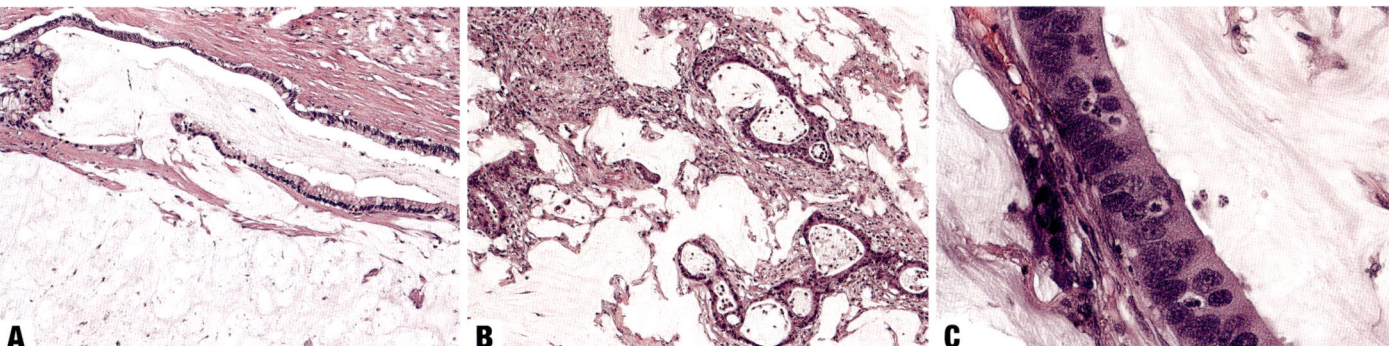

Fig. 1.70 Colloid adenocarcinoma. **A** This tumour shows prominent mucin pools. **B** This colloid adenocarcinoma shows prominent pools of mucin lined by cuboidal tumour cells showing some pseudostratification. **C** The tumour cells lining this mucin pool are cuboidal and show pseudostratification and hyperchromatic nuclei.

exhibiting signet-ring morphology. They can float in mucin pools or focally line residual alveolar walls or fibrous tissue surrounding mucin pools {2816}. Tumour cells can be inconspicuous and well differentiated, making diagnosis difficult, particularly in small biopsies and frozen sections. They may show pseudostratification and cytological atypia; however, typically the mitotic count is low and necrosis is absent. An inflammatory infiltrate with histiocytes and a giant cell reaction to the mucin may be seen. The extremely rare tumours previously classified as mucinous cystadenocarcinoma are now included in colloid adenocarcinoma.

Immunohistochemistry
Colloid adenocarcinoma exhibits admixed intestinal markers (CDX2, MUC2, CK20). However, colloid adenocarcinomas are also consistently CK7-positive. Staining for TTF1, napsin A, and EMA (MUC1) is either negative or weak and focal {2816,2545, 2540}.

Differential diagnosis
The differential diagnosis comprises metastases of mucinous carcinoma from other organs, including the gastrointestinal tract, pancreas, and breast. For lung primary tumours, invasive mucinous adenocarcinoma generally shows preserved alveolar walls lacking the large pools of mucin destroying alveolar walls characteristic of colloid adenocarcinoma. Although colloid adenocarcinoma is rarely mixed with other adenocarcinoma subtypes, ≥ 50% of the tumour should have this appearance to warrant the diagnosis of colloid adenocarcinoma.

Cytology
A predominant background of extracellular mucin contains scant mucin-laden tumour cells, isolated or in small clustered aggregates, usually with bland cytological features.

Diagnostic molecular pathology
About one half of tumours show *KRAS* mutations {1335,2816, 1031}, with molecular similarities to invasive mucinous adenocarcinoma of the lung and mucin-producing gastrointestinal and pancreatic intraductal papillary mucinous neoplasms {2816, 1031,73}. Other frequently detected mutations are in *STK11* and *PARP1* {1335}.

Essential and desirable diagnostic criteria
Essential:
- Abundant pools of extracellular mucin that distend alveolar spaces and destroy their walls
- Tumour cells are mucin-filled, cuboidal to columnar, and either floating within the mucin pools or lining fibrous walls of mucin-filled spaces
- ≥ 50% colloid pattern when mixed with other adenocarcinoma subtypes
- Distinction from metastases from the other organs

Desirable:
- Bland cytology of tumour cells in mucin pools
- Frequent positivity for CK7 and CDX2

Staging
Staging should be performed according to the eighth-edition TNM classification {315}.

Prognosis and prediction
The clinical course is mostly indolent, with a relatively favourable prognosis after complete surgical resection. The presence of signet-ring cells and a non-colloid component signifies worse prognosis, with recurrence and metastasis {2545}. Colloid adenocarcinomas are generally negative for predictive biomarkers such as *EGFR* mutation and *ALK* rearrangement {3476,934}.

Fetal adenocarcinoma of the lung

Jain D
Asamura H
Cardona AF
MacMahon H
Nakatani Y

Definition

Fetal adenocarcinoma of the lung is pulmonary adenocarcinoma resembling developing fetal lung in its pseudoglandular stage.

ICD-O coding

8333/3 Fetal adenocarcinoma

ICD-11 coding

2C25.0 & XH5P16 Adenocarcinoma of bronchus or lung & Fetal adenocarcinoma

Related terminology

Not recommended: pulmonary endodermal tumour resembling fetal lung.

Subtype(s)

Low-grade fetal adenocarcinoma / well-differentiated fetal adenocarcinoma; high-grade fetal adenocarcinoma

Localization

Fetal adenocarcinoma of the lung is mostly located in peripheral lung.

Clinical features

Low-grade fetal adenocarcinomas are often discovered incidentally {249,2638}. On imaging, fetal adenocarcinomas are peripherally located, well-demarcated tumours ranging from 10 to 120 mm in size {249,2935,2475}. Low-grade fetal adenocarcinoma occurs in younger individuals, with an almost equal sex ratio {2475,3495}, whereas high-grade fetal adenocarcinoma is

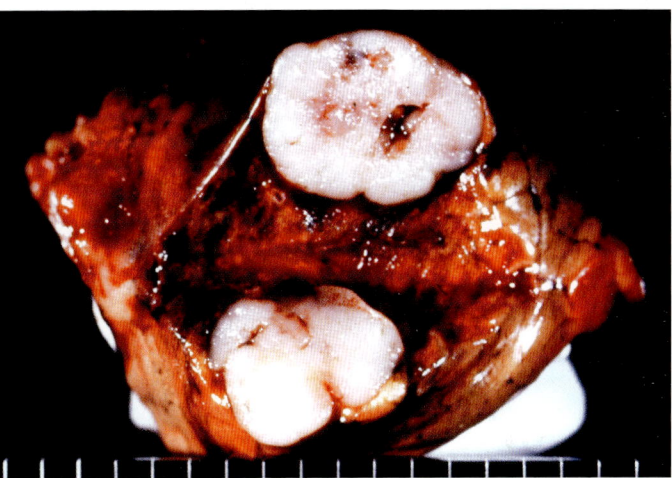

Fig. 1.71 Gross appearance of fetal adenocarcinoma. Low-grade fetal adenocarcinoma. A sharply circumscribed, greyish-white to tan-coloured tumour with scalloped borders.

more common in elderly men who are heavy smokers {2001, 2935,2934,2475}.

Epidemiology

These are rare tumours. Low-grade fetal adenocarcinoma and high-grade fetal adenocarcinoma account for 0.3% {3487,876} and 0.5–1.4% {3487,2934} of pulmonary adenocarcinomas, respectively.

Etiology

See *Tumours of the lung: Introduction* (p. 20).

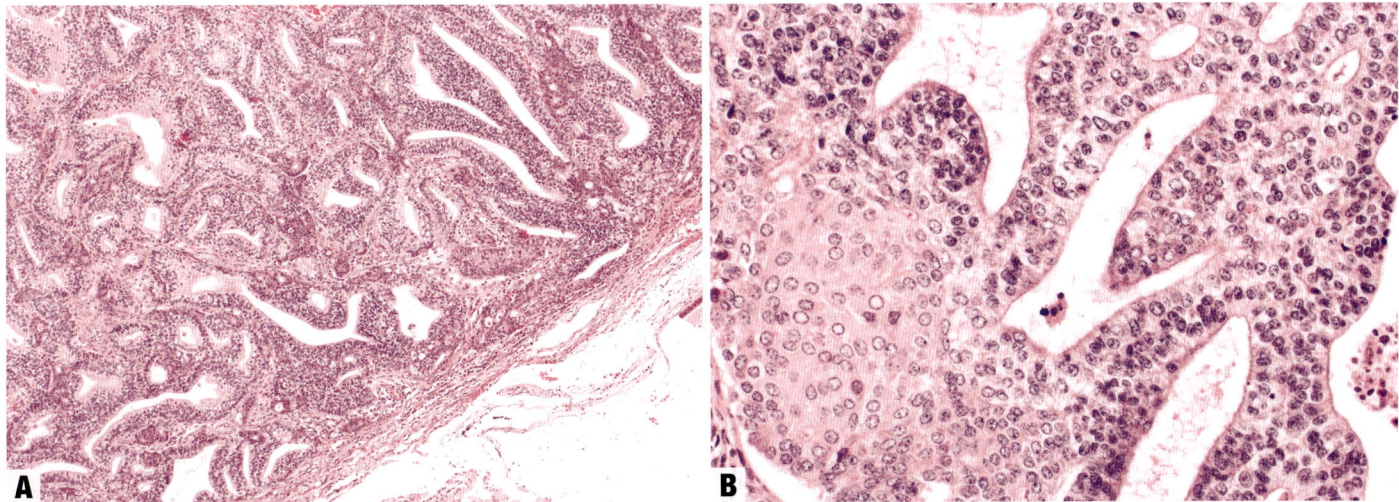

Fig. 1.72 Low-grade fetal adenocarcinoma. **A** Complex glandular structures are tightly packed, with a sharp demarcation from the surrounding lung. **B** Note a morular structure with a few optically clear nuclei. The glandular cells show regular, monotonous round nuclei of low-grade atypia.

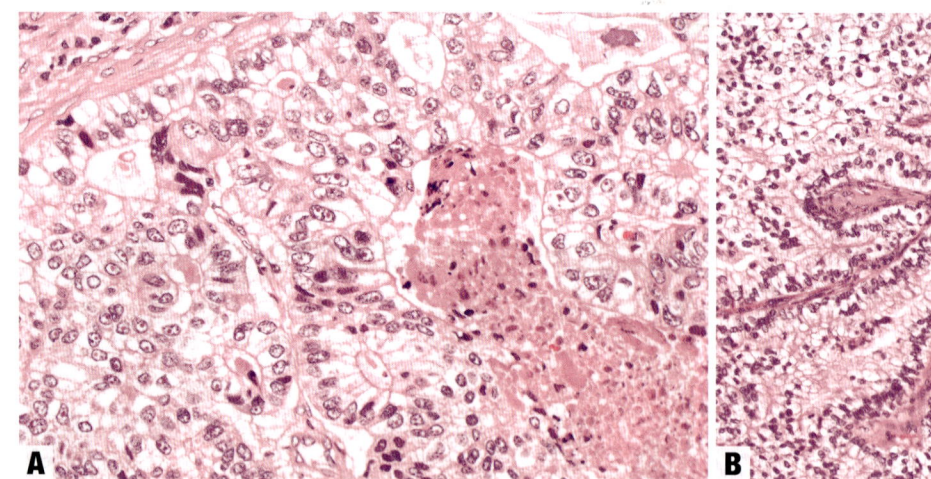

Fig. 1.73 High-grade fetal adenocarcinoma. **A** The tumour cells show severe nuclear atypia. **B** Complex glandular structures composed of pseudostratified columnar cells with subnuclear vacuoles.

Pathogenesis
Abnormalities in β-catenin and aberrations in the WNT signalling pathway are crucial to the development of low-grade fetal adenocarcinoma {2064,2702,2475}.

Macroscopic appearance
Fetal adenocarcinomas typically appear as sharply circumscribed, solid, white to greyish-white or tan-coloured tumours, often with lobulated borders {2062,2063,2934,3495}.

Histopathology
The tumours resemble airway epithelium of the fetal lung, displaying complex glandular, papillotubular, or cribriform structures composed of pseudostratified columnar cells with glycogen-rich clear to mildly eosinophilic cytoplasm forming subnuclear vacuoles {2062,249,2063,2934,2475}. Sheet-like growth may also be present {2062,2935,2934}.

Low-grade fetal adenocarcinomas typically show relatively small, round, and monotonous nuclei and morule formation, with low nuclear atypia and inconspicuous nuclei {2062,249}. Necrosis is usually punctate, if present. High-grade fetal adenocarcinoma displays more diffuse nuclear atypia, absence of morule formation, and broad necrosis. High-grade fetal adenocarcinoma is commonly mixed with other adenocarcinoma patterns, such as hepatoid and enteric, high-grade neuroendocrine, and conventional adenocarcinomas {2063,2001,2935,2934}. At least 50% of the entire tumour should display the histology of high-grade fetal adenocarcinoma for the diagnosis.

Nuclear/cytoplasmic expression of β-catenin is observed in low-grade fetal adenocarcinoma, whereas membranous expression of β-catenin is predominant in high-grade fetal adenocarcinoma {2064}. Low-grade fetal adenocarcinoma is positive for TTF1, whereas approximately 50% of high-grade fetal adenocarcinomas are negative. Both are frequently positive for neuroendocrine markers. High-grade fetal adenocarcinoma commonly expresses oncofetal proteins such as AFP, SALL4, and glypican-3 (GPC3) {2063,2001,2935,3487,2475}.

The differentiation between low-grade fetal adenocarcinoma and high-grade fetal adenocarcinoma is essential because of the marked difference in prognosis. They need to be differentiated from pulmonary blastoma, carcinosarcoma with a high-grade fetal adenocarcinoma component, and metastatic endometrioid carcinoma {1521,2065,933}.

Cytology
Specific cytomorphological features include a two-cell population of columnar and squamoid cells, subnuclear vacuoles, a focal tigroid background, and neuroendocrine differentiation {933}.

Diagnostic molecular pathology
In low-grade fetal adenocarcinoma, *CTNNB1* mutations are common {2064,2702,630,876}. *DICER1* mutation has been reported {630}. Other major driver mutations, including *KRAS*, *EGFR*, *BRAF*, and *PIK3CA* mutations, are rare to absent.

Essential and desirable diagnostic criteria
Essential:
- Adenocarcinoma resembling fetal lung airway epithelium of pseudoglandular stage
- Low-grade fetal adenocarcinoma shows mild nuclear atypia and aberrant nuclear/cytoplasmic β-catenin expression
- High-grade fetal adenocarcinoma shows severe nuclear atypia
- High-grade fetal adenocarcinomas are frequently mixed with other adenocarcinoma patterns and should constitute ≥ 50% of the entire tumour

Desirable:
- Low-grade fetal adenocarcinoma should express TTF1
- High-grade fetal adenocarcinoma should have predominantly membranous β-catenin expression

Staging
Staging should be performed according to the eighth-edition TNM classification {315}.

Prognosis and prediction
Patients with low-grade fetal adenocarcinoma present at early stages with rare lymph node metastasis and fairly good prognosis, whereas high-grade fetal adenocarcinoma has a poor prognosis, with a 5-year overall survival rate of 44% in resected cases {2063,2475,3495,2934}.

Enteric-type adenocarcinoma of the lung

Jain D
MacMahon H
Nakatani Y
Soares FA
Zhang J

Definition
Enteric-type adenocarcinoma is a primary pulmonary adenocarcinoma that resembles colorectal adenocarcinoma.

ICD-O coding
8144/3 Adenocarcinoma, enteric-type

ICD-11 coding
2C25.0 & XH0349 Adenocarcinoma of bronchus or lung & Adenocarcinoma, intestinal type

Related terminology
Not recommended: pulmonary intestinal-type adenocarcinoma; adenocarcinoma with intestinal differentiation.

Subtype(s)
None

Localization
Enteric-type adenocarcinoma of the lung is mostly located in the peripheral lung.

Clinical features
The clinical features are not substantially different from those of other lung adenocarcinomas. According to the few reports available in the literature, most of the patients are elderly men and smokers with advanced-stage disease {1842,1685,3505}. It is crucial to exclude metastatic colorectal carcinoma, which is more common than primary enteric-type adenocarcinoma in the lung, by careful clinical evaluation {1246}.

Epidemiology
The number of reported cases is too small to establish accurate epidemiological data.

Etiology
The etiology is thought to be the same as for other pulmonary adenocarcinomas.

Pathogenesis
The pathogenesis is thought to be the same as for other pulmonary adenocarcinomas.

Macroscopic appearance
Enteric-type adenocarcinomas are well-demarcated, white to grey-white tumours, often with yellowish spotty to geographical necrosis {1246,3196}. The reported sizes range from 10 to 115 mm.

Histopathology
The histological features of this tumour resemble those of colorectal adenocarcinoma. It displays acinar, cribriform, or papillotubular structures with common intraluminal necrotic cellular debris {1246,3196,1842}. The cells are columnar in shape, with cigar-shaped nuclei. The luminal surfaces of tumour glands are flat with occasional brush borders. Mitotic figures are frequently observed. The stroma is often desmoplastic, commonly with prominent inflammatory cell infiltrates. The enteric pattern can be admixed with other patterns of adenocarcinomas; diagnosis of enteric adenocarcinoma should be made when the enteric component is ≥ 50% of the tumour {1246,3196,1842}.

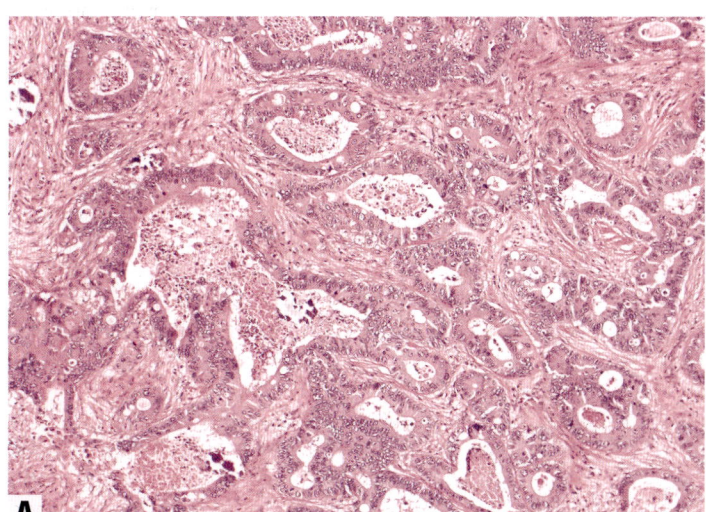 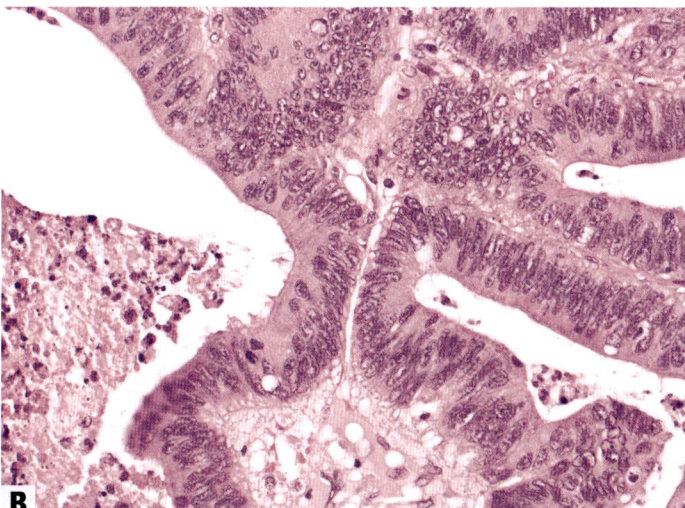

Fig. 1.74 Enteric adenocarcinoma. **A** Note invasive adenocarcinoma in acinar and cribriform patterns associated with marked desmoplasia. Intraluminal necrotic cellular debris is prominent. Resemblance to colorectal carcinoma is striking. **B** Glandular columnar cells show eosinophilic cytoplasm and oval to cigar-shaped nuclei in a palisading pattern.

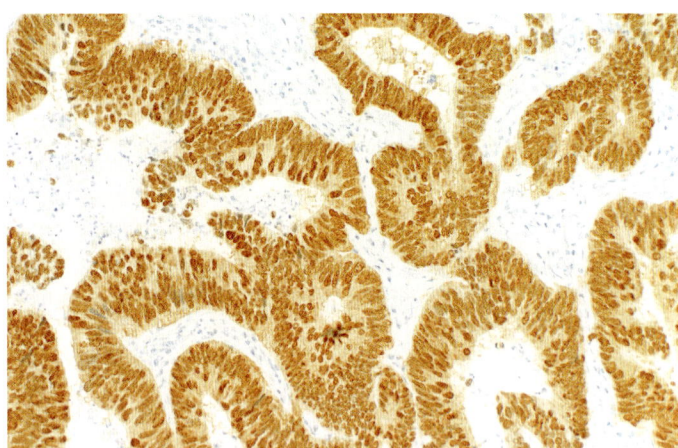

Fig. 1.75 Enteric adenocarcinoma. Immunohistochemistry showing diffuse positivity for CDX2.

Immunohistochemistry

The morphological features are supported by positive intestinal markers; CK20 and MUC2 are expressed in about half and one third of cases, respectively, whereas CDX2, villin, and HNF4α are expressed in the majority {476,3505,2143,1335}. New intestinal markers, SATB2 and cadherin 17, are expressed rarely {476,227,1835}. CK7 expression in > 80% of tumours cells helps differential diagnosis from colorectal adenocarcinoma. TTF1 expression can be absent in more than half of cases {476, 3505,1334,2143,1335}.

Differential diagnosis

Tumours that resemble colorectal carcinoma but express only pneumocytic markers are better classified as pulmonary adenocarcinoma with enteric morphology, and not as enteric adenocarcinoma {3441,3074}.

Cytology

Enteric-type adenocarcinoma of the lung has features similar to those of colorectal carcinoma.

Diagnostic molecular pathology

KRAS mutations are more frequent in enteric adenocarcinoma than in usual adenocarcinoma {3505,476,2143,2142}. Recent reports suggested molecular features shared with lung cancer (mutation profile and DNA methylation pattern), as well as with colorectal cancer (high tumour mutation burden and DNA mismatch repair gene mutations), but without *APC* mutations {476, 1334,3488}.

Essential and desirable diagnostic criteria

Essential:
- Histology resembling that of colorectal adenocarcinoma in ≥ 50% of tumour
- Expression of at least one intestinal marker (CDX2, CK20, HNF4α, or MUC2)
- Clinical exclusion of metastasis from colorectal carcinoma

Desirable:
- A tumour with enteric morphology and expression of intestinal markers (CDX2, CK20, HNF4α, or MUC2) and coexpression of TTF1 or CK7

Staging

Staging should be performed according to the eighth-edition TNM classification.

Prognosis and prediction

There are no consistent data comparing enteric adenocarcinoma with pulmonary adenocarcinoma stage-by-stage. No predictive biomarker exists.

Squamous dysplasia and carcinoma in situ of the lung

Lantuejoul S
Hwang DM
Mascaux C
Remon J
Van Schil PEY
Warth A

Definition

Squamous dysplasia and squamous carcinoma in situ (SCIS) are preinvasive squamous lesions that are precursors of squamous cell carcinoma (SCC), arising in the bronchial epithelium. They are part of a continuum of recognizable neoplastic histological changes in airway epithelium and associated with accumulation of somatic genetic alterations.

ICD-O coding

8070/2 Squamous cell carcinoma in situ
8077/0 Mild squamous dysplasia
8077/2 Moderate squamous dysplasia
8077/2 Severe squamous dysplasia

ICD-11 coding

2E62.2 & XH3EA2 Carcinoma in situ of bronchus or lung; Intraepithelial neoplasia (dysplasia) of bronchus and lung, high grade & Squamous intraepithelial neoplasia, high grade
2F00.Y & XH4611 Other specified benign neoplasm of middle ear or respiratory system & Squamous intraepithelial neoplasia, low grade

Related terminology

Acceptable: preinvasive squamous lesions; high-grade intraepithelial neoplasia.
Not recommended: squamous atypia; bronchial dysplasia; angiogenic squamous dysplasia; bronchial premalignancy; early non-invasive cancer.

Subtype(s)

Mild squamous dysplasia; moderate squamous dysplasia; severe squamous dysplasia; squamous carcinoma in situ

Localization

These lesions may occur anywhere in airways and can be single or multifocal throughout the tracheobronchial tree {860,1108}.

Clinical features

Signs and symptoms

Squamous dysplasia and SCIS are asymptomatic and diagnosed incidentally on bronchoscopy. Squamous dysplasia occurs in 40% of heavy smokers (> 30 pack-years) or in patients with obstructive airway disease {2005,1160}. Preinvasive squamous lesions are more frequent in men {1588} and in patients exposed to asbestos and other occupational carcinogens {2266,2005}.

White-light and autofluorescence endoscopy

Approximately 40% of squamous dysplasia / SCIS can be detected by white-light reflectance bronchoscopy (WLB). Combination of WLB with autofluorescence bronchoscopy (AFB) using a violet or blue light for illumination enables the detection

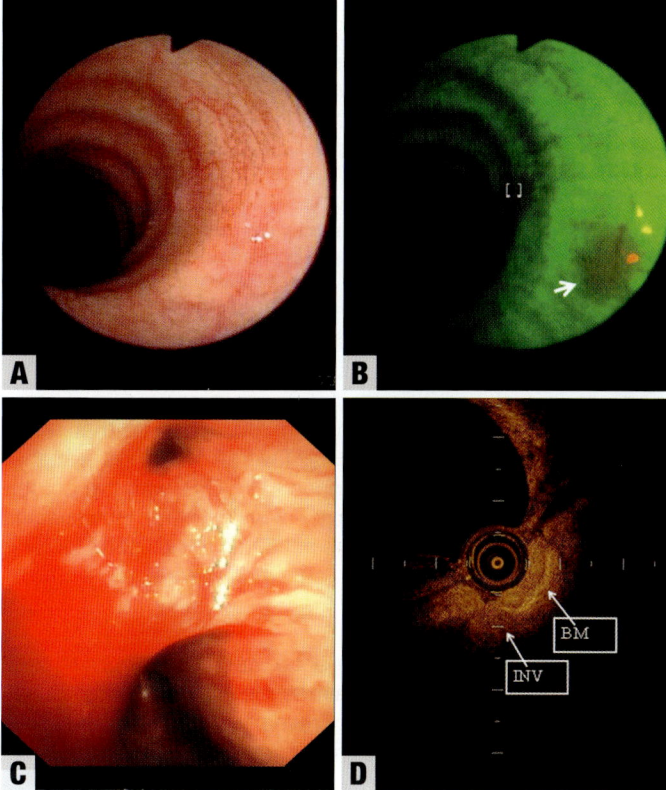

Fig. 1.76 Squamous carcinoma in situ. White-light reflectance bronchoscopy (**A**) and autofluorescence bronchoscopy (**B**) of a squamous carcinoma in situ with microinvasion in the trachea. There was no light abnormality on the white-light reflectance bronchoscopy examination. **C** A plaque-like lesion on white-light reflectance bronchoscopy. **D** Optical coherence tomography showing invasion of the tumour through the basal membrane.

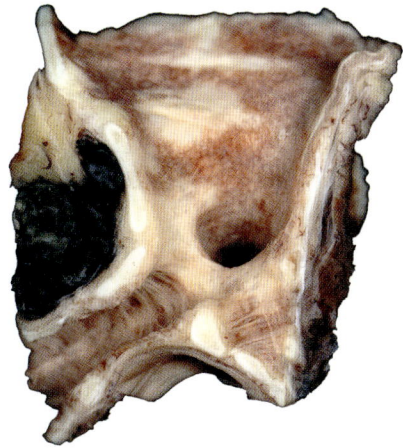

Fig. 1.77 Squamous carcinoma in situ at gross examination. Gross examination showing a squamous carcinoma in situ at bronchial bifurcation. Note the plaque-like greyish lesions.

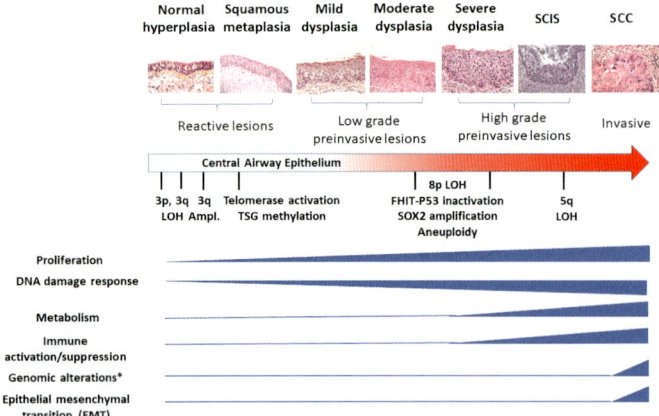

Fig. 1.78 Multistage pathogenesis of squamous cell carcinoma (SCC). Multistage pathogenesis of SCC of the lung is represented by progressive morphological and genetic alterations and pathway deregulation. *Driver mutations, copy-number alteration, structural variants. Ampl., amplification; LOH, loss of heterozygosity; SCIS, squamous cell carcinoma in situ; TSG, tumour suppressor gene.

of lesions as small as 0.5 mm {1868}. Preinvasive and invasive squamous lesions appear brownish red, while normal areas appear green or light blue {1868}. Overall, AFB has a higher sensitivity than WLB for the diagnosis of SCIS, with the combination of both reaching a sensitivity of 85% {2899}. However, its specificity is lower and AFB does not seem to be useful for lung cancer screening {3085}.

Narrow-band imaging
Narrow-band imaging (image-enhanced endoscopy) uses narrow-band range filters to enhance the visualization of abnormal vessels {613,1243}. Blue light reveals superficial dotted and complex tortuous capillaries and green light the deeper submucosal veins {3473,2738}. Narrow-band imaging has a high specificity for the detection of preinvasive lesions, and a higher sensitivity, specificity, and diagnostic yield than AFB {1231, 1133}.

Optical coherence tomography
Illumination of the bronchial surface with infrared light provides near-histological cross-sectional images with a spatial resolution of 3–15 μm and a depth of penetration of 2 mm {1589,1243}.

Radial probe endobronchial ultrasound
Radial probe endobronchial ultrasound provides circumferential images with a resolution of < 1 mm and a penetration depth of 50 mm, in order to investigate the depth of invasion and node metastasis {1034}.

Radiology
Preinvasive lesions are not seen on chest CT or PET.

Epidemiology
The epidemiology is similar to that of lung SCC (see *Tumours of the lung: Introduction*, p. 20).

Etiology
The etiology is similar to that of lung SCC (see *Tumours of the lung: Introduction*, p. 20).

Pathogenesis
Preinvasive squamous lesions result from sequential genetic and epigenetic changes related to cigarette carcinogen exposure, which affects the entire tracheobronchial tree – a phenomenon referred to as field carcinogenesis {1159,860,1108}. Loss of heterozygosity at 3p and 9p21 occurs early, starting from the normal epithelium. Later changes affect 8p21-p23, 13q14 (*RB1* locus), 17p13 (*TP53* locus), and 5q21 (*APC*) regions {1793,3326, 3327,3329}. *TP53* mutations occur at variable times {3326,3329}. Recently, genomic, transcriptomic, and epigenomic analyses of SCIS showed frequent somatic and copy-number alterations in the *TP53*, *CDKN2A*, *SOX2*, and *AKT2* genes, as well as a tobacco mutation signature and chromosomal instability in relation to cell-cycle and DNA repair pathway alterations {3012}. Activation of immune responses and immune escape through immune checkpoints and suppressive interleukins have been shown from high-grade preinvasive squamous lesions {1822}.

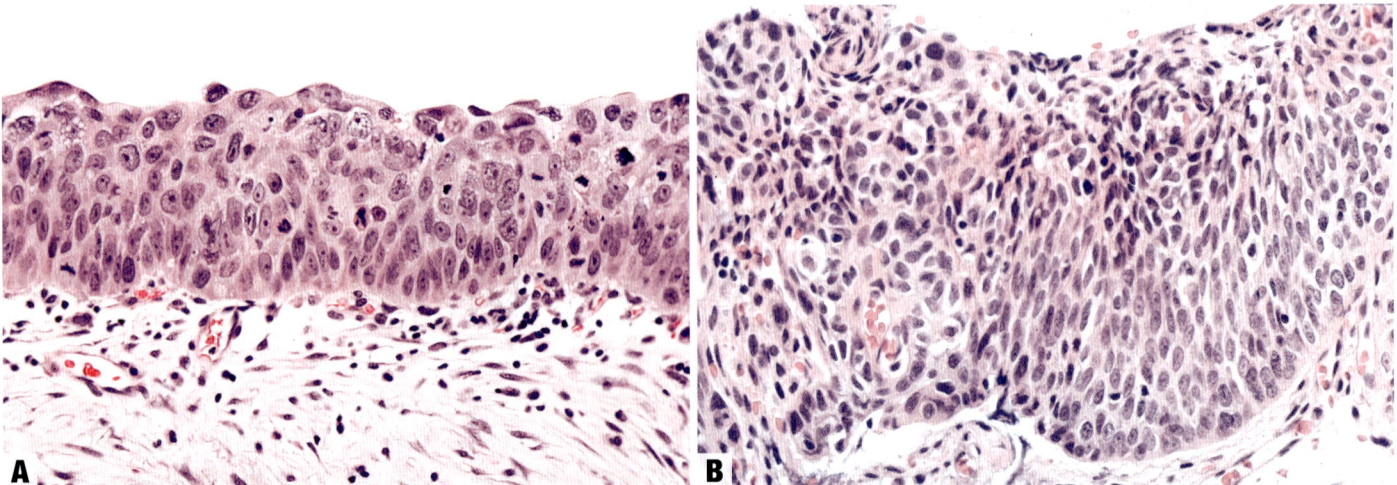

Fig. 1.79 Severe dysplasia. **A** Bronchial mucosa replaced by markedly dysplastic squamous epithelium with full-thickness loss of cellular maturation. **B** Bronchial mucosa replaced by squamous epithelium displaying dysplastic nuclear features but superficial retention of cellular maturation.

Macroscopic appearance

SCIS often arises near bifurcations in the segmental bronchi, subsequently extending into the adjacent lobar and subsegmental branches. The lesions are less common in the trachea. Nodular/polypoid lesions (25% of preinvasive squamous lesions) as small as 1–2 mm in diameter can be observed. Flat lesions (75%) > 10 mm occur as focal thickening with increased vascularity, or marked irregularity of the mucosa, while smaller lesions appear nonspecific, mimicking inflammation or squamous metaplasia {3125,1235}.

Histopathology

In response to irritants and carcinogens, the bronchial epithelium may show basal cell hyperplasia or squamous metaplasia with loss of normal goblet and ciliated cells. These lesions are not considered preneoplastic per se. Further exposure leads to their progression to mild, moderate, and severe dysplasia and ultimately to SCIS. Dysplasia can be graded as low-grade (mild and moderate dysplasia) and high-grade (severe dysplasia) – see Table 1.10 (p. 88). Dysplasia may be angiogenic and papillary {1418,2737}, but these features have no known prognostic significance. Distinction between different subtypes of dysplasia and SCIS is based on cell size and maturation, nuclear features, cell orientation, and epithelial thickness. This grading system is somewhat theoretical, because morphological changes are a continuum, but the reproducibility of histological criteria among trained observers has been good {2102}.

Immunohistochemistry

Preinvasive squamous lesions demonstrate a diagnostic immunohistochemical profile similar to that of invasive SCCs (CK5/6+, p63/p40+). Proliferative activity increases along with severity of dysplasia, as evidenced by expression of Ki-67 {1871,1896, 2821}. Increased expression of p53 protein is often present {208,303,1816,2821,1823,2343}. Expression of markers such as cyclin D1 and cyclin E {304,1297,2438}, VEGF {852,1595}, and MDM2 {1823}, as well as BCL2:BAX ratio {304,303}, reflecting oncogene activation, gradually increases along with the severity of the lesions, whereas expression of tumour suppressor gene markers (i.e. FHIT, p16, p14ARF) is gradually lost {2824,1823}.

Differential diagnosis

Mild dysplasia must be distinguished from basal cell (reserve cell) hyperplasia and squamous metaplasia. The distinction between SCIS and invasive carcinoma may be difficult on small fragments, because SCIS can extend to bronchial gland ducts, mimicking invasion; however, necrosis and the presence of an endoscopic mass favour an invasive process {1422}. Dysplasia and SCIS can coexist with small cell lung carcinoma, with pagetoid migration of small cells within the dysplastic epithelium.

Cytology

Cells of dysplasia and SCIS are defined largely on the basis of progressive nuclear abnormalities. As dysplasia increases in severity, N:C ratio increases, with nuclei demonstrating more membrane contour irregularities, a more darkly stained and coarsely granular chromatin, or a homogeneous (pyknotic-like) appearance {133,2586,2587}. Cytoplasmic keratinization may be present, especially in more severe lesions. It is not possible

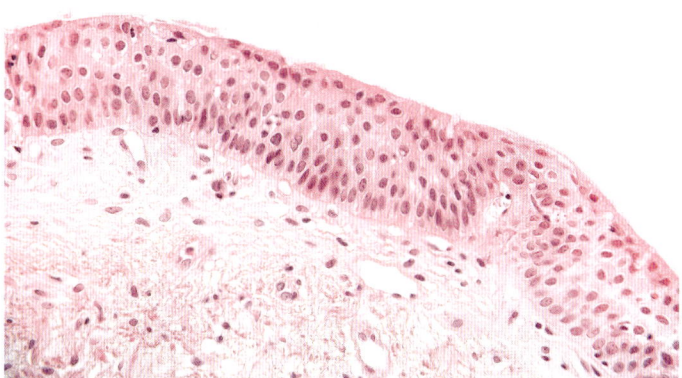

Fig. 1.80 Squamous metaplasia. Squamous metaplasia of a bronchial epithelium. Note the absence of atypical cells; the maturation of the epithelium is respected and no mitoses are observed.

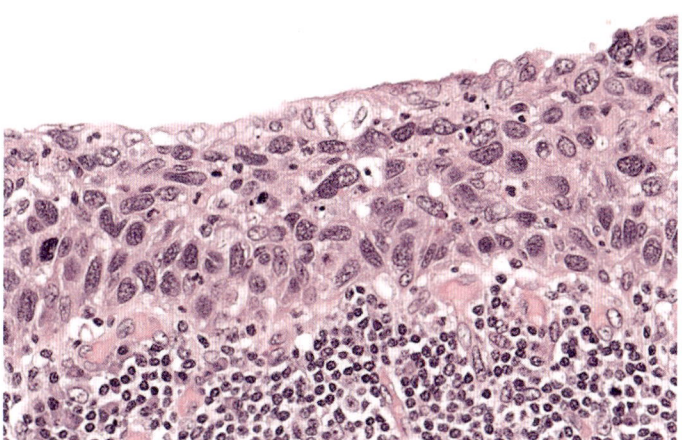

Fig. 1.81 Squamous carcinoma in situ. Squamous carcinoma in situ showing marked cellular atypia, no increased thickness, and no consistent orientation of nuclei in relation to epithelial surface.

to reliably distinguish SCIS from invasive SCC in cytological preparations.

Diagnostic molecular pathology

Not relevant

Essential and desirable diagnostic criteria

Essential:
- Squamous differentiation of bronchial epithelium accompanied by progressive abnormalities in nuclear features, cell size and maturation, cell orientation, and epithelial thickness associated with degree of dysplasia (mild, moderate, severe) and carcinoma in situ

See also Table 1.10 (p. 88).

Staging

Dysplasia has no staging system. SCIS is classified as Tis (SCIS) according to the eighth edition of the TNM classification {315}.

Table 1.10 Diagnostic criteria for squamous dysplasia and squamous carcinoma in situ

Abnormality	Thickness	Cell size	Maturation/orientation	Nuclei
Mild dysplasia	Mildly increased	Mildly increased Mild anisocytosis and pleomorphism	Continuous progression of maturation from base to luminal surface Basilar zone expanded, with cellular crowding in the lower third of epithelium Distinct intermediate (prickle cell) zone present Superficial flattening of epithelial cells	Mild variation of N:C ratio Finely granular chromatin Minimal angulation Nucleoli inconspicuous or absent Nuclei vertically oriented in lower third Mitoses absent or very rare
Moderate dysplasia	Moderately increased	Mildly increased Cells often small May have moderate anisocytosis and pleomorphism	Partial progression of maturation from base to luminal surface Basilar zone expanded, with cellular crowding in the lower two thirds of epithelium Intermediate zone confined to upper third of epithelium Superficial flattening of epithelial cells	Moderate variation of N:C ratio Finely granular chromatin Angulations, grooves, and lobulations present Nucleoli inconspicuous or absent Nuclei vertically oriented in lower two thirds Mitotic figures present in lower third
Severe dysplasia	Markedly increased	Markedly increased May have marked anisocytosis and pleomorphism	Little progression of maturation from base to luminal surface Basilar zone expanded, with cellular crowding well into the upper third of epithelium Intermediate zone greatly attenuated Superficial flattening of epithelial cells	N:C ratio often high and variable Chromatin coarse and uneven Nuclear angulations and folding prominent Nucleoli frequently present and conspicuous Nuclei vertically oriented in lower two thirds Mitotic figures present in lower two thirds
Carcinoma in situ	May or may not be increased	May be markedly increased May have marked anisocytosis and pleomorphism	No progression of maturation from base to luminal surface; epithelium can be inverted, with little change in appearance Basilar zone expanded, with cellular crowding throughout the epithelium Intermediate zone absent Surface flattening confined to the most superficial cells	N:C ratio often high and variable Chromatin coarse and uneven Nuclear angulations and folding prominent Nucleoli may be present or inconspicuous No consistent orientation of nuclei in relation to epithelial surface Mitotic figures present through full thickness

Prognosis and prediction

Prognosis

Up to 37% of severe dysplasia and 88% of SCIS will persist or progress {3012,287,1305,313}. SCIS has understandably a much better prognosis than invasive carcinoma; therefore, early detection is the key to successful management {613}. Resection at this stage results in 100% curability, although frequent multi-focality means that other foci are liable to be present elsewhere in the airways.

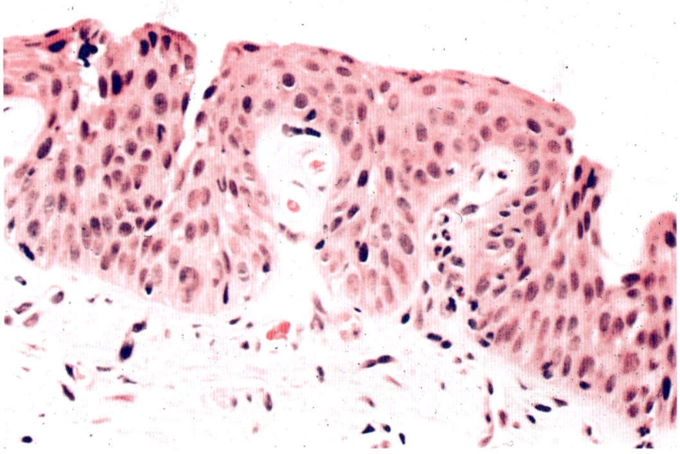

Prediction

The presence of preinvasive squamous lesions, especially high-grade lesions, is a risk marker for lung cancer in both the central airways and the peripheral lung {3134}, and p53 overexpression in squamous metaplasia may predict the presence of carcinoma elsewhere in the respiratory tract {250}. Host factors such as the inflammatory load and levels of anti-inflammatory proteins in the lung influence the progression or regression of preneoplastic lesions {1267,195}. Recently, changes in cell-cycle control, inflammatory activity, and epithelial differentiation / cell–cell adhesion were found in high-risk persistent bronchial dysplasia and may underlie progression to invasive SCC {1895}. Comparative genomic hybridization studies have revealed that multiple copy-number alterations characterized progressive dysplasia {3133,3135}. In a cohort of SCIS longitudinally monitored, progression-specific methylation changes and a chromosomal instability signature were identified to predict lesions that will progress {3012}.

Fig. 1.82 Squamous angiogenic papillary metaplasia. Bronchial mucosa with metaplastic squamous epithelium showing irregular pseudopapillary extension of stroma.

Squamous cell carcinoma of the lung

Warth A
Botling J
Chung JH
Ishii G
Rossi G
Wistuba I

Definition
Squamous cell carcinoma (SCC) is a malignant epithelial tumour characterized by the presence of keratinization, intercellular bridges, or immunohistochemical markers of squamous cell differentiation.

ICD-O coding
8070/3 Squamous cell carcinoma, NOS

ICD-11 coding
2C25.2 Squamous cell carcinoma of bronchus or lung

Related terminology
Not recommended: epidermoid carcinoma.

Subtype(s)
SCC, keratinizing; SCC, non-keratinizing; basaloid SCC

Localization
Pulmonary SCCs usually arise from a main or lobar bronchus and historically at least two thirds are located in the central compartment of the lung. Although precise definitions of "central" and "peripheral" are lacking so far {399}, about one third of cases are peripherally located and their incidence seems to be increasing {1538}. Peripheral SCC is particularly evident in patients with underlying interstitial lung disease {883}.

Clinical features
The signs and symptoms of SCC are similar to those of other non-small cell lung carcinomas (see *Tumours of the lung: Introduction*, p. 20) but are generally related to the tumour location. SCC has a tendency to be locally aggressive, with progressive involvement of peribronchial structures through direct invasion, but distant metastases occur similarly to other non-small cell lung carcinomas. Symptoms are related to endobronchial obstruction, leading to haemoptysis, cough, and recurrent pneumonitis. With central tumours, the proximity to the carina is a crucial factor for planning surgical treatment {3071}. Peripherally, SCC may show cavitation with superimposed fungal and bacterial infections {1601}.

Epidemiology
See *Tumours of the lung: Introduction* (p. 20).

Like all lung cancers, but to a higher degree than adenocarcinoma, SCC is strongly associated with smoking, and worldwide trends in SCC incidence closely mirror changes in smoking patterns {1955}. SCC is the second most prevalent type, accounting for approximately 20% of lung cancer {163}. SCC is the most common histological type of lung cancer arising in patients with idiopathic pulmonary fibrosis and interstitial lung disease {3113, 3413,3415}.

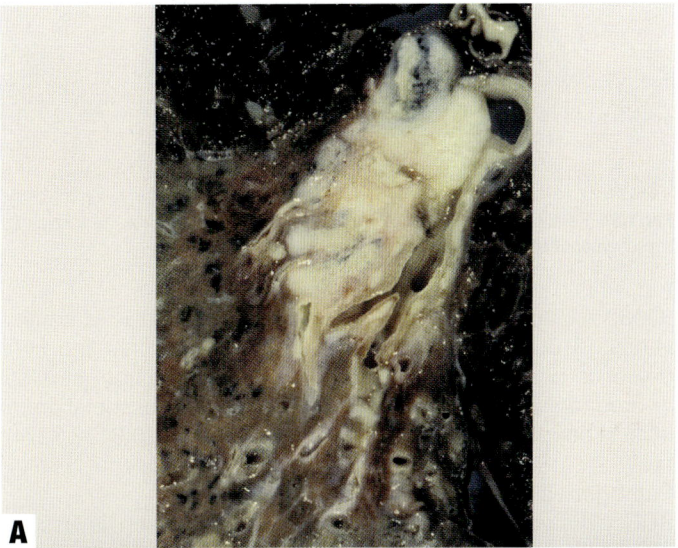

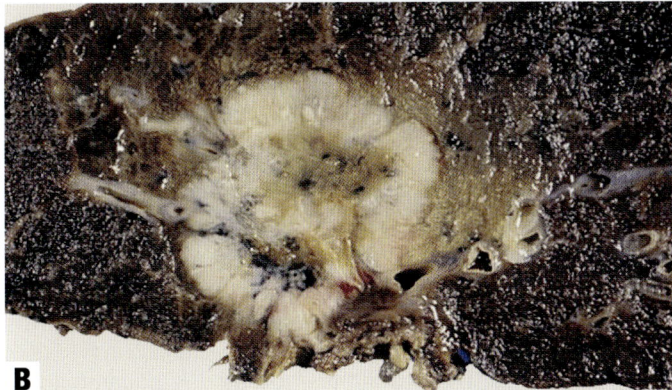

Fig. 1.83 Squamous cell carcinoma. **A** Central squamous cell carcinoma arising in the proximal left lower lobe bronchus. Contiguous intralobar lymph node invasion, obstructive lipoid pneumonia, and mucopurulent bronchiectasis in the basal segments. **B** Central tumour arising in a lobar bronchus with bronchial and parenchymal invasion and central necrosis.

Etiology
See *Tumours of the lung: Introduction* (p. 20).

More than 90% of patients with SCC are current or former heavy smokers, and a male predilection is reported {1128}. Carcinogenic risk factors include exposure to radon gas, metals (arsenic, cadmium, chromium), radiation, air pollution, and infections {723}. Other risk factors for SCC include age, family history, and exposure to secondhand smoke.

Smoking has a relatively predictable mutagenic signature (signature 4), preferentially acting on guanine base pairs and creating C>A substitutions {55}. Rarely, some SCCs develop in never-smokers or light smokers, and these tumours may harbour driver mutations found more commonly in adenocarcinoma, such as *EGFR* and *ALK* mutations {1635,2620,3233,

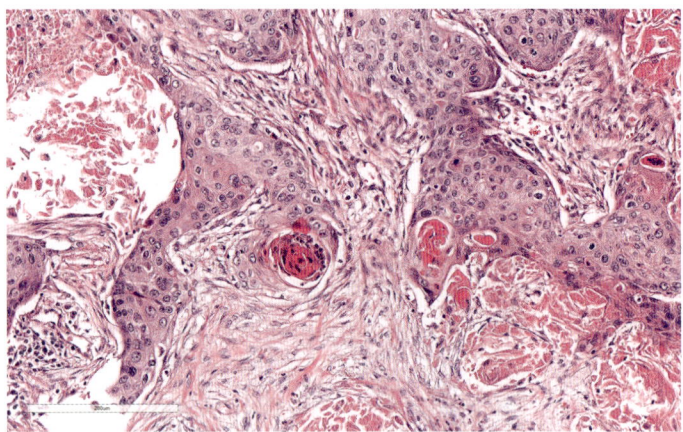

Fig. 1.84 Keratinizing squamous cell carcinoma. Resection specimen of a keratinizing squamous cell carcinoma with formation of keratin pearls.

3203}. A putative role of HPV in SCC pathogenesis is controversial {3106}. Several studies with rigorously controlled HPV detection protocols and exclusion of metastases from cervical or oropharyngeal cancers have questioned the association, at least in populations of European descent {238,1520,3132,3374}.

Pathogenesis

SCC develops via multistep transformation, which is associated with progressive accumulation of genetic and epigenetic aberrations and with increasing morphological dysplasia (see *Squamous dysplasia and carcinoma in situ of the lung*, p. 85). Squamous cell carcinogenesis is linked closely to genomic perturbations, genetic mutations, and/or altered expression of key molecules involved in various stages of squamous cell lineage commitment and/or terminal differentiation {723,1435A}. Comprehensive genomic characterization of SCC revealed complex genomic alterations, with a mean of 360 exonic mutations, 165 genomic rearrangements, and 323 segments of copy-number alteration per tumour {369}. Two pathways appear to be preferentially involved by genetic alterations. The first involves the oxidative stress pathway and includes mutations in *NFE2L2*, *KEAP1*, or *CUL3*. The second is implicated in squamous differentiation and includes overexpression and amplification of *SOX2* and *TP63*; loss-of-function mutations in *NOTCH1*, *NOTCH2*, and *ASCL4*; and focal deletions in *FOXP1*.

Frequent molecular alterations found in pulmonary SCC include gain/amplification of chromosomes 3q (*SOX2*, *TP63*) {165,3051}, 7p (*EGFR*), and 8p (*FGFR1*), as well as frequent deletion of chromosome 9p (*CDKN2A*) {1158,543}. Commonly mutated genes include *TP53*, *CDKN2A*, *PTEN*, *PIK3CA*, *KEAP1*, *KMT2 (MLL2)*, *HLA-A*, *NFE2L2*, *NOTCH1*, and *RB1* {369,1455}. Gene expression profiling has identified four subtypes: primitive, classic, secretory, and basal {3310,369}. However, there is no correlation between the basal gene expression subtype and the basaloid histological subtype {369}.

Basaloid SCC shares most of the mutation and copy-number alteration landscape of classic SCCs. However, transcriptomic analyses compared with non-basaloid squamous carcinoma revealed differential upregulation of genes related to cell cycle, embryonic development, mRNA splicing, chromatin modification pathways, and downregulation of the squamous differentiation, in line with the aggressiveness and poor differentiation of this tumour {301}.

Macroscopic appearance

Pulmonary SCC has a firm white, light-brown, or grey cut surface, occasionally with carbon pigment deposits in the centre and star-like retractions on the periphery. Focal haemorrhage may be present. In larger tumours, central cavitation due to necrosis may occur. Central tumours are often endobronchial with exophytic papillary growth. Obstruction of bronchi is common, often with adjacent atelectasis and obstructive pneumonia, which might be superimposed by fungal and/or bacterial infections.

Histopathology

Keratinizing, non-keratinizing, and basaloid SCC subtypes are recognized, with the same histomorphological features as SCCs at other anatomical regions.

Keratinizing SCC is characterized by morphological features of keratinization (presence of keratinization, pearl formation, and/or intercellular bridges). The extent of keratinization varies with the degree of differentiation: it is prominent in better-differentiated tumours where there is typically widespread keratinization, although it may be present only focally or be less apparent in those that are more poorly differentiated.

Non-keratinizing SCC is a solid non-small cell carcinoma that lacks keratinization. In these tumours, the squamous cell differentiation requires confirmation by immunohistochemical markers (see below). The presence of intracellular mucin in a few cells does not exclude tumours from this category. The issue of small-sample diagnosis is addressed in *Small diagnostic samples* (p. 29). Some non-keratinizing SCCs may morphologically resemble urothelial transitional cell carcinoma.

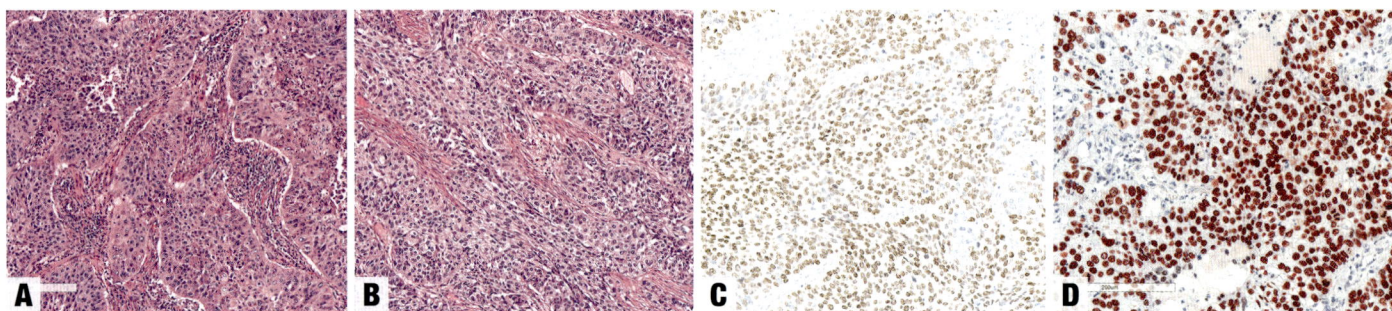

Fig. 1.85 Non-keratinizing squamous cell carcinoma. **A** Resection specimen of a non-keratinizing squamous cell carcinoma. **B** This poorly differentiated carcinoma shows a solid pattern with no keratinization. **C** Squamous differentiation is confirmed by diffuse strongly positive nuclear p40 staining. **D** Immunohistochemical expression of p40.

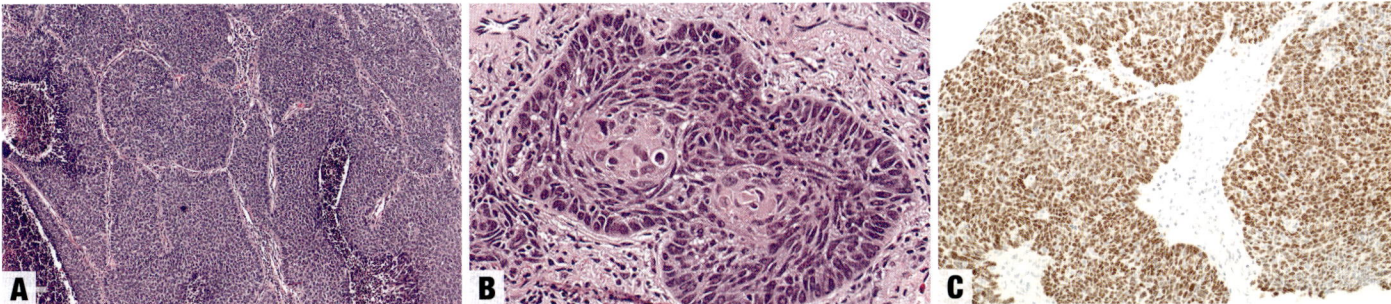

Fig. 1.86 Basaloid squamous cell carcinoma. **A** Resection specimen of a basaloid squamous cell carcinoma. **B** This tumour shows abrupt keratinization, with typical basaloid carcinoma morphology merging with a focus of keratinizing squamous cell carcinoma. **C** Expression of p40 in a biopsy of a basaloid squamous cell carcinoma.

Basaloid SCC is characterized by small to intermediate-sized cells with lobular architecture and peripheral palisading that lack squamous morphology, but it shows immunohistochemical expression of squamous markers. Cytoplasm is scant but well defined. Mitotic count is high (15–50 mitoses/2 mm²) and the Ki-67 index is very high (50–80%). Keratin pearl formation may be seen. Rosettes can be seen. Stroma may show a hyaline or mucoid appearance. Carcinoma in situ is frequent. SCCs (whether keratinizing or non-keratinizing) with a basaloid component of ≥ 50% are classified as basaloid SCC.

Other histological features
All histological subtypes of SCC can show a variety of unusual patterns, including spindle cell morphology and clear cell cytological changes, as well as papillary, pseudovascular, or alveolar-filling patterns.

There is currently no established grading system for SCC of the lung.

Immunohistochemistry
Diffuse positive staining with a squamous cell marker and negative staining for TTF1 confirm the diagnosis of SCC, although some markedly keratinized tumours may show lack of staining with squamous cell markers. In biopsies, the p40-positive staining rate of tumours cells should be > 50% {3390}. p40 is considered the most specific marker for SCCs, whereas high-molecular-weight cytokeratins (CK5/6, 34βE12), desmocollin, desmoglein, and p63 are less specific markers of squamous cell differentiation {2546,2314,3390}. Neuroendocrine markers can occasionally be positive (especially CD56), but if p40 is diffusely positive, the tumour is classified as SCC.

Differential diagnosis
The differential diagnosis of SCC varies depending on the histological subtype.

The main differential diagnoses are between poorly differentiated or basaloid SCC versus poorly differentiated non-small cell lung carcinoma NOS, particularly on small biopsy specimens with limited tumour tissue (see *Small diagnostic samples*, p. 29), or large cell carcinoma with a null phenotype in resection specimens. In these cases, phenotyping by a limited panel of immunomarkers, including the most specific and sensitive primary antibodies indicating squamous cell (p40) and adenocarcinoma (TTF1) histology, is required {2546,2314,3390}. Mucin stains may be misleading, because SCC cells may be focally positive. Tumour entrapment of bronchial cells or peribronchial salivary glands may erroneously lead to a diagnosis of adenocarcinoma or adenosquamous carcinoma. It is well known

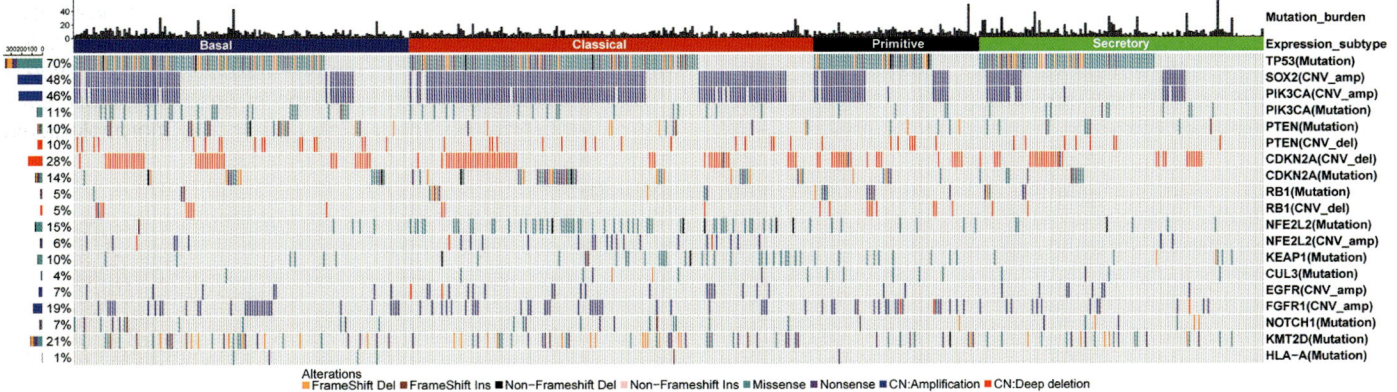

Fig. 1.87 Molecular profile of lung squamous cell carcinoma. Genetic profile of squamous cell carcinoma. The frequencies of significantly altered genes were identified by whole-exome sequencing and gene copy-number variation (CNV) analyses of 501 resected lung squamous cell carcinomas in The Cancer Genome Atlas (TCGA) project {367}. The OncoPrint plot displays the frequency (on the left) of various genomic aberrations, including mutation, amplification (amp), and deletion (del), involving *TP53*, *SOX2*, *PIK3CA*, *PTEN*, *CDKN2A*, *RB1*, *NFE2L2*, *KEAP1*, *CUL3*, *EGFR*, *FGFR1*, *NOTCH1*, *KMT2D*, and *HLA-A*. Samples were grouped according to their respective expression subtype (basal, classical, primitive, secretory), as identified by Wilkerson et al. {3310}. The OncoPrint is generated using data available from the TCGA Research Network (https://portal.gdc.cancer.gov/projects/TCGA-LUSC). CN, copy number; Del, deletion; Ins, insertion.

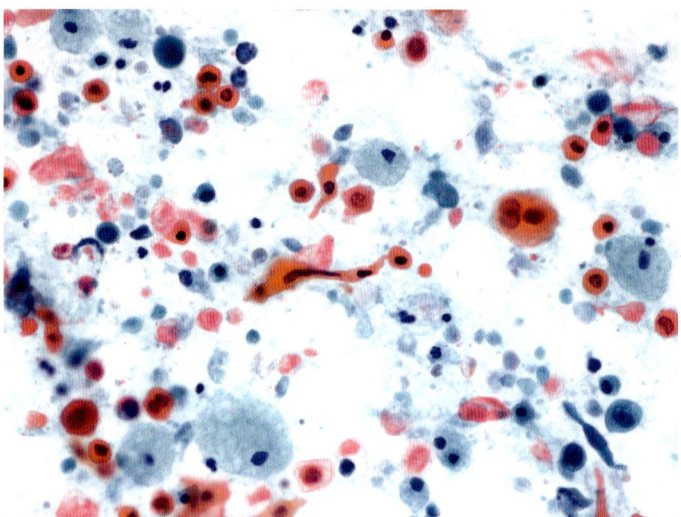

Fig. 1.88 Keratinizing squamous cell carcinoma. Cytology specimen of keratinizing squamous cell carcinoma. Tumour cells are characterized by marked pleomorphism and keratinization. Isolated malignant squamous cells with a bizarrely shaped keratinized cell (tadpole cell). Aspiration cytology (Pap stain).

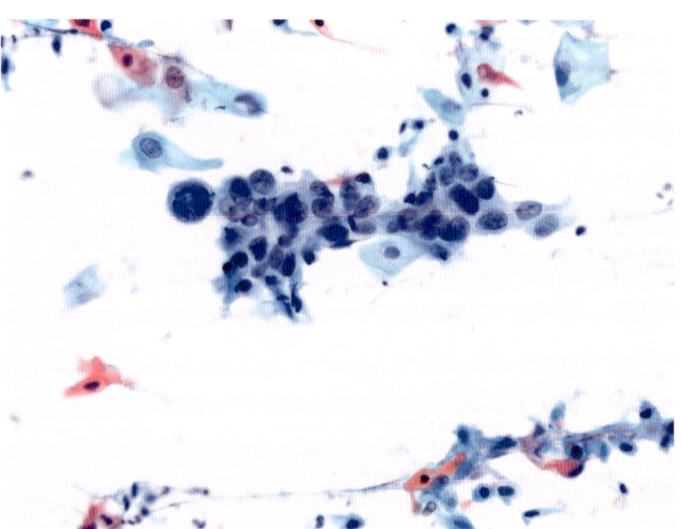

Fig. 1.89 Non-keratinizing squamous cell carcinoma. Cytology of a non-keratinizing squamous cell carcinoma. The malignant cells are present in sheets and as single cells. The tumour cells are more uniform than those of keratinizing squamous cell carcinoma, with higher N:C ratios. The nuclear membrane is irregular and chromatin is coarse and hyperchromatic. Endobronchial ultrasound FNA (Pap stain).

that a subset of adenocarcinomas can show (although rarely) a pseudosquamous appearance, and some SCC has a pseudoadenocarcinomatous morphology {1908}.

Mucoepidermoid carcinoma may be challenging in small biopsy or cytology. However, it should show a mucin-producing glandular component and/or a *MAML2* translocation {273}.

Basaloid SCC must be differentiated from large cell neuroendocrine carcinoma (LCNEC), small cell carcinoma (small cell lung carcinoma), high-grade adenoid cystic carcinoma, NUT carcinoma, and poorly differentiated squamous cell or adenocarcinoma. Palisading and rosette-like structures, as well as some degree of neuroendocrine marker expression, can be seen in basaloid SCCs mimicking LCNEC. Some basaloid SCCs have very small tumour cells, morphologically resembling

or identical to small cell lung carcinoma. However, diffuse p40 expression favours basaloid SCC and excludes LCNEC or small cell lung carcinoma. High-grade adenoid cystic carcinomas can express SOX10, and if better-differentiated areas are present, these may show dual staining of CAM5.2, which is strong in ductal/luminal cells but weak in myoepithelial cells, with positive p63 and S100 in myoepithelial cells. Adenoid cystic carcinomas also can have *MYB-NFIB* or *MYBL1-NFIB* fusions by FISH (see *Adenoid cystic carcinoma of the lung*, p. 117). NUT carcinomas express positive staining with the NUT antibody or NUT gene fusion by molecular analysis (see *NUT carcinoma of the thorax*, p. 364) {1331,237} and are more likely to be encountered in young and/or never-smoker patients.

Lymphoepithelial carcinoma has a squamous phenotype but is usually clearly recognized by the dense intratumoural inflammatory cells, positive in situ hybridization for EBV, and frequent lack of strong smoking history in most cases (see *Lymphoepithelial carcinoma of the lung*, p. 94).

SMARCA4-deficient tumours (see *Thoracic SMARCA4-deficient undifferentiated tumour*, p. 111) are undifferentiated neoplasms, mostly representing smoking-related poorly differentiated carcinomas characterized by SMARCA4 (BRG1) deficiency that can express focal p40 staining in some cases {1886,2460}.

Metastatic tumours (see *Metastasis to the lung*, p. 452) with squamous and/or squamoid differentiation are particularly difficult to differentiate from primary pulmonary SCC. Clinical and radiological correlation is most important in addressing this question. Urothelial carcinomas more often stain positively with GATA3, uroplakin-3, and CK20 {1011A}. Immunohistochemical stains against CD5 and KIT (CD117) are helpful to demonstrate a thymic origin {1535}. Distinguishing primary lung SCC from a metastasis in patients with a history of SCC elsewhere (e.g. head and neck region, oesophagus, uterine cervix) can also be challenging. The presence of associated precursor lesions helps to confirm lung primaries. Molecular comparison using multigenic panel and HPV testing/genotyping of lung tumour and extrathoracic SCC can be helpful in these cases.

Florid squamous cell metaplasia – due to infarction, diffuse alveolar damage, postinflammatory processes (infections and radiation), or benign lesions (granular cell tumour) – should always be considered by integrating morphology with clinical and imaging findings. Squamous papilloma/papillomatosis should be excluded in the presence of endobronchial lesions with or without condylomatous changes.

Cytology

The cytological features of SCC vary depending on the degree of squamous differentiation and the sampling method {1228, 2584}. The classic pattern of SCC shows singly scattered or clusters of atypical cells in the background of necrotic debris: a granular, amorphous precipitate with nuclear debris and red blood cells called tumour diathesis. In a well-differentiated SCC, the malignant cells are usually non-cohesive and show a variety of shapes (polygonal, rounded, spindle, tadpole), with abundant smooth, dense cytoplasm filled with keratin. The cytoplasm stains green, yellow, or orange with the Pap stain and robin's egg blue with Romanowsky stains. Nuclei are usually small, hyperchromatic, and smudgy, and nucleoli are often inconspicuous.

In moderately and poorly differentiated SCC, keratinization is less apparent, cytoplasm is scant, and tumour cells appear in cohesive aggregates with elongated or spindle nuclei.

Nuclei are hyperchromatic and they have a prominent nucleolus and a highly irregular pattern of chromatin distribution. The basaloid subtype of SCC shows prominent palisading of nuclei around the perimeter of cell groups.

In exfoliative samples, surface tumour cells predominate and occur as individually dispersed cells with prominent cytoplasmic keratinization and dark pyknotic nuclei. In contrast, in brushings, cells from deeper layers are sampled, showing a much greater proportion of cohesive aggregates.

Centrally located SCC may exfoliate tumour cells that can be identified in sputum cytology.

Diagnostic molecular pathology

EGFR mutation or *ALK* rearrangement can occur in lung SCC. This possibility should be considered in young never-smoking patients, in particular those with a history of lung adenocarcinoma with one of these genetic alterations {1691,1692,3363A,2461}.

Essential and desirable diagnostic criteria

Essential:

- Definitive morphological features such as intercellular bridges and/or keratinization, or a poorly differentiated tumour with immunohistochemical evidence of squamous cell differentiation (positive p40 and negative TTF1)
- Keratinizing SCC can be diagnosed without the use of immunostains {3390}
- The basaloid component should be ≥ 50% for the diagnosis of basaloid SCC

Desirable:

- Exclusion of possible metastasis from SCC at extrapulmonary sites or other primary neoplasms with squamous cell differentiation (e.g. NUT carcinoma, mucoepidermoid carcinoma, SMARCA4-deficient tumour, or thymic SCC)

Staging

SCCs are staged according to the eighth edition of the Union for International Cancer Control (UICC) / American Joint Committee on Cancer (AJCC) TNM classification (see *TNM staging of carcinomas of the lung*, p. 11 {315}). Superficial spreading tumours with an invasive component limited to the bronchial wall are classified as T1a.

Prognosis and prediction

The prognosis of a SCC patient depends mainly on the patient's performance score and the clinical/tumour stage at time of diagnosis. Although clinicopathological characteristics may differ, the prognoses of central and peripheral SCCs seem to be comparable {1686}. There are no validated clinical factors or biomarkers that are predictive of tumour response to local or systemic therapies. Histological subtyping does not correlate with prognosis.

Lymphoepithelial carcinoma of the lung

Chou TY
Chang YL
Wong MP

Definition

Lymphoepithelial carcinoma is a poorly differentiated squamous cell carcinoma (SCC) admixed with variable amounts of lymphoplasmacytic infiltrate, frequently associated with EBV.

ICD-O coding

8082/3 Lymphoepithelial carcinoma

ICD-11 coding

2C25.2 & XH1E40 Squamous cell carcinoma of bronchus or lung & Lymphoepithelial carcinoma

Related terminology

Not recommended: lymphoepithelioma-like carcinoma; lymphoepithelioma; lymphoepithelial-like carcinoma.

Subtype(s)

None

Localization

These tumours are often peripherally located. Intrabronchial components are noted in a minority of cases {448}.

Clinical features

Signs and symptoms

As many as one third of cases are identified by an incidental radiographic finding {1673}. Cough with or without blood-tinged sputum is the most common presenting symptom {448}. Others include chest pain, body-weight loss, and haemoptysis {448, 1673}.

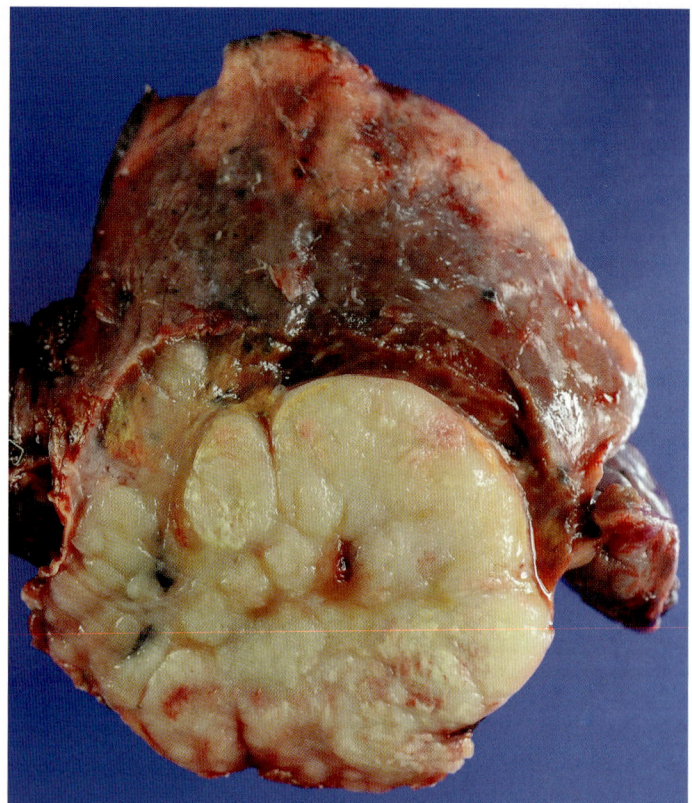

Fig. 1.90 Lymphoepithelial carcinoma. A well-circumscribed solid and firm lesion demonstrates a homogeneous, fish-flesh appearance on cut surface.

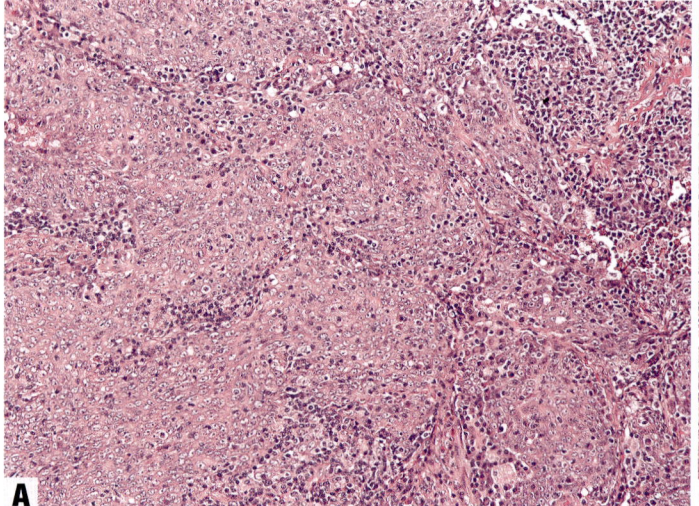
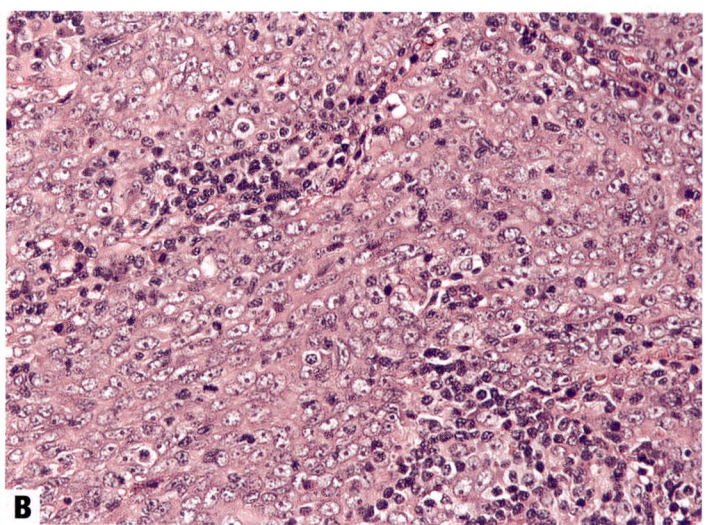

Fig. 1.91 Lymphoepithelial carcinoma. **A** Lymphoepithelial carcinoma shows a syncytial growth pattern of tumour cells with large vesicular nuclei, prominent nucleoli, and a heavy lymphocytic infiltrate. **B** At higher power.

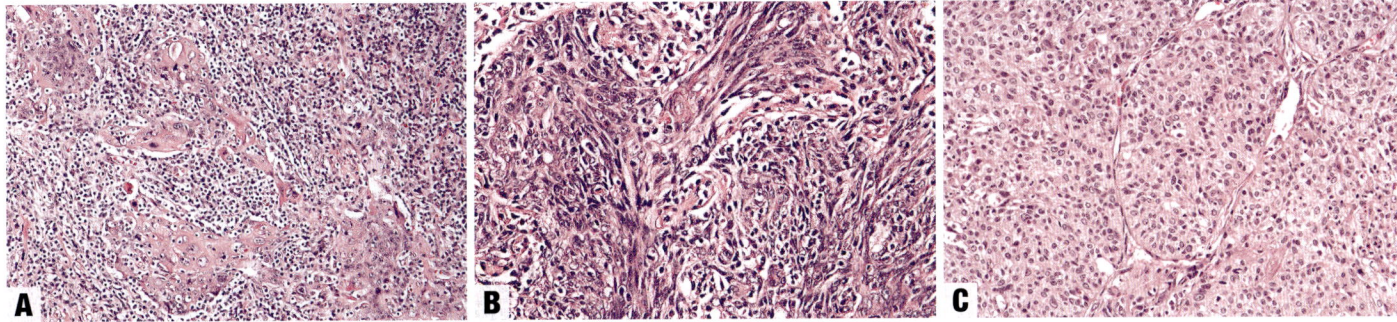

Fig. 1.92 Lymphoepithelial carcinoma. **A** This lymphoepithelial carcinoma shows focal squamous differentiation. Nests of squamous cell carcinoma are accompanied by a prominent lymphocytic stroma. **B** This lymphoepithelial carcinoma shows prominent spindly tumour cells surrounded by a lymphocytic stroma. **C** This tumour consists of sheets and nests of poorly differentiated tumour cells, with little lymphocytic cell infiltrate.

Imaging

Tumours usually form a discrete coin lesion on imaging. Thin-walled cavitary lesions {1143,3478} and pleural effusions are uncommon {448}.

Epidemiology

These tumours are rare (0.92% of non-small cell lung carcinomas), predominantly affecting younger, Asian, non-smokers, with a median age of 51 years (range: 9–74 years) {3398,449, 450,1682,190}. Most studies {3398,449,450,1682}, but not all {1673,1105}, show a female predominance.

Etiology

Association with EBV is found in > 90% of cases occurring in Asian patients, but at a much lower frequency in patients of European descent. The clinicopathological manifestations, as well as patients' EBV serological profile, the presence of EBV-encoded small RNA 1 (EBER1), expression of LMP1 and BCL2 in the tumour cells, and intratumoural infiltration of CD8+ T lymphocytes suggest a role of EBV in the genesis of the EBV-associated subtype of lymphoepithelial carcinoma {448,1673, 1143}. There is a parallel correlation between the EBV serology titre and both tumour burden and stage {448}.

Pathogenesis

TP53, *KRAS*, and *EGFR* mutations as well as *ALK* and *ROS1* translocations are typically absent, suggesting a molecular tumorigenesis distinct from that of conventional non-small cell lung carcinomas {448,1673,450,3398,1059}.

Macroscopic appearance

The tumours appear to be solitary, round to ovoid, and circumscribed, ranging in size from 10 to 110 mm. The cut surfaces are pink-white and fleshy {448,3398}.

Histopathology

Histology

Most tumours show a syncytial pattern of growth and a marked lymphoplasmacytic infiltration within and between the tumour islands. In a minority of cases, lymphoplasmacytic infiltration is not so prominent, resulting in a morphology resembling that of non-keratinizing SCC {3398,3195}. Tumour cells show a moderate amount of eosinophilic cytoplasm, large vesicular nuclei, and prominent eosinophilic nucleoli. Focal keratinization, spindle cell growth, and intratumoural amyloid deposition can occur

{3398,1188,442,448,1102}. The mitotic count is variable {1102}. The tumour mostly has pushing borders at the interface with the adjacent lung parenchyma and grows in the form of irregularly shaped islands or diffuse sheets with infrequent necrosis {448, 1673,1188}. Spread through alveolar spaces (spread through airspaces) of the tumour cells can be observed {3398}. The stroma may show a non-necrotizing granulomatous reaction {3398,1059}.

Immunohistochemistry

The tumour cells show diffuse staining for pancytokeratin, CK5/6, p40, and p63, indicating squamous differentiation. Diffuse positive staining for p40/p63 is characteristic, and negative staining for these markers is exceptional. The accompanying lymphoid infiltrate comprises a mixture of CD3-positive T cells and CD20-positive B cells.

Differential diagnosis

The tumour can mimic metastatic non-keratinizing SCC of the nasopharynx, poorly differentiated non-small cell carcinoma and NUT carcinoma arising in the lung, and non-Hodgkin lymphomas. This diagnosis should be considered when a pulmonary non-keratinizing SCC is encountered in a young never-smoker,

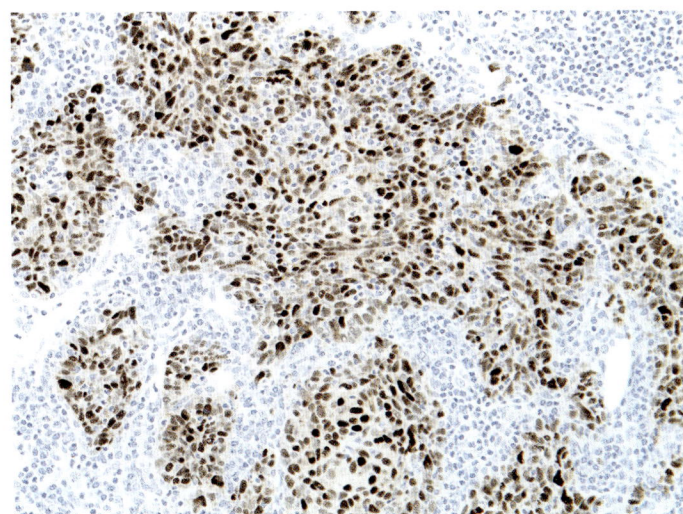

Fig. 1.93 Pulmonary lymphoepithelial carcinoma. In situ hybridization for EBV-encoded small RNA (EBER) selectively labels the carcinoma cells, while the lymphoid cells are negative.

particularly if the patient is from Asia. Metastatic carcinoma must be excluded by careful evaluation of the nasopharynx in addition to correlation with a history of any known previous neoplasm. NUT carcinoma can show prominent infiltrating neutrophils and positivity for NUT by immunohistochemical staining (see *NUT carcinoma of the thorax*, p. 364). Lymphoma is negative for epithelial markers but positive for lymphoid markers (see the sections on haematolymphoid tumours, beginning on p. 174) {448,3195}.

Cytology

Tumours show cohesive sheets and clusters of large uniform tumour cells with a syncytial appearance, round or oval vesicular nuclei, and conspicuous nucleoli. Lymphocytic infiltration is typically extensive but can be sparse in some cases {3416}. Occasionally, spindle cell growth, prominent mitotic figures, and finely granular to flocculent cytoplasm are identified {1102, 3416}.

Diagnostic molecular pathology

Demonstration of EBV is usually by in situ hybridization for EBER.

Essential and desirable diagnostic criteria

Essential:
- Non-keratinizing SCC with syncytial-appearing tumour cells, vesicular nuclei, and distinct nucleoli
- Lymphoplasmacytic infiltrate between and within tumour islands
- Exclusion of metastatic nasopharyngeal carcinoma clinically

Desirable:
- EBER in situ hybridization positive in EBV-associated tumours, but negative in EBV-independent tumours

Staging

Tumours are staged according to the eighth-edition TNM system. Metastases occur most frequently in hilar or mediastinal lymph nodes, followed by pericardium, liver, bone, and brain {448}.

Prognosis and prediction

The survival rates are better for patients with lymphoepithelial carcinoma than patients with conventional non-small cell lung carcinomas, at both early and late stages. Complete resection is the primary approach to obtain a cure for early-stage patients {1673,3478}. Patients with locally advanced disease can receive neoadjuvant or adjuvant chemotherapy/chemoradiotherapy or immunotherapy {448,1673,450}. Tumour necrosis, low lymphocytic infiltration, and recurrence are poor prognostic factors {1059,3398}. The presence of abundant CD8+ cytotoxic T lymphocytes adjacent to tumour cells, low expression of the p53 and ERBB2 oncoproteins in tumour cells, and granulomatous inflammation may be associated with better prognosis {448,1673,3398,1188,1102}. The presence of PDL1 expression is associated with increased disease-free survival {3457}. Conversely, high baseline plasma EBV DNA concentration is an independent poor prognostic factor {3457,3350}.

Large cell carcinoma of the lung

Rossi G
Leighl NB
Lu S
Nicholson AG
Smit EF

Definition
Large cell carcinoma (LCC) is an undifferentiated non-small cell carcinoma (NSCC) that lacks the cytological, architectural, immunohistochemical, and histochemical features of small cell carcinoma, adenocarcinoma, or squamous cell carcinoma (SCC), in addition to giant cell, spindle cell, or pleomorphic carcinoma. The diagnosis requires a thoroughly sampled resected tumour and cannot be made on non-surgical biopsy or cytology.

ICD-O coding
8012/3 Large cell carcinoma

ICD-11 coding
2C25.3 Large cell carcinoma

Related terminology
Not recommended: large cell anaplastic carcinoma; large cell undifferentiated carcinoma.

Subtype(s)
None

Localization
LCCs are typically peripheral masses.

Clinical features
The symptoms, imaging, and tumour spread {3256,2758,226} of LCC are similar to those of other NSCCs (see *Tumours of the lung: Introduction*, p. 20).

Epidemiology
In the 1990s, LCC accounted for approximately 10% of all lung cancers {3080}, but according to data from the US National Cancer Institute (NCI)'s SEER Program, in the USA the rate of LCC has since dropped precipitously, to about 1.5% of all lung carcinomas (see Fig. 1.02, p. 23), which is probably due to the introduction of TTF1 immunohistochemistry around 1990, followed by immunostaining for p63/p40 and subsequently molecular testing, into clinical practice by pathologists {2139, 489,1660,1903,1690,1739,2280,2465}. The average age at diagnosis is about 65 years, and most patients are male.

Etiology
The etiology of LCC is similar to that of other NSCCs (see *Tumours of the lung: Introduction*, p. 20). The majority of patients are current or former smokers.

Pathogenesis
The pathogenesis of LCC is similar to that of other lung cancers (see *Tumours of the lung: Introduction*, p. 20). About two thirds of all LCCs harbour alterations in oncogenic drivers, similar to adenocarcinoma {2045,2464,2544,1712,1387,2462}.

Genomic analyses have provided a basis for potential refinement of LCC, but these features are not yet disease-defining criteria. Of greatest relevance is the fact that genetic alterations commonly associated with adenocarcinoma (*KRAS*, *EGFR*, *BRAF* mutations and *ALK* rearrangements) may be observed in LCC with a null immunophenotype {731,2464,2301,2303,2544, 1712,157,2045,1387,2462,441}. Gene expression profiling has also shown evidence of epithelial–mesenchymal transition as a frequent finding in LCCs, reflecting their poor differentiation compared with other NSCCs {2303,150}.

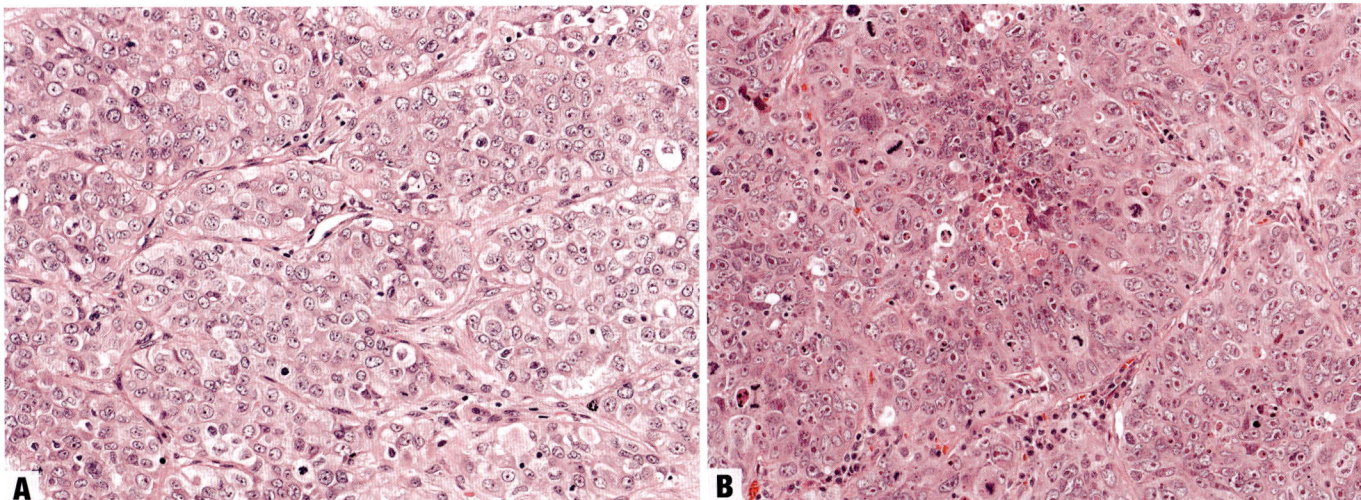

Fig. 1.94 Large cell carcinoma. **A** Undifferentiated non-small cell carcinoma with negative staining with TTF1 and p40, subsequently classified as large cell carcinoma with null phenotype. **B** Large cell carcinoma consisting of sheets/nests of large polygonal cells with prominent nucleoli and a moderate amount of cytoplasm.

Table 1.11 Immunohistochemical typing of cytokeratin-positive, undifferentiated non-small cell carcinoma (NSCC)

TTF1[a]	p40	Mucin stains	Diagnosis on resection	Diagnosis on biopsy / cell block / cytology
Positive (focal or diffuse)	Negative	Positive	Adenocarcinoma	NSCC, favour adenocarcinoma
Positive (focal or diffuse)	Positive (focal)	Positive	Adenocarcinoma	NSCC, favour adenocarcinoma
Negative	Positive (diffuse)	Negative	Squamous cell carcinoma	NSCC, favour squamous cell carcinoma
Negative	Negative	Negative	LCC	NSCC-NOS
Negative	Positive (focal)	Negative	LCC, unclear[b]	NSCC-NOS
No stain available	No stain available	Negative	LCC, with no additional stains[c]	NSCC-NOS (no stains available)

Diffuse, > 10% of positive tumour cells; focal, 1–10% of positive tumour cells; LCC, large cell carcinoma; NSCC, non-small cell carcinoma.
[a]Napsin A may be used as an alternative to TTF1.
[b]Negativity for TTF1 and focal positivity with p40 point to adenocarcinoma cell lineage once large cell neuroendocrine carcinoma is excluded.
[c]Sarcomatoid carcinoma and large cell neuroendocrine carcinoma should be excluded.

Macroscopic appearance

LCCs are usually large, circumscribed, solid masses, often with necrosis and rarely with cavitation.

Histopathology

LCC is a diagnosis of exclusion in a surgically resected NSCC with no clear-cut small cell carcinoma, SCC, or adenocarcinoma in addition to giant cell, spindle cell, or pleomorphic carcinoma on morphology or after immunohistochemistry and/or mucin stains. The tumour comprises sheets or nests of large polygonal cells with vesicular nuclei, prominent nucleoli, and moderate amounts of cytoplasm. Clear cell and/or rhabdoid cytological features may be present, and these should be documented in percentage increments within the LCC {2543,3082,3256,2758, 2301,2544,3064}.

Immunohistochemistry and histochemistry

Immunohistochemistry should be undertaken, unless not feasible for logistical reasons. In regard to sensitivity and specificity, the immunohistochemical markers of first choice to detect adenocarcinomatous and squamous cell differentiation are TTF1 and p40, respectively {2543,2483,2045,2464,2544,1712, 1387,2462,668,2463,1945,2774}. The diagnosis also requires mucin staining to be negative or show < 5 positive cells in two high-power fields (~0.4 mm^2). Cytokeratin staining should also be undertaken to confirm epithelial differentiation as required. Cases that are negative for TTF1 and p40 should be termed

"LCC (null immunophenotype)". If staining does not provide a clear answer (see Table 1.11), then cases should be termed "LCC (unclear immunophenotype)". If immunohistochemistry cannot be undertaken due to lack of available blocks or unstained slides, cases should be termed "LCC (additional stains unavailable)".

Differential diagnosis

The main differential diagnosis of LCC is presented in Table 1.12. Adenocarcinomas with a solid pattern, which stain with TTF1 (and/or napsin A), and non-keratinizing SCC, which stains with p40 (and/or CK5/6), require exclusion. Negative mucin stains are also needed to exclude solid adenocarcinoma with mucin. Most cases of adenosquamous carcinoma show morphological evidence of both lines of differentiation, but rare cases may show separate areas of TTF1 and p40 expression in a morphologically undifferentiated NSCC. Large cell neuroendocrine carcinoma (LCNEC) is excluded through recognition of neuroendocrine morphology and positive immunohistochemical staining for neuroendocrine markers (chromogranin, synaptophysin, and/or CD56). Neuroendocrine markers are not recommended on cases lacking neuroendocrine morphology. However, if a morphologically undifferentiated NSCC is stained and shows a profile of cytokeratin+, TTF1–, p40–, and neuroendocrine marker+, it should be termed "LCC with neuroendocrine differentiation (or LCC with neuroendocrine immunophenotype)" (see *Lung neuroendocrine neoplasms: Introduction*, p. 127) {2045, 2464,

Table 1.12 Subtyping of resected morphologically undifferentiated non-small cell carcinoma (formerly large cell carcinoma)

Tumour type	Immunohistochemistry findings
Adenocarcinoma, solid subtype[a]	Positive TTF1 and/or napsin A and/or mucin Negative (or focal staining in scattered tumour cells) p40, p63[b], CK5/6
Non-keratinizing squamous cell carcinoma[a]	Negative TTF1, napsin A, mucin Diffusely positive p40, p63[b], CK5/6
Adenosquamous carcinoma[a]	Positive adenosquamous and squamous markers in geographically distinct cell populations, each representing ≥ 10% of tumour cells
Large cell carcinoma (null immunophenotype)	Positive cytokeratins Negative lineage-specific markers
Large cell carcinoma (unclear immunophenotype)	Positive cytokeratins Unusual immunoprofiles

[a]In cases where there is morphological evidence of either squamous cell carcinoma or adenocarcinoma, immunohistochemistry is not needed to assess undifferentiated areas.
[b]p63 (4A4) can rarely be diffusely positive in some TTF1-positive tumours – these should be classified as adenocarcinomas.

2544, 1712, 1387, 2462, 668, 2463, 1945, 2774}. Rhabdoid cells sometimes raise the possibility of a carcinosarcoma showing areas of rhabdomyosarcomatous differentiation, but LCC with rhabdoid cytology is positive for cytokeratins and negative for desmin and myogenin {409,2748,2978}. The presence of rhabdoid morphology in a tumour resembling LCC should raise the consideration of thoracic SMARCA4-deficient undifferentiated tumour (see *Thoracic SMARCA4-deficient undifferentiated tumour*, p. 111). Cytokeratin positivity and other markers, as well as clinicoradiological correlation, are often needed, on a case-by-case basis, to exclude the possibility of extrathoracic unsuspected poorly differentiated carcinoma, lymphoma, melanoma, or mesothelioma. Metastatic carcinoma from elsewhere should be excluded, depending on patient sex and tumour morphology, on the basis of clinical correlation (see Chapter 9: *Metastases*). A tumour showing > 10% of pleomorphic features (spindle and/or giant cells) should be classified as a pleomorphic carcinoma.

Cytology

The diagnosis of LCC should not be rendered in cytological specimens. "NSCC-NOS" is the preferred terminology if clear-cut morphological or immunohistochemical differentiation is lacking. At cytology, the tumour cells have high-grade, overtly malignant cytological features, similar to those of other poorly differentiated NSCCs. Malignant cells with rhabdoid cytology show voluminous cytoplasm with eccentrically located nuclei and massive nucleoli. The presence of rhabdoid features on cytology is usually related to tumour cell discohesion {2680, 2978,1940,1101}.

Diagnostic molecular pathology

In tumours diagnosed as LCC on surgical resection but that relapse with advanced disease, molecular testing aimed at identification of targetable genetic therapy is recommended if it was not carried out at the time of initial surgical resection and diagnosis.

Essential and desirable diagnostic criteria

Essential:

- Undifferentiated NSCC, lacking any evidence of glandular, squamous cell, or neuroendocrine differentiation
- The diagnosis should only be rendered on surgical resection and cannot be made on small biopsy or cytology
- Negative immunohistochemistry with markers associated with adenocarcinoma (TTF1 or napsin A), SCC (p40 or CK5/6), and neuroendocrine carcinoma (NEC; only when there is neuroendocrine morphology as well as positive chromogranin, synaptophysin, CD56)

Desirable:

- If available, molecular analysis to look for genetic alterations that may guide therapy

Staging

Staging of LCC is similar to that of other NSCCs, according to the eighth-edition TNM classification {315}.

Prognosis and prediction

Like in other NSCCs, the prognosis is based on performance status at diagnosis, and the disease extension reflected by the TNM stage. Histopathological marker–null LCCs may be associated with inferior disease-free and overall survival compared with solid-predominant adenocarcinomas and non-keratinizing SCCs that would previously have been classified as LCC {2464}. Rhabdoid features are related to poorer prognosis (see *Thoracic SMARCA4-deficient undifferentiated tumour*, p. 111) {2680,2978,1940,1101}. Systemic therapy is similar to that used for other NSCCs. On the basis of the presence of predictive genetic abnormalities and PDL1 immunohistochemistry, tyrosine kinase inhibitors, single-agent immunotherapy, or chemoimmunotherapy combinations may be administered {2484,2308}.

Adenosquamous carcinoma of the lung

Moreira AL
MacMahon H
Mino-Kenudson M
Soo RA
Yatabe Y

Definition

Adenosquamous carcinoma is a carcinoma showing components of both squamous cell carcinoma (SCC) and adenocarcinoma, with each accounting for ≥ 10% of the tumour.

ICD-O coding

8560/3 Adenosquamous carcinoma

ICD-11 coding

2C25.Z & XH7873 Malignant neoplasms of bronchus or lung, unspecified & Adenosquamous carcinoma

Related terminology

None

Subtype(s)

None

Localization

Adenosquamous carcinoma usually forms a nodule, similar to other conventional non-small cell carcinomas (NSCCs) of the lung.

Clinical features

Patients with adenosquamous lung cancers present with manifestations similar to those of patients with other NSCCs (see *Tumours of the lung: Introduction*, p. 20); adenosquamous lung cancers are more commonly peripheral than central, and they have heterogeneous attenuation on contrast CT {3236,3452, 1646}. Peripheral tumours may show central scarring and spiculation or pleural indentation, and some may have a peripheral ground-glass opacity and air bronchogram {3236,1413}. None of these features are specific.

Epidemiology

Adenosquamous carcinoma is estimated to account for about 2–3% of all lung cancers, with little change over past decades {3206,2180,2645,3215}. Adenosquamous carcinoma has a male predominance, and the median age at presentation is about 65–67 years, similar to patients with other histological

subtypes {2959,3236,1760,569,3158,3483}. Adenosquamous carcinoma is associated with a history of smoking {3236,1760, 3483,1990,924}. It may, however, also occur in never-smokers, more often in women {3236}. Otherwise the epidemiology is similar to that of other non-small cell lung carcinomas (see *Tumours of the lung: Introduction*, p. 20).

Etiology

Adenosquamous carcinoma is associated with smoking, but like adenocarcinoma, it can also occur in never-smokers (see *Tumours of the lung: Introduction*, p. 20, and *Invasive non-mucinous adenocarcinoma of the lung*, p. 64).

Pathogenesis

Although adenosquamous carcinoma has morphologically distinct components, i.e. squamous and adenocarcinoma components, the two components share driver mutations, suggesting a clonally identical tumour {3158,3215,74}, not a collision of two different types of cancer. Two potential pathogenetic mechanisms have been proposed: multipotent tissue stem cell origin {1830} and transdifferentiation from either adenocarcinoma or SCC {1061,1511}.

Macroscopic appearance

Adenosquamous carcinomas appear as grey-tan irregular masses that arise either in the periphery {3236,3512} or centrally in the lungs {3236}. Peripheral tumours can be associated with pleural puckering. Cavitation can occur. Their gross pathological features are similar to those of other non-small cell lung carcinomas.

Histopathology

Adenosquamous carcinoma is composed of a mixture of variable proportions of adenocarcinoma and SCC components, with each accounting for ≥ 10% of the tumour. This can occur in four different ways, depending on whether the differentiation is detectable by H&E light microscopy and/or immunohistochemistry (see Table 1.13). Any histological pattern of adenocarcinoma can be seen in the adenocarcinoma component, and the squamous component can be of keratinizing or non-keratinizing

Table 1.13 Four combinations of adenocarcinoma and squamous cell carcinoma elements in adenosquamous carcinoma

Adenocarcinoma component	Squamous cell carcinoma component
Glandular morphology on H&E stain	Keratinizing squamous cell carcinoma on H&E stain
Glandular morphology on H&E stain	Non-keratinizing or basaloid squamous cell carcinoma requiring IHC (usually p40)
Solid-pattern adenocarcinoma requiring TTF1 IHC or mucin stains showing > 5 intracytoplasmic mucin droplets in at least two high-power fields	Keratinizing squamous cell carcinoma on H&E stain
Solid-pattern adenocarcinoma requiring TTF1 IHC or mucin stains showing > 5 intracytoplasmic mucin droplets in at least two high-power fields	Non-keratinizing or basaloid squamous cell carcinoma requiring IHC (usually p40)

IHC, immunohistochemistry.

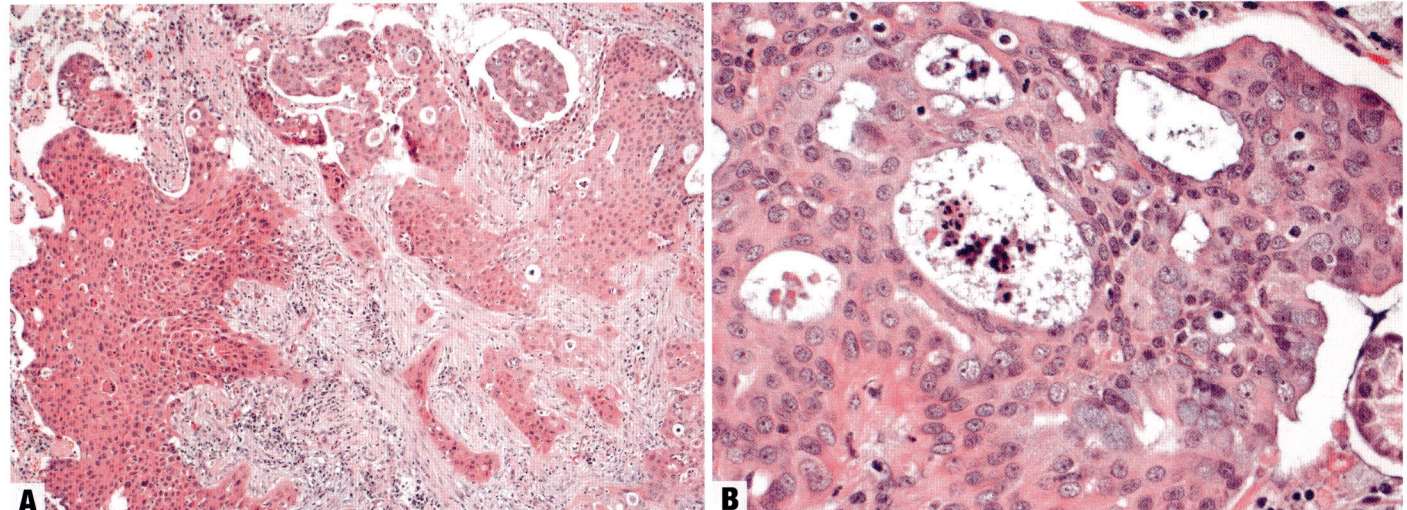

Fig. 1.95 Adenosquamous carcinoma. **A** This tumour contains two components: squamous cell carcinoma and adenocarcinoma. **B** This component shows adenocarcinoma with an acinar pattern and mucin production.

subtype. It is easier to diagnose adenosquamous cell carcinoma if well-differentiated components of each carcinoma are present. Diagnosis is more difficult if the tumour has a partly solid adenocarcinoma component or a non-keratinizing SCC component. Diagnosis is easier if the components are regionally discrete within the tumour, more difficult if they are merged and intermingled.

The criterion of 10% for each component is arbitrary, but if a minor component of adenocarcinoma that does not reach the threshold of 10% is present, it should be reported, because the tumour may carry actionable mutations regardless of the adenocarcinoma proportion {3215,2461,2252}. The identification of both components is dependent on the extent of histological sampling of the tumour. For tumours < 30 mm it is appropriate to sample the entire tumour and for larger tumours at least one section per 10 mm of tumour diameter. Definitive diagnosis requires a resection specimen, although it may be suggested on the basis of findings in small biopsies or cytology or excisional biopsies.

Immunohistochemistry

Each component shows the immunoprofile of conventional adenocarcinoma or SCC, respectively, although if the morphology is unequivocal on H&E stains, immunohistochemistry is not required for diagnosis. The best immunohistochemical marker for adenocarcinoma is TTF1 and for SCC p40. Because 10–20% of lung adenocarcinomas are TTF1-negative, positive mucin stains would be required to confirm adenocarcinoma differentiation in a solid, TTF1-negative component. It is not clear how to classify the exceptionally rare tumours where there is coexpression of TTF1 and p40 in the same tumour cells; however, these cases do not meet the current criteria for adenosquamous carcinoma {2832,2304,1103}. Some poorly differentiated, solid adenocarcinomas may focally express p40 as well as TTF1. An additional partly solid component with a null immunoprofile may exist in a tumour that is otherwise adenosquamous carcinoma, but its presence does not change the diagnosis.

The topic of NSCCs with adenocarcinoma and SCC components in small biopsies and/or cytology specimens is addressed in *Small diagnostic samples* (p. 29).

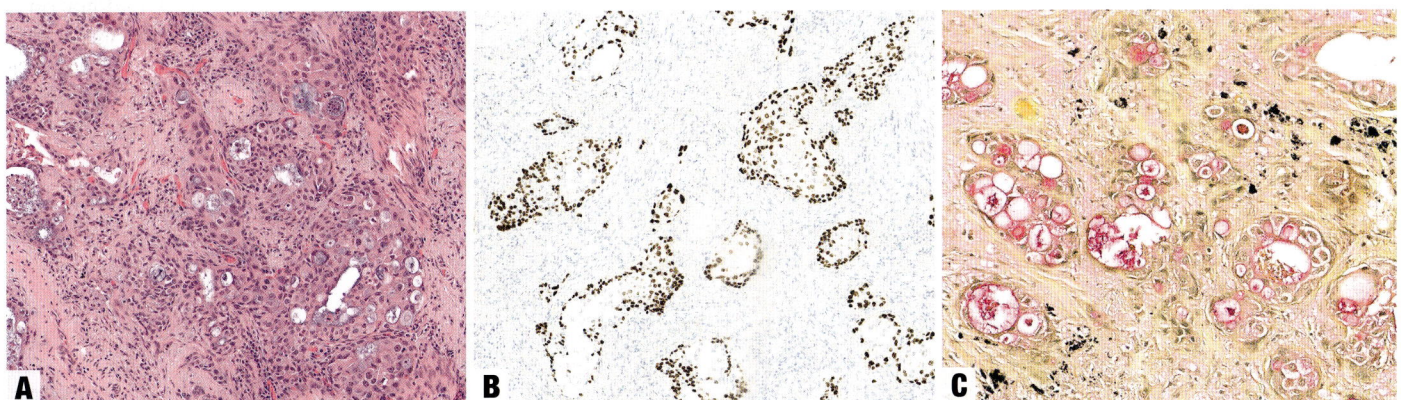

Fig. 1.96 Adenosquamous carcinoma with mucoepidermoid-like features. **A** This adenosquamous carcinoma has features resembling those of mucoepidermoid carcinoma. It contains squamous cell carcinoma as well as adenocarcinoma with prominent intracytoplasmic mucin. MAML1-negative. **B** p40 highlights the squamous cells, some of which are at the periphery of the tumour cell nests. **C** This mucin stain highlights the abundant mucin-producing adenocarcinoma component.

Differential diagnosis

The differential diagnosis includes SCC, adenocarcinoma, high-grade mucoepidermoid carcinoma, and reactive non-neoplastic lesions. When SCCs or adenocarcinomas have an extensive solid (undifferentiated) component, it can be useful to perform TTF1 and/or a mucin stain or p40 to investigate whether this may represent a second component, thus qualifying for adenosquamous carcinoma. If this solid component is negative for all of these markers, the tumour should be classified according to the glandular or keratinizing squamous component. In addition, entrapped TTF1-positive pneumocytes and squamous metaplasia of entrapped bronchiolar structures should be differentiated from a possible adenosquamous carcinoma component. A distinction should be made from morules or morule-like components that can be seen in association with papillary-pattern adenocarcinoma {3103}, and immunohistochemical stains are particularly important to differentiate from mimics, such as solid-type adenocarcinoma with squamoid features {1341,2461} and pseudogland formation in SCC {3440,2430}.

Mucoepidermoid carcinoma, in particular high-grade type, constitutes a major differential diagnosis for adenosquamous carcinoma. Mucoepidermoid carcinoma more often shows (1) a characteristic mixed cellular composition of mucinous, squamoid, and intermediate cells; (2) a proximal exophytic endobronchial location; (3) areas of classic low-grade mucoepidermoid carcinoma; (4) a lack of keratinization or squamous pearl formation; (5) no overlying SCC in situ {3443,2614}; and (6) absence of a tubular, acinar, and papillary growth pattern. A lack of TTF1 in a mucoepidermoid carcinoma may also be useful for differential diagnosis {2742}. MAML2 rearrangement is exclusively seen in mucoepidermoid carcinoma {12}. Rare adenosquamous carcinomas have morphological overlap with mucoepidermoid carcinomas in that they have a squamous component with cells positive for p63 or p40 at the periphery of tumour cell nests and a mucin-producing adenocarcinoma component showing a cribriform or tubular pattern that lacks TTF1 or napsin A, and MAML2 rearrangement {3367}. Some of these tumours have ALK rearrangements {1212}.

Cytology

The cytological diagnosis of adenosquamous carcinoma can be suggested only when both components have been sampled abundantly. Such instances are, however, rare; most samples from true adenosquamous carcinoma contain only one of the components, and a smaller component, if present, may be overlooked or misinterpreted as a reactive process. In small biopsy/cytology specimens, the diagnosis of SCC in a never-smoker should at least raise for consideration the possibility of adenosquamous carcinoma. The diagnosis of each component, if present, follows the same criteria as for their monotypic counterparts.

Diagnostic molecular pathology

The genetic characteristics of adenosquamous carcinoma are intermediate between those of adenocarcinoma and SCC; thus, adenosquamous carcinoma does not have definite diagnostic molecular findings. Adenosquamous carcinoma may harbour gene rearrangements in ALK {3215,429}, ROS1 {3422}, or RET {3215,3214}; gene mutations in EGFR {3215,2004}, KRAS {3215}, AKT1 {3215}, ERBB2 (HER2) {3215,3049}, PIK3CA {3215}, or STK11 (LKB1) {1502}; or FGFR1 amplification {2385}.

Essential and desirable diagnostic criteria

Essential:
- A tumour with distinct cell populations of adenocarcinoma and SCC, each accounting for ≥ 10% of tumour cells
- Immunohistochemistry and/or mucin stains are required when the tumour contains a non-keratinizing or basaloid squamous component (i.e. p40) or a solid adenocarcinoma component (i.e. TTF1 or mucin stains)

Desirable:
- Exclusion of mucoepidermoid carcinoma and other mimics with immunohistochemistry and molecular testing
- Molecular testing for lung adenocarcinoma driver mutations may be useful

Staging

Staging of adenosquamous carcinoma is similar to that of other NSCCs, according to the eighth-edition TNM classification {315}.

Prognosis and prediction

Adenosquamous carcinoma has aggressive biology, with a poorer prognosis reported compared with other non-small cell lung carcinoma histological subtypes; the 5-year survival rate following surgical resection has been reported to be 37–60% {569,1990,2645}. The predominant component within individual tumours has not been shown to affect prognosis {3236,1760}. Prediction of response to molecular targeted therapy in patients with advanced adenosquamous carcinoma is based on the presence of the same genetic abnormalities found in lung adenocarcinomas.

Pleomorphic carcinoma of the lung

Rossi G
Boland JM
Pelosi G
Roden AC

Definition

Pleomorphic carcinoma is a poorly differentiated non-small cell lung carcinoma (non-small cell carcinoma [NSCC], including adenocarcinoma, squamous cell carcinoma [SCC], and/or large cell carcinoma [LCC]) containing at least a 10% component of spindle and/or giant cells, or a carcinoma that consists entirely of spindle and/or neoplastic giant cells. The definitive diagnosis of pleomorphic carcinoma may be rendered only in surgical specimens.

ICD-O coding

8022/3 Pleomorphic carcinoma

ICD-11 coding

2C25.Y & XH35G0 Other specified malignant neoplasms of bronchus or lung & Pleomorphic carcinoma
2C25.Y & XH3RZ4 Other specified malignant neoplasms of bronchus or lung & Spindle cell carcinoma, NOS
2C25.Y & XH1JZ2 Other specified malignant neoplasms of bronchus or lung & Giant cell carcinoma

Related terminology

Acceptable: "sarcomatoid carcinoma" is an overarching term that encompasses pleomorphic carcinoma, carcinosarcoma, and pulmonary blastoma.
Not recommended: monophasic or biphasic carcinomas, with or without heterologous components; metaplastic carcinomas (obsolete).

Subtype(s)

Pleomorphic carcinoma; giant cell carcinoma; spindle cell carcinoma

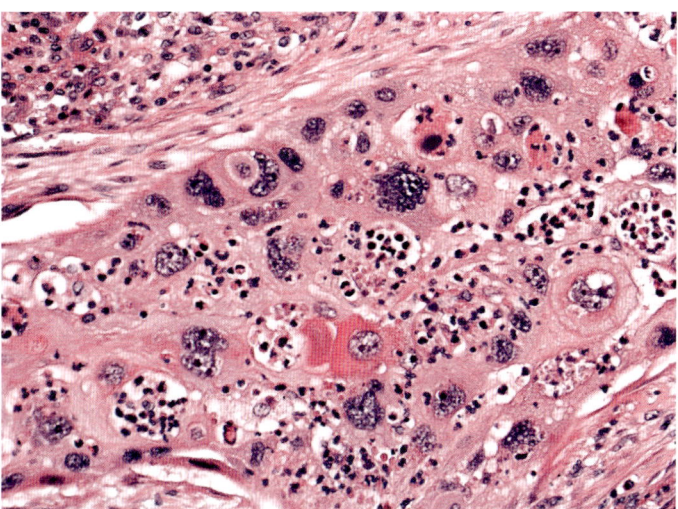

Fig. 1.97 Pleomorphic carcinoma. Histology shows tumour giant cells and neutrophil emperipolesis.

Localization

Pleomorphic carcinoma is more prevalent in the right lung and upper lobes, and it is frequently peripheral with invasion of the chest wall {2542,839,2316,2305}. An endobronchial location is uncommon {839,2316,2542}.

Clinical features

The signs and symptoms of pleomorphic carcinoma are similar to those of other NSCCs (see *Tumours of the lung: Introduction*, p. 20). Presenting symptoms include cough, pain, haemoptysis, and dyspnoea {1454,1781,3259}. Imaging shows a large central or peripheral mass, usually in the upper lobe, showing

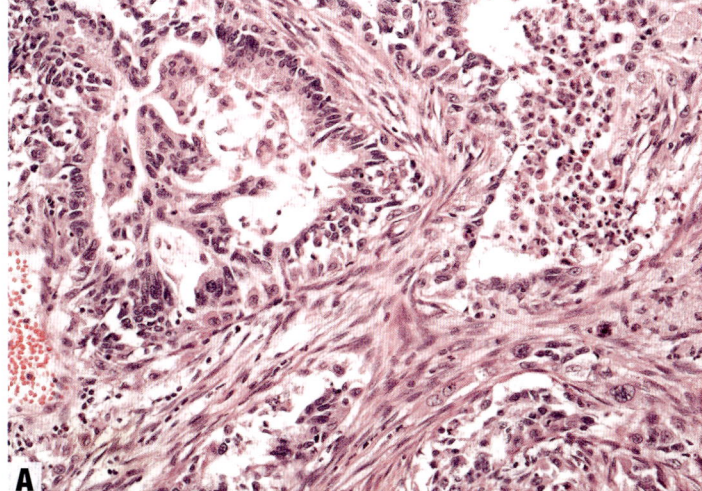
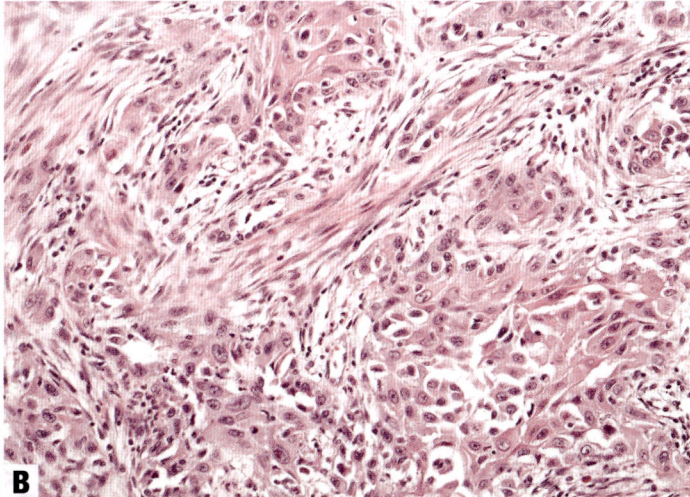

Fig. 1.98 Pleomorphic carcinoma. **A** There is an adenocarcinoma component closely intermingled with a spindle cell carcinoma. **B** Pleomorphic carcinoma consisting of a squamous cell carcinoma component closely intermingled with a spindle cell carcinoma.

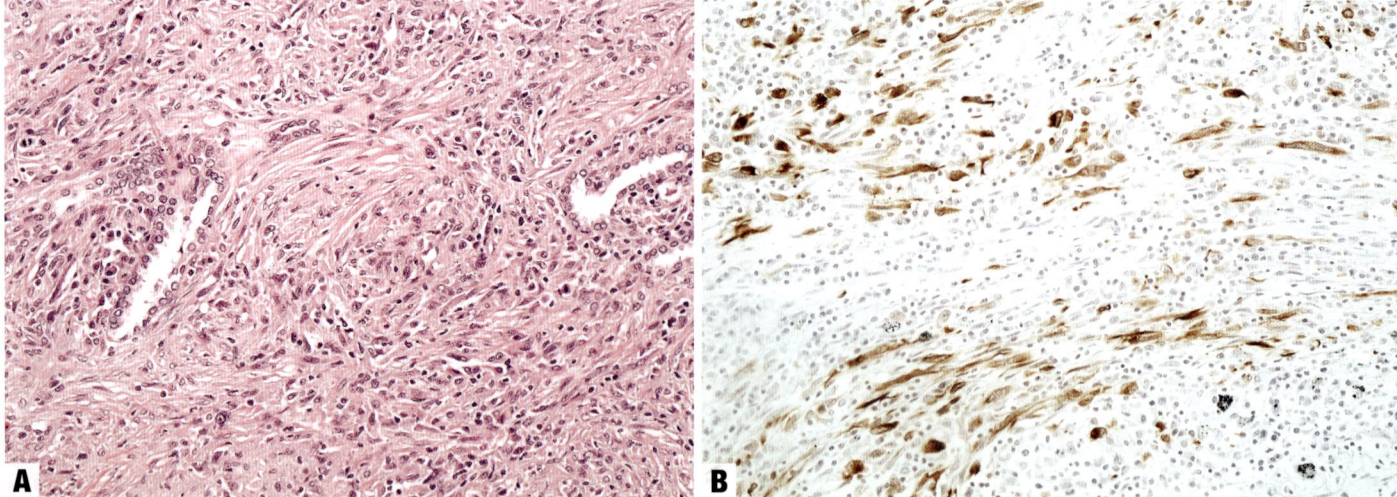

Fig. 1.99 Spindle cell carcinoma. **A** The tumour shows entrapping alveolar structures with hyperplastic pneumocytes. The tumour is positive for pancytokeratins (**B**) and TTF1 (not shown).

low-attenuation central necrosis, frequent pleural invasion, ill-defined borders with a ground-glass halo, and intense PET avidity {1454,1453,3347,2435}.

Epidemiology

These tumours account for 2–3% of all NSCC cases in surgical series, but they constitute < 1% in epidemiological studies {2790,3401,839,1948}. Peak incidence is in the seventh decade of life (age range: 29–83 years), with male predominance {3401, 1942,2773,2542}. The majority of the patients are current or former smokers {3401,1781,3259}.

Etiology

Active and heavy exposure to cigarette smoke is the main etiological factor. Lung cancer carcinogens such as asbestos, radon, and other chemical agents have also been implicated (see *Tumours of the lung: Introduction*, p. 20) {123}.

Pathogenesis

The mesenchymal-like or sarcomatoid component of pleomorphic carcinoma is thought to derive from carcinoma cells through activation of a stable epithelial–mesenchymal transition programme {2316,2305,2460}. The sarcomatoid phenotype may be lost at metastatic sites through reverse mesenchymal–epithelial transition {2316}. *MET* mutations leading to exon 14 skipping might play a causative role {1714,2316,3181,2460}.

Macroscopic appearance

Pleomorphic carcinomas are usually well-circumscribed masses with a grey-white and sometimes gelatinous cut surface, with a mean diameter of 50 mm (range: 10–180 mm). Some tumours have central necrosis and/or cavitation {3410,2046,1942,1948}. They often invade the chest wall or mediastinum {446}.

Histopathology

Pleomorphic carcinoma is composed of ≥ 10% spindle and/or giant cells admixed with components of adenocarcinoma (31–72% of cases), SCC (12–26%), or LCC (up to 43%) {2542,2305, 2316}. Some tumours are composed only of spindle cells and/or tumour giant cells. The epithelial and spindle/giant cells may

be intimately admixed or sharply demarcated from one another. When present, adenocarcinoma, SCC, or LCC components should be mentioned in the pathology report (e.g. "pleomorphic carcinoma with adenocarcinoma"). Sometimes, osteoclast-type giant cells are scattered throughout the tumour, and these may be keratin-negative and positive for macrophage markers {2316, 247}. Variable amounts of stroma are present in pleomorphic carcinoma, which may be collagenous or myxoid. Necrosis, haemorrhage, and vascular invasion are common. Pleomorphic carcinoma may exhibit spread through airspaces {3410}. Giant cell carcinoma consists solely of highly pleomorphic giant cells with multiple irregular, sometimes multilobate nuclei and abundant eosinophilic to granular cytoplasm with frequent leukocyte emperipolesis. Spindle cell carcinoma consists solely of neoplastic spindled cells of variable morphology, lacking differentiated elements. The elongated tumour cells may be markedly atypical or deceptively bland, featuring fascicular or storiform growth along with variable chronic inflammation sometimes resembling inflammatory myofibroblastic tumour {2542,3303}. The approach to tumours with these features found in small biopsies and cytology specimens is discussed in *Small diagnostic samples* (p. 29) {2313,2315,150}.

Immunohistochemistry

Immunohistochemistry is helpful to highlight the different cell components. The NSCC components are usually positive for pancytokeratin while the spindle and giant cell components are variably reactive or negative for pancytokeratin {2316,2305, 2310}. In some cases, multiple keratins may be needed to confirm epithelial differentiation. Other lineage markers, such as napsin A, TTF1, or p40, are variably expressed depending on the direction of differentiation and are usually more prominent in the NSCC component, if present {150,2310,2305,2316}.

Differential diagnosis

The differential diagnosis includes carcinosarcoma, pulmonary blastoma, metastatic sarcomatoid carcinoma from various sites (breast, gastrointestinal tract, bladder, uterus, ovary), sarcoma (synovial sarcoma, epithelioid haemangioendothelioma, myxoid sarcoma, rhabdomyosarcoma), inflammatory myofibroblastic tumour, germ cell tumours, melanoma, dendritic cell sarcoma, and biphasic/sarcomatoid mesothelioma {150,2316}. If definite adenocarcinoma, SCC, or LCC components are present, even if keratins are completely negative in the spindle and/or giant cell component, the tumour is regarded as pleomorphic carcinoma, because malignant heterologous elements such as osteosarcoma, chondrosarcoma, or rhabdomyosarcoma are needed to diagnose carcinosarcoma (see *Carcinosarcoma of the lung*, p. 109). In contrast to the conventional adenocarcinoma morphology of pleomorphic carcinoma, the adenocarcinoma component of pulmonary blastoma should show endometrioid morphology (see *Pulmonary blastoma*, p. 106). Strong diffuse positivity for GATA3 may support the diagnosis of sarcomatoid/desmoplastic mesothelioma over pleomorphic carcinoma, but it is not entirely specific {213}. Infrequently, reactive fibrotic processes (i.e. organizing pneumonia, scar, etc.) may also enter the differential diagnosis of bland-looking spindle cell carcinoma with prominent inflammation {560,84}. If tumours with spindle and/or giant cell components have components of small cell lung carcinoma or large cell neuroendocrine carcinoma (LCNEC), rather than pleomorphic carcinoma, the tumours should be classified as combined small cell lung carcinoma or LCNEC with mention of the additional histological components.

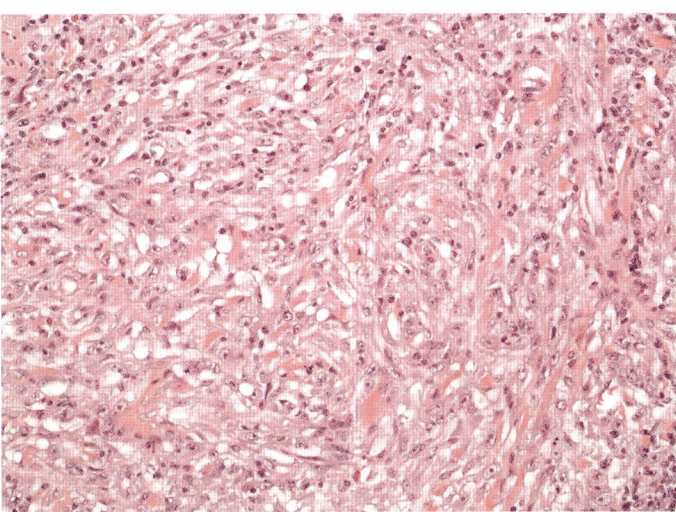

Fig. 1.100 Inflammatory-type spindle cell carcinoma. Inflammatory-type spindle cell carcinoma with atypical spindle-shaped cells intermingled with inflammatory infiltrate.

Cytology
On cytology, the neoplastic cells are discohesive, enlarged, and highly pleomorphic, with prominent eosinophilic cytoplasm and evident nucleoli. A background of necrotic debris, inflammatory infiltrate, and myxoid or collagen-rich stroma is often noted {1208,513,172}.

Diagnostic molecular pathology
Genetic events mirror those found in other NSCCs, particularly pulmonary adenocarcinoma {3022,795,2679}. Complex chromosomal abnormalities and *TP53* mutations are common {3022,795,244,1792}. The frequency of *KRAS* and *EGFR* mutations is similar to pulmonary adenocarcinoma, when patient ethnicity and smoking history are taken into account {3022, 1313,1714,795}. *ALK* rearrangements rarely occur {3022}. *MET* exon 14 skipping mutations are present in a subset {1572,1714, 1792}. Pleomorphic carcinomas have a high incidence of PDL1 expression (60–90%), which is often stronger in the sarcomatoid areas {2058,1450,3347,1724,2679}.

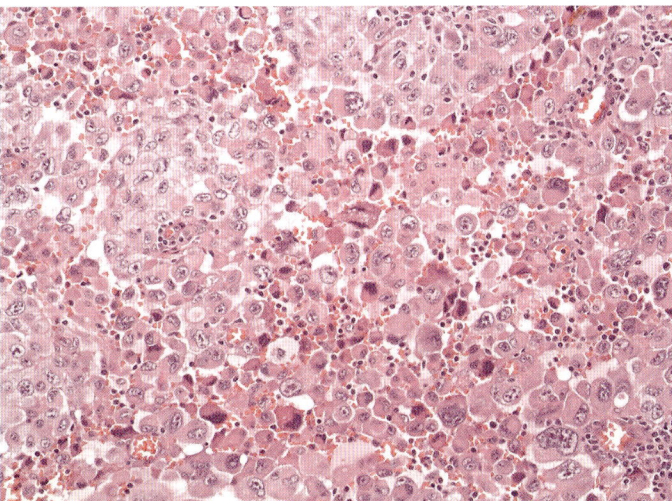

Fig. 1.101 Giant cell carcinoma. Giant cell carcinoma with discohesive, large tumour cells showing emperipolesis.

Essential and desirable diagnostic criteria
Essential:
- Resection specimen showing NSCC including adenocarcinoma, SCC, and/or LCC, composed of ≥ 10% spindled and/or tumour giant cells or a carcinoma consisting entirely of spindle and giant cells
- Spindle cell carcinoma consists purely of malignant spindle cells
- Giant cell carcinoma consists purely of malignant giant cells with or without multinucleated giant cells

Staging
Staging of pleomorphic carcinoma is similar to that of other NSCCs, according to the eighth-edition TNM classification {315}.

Prognosis and prediction
Pleomorphic carcinoma has a worse outcome than other NSCCs. The 5-year survival rate is stage-dependent {1118}, and the reported 5-year overall survival rate is 25–68% {2046,3401, 1948,1722}. Metastases occur in the lungs, bone, brain, pleura, liver, thoracic and neck lymph nodes, adrenal glands, and (rarely) gastrointestinal tract and skin {1948}. Worse outcome has been associated with older age, comorbidities, higher T and N stages, vascular invasion, and spread through airspaces {3401,1942,471,3410,1722}. Tumours with *MET* exon 14 skipping mutations may respond to tyrosine kinase inhibitors {2307,1714,2242A,3333A}.

Pulmonary blastoma

Nakatani Y
Boland JM

Definition

Pulmonary blastoma is a biphasic tumour that consists of low-grade fetal adenocarcinoma / well-differentiated fetal adenocarcinoma and primitive mesenchymal stroma. Foci of specific mesenchymal differentiation (osteosarcoma, chondrosarcoma, or rhabdomyosarcoma) may also be present but are not required for the diagnosis.

ICD-O coding

8972/3 Pulmonary blastoma

ICD-11 coding

2C25.Y & XH5VH1 Other specified malignant neoplasms of bronchus or lung & Pulmonary blastoma

Related terminology

None

Subtype(s)

None

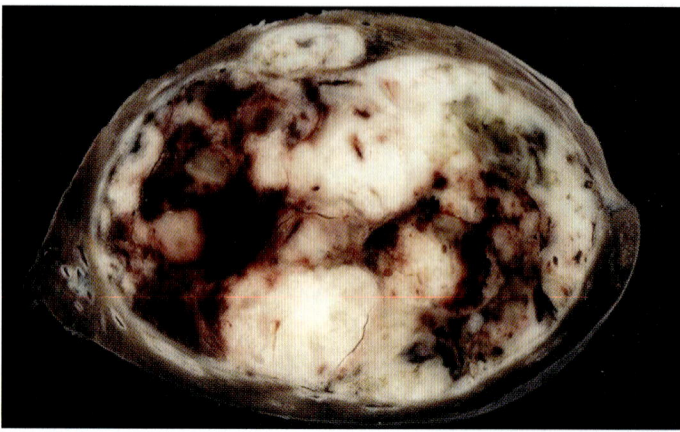

Fig. 1.102 Pulmonary blastoma. Gross photo. A white to greyish large mass with extensive haemorrhage and necrosis.

Localization

Pulmonary blastomas are more common in the peripheral lung. Despite the similar name, they are a completely separate entity from pleuropulmonary blastoma (see *Pleuropulmonary blastoma*, p. 160).

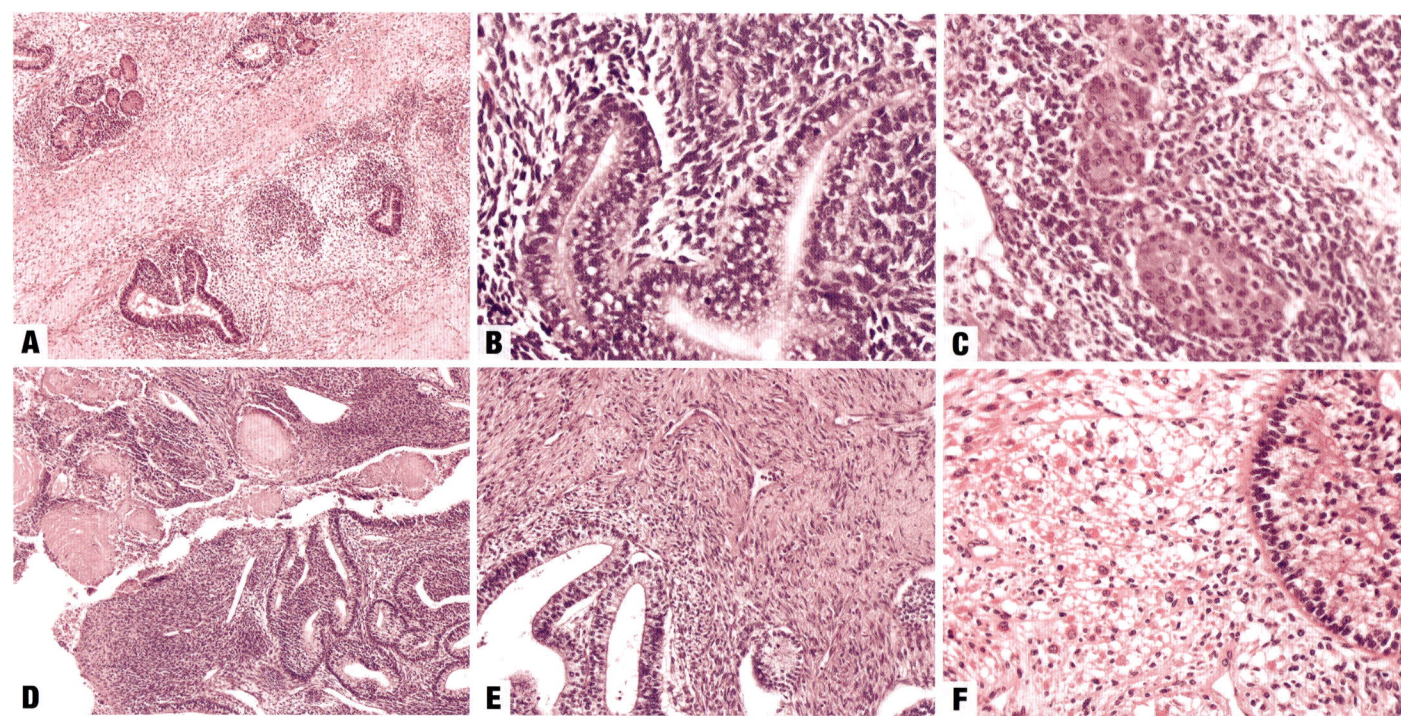

Fig. 1.103 Pulmonary blastoma. **A** Low magnification, showing scattered glands with endometrioid appearance and mesenchymal cells of various densities and maturation. **B** High magnification, showing the low-grade fetal adenocarcinoma / well-differentiated fetal adenocarcinoma component and closely packed blastemal cells. **C** Morule-like structures surrounded by primitive blastemal cells. **D** Foci resembling the so-called wet keratin of craniopharyngioma may be present. **E** Broad area of relatively mature fibroblastic cells associated with collagen, admixed with the low-grade fetal adenocarcinoma / well-differentiated fetal adenocarcinoma component. **F** The stroma may show scattered rhabdomyoblastic cells with eosinophilic cytoplasm.

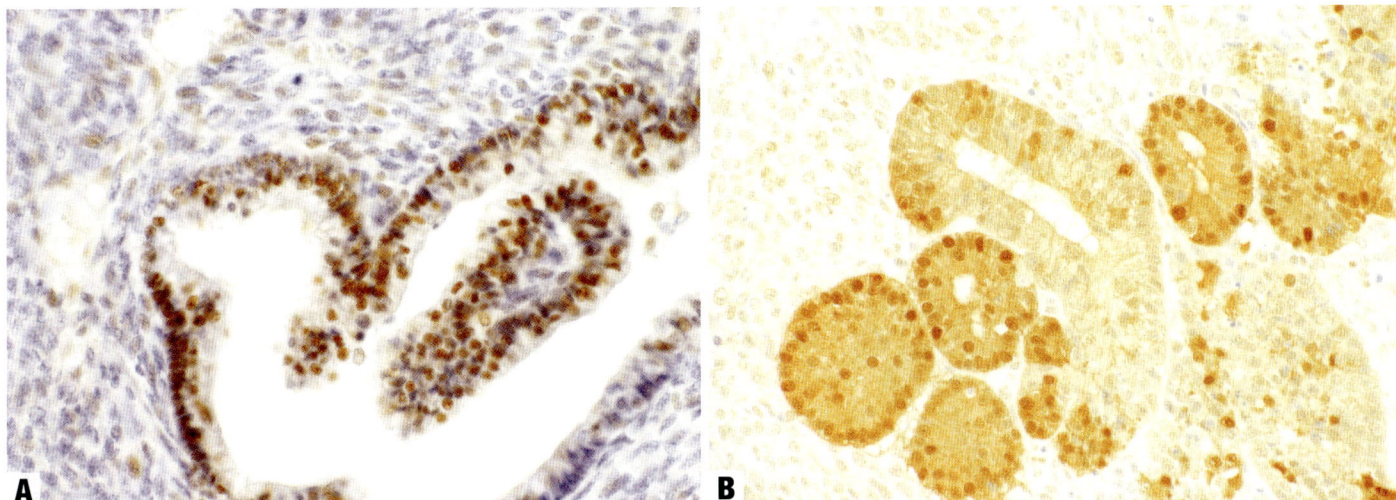

Fig. 1.104 Pulmonary blastoma. **A** The epithelial component expresses TTF1. **B** Note the predominantly nuclear/cytoplasmic localization of β-catenin.

Clinical features

The signs, symptoms, and imaging are similar to those of other non-small cell lung carcinomas (see *Tumours of the lung: Introduction*, p. 20). Cough, pain, and haemoptysis are common presenting symptoms {1523}. On imaging, pulmonary blastomas typically appear as well-demarcated large masses. Pulmonary blastomas are aggressive and may extend to the mediastinum or show intrapulmonary metastases {2426,96}. Lymph node involvement is relatively uncommon (~10%) at presentation {1523}.

Epidemiology

Pulmonary blastoma is a very rare subtype of sarcomatoid carcinoma, constituting < 0.1% of resected lung cancers {2542}. These tumours are most common in the fourth to fifth decades of life, without obvious sex predilection, and they rarely occur in children {1523,470}.

Etiology

Smoking is an important risk factor {1523}.

Pathogenesis

Pulmonary blastomas frequently harbour missense mutations in exon 3 of *CTNNB1*, leading to activation of the WNT pathway through aberrant nuclear localization of β-catenin protein, which may be detected by immunohistochemistry {1755,2065, 2306,2702}. Similar mutations are observed in low-grade fetal adenocarcinoma / well-differentiated fetal adenocarcinoma {2702,2064}. *TP53* mutations also occur in pulmonary blastoma {249,2306,1174}. Other gene alterations that occur in pulmonary adenocarcinomas (*ROS1*, *EGFR*) can also be observed in combination with *CTNNB1* mutation in pulmonary blastoma {1302,1755}. Some adult cases of pulmonary blastoma harbour somatic *DICER1* mutations coupled with *CTNNB1* mutations, indicating a potential genetic link to paediatric pleuropulmonary blastoma {629}.

Macroscopic appearance

Tumours are generally large, averaging 100 mm in diameter {1523}. The tumour is typically a peripheral, well-demarcated solid mass with a variegated grey, white, yellow, and/or pink appearance. Necrosis and haemorrhage are common.

Histopathology

Pulmonary blastoma shows a biphasic pattern including branching glandular structures and primitive mesenchymal cells. The tumour may show extensive intermingling of these two components or may be composite with areas of solely epithelial differentiation. The glandular structures consist of pseudostratified columnar cells with relatively small, uniform, round to oval nuclei and clear to slightly eosinophilic cytoplasm, resembling endometrioid carcinoma {1523,3446,2065}. The cells may demonstrate subnuclear cytoplasmic vacuoles, reminiscent of secretory endometrium. Morule formation is seen in about 40% of cases {1523}. Focal keratinization is rarely observed {3446, 2065}. These features are essentially identical to those of low-grade fetal adenocarcinoma / well-differentiated fetal adenocarcinoma {1523,2065,150}. One third to half of cases display areas of high-grade progression with more atypical glands resembling conventional adenocarcinoma or poorly differentiated sheet-like growth {1523,150}. The mesenchymal component shows closely packed primitive, oval to spindle-shaped, small blastema-like cells, with various amounts of more mature and loosely arranged fibroblast-like cells in gradual transition with the blastemal cells. The mesenchymal cells may focally show bizarre nuclei. Foci of immature striated muscle, cartilage, and bone are observed in 25% {1523}. Rare cases with unusual differentiation have been reported, including elements of various germ cell tumours, small cell carcinoma, and melanoma {2769,96,554}.

Immunohistochemistry

The epithelial component shows an immunophenotype identical to that of low-grade fetal adenocarcinoma / well-differentiated fetal adenocarcinoma, with expression of keratin (AE1/AE3, CAM5.2, CK7), EMA, and TTF1 {3446,913,2068}. Neuroendocrine markers are commonly expressed in scattered cells. The mesenchymal component expresses vimentin, and tissue-specific antigens such as S100 and desmin are expressed in chondrosarcomatous and rhabdomyosarcomatous elements,

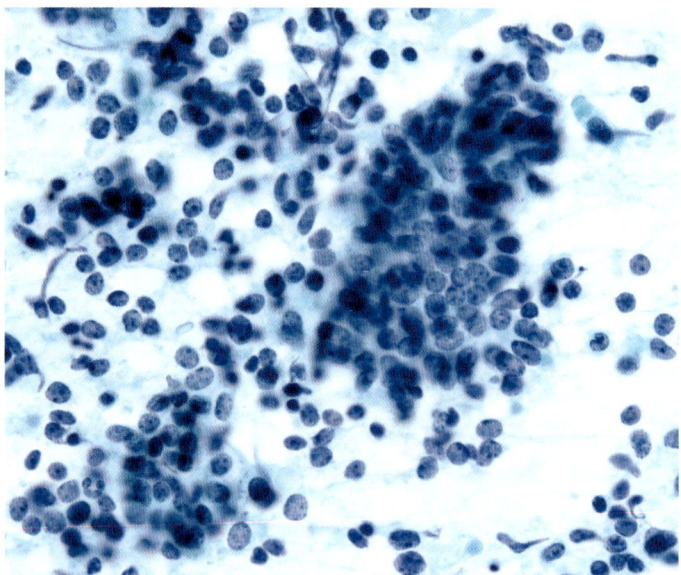

Fig. 1.105 Pulmonary blastoma. Cytological smear. Note clusters of epithelial cells with regular round to oval nuclei and scattered, isolated cells with small bare nuclei.

respectively. Glandular elements, morules, and blastema show cytoplasmic and nuclear expression of β-catenin.

Differential diagnosis

The differential diagnosis includes fetal adenocarcinoma {2475}, carcinosarcoma {2065,1521,1401,2605}, pleomorphic carcinoma, and even endometriosis. Carcinosarcoma with an adenocarcinoma component resembling high-grade fetal adenocarcinoma may be easily mistaken for pulmonary blastoma; careful examination of morphology (high-grade atypia and absence of morules) and immunohistochemistry (predominantly membranous expression of β-catenin and absence/reduction of TTF1 expression), as well as genetic analysis (no *CTNNB1* mutation), may be useful in this distinction {2065,1401,1755}.

Cytology

Cytological smears are highly cellular, with two cell types {577, 1765}; there are loosely cohesive or singly scattered oval to spindle cells with uniform nuclei, fine chromatin, and indistinct nucleoli, as well as slightly larger round to ovoid or columnar epithelial cells with cyanophilic or amphophilic cytoplasm in cohesive clusters. The nuclear features of the two cell types are very similar.

Diagnostic molecular pathology

Pulmonary blastomas frequently harbour missense mutations in exon 3 of *CTNNB1*; this may be helpful in diagnosis and is the cause of aberrant nuclear localization of β-catenin protein, which may be detected by immunohistochemistry {1755,2065, 2306,2702}.

Essential and desirable diagnostic criteria

Essential:
- Biphasic morphology including low-grade fetal adenocarcinoma / well-differentiated fetal adenocarcinoma and primitive mesenchymal stroma

Desirable:
- Expression of TTF1 and nuclear/cytoplasmic localization of β-catenin in the fetal adenocarcinoma component
- *CTNNB1* mutation
- Malignant heterologous elements such as osteosarcoma, chondrosarcoma, or rhabdomyosarcoma may be present

Staging

Staging of pulmonary blastoma is similar to that of other non-small cell carcinomas, according to the eighth-edition TNM classification {315}.

Prognosis and prediction

Distant metastases and tumour recurrence are common and prognosis is poor, which correlates with stage {1523}. Death rates are especially high within 2 years after initial treatment {1523}. No predictive factors have been identified.

Carcinosarcoma of the lung

Borczuk AC
Dacic S

Definition
Carcinosarcoma is a malignant tumour consisting of non-small cell carcinoma (NSCC) components (usually squamous carcinoma or adenocarcinoma) combined with at least one sarcomatous heterologous element such as rhabdomyosarcoma, chondrosarcoma, or osteosarcoma.

ICD-O coding
8980/3 Carcinosarcoma

ICD-11 coding
2C25.Y & XH2W45 Other specified malignant neoplasms of bronchus or lung & Carcinosarcoma, NOS

Related terminology
Not recommended: heterologous sarcomatoid carcinoma; biphasic sarcomatoid carcinoma.

Subtype(s)
None

Localization
Tumours are central (most commonly), endobronchial, or peripheral.

Clinical features
Patients with carcinosarcoma may present with cough. Haemoptysis is reported for central tumours, and chest wall pain for peripheral tumours {1521,2542}. Imaging is similar to that for other NSCCs (see *Tumours of the lung: Introduction*, p. 20). It typically shows a large, inhomogeneous tumour with contrast enhancement, necrosis, and occasionally calcification {1448}. Most patients (> 75%) have more than locoregional disease at presentation {781}.

Epidemiology
Carcinosarcomas are rare tumours representing < 0.2% of lung cancers {620}. They are more common in males than females (M:F ratio: 7:1) {1521}. They occur at a median age of 65 years, with a range similar to that seen with other NSCCs {781,3266, 1521,620,2542}.

Etiology
Most patients are either current or former heavy smokers {1521, 2542}.

Pathogenesis
Equivalent allelic loss {600} and oncogenic *EGFR* mutations in the two components support that these tumours arise from a single clonal origin {1490,3058}. From a molecular perspective, these tumours are carcinomas with heterologous sarcomatous

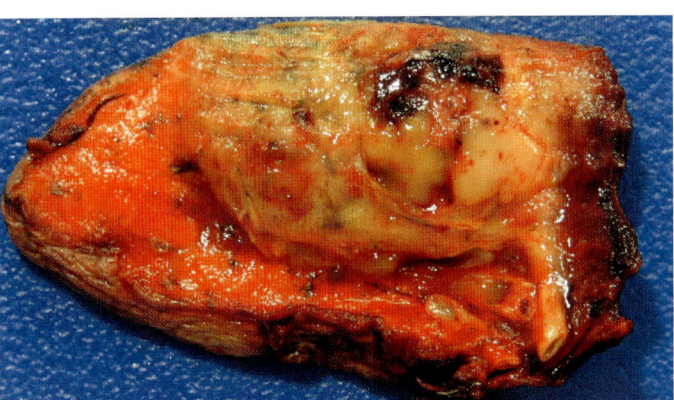

Fig. 1.106 Carcinosarcoma. Gross photograph showing heterogeneous cut surface with areas of fish-flesh appearance, haemorrhage, and umbilication

differentiation. *TP53* mutations are described {1174,1490,2652}, but *KRAS* mutations less frequently {1174}; however, these rare tumours more often contain squamous carcinoma than adenocarcinoma.

Macroscopic appearance
Tumours are often bulky, with necrotic and haemorrhagic areas {1521}.

Histopathology
These biphasic tumours are primarily carcinomas containing histological elements of both carcinoma and sarcoma, the latter demonstrating specific heterologous elements. A minimum proportion for the minority component is not described. Carcinomatous components include squamous cell carcinoma most commonly, followed by adenocarcinoma and large cell carcinoma {1521}. Small cell carcinoma and large cell neuroendocrine carcinoma (LCNEC) are rare in tumours with heterologous elements {2129} and should be classified as combined small cell carcinoma or LCNEC, not carcinosarcoma.

The sarcomatous component includes rhabdomyosarcoma, chondrosarcoma, and osteosarcoma {2804,299}, alone or in combination, and rarely liposarcoma {1473} or angiosarcoma {333}. These components are distinctive in H&E-stained sections by light microscopy, but they may require extensive sampling to be identified. Heterologous elements distinguish carcinosarcoma from pleomorphic carcinoma.

High-grade fetal-type or clear cell adenocarcinoma with heterologous elements and lacking the molecular features of blastoma has been described as "blastomatoid variant of carcinosarcoma"; however, the term "blastomatoid" is not encouraged, because it could lead to confusion with pulmonary blastoma {2065,2605}. The diagnosis of carcinosarcoma should be rendered with a comment about which specific epithelial and sarcomatous elements are present.

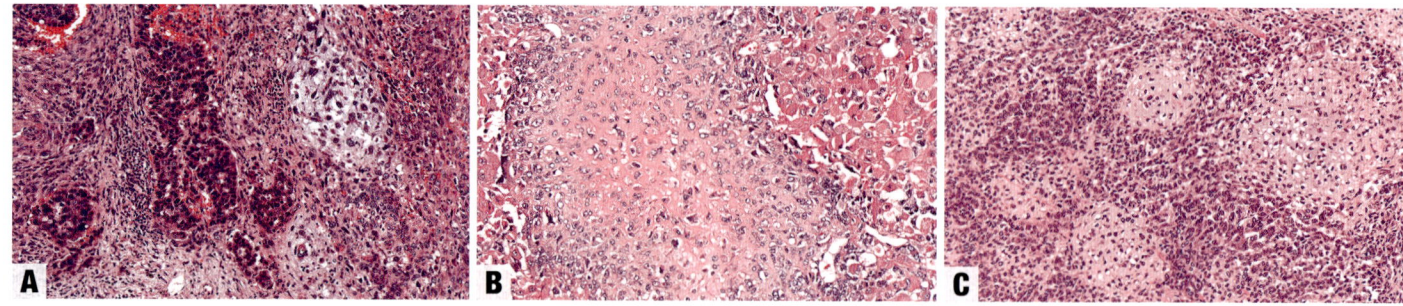

Fig. 1.107 Carcinosarcoma. **A** Poorly differentiated adenocarcinoma alongside an immature matrix-producing cartilaginous focus. **B** Histological image focused on heterologous elements in a carcinosarcoma, with cartilaginous and rhabdomyosarcomatous elements. **C** This tumour has components of large cell carcinoma and chondrosarcoma.

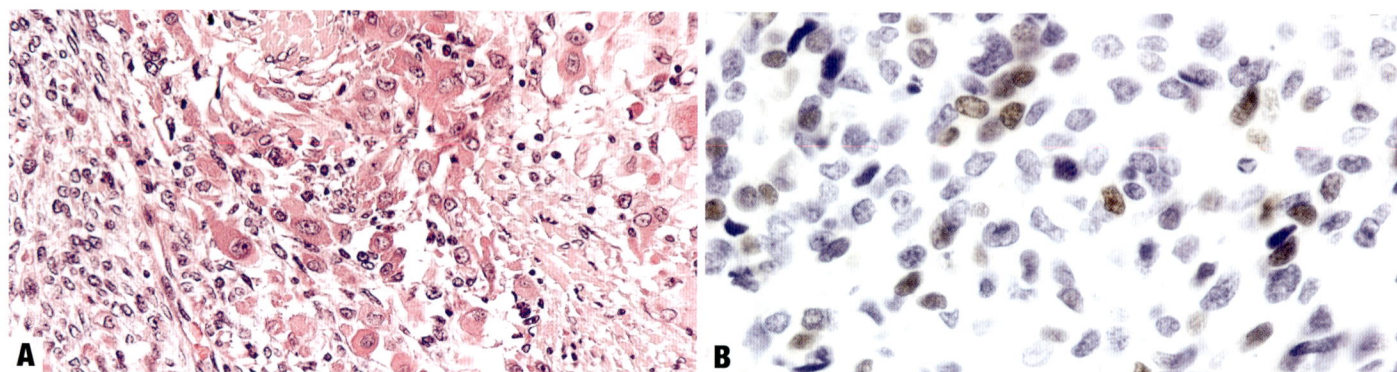

Fig. 1.108 Carcinosarcoma: rhabdomyosarcoma component. **A** Numerous rhabdomyoblasts are present in this rhabdomyosarcomatous component of a carcinosarcoma. **B** This rhabdomyosarcoma component of a carcinosarcoma shows positive nuclear staining for myogenin.

Immunohistochemistry

The immunohistochemistry of the carcinomatous component is that of the conventional tumours of the same type: TTF1 and napsin A in adenocarcinoma and p40 in squamous carcinoma {2542,3390}. Heterologous sarcomatous components can be highlighted by desmin or myogenin for rhabdomyosarcoma or by S100 for chondrosarcoma, but care must be taken not to overinterpret spurious staining in undifferentiated tumour cells. The spindled areas may stain for cytokeratin or may be cytokeratin-negative. These areas are usually negative for TTF1, napsin A, or p40/p63; however, given some reactivity of sarcomas for p63, p40 may perform better, avoiding this pitfall.

Pulmonary blastomas show nuclear staining for β-catenin in fetal-type and mesenchymal areas; carcinosarcomas show membranous staining, including cases with high-grade areas and clear cells, resembling fetal-type adenocarcinoma {2065}. These areas may be CDX2-positive {2935}.

Differential diagnosis

The differential diagnosis includes pleomorphic carcinoma, pulmonary blastoma, sarcoma, and mesothelioma. Pleomorphic carcinomas lack heterologous elements. Pulmonary blastomas have fetal adenocarcinoma (β-catenin nuclear-positive) and blastema-like areas. Sarcomas can have high-grade epithelioid areas, but no glands or keratinization. Mesenchymal tumours can have reactive pneumocyte entrapment, mimicking carcinoma. A notable exception is the biphasic synovial sarcoma; however, the glandular elements of these tumours lack TTF1, and the spindle component is not generally heterologous. If doubt remains, demonstration of SS18-SSX fusion would favour synovial sarcoma.

Mesotheliomas that enter the differential diagnosis will be biphasic, and mesothelial markers will be demonstrable in the epithelioid elements. It is important to perform the immunohistochemistry on sections with significant amounts of the epithelioid component.

Cytology

The diagnosis can be suggested if both components are identified. The epithelial component is more commonly squamous than adenocarcinoma, although both are encountered. The malignant sarcomatous component frequently manifests as spindle cells admixed with chondrosarcoma, osteosarcoma, and/or rhabdomyosarcoma.

Diagnostic molecular pathology

An adenocarcinoma component may require predictive molecular profiling to identify actionable mutations.

Essential and desirable diagnostic criteria

Essential:
- Elements of both NSCC (usually squamous cell carcinoma or adenocarcinoma) and sarcoma with heterologous elements (rhabdomyosarcoma, chondrosarcoma, and osteosarcoma) must be present

Staging

Staging uses the eighth edition of the lung TNM classification {315}.

Prognosis and prediction

Carcinosarcomas have a poor prognosis, like other sarcomatoid carcinomas {1014} with high T and overall TNM stage at presentation {1521,3266}. Resection for localized disease has prognostic benefit {781}.

Thoracic SMARCA4-deficient undifferentiated tumour

Yoshida A
Boland JM
Jain D
Le Loarer F
Rekhtman N

Definition

Thoracic SMARCA4-deficient undifferentiated tumour (SMARCA4-UT) is a high-grade malignant neoplasm that significantly involves the thorax of adults and shows undifferentiated or rhabdoid phenotype and deficiency of SMARCA4, a key member of the BAF chromatin-remodelling complex.

ICD-O coding

8044/3 Thoracic SMARCA4-deficient undifferentiated tumour

ICD-11 coding

2C25.Y Other specified malignant neoplasms of bronchus or lung

Related terminology

Not recommended: SMARCA4-deficient thoracic sarcoma; SMARCA4-deficient thoracic sarcomatoid tumour.

Subtype(s)

None

Localization

SMARCA4-UTs involve the mediastinum, pulmonary hilum, lung, and/or pleura, with or without chest wall invasion. The lung is at least focally involved in most cases, but it may be overshadowed by prominent mediastinal involvement. Rare cases seem to lack pulmonary involvement {3421,2070}.

Clinical features

Presenting symptoms include dyspnoea, pain, superior vena cava syndrome, weight loss, and symptoms referable to metastasis. Imaging typically shows a large, ill-defined and invasive PET-avid mass that compresses adjacent structures, especially when centred in the mediastinum, but primary lung tumours may rarely be small {1617,2643,2324,588}. The tumour is aggressive, with frequent metastases at initial presentation, to lymph nodes, bones, adrenal glands, brain, and abdominal cavity/pelvis {3421,2643,588,2460}. Coexisting bulky abdominal disease may make determination of primary site difficult {3421}.

Epidemiology

SMARCA4-UTs often affect young to middle-aged adults, with a median age of 48 years, but a wide age range is observed (27–90 years) {1617,3421,2643,2324}. There is a striking male predominance.

Etiology

The vast majority of tumours affect heavy smokers, and most harbour a genomic smoking signature {2460}. Smoking-related bullous emphysema is present in more than half of cases {3421, 588,2460}, even in young patients, suggesting increased

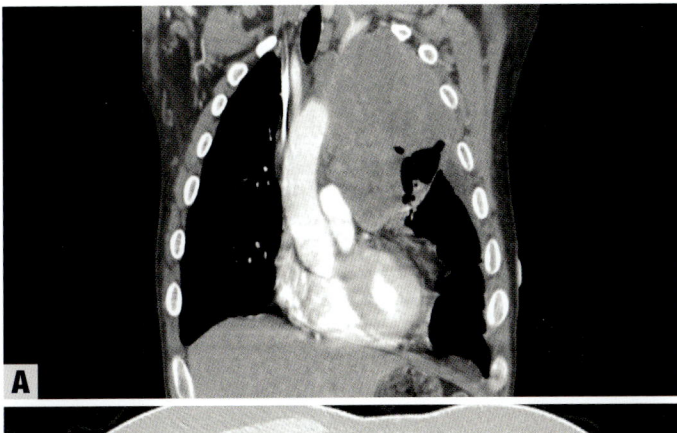

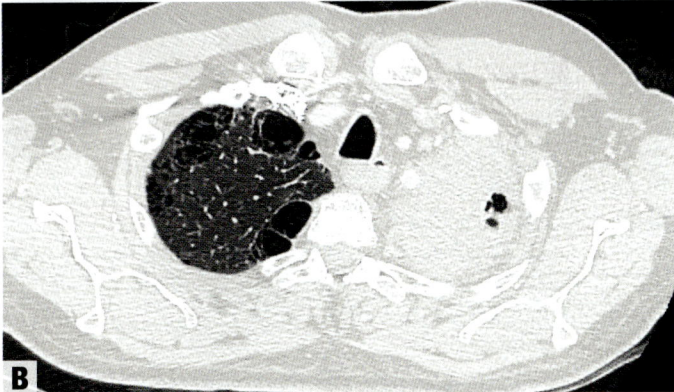

Fig. 1.109 SMARCA4-deficient undifferentiated tumour. **A** Contrast-enhanced CT showing a large compressive mass in the left thoracic cavity. **B** Contrast-enhanced CT showing a tumour in the left thorax. The lung shows emphysematous change.

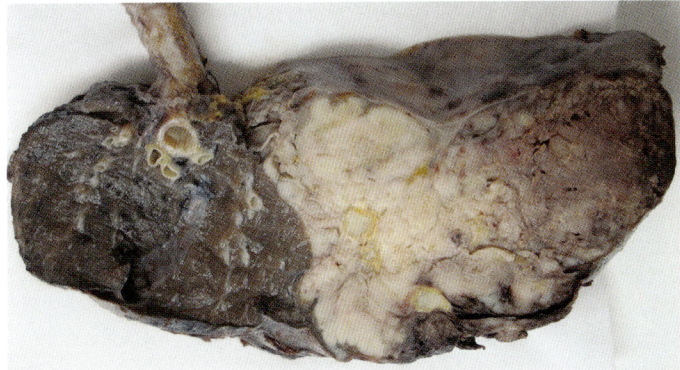

Fig. 1.110 Thoracic SMARCA4-deficient undifferentiated tumour. Macroscopic appearance.

vulnerability to smoking-related injury. Approximately 10% of the patients are never-smokers, who may also have bullous and interstitial lung diseases {3421,2460}. No germline mutation of *SMARCA4* has been reported in these tumours {1617}.

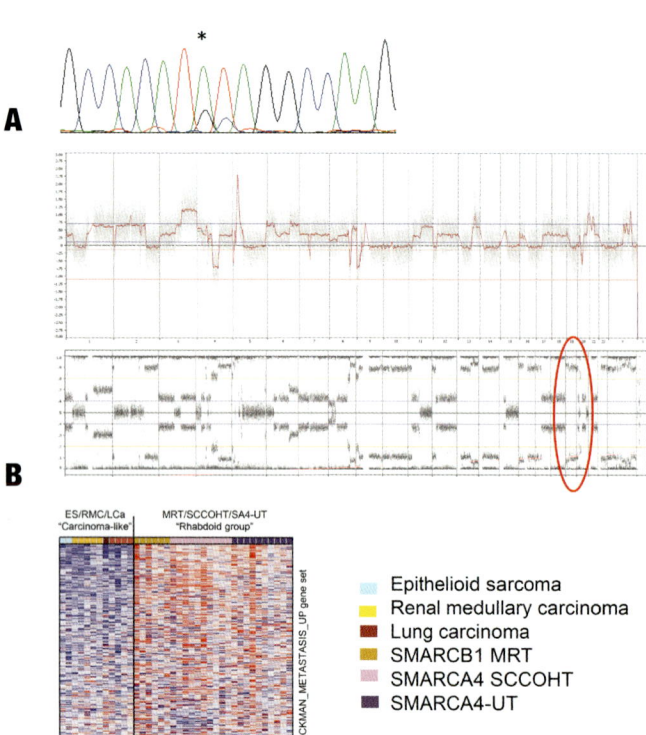

Fig. 1.111 Thoracic SMARCA4-deficient undifferentiated tumour, molecular genetic findings. **A** Sanger sequencing detecting an inactivating *SMARCA4* mutation of dinucleotide substitution exon21:c.3033_3034delinsAT (asterisk) (NM_003072). **B** Array comparative genomic hybridization showing complex genomic profiles with numerous copy-number alterations across the tumour genome (upper panel) and loss of heterozygosity of chromosome 19 encompassing the *SMARCA4* locus (lower panel, red oval). **C** The expression profiles of thoracic SMARCA4-deficient undifferentiated tumours (SMARCA4-UT) using whole-RNA sequencing. These tumours cluster together with SMARCB1-deficient malignant rhabdoid tumours (SMARCB1 MRT) and SMARCA4-deficient small cell carcinoma of the ovary, hypercalcaemic type (SMARCA4 SCCOHT), but not with SMARCA4-deficient lung carcinomas. Their profiles are enriched in genes involved in neural development and stem cell pathways, as well as genes related to metastasis. Data courtesy of Dr Franck Tirode's laboratory.

Pathogenesis

Tumorigenesis is driven by biallelic inactivation of *SMARCA4*, including mainly nonsense and frameshift mutations, with missense mutations, splice-site mutations, or deletions being less common. They are combined with loss of heterozygosity or, uncommonly, deletion or a second mutation {1617,2460}. Multiple, mostly non-recurrent copy-number alterations are present across the tumour genome. *TP53* inactivation is common {1617}. The transcriptional profiles of these tumours are distinct from those of SMARCA4-deficient non-small cell lung carcinoma (NSCLC) but similar to those of malignant rhabdoid tumour {1617}. However, the genomic landscape is different, because malignant rhabdoid tumours lack a complex genomic profile and *TP53* mutation.

As many as 44% of cases show additional mutations in *KRAS*, *STK11*, and/or *KEAP1*, which are common drivers of smoking-associated NSCLC {1617,3421,2460}. *NF1* mutation is present in a subset {3421,2460}. Most tumours also have genomic smoking mutation signatures and high tumour mutation burden {1617,2460}, supporting the notion that they are genomically closely related to conventional NSCLC. The existence of rare (~5%) combined tumours with conventional NSCLC further suggests that even pure undifferentiated tumours may derive from epithelial precursors and may represent undifferentiated/dedifferentiated carcinoma {2460}. However, these tumours have significant phenotypic and clinical differences from conventional NSCLC, making them a distinct entity.

A small subset of tumours (~10%) affect never-smokers, lack the smoking genomic signature, or apparently spare lung parenchyma {1617,2070,2460}, suggesting that alternative pathogenetic pathways may exist.

Macroscopic appearance

The tumours are usually large, white-grey, and soft, with massive necrosis {3421}.

Histopathology

SMARCA4-UTs consist of diffuse sheets of variably discohesive, large round to epithelioid cells with vesicular chromatin and prominent nucleoli. The nuclei are relatively monotonous,

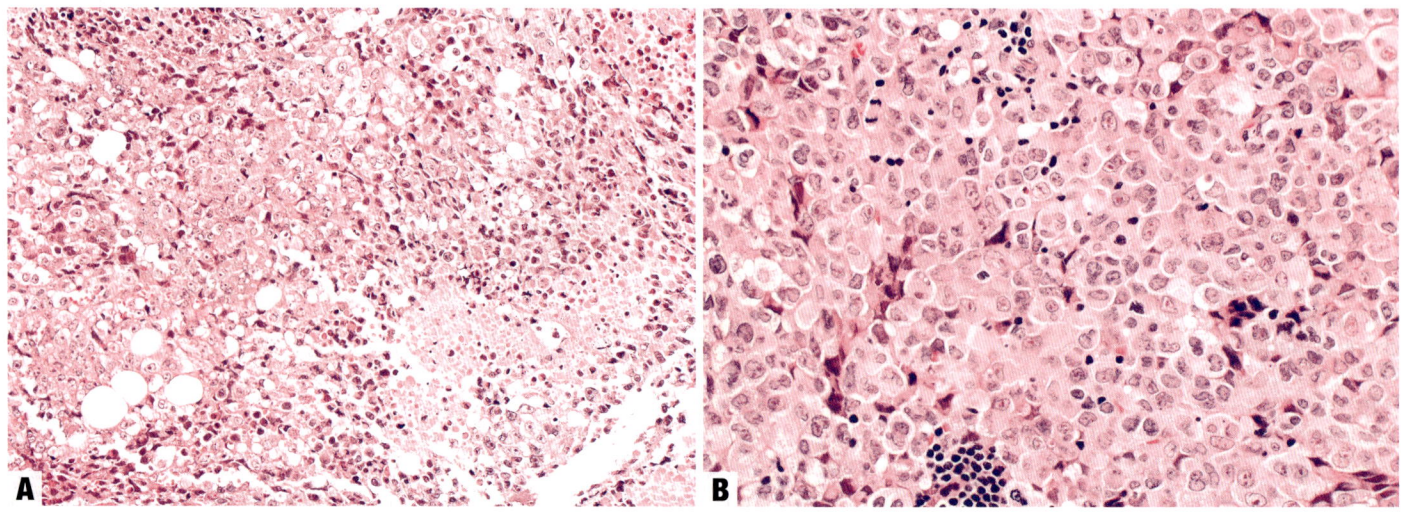

Fig. 1.112 Thoracic SMARCA4-deficient undifferentiated tumour, histology. **A** There are diffuse sheets of round to epithelioid cells infiltrating mediastinal fat. Necrosis is present. **B** The epithelioid tumour cells show relatively uniform nuclei with prominent nucleoli.

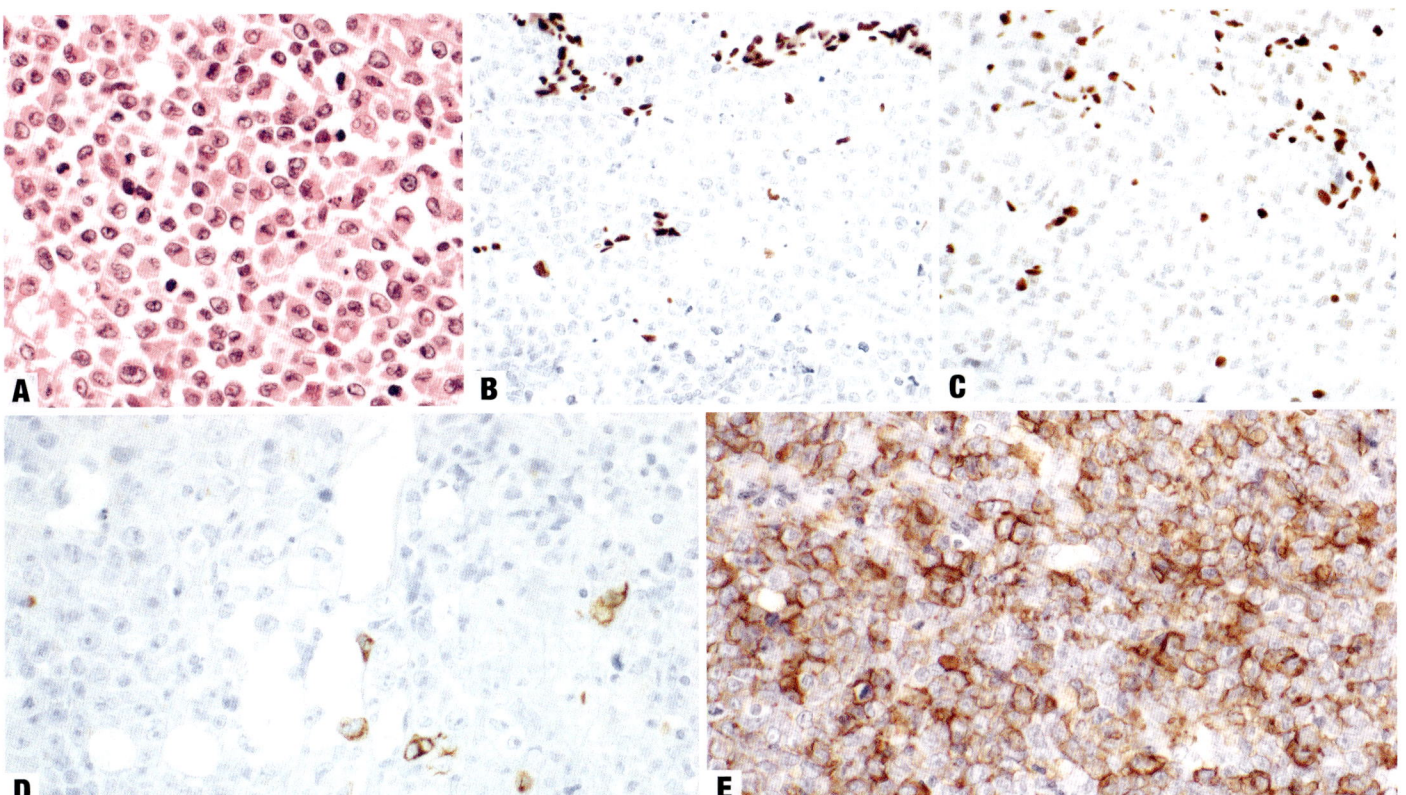

Fig. 1.113 Thoracic SMARCA4-deficient undifferentiated tumour. **A** The tumour cells showing discohesive growth of round and rhabdoid cells. **B** Most tumours show complete loss of SMARCA4 staining. **C** A minor subset of tumours show markedly reduced but still visible SMARCA4 expression. **D** Cytokeratin is focally expressed in more than half of cases. **E** CD34 can be expressed.

with occasional cells displaying mild to moderate pleomorphism. Rhabdoid cells may be present, although they are often a focal finding and may be absent in small specimens. Mitoses are numerous and necrosis is common. Rare findings include spindling, myxoid change, sclerosis, alveolar pattern, and clear cell change {3421,2324,2460}. Unequivocal evidence of epithelial differentiation (e.g. gland, papilla, or keratinization) is absent in most cases, but about 5% of cases show a combined histology with juxtaposed conventional NSCLC {2460}.

Immunohistochemistry
Complete loss of SMARCA4 (BRG1) expression is typical. However, about 25% of cases show diffuse severe reduction of SMARCA4 staining rather than complete loss {3421,2460}. SMARCA2 (BRM) staining is lost in most cases {3421,2324}. SMARCB1 (INI1) expression is retained. Many cases express CD34, SOX2, and/or SALL4 {3421,2643,2324,2460}. p53 is overexpressed in the majority of cases {3421}. Cytokeratins are often expressed in a focal or weak manner and may be entirely negative, whereas strong and diffuse expression is lacking. Synaptophysin expression may be prominent {588,2460}. Claudin-4 is negative or only focally positive in virtually all cases {3421,2324,2460}. Rare cases may focally express TTF1, p63, p40, or WT1 {1617,3421,2460}. Mismatch repair proteins show a proficient pattern {3421}.

Differential diagnosis
Differential diagnosis includes lymphoma, NUT carcinoma, germ cell tumour, neuroendocrine carcinoma (NEC), large cell carcinoma, and melanoma, as well as various types of sarcomas, such as *CIC*-rearranged sarcoma, malignant rhabdoid tumour, and epithelioid sarcoma. SMARCA4 deficiency is observed in about 5% of conventional NSCLCs {1833,2171, 3430,1131,2071,602}, which should be distinguished by epithelial architecture (e.g. glands), cellular cohesion, and diffuse strong keratin expression. Ancillary markers (SMARCA2, claudin-4, CD34, SALL4, and SOX2) may also be helpful, although none is entirely sensitive or specific. Because SMARCA4-UTs with a similar phenotype may metastasize to the thorax from extraneous sites (e.g. uterus, ovary, stomach, kidney, and pancreas), clinical correlation is mandatory.

Cytology
Smears are typically cellular in a necrotic background, with cells appearing singly or in loosely cohesive groups. Cells are round to ovoid, with typically eccentric nuclei and prominent nucleoli. Despite overall monomorphism, isolated pleomorphic cells are common. Hyaline inclusions are not well demonstrated in cytological smears, but dense cytoplasm with indentation of nuclei is apparent in some cells {2963,1874,1843}.

Diagnostic molecular pathology
Sequencing can confirm the presence of *SMARCA4* mutation, but it is not necessary for the diagnosis, because immunohistochemistry shows complete loss in most cases and is sufficient to document SMARCA4 deficiency. However, sequencing can be helpful to clarify the significance of reduced expression of SMARCA4. The mutation may not be detectable, depending on

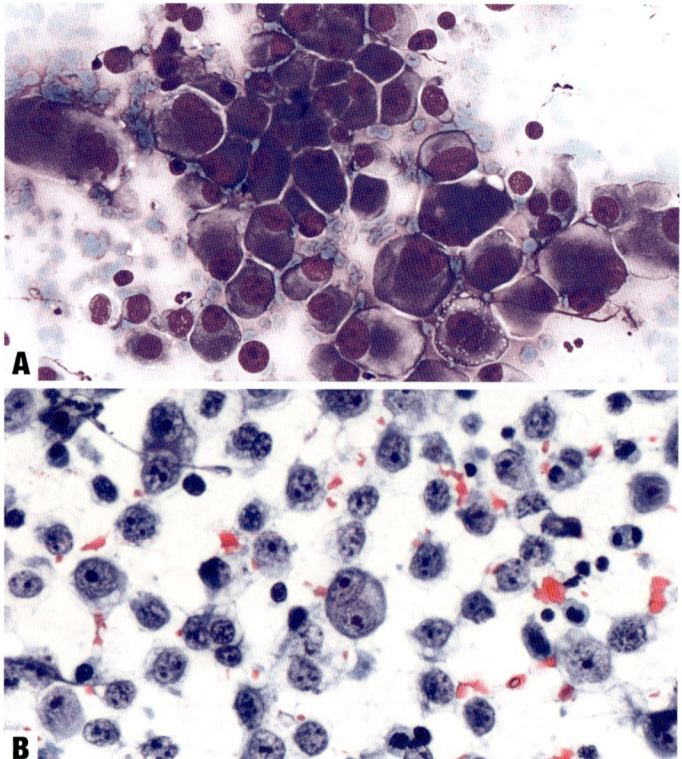

Fig. 1.114 Thoracic SMARCA4-deficient undifferentiated tumour, cytology. Air-dried Diff-Quik (Giemsa)-stained smear (**A**) and alcohol-fixed Pap-stained smear (**B**) illustrate monomorphic discohesive single cells or loosely cohesive clusters comprising epithelioid cells with eccentric nuclei and prominent nucleoli. Binucleation is commonly seen. The appearance resembles that of melanoma or large cell lymphoma. Prototypical rhabdoid inclusions are inconspicuous in cytological smears, but dense cytoplasm and nuclear indentation are at least focally apparent.

the methods used, despite SMARCA4 immunohistochemical loss {2460}. Because the second hit is often copy-neutral loss of heterozygosity, *SMARCA4* FISH assay is of limited utility {2460}.

Essential and desirable diagnostic criteria
Essential:
- Tumour in adults, with significant thoracic involvement
- Diffuse sheets of variably discohesive, round to epithelioid, relatively monotonous cells with vesicular nuclei and prominent nucleoli
- No clear evidence of epithelial differentiation (except juxtaposed carcinoma in combined cases)
- SMARCA4 (BRG1) deficiency by immunohistochemistry

Desirable:
- SMARCA2 (BRM) deficiency by immunohistochemistry
- Expression of CD34, SOX2, and/or SALL4
- Absent or focal claudin-4 expression

Staging
American Joint Committee on Cancer (AJCC) or Union for International Cancer Control (UICC) staging for lung cancer has been applied, although its utility for prognostic stratification has not been validated, because virtually all cases are stage IV.

Prognosis and prediction
SMARCA4-UTs show universally aggressive behaviour and poor prognosis, with a median overall survival of 4–7 months {1617,3421,2643,2460}. They have a poorer outcome than SMARCA4-deficient conventional NSCLCs {1617,2460}. Cytotoxic chemotherapy regimens have been reported as generally ineffective, and novel treatment strategies are awaited, including immune checkpoint inhibition {1121}.

Pleomorphic adenoma of the lung

Mehrad M
Farver CF
Nicholson AG

Definition

Pleomorphic adenoma is a benign tumour with epithelial and modified myoepithelial cells intermingled with a chondromyxoid stroma.

ICD-O coding

8940/0 Pleomorphic adenoma

ICD-11 coding

2F00.Y & XH2KC1 Other specified benign neoplasm of middle ear or respiratory system & Pleomorphic adenoma

Related terminology

Not recommended: benign mixed tumour.

Subtype(s)

None

Localization

Most pleomorphic adenomas arise in proximal bronchi or the trachea.

Clinical features

Patients with endobronchial tumours may present with dyspnoea or haemoptysis, often associated with postobstructive pneumonia and/or atelectasis {794}. Intraparenchymal tumours are frequently asymptomatic. Imaging shows well-circumscribed solid masses {393,1067}. The heterogeneity of CT and MRI corresponds to different histological elements. Tumours may be PET-positive {1067}.

Epidemiology

Pleomorphic adenoma occurs within an age range of 8–74 years {136}, but mostly in adults. There is no sex predominance.

Etiology

Unknown

Pathogenesis

Reports of molecular studies in pulmonary pleomorphic adenomas are rare {2969}, without documentation yet of the *PLAG1* and/or *HMGA2* fusions known to occur in salivary gland counterparts {1393}.

Macroscopic appearance

Pleomorphic adenoma ranges from 10 to 160 mm {794}. Endobronchial pleomorphic adenoma is polypoid; parenchymal tumours are well-circumscribed nodules. The cut surface is white-grey, myxoid, and soft to rubbery.

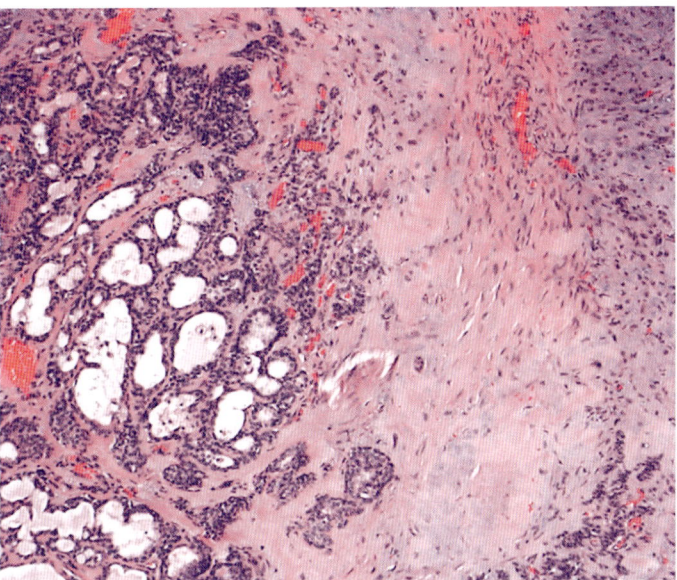

Fig. 1.115 Pleomorphic adenoma. Prominent ductular structures are present within a chondroid and hyalinized stroma.

Histopathology

Pulmonary pleomorphic adenomas are histologically similar to pleomorphic adenomas in salivary glands. They have a prominent tubular or ductal component associated with spindled to plasmacytoid myoepithelial cells embedded in a chondromyxoid stroma. Squamous metaplasia may also be seen {794}. Solid islands of epithelial cells with a focal myxoid stroma can be seen. Immunohistochemistry is not specific but supports a biphasic tumour. A panel of cytokeratin, S100, GFAP, p40, p63, calponin, α-SMA, and SMMHC will be variably positive. The key differential diagnosis is a metastatic salivary gland tumour (so-called benign metastasizing pleomorphic adenoma). Other differential diagnoses include pulmonary hamartoma and carcinosarcoma. Hamartomas comprise well-developed mesenchymal elements. Pulmonary carcinosarcomas have overtly malignant elements. Exceptionally, a malignancy may arise within a pleomorphic adenoma. The carcinoma component can be epithelial, myoepithelial, or mixed in origin and shows malignant features including necrosis, cellular atypia, ≥ 5 mitoses/2 mm², and vascular and/or perineural invasion. These tumours should be called carcinoma ex pleomorphic adenoma, and the type of carcinoma should be reported {794}.

Cytology

Although not reported in the pulmonary system, the finding of a combination of bland ductal epithelial cells and myoepithelial cells blended intimately with a chondromyxoid stroma would be expected.

Diagnostic molecular pathology

Not clinically relevant

Essential and desirable diagnostic criteria

Essential:

- A benign mixed salivary gland–type neoplasm with ductal cells, myoepithelial cells, and a chondromyxoid stromal component

Staging

Not clinically relevant

Prognosis and prediction

Small, well-circumscribed tumours are benign. Tumours with infiltrative borders may recur and metastasize, and they behave as low-grade malignancies {3272}.

Adenoid cystic carcinoma of the lung

Mehrad M
Farver CF
Nicholson AG

Definition

Adenoid cystic carcinoma is a malignant biphasic salivary gland–type tumour consisting of epithelial and myoepithelial cells. There are three main architectural growth patterns: tubular, cribriform, and solid.

ICD-O coding

8200/3 Adenoid cystic carcinoma

ICD-11 coding

2C25.Y & XH4302 Other specified malignant neoplasms of bronchus or lung & Adenoid cystic carcinoma

Related terminology

Not recommended: cylindroma; adenocystic carcinoma.

Subtype(s)

None

Localization

Adenoid cystic carcinoma typically arises as an endobronchial tumour.

Clinical features

Common symptoms include shortness of breath, cough, wheezing, and haemoptysis due to airway obstruction {794}. Imaging typically shows a centrally located mass that may have an endobronchial component. Adenoid cystic carcinomas are larger, more frequently involve the central airways, and have a higher median FDG uptake than mucoepidermoid carcinomas {762}. Adenoid cystic carcinoma grows insidiously and infiltratively, sometimes extending to the lung parenchyma and mediastinum. Perineural invasion makes complete surgical resection difficult, and local recurrence is common. Metastases to remote organs are uncommon.

Epidemiology

Adenoid cystic carcinoma accounts for < 1% of all lung tumours, with no sex predominance.

Etiology

There is no evidence of an association with smoking.

Pathogenesis

The main genomic alterations, including a fusion of the *MYB* oncogene and *NFIB* transcription factor t(6;9)(q22-q23;p23-p24) and less commonly t(8;9)/*MYBL1-NFIB* gene fusion, can occur in 30–100% of adenoid cystic carcinomas of the head and neck and tracheobronchial tree {548,2326,2296,2507}. Loss of heterozygosity of chromosomes 3p14 and 9p has been reported rarely in bronchial adenoid cystic carcinoma {2893}. High-resolution comparative genomic hybridization analysis

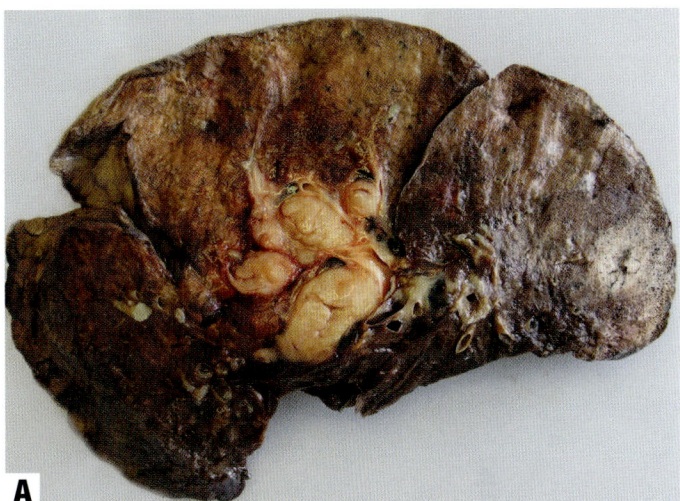

A

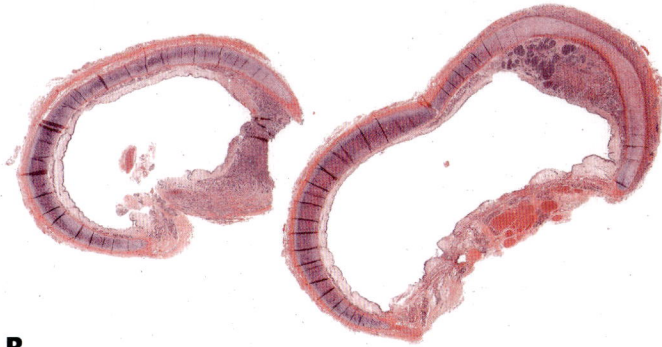

B

Fig. 1.116 Adenoid cystic carcinoma. **A** Macroscopy of an adenoid cystic carcinoma arising within the bronchus. **B** Tumour growing in an endobronchial manner, with infiltration of the peribronchial soft tissue.

showed losses at 3p, 4p, and 15q and gains at 12q15 (the *MDM2* site) {217}. Despite immunoreactivity for KIT, *KIT* mutations are absent {124,3291}. Although whole-exome sequencing of head and neck adenoid cystic carcinoma identified mutations in *PIK3CA, ATM, CDKN2A, SF3B1, SUFU, TSC1, CYLD, NOTCH1/2, SPEN,* and *FGFR2* {2857}, there are no similar studies for bronchopulmonary adenoid cystic carcinoma.

Macroscopic appearance

The tumours are usually < 40 mm in size, with a greyish-white, homogeneous cut surface. Sampling of peribronchial soft tissue is recommended, because there is often microscopic spread beyond visible macroscopic margins.

Histopathology

Adenoid cystic carcinoma is composed of small, angulated cells with scant cytoplasm and usually homogeneous

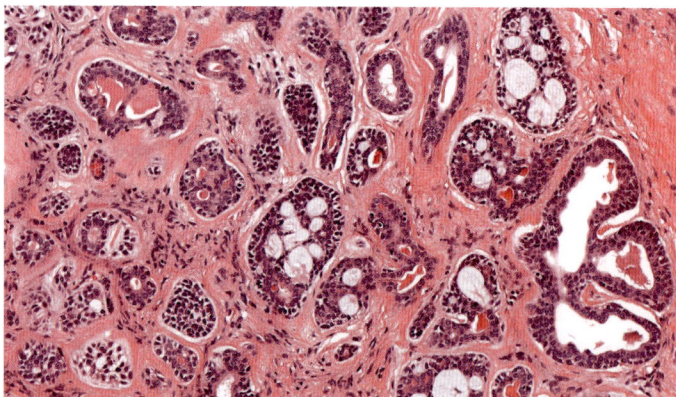

Fig. 1.117 Adenoid cystic carcinoma. Cribriform nests with sharply demarcated round spaces filled with lightly basophilic myxoid ground substance and occasional ductal formation.

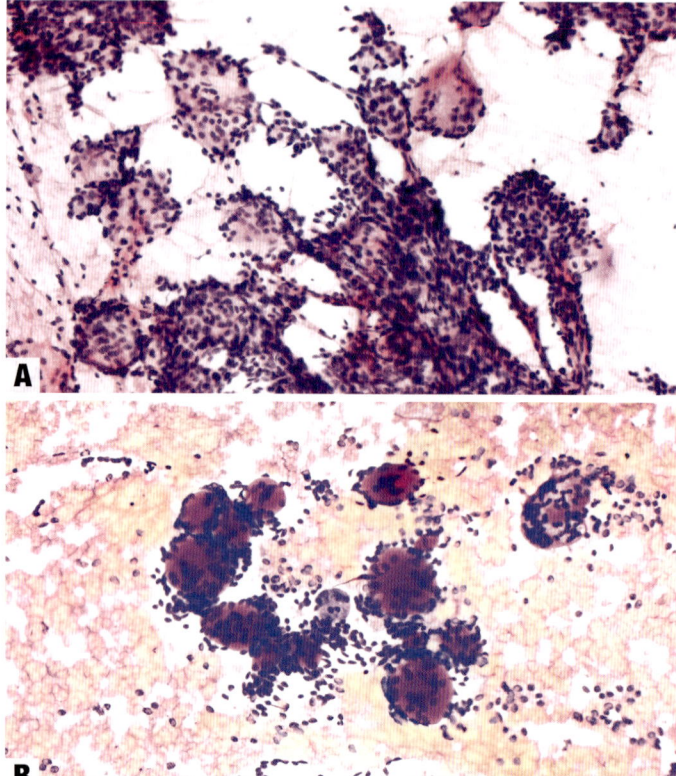

Fig. 1.118 Adenoid cystic carcinoma. **A** Cytology smear showing the lightly stained basement membrane–like material surrounded by uniform basaloid cells. **B** Diff-Quik staining shows metachromatic matrix spheres surrounded by small basaloid epithelial cells.

hyperchromatic nuclei, showing frequent perineural invasion and infrequent mitosis. Architecturally, it shows three growth patterns: cribriform, tubular, and solid. The most common pattern is the cribriform, characterized by nests of tumour cells with punched-out luminal spaces containing basophilic matrix. When forming tubules with two layers of cells, the luminal cells show a cuboidal appearance and the peripheral cells form a myoepithelial layer. The solid pattern consists of tumour nests without lumen formation.

Immunohistochemistry demonstrates both ductal and myoepithelial phenotypes, including cytokeratin, vimentin, actin, S100, and KIT. The matrix recapitulates basement membrane–like characteristics such as collagen IV, laminin, and heparin sulfate. The differential diagnoses include carcinoid tumours, basaloid squamous cell carcinoma, and small cell carcinoma – all of which can typically be distinguished by immunohistochemical staining. Additionally, basaloid squamous cell carcinoma has a high proliferation rate, unlike most adenoid cystic carcinomas. Pleomorphic adenoma with a focally cribriform architecture may resemble adenoid cystic carcinoma. Metastasis from other organs should be carefully ruled out.

Cytology
3D microacinar patterns are seen, with pink to pale opaque globules corresponding to intraluminal basement membrane–like material {726}.

Diagnostic molecular pathology
Testing for *MYB-NFIB* and *MYBL1-NFIB* gene fusions by FISH or next-generation sequencing can help to establish the diagnosis of adenoid cystic carcinoma {548,2326,2296,2507}.

Essential and desirable diagnostic criteria
Essential:
- Adenoid cystic carcinoma is a biphasic salivary gland–type carcinoma with hyperchromatic and angulated nuclei demonstrating both ductal and myoepithelial phenotypes
- Metastasis from other organs should be carefully ruled out {1193,794}

Desirable:
- Demonstration of *MYB-NFIB* gene fusion

Staging
Staging is according to the Union for International Cancer Control (UICC) TNM classification.

Prognosis and prediction
Tumours behave in an indolent fashion, and local recurrence (often multiple) may occur over a 10–15 year period after resection {3520}. Distant metastases may eventually occur. Poor prognosis relates to stage of the tumour at diagnosis, positive margins at surgery, older patient age, and a solid growth pattern {1551,2402}.

Epithelial-myoepithelial carcinoma of the lung

Husain AN
Farver CF
Nicholson AG

Definition

Epithelial-myoepithelial carcinoma is a biphasic malignant salivary gland–type tumour composed of an inner layer of epithelial cells forming duct-like structures and an outer layer of myoepithelial cells.

ICD-O coding

8562/3 Epithelial-myoepithelial carcinoma

ICD-11 coding

2C25.Y & XH9JP2 Other specified malignant neoplasms of bronchus or lung & Epithelial-myoepithelial carcinoma

Related terminology

Not recommended: adenomyoepithelioma; pneumocytic adenomyoepithelioma; epimyoepithelial carcinoma; epithelial-myoepithelial tumour; malignant mixed tumour comprising epithelial and myoepithelial cells.

Subtype(s)

None

Localization

Epithelial-myoepithelial carcinoma is most often centrally located in the lung, involving a major bronchus; about 20–30% of cases are purely intraparenchymal {2725,2061}.

Clinical features

Owing to the common central location of epithelial-myoepithelial carcinoma of the lung, the presenting symptoms are those of bronchial obstruction, including productive cough, fever, and dyspnoea. Epithelial-myoepithelial carcinoma may also be asymptomatic, especially if located in the parenchyma. Imaging shows a well-demarcated homogeneous tumour, most often with no FDG uptake on FDG PET-CT {2061}.

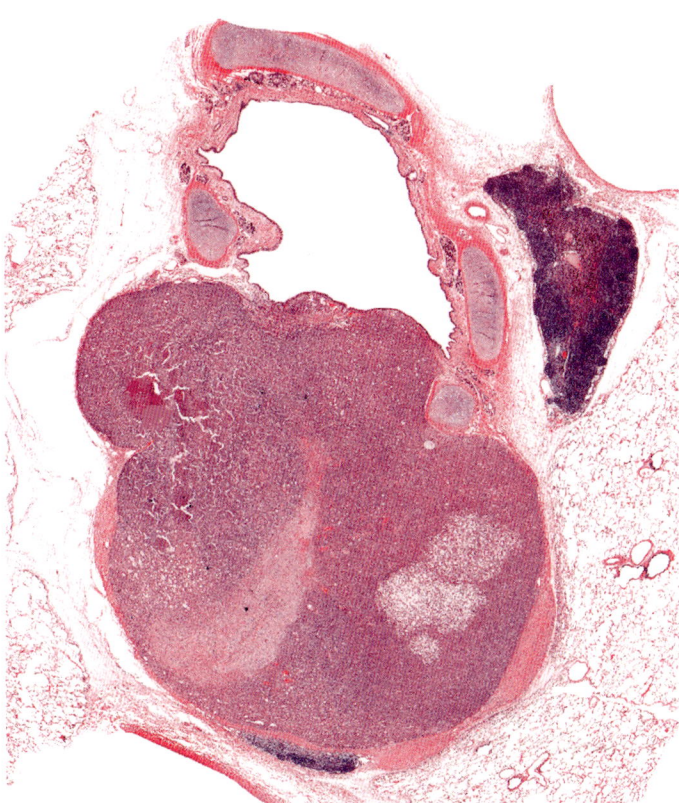

Fig. 1.119 Epithelial-myoepithelial carcinoma. This low-power image demonstrates a lobulated, well-circumscribed tumour located in the submucosa of a central bronchus.

Epidemiology

Epithelial-myoepithelial carcinoma is a rare tumour, accounting for only 3.8% of primary salivary gland–type tumours of the lung {916,2061}. The age range of patients is 7–81 years, with an average age of 56 years. There is no sex predominance.

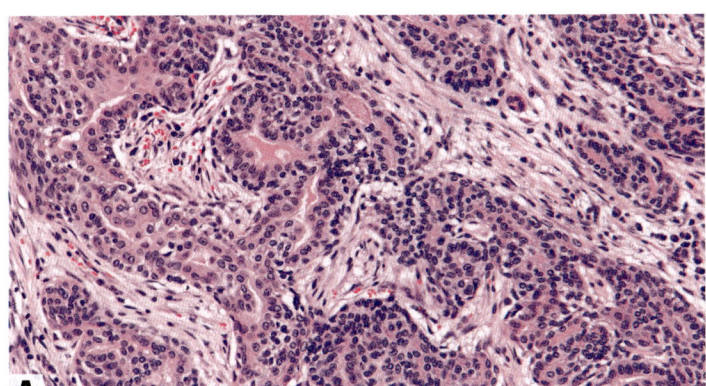
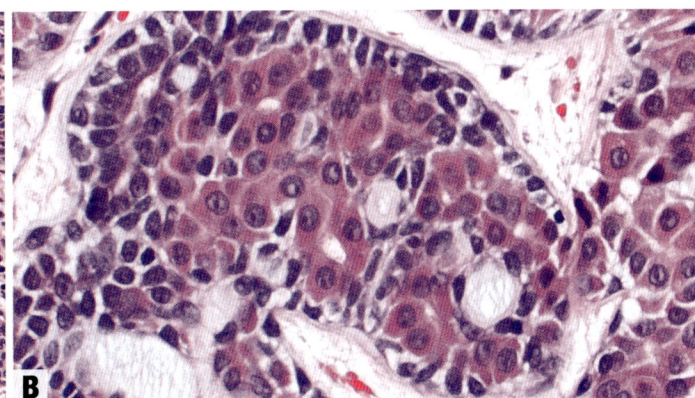

Fig. 1.120 Epithelial-myoepithelial carcinoma. **A** The tumour has a biphasic morphology, with an inner layer of epithelial cells forming duct-like structures and an outer layer of smaller uniform cells that are myoepithelial. **B** This example shows more eosinophilic epithelial cells and clear myoepithelial cells.

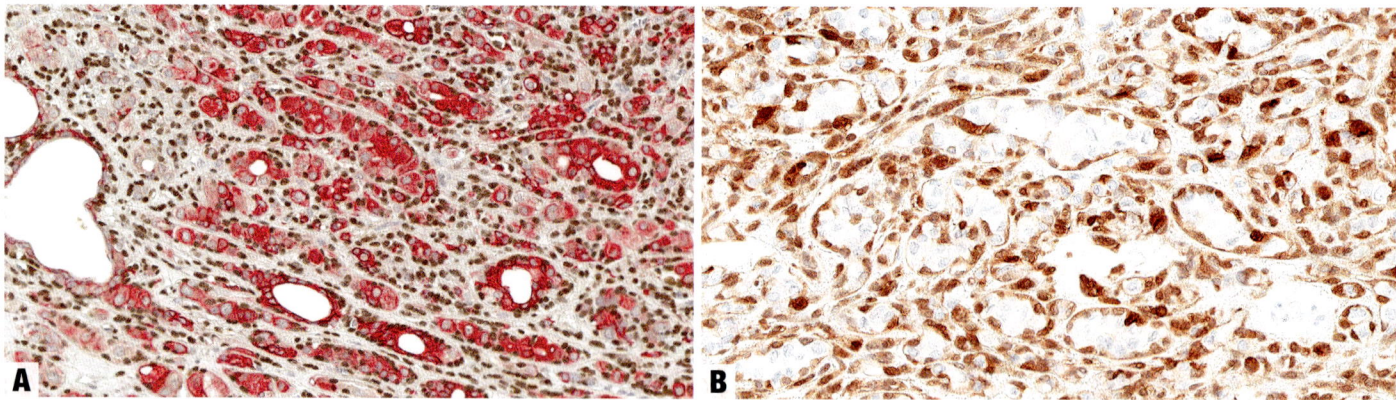

Fig. 1.121 Epithelial-myoepithelial carcinoma. **A** Double staining shows epithelial cells positive for cytokeratin (red) while the myoepithelial cells are positive for p63 (brown). **B** The myoepithelial cells stain with S100.

Etiology
There is no association with smoking or other causes of lung carcinoma.

Pathogenesis
Unknown

Macroscopic appearance
Epithelial-myoepithelial carcinoma is usually a well-circumscribed, solid, homogeneous, white to tan-grey tumour. A case of cavitary tumour has been described {1993}.

Histopathology
Epithelial-myoepithelial carcinoma is biphasic, with epithelial and myoepithelial components. The most common pattern consists of an inner layer of cuboidal epithelial cells forming duct-like structures and an outer layer of myoepithelial cells. The epithelial cells have uniform small nuclei surrounded by eosinophilic cytoplasm. The outer myoepithelial cells often have clear cytoplasm. Mitoses are rare and there is no necrosis. In the second most common pattern, the myoepithelial cells are more eosinophilic and spindled, and they form solid areas. In the least common pattern, the myoepithelial cells predominate, with increased nuclear atypia (called myoepithelial anaplasia), which tends to correlate with a more malignant behaviour {2061}.

The inner epithelial cells are strongly positive for cytokeratins and negative for myoepithelial markers. The myoepithelial cells are usually strongly positive for S100 (although S100-negative cases have been reported), p40, p63, and actins and negative for CEA and HMB45 {2810}. Occasionally, there is exuberant pneumocytic hyperplasia associated with myoepithelial neoplasms (originally termed pneumocytic adenomyoepitheliomas) {3458}.

Cytology
Cytological material obtained by FNA shows tight 3D clusters of basaloid cells with scant cytoplasm and occasional clusters of epithelioid cells with large, overlapping nuclei. Naked nuclei are seen in the background.

Diagnostic molecular pathology
Not clinically relevant

Essential and desirable diagnostic criteria
Essential:
- Low-grade salivary gland–type tumour
- Biphasic morphology with inner epithelial cells forming ducts and outer myoepithelial cells in varying proportions

Desirable:
- Myoepithelial cell positivity for S100, p40/p63, and actins

Staging
Staging is according to the Union for International Cancer Control (UICC) TNM classification.

Prognosis and prediction
Most epithelial-myoepithelial carcinomas are low-grade, with no recurrence after complete resection {3520}. Few cases of mediastinal lymph node or distant metastasis have been reported. Tumours may recur and/or metastasize to mediastinal lymph nodes {2061}. A high mitotic count, tumoural necrosis, nuclear pleomorphism, and predominance of the myoepithelial component with atypia appear to be adverse prognostic factors {891, 2948}.

Mucoepidermoid carcinoma of the lung

Husain AN
Farver CF
Nicholson AG

Definition
Mucoepidermoid carcinoma (MEC) is a malignant salivary gland–type tumour that is composed of mucin-secreting cells, squamoid cells, and intermediate-type cells.

ICD-O coding
8430/3 Mucoepidermoid carcinoma

ICD-11 coding
2C25.Y & XH1J36 Other specified malignant neoplasms of bronchus or lung & Mucoepidermoid carcinoma

Related terminology
Not recommended: mucoepidermoid tumour.

Subtype(s)
None

Localization
MECs are usually endobronchial and are more common in central airways.

Clinical features
Presentation is usually secondary to obstruction or irritation of the airways, with symptoms of cough, haemoptysis, and recurrent infection. Symptoms are sometimes mistaken for asthma. Some patients are asymptomatic. On CT, the tumours are rounded or lobulated masses, with features of associated obstruction commonly seen {488,3443,2614,1954,2402}.

Epidemiology
MECs account for < 1% of lung carcinomas. There is a female predominance in some series and a wide age range {3443, 2614,1954,2402}.

Etiology
The etiology is unknown. There is no association with smoking.

Pathogenesis
The t(11;19)(q21;p13) involves the *CRTC1* and *MAML2* genes, located on chromosomes 19p13 and 11q21, respectively. *CRTC1-MAML2* fuses exon 1 of *CRTC1* with exons 2–5 of *MAML2* {3050}.

Macroscopic appearance
Low-grade tumours are well demarcated and sometimes polypoid within the airways, with an average size of 30 mm. High-grade tumours are more infiltrative. The cut surface varies from soft to firm and white/grey to yellow, depending on the extent of fibrosis and mucin-filled cells. Tumours may sometimes be cystic.

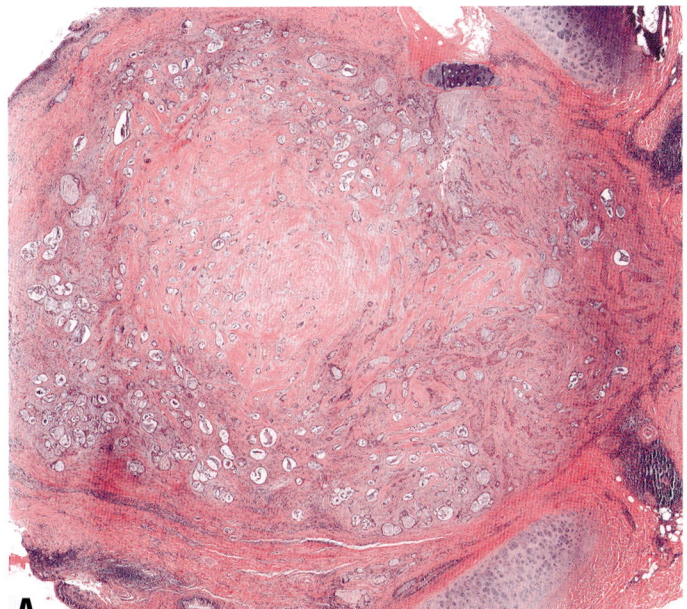

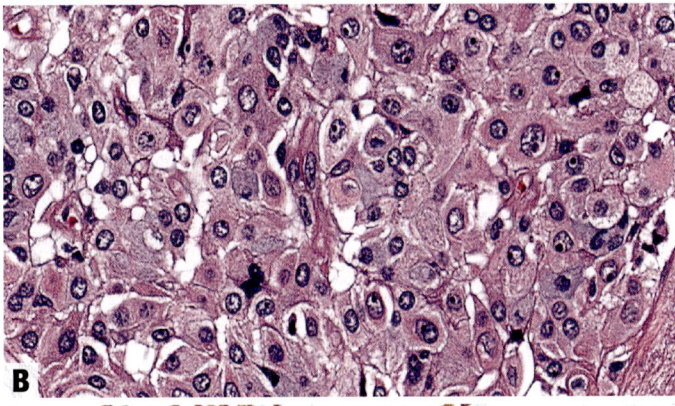

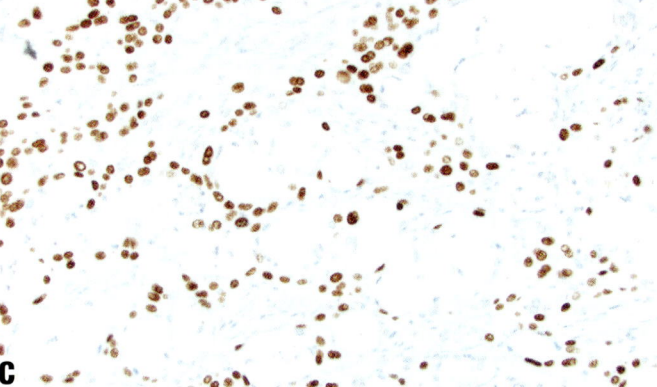

Fig. 1.122 Mucoepidermoid carcinoma. **A** Whole-mount section shows a tumour growing in an endobronchial manner. **B** High-grade mucoepidermoid carcinoma shows cells with atypical nuclei and prominent nucleoli. **C** p63-positive staining in the epidermoid component of the tumour.

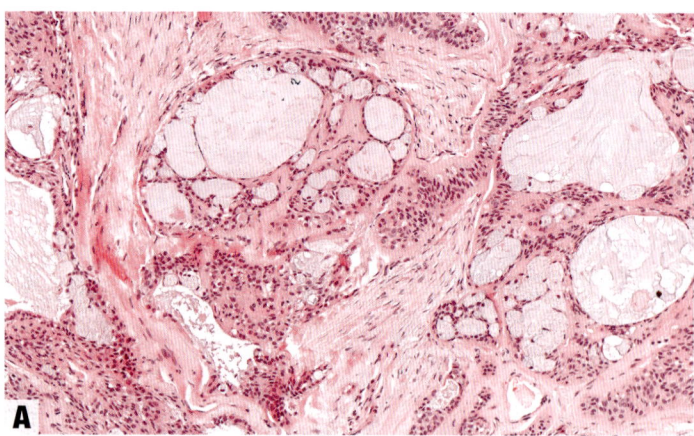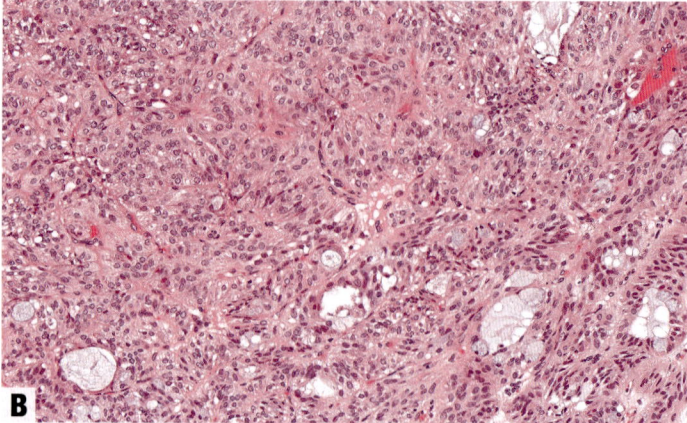

Fig. 1.123 Low-grade mucoepidermoid carcinoma. **A** Mucin-filled glands predominate, lying in dense fibrous stroma. **B** The tumour consists mainly of intermediate cells, with scattered mucin-filled glands and mucinous cells.

Histopathology

Low-grade tumours comprise varying numbers of mucin-secreting, squamoid, and intermediate cells. Cystic areas are typically lined by mucin-secreting cells. Solid areas comprise intermediate cells and/or non-keratinizing squamoid cells. Clear cell and oncocytic changes are often focally seen and may rarely predominate. Mitoses are rare. Background stroma may show calcification, ossification, a granulomatous reaction to extravasated mucin, and sometimes a florid inflammatory host response. High-grade tumours are rare and are mainly composed of atypical squamoid and intermediate cells, with frequent mitosis and necrosis, accompanied by variable numbers of mucin-secreting cells. All cell types are positive for cytokeratins and negative for TTF1, napsin A, SMA, and S100 {2506, 1212}. Squamoid cells are positive for p40, p63, and CK5/6.

The important differential diagnosis is metastasis from a head and neck salivary gland tumour. Clinical correlation is necessary because MECs arising in other anatomical sites show *MAML2* gene rearrangement and a similar morphology. *MAML2* gene rearrangement is seen almost exclusively in MEC and can exclude adenosquamous carcinoma in some cases {12}. Criteria more typical of high-grade MEC than adenosquamous carcinoma include (1) proximal exophytic endobronchial location; (2) transitional areas from low grade to high grade; (3) no overlying squamous cell carcinoma in situ; (4) lack of individual cell keratinization or squamous pearl formation; and (5) absence of tubular, acinar, and papillary growth pattern {3443,2614}. The lack of intermediate and squamoid cells discriminates mucous gland adenoma from low-grade MEC.

Cytology

All three cell types (squamoid, glandular, and intermediate) may be intermingled {2695,2589}. Glandular cells may be present singly or in acinar formations. Intermediate cells are round to elongated, with dense homogeneous cytoplasm. Squamoid cells are larger, with centrally located round nuclei.

Diagnostic molecular pathology

Testing for *CRTC1-MAML2* gene fusion by FISH can help to establish the diagnosis of MEC {12,2506}.

Essential and desirable diagnostic criteria

Essential – low-grade:
- Cytologically bland mucin-secreting, squamoid, and intermediate cells

Essential – high-grade:
- Atypical mucin-secreting, squamoid, and intermediate cells
- Transition from low-grade to high-grade areas, absence of keratinization, central location, and absence of carcinoma in situ

Desirable:
- Identification of *CRTC1-MAML2* gene fusion.

Staging

Staging is according to the Union for International Cancer Control (UICC) TNM classification.

Prognosis and prediction

Low-grade MECs have a good prognosis. High-grade tumours have a prognosis similar to that of other non-small cell carcinomas. Incomplete resection and nodal metastases are poor prognostic factors {3443,2614,1954}. *CRTC1-MAML2* fusion–positive cases are associated with better survival {193}.

Hyalinizing clear cell carcinoma of the lung

Husain AN
Farver CF
Nicholson AG

Definition

Hyalinizing clear cell carcinoma is a low-grade malignant epithelial tumour with cords, trabeculae, and nests of clear and eosinophilic cells infiltrating within a background of myxohyaline and cellular fibrous stroma.

ICD-O coding

8310/3 Hyalinizing clear cell carcinoma

ICD-11 coding

2C25.Y Other specified malignant neoplasms of bronchus or lung & XH6L02 Clear cell adenocarcinoma

Related terminology

None

Subtype(s)

None

Localization

Hyalinizing clear cell carcinomas are endobronchial in central airways.

Clinical features

The central location predominantly causes symptoms of obstruction, cough, and dyspnoea. Haemoptysis is rare {726}.

Epidemiology

Hyalinizing clear cell carcinomas are rare lung cancers, with only 11 reported cases. The age range is 30–66 years, with a slight female predominance {1298,1224,794,2711}.

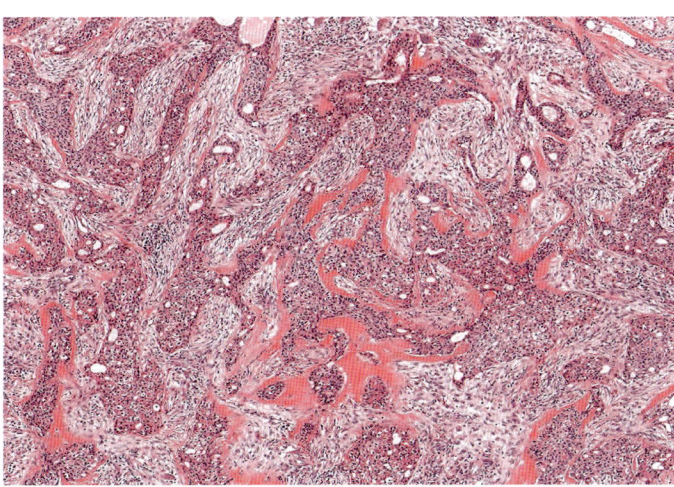

Fig. 1.124 Hyalinizing clear cell carcinoma. Cells infiltrating in trabeculae and nests through a background with dense, eosinophilic, hyalinizing stroma adjacent to areas of a myxoid fibrosis.

Etiology

Unknown

Pathogenesis

Unknown

Macroscopic appearance

Hyalinizing clear cell carcinomas are tan-white, relatively circumscribed, unencapsulated tumours. Invasion into bronchial cartilage can occur {2711}. Sizes range from 9 to 35 mm {794, 2957}.

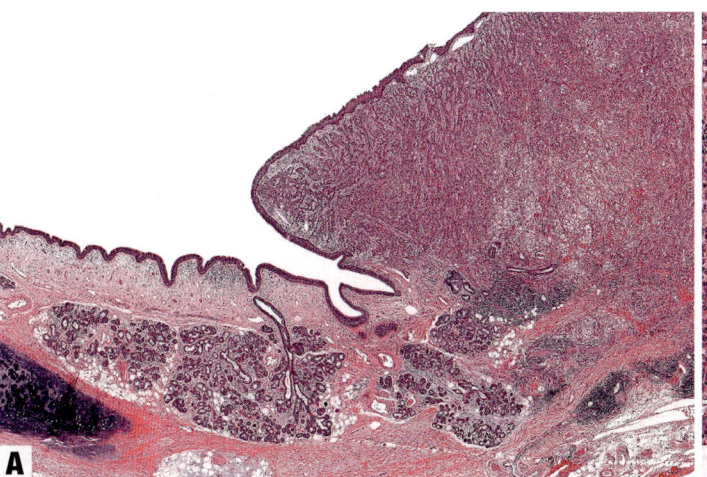
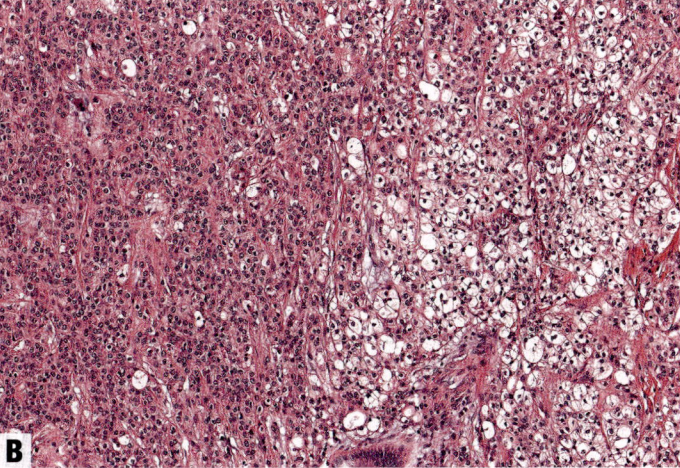

Fig. 1.125 Hyalinizing clear cell carcinoma. **A** Whole-mount section shows a hyalinizing clear cell carcinoma arising within the bronchus, growing in an endobronchial manner. The tumour infiltrates into the peribronchial soft tissue, causing a lymphocytic inflammatory response. **B** The characteristic two cell populations are demonstrated, with cells containing eosinophilic cytoplasm (left) and cells with clear cytoplasm (right).

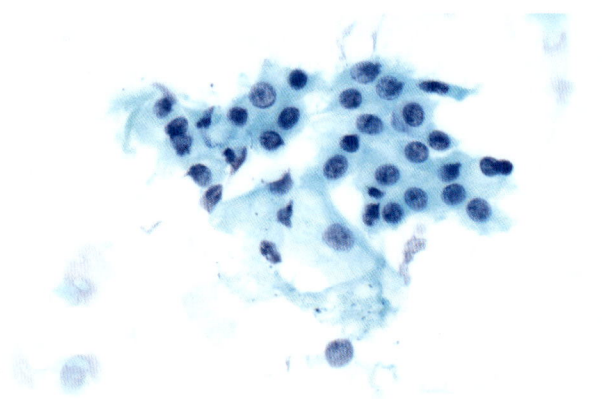

Fig. 1.126 Hyalinizing clear cell carcinoma. Pap staining of an FNA specimen demonstrating clusters of cells with round, uniform nuclei and some prominent nucleoli. The background reveals rare single cells and wispy cytoplasm.

Histopathology

Hyalinizing clear cell carcinomas are composed of small to medium-sized cells with clear or pale eosinophilic cytoplasm infiltrating in cords, nests, and trabeculae. The cells infiltrate within a background of alternating myxohyaline and fibrous stroma. Mitotic activity is minimal and necrosis is not seen. Occasional cells have intracytoplasmic mucin. Perineural invasion can be present, and peritumoural lymphocytic infiltrations are seen {794,911,2714,2711,2957}. Tumour cells are positive for CK7, high-molecular-weight cytokeratin (34βE12), CK5/6, p63, and p40. Positivity for EMA, CAM5.2, CK19, and CK14 has been reported {794}. Tumour cells are negative for TTF1, napsin A, CK20, S100, SMA, synaptophysin, and chromogranin {2711,2957}.

Cytology

Tumour cells are small to medium-sized, with either clear or pale eosinophilic cytoplasm; they are present as loose clusters and single cells with round uniform nuclei, small prominent nucleoli, and abundant wispy cytoplasm {726}.

Diagnostic molecular pathology

The *EWSR1-ATF1* fusion is present in all reported cases {2957}. One case reports an *EWSR1-CREM* fusion by FISH, which is also found in head and neck primaries {454}.

Essential and desirable diagnostic criteria

Essential:
* Low-grade epithelial cells with variable areas of cells with clear cytoplasm and cells with eosinophilic cytoplasm, within myxohyaline and sclerotic stroma

Desirable:
* Demonstration of *EWSR1-ATF1* fusion

Staging

Staging is according to the Union for International Cancer Control (UICC) TNM classification.

Prognosis and prediction

Hyalinizing clear cell carcinomas are low-grade, with an indolent course. No recurrences have been reported after resection {911,2714}.

Myoepithelioma and myoepithelial carcinoma of the lung

Husain AN
Hornick JL

Definition

Myoepithelial neoplasms of the thoracic cavity are very rare tumours that share morphological, immunophenotypic, and genetic features with their counterparts in soft tissue, salivary gland, bone, and skin. The term "myoepithelioma" is applied to benign myoepithelial tumours, whereas malignant myoepithelial tumours are designated "myoepithelial carcinoma".

ICD-O coding

8982/0 Myoepithelioma
8982/3 Myoepithelial carcinoma

ICD-11 coding

2C25.Y & XH3CQ8 Other specified malignant neoplasms of bronchus or lung & Myoepithelioma
2C25.Y & XH43E6 Other specified malignant neoplasms of bronchus or lung & Malignant myoepithelioma

Related terminology

Acceptable: myoepithelial tumour.

Subtype(s)

None

Localization

About half of pulmonary myoepithelial neoplasms are located in the large airways (endobronchial or endotracheal), with the remaining being intraparenchymal {1623}. Myoepithelial tumours may also arise in the chest wall, mediastinum, and heart {1179,970}.

Clinical features

Imaging shows central endobronchial tumours to be well circumscribed, homogeneous, polypoid, and sessile, whereas intraparenchymal tumours are either well-defined nodules or irregular masses with calcifications. Presenting features include cough with or without haemoptysis and dyspnoea, indicating obstruction in central tumours. Intraparenchymal tumours may be asymptomatic.

Epidemiology

Thoracic myoepithelial tumours are very rare, most often occurring in adults (mean age: 52 years) {1623}. Myoepithelial carcinomas predominate in children {970}.

Etiology

There is no association with smoking or other carcinogens.

Pathogenesis

EWSR1 gene rearrangements are common in myoepithelial tumours, identified in about 50% of cases, with diverse fusion partners, including *POU5F1*, *PBX1*, *ZNF444*, *KLF17*, *PBX3*, and *ATF1* {91,22,1623}; occasional cases show alternative *FUS* gene rearrangements {1201,1623}. A subset of myoepithelial carcinomas harbour homozygous deletions of *SMARCB1* {1618}.

Macroscopic appearance

Myoepithelial tumours can be well circumscribed or infiltrative, with a yellow-tan cut surface {1623}. They vary in size from 15 to > 130 mm, with a larger size seen in malignant tumours {794}. Malignant tumours may show necrosis and/or haemorrhage.

Histopathology

In contrast to mixed tumours, myoepitheliomas and myoepithelial carcinomas are composed exclusively of myoepithelial cells, without ductal or tubular structures. Myoepithelial tumours are multilobulated, with cells that vary from epithelioid or round and clear to plasmacytoid to spindled and that may be arranged in sheets or nests or have a reticular or trabecular pattern, embedded in myxoid, myxochondroid, or hyalinized matrix. Entrapped type II pneumocytes can be hypertrophic and resemble glands {3458}. Myoepithelial carcinomas often show marked nuclear

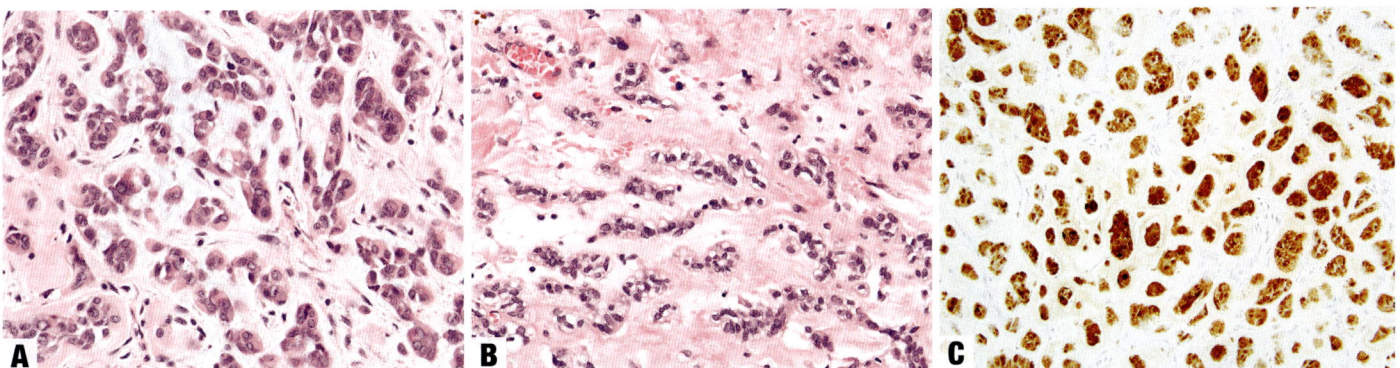

Fig. 1.127 Myoepithelioma. **A** Epithelioid tumour cells with rounded nuclei and eosinophilic cytoplasm embedded in myxoid stroma. **B** This chest wall tumour shows a nested and trabecular growth pattern. Note the collagenous stroma. **C** Immunoreactivity for S100 is characteristic.

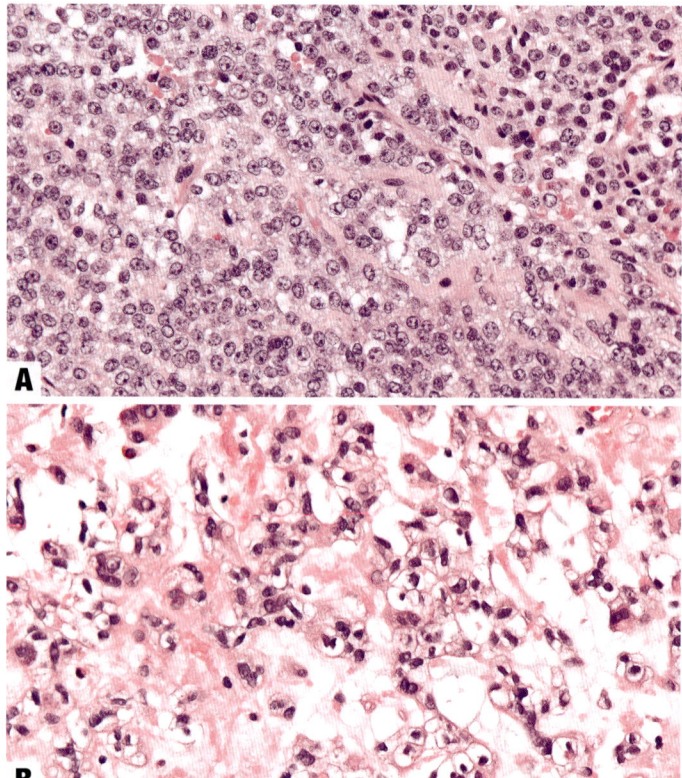

Fig. 1.128 Myoepithelial carcinoma. **A** Paediatric myoepithelial carcinomas often contain areas with a highly cellular, round cell appearance. **B** The tumour cells show a vacuolated, chordoma-like appearance.

atypia, significant pleomorphism, increased mitoses, necrosis, and infiltrative growth {794}; some paediatric examples contain sheets of round cells {970}. The tumour cells express keratins, EMA, and S100 and variably p63, p40, SOX10, SMA, and GFAP.

Cytology
Not relevant

Diagnostic molecular pathology
Rearrangements of *EWSR1* or *FUS* can be detected.

Essential and desirable diagnostic criteria
Essential:
- Trabecular, reticular, nested, and/or solid growth of variably epithelioid or spindled cells, with a frequent myxoid or hyalinized stroma
- Myoepithelial carcinomas show increased nuclear atypia, mitotic activity, and necrosis
- Positivity for EMA/keratins and S100, SOX10, or GFAP
- Exclusion of metastasis from other sites

Desirable:
- *EWSR1* rearrangements may be helpful in selected cases

Staging
Not clinically relevant

Prognosis and prediction
The presence of necrosis and ≥ 5 mitoses/2 mm² correlates with worse prognosis {1623}.

Lung neuroendocrine neoplasms: Introduction

Travis WD
Beasley MB
Cree IA
Papotti M
Rekhtman N
Rossi G

Lung neuroendocrine neoplasms (NENs) are classified as neuroendocrine tumours (NETs), comprising low-grade typical carcinoid (TC) and intermediate-grade atypical carcinoid (AC), and neuroendocrine carcinomas (NECs), comprising large cell carcinoma and small cell (lung) carcinoma (SCLC). The diagnostic criteria used in this volume are similar to those used since the 1999 WHO classification (see Table 1.14) {3068,3069,3076, 2490}. In 2015, this approach was also endorsed by an international multidisciplinary panel of the European Neuroendocrine Tumor Society (ENETS) {379} and confirmed at a consensus meeting convened by the International Agency for Research on Cancer (IARC) in 2017 {2490}. In line with this common classification framework for NENs {2490} and the 2019 WHO classification of pancreatic NETs (PanNETs), the low-grade TC and intermediate-grade AC fit into the well-differentiated category and generally correspond to grade 1 (G1) and grade 2 (G2) PanNET, respectively, whereas large cell NEC (LCNEC) and SCLC are poorly differentiated and correspond to pancreatic NEC (PanNEC) {3297}. In reporting these tumours in the lung, however, the diagnostic terms "small cell lung carcinoma" and "large cell neuroendocrine carcinoma" should be used rather than the term "neuroendocrine carcinoma" followed by the subtype.

As many as 25% of surgically resected SCLCs and LCNECs have histological components of other non-small cell carcinomas (NSCCs), such as adenocarcinoma or squamous cell carcinoma, and these tumours are classified as combined SCLC or combined LCNEC, respectively (see Table 1.14) {2631}. These cases are much more common than in the digestive tract and

pancreas, where the terms "mixed neuroendocrine–non-neuroendocrine neoplasm (MiNEN)" and "mixed adenoneuroendocrine carcinoma (MANEC)" are used {3297}. However, these terms are not recommended for combined SCLC and LCNEC. In contrast to SCLC and LCNEC, carcinoids characteristically do not have components of NSCC {2490,3068}.

Criteria and terminology for surgical resection and biopsy specimens of primary lung tumours vs biopsies of metastases of lung carcinoid tumours

Two issues need to be considered with the pathological diagnosis of NETs of the lung. The first is the difference in the approach to diagnosis in pathological specimens from primary lung tumours versus metastases. The second is the different approach to diagnosis in resected primary lung tumours versus non-resection specimens (small biopsy, cytology, or excisional biopsy), which can be obtained from either metastatic or recurrent tumours in the lung or extrapulmonary metastatic sites.

Because > 90% of carcinoid tumours are resectable, virtually all these tumours are evaluated for definitive diagnosis on a resection specimen. In addition, until recently the diagnosis of LCNEC was very difficult without a resection specimen. As a result, most of the published pathological, genetic, and clinical outcome data on carcinoid tumours and LCNEC are based on resected specimens, including the pathological criteria for diagnosing and distinguishing TC from AC. However, in non-resection specimens, the situation differs, as described below and in detail in *Carcinoid/neuroendocrine tumour of the lung*

Table 1.14 Major clinicopathological features of lung neuroendocrine tumours

	Typical carcinoid	Atypical carcinoid	LCNEC	SCLC
Average age	Sixth decade	Sixth decade	Seventh decade	Seventh decade
Sex predominance	Female	Female	Male	Male
Diagnostic criteria				
Mitoses per 2 mm^2	< 2	2–10	> 10 (median: 70)	> 10 (median: 80)
Necrosis	No	Focal, if any	Yes	Yes
Neuroendocrine morphology	Yes	Yes	Yes	Yes
Ki-67 proliferation index	Up to 5%	Up to 30%	30–100%	30–100%
TTF1 expression	Mostly positive in peripheral, mostly negative in central tumours	Mostly positive in peripheral, mostly negative in central tumours	Positive (70%)	Positive (85%)
p40 expression	Negative	Negative	Negative	Negative
Combined with NSCC component	No	No	Up to 25% of resected LCNEC	Up to 25% of resected SCLC

LCNEC, large cell neuroendocrine carcinoma; NSCC, non-small cell carcinoma; SCLC, small cell lung carcinoma.

Box 1.08 Criteria for the diagnosis of lung neuroendocrine tumours

Typical carcinoid
- A tumour ≥ 5 mm with carcinoid morphology and < 2 mitoses/2 mm², lacking necrosis

Atypical carcinoid
- A tumour with carcinoid morphology and 2–10 mitoses/2 mm² and/or necrosis (often punctate) or both

Large cell neuroendocrine carcinoma
- A tumour with neuroendocrine morphology (organoid nesting, palisading, rosettes, trabeculae)
- High mitotic count: > 10 mitoses/2 mm², median of 70 mitoses/2 mm²
- Necrosis (often in large zones)
- Cytological features of a non-small cell carcinoma, as well as large cell size; low N:C ratio; vesicular, coarse, or fine chromatin; and/or frequent nucleoli; some tumours have fine nuclear chromatin and lack nucleoli but qualify as non-small cell carcinoma because of large cell size and abundant cytoplasm
- Positive immunohistochemical staining for one or more neuroendocrine markers (other than NSE) and/or neuroendocrine granules by electron microscopy

Small cell lung carcinoma
- Small size (generally less than the diameter of 3 small resting lymphocytes)
- Scant cytoplasm
- Nuclei: finely granular nuclear chromatin, absent or faint nucleoli
- High mitotic count: > 10 mitoses/2 mm², median of 80 mitoses/2 mm²
- Frequent necrosis (often in large zones)

(p. 133), *Small cell lung carcinoma* (p. 139), and *Large cell neuroendocrine carcinoma of the lung* (p. 144).

Introduction of the term "carcinoid tumour NOS"

The term "carcinoid tumour NOS" is introduced to be used in three settings where the distinction between typical carcinoid (TC) and atypical carcinoid (AC) may not be possible or appropriate. In such cases, rather than specifying TC or AC, it is suggested to record the mitotic count, the presence or absence of necrosis, and (if available) the Ki-67 index {2458}. First, in small biopsies or cytology, the distinction between TC and AC is not possible in most cases because of the limited sampling of tumour. Second, this term should be used for metastatic carcinoids. The diagnostic criteria for distinguishing TC from AC were established on lung resection specimens and not on specimens from metastatic sites {2458}. Metastatic pulmonary carcinoid patients are often treated by medical oncologists who also manage gastrointestinal/pancreatic NETs, where Ki-67 is used to stratify patients for therapeutic decisions {2712,173,1368}. So documenting Ki-67 may be useful in the metastatic setting, although mitotic counts and necrosis remain the main diagnostic criteria in resected pulmonary carcinoids. In metastatic pulmonary carcinoids, further study is needed to determine the role of Ki-67 in classification, prognostication, and therapeutic management {2712,2500,173,1368,1807,379,2458}. This topic is addressed in more detail in *Carcinoid/neuroendocrine tumour of the lung* (p. 133). Third, in some cases, only representative slides of a resected carcinoid tumour are provided for review, rather than the entire set of tumour slides. In such cases, it is not possible to exclude the presence of an increased mitotic count or necrosis on slides not provided, to fully address the differential diagnosis of TC versus AC.

Comparative frequency and epidemiology

Within the lung, 95% of NENs are high-grade poorly differentiated tumours, including SCLC (79%) and LCNEC (16%), with carcinoids accounting for only a small proportion (2–5% TC and 0.2–0.5% AC) {3065,2770}. Poorly differentiated NECs typically occur in older patients, with a strong association with cigarette smoking and a very poor prognosis. A reported 3–10% of patients on treatment for *EGFR*-mutated adenocarcinomas with

EGFR inhibitors experience recurrence with SCLC, suggestive of clonal evolution towards neuroendocrine differentiation {1808,3449}.

Clinical and therapeutic considerations

Clinically, SCLC is distinct from all other non-small cell lung carcinomas and the other NENs in that it consistently shows an initial clinical response to chemotherapy with cisplatin in combination with etoposide, a TOP2A inhibitor {1351}. Responsiveness to SCLC chemotherapy regimens has been reported in some LCNEC series, but this is not a consistent finding {2631, 2539,2900}. TC and AC occur in younger patients than SCLC or LCNEC, and in contrast to these high-grade NECs, they do not show a strong association with cigarette smoking {3065}. Optimal therapy for metastatic carcinoids is not established, because these tumours do not show a consistent response to cisplatin/etoposide or other forms of chemotherapy. Therapeutic options include somatostatin analogues, peptide receptor radionuclide therapy, and everolimus {3056}.

Method of counting mitoses

NENs are primarily distinguished on the basis of mitotic counts per 2 mm², the presence or absence of necrosis, and (for NEC) whether the tumour has small cell or large cell cytological features (see Box 1.08) {3068}. Since the 1999 WHO classification, WHO has recommended that mitotic counts be expressed per 2 mm², rather than 10 HPF {3068,3069,3076}. This is an important standard because field of view varies between different microscopes {2490,2588,584,3084}. Mitoses should be counted in the areas of highest mitotic activity and in areas in which the entire microscopic field consists of tumour cells rather than fibrotic or inflammatory stroma and necrosis. In tumours that are near the cut-off point of 2 or 10 mitoses/2 mm², the mitotic count reported should be the average of counts in at least three sets of 2 mm² rather than the single highest count, even if the single highest count is in a hotspot {3068}. Features favouring a mitotic figure rather than a pyknotic cell include absence of a nuclear membrane, absence of a clear zone in the centre, presence of hairy rather than triangular or spiky projections, and basophilia of the surrounding cytoplasm rather than eosinophilia. Only definite mitoses should be counted;

questionable ones should be excluded {3084}. Mitotic counts and the presence or absence of necrosis should be included in pathology reports.

Role of Ki-67

The main role of Ki-67 in lung NENs is to help distinguish carcinoid tumours (NETs) from LCNEC and SCLC, especially in small biopsies with crush artefact, where carcinoids can be mistaken for SCLC {2490,2311,2312}. Although in general Ki-67 correlates with prognosis in surgically resected lung NENs, unlike in gastrointestinal and pancreatic NENs, data have not consistently supported a primary role for Ki-67 in diagnosis and classification for the following reasons:

(1) In addition to widely varying methodology for staining and interpretation of Ki-67 in published studies, no consistent threshold has been found for Ki-67 proliferation index to separate TC (G1 NET) from AC (G2 NET).

(2) Although some studies have indicated prognostic usefulness of Ki-67 in grading lung carcinoids {671,2489}, others have shown that Ki-67 is not a better predictor of patient outcome than mitotic counts {2311,2938,3192}.

(3) It has been difficult to establish definitive Ki-67 proliferation index cut-off points for separating TC from AC and for distinguishing carcinoids from SCLC or LCNEC, because the published data do not show consistent results. In carcinoids, the cut-off points range from 2.3% to 4.15% for TC and 9% to 17.8% for AC {2311,2489}. Similarly, for separating carcinoids from SCLC or LCNEC, the published cut-off points range widely, from 2.5% to 30% {2311}.

Although the published evidence has not allowed for definitive cut-off points to be determined, based on expert opinion, we suggest that tumours with a Ki-67 proliferation index > 5% are more likely to be AC than TC, and those with an index > 30% are more likely to be high-grade (LCNEC or SCLC) than AC. However, in the metastatic setting, Ki-67 can exceed these values {2458,2309}. Although Ki-67 may be useful in lung NENs, and documenting this in reports is considered desirable, the primary diagnostic criterion for separating these tumours remains mitotic count per 2 mm².

More-definitive cut-off points need more validation with future studies. Some studies focus only on carcinoids {671,1327,1806}, whereas others have evaluated the entire spectrum of neuroendocrine lung neoplasms, with various proposals of how to incorporate Ki-67 proliferation index and mitotic counts, but there is no consensus on the optimal approach {379,2311,2489,3146, 917}. Ki-67 has been shown to be useful in the setting of metastatic carcinoids of the lung to separate these tumours from SCLC or LCNEC {2458}. However, for the distinction between TC and AC in metastatic sites, Ki-67 is not recommended, because these criteria were established only in resection specimens. In the metastatic setting, the term "metastatic carcinoid NOS" is recommended, with specification of the key features of mitoses per 2 mm², necrosis, and Ki-67 proliferation index {2458}. In this setting, more investigations are needed before incorporating Ki-67 into the classification of resected lung NETs.

Carcinoid tumours with elevated mitotic counts and/or Ki-67 proliferation index

Recent literature has documented the existence of lung NETs with morphological features of AC but higher mitotic counts (> 10 mitoses/2 mm²) than in the currently defined 2015 WHO criteria and/or with Ki-67 proliferation index values that are higher than would be expected (> 30%) {1806,2405,1391,2463, 2173,1240}. Such tumours are very rare at primary sites but are not uncommon in the metastatic setting. These tumours were recognized in the 1999 WHO classification, but due to lack of enough data, it was proposed they be called LCNEC {3076}. Since that time, only a few papers have been published on this topic, with varying pathological features and limited genetic and outcome data {1806,2405,1391,2463,2173,1240}. These tumours generally correspond to those regarded as grade 3 (G3) NETs in the pancreas (PanNET). This topic is discussed in more detail in *Carcinoid/neuroendocrine tumour of the lung* (p. 133).

Genetics

NECs (SCLC and LCNEC) have many more genetic alterations, consisting of amplifications, deletions, and mutations, than do lung carcinoids {543}. Biallelic inactivation of *TP53* and *RB1* is characteristic of SCLC, and 25% of cases show inactivating mutations of genes in the NOTCH family {937,2563}. However, LCNEC shows more genetic heterogeneity than SCLCs, with an SCLC-like group that shows biallelic inactivation of *TP53* and *RB1* and an NSCC-like group with mutations in *KRAS* and *STK11/KEAP1* {2463,938,668}. Lung carcinoids (NETs) are very different from high-grade NECs in that they lack mutations in *TP53*, *RB1*, *KRAS*, and *STK11/KEAP1*. However, in 40% of cases they have mutations in chromatin-remodelling genes, such as covalent histone modifiers, and in 22% of cases they have mutations in subunits of the SWI/SNF complex, including the *MEN1*, *PSIP1*, and *ARID1A* genes {816}. Rare tumours with carcinoid-like morphology and genetic features such as *MEN1* mutations can occur and have been suggested to correspond to tumours with carcinoid morphology but elevated mitotic counts and Ki-67 index {2463}.

In summary, there are major clinical, epidemiological, histological, genetic, and prognostic differences between the carcinoids/NETs (TC and AC) and high-grade NECs (both SCLC and LCNEC).

NSCCs with neuroendocrine differentiation

Some non-small cell lung carcinomas lacking neuroendocrine morphology by light microscopy demonstrate immunohistochemical and/or ultrastructural features of neuroendocrine differentiation. This differentiation can be found by immunohistochemistry in 10–20% of squamous cell carcinomas, adenocarcinomas, and large cell carcinomas, although more often found in adenocarcinomas {3068}. These tumours are regarded as NSCCs with neuroendocrine differentiation. No consistent data have demonstrated significant clinical differences from tumours lacking neuroendocrine differentiation {3074}. Therefore, it is not recommended to perform neuroendocrine immunohistochemical stains or electron microscopy in the absence of neuroendocrine morphology {3068}.

Diffuse idiopathic pulmonary neuroendocrine cell hyperplasia

Rossi G
MacMahon H
Marchevsky AM
Nicholson AG
Snead DRJ

Definition

Diffuse idiopathic pulmonary neuroendocrine cell hyperplasia (DIPNECH) is a multifocal hyperplasia of pulmonary neuroendocrine cells associated with tumourlets. It is a preinvasive condition that may develop into carcinoid tumours. DIPNECH may be accompanied by bronchiolar fibrosis with constrictive features.

ICD-O coding

8040/0 Diffuse idiopathic neuroendocrine cell hyperplasia

ICD-11 coding

2F00.Y Other specified benign neoplasm of middle ear or respiratory system

Related terminology

DIPNECH was originally recognized in 1992 and termed Aguayo's syndrome {31}. The term "DIPNECH syndrome" has been proposed to distinguish symptomatic cases with constrictive bronchiolitis {2541}.

Subtype(s)

None

Localization

DIPNECH is a bronchiolar / small airway disease involving secondary lobules {31,619,1514,2078,2541,1887}.

Clinical features

DIPNECH manifests as a continuous spectrum of pathological {2078,1805,3324,1803}, clinical, and radiological features {31, 619,2541,1887}.

Signs and symptoms

There are two major clinical presentations: DIPNECH presenting with clinical symptoms and DIPNECH presenting in asymptomatic patients.

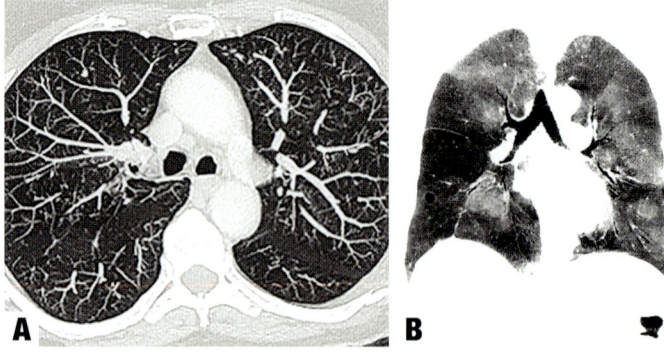

Fig. 1.129 Diffuse idiopathic pulmonary neuroendocrine cell hyperplasia. **A** Maximum intensity projection CT with multiple small lung nodules consistent with tumourlets. **B** Coronal minimum intensity projection CT showing mosaic perfusion pattern secondary to air trapping, consistent with diffuse idiopathic pulmonary neuroendocrine cell hyperplasia.

DIPNECH presenting with clinical symptoms is associated with constrictive bronchiolitis. It manifests with a long history of cough, breathlessness, and wheezing, and it is often misdiagnosed as asthma {31,619,2541,1887}. It shows characteristic imaging, and definitive diagnosis is made on the basis of lung biopsy that shows lesions of pathological DIPNECH. In addition, even without a biopsy, the diagnosis may be suspected in patients with characteristic clinical and imaging characteristics.

DIPNECH presenting in asymptomatic patients is typically an incidental finding, on high-resolution CT performed for a different reason. These patients are often suspected to have metastases due to multiple bilateral lung nodules {31,619,1514,2078, 2541,1887}.

Rarely, DIPNECH is a component of multiple endocrine neoplasia type 1 {2078}.

Imaging

On CT, DIPNECH syndrome is characterized by mosaic perfusion due to air trapping, bronchiolar wall thickening, and

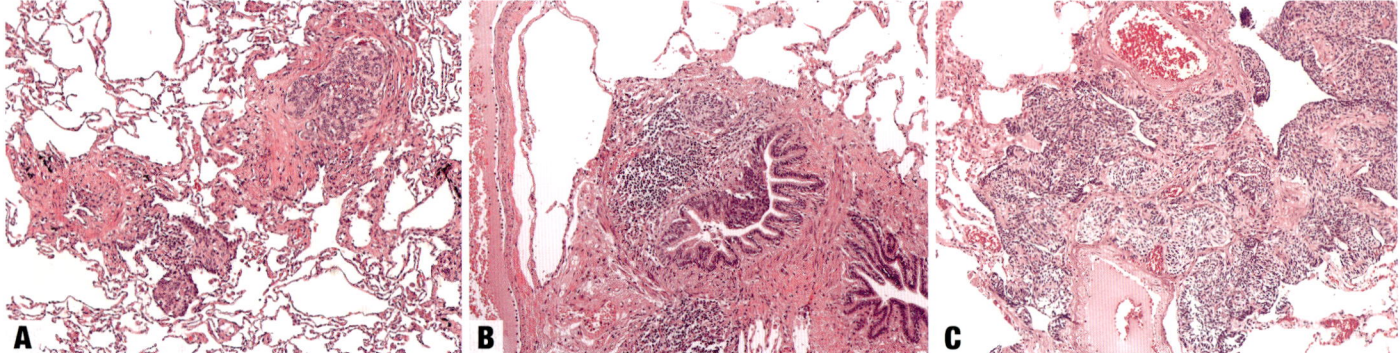

Fig. 1.130 Diffuse idiopathic pulmonary neuroendocrine cell hyperplasia. **A** Proliferation of neuroendocrine cells within a terminal bronchiole associated with constrictive bronchiolitis. **B** Intramucosal linear proliferation of neuroendocrine cells in a terminal bronchiole with a tiny tumourlet spreading through the basement membrane. **C** A tumourlet characterized by an invasive bronchiolocentric neuroendocrine cell proliferation of < 5 mm with fibrotic stroma.

bronchiectasis with mucus plugging {1514,459}. Identification of a mosaic pattern may require expiration high-resolution CT. In addition, multiple bilateral small nodules (< 5 mm) corresponding to tumourlets are frequent. Nodules measuring ≥ 5 mm may represent carcinoid tumours. DIPNECH syndrome may be suspected on the basis of CT before biopsy if all of the above features are present, particularly in a symptomatic middle-aged female patient {459}.

Epidemiology

DIPNECH syndrome typically occurs in non-smokers in their fifth or sixth decade of life and is more common in women {31, 619,2541,1887}. Histological evidence of DIPNECH is often readily evident when associated with peripheral-type carcinoid tumours; however, it may require extensive sampling of lung adjacent to carcinoids {1887}.

Etiology

DIPNECH syndrome is idiopathic, but neuroendocrine cell hyperplasia may be a consequence of unrecognized chronic pulmonary injuries. However, in DIPNECH syndrome, it is more likely that these changes are secondary to an autocrine/paracrine stimulation of molecules released by the proliferating neuroendocrine cells {31,619,2078,1805,3324,1803,2541}.

Pathogenesis

Although the pathogenesis of DIPNECH remains unclear, several conditions may induce neuroendocrine cell hyperplasia, including chronic pulmonary diseases, interstitial fibrosis, airway inflammation and/or fibrosis, infections, and hypoxaemic status {31,619,2078,1805,3324,1803,2541}. Rare cases are associated with multiple endocrine neoplasia type 1 {619}.

Reproducible genetic alterations of DIPNECH are lacking, although occasional association with multiple endocrine neoplasia type 1 is described {619,2537}. CD10, GRP (bombesin), mTOR and p70S6K, and SSTR2 are commonly upregulated in DIPNECH, while a focal expression is noted with p53, p16, and Ki-67 {992, 1887}. No gene alterations have been reported in *EGFR, KRAS, KIT*, PDGFR genes, *MET*, or *ALK* {1887}. Heterozygous mutation of the *NKX2-1* gene (encoding TTF1) is reported in a rare childhood disease, neuroendocrine cell hyperplasia of infancy {3438}.

Tumour development

DIPNECH arises in terminal bronchioles as a proliferation of single or clusters of neuroendocrine cells. When tumourlets develop, they invade locally into and through the bronchiolar wall, sometimes into adjacent parenchyma. DIPNECH is considered to be a preinvasive lesion in a subset of carcinoids, mostly typical carcinoids {619,2078}. High-grade neuroendocrine carcinomas (NECs) are not associated with DIPNECH.

Macroscopic appearance

The neuroendocrine cell hyperplasia of DIPNECH is not visible macroscopically, but tumourlets may be seen as grey-white nodules as large as 5 mm.

Histopathology

Pathological DIPNECH is characterized by proliferation of neuroendocrine cells and/or tumourlets involving small airways. Neuroendocrine cell hyperplasia consists of individual cells

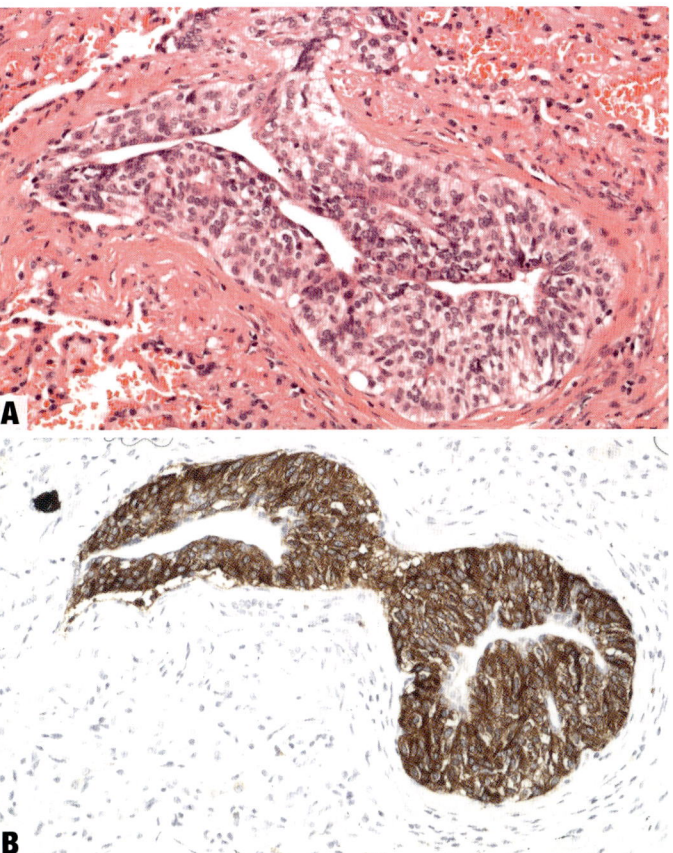

Fig. 1.131 Diffuse idiopathic pulmonary neuroendocrine cell hyperplasia. **A** Intramucosal linear proliferation of neuroendocrine cells in a respiratory bronchiole with increased thickening of the epithelium. **B** Chromogranin staining highlights the neuroendocrine cell hyperplasia.

or cellular aggregates designated as neuroendocrine bodies within the bronchiolar mucosa. The neuroendocrine cells have round, oval, or spindle-shaped nuclei with salt-and pepper chromatin and a moderate amount of amphophilic or eosinophilic cytoplasm. Nodular proliferations of neuroendocrine cells that invade beyond the bronchiolar wall measuring < 5 mm are classified as tumourlets. It has been proposed that neuroendocrine cell hyperplasia consists of the presence of ≥ 5 neuroendocrine cells, singly or in clusters, located within the basement membrane of the bronchiolar epithelium, and that there is multifocal neuroendocrine cell hyperplasia when ≥ 3 bronchioles are involved {1805}, but this requires further validation. In DIPNECH syndrome, bronchiolar fibrosis with luminal narrowing or constrictive bronchiolitis is present. DIPNECH associated with carcinoid tumours shows one or more carcinoid tumours in the lung parenchyma in addition to neuroendocrine cell hyperplasia and tumourlets meeting the above criteria {1805,1887}. Pathological confirmation of DIPNECH requires a surgical lung biopsy or resection specimen; a definitive pathological diagnosis cannot be made on small biopsies.

Immunohistochemistry

DIPNECH expresses neuroendocrine markers (chromogranin, synaptophysin, CD56), pancytokeratins, and TTF1 (generally less intensively than pneumocytes), while negative for p40/p63 and high-molecular-weight cytokeratins.

Differential diagnosis

DIPNECH must be separated from localized reactive neuroendocrine cell hyperplasia associated with carcinoid tumours or with neuroendocrine cell hyperplasia/tumourlets secondary to airway inflammation, granulomas, fibrosis, or high altitude. Incidental tumourlets and/or neuroendocrine cell hyperplasia can be seen in the non-neoplastic lung parenchyma surrounding 75% of carcinoid tumours {1925}. Nodular proliferations of neuroendocrine cells measuring ≥ 5 mm are diagnosed as carcinoid tumours. DIPNECH should be distinguished from neuroendocrine cell hyperplasia of infancy, which occurs in young children {3437}.

Cytology

Normal or hyperplastic neuroendocrine cells are usually not seen in cytological specimens. When observed, they can present a potential diagnostic pitfall, because they can be mistaken for carcinoid or small cell carcinoma cells {1795,103}. Therefore, DIPNECH cannot be diagnosed on cytology alone.

Diagnostic molecular pathology

Not clinically relevant

Essential and desirable diagnostic criteria

Clinicopathological DIPNECH can be suspected without biopsy in patients with characteristic clinical and radiological findings. The diagnosis of DIPNECH may also be primarily based on pathological findings rather than clinical or imaging findings; this usually occurs in asymptomatic patients.

Pathological DIPNECH

Essential:
- Neuroendocrine cell hyperplasia and/or tumourlets, both usually multifocal

Desirable:
- Constrictive bronchiolitis is frequent, particularly in clinical DIPNECH
- Carcinoid tumours, single or multiple, may be present
- Multidisciplinary exclusion of reactive neuroendocrine cell hyperplasia and tumourlets either associated with lung neoplasms other than carcinoids or due to non-neoplastic lung disorders such as interstitial fibrosis or small airway disease other than constrictive bronchiolitis

Clinical DIPNECH

Essential:
- Symptoms related to airway obstruction such as cough, breathlessness, and wheezing, often misdiagnosed as asthma
- CT findings of mosaic attenuation with or without bilateral pulmonary nodules < 5 mm (i.e. probable tumourlets) or ≥ 5 mm (probable carcinoid tumours)

Desirable:
- Middle-aged women with dyspnoea
- Pathological confirmation of multifocal neuroendocrine cell hyperplasia and/or tumourlet(s)

Staging

DIPNECH is preinvasive. Carcinoid tumours are staged according to the TNM scheme, and multiple carcinoids in the setting of DIPNECH should not be regarded as intrapulmonary metastases, but as independent primaries {3078,2421}.

Prognosis and prediction

DIPNECH syndrome associated with constrictive bronchiolitis is usually treated with steroids and/or beta agonists {3324}. Progression requiring lung transplantation can occur {2078, 3324,1805}. Patients with DIPNECH associated with neuroendocrine proliferations have a good prognosis, with slow growth of the pulmonary nodules. Somatostatin analogue therapy does not appear to control tumour progression, although there are reports of response to somatostatin analogues, azithromycin, and everolimus in the management of debilitating symptoms {2078,990,2041,68}. There are no reports of DIPNECH patients developing high-grade neuroendocrine neoplasms (NENs) of the lung such as large cell NEC (LCNEC) or small cell carcinoma.

Carcinoid/neuroendocrine tumour of the lung

Papotti M   MacMahon H
Brambilla E   Osamura RY
Dingemans AC   Pelosi G
Fernandez-Cuesta L Rekhtman N
Lantuejoul S

Definition

Carcinoid tumours are neuroendocrine malignancies with a well-differentiated organoid architecture. There are two subtypes: *typical carcinoids* (TCs; carcinoid tumours with < 2 mitoses/2 mm² and lacking necrosis) and *atypical carcinoids* (ACs; carcinoid tumours with 2–10 mitoses/2 mm² and/or foci of necrosis, usually punctate).

ICD-O coding

8240/3 Carcinoid tumour, NOS / neuroendocrine tumour, NOS
8240/3 Typical carcinoid / neuroendocrine tumour, grade 1
8249/3 Atypical carcinoid / neuroendocrine tumour, grade 2

ICD-11 coding

2C25.4 & XH9LV8 Carcinoid or other malignant neuroendocrine neoplasms of bronchus or lung & Neuroendocrine tumour, grade 1
2C25.4 & XH51K1 Carcinoid or other malignant neuroendocrine neoplasms of bronchus or lung & Neuroendocrine tumour, grade 2

Related terminology

"Neuroendocrine tumour (NET)" is a related term, according to the unifying nomenclature proposed by the International Agency for Research on Cancer (IARC) and the WHO Classification of Tumours Group {2490}, that includes well-differentiated grade 1 (G1) NET and grade 2 (G2) NET, which generally correspond to TC and AC, regarded as low-grade and intermediate-grade, respectively.

The terminology "well-differentiated neuroendocrine tumour, grades 1 and 2" is not recommended for lung carcinoid tumours.

Subtype(s)

Typical carcinoid; atypical carcinoid

Localization

Pulmonary carcinoids may be central or peripheral lesions, with TC and AC situated more often centrally and peripherally, respectively {1047,2800,832,2260,182}. Different location of carcinoids could imply different precursors and/or development mechanisms {1582,1927}.

Clinical features

Signs and symptoms

Patients with central carcinoids involving segmental and larger airways may present with symptoms related to bronchial obstruction, including cough, wheezing, haemoptysis, and recurrent pneumonia. In addition, symptoms may mimic asthma. At bronchoscopy, central carcinoids appear as endobronchial, polypoid, and hypervascular lesions. Peripheral carcinoids are generally asymptomatic and are typically detected as an incidental finding on chest imaging. Symptoms related to hormone secretion (e.g. carcinoid syndrome or Cushing syndrome) are rare {1055,1856}.

Imaging

TCs usually form central nodules or masses with lobulated, well-circumscribed contours. Due to their vascular nature, they show pronounced attenuation increase on contrast-enhanced CT. Calcification resulting from stromal ossification is detectable by CT in a minority of cases {1308,1877,3528}. When an endobronchial component is present, secondary distal effects can include recurrent pneumonia, atelectasis, bronchiectasis, and hyperlucency on CT {1877}. Peripheral carcinoids form sharply circumscribed intraparenchymal lesions and are more often atypical. FDG PET usually shows some abnormal uptake in TCs, but with lower average standardized uptake values than other solid lung cancers {1541,3528}. ACs show greater FDG avidity. Both FDG PET and 68Ga-DOTATOC PET (targeting the somatostatin receptor) are useful in the staging of carcinoids, with the highest sensitivity for 68Ga-DOTATOC PET (90% vs 71%) {1314}.

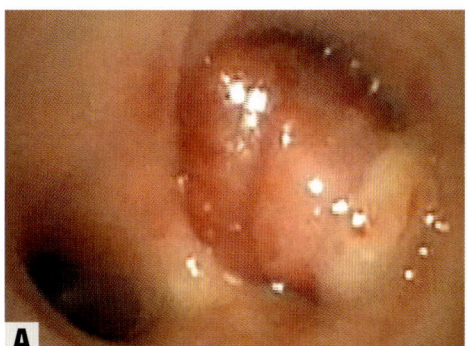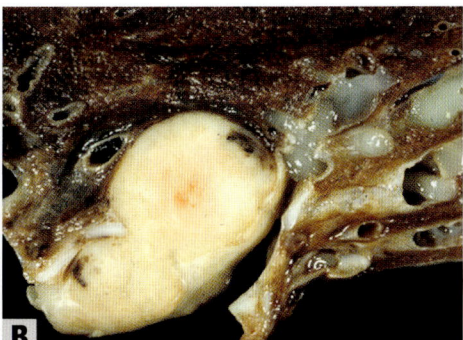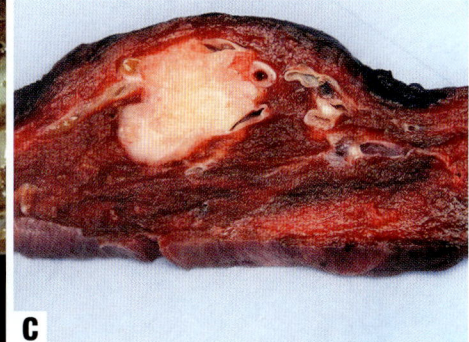

Fig. 1.132 Typical carcinoid. **A** Bronchoscopic image of a typical carcinoid forming a polypoid endobronchial mass. **B** A circumscribed endobronchial mass causing complete obstruction of the bronchus and postobstructive dilation of the distal bronchial segment. **C** A peripheral subpleural well-circumscribed whitish mass.

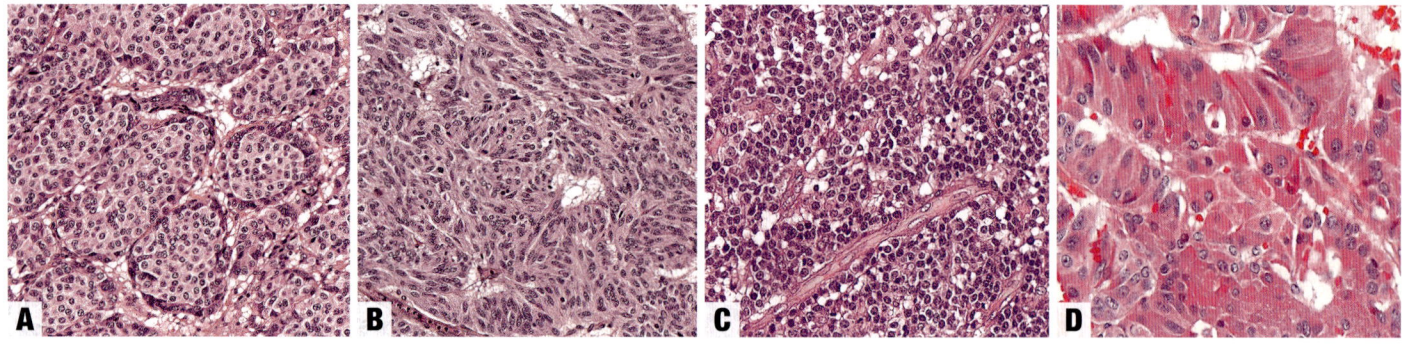

Fig. 1.133 Typical carcinoid. Various growth patterns are identifiable, including nests (**A**), spindle (**B**), and solid (**C**). Diffuse oncocytic changes (**D**) are rarely observed.

Tumour spread

Distant metastases are rare for TCs (< 5%) but are common for ACs (20–30%) {2454}. Typical sites of distant metastasis for lung carcinoids include liver, bone, and brain. In particular, brain metastases are present in 20–30% of patients with stage IV lung carcinoids {515,2458}. Lung carcinoids also have a propensity to metastasize to unusual sites, including skin, eye, and ovary {2458}. Regional lymph node metastases occur in approximately 10% and 50% of TC and AC cases, respectively {2454,2412}.

Epidemiology

Pulmonary carcinoids are rare tumours, accounting for ≤ 2% of all lung malignancies {379}. The ratio of TCs to ACs is about 8–10:1 {2800,3417,1047,173,831}. The age-adjusted incidence rate ranges from 0.2 to 2 cases per 100 000 person-years {379}. This is slightly higher in women {819}, white populations {1950, 3387,2323}, and in the fifth and sixth decades of life (median age: 45 years for TC and one decade later for AC) {791,1090, 182}. Pulmonary carcinoids account for a substantial portion of childhood lung tumours, occurring mostly in late adolescence {2499,3447,1675}.

Etiology

No risk factors are recognized for carcinoid tumour. Tobacco smoking has been proposed, but no genetic signature of tobacco damage has so far been recognized, indicating that a link is questionable. Genetic causes include *MEN1* gene mutations in the setting of hereditary multiple endocrine neoplasia type 1, in which ACs are most common.

Pathogenesis

Diffuse idiopathic pulmonary neuroendocrine cell hyperplasia is recognized as a preinvasive condition for carcinoids (see *Diffuse idiopathic pulmonary neuroendocrine cell hyperplasia*, p. 130) {2454,619}, although the rate of progression to carcinoid is presumably low {125}. Localized and diffuse neuroendocrine cell hyperplasia can be seen in association with 60–75% of peripheral carcinoids {1925,2498}. Neuroendocrine cell hyperplasia can be a secondary reaction to airway fibrosis and inflammation, and carcinoids can develop in this setting {2498, 2318}. Orthopedia homeobox protein (OTP), a key player in the development of the hypothalamic neuroendocrine system, is expressed in diffuse idiopathic pulmonary neuroendocrine cell hyperplasia and carcinoids, while not in normal neuroendocrine cells {2134}, suggesting a role for the *OTP* gene along with deregulated proliferation in the development of pulmonary carcinoids {1964}.

The distinct epidemiological, clinical, morphological, and molecular profiles of pulmonary carcinoids – NETs – versus the high-grade small cell lung carcinoma (SCLC) and large cell neuroendocrine carcinoma (LCNEC) – neuroendocrine carcinomas (NECs) – support two separate tumour groups with different carcinogenic processes (see Table 1.14, p. 127). In the uncommon advanced-stage metastatic setting, pulmonary carcinoids can show an increased mitotic count and Ki-67 index compared with the primary tumour {2458,2309}.

Research genomic studies show that pulmonary carcinoids (NETs) have a low mutation rate {816,2775,543}. Significantly mutated genes include *MEN1*, *EIF1AX*, and *ARID1A* {816,1582}. Mutations in chromatin-remodelling genes such as those involved

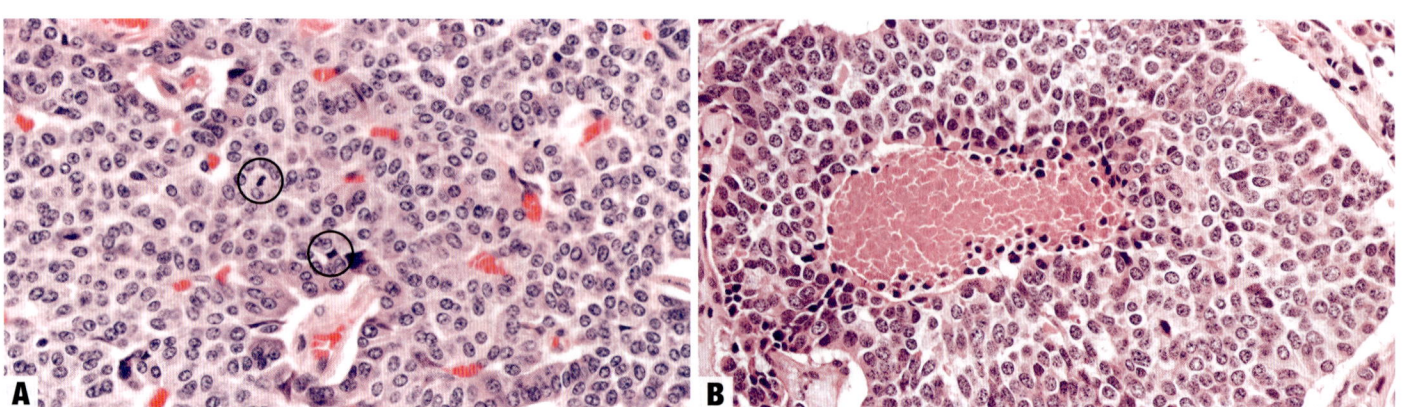

Fig. 1.134 Atypical carcinoid. **A** Solid growth pattern with minimal atypia. Two mitoses are present (circled). **B** This atypical carcinoid tumour shows punctate necrosis.

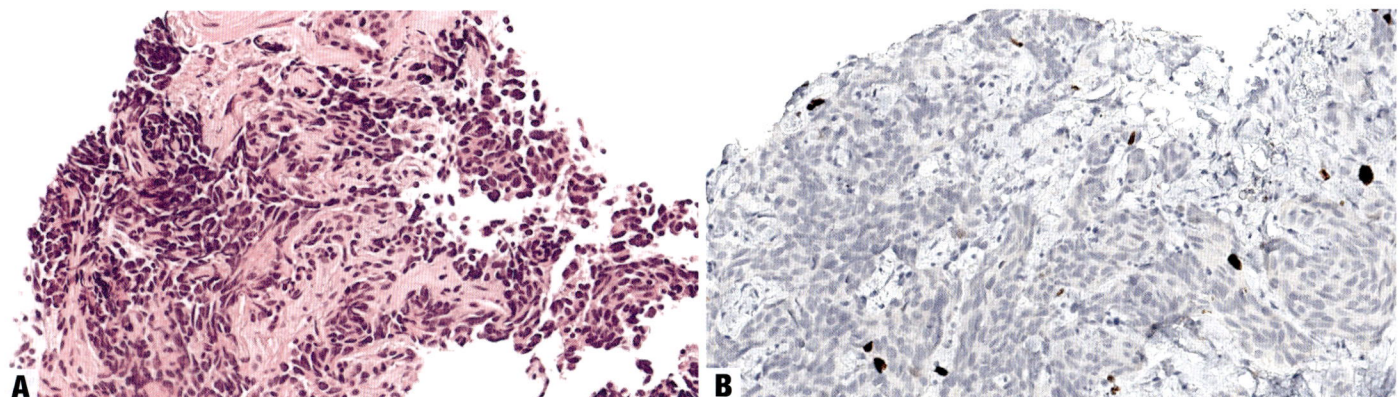

Fig. 1.135 Carcinoid. **A** Bronchial biopsy of a lung tumour made of small uniform cells. **B** Ki-67 index is quite low in tumour cells, excluding the possibility of a small cell carcinoma.

in histone methylation and acetylation, as well as members of the SWI/SNF complex, are present in 50% of cases {816,2775}. Overall, *MEN1* is the most frequently mutated gene, with somatic mutations in 11–22% of cases {816,2775,2939,644}. Unlike in SCLC and LCNEC, mutations in the *TP53* and *RB1* tumour suppressor genes are extremely rare in pulmonary carcinoids (NETs) {816,2775}, and the minority of ACs that show *TP53* mutations lack the smoking-related G>T and C>A transversions typically found in SCLC and LCNEC {2194}.

Three molecular groups have been identified among lung carcinoids {50,1582}. All *MEN1* mutations are found in the group that is enriched for ACs and has high levels of UGT and CYP genes, high levels of *ANGPTL3* and *ERBB4*, and low levels of *OPT* and *TTF1*. The other two groups consist mostly of TCs: one shows high levels of *ASCL1* and *DLL3*, with *EIF1AX* mutations; the other has low levels of *SLIT1* and *ROBO1*, with expression of *HNF1A* and *FOXA3*.

A small number of carcinoids (NETs) have unusual genetic findings, with high levels of immune checkpoint receptors and ligands (including PDL1 and CTLA-4) similar to – or even higher than – those of LCNEC and SCLC {50}. More study is needed to validate and determine the clinical relevance of these genetic findings.

Macroscopic appearance

Central carcinoids are well-circumscribed, round to ovoid masses that are often endobronchial and may be pedunculated.

Tumours may grow between the cartilaginous plates into adjacent tissues. Peripheral tumours may not be clearly associated with an airway. An endobronchial component can be seen in 50% of cases. By definition, neuroendocrine proliferations ≥ 5 mm are classified as carcinoid tumours, and if < 5 mm they are classified as tumourlets (see Box 1.08, p. 128). TCs are generally smaller than the ACs, but size is not a distinguishing criterion {3130,990,2469}. Carcinoids are grey to yellow and may show haemorrhagic areas. They may be soft or firm and can be hard if they contain bone. Tumours causing bronchial obstruction may be associated with secondary abscesses and/or bronchiectasis.

Histopathology

TCs and ACs are well-differentiated NETs at the level of both tumour architecture and cytological features. However, clinically, TCs are low-grade and ACs are intermediate-grade. Differences are only related to mitosis and/or necrosis. TCs (G1 NETs) have a mitotic count of < 2 mitoses/2 mm^2 and lack necrosis. ACs (G2 NETs) have 2–10 mitoses/2 mm^2 and/or may have necrosis, which is usually focal and punctate. See *Lung neuroendocrine neoplasms: Introduction* (p. 127) for details on methods of counting mitoses. Neuroendocrine morphology is defined by organoid patterns of growth with trabecular, rosette formation, insular, palisading, ribbon, follicular, pseudoglandular, or solid arrangements, while true glandular spaces or papillae are uncommon. Oncocytic, clear cell, and melanin-laden

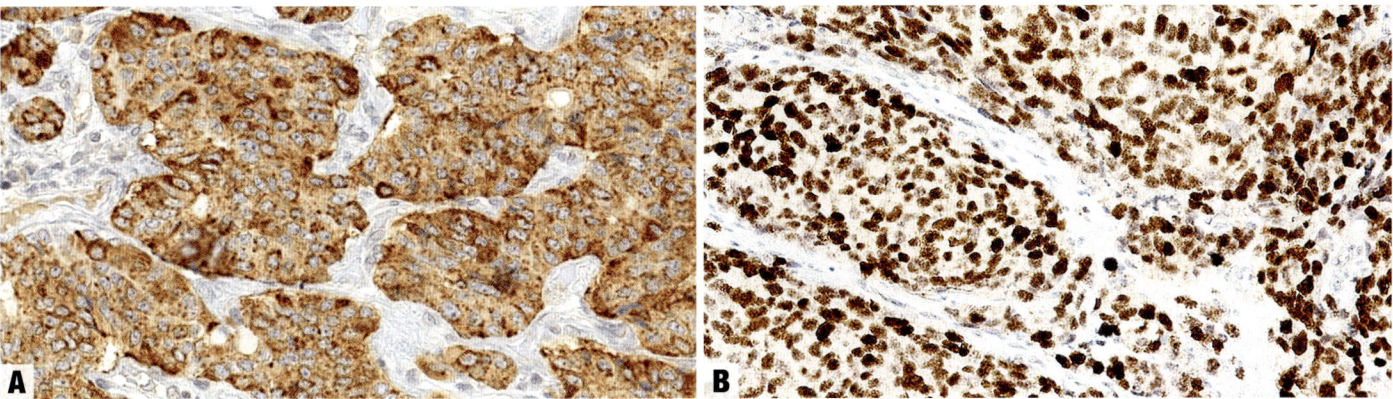

Fig. 1.136 Carcinoid. Chromogranin A (**A**) and INSM1 (**B**) strong reactivity is present in most tumour cell cytoplasm and nuclei of a typical carcinoid and an atypical carcinoid, respectively.

carcinoids can occur. Tumour cells are uniform, featuring finely granular nuclear chromatin, moderate to abundant eosinophilic cytoplasm, inconspicuous to variably evident nucleoli, and fine to coarsely granular chromatin texture. Tumour cells are small to intermediate in size and cuboidal to polygonal or fusiform. Fusiform cells are especially seen in peripheral lesions {2260}. Unlike for SCLC and LCNEC, the combination of carcinoids with adenocarcinoma or squamous cell carcinoma is exceptional {833,831,2490,2631,2442,182,2108,543,816,2463,938,3084, 3068}. In addition, carcinoid tumours characteristically do not occur in combination with SCLC and LCNEC {833,831,2490, 2631,2442,182,2108,543,816,2463,938,3084,2682,3068}.

Carcinoid tumours / NETs with elevated mitotic counts and/or Ki-67 proliferation index

Rare lung carcinoids (NETs) have morphological features of AC but higher mitotic counts (> 10 mitoses/2 mm^2) than defined in the present WHO classification and/or a higher Ki-67 proliferation index than expected (> 30%) {1806,2405,1391,2463, 1240}. Genomic analysis is available for only a few such cases, but it supports a relationship with carcinoids rather than SCLC or LCNEC, based on lack of *RB1* or *TP53* mutations, low total mutation burden, and/or presence of *MEN1* mutations {2463}. These tumours generally correspond to those regarded as grade 3 (G3) NETs in the pancreas (PanNET); however, in the lung, more clinical, pathological, and genetic studies are needed to determine how to fit these tumours into the classification. Currently, such tumours are usually classified as LCNEC, but their prognosis has been suggested to be different from that of conventional LCNEC. Until these tumours are better defined, we suggest adding a note stating the presence of histological features of a carcinoid tumour and documenting the mitotic counts and if available the Ki-67 index. The optimal approach to systemic management (e.g. the effectiveness of immunotherapies) needs to be addressed. Careful attention to the method of mitosis counting is needed, as outlined in *Lung neuroendocrine neoplasms: Introduction* (p. 127), because mitotic counts can be artefactually elevated by failure to adjust for the varying microscope fields of view depending on the microscope

manufacturer and model or by lack of a strict definition of a mitotic figure {2490,2588,584,3084}.

Immunohistochemistry

Carcinoid tumours are positive for low-molecular-weight cytokeratins, but they lack reactivity to high-molecular-weight cytokeratins {2884}. They are strongly reactive for neuroendocrine markers such as chromogranin A, synaptophysin, CD56, and INSM1 {2022,2523,881}. TTF1 tends to be positive in peripheral but negative in central tumours {732}.

The proliferation marker Ki-67 is not part of the diagnostic criteria for lung carcinoids, particularly in the distinction of TC from AC {2938,3192}. Although tumours with a Ki-67 index > 5% are more likely to be ACs, this is not an absolute cut-off value {1806}. The main role of Ki-67 is in crushed cytology or biopsy samples to exclude SCLC or LCNEC {2312}. Further work is needed to address the clinical significance and optimal role of Ki-67 index in the diagnosis and prognostic evaluation of pulmonary carcinoids {2317,1799,1806,2309,2311}.

Differential diagnosis

The differential diagnosis of pulmonary carcinoids includes metastatic carcinoids from elsewhere, especially those originating in the gastrointestinal tract {2835}. Glandular structures are unusual in pulmonary carcinoids but a frequent finding in gastrointestinal carcinoids. Gastrointestinal and pancreatic carcinoids are usually negative for TTF1 but frequently express CDX2 or PAX8 {2835,1727}. Mitotic counts are the most important morphological feature for distinguishing carcinoids from SCLC and LCNEC (see *Lung neuroendocrine neoplasms: Introduction*, p. 127), but they may be difficult to determine in small crushed biopsies. In this setting, Ki-67 plays an important role, because tumours with a high labelling index (> 30%) are more likely to be SCLC or LCNEC, and tumours with a Ki-67 proliferation index < 30% are more likely to be carcinoids {2312,118}. The monotonous nuclear appearance of carcinoids may also be seen in salivary gland–type tumours, metastases of lobular breast carcinoma, paraganglioma, melanoma, and glomus tumours. Salivary gland–type tumours are usually negative for

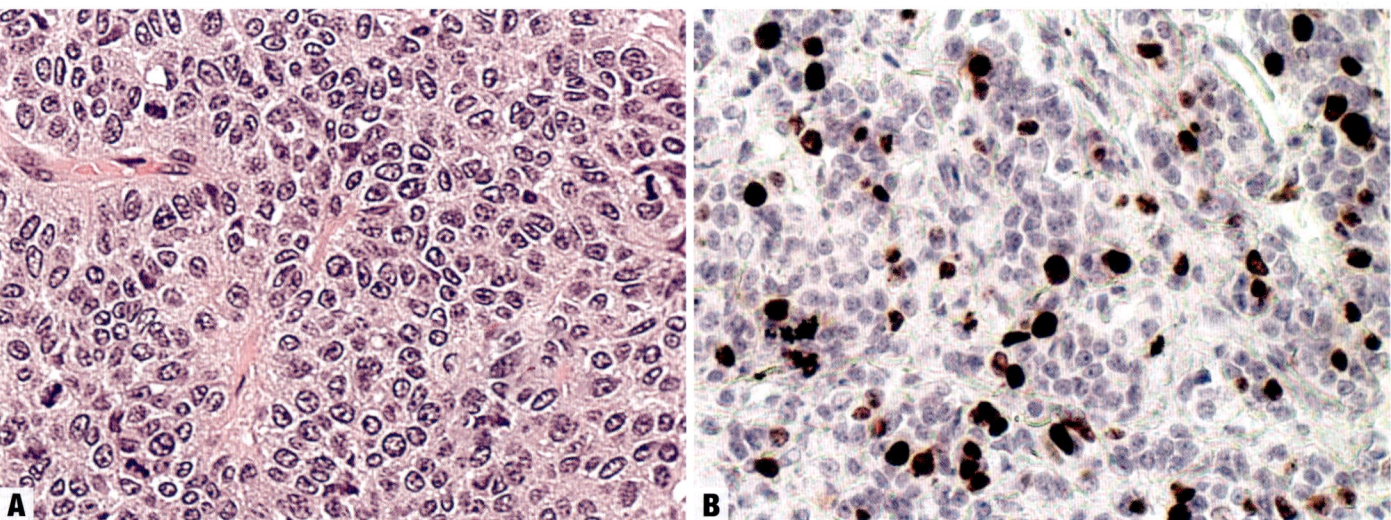

Fig. 1.137 Large cell neuroendocrine carcinoma (LCNEC) with morphological features of carcinoid / neuroendocrine tumour (NET) with high proliferation. Solid growth pattern in an area with high mitotic activity (21 mitoses/2 mm^2) (**A**), associated with a Ki-67 index of 20% (**B**).

neuroendocrine markers. Mucoepidermoid carcinomas usually express p40 and have intracytoplasmic mucin. Adenoid cystic carcinomas show a dual pattern of cellular staining with CAM5.2, which is strong in ductal/luminal cells but weak in myoepithelial cells, and both p63 and S100 are positive in myoepithelial cells. Adenoid cystic carcinomas also have *MYB-NFIB* or *MYBL1-NFIB* fusions by FISH in 60–90% of cases (see *Adenoid cystic carcinoma of the lung*, p. 117). Breast carcinomas may be positive for ER and/or PR, and they are usually negative for neuroendocrine markers. However, positive staining for ER and PR has been reported in some carcinoid tumours {2764}. Metastases from thyroid carcinoma are positive for TTF1, thyroglobulin, and PAX8. The distinction of carcinoids from paragangliomas is based mainly on morphology; although paragangliomas are pancytokeratin-negative, so are about 20% of carcinoid tumours, and S100-positive sustentacular cells can be seen in both entities {2454,3081}. Melanomas are positive for melanoma markers (HMB45, S100, and SOX10) but negative for neuroendocrine markers, although melanocytic carcinoids may express both {153}. Glomus tumours are positive for SMA but negative for neuroendocrine markers.

Diagnosis in non-resection specimens and metastases

The diagnosis of carcinoid tumours can be readily made on the basis of small biopsies and cytology specimens in most cases. The distinction between TC and AC cannot be made in small biopsies, and resection is required. In this setting, the term "carcinoid tumour NOS" is recommended. If a few mitotic figures and/or foci of punctate necrosis are identified, this may be suggestive of AC, and this can be mentioned in a comment. If there is any doubt about the diagnosis of carcinoid tumour, immunohistochemistry should be performed. Ki-67 may be helpful in the distinction from SCLC and LCNEC, particularly in small crushed specimens. Notably, in metastatic carcinoids, Ki-67 may occasionally exceed 30%, usually in hotspots {2458}.

In pathological specimens from patients with metastatic pulmonary carcinoids, the term "metastatic carcinoid tumour NOS" (NET) should be used rather than specifying TC or AC, because proliferation rates may vary at different sites and many core biopsies from metastatic tumours may be too small to allow accurate mitotic counts per 2 mm² {2458,2309}. These tumours should be reported as "metastatic carcinoid tumour NOS", and the mitotic counts and presence of any necrosis should be documented. Metastatic pulmonary carcinoid (NET) patients are often treated by medical oncologists who also manage gastrointestinal/pancreatic carcinoids (NETs), where Ki-67 is used to stratify patients for therapeutic decisions {2712,173,1368}. In summary, documenting Ki-67 may be useful in metastatic pulmonary carcinoids (NETs), although mitotic counts and necrosis remain the main diagnostic criteria in primary resected tumours. In metastatic pulmonary carcinoids (NETs), further study is needed to determine the role of Ki-67 in classification, prognostication, and therapeutic management {2712,2500,173,1368,1807,379,2458}.

Cytology

The hallmark cytological features of carcinoid tumours include bland, monotonous nuclei with smooth contours and salt-and-pepper chromatin (indicating a mixture of fine and larger granules), lacking prominent nucleoli. In smears, cells tend to be loosely cohesive, yielding single-cell patterns or loosely

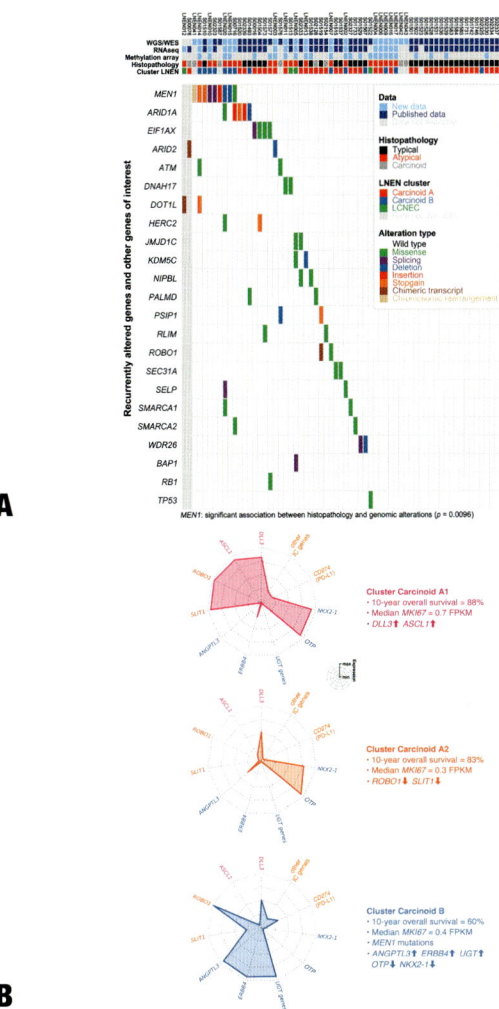

Fig. 1.138 Molecular characteristics of pulmonary carcinoids. **A** Recurrently altered and cancer-relevant genes found in pulmonary carcinoids by whole-genome/exome sequencing (WGS/WES). **B** Clinical characteristics and radar charts of the expression level of the characteristic genes of each molecular group of pulmonary carcinoids. FPKM, fragments per kilobase million; IC, immune checkpoint; LCNEC, large cell neuroendocrine carcinoma; LNEN, lung neuroendocrine neoplasm; RNAseq, RNA sequencing.

cohesive groups. Cells are frequently plasmacytoid {564,2584}. Rosettes may be preserved in some specimens and should not be mistaken for glandular structures of adenocarcinoma. In air-dried Diff-Quik preparations, cytoplasm may be inconspicuous, and dispersed naked nuclei may mimic a haematolymphoid neoplasm. Spindle cell carcinoids in cytological preparations may mimic a mesenchymal neoplasm. TCs and ACs generally cannot be reliably distinguished in cytological preparations. In some cases, carcinoids enter in the differential diagnosis with small cell carcinoma or LCNEC. This distinction can be aided by Ki-67, with a low index (< 30%) supporting the diagnosis of carcinoid tumour {1687}, although some cytological fixatives inhibit Ki-67 reactivity and this may be a pitfall {336}. There are no established criteria for distinguishing TC from AC on the basis of Ki-67 in cytology specimens.

Diagnostic molecular pathology

There is no recognized molecular test for lung carcinoids.

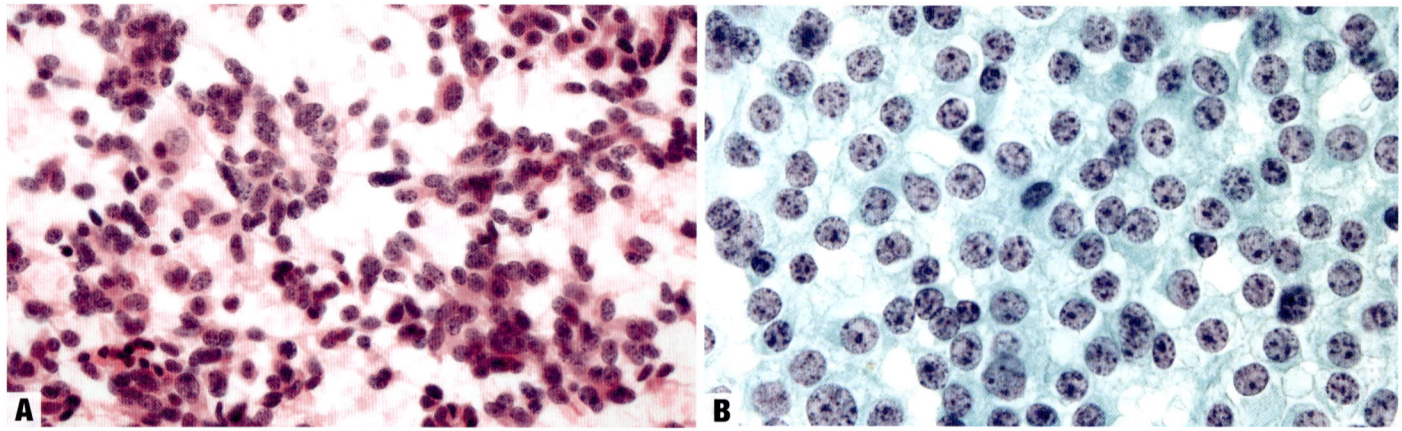

Fig. 1.139 Carcinoid. **A** Alcohol-fixed, haematoxylin-stained smear. Discohesive, bare round or ovoid nuclei similar in size, with salt-and-pepper chromatin and occasional rosette-like formations. **B** Pap-stained smear with uniform plasmacytoid cells having salt-and-pepper chromatin.

Essential and desirable diagnostic criteria

Essential:

- A NET with a well-differentiated architecture, often consisting of organoid nesting, trabeculae, rosettes, and palisading arrangements
- Tumour cells with moderate to abundant cytoplasm with an eosinophilic hue and finely granular nuclear chromatin
- Low-grade TC has < 2 mitoses/2 mm² and lacks necrosis, and intermediate-grade AC has 2–10 mitoses/2 mm² and/or foci of necrosis
- The number of high-power fields used for mitosis counting should be adjusted to achieve 2 mm² according to the microscope field of view, which varies depending on the microscope manufacturer and model (see Table A, p. xii)

Desirable:

- Neuroendocrine marker immunoexpression (chromogranin A, synaptophysin, CD56, INSM1)
- Ki-67 can be useful in distinguishing carcinoids from high-grade LCNEC and SCLC, particularly in small crushed biopsies
- Although Ki-67 may be useful in lung carcinoids (NETs) and documenting it in reports is considered desirable, the primary diagnostic criteria for separating these tumours remain mitotic count per 2 mm² and/or presence of necrosis
- In non-resection specimens, including biopsies of metastases, the diagnosis of "carcinoid tumour NOS" rather than TC or AC is recommended, with specification of the mitotic counts per 2 mm², presence or absence of necrosis (including extent – punctate or extensive), and (if available) Ki-67 index; the distinction between TC and AC requires a resection specimen

Staging

The eighth edition of the TNM classification applies to carcinoids with the same criteria as for other lung cancers. Multiple carcinoids in the setting of diffuse idiopathic pulmonary neuroendocrine cell hyperplasia should be considered separate primaries and not metastases, mentioning T size of the largest (m) {681,2099}. However, some overlaps in combined stages and subcategories have been reported with this new edition regarding disease-specific survival {3417}.

Prognosis and prediction

The distinction between TC and AC is a critical prognostic factor {1483,1203}, as evidenced by the 5-year survival rates of 82–100% and 50–68%, respectively. Mitotic counts are the most important predictor of outcome {2800,3084}. In addition, 10–23% of TCs and 40–50% of ACs have nodal metastases {1807}. Age, sex, TNM stage according to the eighth-edition TNM classification, existence of previous malignancies, peripheral location, and Eastern Cooperative Oncology Group (ECOG) performance status are additional reported prognostic factors, as are surgery and regional lymph node examination {482,3417,2865,831,670,599}. Lymph node metastasis as part of TNM staging is an independent prognostic factor associated with worse survival for TCs > 20 mm and ACs {1483}, encouraging radical lymphadenectomy during surgical resections, particularly for ACs {373}. Spread through airspaces is correlated with high tumour stage, positive nodal status, high Ki-67 index, presence of angioinvasion, and shorter overall survival and time to progression {67,69}. Ki-67 index values of ≥ 5% and ≥ 10% were reported as prognostic factors in TCs and ACs, respectively {640,1806}, but more data are needed to define their use in practice {2302,3399}.

Several prognostic markers have been identified in research settings, but they are not yet recommended for routine clinical practice because they have not been tested in comparison with the above parameters. High coexpression of CD44 and nuclear OTP, mainly observed in TCs, was associated with a higher recurrence-free survival rate {2261}, whereas low CD44 and nuclear OTP expression and high RET expression were associated with a low 20-year survival rate {2937}.

The expression of SSTR2A could predict response to somatostatin analogue therapy, and high levels of phosphorylated mTOR and S6K were associated with a better response to rapalogues in experimental models, but these have yet to be validated in the clinical setting {2485}. Preliminary data suggest that methylation of the *MGMT* promoter could be a predictive factor of objective response to temozolomide-based therapies, in addition to its prognostic significance {366}.

Small cell lung carcinoma

Beasley MB
Brambilla E
MacMahon H
Osamura RY
Papotti M
Rekhtman N

Rossi G
Scagliotti GV
Snead DRJ

Definition

Small cell lung carcinoma (SCLC) is a malignant epithelial tumour composed of small cells with scant cytoplasm, finely granular nuclear chromatin, and absent or inconspicuous nucleoli, with a high mitotic count and frequent necrosis. Most SCLCs express neuroendocrine markers. Combined SCLC has an additional component of non-small cell carcinoma (NSCC), which may include large cell neuroendocrine carcinoma (LCNEC), adenocarcinoma, squamous cell carcinoma (SCC), large cell carcinoma (LCC), spindle cell carcinoma, or giant cell carcinoma.

ICD-O coding

8041/3 Small cell carcinoma
8045/3 Combined small cell carcinoma

ICD-11 coding

2C25.1 Small cell carcinoma of bronchus or lung

Related terminology

Not recommended (obsolete): oat cell carcinoma; undifferentiated SCLC; intermediate cell–type SCLC; mixed small cell / large cell carcinoma.

Subtype(s)

Small cell carcinoma; combined small cell carcinoma

Localization

SCLC is usually located centrally in the major airways, frequently also involving the mediastinal lymph nodes, but it may occur peripherally in the lungs in about 5% of cases {3065}. Metastatic spread, most frequently to the liver, bone, brain, ipsilateral and contralateral lung, and adrenal glands, is commonly present at the time of presentation. Malignant pleural and pericardial effusions are also common.

Clinical features

Signs and symptoms

Patients often present with rapid-onset signs or symptoms due to local intrathoracic tumour growth, extrapulmonary distant spread, paraneoplastic syndromes, or a combination of these features. The symptoms of SCLC are similar to those of other lung cancers (see *Tumours of the lung: Introduction*, p. 20). Paraneoplastic effects are more frequent in SCLC than in other histological types, and they can be the presenting symptoms. Ectopic hormone secretion can cause hyponatraemia or Cushing syndrome, and immune-mediated paraneoplastic syndromes can cause Lambert–Eaton myasthenic syndrome, peripheral neuropathy, or limbic encephalopathy {3150}. Serum tumour markers for diagnosis, monitoring, and evaluation of SCLC response to therapy have had little clinical impact to date.

Radiographic findings

Patients with SCLC present with the full spectrum of imaging findings of lung cancer (see *Tumours of the lung: Introduction*, p. 20), but because of rapid growth, the tumour at presentation tends to be larger and at a more advanced stage than non-small cell lung carcinoma {2099}, typically occurring as a large hilar mass and bulky mediastinal lymph nodes. Approximately 15% of neurologically asymptomatic patients will have metastases detected on brain MRI {1169,3464}.

Epidemiology

SCLC accounts for approximately 15% of all lung carcinomas diagnosed worldwide. In the USA, the incidence in both sexes appears to have peaked in the mid-1980s / late 1990s and has been declining {1186,1187}. Although the rates in certain countries in Asia and eastern Europe with high smoking rates continued to increase into the 2000s, a stabilization or slight decline has more recently been reported {3380,3477,1}.

Etiology

The majority of SCLCs arise in patients with a history of heavy smoking, although de novo SCLC can rarely occur in never-smokers {3153}. SCLC can also occur as a resistance mechanism secondary to tyrosine kinase inhibitor therapy for treatment of *EGFR*-mutated lung adenocarcinomas or other oncogene-driven non-small cell lung carcinomas {2708,2360}.

The smoking-related etiology is supported by the characteristic tobacco carcinogen-associated molecular signature, with a high frequency (28%) of G>T and C>A transversions and an extremely high mutation frequency {2297,937}. Like in SCLC in general, *RB1* loss is a common feature in SCLCs arising in the setting of acquired resistance to tyrosine kinase inhibitor therapy for *EGFR*-mutant adenocarcinoma. The *EGFR* mutations are typically maintained, suggesting a common cell lineage and a role for *RB1* loss in the pathogenesis of SCLC {45,3153,2219}.

Pathogenesis

TP53 and *RB1* biallelic loss of function is obligatory in SCLC, as supported by its requirement in mouse models {597,2654, 2563,937}. *TP53* mutations affect the functional domain, but *RB1* mutations are more complex, with multiple incompletely detected rearrangements. In addition, significantly mutated genes are *CRACD* (*KIAA1211*) and *COL22A1*, *RGS7*, and *FPR1*, involved in G protein–coupled receptor signalling. Inactivating mutations of two histone acetylases (*CREBBP* and *EP300*) and damaging mutations of *FMN2* and NOTCH-family genes are often seen. Significant clustered mutations occur in the *ASPM*, *ALMS1*, and *PDE4DIP* genes (involved in centrosome function) and in *XRN1* (involved in RNA regulation). The *TP73* homologue of *TP53* is affected by clustered somatic rearrangements/

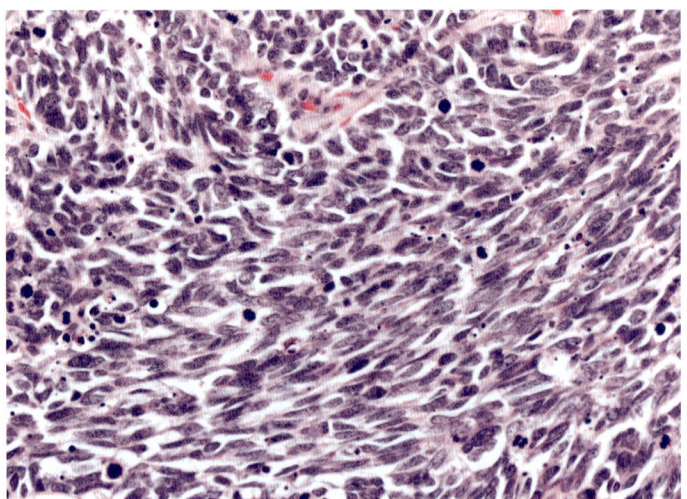

Fig. 1.140 Small cell lung carcinoma. This tumour consists of sheets of spindle and oval-shaped tumour cells with scant cytoplasm, finely granular nuclear chromatin, lack of nucleoli, and frequent mitoses.

breaks creating N-terminally truncated transcript p73 variants, which include p73 delta ex2, delta ex2/3, and delta ex10, all of which lack fully competent transactivation domains, as inferred from transcriptome sequencing. *CREBBP*, *EP300*, *TP73*, *RBL1*, *RBL2*, and NOTCH-family gene mutations are largely mutually exclusive {937,2297,2563}.

The majority of SCLCs have downregulated Notch signalling. *TP53*/*RB1* knock-out mouse models with an activated extramembrane Notch domain (NICD) are found to have a decreased number of tumours, with a lower proliferation rate, decreased neuroendocrine expression, and increased survival time. These findings confirm Notch signalling as a tumour suppressor in SCLC and a regulator of neuroendocrine differentiation {2654, 937}.

Reported somatic gene copy-number alterations include amplification of the MYC-family genes *MYCL* (*MYCL1*), *MYCN*, *MYC*, *FGFR1*, and *IRS2* and genomic losses of 3p genes: *FHIT* (3p14) and *ROBO1* (3p12) {2297,927}.

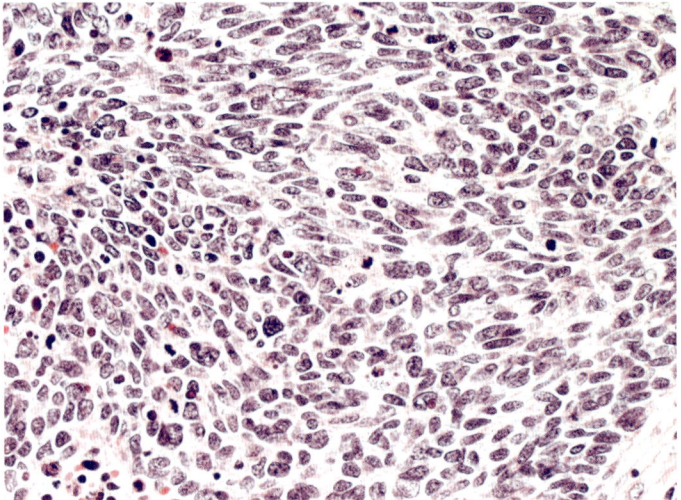

Fig. 1.141 Small cell carcinoma. The tumour is characterized by small to intermediate-sized cells with finely granular chromatin and scant cytoplasm. Cells are often oval to spindle in shape. Nucleoli are inconspicuous or absent. Mitotic figures are numerous.

In contrast with carcinoids, SCLC does not occur in the context of multiple endocrine neoplasia type 1 disease, and it has no constitutive or somatic *MEN1* mutations {644,645}. The neuroendocrine nature of SCLC is thought to be driven by ASCL1, with or without NeuroD1 participation {2564}.

Additionally, SCLC may show greater heterogeneity than previously thought. A recent comprehensive study of animal models, xenografts, cell lines, and human primaries of untreated or treated tumours identified four SCLC classes according to expression of four predominant transcription factors (opening consideration of new concepts of pathogenesis and therapeutic options): ASCL1 is dominant in SCLC type A, NeuroD1 in type D, YAP1 in type Y, and POU2F3 in type P. It was recognized, however, that the vast majority of human untreated SCLCs belong to type A and a minority to type D, enriched in pretreated SCLC and rarely others {2564,143A}. Further study is needed to elucidate how this might translate to disease management.

A defined precursor lesion for SCLC has not been identified in humans, and, unlike carcinoids, SCLC is not associated with the precursor lesion of diffuse idiopathic pulmonary neuroendocrine cell hyperplasia. Precursor lesions have been reported in mouse models, typically associated with *Tp53*/*Rb1* double knock-out, in some studies by adding *Pten* and/or *Rbl2* (*p130*) ablation {597,2654} or by introducing a *Myc* mutant allele {1957}. Genetically engineered mouse models have identified a minimum of two gene ablations (of *Tp53* and *Rb1*) as being required and sufficient for initiation and progression of SCLC {926}.

Although a precursor cell has not been definitely characterized in humans, putative cells of origin can be any lung epithelial cell: a basal cell, a neuroendocrine cell, or a totipotent epithelial cell with plasticity towards different phenotypes. This is supported by the reported effect of chemotherapy in human SCLC {305,2696}, with reports describing posttherapy morphological changes towards a larger size, combined SCLC, and multiple differentiation in the same tumours and/or individual cells {2696,305}, which would also support a common lineage for combined SCLC.

Macroscopic appearance

SCLC typically occurs as an unresectable large perihilar mass, which may be associated with bronchial compression and nodal involvement. The tumour has a tan, necrotic cut surface and may spread along bronchi in a subepithelial pattern. Approximately 5% of carcinomas occur as a circumscribed peripheral nodule {3065}.

Histopathology

Tumour cells have scant cytoplasm, poorly defined cell borders, and finely granular nuclear chromatin. The cells are usually less than the diameter of 3 small resting lymphocytes and are oval to spindle in shape. Nucleoli are absent or inconspicuous. Nuclear moulding is common. The tumour cells are usually densely packed and commonly grow in a sheet-like pattern. Necrosis and apoptotic cells are frequent and often extensive. Crush artefact and encrustation of basophilic nuclear DNA around blood vessels (the Azzopardi effect) may be encountered. Neuroendocrine growth patterns (organoid, trabecular, rosette formation, etc.) are typically absent in biopsies but may be prominent in resected tumours {180}. Occasional larger cells, including pleomorphic tumour giant cells, may be admixed but should not make up > 10% of the tumour. Mitotic count is high; by definition, it is > 10 mitoses/2 mm², but the average is 60 mitoses/2 mm² and the median is 80 mitoses/2 mm² {3065}.

Combined SCLCs are tumours consisting of SCLC with an additional component of NSCC, including LCNEC. Most commonly, the second component is LCC, adenocarcinoma, or SCC, but it rarely may consist of spindle or giant cell carcinoma {2108,3066}. A diagnosis of combined SCLC should include mention of each of the NSCC components present. As noted above, SCLC may show occasional larger cells. Therefore, large cells should make up ≥ 10% of the tumour for a tumour to be classified as combined SCLC/LCNEC or combined SCLC and LCC. The percentage requirement is not applicable to other non-small cell elements, such as adenocarcinoma and SCC. The presence of an adenocarcinoma component in a combined SCLC or a new diagnosis of SCLC in a never-smoker should prompt molecular testing and consideration of a driver mutation such as an *EGFR* mutation or *ALK* rearrangement. This occurs most often as a manifestation of resistance to targeted therapy in known *EGFR*-mutated or *ALK*-rearranged lung adenocarcinomas, but it can be found de novo in untreated patients. Tumours with mixtures of SCLC and equal or greater amounts of spindle cell and/or giant cell carcinoma or heterologous sarcomatous components should be classified as combined SCLC with mention of the various histologies identified.

Immunohistochemistry

Classically, SCLC is considered a light-microscopic diagnosis, and immunostains are not required to confirm a diagnosis of SCLC. However, immunostains are commonly used and are of particular utility in excluding or confirming an alternate diagnosis.

SCLC typically stains for cytokeratins such as AE1/AE3 and CAM5.2, often with a rim-and-dot–type pattern, but it is negative for high-molecular-weight cytokeratins {2885}. CK7 is positive in < 50% of cases and CK20 is usually negative {522}. Most SCLCs will stain for neuroendocrine markers such as chromogranin, synaptophysin, and CD56 (NCAM), the last of which is most sensitive but less specific {2523,2317}. Staining for chromogranin may be weak and focal {3390}. SCLC may be negative for all three of these markers in approximately 5–10% of cases. Studies have shown variable results in regard

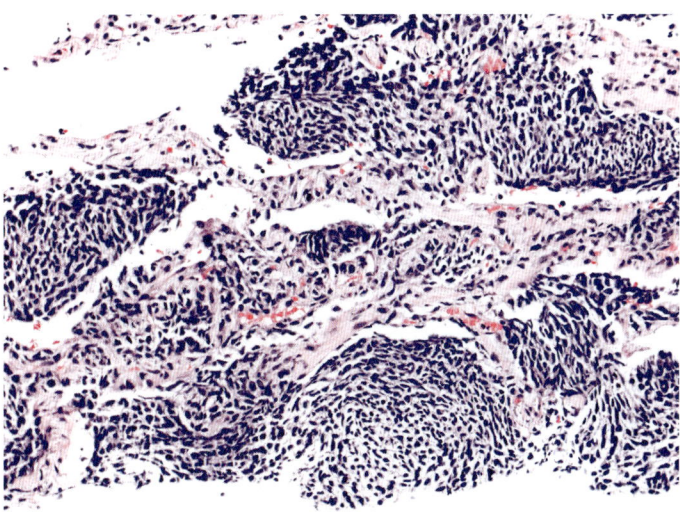

Fig. 1.142 Small cell lung carcinoma. This lung core biopsy is from a patient with an *EGFR* p.L858R–mutated lung adenocarcinoma 1 year previously. The tumour shows typical features of small cell carcinoma, with a high mitotic count, sheets of small cells with scant cytoplasm, and lack of nucleoli. Immunohistochemistry showed RB1 was lost and the Ki-67 index was 90%. By next-generation sequencing, this tumour also showed the same *EGFR* mutation, as well as alterations in *TP53* and *RB1*.

to whether INSM1 is more or less specific than a combination of chromogranin, synaptophysin, and CD56, but INSM1 has been shown to be a consistently reliable marker, particularly in the setting of SCLC {1533,2022}. ASCL1 (hASH1) is emerging as an additional marker of neuroendocrine differentiation, but its value in SCLC needs further evaluation {1917,3396}. TTF1 expression has been reported in 90–95% of SCLCs, depending on the clone used, but it is not specific for pulmonary origin in the setting of a small cell carcinoma {1398,1831}. Napsin A is negative in SCLC {2462}. p63 and p40 are generally negative in SCLC. Focal staining has been reported in some series, but diffuse nuclear staining is not observed {2463}. The vast majority of SCLCs show loss of RB1 protein and p53 overexpression or null expression {181,2194}. Ki-67, although not part of the diagnostic criteria for SCLC or neuroendocrine tumours (NETs) in general, may be useful in the setting of crushed biopsies to avoid misdiagnosing carcinoid tumours, which may also show crush artefact. The reported Ki-67 index for SCLC is 65–100% and for

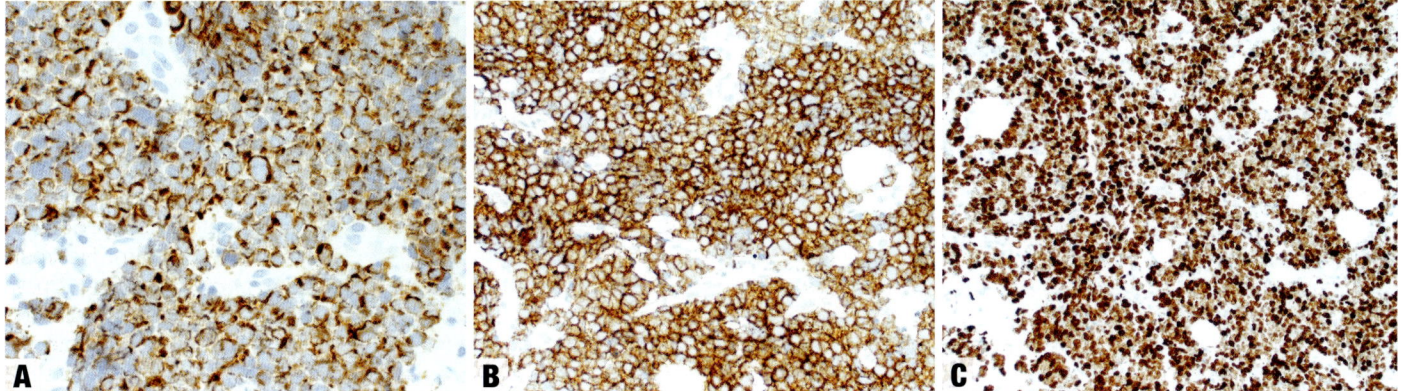

Fig. 1.143 Small cell carcinoma. **A** The tumour is typically positive for cytokeratin and may sometimes show a rim-and-dot–type staining pattern (CAM5.2). **B** Small cell carcinoma is a high-grade neuroendocrine carcinoma and is usually positive for one of more neuroendocrine markers, such as CD56 in this example. **C** Small cell carcinoma typically has a high proliferation rate, as reflected by extensive nuclear staining with Ki-67 (MIB1 clone)

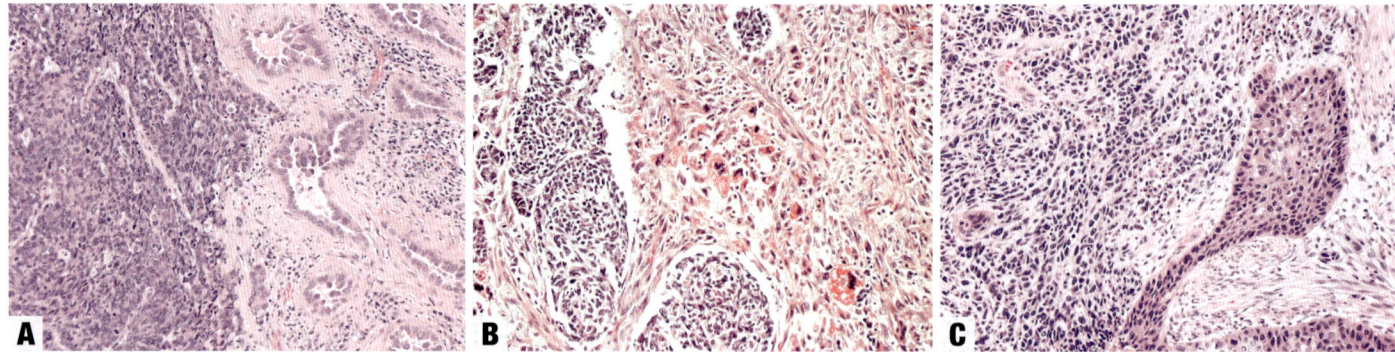

Fig. 1.144 Combined small cell carcinoma. **A** This tumour shows small cell carcinoma (left) and adenocarcinoma with an acinar and micropapillary pattern (right). **B** Small cell carcinoma may be combined with any type of non-small cell lung carcinoma. In this example, small cell lung carcinoma is combined with pleomorphic carcinoma composed of spindle and giant cells. **C** This tumour shows small cell carcinoma (left) and squamous cell carcinoma (right).

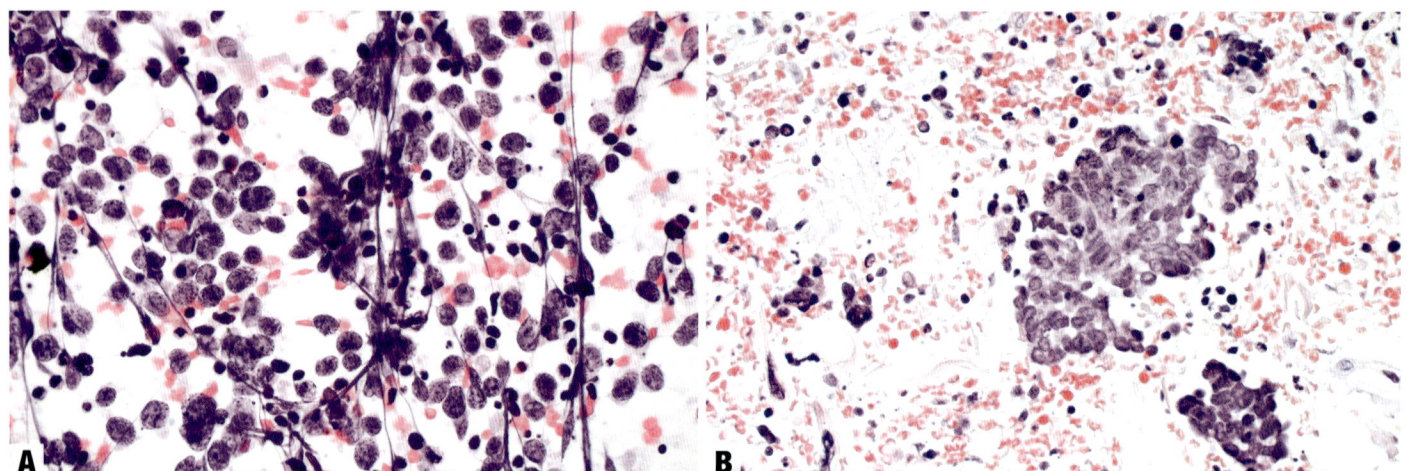

Fig. 1.145 Small cell carcinoma. **A** Alcohol-fixed cytology smear shows single and loosely cohesive cells with a minimal amount of stripped cytoplasm, granular chromatin without prominent nucleoli, and multiple dark apoptotic/pyknotic cells. Nuclear streaking is prominent. **B** Formalin-fixed transbronchial needle aspirate shows cohesive and single cells with scant cytoplasm and identifiable mitoses. Occasional lymphocytes are present in the background for size comparison.

typical carcinoids is < 5%, although proliferation rates as high as 30% have been reported in atypical carcinoid (see *Lung neuroendocrine neoplasms: Introduction*, p. 127) {2311,2312}. In virtually all cases, a very high proliferation rate would exclude a carcinoid tumour, whereas a very low rate would exclude SCLC {2490,2311}. In cytology specimens, it has been reported that CytoLyt fixation reduces Ki-67 when the MIB1 clone is used, but not with the Ki-67 30-9 antibody {336}. Orthopedia homeobox protein (OTP) has been shown to preferentially stain carcinoids as opposed to high-grade tumours {1064,3175}.

Differential diagnosis

The differential diagnosis of SCLC includes other neuroendocrine carcinomas (NECs), particularly LCNEC, as well as basaloid SCC, small round cell sarcomas, and lymphoma.

SCLC should be differentiated from other pulmonary NETs (i.e. carcinoids and LCNEC). Immunostains are generally not useful in this regard, because all of these tumours will be positive for cytokeratins and neuroendocrine markers. The differentiation from carcinoid tumours is based primarily on morphology and mitotic count (see Table 1.14, p. 127), although, as noted above, Ki-67 may aid in discriminating SCLC from carcinoid tumours in crushed biopsies. The discrimination of SCLC from LCNEC is based primarily on light-microscopic features, with LCNEC usually having more abundant cytoplasm, polygonal cell shape, distinct cell borders, and vesicular nuclear chromatin (often with nucleoli). Owing to the spectrum of cell sizes that may occur in both tumours, discriminating SCLC from LCNEC may be particularly challenging, and there is currently no immunohistochemical stain or genetic marker to discriminate between the two {2454,3065}. Because the diagnosis depends primarily on morphological features, good-quality H&E sections elucidating these features are critical. Merkel cell carcinoma, a NEC of the skin, is typically positive for CK20, NFP, and Merkel cell polyomavirus but negative for TTF1, which can help distinguish it from SCLC {494}.

Basaloid squamous carcinoma is characterized by nests of basaloid cells, often with peripheral palisading around tumour nests and a high mitotic count. Although most tumours show cytological features of an NSCC, some have small tumour cell size along with palisading and focal rosette-like structures morphologically identical to SCLC. Basaloid squamous carcinoma is characterized by strong diffuse staining for p40 or p63 (which are only rarely focally positive in SCLC {2463}) and is positive for keratin 34βE12, which is negative in SCLC {2885,2884}. Of note, CD56 may rarely be diffusely and strongly positive in basaloid SCC. In TTF1-negative tumours that appear to be SCLC, a p40 stain should be performed to exclude basaloid SCC.

SMARCA4-deficient thoracic undifferentiated tumours may have small-sized tumour cells. These tumours frequently express synaptophysin and may have focal TTF1 expression (see *Thoracic SMARCA4-deficient undifferentiated tumour*, p. 111) {2460}. Diagnosis is facilitated by immunohistochemistry demonstrating loss of SMARCA4 protein (also known as BRG1).

Small round cell sarcomas, both in the Ewing sarcoma family (e.g. Ewing sarcoma) and recently described morphologically similar tumours lacking *EWSR1* gene rearrangement (e.g. *CIC-DUX4*–rearranged and *BCOR-CCNB3*–rearranged tumours {88,586,1811}), may enter the differential diagnosis because they may occasionally show positive staining for neuroendocrine markers, particularly CD56. Patient age, tumour morphology, and smoking history, as well as lack of cytokeratin immunoreactivity, should raise the index of suspicion for an alternate diagnosis from SCLC. Appropriate FISH studies should confirm the diagnosis in most cases.

SCLC may occasionally have greater than expected loss of cell cohesion, raising the possibility of lymphoma. The absence of keratin staining and the presence of lymphoid markers readily discriminate lymphoma from SCLC.

Rare SCLCs are keratin-negative. Tumours suspected to be SCLC that are keratin-negative should be carefully evaluated with markers to exclude lymphoma, sarcoma, and melanoma. The diagnosis in such cases would also require classic morphology in addition to immunohistochemical markers showing characteristic features such as neuroendocrine markers, RB1 loss, and aberrant p53 expression.

Cytology
Cytology preparations serve as an important diagnostic tool in the diagnosis of SCLC, and in many cases they highlight nuclear features that may be difficult to evaluate on crushed tissue biopsies.

Smears show loosely cohesive round, oval, or occasionally spindle cells with minimal cytoplasm, present singly or in small clusters. Abundant apoptotic or pyknotic dark nuclei are commonly seen, although mitotic figures are poorly preserved in smears. Necrotic background is usually evident. Chromatin streaking is a prominent feature. In alcohol-fixed preparations, chromatin has a distinctive finely or coarsely granular quality, lacking prominent nucleoli. Nuclear moulding can be seen. In air-dried Diff-Quik (Giemsa)-stained preparations, single-cell pattern with round cells containing minimal or stripped cytoplasm closely mimics haematolymphoid malignancies.

Diagnostic molecular pathology
There is no established role for molecular testing in the diagnosis of SCLC. Whole-genome sequencing of SCLC {937,2297, 2563} demonstrates biallelic alteration of both *TP53* and *RB1*.

Essential and desirable diagnostic criteria
Essential – SCLC:
- Tumour composed of small cells (usually less than the size of 3 resting lymphocytes) with scant cytoplasm, oval to spindle shape, and high mitotic count (> 10 mitoses/2 mm² but usually higher, ~60 mitoses/2 mm²), often with necrosis
- Tumour cells have finely granular nuclear chromatin
- Nucleoli are absent or inconspicuous

Essential – combined SCLC:
- Features of SCLC but with a component of a non-small cell lung carcinoma (LCC, LCNEC, adenocarcinoma, SCC, or less commonly spindle and/or giant cell carcinoma)
- In the case of SCLC combined with LCNEC or LCC, but not the other histological types, the second component should make up ≥ 10% of the tumour

Desirable:
- Positive immunohistochemistry for low-molecular-weight cytokeratin
- Frequent expression of neuroendocrine markers (> 90% of cases)
- Lack of diffuse p40 expression, unless in areas of SCC in a combined SCLC

Staging
SCLC and combined SCLC should be staged according to the TNM system for lung carcinomas. The Veterans Administration Lung Study Group (VALSG) system is often used to stage SCLC as limited-stage or extensive-stage; however, the TNM staging system is prognostically significant and its use is recommended {2099}.

Prognosis and prediction
Stage IV SCLC has a poor prognosis, with survival rates with conventional chemotherapy using cisplatin and etoposide of approximately 8% at 2 years {2099} and 2% at 5 years, which has remained unchanged between 1992 and 2007 {920}. However, two phase III studies demonstrated a modest but consistent 2–3 month survival benefit to patients with metastatic SCLC treated with first-line chemotherapy with a PDL1 inhibitor compared with chemotherapy alone {2293,1178}. There are no prospectively validated predictive biomarkers of response to combination chemotherapy and PDL1 inhibition used for clinical practice {1178}; in retrospective studies, PDL1 combined positive score > 1 and high tumour mutation burden are associated with improved outcomes among patients treated with immune checkpoint inhibitors {527,1114}. In patients with limited-stage SCLC, concurrent chemotherapy and radiation is the standard of care, with median overall survival of 25–30 months and a 5-year overall survival rate of 31–34% {792}. Surgical resection is an option for T1–T2 SCLC without lymph node involvement, and patients are likely to benefit from adjuvant chemotherapy {2667,3377}. Younger age, female sex, and surgery for limited disease are favourable prognostic features {920}.

Large cell neuroendocrine carcinoma of the lung

Rekhtman N
Beasley MB
Brambilla E
Farago AF
MacMahon H
Osamura RY
Papotti M
Rossi G
Scagliotti GV
Snead DRJ

Definition

Large cell neuroendocrine carcinoma (LCNEC) is a high-grade non-small cell carcinoma with neuroendocrine morphology and a mitotic count of > 10 mitoses/2 mm², that expresses one or more neuroendocrine immunohistochemical markers. Combined LCNEC is an LCNEC with components of adenocarcinoma, squamous cell carcinoma, or spindle or giant cell carcinoma.

ICD-O coding

8013/3 Large cell neuroendocrine carcinoma
8013/3 Combined large cell neuroendocrine carcinoma

ICD-11 coding

2C25.4 & XH0NL5 Carcinoid or other malignant neuroendocrine neoplasms of bronchus or lung & Large cell neuroendocrine carcinoma

Related terminology

None

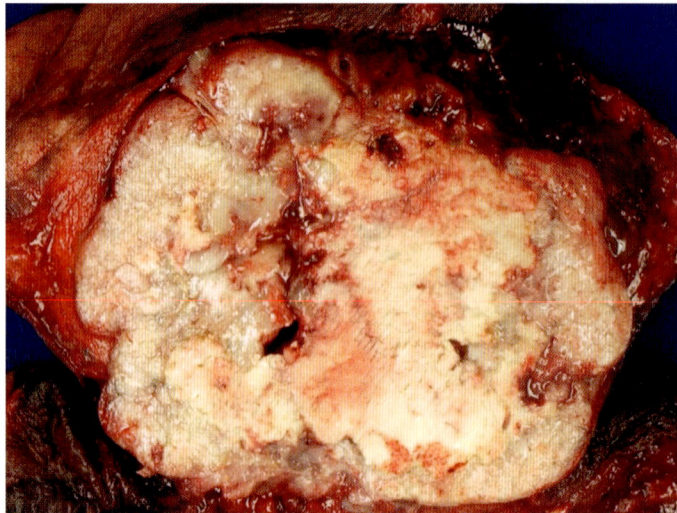

Fig. 1.146 Large cell neuroendocrine carcinoma (LCNEC). Macroscopic view of a peripheral well-circumscribed tumour with tan-yellow cut surface containing foci of haemorrhage and necrosis.

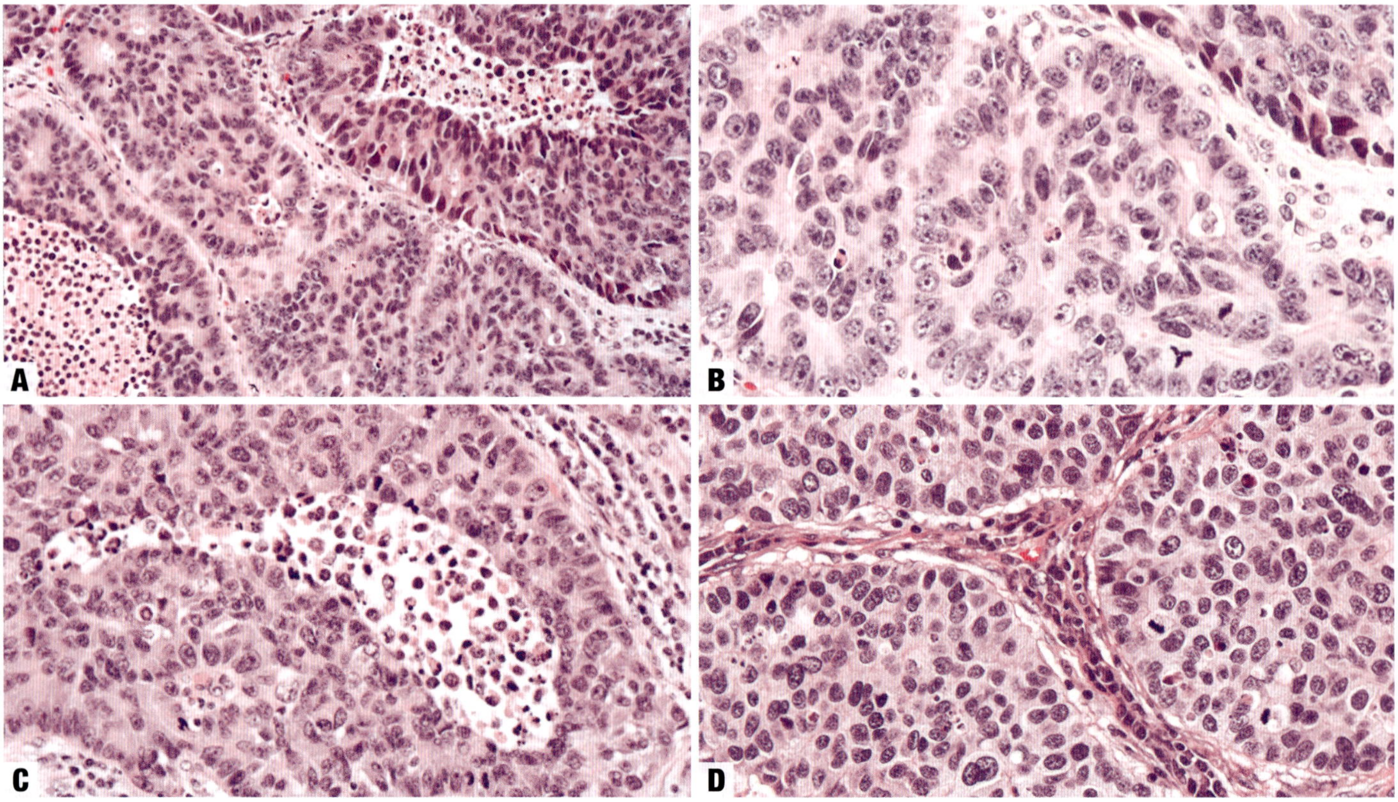

Fig. 1.147 Large cell neuroendocrine carcinoma (LCNEC). **A** Organoid nesting with peripheral palisading and rosettes associated with necrosis. **B** Higher power shows cells with coarse/stippled chromatin with easily identifiable nucleoli, a moderate amount of cytoplasm, frequent mitotic figures, and apoptotic bodies. **C** LCNEC with variably granular to vesicular chromatin. **D** LCNEC entirely lacking nucleoli but with a moderate amount of cytoplasm, making intercellular membranes readily visible.

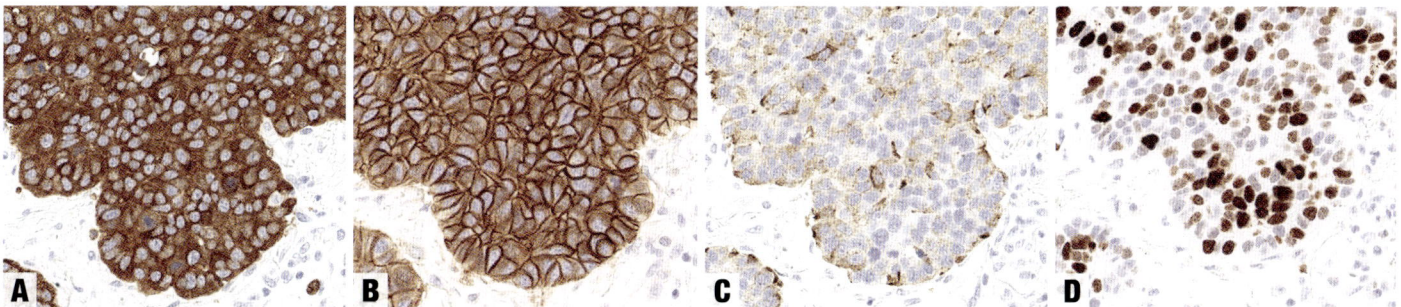

Fig. 1.148 Large cell neuroendocrine carcinoma (LCNEC). Immunohistochemistry illustrates ldiffuse strong staining for synaptophysin (**A**) and CD56 (**B**), with weak staining for chromogranin A (**C**); Ki-67 shows nuclear staining of 80% of the tumour cells (**D**).

Subtype(s)

Large cell neuroendocrine carcinoma; combined large cell neuroendocrine carcinoma

Localization

The majority (> 75%) of LCNECs are located in the lung periphery, but some tumours arise in the central compartment adjacent to or involving central airways {2220,1641}.

Clinical features

Signs and symptoms

The clinical presentation of LCNEC is usually similar to that of non-small cell lung carcinoma (NSCLC; see *Tumours of the lung: Introduction*, p. 20). Patients with LCNEC are more likely to present with operable disease (~50%) than patients with small cell lung carcinoma (SCLC). Distant metastases are present in 40–50% of patients at presentation {3207,1467}. Common sites of metastasis include brain, liver, and bone, and metastases may result in constitutional symptoms such as weight loss or fatigue, or symptoms such as pain or neurological deficits attributable to specific metastatic sites {2045}. Brain metastases occur in approximately 50% of patients with LCNEC, which is similar to the frequency in SCLC {2045}. Although associated paraneoplastic syndromes are a feature of small cell carcinoma, they are rare in LCNEC.

Radiographic findings

LCNEC is generally radiologically similar to NSCLC (see *Tumours of the lung: Introduction*, p. 20). On CT, most tumours are peripherally located, exhibiting expansive growth and irregular margins. Cavitation is uncommon. Hilar or mediastinal lymph nodes are commonly involved, but bulky lymphadenopathy is rare. Airway obstruction resulting in postobstructive pneumonia occurs in approximately 25% of patients {2220,38,1641}.

Epidemiology

LCNEC accounts for approximately 3% of resected lung carcinomas {3065}. There has been an increase in the incidence of LCNEC in various countries in recent epidemiological studies {666,3381,660,1467}, which could be related to better pathological recognition of this entity. LCNEC tends to occur more commonly in males and in people aged > 65 years, and ≥ 90% of patients are heavy smokers {2045,2631}.

Etiology

The major etiological factor for LCNEC is smoking, as supported by a high exonic mutation rate (8.6 non-synonymous mutations per 1 million bp) and a mutation signature strongly associated with smoking, characterized by G>T and C>A transversions {938}. A distinct etiological pathway for LCNEC development in recent years is transformation from pre-existing *EGFR*-mutated adenocarcinoma after treatment with EGFR (HER1) inhibitors. Although such transformation predominantly occurs in the form of SCLC, instances of LCNEC transformation have been described {1500,3503,1997}.

Pathogenesis

Recent studies using comprehensive next-generation sequencing revealed a high frequency of *TP53* and *RB1* inactivation in LCNEC {2463,1945,2537,667,938}. Tumours largely comprise two distinct genomic subsets: one with an SCLC-like genomic profile (*RB1*/*TP53* inactivation, *MYCL* [*MYCL1*] amplification) and the other with an NSCLC-like genomic profile with predominant similarity to that of adenocarcinoma, characterized by *STK11* (*LKB1*), *KEAP1*, *KRAS*, and other RAS pathway gene alterations {2463,667,938}. Notably, by transcriptomic analysis, the SCLC-like and the NSCLC-like genomic subsets of LCNEC are distinct from conventional SCLC and NSCLC, respectively. In particular, the NSCLC-like genomic subset was associated with an ASCL1-high/DLL3-high/Notch-low expression profile (typical of SCLC), whereas the SCLC-like genomic subset was associated with an ASCL1-low/DLL3-low/Notch-high profile {938}. These molecular data indicate that LCNEC harbours a unique combination of genomic and transcriptional programs compared with both SCLC and NSCLC, supporting that it represents a distinct entity. These data also highlight the heterogeneity of LCNEC, potentially reflecting phenotypic convergence of tumour groups derived from distinct cells of origin. Molecular subsets cannot be reliably distinguished by histopathological examination alone, although SCLC-like (RB1-deficient) tumours tend to exhibit higher proliferation rates {2463} and central location {3513}.

Although the cell of origin and pathogenesis of LCNEC are not known, a relationship with both SCLC and NSCLC is suggested in experimental models {1870,667}. In genetically engineered mouse models of small cell carcinoma arising primarily from neuroendocrine precursors, there are frequent subpopulations of LCNEC {926}. The close pathogenetic link of at least a subset of LCNEC with SCLC is in line with the observation that

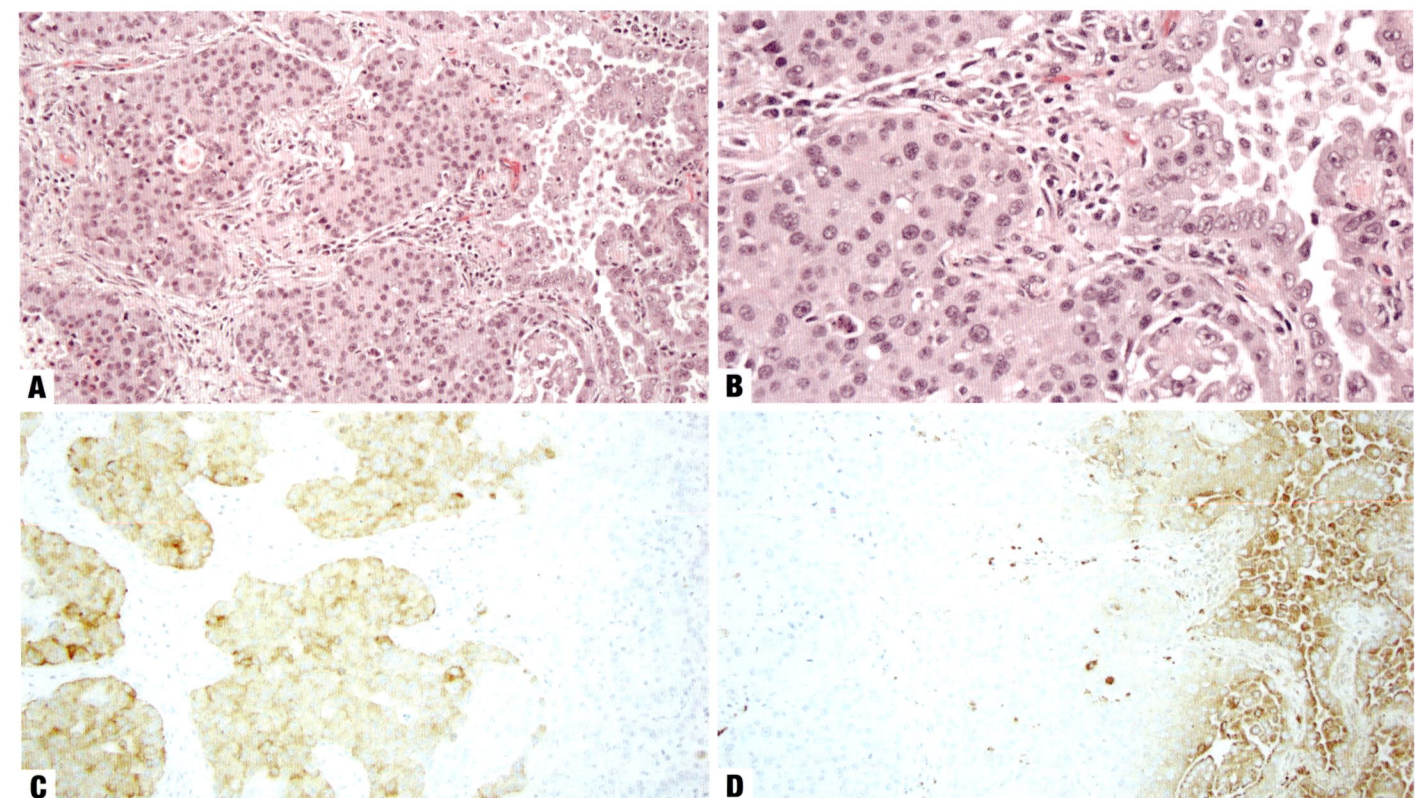

Fig. 1.149 Large cell neuroendocrine carcinoma (LCNEC) combined with adenocarcinoma. **A** Adenocarcinoma with micropapillary pattern (right) juxtaposed with solid nests of LCNEC with peripheral palisading and rosettes (left). **B** More amphophilic cytoplasm and more granular chromatin in LCNEC can be appreciated in this higher-power image. **C,D** Synaptophysin (**C**) and napsin A (**D**) show strikingly dichotomous expression in LCNEC versus adenocarcinoma components, respectively.

some human SCLCs are combined with LCNEC, and that cytotoxic chemotherapy may induce evolution of SCLC to LCNEC {305}. An alternative pathway of LCNEC development from non-neuroendocrine precursors has also been suggested in mouse models {39,1610}, consistent with the observation of combined LCNEC with other histological types of NSCLC, as well as the transformation of lung adenocarcinoma to SCLC/LCNEC after EGFR inhibitor therapy {1500,3503,1997}. The potential derivation of LCNEC from different cells of origin may underlie recent genomic data revealing distinct subsets of LCNEC with SCLC-like and NSCLC-like genomic profiles. Conversely, the combination of LCNEC with conventional carcinoids is not an established phenomenon, and, unlike carcinoids, LCNECs do not arise in the setting of diffuse idiopathic pulmonary neuroendocrine cell hyperplasia {1803}.

Macroscopic appearance

LCNECs are usually peripheral tumours with a size range of 10 to > 100 mm {2220,38,1641}. The cut surface is generally well circumscribed, tan-red, and necrotic.

Histopathology

Histology

LCNEC is characterized by an organoid nesting trabecular growth pattern, peripheral palisading, and rosettes – the patterns that can be encountered in other neuroendocrine tumours {3079,2454,3065,1157}. The cytological characteristics of LCNEC are those of NSCLC, which include frequent moderate to prominent nucleoli and/or moderate to abundant cytoplasm

with distinct cell borders such that intercellular membranes are visible. Cell size of LCNEC is usually more than the size of 3 small resting lymphocytes, exceeding that of SCLC. Chromatin is generally coarsely granular/stippled, but it may be vesicular or have intermediate quality. Some LCNECs have nuclear characteristics that are analogous to SCLC (granular chromatin without prominent nucleoli), but they qualify for the diagnosis of LCNEC by virtue of abundant cytoplasm. Necrosis is present in virtually all LCNECs and is typically extensive, with large confluent areas, but in some cases necrosis may be more limited. Associated stromal desmoplasia and marked stromal inflammation are common. By definition, mitotic counts in LCNEC are > 10 mitoses/2 mm², and generally they are substantially above this threshold (median: 70 mitoses/2 mm²), although less commonly LCNECs can have < 30 mitoses/2 mm² {3079,3084}.

Immunohistochemistry

Expression of a neuroendocrine marker is required for the diagnosis of LCNEC. Most tumours express two or three of the three standard neuroendocrine markers (synaptophysin, chromogranin A, CD56 [NCAM1]), and expression of at least one marker is typically diffuse {665,3390}. However, if morphological features are convincing for LCNEC, any extent of expression of even a single neuroendocrine marker is accepted to support the diagnosis {3390}. Caution should be exercised in interpreting cases labelling for CD56 alone because of its lower specificity {3390}. Although additional neuroendocrine markers have been emerging in recent years, especially ASCL1 (hASH1) and INSM1, their role in the diagnosis of LCNEC remains to be

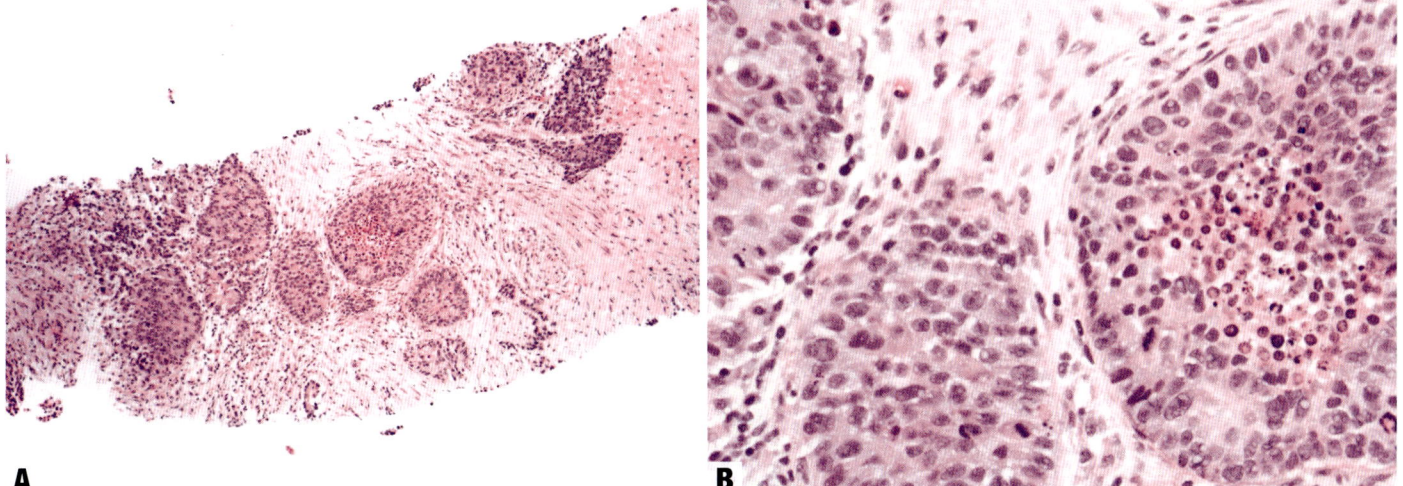

Fig. 1.150 Large cell neuroendocrine carcinoma (LCNEC), core biopsy. **A** Low-power view shows a tumour with extensive necrosis, nested pattern, peripheral palisading, and rosettes. **B** Higher magnification shows non-small cell lung carcinoma cytology (conspicuous nucleoli, moderate amount of cytoplasm), variably granular to vesicular chromatin, and frequent mitotic figures. The tumour stained positively with neuroendocrine immunohistochemical markers.

clarified. Importantly, NSE should not be used, because of its low specificity {3390}.

Approximately 50% of LCNECs express TTF1. Napsin A is usually entirely negative, but it is expressed weakly/focally in a minority of LCNECs {2462,145}. The combination of diffuse/strong TTF1 with negative or minimal napsin A is a distinctive feature of LCNEC (or SCLC), given that such a profile is uncommon for lung adenocarcinoma {2462}. Labelling for squamous markers (p40/p63, CK5/6, 34βE12) can be seen in scattered cells in LCNEC, but diffuse labelling is not expected unless there is a combined LCNEC with squamous cell carcinoma {2884,2463}. Pankeratins usually have strong and diffuse labelling in LCNEC; however, some LCNECs have granular (dot-like) labelling analogous to that of SCLC {3038}. The Ki-67 proliferation index in LCNEC is consistently > 30% and usually > 40%, with some cases reaching the typical range of SCLC, of ≥ 80% {3235,2463,145}.

Differential diagnosis

LCNEC is distinguished from SCLC by the presence of prominent nucleoli and/or abundant cytoplasm, and in most cases by larger cell size. Nested architecture or larger cell size alone should not be used as the sole criterion for the diagnosis of LCNEC over SCLC {2108,3066,144}. Due to the spectrum of nucleocytoplasmic morphology that exists in both tumours, distinguishing LCNEC from SCLC can be challenging in a subset of cases, and there is no immunohistochemical or genetic marker that can reliably distinguish LCNEC from SCLC {2454, 3065}. The presence of any amount of SCLC in a predominant LCNEC qualifies a tumour for the diagnosis of combined SCLC and LCNEC (see *Small cell lung carcinoma*, p. 139).

LCNEC is distinguished from pulmonary adenocarcinomas with a solid/nested or cribriform pattern and solid/nested large cell carcinoma by the presence of nuclear palisading and rosettes and by neuroendocrine marker expression. Although 10–20% of NSCLCs lacking neuroendocrine morphology express neuroendocrine markers, such expression is usually focal and limited to a single marker {665,145,144}.

LCNEC is distinguished from atypical carcinoid by a higher mitotic count (> 10 mitoses/2 mm²) together with greater nuclear membrane irregularities, moderate to prominent nucleoli, and in most cases extensive necrosis. Tumours with carcinoid morphology that qualify as LCNEC due to mitotic counts exceeding 10 mitoses/2 mm² – usually only mildly – occur rarely as lung primary tumours, but they are relatively common in the metastatic setting {2463,2405,1240}. Emerging data suggest that such tumours have genomic and clinical characteristics similar to those of carcinoid tumours {2463}, but more data are needed (see *Lung neuroendocrine neoplasms: Introduction*, p. 127, and *Carcinoid/neuroendocrine tumour of the lung*, p. 133).

Basaloid squamous cell carcinomas can have nests, palisading, and rosette-like structures. They are distinguished from LCNEC by consistent expression of squamous markers (p40/p63, high-molecular-weight cytokeratin 34βE12) even though some neuroendocrine markers (especially CD56) may be occasionally positive {2631,3390,144}.

Thoracic SMARCA4-deficient undifferentiated tumours commonly express synaptophysin and may mimic LCNEC clinically and pathologically, especially in small biopsies {1617,3421, 2460,144}. They are distinguished from LCNEC by the loss of SMARCA4 (BRG1) expression and by several other distinctive morphological and immunohistochemical features (see *Thoracic SMARCA4-deficient undifferentiated tumour*, p. 111).

Diagnosis in small biopsies

The definitive diagnosis of LCNEC is possible in small biopsies provided that biopsy size is sufficient to assess neuroendocrine morphology and immunohistochemical markers {3235,145}. In scant or disrupted samples of NSCLC where neuroendocrine morphology and/or marker expression is not definitive, the diagnosis of "non-small cell lung carcinoma, possible large cell neuroendocrine carcinoma" is appropriate. Historically, the diagnosis of LCNEC was considered rarely feasible in small biopsies {3074}. However, with the recent trend of obtaining larger volumes of tissue in thoracic biopsies for molecular testing, the diagnosis is possible more often {2045,665,3522,3064}.

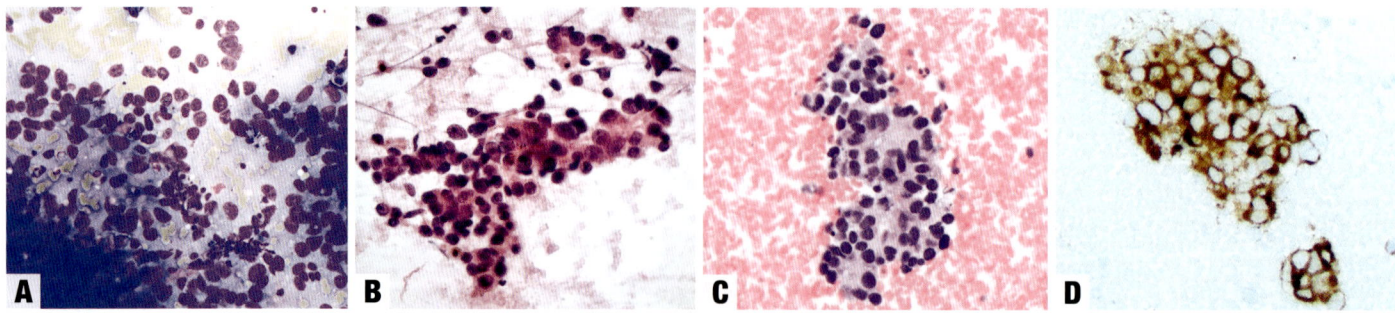

Fig. 1.151 Large cell neuroendocrine carcinoma (LCNEC), cytology. Diff-Quik (Giemsa) stain of air-dried smear (**A**) and H&E-stained alcohol-fixed smear (**B**) demonstrate combination of groups and single cells, with many naked nuclei and subtle suggestion of rosette-like structures. Granular chromatin with nucleoli is visible in panel B. **C** Cell block preparation, in which clusters are preserved and rosettes are most apparent. **D** Synaptophysin shows diffuse labelling in the cell block.

The distinction of LCNEC from SCLC in biopsies can be limited by crush artefact and extensive necrosis. In the absence of well-preserved areas to allow evaluation of cytological features, the diagnosis of "high-grade neuroendocrine carcinoma NOS" is appropriate. However, this term should be used as infrequently as possible. In such difficult cases, correlation with a concurrent cytology specimen may be helpful, because the morphology may be clearer than on the biopsy.

The distinction of LCNEC from other NSCLCs requires neuroendocrine morphology and immunohistochemical marker expression, which can be appreciated in most but not all biopsies of LCNECs {145}, depending in part on the biopsy size {665}. A semiquantitative score based on a combination of morphological features, expression of neuroendocrine markers, and Ki-67 index > 40% allowed the distinction of LCNEC from other NSCLCs on biopsies with high sensitivity and specificity {145}. Labelling for ≥ 2 neuroendocrine markers is substantially more common in LCNECs (≥ 80%) than NSCLCs (1% to ~4%)

{665}; however, because occasionally such expression does occur in non-neuroendocrine NSCLC, the diagnosis of LCNEC should only be made in the context of appropriate morphology.

Combined LCNEC

Combined LCNECs occur most commonly with adenocarcinoma, but any non-neuroendocrine NSCLC histological type may be present. Combined tumours account for approximately 20–25% of resected LCNECs {2631}. LCNEC and NSCLC components are clonally related, as revealed by genomic studies, supporting the concept of phenotypic divergence rather than a collision phenomenon {1945}.

NSCLC with isolated neuroendocrine morphology or neuroendocrine marker expression

The term "large cell carcinoma with neuroendocrine morphology" refers to rare tumours that have the morphology of LCNEC but lack demonstrable neuroendocrine marker expression by

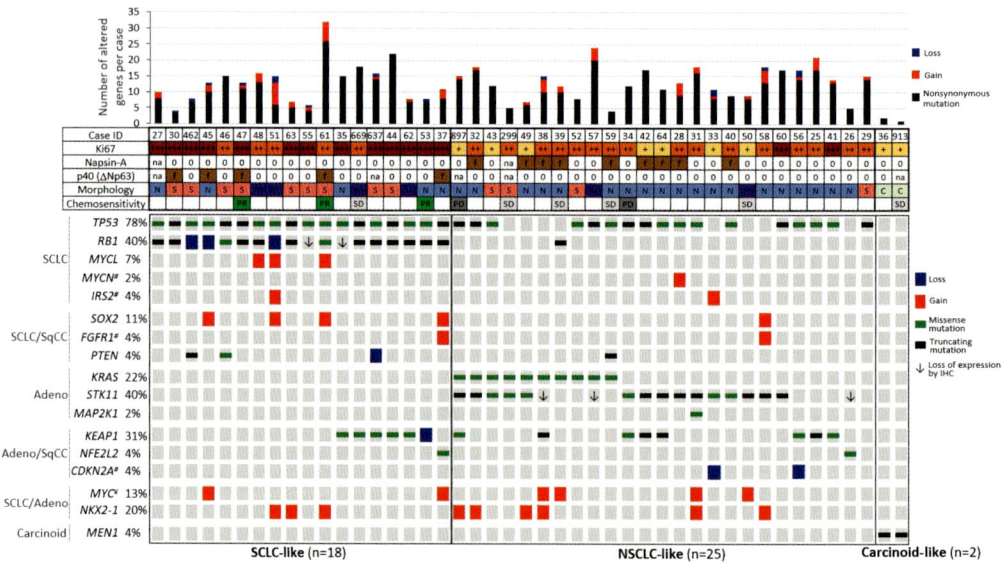

Fig. 1.152 Molecular subsets of large cell neuroendocrine carcinoma (LCNEC). OncoPrint depicting co-alterations in selected genes in LCNEC, with presence or absence of *RB1+TP53* co-alteration defining the major small cell lung carcinoma (SCLC)-like and non-small cell lung carcinoma (NSCLC)-like subsets, respectively, and *MEN1* mutations and low total mutation burden defining a carcinoid-like subset. At the left, conventional lung cancer types characteristically associated with the indicated gene alterations are shown. ¥, *MYC* amplifications also occur in squamous cell carcinoma (SqCC). #, genes for which only copy-number alterations are shown. Loss of RB1 (pRB) and STK11 expression by immunohistochemistry (IHC) (↓) is only shown for cases without gene mutations/losses. For all other cases, loss of expression and molecular results were concordant. No RB1 (pRB) IHC available for cases 27, 897, and 299; no STK11 IHC available for cases 27, 55, 637, 299, and 913. Selected clinicopathological features are designated as follows: Ki-67: +++, > 80%; ++, 60–80%; +, 40–50%. Napsin A and p40: f, focally expressed by IHC; 0, no expression; na, not available. Morphology: S, SCLC spectrum; N, NSCLC spectrum; M, mixed; C, carcinoid-like. Chemosensitivity: PR, partial response; SD, stable disease; PD, progressive disease.

immunohistochemistry. Clinical data are limited but suggest aggressive behaviour similar to that of LCNEC {1278,3463}. The term "non-small cell lung carcinoma with neuroendocrine differentiation" refers to pulmonary adenocarcinoma; squamous cell carcinoma; and large cell, spindle cell, or giant cell carcinomas that express neuroendocrine marker(s) in the absence of neuroendocrine morphology. As mentioned above, this occurs in 10–20% of NSCLCs, most commonly adenocarcinomas. Given the lack of consistent data to support clinical relevance {1259, 2859}, staining for neuroendocrine markers in the absence of neuroendocrine morphology is not recommended {3070,3390} (see *Lung neuroendocrine neoplasms: Introduction*, p. 127).

Cytology

The definitive diagnosis of LCNEC is difficult in cytology samples, but the diagnosis may be suggested in cases with cellular cell blocks that allow for the assessment of neuroendocrine morphology (palisading, rosettes) and immunohistochemistry. In smears, LCNECs exhibit intermediate to large cells containing variable nucleoli, frequently in a necrotic background {3299, 3383,1812,1317,1196,1242}. Key features distinguishing LCNEC from other NSCLCs include a prominent single-cell component and frequent crush artefact with nuclear streaming that on low power may resemble SCLC {1317}. Naked nuclei are common in air-dried preparations and can also mimic SCLC or haematolymphoid neoplasms. The distinction from SCLC relies on the same criteria as applied to histological specimens, including the presence of nucleoli and/or more abundant cytoplasm and overall larger cell size. Marked nuclear membrane irregularities, including nuclear notching, are more characteristic of LCNEC than SCLC, whereas cell spindling is uncommon.

Diagnostic molecular pathology

Given that the effect on patient management and the tools of distinguishing LCNEC subsets remain investigational, performing molecular studies or RB1/p53 immunohistochemistry to identify subtypes of LCNEC in routine practice is not currently recommended. The prevalence of targetable NSCLC oncogenic drivers, such as *EGFR* and *ALK* alterations, is low in LCNEC, but such alterations do occur, and patients with these alterations may respond to targeted therapies {634,3511,1100}.

Essential and desirable diagnostic criteria

Essential:

- Neuroendocrine morphology: organoid nesting, trabeculae, peripheral palisading, rosettes
- Non-small cell cytology: prominent nucleoli and/or moderate to abundant cytoplasm, larger cell size than SCLC (> 3 lymphocytes), and chromatin may be either granular/stippled or vesicular
- High proliferation rate: > 10 mitoses/2 mm^2, with a median of 70 mitoses/2 mm^2
- Positive immunohistochemical staining for one or more neuroendocrine markers (other than NSE)

Desirable:

- Necrosis: generally in large confluent zones but may be limited to the centres of tumour nests
- High Ki-67 index: > 30%, generally 40–80%
- Negative p40 immunohistochemistry

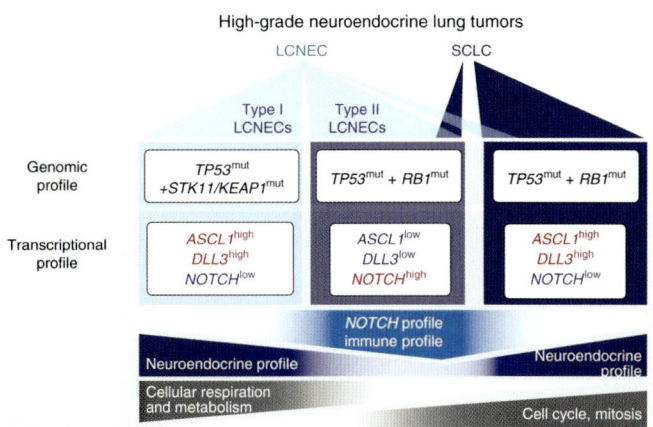

Fig. 1.153 Molecular subsets of large cell neuroendocrine carcinoma (LCNEC). Schematic overview of somatic alterations and expression profiles in high-grade neuroendocrine lung tumours: LCNEC and small cell lung carcinoma (SCLC). Significantly mutated (mut) genes are shown in black, and differentially expressed genes are shown in red and blue, describing higher and lower expression, respectively. Upregulated expression profiles and signalling pathways are indicated by colour gradients.

Staging

Staging should be performed according to the eighth-edition TNM classification.

Prognosis and prediction

LCNEC is a clinically aggressive disease. Patients with resected tumours are more likely to develop locally recurrent or metastatic disease and have shorter survival than patients with other histological subtypes of NSCLC (40–70% recurrence rate), even with stage I tumours {2539,815,1277,2631,830}. In a nonsurgical metastatic setting, outcomes are generally similar to those of SCLC, with median survival times of approximately 10 months {2045,3207,1467}. Adjuvant chemotherapy is suggested as potentially beneficial even for patients with stage I disease, but this requires clinical validation {2539,1277,830}. Treatment of stage IV LCNEC is controversial, with both SCLC and NSCLC chemotherapy regimens commonly used in practice {2045}. Several recent studies suggest that selection of systemic therapies may be aided by identification of genomic subsets of LCNEC {2463,668,3522}; however, further validation is needed.

Activity of immunotherapy in LCNEC in not well established, but robust responses to checkpoint inhibitors have been reported in isolated cases {3217,1849}. PDL1 is expressed in about 15% of LCNECs (5% with > 50% of cells labelled), with equal distribution in *RB1*-mutated and wildtype tumours {3100, 756,1130}. Clinical data on the predictive value of PDL1 specifically in LCNEC is lacking.

Melanoma of the lung

Scolyer RA
de la Fouchardière A
Travis WD

Definition
Melanoma of the lung is a malignant melanocytic neoplasm arising in the lung.

ICD-O coding
8720/3 Melanoma

ICD-11 coding
2C25.Y & XH4846 Other specified malignant neoplasms of bronchus or lung & Melanoma
2C25.Y & XH5QP3 Other specified malignant neoplasms of bronchus or lung & Mucosal lentiginous melanoma
2C25.Y & XH4QG5 Other specified malignant neoplasms of bronchus or lung & Nodular melanoma

Related terminology
Acceptable: mucosal melanoma; mucosal lentiginous melanoma; pulmonary melanoma; lung melanoma.

Subtype(s)
None

Localization
Primary pulmonary melanoma can arise anywhere in the lower respiratory tract, including in the large airways or periphery of the lung.

Clinical features
Primary pulmonary melanoma usually occurs either as a unifocal polypoid obstructing lesion within the tracheobronchial tree or as a mass within the lung parenchyma {3354}. The presenting

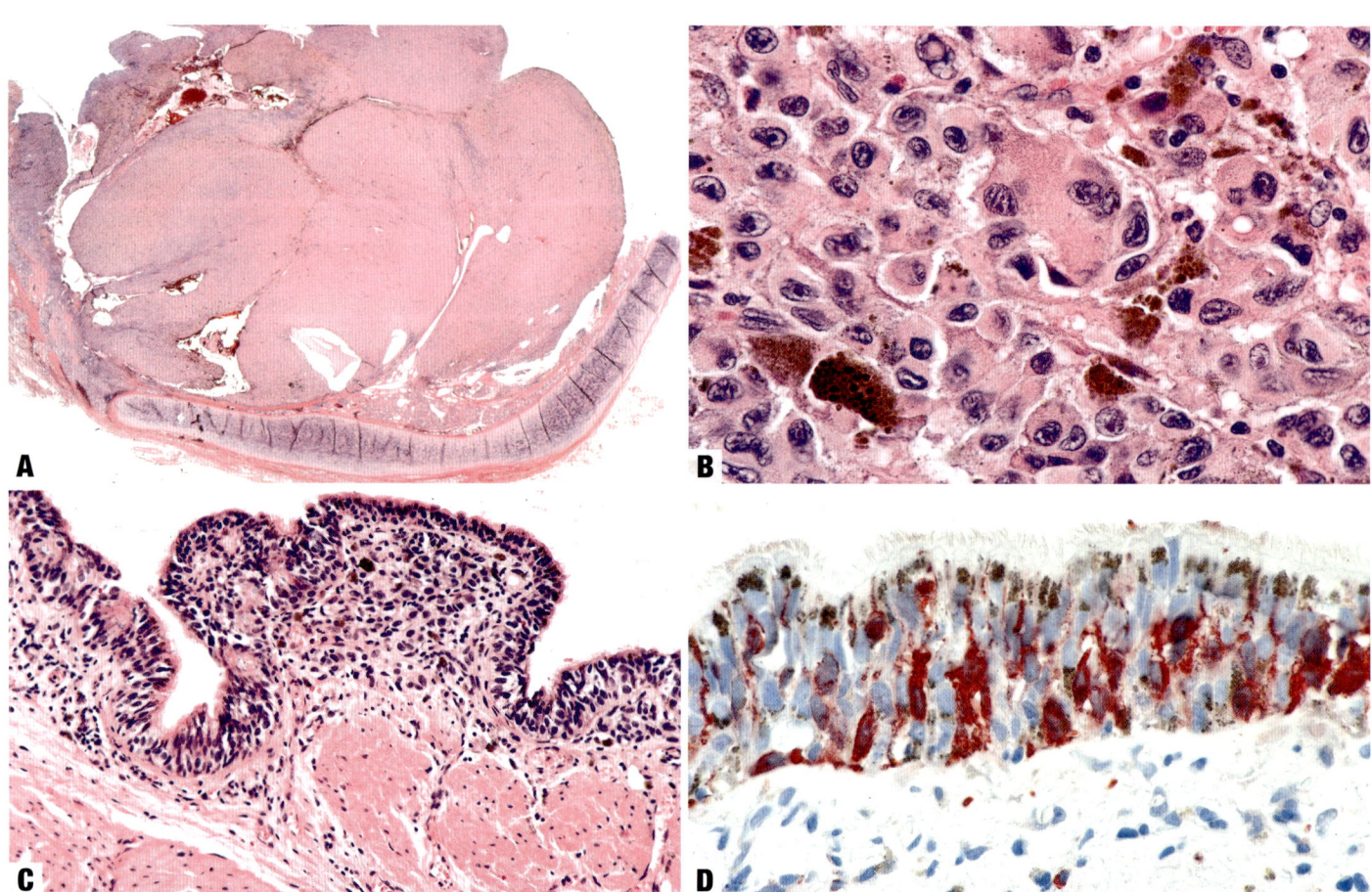

Fig. 1.154 Melanoma. **A** A polypoid endobronchial mass protrudes into the lumen of this bronchus. **B** The tumour consists of nests of cytologically malignant cells with large atypical nuclei, prominent nucleoli, and focally abundant melanin pigment. **C** The bronchial submucosa shows nests of cytologically bland melanocytic cells, some of which contain brown melanin pigment. **D** S100 staining highlights melanocytic cells growing within the bronchial mucosa in a pagetoid manner.

symptoms are determined by the site and size of the tumour {1676}. Pigment in sputum has been reported {828}. Careful clinical evaluation is necessary to assess the possibility of previous or current extrapulmonary primary melanoma, including cutaneous and extracutaneous melanomas.

Epidemiology

Primary melanoma involving the respiratory tract is extremely rare and accounts for < 0.1% of all lung malignancies {1921, 2701}. There is no racial predisposition. Primary melanomas of the lung represent < 0.1% of all melanomas.

Etiology

The etiology of primary melanomas of the lung is unknown.

Pathogenesis

Because melanocytes are not normally found in the tracheobronchial tree, it is difficult to explain the pathogenesis of primary melanomas of the lung. They may arise from neuroendocrine precursor cells in lung tissue {2352} or from a melanoblast with aberrant migration from the neural crest to the pulmonary anlage {353}. It has been questioned whether the condition actually exists. The difficulty arises because an unrecognized primary cutaneous melanoma can occasionally undergo complete regression and disappear without a trace, while a lung metastasis that has arisen from it continues to grow and may eventually be detected as an apparently isolated focus of melanoma {1281}. This hypothesis is supported by data from a recent study of patients with lung-only melanoma using next-generation sequencing, which showed that all cases had a dominant ultraviolet (UV) light mutation signature, suggesting they represented metastases from occult or unrecognized regressed skin primary melanomas rather than primary lung tumours {3376}.

Macroscopic appearance

Primary melanoma of the lung usually occurs as a polyp in a bronchus or as a circumscribed nodular mass within the lung parenchyma {721,2733}. Polyps usually show surface ulceration. The cut surface is often tan and haemorrhagic.

Histopathology

The tumour is usually formed by sheets or expansive nodules of large pleomorphic epithelioid or, less commonly, spindle malignant melanocytic cells {641}. The bronchial epithelium is unusually ulcerated. Necrosis is often present. The nuclei often have vesicular chromatin and prominent nucleoli {62}. An intramucosal in situ component with pagetoid scatter may be seen in the bronchial or tracheal epithelium adjacent to the invasive component {3320}. This feature has also been reported in the vicinity of metastases {1701}. However, an intramucosal component is lacking in many reported cases.

Cytology

FNA specimens of melanomas in the lung are usually obtained from metastases. Similar to those of melanomas occurring elsewhere, typical cytological appearances include a dissociated population of large epithelioid or sometimes spindle cells {2030}. Occasional giant cells and intranuclear pseudoinclusions are often present. Melanin pigment can be present either in the cytoplasm of tumour cells or within pigmented macrophages.

Diagnostic molecular pathology

A recent study of lung-only melanomas showed frequent mutations known to be associated with cutaneous melanoma, including *BRAF*, *NRAS*, *NF1*, *KIT*, and *KRAS* mutations and UV mutation signatures, suggesting that these neoplasms represented cutaneous melanoma metastases to the lung {3376}. Previous studies reported that most cases lack *BRAF*, *NRAS*, or *KIT* mutations, although one case harbouring an oncogenic *NRAS* mutation has been described {1140,3234}.

Essential and desirable diagnostic criteria

Essential:

- Demonstration of malignancy and melanocytic differentiation
- Relation to mucosa of the lung
- Absence of evidence for previous or synchronous melanoma outside the lung

Staging

There are no Union for International Cancer Control (UICC) staging criteria for primary melanoma of the lung.

Prognosis and prediction

Unlike for cutaneous melanoma patients, the very limited information that can be gleaned from published reports indicates that the prognosis for patients with melanoma of the lung is generally very poor {1575,3364,2733}. The principal determinant of outcome is the presence or absence of local (peribronchial and hilar) lymph node and distant metastases. However, in one series of 15 patients who presented with isolated pulmonary melanoma with no known primary tumour, the overall actuarial survival rate was 42% {641}. A case has been reported that responded to anti-PD1 immunotherapy {1152}.

Meningioma of the lung

Motoi N
Duhig EE

Definition

Pulmonary meningiomas are identical to meningothelial (arachnoidal) cell neoplasms that typically arise from dura mater of the CNS but are without a demonstrable CNS lesion.

ICD-O coding

9530/0 Meningioma

ICD-11 coding

2F71.3 & XH11P5 Neoplasms of uncertain behaviour of trachea, bronchus, or lung & Meningioma, NOS

Related terminology

None

Subtype(s)

None

Localization

There is no predilection for a specific anatomical site in the lung {1967}.

Clinical features

Most cases are incidental, although some patients present with respiratory symptoms including haemoptysis {1247}. Images shows slow-growing, well-circumscribed nodules on CT, with high metabolic activity on FDG PET {1247}.

Epidemiology

There is a slight female predominance. The median age is 56 years (range: 18–108 years) {1280,3244,2158}.

Etiology

Hypotheses include origin from pluripotent cells, heterotopic embryonic rests, and meningothelioid nodules {1967,1247}. Although isolated meningothelioid nodules {1258} lack mutation damage, multiple meningothelioid nodules show increased genetic alterations and may represent transition to neoplasia. Occasional meningiomas occur in the setting of multiple meningothelioid nodules {986}.

Pathogenesis

Unknown

Macroscopic appearance

Most are solitary, well circumscribed, and firm, with a yellow-tan to grey cut surface. Size is markedly variable (median: 24 mm; range: 4–150 mm) {2158,3117A}.

Histopathology

Most tumours are well circumscribed and consist of a solid proliferation of tumour cells growing in whorls and lobular nests, most often with transitional or fibrous patterns. Rare examples of anaplastic {3244,1653} and chordoid meningiomas are reported {2557,2340,135}. CNS criteria have been used for grading. Cells are positive for vimentin, EMA, PR, SSTR2A {1740}, and (rarely) S100 {2158}. CD56 can be positive. Cytokeratin, other melanoma markers, and neuroendocrine markers are negative. Increased proliferation may be seen in anaplastic meningiomas {3244}. Metastatic meningioma requires exclusion, as do spindle cell thymoma, solitary fibrous tumour, and monophasic synovial sarcoma, using appropriate immunohistochemistry {1967}. Meningothelioid nodules are distinguished from meningiomas by their interstitial and frequently perivenular pattern of growth and ill-defined borders. In contrast to

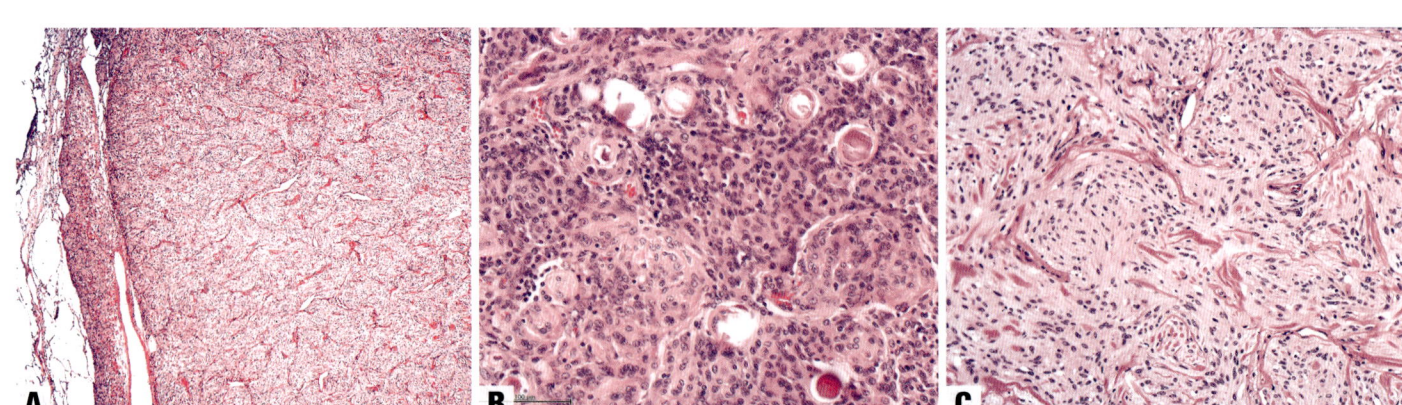

Fig. 1.155 Meningioma. **A** This tumour is circumscribed, with a sharp border to the adjacent lung parenchyma. The tumour shows whorled nests of spindle cells surrounded by a fine fibrovascular stroma. **B** Pulmonary meningotheliomatous meningioma shows solid sheet-like growth of spindle to round-shaped tumour cells, with whorl formation. Tumour cells have small fusiform or round nuclei and numerous intranuclear cytoplasmic inclusions. Note scattered psammoma bodies. **C** This tumour consists of whorled nests of spindle cells surrounded by a fine fibrovascular stroma.

meningiomas, they typically lack a solid growth pattern and a sharply circumscribed border. Most meningothelioid nodules are ≤ 3 mm in size, but they can be as large as 5 mm {2916, 898}.

Cytology

Tumours can rarely be diagnosed by FNA {986}. The presence of intranuclear inclusions and psammoma bodies can create confusion with thyroid carcinoma {2158}.

Diagnostic molecular pathology

In the CNS, most meningiomas have allelic loss on chromosome 22 and *NF2* mutations {1740}.

Essential and desirable diagnostic criteria

Essential:

- A circumscribed solid proliferation of tumour cells growing in whorls and lobular nests, most often with transitional or fibrous patterns
- Absence of CNS disease with histological and immunohistochemical features of CNS meningioma
- Lack of predominant interstitial or perivenular distribution, ill-defined borders
- Size usually > 4 mm

Staging

Not clinically relevant

Prognosis and prediction

Most tumours show indolent growth. Rare aggressive behaviour is associated with atypical or anaplastic features (WHO grades II–III) {2384,3244}.

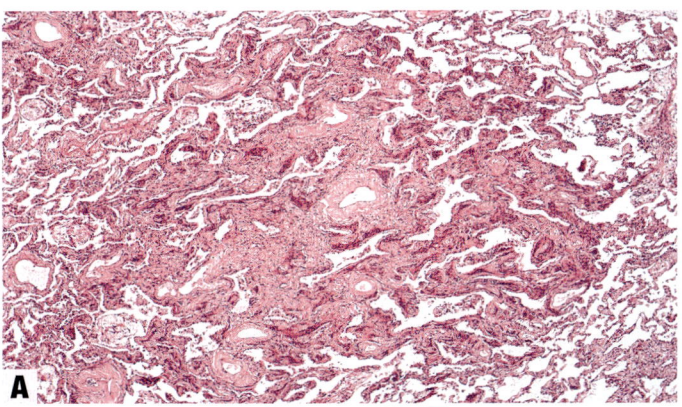

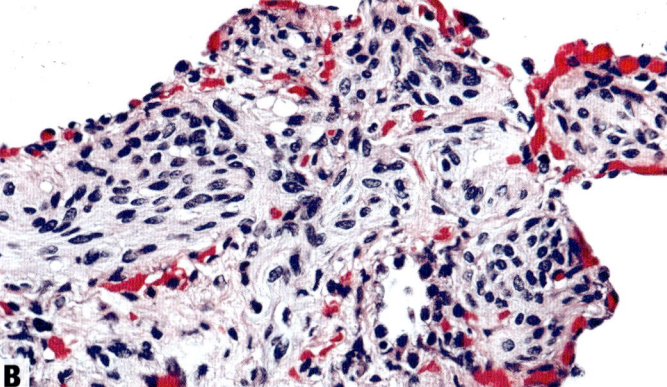

Fig. 1.156 Meningothelioid nodule. **A** This differs from meningioma in that it has ill-defined borders and shows an interstitial pattern of growth. **B** Organoid nests of cytologically bland round to oval tumour cells with a moderate amount of eosinophilic cytoplasm. Nuclear chromatin is finely granular. Some cells show faint nucleoli. Morphology is similar to the tumour cells of meningioma.

Pulmonary hamartoma

Boland JM
Aubry M-C

Definition

Pulmonary hamartomas are benign mesenchymal neoplasms with variable amounts of at least two mesenchymal elements and entrapped respiratory epithelium.

ICD-O coding

8992/0 Pulmonary hamartoma

ICD-11 coding

2F00.Y & XH3UD9 Other specified benign neoplasm of middle ear or respiratory system & Pulmonary hamartoma

Related terminology

Not recommended: chondroid hamartoma; mesenchymoma.

Subtype(s)

None

Localization

Most are peripheral, with approximately 10% located centrally in a bronchus. Hamartomas occur in all lobes {3138}.

Clinical features

Peripheral pulmonary hamartomas are usually asymptomatic, solitary, well-circumscribed nodules; multifocality is rare {3138}. Endobronchial hamartomas often produce signs and symptoms of obstruction {3138,578}.

Imaging

Popcorn calcification is a helpful radiographic feature but is present in a minority of cases {1168}. Presence of adipose tissue on CT is a specific feature {1168,972}. Hamartomas have low FDG avidity (mean maximum standardized uptake value: 1.5) {1311}.

Epidemiology

Hamartomas are the most common benign pulmonary neoplasm, accounting for 8% of radiographically detected coin lesions {3052}. Hamartomas have a male predominance, with peak incidence in the sixth decade of life, and they rarely occur in children {3138,578}.

Etiology

Molecular and cytogenetic data suggest a neoplastic origin, with recurrent translocations leading to fusion genes that drive tumorigenesis {2515,2674}.

Pathogenesis

Pulmonary hamartomas frequently have the translocation t(3;12) (q27-q28;q14-q15). The resulting *HMGA2-LPP* fusion gene usually consists of exons 1–3 of *HMGA2* and exons 9–11 of *LPP*, and it is consistently expressed in tumours with this translocation

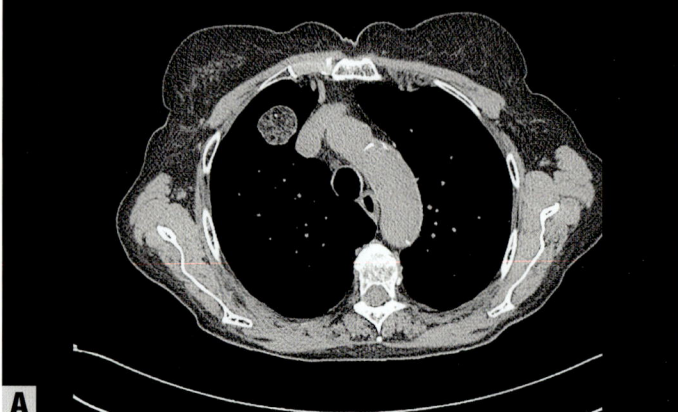

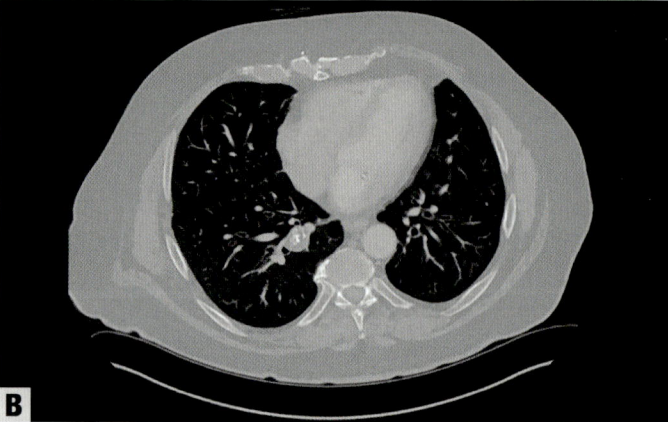

Fig. 1.157 Pulmonary hamartoma. **A** Classic CT findings of pulmonary hamartoma include fat attenuation (mediastinal window). **B** The classic CT finding of popcorn calcification is pictured in a pulmonary chondroma (bone window), but this is present in only a minority of cases.

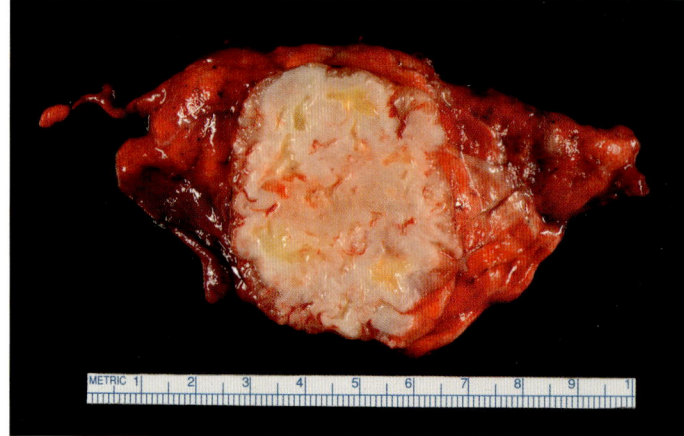

Fig. 1.158 Pulmonary hamartoma. Grossly, hamartomas are usually circumscribed, lobulated, firm, and white.

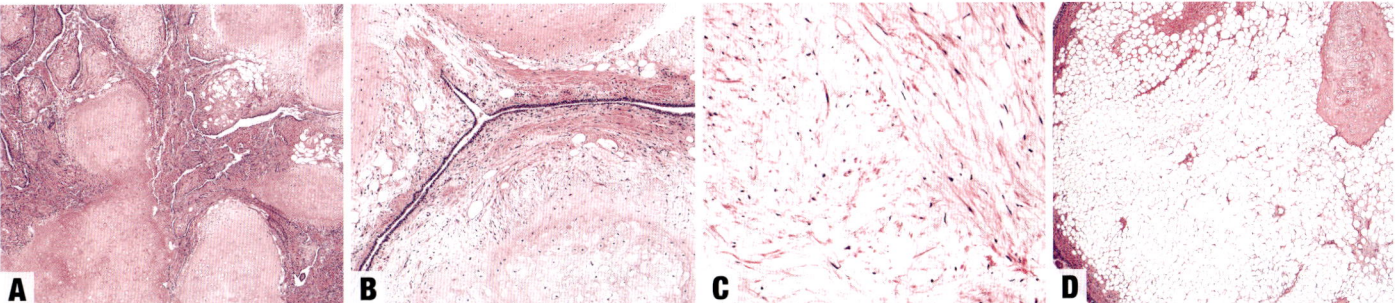

Fig. 1.159 Pulmonary hamartoma. **A** Hamartoma showing the typical admixture of hyaline cartilage, adipose tissue, and invaginated bronchial epithelium. **B** Entrapped bronchial epithelium surrounded by myxoid spindle cells, fat, and hyaline cartilage. **C** Myxoid area of hamartoma, with low cellularity and bland spindle cells. **D** Adipose-rich hamartoma with little hyaline cartilage, a so-called lipomatous hamartoma.

{607,2515,3180,1414}. The same translocation and fusion gene are common in lipomas {2515,2674,842}.

Macroscopic appearance

Hamartomas are firm, round to multilobulated, well-circumscribed nodules that often shell out from the surrounding lung. They are white to bluish and may be gritty. Most are < 40 mm, but they may uncommonly reach a large size (> 90 mm) {1311,3138,1168}. Cystic change is uncommon. Endobronchial hamartomas are often yellow to grey and sessile.

Histopathology

Pulmonary hamartomas are usually composed predominantly of hyaline cartilage, which may show myxoid change, intermixed with variable amounts of other mesenchymal components, including fat, bland myxoid spindle cells, smooth muscle, fibrous tissue, and bone {3138}. Clefts of entrapped respiratory epithelial cells invaginate between the lobules of cartilage and connective tissue. Endobronchial hamartomas may have prominent adipose tissue (termed lipomatous hamartoma), whereas epithelial inclusions tend to be inconspicuous {3138}. In some cases, other mesenchymal elements may dominate, such as smooth muscle (termed adenoleiomyomatous hamartoma) or rarely fibrous tissue. Immunohistochemistry is usually not necessary, because hamartomas would show the expected staining pattern for the represented mesenchymal elements.

Differential diagnosis

Pulmonary hamartomas are differentiated from monomorphic soft tissue tumours by the presence of more than one mesenchymal component. Other soft tissue neoplasms may enter the differential diagnosis on small biopsies where only one mesenchymal component is represented. Pulmonary chondromas typically arise in patients with Carney triad (i.e. gastrointestinal stromal tumours, pulmonary chondromas, paragangliomas); sporadic examples are very uncommon. Chondromas lack entrapped epithelium, frequently show calcification / bone metaplasia, and are bounded by a fibrous pseudocapsule

{2512}. SDHB immunohistochemistry may be useful; it shows abnormal loss in Carney-associated chondromas but not in hamartomas {461}. Endobronchial lipoma may show overlapping morphological and genetic features with hamartoma {261}, but the distinction between hamartoma and lipoma is generally not critical. The differential diagnosis may be particularly challenging if only the myxoid spindle cell component is sampled, which could lead to consideration of myxoid peripheral nerve sheath tumour or even myxoid sarcoma; however, unlike those of sarcomas, the spindle cells of hamartoma are generally very bland, without atypia, and they have very low cellularity.

Cytology

Cytological preparations commonly include abundant fibromyxoid stroma with cartilage, as well as benign reactive epithelial cells {3337,2628}. Mesenchymal elements may be subtle on a Pap stain, and epithelial cells may be abundant, leading to false positive diagnoses of malignancy {1205}.

Diagnostic molecular pathology

Not relevant

Essential and desirable diagnostic criteria

Essential:

- At least two types of benign mesenchymal tissue, most commonly hyaline cartilage, fat, and/or myxoid spindle cells, with entrapped invaginated bronchial epithelium

Staging

Not relevant

Prognosis and prediction

Pulmonary hamartomas are slow-growing neoplasms with excellent prognosis {3138}. Surgical resection is the optimal treatment for endobronchial lesions and parenchymal tumours that are large/symptomatic. Recurrence and malignant transformation are very rare {3138,164}.

Pulmonary chondroma

Aubry M-C
Boland JM

Definition
Chondroma is a benign neoplasm of hyaline cartilage.

ICD-O coding
9220/0 Chondroma

ICD-11 coding
2F00.Y & XH0NS4 Other specified benign neoplasm of middle ear or respiratory system & Chondroma, NOS

Related terminology
None

Subtype(s)
None

Localization
Chondromas usually occur in the peripheral lung; rarely they may be endobronchial.

Clinical features
Patients are usually asymptomatic, but reported symptoms include cough, chest pain, dyspnoea, and pneumonia {2512}. Chondromas occur in all pulmonary lobes; they tend to be multiple (averaging three) in Carney triad and solitary in sporadic

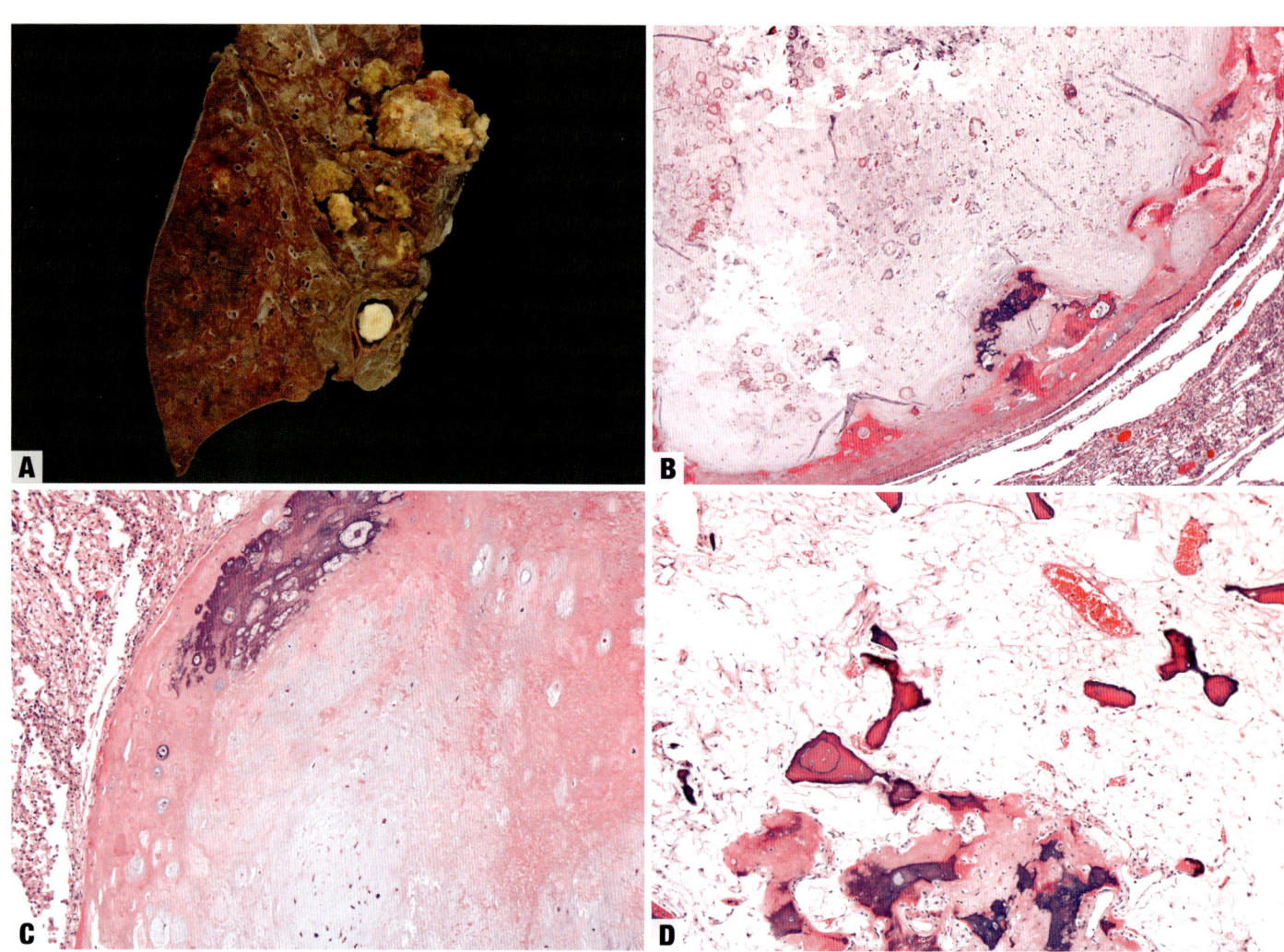

Fig. 1.160 Multiple chondromas in a patient with Carney triad. **A** Gross photo showing multiple well-circumscribed nodules. Most of these nodules are calcified and ossified, with a pale-grey, gritty cut surface. One nodule, mainly composed of cartilage, has a whiter and smoother cut surface. **B** Chondroma is mostly composed of cartilage, with focal calcification and ossification. Note the well-circumscribed contour, with no invagination, in contrast to hamartoma. **C** Although the cartilage is typically hyaline, myxoid changes are often seen and can occasionally be prominent. **D** When ossification occurs, it is often associated with prominent adipose tissue, as would be seen in bone marrow. This is to be distinguished from the adipose tissue seen in hamartoma.

cases {2512,461}. Imaging shows well-delineated nodules that may be calcified, most commonly with a popcorn-like or central pattern {2512}.

Epidemiology
Chondromas are typically found in young woman (aged < 30 years) affected by Carney triad {2512,461,389}. Rare sporadic examples have male predominance and older average age (mean: 53 years) {2512}.

Etiology
Most affected patients have Carney triad, a non-hereditary tumour syndrome characterized by gastrointestinal stromal tumours, pulmonary chondromas, and paragangliomas {389, 2869}.

Pathogenesis
Gain of chromosome 6 and loss of 1q have been reported in pulmonary chondroma {2869}. Functional deficiency of succinate dehydrogenase is the underlying mechanism of Carney triad, driven by hypermethylation of *SDHC* {2710}.

Macroscopic appearance
Chondromas are well circumscribed and lobulated and have a grey-white to bluish gritty cut surface {2512}. The average size is 28 mm (range: 8–75 mm) {2512}.

Histopathology
Chondromas are circumscribed nodules of pure hyaline cartilage with frequent myxoid change. The cartilage is moderately cellular without atypia and is surrounded by a fibrous pseudocapsule without invagination of the overlying bronchial epithelium. Calcification and ossification are common, and ossification may be accompanied by adipose tissue.

The differential diagnosis includes pulmonary hamartoma and chondrosarcoma. Hamartomas have entrapped respiratory epithelium between the lobules of cartilage, and they frequently contain other mesenchymal elements (fat, smooth muscle, myxoid spindle cells). Primary pulmonary chondrosarcomas are exceptionally rare; chondrosarcomas in the lung are more often metastases from high-grade skeletal tumours, with significantly increased cellularity and atypia {240,1356}.

Carney-associated chondromas show frequent loss of SDHB by immunohistochemistry, in contrast to hamartomas {461}, and this can be a useful diagnostic adjunct when the distinction is difficult.

Cytology
Not clinically relevant

Diagnostic molecular pathology
Not clinically relevant

Essential and desirable diagnostic criteria
Essential:
- Bland cartilaginous stroma
- Absence of invaginated epithelium
- Absence of other mesenchymal components

Desirable:
- Carney triad

Staging
Not relevant

Prognosis and prediction
No metastasis or death has been reported {2512}.

Diffuse pulmonary lymphangiomatosis

Yi ES
Calonje JE

Definition
Diffuse pulmonary lymphangiomatosis is a diffuse proliferation of lymphatic channels and smooth muscle along otherwise normal lymphatic vessels of the lungs, pleura, and mediastinum.

ICD-O coding
9170/3 Diffuse lymphangiomatosis

ICD-11 coding
LA75.Y & XH9MR8 Other specified structural developmental anomalies of lungs & Lymphangioma, NOS

Related terminology
Not recommended: lymphangiomatosis; lymphatic dysplasia.

Subtype(s)
None

Localization
Lymphangiomatosis within the thorax frequently involves the mediastinum, with or without involvement of the heart. It may be limited to the lung and pleura.

Clinical features
Diffuse pulmonary lymphangiomatosis usually presents in children. It can result in mass effect from infiltrative disease, restrictive and obstructive pulmonary physiology, chylous effusions, and respiratory failure. In paediatric patients the disease has an aggressive course, with progressive respiratory failure and death. Adult patients may present with mild wheezing, non-productive cough, recurrent chylous pleural effusions, or respiratory failure {1336,1715}.

Imaging
On imaging, chest radiographs may show increased interstitial marking and pleural effusions. CT shows mediastinal soft tissue infiltration, pleural thickening (with effusions), thickening of peribronchovascular bundles, and interlobular septa {1336}.

Epidemiology
Diffuse pulmonary lymphangiomatosis is typically diagnosed shortly after birth or during childhood, but also rarely during adulthood {264,3456}. It affects both sexes equally.

Etiology
Unknown

Pathogenesis
Unknown

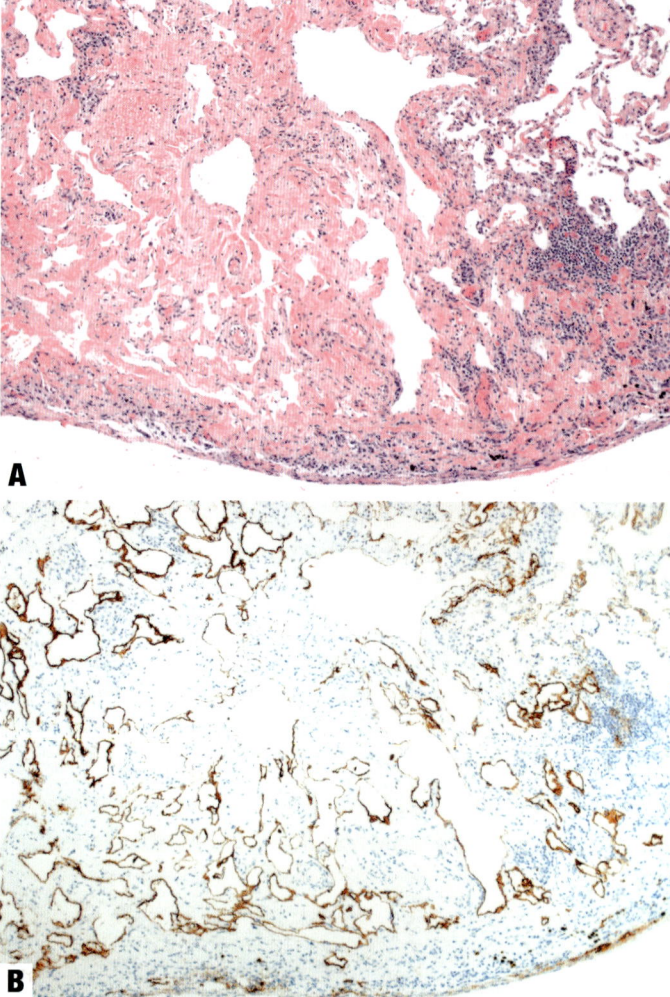

Fig. 1.161 Diffuse pulmonary lymphangiomatosis. **A** There is lymphatic proliferation along the interlobular septa. **B** D2-40 stain highlights the lining lymphatic endothelial cells.

Macroscopic appearance
Obvious cysts or mass lesions may not be present. Diffuse pulmonary lymphangiomatosis shows lymphatic distribution as evidenced by prominence of visceral pleural, interlobular septa, and bronchovascular bundles {3002}.

Histopathology
Increased numbers of anastomosing, variably sized, endothelial-lined spaces containing acellular eosinophilic material are distributed along the lymphatic routes and lined by a layer of flattened lymphatic endothelial cells. Collagen layers or spindle cells resembling smooth muscle cells are present between

channels. The adjacent lung tissue shows various quantities of haemosiderin-laden macrophages {3002,264}.

The lining cells are positive for D2-40, CD31, and ERG, and the stromal spindle cells express vimentin, desmin, actin, and PR but not ER, keratin, or HMB45 {3002,264}.

The differential diagnoses include lymphangioleiomyomatosis, lymphangiectasis, haemangiomatosis, and Kaposi sarcoma. Lymphangioleiomyomatosis contains HMB45-positive spindle cells. Lymphangiectasis does not show an increased number of anastomosing lymphatic vessels. Kaposi sarcoma does not show the complex anastomosing lymphatic canals. In haemangiomatosis, vascular spaces are blood-filled.

Cytology
In the setting of chylous effusions where there is milky pleural fluid, cytology can show lymphocytes within lymphatic fluid, although this is not specific for diagnosis {3456}.

Diagnostic molecular pathology
Not clinically relevant

Essential and desirable diagnostic criteria
Essential:
- Increased numbers of cytologically bland anastomosing lymphatic channels distributed along the lymphatic routes
- Positive staining for lymphatic markers (e.g. D2-40)
- No cytological features of malignancy

Staging
Not clinically relevant

Prognosis and prediction
Prognosis is poor; there is no established curative treatment. However, recent case studies have reported improved outcome with bevacizumab and sildenafil {2196,1850}.

Pleuropulmonary blastoma

Hill DA

Definition
Pleuropulmonary blastoma (PPB) is an embryonal tumour that forms a cystic and/or solid mass in the lung in infants and young children.

ICD-O coding
8973/3 Pleuropulmonary blastoma

ICD-11 coding
2C25.Y & XH2FY9 Other specified malignant neoplasms of bronchus or lung & Pleuropulmonary blastoma

Related terminology
Not recommended: rhabdomyosarcoma arising in congenital cystic adenomatoid malformation; pulmonary blastoma of childhood; pulmonary sarcoma arising in mesenchymal cystic hamartoma; embryonal rhabdomyosarcoma arising within congenital bronchogenic cyst; pulmonary blastoma associated with cystic lung disease; pleuropulmonary blastoma in congenital cystic adenomatoid malformation.

Subtype(s)
Types I, Ir, II, and III

Localization
PPB occurs in the lung and derives from lung mesenchyme or subpleural mesenchyme {1784}.

Clinical features
Signs and symptoms
The clinical presentation of PPB varies by age and tumour type. Children with type I PPB present at a median age of 9 months, with shortness of breath with or without pneumothorax secondary to cyst rupture. Some children are asymptomatic, and a cyst is diagnosed as an incidental finding on chest X-ray. Children with

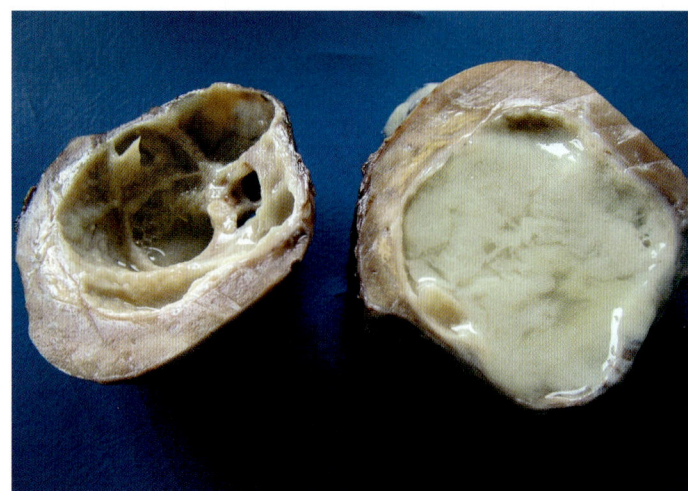

Fig. 1.162 Pleuropulmonary blastoma. A type I pleuropulmonary blastoma showing a typical loculated cystic architecture (left) after removal of purulent fluid from superimposed infection (right).

type II or III PPB are typically older (median: 36 and 42 months, respectively) and present with shortness of breath, weight loss, and fever {1898}.

Imaging
CT is the preferred imaging modality to detect tumours/cysts, determine site(s) of disease, and help classify tumours as purely cystic (type I), cystic and solid (type II), or purely solid (type III). Plain X-ray images are insensitive to small changes and cannot reliably distinguish between masses and consolidations.

Epidemiology
PPB is the most common primary lung neoplasm of childhood.
The prevalence of germline pathogenic *DICER1* variation is between 1 in 3000 and 1 in 10 600 individuals {1445}. There are

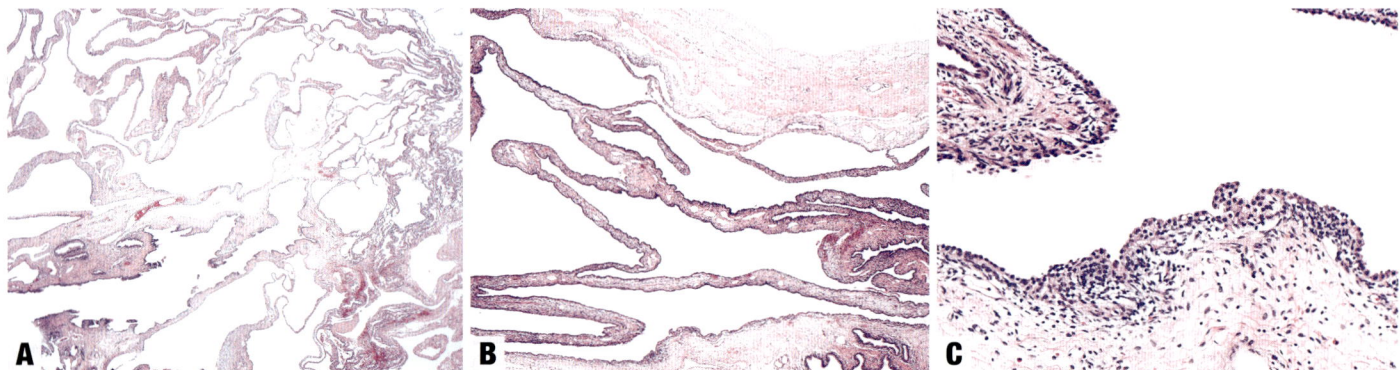

Fig. 1.163 Type I pleuropulmonary blastoma. **A** Low-power view of the multilocular cystic architecture of a type I pleuropulmonary blastoma. Expanded airspaces are separated by septa of variable thickness. **B** Medium-power view showing intersecting septa lined by bronchiolar epithelium. Small areas of subepithelial mesenchyme in the cyst wall at the bottom of the picture (higher power featured in panel C). **C** High-power view of a cyst wall shows focal subepithelial collections of primitive cells in a pale-blue matrix. This portion of the cyst is lined by cuboidal alveolar type II pneumocytes.

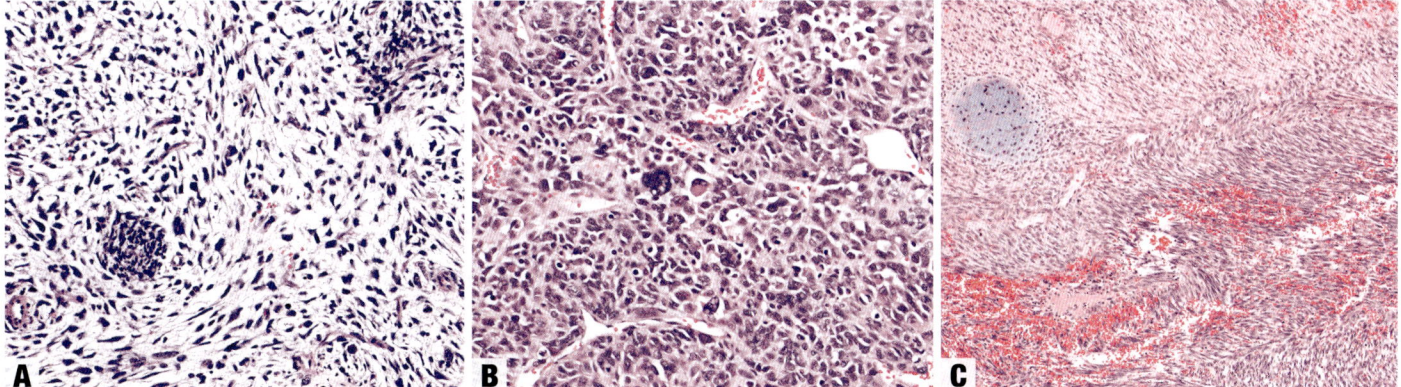

Fig. 1.164 Solid pleuropulmonary blastoma. **A** Solid sarcomatous portions of type II and III pleuropulmonary blastomas commonly have spindled, ovoid, and stellate cells in a pale-blue matrix, resembling embryonal rhabdomyosarcoma. These areas are often associated with more tightly packed blastemal nests of cells with hyperchromatic nuclei and high N:C ratio. A small round blastemal nest is seen in the lower-left portion of this photomicrograph. **B** High-grade malignant cells with hyperchromatic and enlarged nuclei are common in solid portions of type II and III pleuropulmonary blastomas. Regions of anaplasia seen here are associated with *TP53* mutations. **C** Spindle cell sarcoma and malignant cartilage are two other patterns seen in solid portions of type II and III pleuropulmonary blastomas.

no known ethnic or geographical differences in the incidence of PPB. Using the more conservative estimate, there are probably > 38 000 individuals in the USA and > 765 000 individuals worldwide with *DICER1* pathogenic variation. Thyroid neoplasia and lung cysts appear to be the most common phenotype for these individuals {1427,2862}. In addition to individuals with pathogenic germline variation, approximately 16% of children with PPB develop these cancers in the absence of identifiable genetic predisposition, through biallelic tumour-specific *DICER1* mutations {312}.

Etiology

PPB was first recognized as a distinct clinicopathological entity in 1988 {1784}, and the International Pleuropulmonary Blastoma Registry (https://www.ppbregistry.org/) was subsequently created to register and study cases. One of the early observations in children with PPB was that disease could be multifocal, could run in families, and co-occurred with other uncommon conditions, such as cystic nephroma, embryonal rhabdomyosarcoma, and Sertoli–Leydig cell tumour {2387}. A linkage study performed on families with multiple affected individuals led to identification of germline mutations in *DICER1* (MIM number: 606241) as the major genetic factor in this predisposition, now known as *DICER1* syndrome {1146}. *DICER1* encodes a key enzyme that is required to cleave precursor microRNAs into their mature, active form. MicroRNAs modulate gene expression and are critical in organ formation in the embryo and in prevention of cancer {218}. *DICER1* syndrome thus became the first familial cancer predisposition linked to a systemic defect in microRNA biogenesis. This gene discovery has led to imaging-based surveillance of children/families that carry pathogenic *DICER1* variation {174}.

Pathogenesis

PPB is analogous to other organ-based tumours of childhood, such as Wilms tumour, neuroblastoma, and hepatoblastoma. The malignant component of PPB derives from immature lung mesenchyme, which has the capacity to differentiate into multiple sarcomatous lineages, including rhabdomyosarcoma, fibrosarcoma, and chondrosarcoma.

Germline pathogenic *DICER1* variants that define the syndrome are always loss-of-function variants, mostly nonsense or frameshift mutations that truncate the *DICER1* coding sequence {1146,312}. Like other tumour suppressor genes, germline allelic loss-of-function mutations in *DICER1* create tumour susceptibility but appear to be insufficient to initiate tumorigenesis. In addition to the germline allelic loss of function, virtually all PPBs acquire a pathogenic *DICER1* missense variant in the second *DICER1* allele, affecting one of five codons: E1705, D1709, G1809, D1810, or E1813 in the RNase IIIb domain of the DICER1 protein {1125,2698,2394}. Amino acid substitutions at any one of these five positions can disable the RNase IIIb catalytic domain and prevent an entire class of microRNAs (those from the 5p arm of the precursor hairpin) from being produced {2394}. Among the 5p microRNAs absent in PPB is the let-7 family, which modulates expression of oncofetal gene networks during early development. In addition to this unique combination of biallelic loss of function plus hotspot mutations in *DICER1*, mutations and/or loss in *TP53* are also very common {2394,2698}.

Macroscopic appearance

There are three main pathological types of PPB, defined by their macroscopic appearance {1784,2386}. Type I PPB is completely cystic in nature. Grossly, the cysts are air-filled and multilocular, with thin, delicate septa. About 40% of type I tumours are multifocal. Type II tumours also have a cystic component but in addition have grossly visible thickening of the septa or formation of a solid mass. Type III PPB is purely solid.

Histopathology
Pathology of type I PPB

Microscopically, type I PPB has a characteristic architecture of expanded airspaces and wider-than-normal alveolar septa lined by alveolar or bronchiolar-type epithelium {1147}. In classic cases, small nodules of primitive mesenchymal cells are found beneath the epithelium in the cyst wall. These cells may be localized to a single focus or several foci or can be arranged more diffusely in layers beneath the epithelium, as seen in botryoid-type embryonal rhabdomyosarcoma. The primitive small

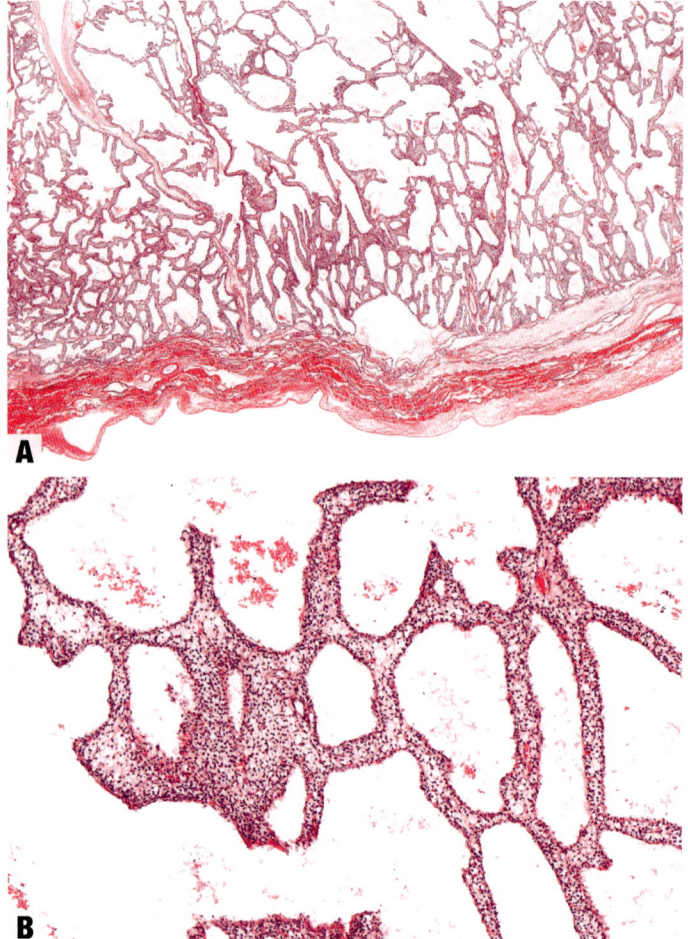

Fig. 1.165 Fetal lung interstitial tumour. **A** A localized mass shows spongiform alveoli-like structures resembling lung of 20–24 weeks' gestation. Note the thick capsule. **B** Interstitial cells are monotonous and uniformly distributed, with the walls covered by native epithelium.

cells may display cytoplasmic tails of pink cytoplasm with striations (rhabdomyosarcomatous differentiation), which is more prominent in the layers most distant from the epithelium. Small nodules of immature cartilage or mature spindle cells may also be found in the septa and are not necessarily accompanied by the small primitive cells. Because the small primitive cells or nodules of cartilage are present only focally in some cases, it may be necessary to submit an entire cyst specimen for microscopic examination.

Pathology of type Ir PPB

In the course of the family linkage study, it became apparent that there were relatives of children with PPB who had lung cysts for years, sometimes decades, without malignant transformation. Some of these cysts from older relatives had been resected and were available for microscopic examination {1147}. These purely cystic lesions show the architecture of type I PPB but lack primitive mesenchymal elements. These cysts were termed "type I regressed", although it is not known whether these lesions ever contained a primitive mesenchymal component. Given the lack of a primitive mesenchymal component, it is thought that the biological potential of type Ir PPB is limited. Differentiating type Ir PPB from blebs or postinfectious cysts can be difficult.

Pathology of type II and III PPBs

Type II PPBs differ from type I tumours in that the primitive tumour cells are no longer limited to a subepithelial distribution and expand the septa to form solid sarcomatous nodules {1147}. Type III tumours represent complete overgrowth of the cystic portions of the tumour and are purely solid. Microscopically, the solid portions of a type II PPB and type III PPB show a multipatterned sarcoma that typically includes areas with (1) solid, cohesive nests of undifferentiated cells with nuclear hyperchromatism and high N:C ratios (blastemal pattern); (2) spindle-shaped, stellate, and ovoid cells with variable amounts of eosinophilic cytoplasm in a pale-blue, myxoid matrix (embryonal rhabdomyosarcoma pattern); (3) compact arrangements of spindle cells with hyperchromatic nuclei in fascicular or herringbone pattern (spindle cell or fibrosarcoma pattern); and/or (4) cartilage, often with immature or overtly chondrosarcomatous features. One or more of these elements may predominate in any one tumour. Anaplasia, defined as in Wilms tumour, occurs in 75% of type II and 90% of type III tumours.

Differential diagnosis

Chest wall or mediastinal rhabdomyosarcoma can be challenging to distinguish from PPB. Limited core biopsies of PPB may show a rhabdomyosarcomatous pattern. Attention to the primary location of the mass in the chest wall, diaphragm, or mediastinum rather than lung parenchyma may help to determine the correct diagnosis, because the lung parenchyma is a rare site for a primary embryonal rhabdomyosarcoma. *DICER1* mutation testing of tumour tissue can also be used to confirm a diagnosis of PPB. Almost all PPBs in infancy are purely cystic. Nevertheless, spongy tumours such as the fetal lung interstitial tumour {713} and solid tumours such as the congenital peribronchial myofibroblastic tumour, which occur in infants, may present a diagnostic challenge. One of the more common diagnostic dilemmas occurs when a cystic mass is encountered with a subepithelial spindle cell component in an adolescent. It is uncommon for PPBs with a primitive cell component to occur in adolescence or adulthood. The primary differential diagnosis for this situation is with cystic synovial sarcoma. PPBs are typically more heterogeneous than synovial sarcomas, but the spindle cell components of PPB and synovial sarcoma can be remarkably similar. Immunohistochemistry demonstrating epithelial markers or identification of a fusion protein involving the gene product SS18 (SYT) is helpful for making a diagnosis of synovial sarcoma.

Cytology

FNA has been used to diagnose PPBs, typically showing primitive malignant mesenchymal and small ovoid blastemal elements {2750}. Pleural effusion cytology is rarely helpful in making a diagnosis, because tumour cells are rarely shed except in cases of tumour rupture {2109}.

Diagnostic molecular pathology

Identification of pathogenic loss of function and RNase IIIb missense *DICER1* variation in tumour tissue is diagnostic of PPB. In older children with cystic sarcomatous masses, RT-PCR or FISH for synovial sarcoma gene fusions may also be helpful to rule out PPB.

Essential and desirable diagnostic criteria

Essential – purely cystic tumours:
- Young age (usually < 1 year)
- Identification of a subepithelial collection of primitive cells or a nodule of cartilage in a multilocular cyst that has been adequately sampled
- For those that lack a primitive cellular component, the type Ir tumour, the diagnosis may remain challenging

Essential – cystic and solid / solid lung mass:
- Young age
- Primitive sarcoma with multiple patterns, including rhabdomyosarcoma, cartilage, blastema, and anaplasia

Desirable:
- Evidence of germline *DICER1* mutation

Staging

There is no formal staging system for PPB. For patients with type II or type III disease, both head MRI and bone scan are recommended to evaluate for metastatic disease; plain radiographs can be used for areas of concern seen on bone scan. Echocardiography may be necessary to define intracardiac extension of tumour, tumour thrombi, or pericardial effusion.

Prognosis and prediction

Pathological type is the only independent prognostic factor currently known. Survival rates decrease as PPB type progresses. Type I PPBs are limited to the lung and are treated with complete surgical resection with or without adjuvant chemotherapy. Type II and III tumours are treated with complete surgical excision whenever possible and high-dose sarcoma-based chemotherapy. Type II and III tumours can recur locally after incomplete or piecemeal excision. The most common metastatic site is the brain, to which as many as 40% of children with type III tumours experience brain metastasis. Tumours may also metastasize to bone, but tumour spread to other sites is rare {1898}. Radiation therapy is typically reserved for local recurrence and brain metastatic disease. For type I tumours, the survival rate is 91%. However, survival rates decrease to 74% for type II and 53% for type III tumours {1898}.

Pulmonary artery intimal sarcoma

Tavora F
Mahar AM
Yi ES

Definition

Pulmonary artery intimal sarcoma is a malignant mesenchymal tumour arising in the large vessels of the pulmonary circulation with predominantly intraluminal growth, obstruction of the lumen of the vessel of origin, and seeding of emboli to peripheral organs.

ICD-O coding

9137/3 Intimal sarcoma

ICD-11 coding

2C25.Y & XH36H7 Other specified malignant neoplasms of bronchus or lung & Intimal sarcoma

Related terminology

None

Subtype(s)

None

Localization

Pulmonary artery intimal sarcomas occur in the proximal elastic arteries, from the level of the pulmonary valve to the lobar branches. Most cases have bilateral involvement, although one side is usually dominant {2138,347}. Cardiac involvement occurs in some cases {2089,341}.

Clinical features

The most common presenting symptom is dyspnoea, followed by chest or back pain, cough, haemoptysis, weight loss, malaise, syncope, and fever. The clinical manifestations mimic those of acute or chronic thromboembolism and pulmonary

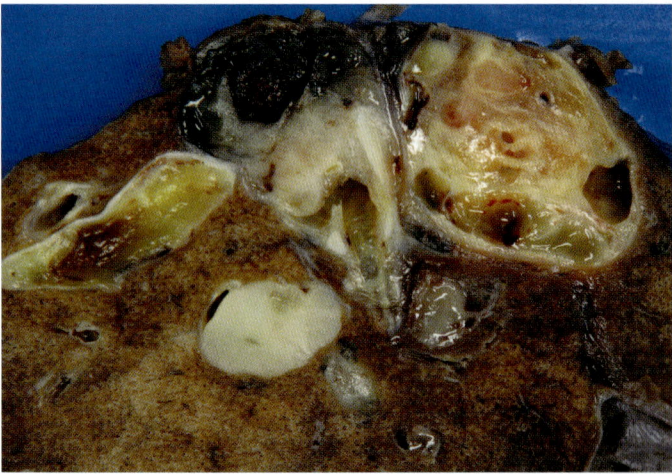

Fig. 1.166 Pulmonary artery intimal sarcoma. A large pulmonary artery is filled with tumour showing solid, gelatinous, and haemorrhagic areas.

hypertension, because of obstruction of the pulmonary circulation {2268}. Recurrent pulmonary embolic disease is the most common primary diagnosis, with diagnosis of malignancy often delayed or made after death.

Imaging

Imaging is largely nonspecific; however, the neoplastic nature of the tissue occluding the lumen can be suspected on CT, MRI, or PET {1437,2693,2222,3323}. Invasion into the surrounding lung parenchyma or mediastinal structures can be a diagnostic finding of intimal sarcoma {3000}. Also, a unilateral lesion within a pulmonary branch is more likely to be malignant, because chronic thromboemboli are usually multifocal {3309}.

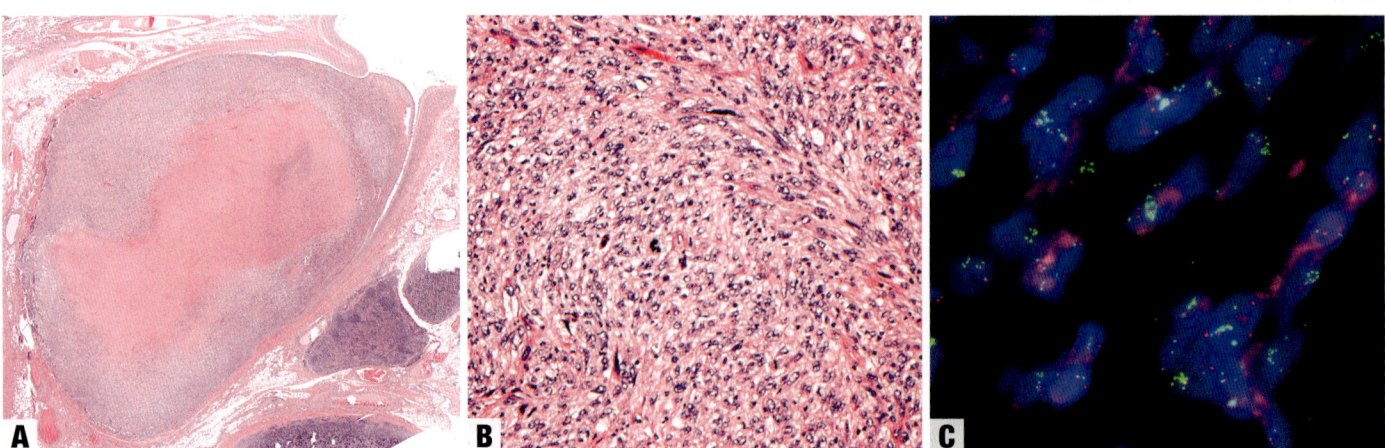

Fig. 1.167 Pulmonary artery intimal sarcoma. **A** Low-power photomicrograph of intimal sarcoma within lumen of a hilar pulmonary artery branch. Note central necrosis. **B** Features of an undifferentiated spindle cell sarcoma on high power, with brisk mitotic activity. **C** MDM2 FISH performed on intimal sarcoma demonstrating MDM2 amplification (green, MDM2 probe; red, CEN12 probe).

Epidemiology

Pulmonary artery intimal sarcomas are rare and occur at approximately twice the rate of aortic intimal sarcomas. They are slightly more common in females (M:F ratio: ~0.7:1) {2836}. The median age at diagnosis of intimal sarcoma of the pulmonary artery is 48 years {1437,347}. Pulmonary artery intimal sarcoma is present in 1–4% of pulmonary thromboendarterectomy specimens from patients thought to have chronic thromboembolic pulmonary hypertension.

Etiology

Unknown

Pathogenesis

Discovery of frequent amplifications and gains in the 12q13-q14 region (containing MDM2 and CDK4) and amplification of PDGFRA and KIT (at 14q12), as detected by a range of molecular techniques including comparative genomic hybridization, array comparative genomic hybridization, FISH, and quantitative PCR, suggests that the MDM2 and PDGFR pathways may play a role in the pathogenesis of intimal sarcoma {248,2551,690, 3139}. Amplification/polysomy of EGFR has also been reported {2979}.

In a series of cardiac sarcomas, intimal sarcoma was identified as the most frequent subtype, mainly on the basis of MDM2 amplification using FISH, PCR, and array comparative genomic hybridization {2089}.

Macroscopic appearance

Intimal sarcomas are polypoid intraluminal masses attached to the wall and can resemble mucoid or gelatinous clots filling vascular lumina. Distal extension may show smooth tapering of the mass {3000,2834}. Solid, fleshy tumour that completely occludes the vascular lumen is common in high-grade tumours, along with areas of haemorrhage and necrosis {2692}.

Histopathology

Intimal sarcomas are mesenchymal neoplasms composed of spindle cells with varying degrees of atypia and variable cellularity. Higher-grade components show a high mitotic count, necrosis, and nuclear pleomorphism. Epithelioid morphology may be seen {2692}. Lower-grade components are less cellular and can show myxoid change {983}. A small proportion of cases show heterologous elements in the form of osteosarcoma or chondrosarcoma. Rare tumours contain rhabdomyosarcomatous or angiosarcomatous features {347,983,1185,2138}. Variable positivity for SMA is found, and some tumours exhibit positivity for desmin. Overall, the diagnosis does not require immunohistochemistry, but nuclear expression of MDM2 can be observed in ≥ 70% of cases and may be a defining feature {248,690}.

Cytology

FNA specimens of intraluminal sarcomas contain pleomorphic malignant spindled cells arranged in loosely cohesive clusters. Cell block material may be used for immunohistochemistry, FISH, or other ancillary techniques {1069}.

Diagnostic molecular pathology

MDM2 amplification has been observed in most pulmonary artery intimal sarcomas, along with immunohistochemical overexpression of the protein product, often coexisting with amplification of PDGFRA {248,2551,3139,341,1315}.

Essential and desirable diagnostic criteria

Essential:
- Presentation in the lumen of a large vessel of the pulmonary circulation
- Primary high-grade sarcoma, with or without heterologous elements

Desirable:
- MDM2 amplification (in selected cases)

Staging

Not clinically relevant

Prognosis and prediction

The prognosis of pulmonary artery sarcoma is generally poor, with a mean survival time of 1–3 years {248,347,2138,2320}. Rare intraluminal myofibroblastic tumours have a relatively good prognosis {3000}.

Congenital peribronchial myofibroblastic tumour

Hill DA
López-Terrada DH
Vargas SO

Definition

Congenital peribronchial myofibroblastic tumour is a solid fibroblastic/myofibroblastic tumour developing in utero or in infancy, composed of mitotically active but histologically bland myofibroblasts arranged in fascicles and resembling congenital mesoblastic nephroma / infantile fibrosarcoma.

ICD-O coding

8827/1 Congenital peribronchial myofibroblastic tumour

ICD-11 coding

2F00.Y & XH85R1 Other specified benign neoplasm of middle ear or respiratory system & Myofibroblastic tumour, peribronchial

Related terminology

Not recommended: bronchopulmonary fibrosarcoma; NTRK-rearranged mesenchymal tumour; congenital bronchopulmonary leiomyosarcoma.

Subtype(s)

None

Localization

Congenital peribronchial myofibroblastic tumour occurs in the lung, with peribronchovascular distribution.

Clinical features

The tumour may be evident on antenatal imaging, and it may be associated with hydrops fetalis. Other presentations range from fetal demise to respiratory distress in the newborn period to incidental radiological mass in an asymptomatic infant. Large size (> 50 mm) and unilateral involvement are typical.

Epidemiology

The tumour is extremely rare, reported only in case reports. There are no known predisposing factors or syndromic associations.

Etiology

Unknown

Pathogenesis

The resemblance to NTRK-rearranged mesenchymal tumour suggests the possibility of an NTRK or other kinase gene fusion. To date, 3 lung tumours called congenital peribronchial myofibroblastic tumours have been reported to harbour *ETV6-NTRK3* rearrangement {2845A}, but these tumours were not illustrated histologically, and the finding has not been confirmed in other histologically convincing cases {442B}. Of note, there is debate about whether such a finding should instead automatically classify this tumour as a primary pulmonary infantile fibrosarcoma {442B,2845A,1184A}. Although congenital peribronchial myofibroblastic tumour bears some morphological similarity to congenital *A2M-ALK*–fused tumours reported as fetal lung interstitial tumour {2192B} and inflammatory myofibroblastic tumour {2984A}, cartilage proliferation has not been described in these congenital *ALK*-fused mesenchymal tumours, and their relationship to peribronchial myofibroblastic tumour remains unknown at the moment.

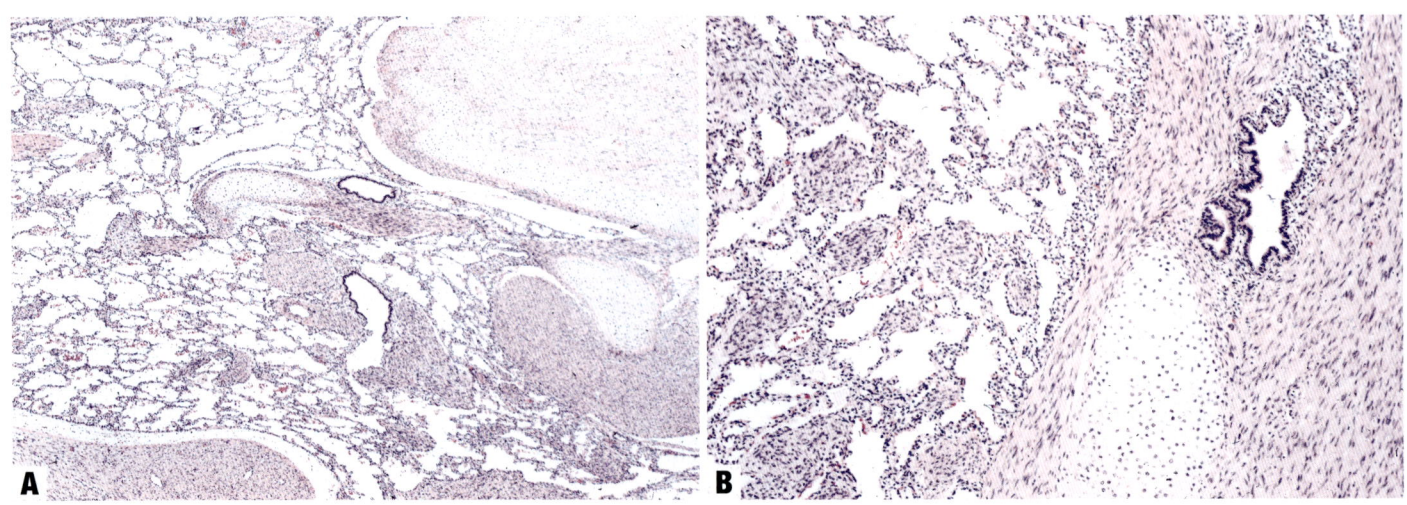

Fig. 1.168 Congenital peribronchial myofibroblastic tumour. **A** The lung shows nodular infiltrates of spindle cells around bronchial cartilage and epithelium. **B** The spindle-shaped tumour cells are cytologically bland and infiltrate around the bronchial epithelium and cartilage. There is also extension of tumour cells into the interstitium of surrounding alveolar walls.

Macroscopic appearance

The tumour is pale tan and firm, and it typically occupies a substantial portion of a lobe or lobes of fetal/infant lung; it surrounds large airways and may connect to the pleura.

Histopathology

The tumour is composed of interlacing fascicles of uniform spindle cells with eosinophilic cytoplasm and ill-defined cell borders. Nuclei are mitotically active but histologically bland; a rare atypical mitosis has been reported {64A,1212A,1860A,633A}. Growth mainly surrounds bronchi and extends along interlobular septa and the pleura; there is some extension into alveolar septa. Large islands of benign cartilage located mainly within peribronchial regions are characteristic. The spindle cells are generally positive for SMA; they may also be positive for desmin and S100. Congenital peribronchial myofibroblastic tumour lacks the epithelium-lined cysts and small islands of primitive cartilage that can be observed in the cyst walls of type I pleuropulmonary blastoma; it also lacks the subepithelial condensation of cells ("cambium layer"), areas of dense cellularity, myogenic differentiation, and anaplasia that can be observed in types II and III pleuropulmonary blastoma. The cells of congenital peribronchial myofibroblastic tumour lack the pulmonary interstitial glycogenosis–like appearance of the spindle cells in fetal lung interstitial tumour, which have small delicate nuclei and variably clear cytoplasm {713}.

Cytology

Not relevant

Diagnostic molecular pathology

No firm molecular diagnostic criteria are available, although demonstration of *ETV6-NTRK3* rearrangement may be helpful.

Essential and desirable diagnostic criteria

Essential:

- Interlacing fascicles of uniform histologically bland spindle cells that are mitotically active
- Peribronchial accentuation of growth
- Associated proliferation of benign-appearing bronchial cartilage

Staging

Not clinically relevant

Prognosis and prediction

The tumour is proposed to be benign due to a lack of documented recurrence; however, there are limited numbers of reported patients, and it is difficult to rule out the possibility of borderline malignant / rarely metastasizing behaviour as can be observed in soft tissue infantile fibrosarcoma, cellular mesoblastic nephroma of the kidney, and other NTRK-associated mesenchymal tumours.

Primary pulmonary myxoid sarcoma with *EWSR1-CREB1* fusion

Thway K
Yoshida A

Definition

Primary pulmonary myxoid sarcoma (PPMS) is a low-grade malignant tumour of the lung that consists of multinodular growth of typically uniform spindle, stellate, or rounded cells in a reticular pattern within a prominent myxoid stroma. Most cases harbour *EWSR1-CREB1* gene fusions.

ICD-O coding

8842/3 Pulmonary myxoid sarcoma with *EWSR1-CREB1* fusion

ICD-11 coding

2C25.Y & XH51Y9 Other specified malignant neoplasms of bronchus or lung & Pulmonary myxoid sarcoma with *EWSR1-CREB1* translocation

Related terminology

Acceptable: primary pulmonary myxoid sarcoma.
Not recommended: low-grade malignant myxoid endobronchial tumour.

Subtype(s)

None

Localization

PPMSs are frequently related to the bronchus and are often predominantly endobronchial.

Clinical features

Patients may present with cough, haemoptysis, systemic symptoms such as weight loss, or (more rarely) symptoms from metastases {3041}. The tumour may be detected incidentally {3041,1304,2098}. Imaging studies typically show a well-circumscribed mass, often with an endobronchial component. Obstructive changes may be present {3041}. Clinical and radiological correlation is needed to exclude a metastasis from an extrapulmonary site such as the soft tissue.

Epidemiology

The tumour often affects middle-aged adults, with a median age of 49 years (range: 26–80 years) and a slight female predominance {2388}.

Etiology

The causative role of smoking has not been established. No relationship is known with inherited cancer predisposition syndromes.

Pathogenesis

In more than 80% of cases, PPMS harbours *EWSR1-CREB1* fusion transcripts, in which *EWSR1* (exon 7) is fused to *CREB1* (exon 7 or uncommonly exon 8 or 5) {3041,1497}. Myxoid tumours with overlapping histology and *EWSR1*-CREB family gene fusions have been reported at various sites, including the CNS, soft tissues, pulmonary artery, and even the lung, using different terminologies (e.g. myxoid subtype of angiomatoid fibrous histiocytoma) {2650,1379,2200,3425,3042}. However, the exact nosological relationship between PPMS and these tumours is not clear, and there are distinct differences between them (e.g. the pronounced reticular morphology of PPMS and the consistent lack of desmin expression, unlike in myxoid angiomatoid fibrous histiocytoma). The subset of PPMSs that lack *EWSR1-CREB1* fusion has not been genetically characterized {3041,2793}.

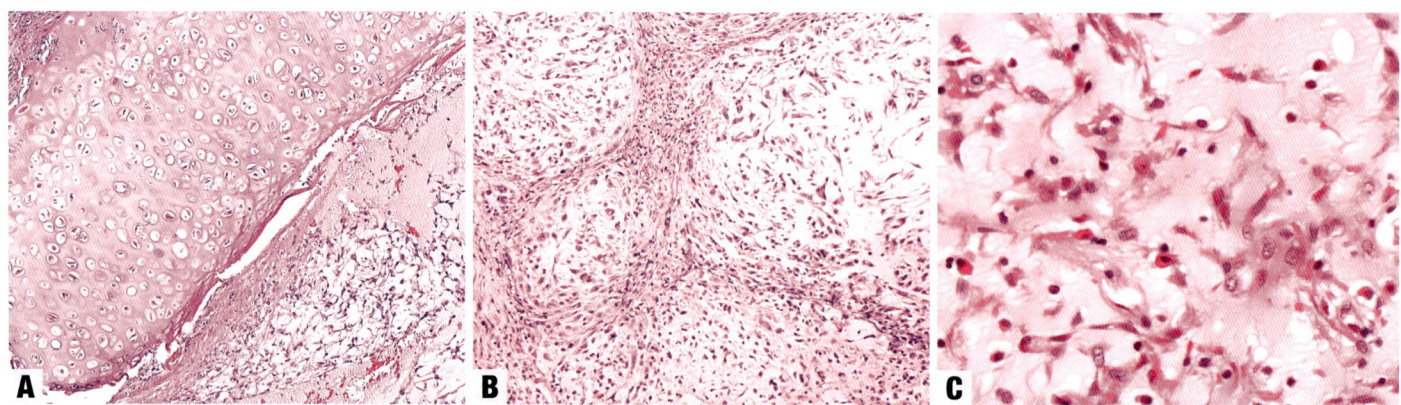

Fig. 1.169 Primary pulmonary myxoid sarcoma. **A** Myxoid tumour is seen to abut the bronchial cartilage. The reticulated distribution of tumour cells is appreciable. **B** The lobulated architecture is striking, with cords and strands of spindle and stellate cells dispersed in the prominent myxoid stroma. **C** At high magnification, the cells are typically bland and are most frequently spindled to stellate, with relatively small vesicular nuclei and fibrillary cytoplasm. They are dispersed as cords and strands within the abundant, lightly basophilic myxoid stroma.

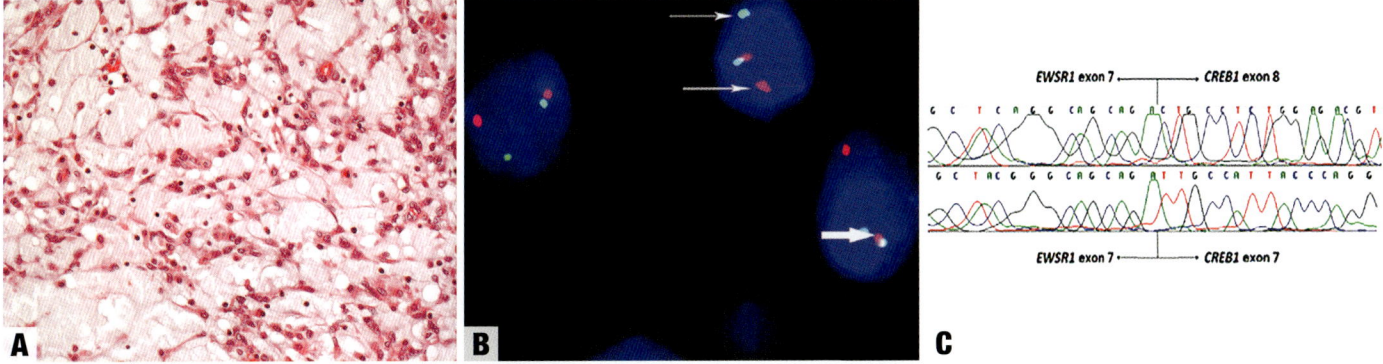

Fig. 1.170 Primary pulmonary myxoid sarcoma. **A** Spindle and rounded cells with typically bland nuclei show a lace-like or reticular architecture within sparsely cellular myxoid stroma, with a mixed chronic inflammatory infiltrate. **B** FISH shows split red and green signals (thin arrows) with *EWSR1* break-apart probes in tumour nuclei, consistent with the presence of rearrangements of this gene, contrasting with the fusion signal in a non-rearranged gene (thick arrow). **C** Direct sequencing confirms the presence of *EWSR1-CREB1* fusions, which predominantly involve exon 7 of each gene (lower diagram) or more rarely occur between exon 7 of *EWSR1* and exon 8 of *CREB1* (upper diagram).

Macroscopic appearance

The tumours measure 15 to > 100 mm and are well circumscribed or nodular, pale, and glistening or gelatinous on cut surface, ranging in colour from white/grey to yellow {3041}.

Histopathology

PPMSs have a lobulated architecture, often with an endobronchial location. A partial fibrous pseudocapsule may be present. Tumours are composed of spindle, round, stellate, or polygonal cells, with a predominant reticular network of delicate lace-like strands and cords within prominent myxoid stroma. The myxoid stroma is positive with Alcian blue, with staining sensitive to treatment with hyaluronidase {2098}. More compact areas may be found, which may have collagenous stroma. A minority have a predominantly compact architecture, with a more patternless distribution of cells. Cellular atypia is generally mild to sometimes focally moderate, and mitotic counts are < 5 mitoses/2 mm². Focal necrosis can be present. Most cases have a chronic inflammatory cell infiltrate of mainly lymphocytes and plasma cells. Vascular invasion is rare. Unusual histology has been reported in a small subset of cases lacking *EWSR1-CREB1*, including focal multinucleation, severe nuclear atypia, and high mitotic activity with atypical forms {3041,2793, 19A}. About 60% show typical weak and focal expression of EMA. The tumour is consistently negative for cytokeratin, S100, desmin, CD34, and neuroendocrine markers.

Cytology

Cytology is not relevant for diagnosis.

Diagnostic molecular pathology

The *EWSR1-CREB1* fusion is detectable by a variety of molecular methods and is helpful to confirm the diagnosis, although occasional tumours may harbour a different genetic alteration.

Essential and desirable diagnostic criteria

Essential:
- Primary involvement of the lung
- Spindle to round cells in a reticular pattern within prominent myxoid stroma
- Exclusion of other tumour types with similar histology, such as extraskeletal myxoid chondrosarcoma and myoepithelial tumours

Desirable:
- Presence of an endobronchial component
- Demonstration of *EWSR1-CREB1* fusion

Staging

No staging system is applicable.

Prognosis and prediction

PPMSs are treated with resection, and about 90% of patients remain free of disease. However, uncommon cases show metastatic spread {3041,1304} to the lung, kidney, or brain, and lethal cases have been rarely reported {3041,2388}.

Lymphangioleiomyomatosis of the lung

Jain D
Hornick JL

Definition

Pulmonary lymphangioleiomyomatosis (LAM) is a locally destructive mesenchymal neoplasm consisting of abnormal smooth muscle proliferation along lymphatic routes, producing a bilateral interstitial infiltrate that results in cystic transformation of airspaces and respiratory failure.

ICD-O coding

9174/3 Lymphangioleiomyomatosis

ICD-11 coding

CB07.Z Lymphangioleiomyomatosis, unspecified

Related terminology

None

Subtype(s)

None

Localization

LAM manifests as uniformly distributed cysts throughout the lungs. Retroperitoneal and abdominal lymph nodes may also be involved {1839A}.

Clinical features

Most affected patients experience progressive exertional dyspnoea and pneumothorax; chylous pleural effusions and haemoptysis are less common findings {1893,1322,1038}. Patients with LAM may have renal angiomyolipomas. Associated retroperitoneal lymphadenopathy is common {2581A}.

Imaging

Characteristic findings on high-resolution CT include diffuse, thin-walled, round lung cysts.

Epidemiology

LAM is rare, with an incidence of 5 cases per 1 million person-years {1858}. This disorder nearly exclusively affects adult women; men with tuberous sclerosis (TS) may also occasionally develop LAM {17}. LAM has a peak incidence among women of reproductive age.

Etiology

LAM may arise sporadically or in patients with TS.

Pathogenesis

Sporadic LAM characteristically harbours biallelic inactivating mutations in *TSC2* (less often *TSC1*), which result in activation of the mTOR signalling pathway {395,1249}. TS is an autosomal dominant disorder. Affected patients harbour germline (or somatic mosaic) mutations in *TSC1* or *TSC2*; a somatic mutation

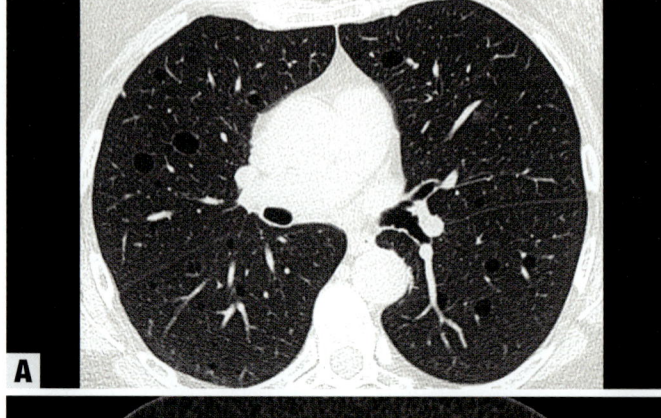
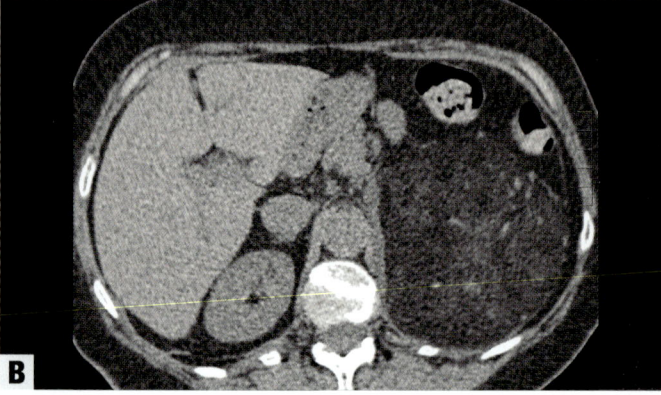

Fig. 1.171 Lymphangioleiomyomatosis. **A** Multiple thin-walled cysts in a 72-year-old woman. **B** A large incidental left adrenal angiomyolipoma in the same patient.

or loss of heterozygosity (second hit) precedes the development of LAM and other TS-associated tumours {3450,1124,1587}.

Macroscopic appearance

Thin-walled cysts are seen throughout the lungs.

Histopathology

The lung contains variably sized cysts. Within the cyst walls, there are nodules or a subtle interstitial distribution of spindle cells with fine chromatin, small nucleoli, and granular eosinophilic cytoplasm {1839}. The spindle cells may infiltrate the walls of veins. Interstitial or intra-alveolar haemosiderin-laden macrophages may be seen. LAM in TS patients may be associated with micronodular type II pneumocyte hyperplasia {1817,1512}.

By immunohistochemistry, the spindle cells are consistently positive for SMA and HMB45 {826}, although the extent of staining for HMB45 may be limited. ER, PR, and melan-A are also often positive, whereas S100 is negative.

Cytology

Not relevant

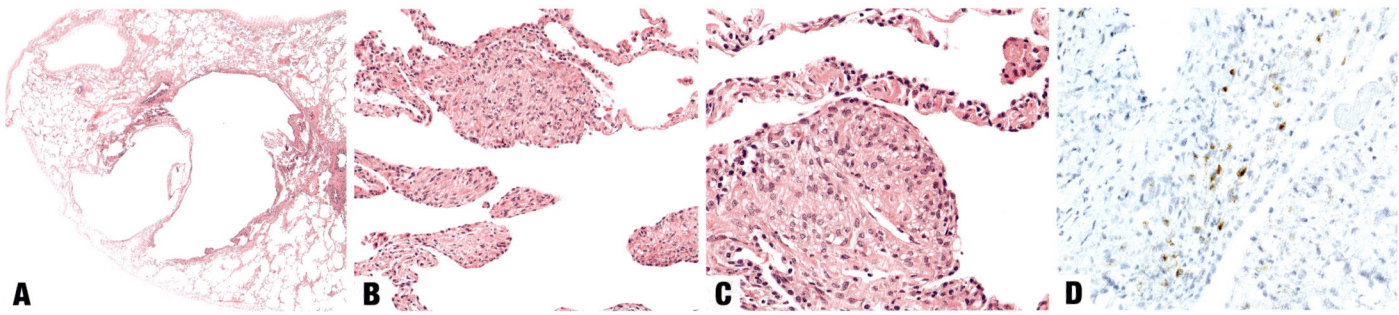

Fig. 1.172 Lymphangioleiomyomatosis. **A** The lung contains large cystic airspaces; within the walls of the cysts, there is a nodular and interstitial infiltrate of lesional cells. **B** The nodules within the cyst walls are composed of eosinophilic spindle cells undermining alveolar epithelium. **C** The lesional spindle cells contain granular eosinophilic to clear cytoplasm. The cells undermine the endothelial lining of a vein in the centre of this nodule. **D** Immunohistochemistry for HMB45 is characteristically positive in the cytoplasm of scattered cells.

Diagnostic molecular pathology
Not relevant

Essential and desirable diagnostic criteria
Most cases are diagnosed clinically without the need for biopsy, via the following:

Essential:
- Characteristic findings on high-resolution CT of uniform diffuse, thin-walled cysts, accompanied by any of the following clinical features: TS, renal angiomyolipoma, chylous pleural effusions, or cystic lymphangioleiomyoma {1858}
- When these clinical features are absent, elevated serum levels of VEGF-D {3436}

When biopsied
Essential:
- Lung cysts with nodules or bundles of cytologically bland myoid spindle cells with granular eosinophilic cytoplasm in the cyst walls

Desirable:
- Expression of SMA and HMB45

Staging
Not relevant

Prognosis and prediction
LAM typically progresses slowly, with increasing cystic destruction and declining lung function that often results in hypoxia requiring supplemental oxygen within 10 years of first symptoms; the 10-year survival rate without transplantation is 85% {2201}. The prognosis of patients with pulmonary LAM correlates with the extent of cysts and/or LAM smooth muscle cell infiltration in surgical lung biopsies {1839}. Patients may be treated by transplantation. The mTOR inhibitor sirolimus stabilizes lung function and results in decreased symptoms and improved quality of life in LAM patients {1859}.

PEComa of the lung

Jain D
Doyle LA

Definition
Perivascular epithelioid cell tumours (PEComas) are neoplasms with perivascular epithelioid-cell differentiation: mesenchymal tumours composed of distinctive cells that are often associated with blood vessel walls and usually express melanocytic and smooth muscle markers.

ICD-O coding
8714/0 PEComa, benign
8714/3 PEComa, malignant

ICD-11 coding
2F00.Y & XH4CC6 Other specified benign neoplasm of middle ear or respiratory system & Perivascular epithelioid tumour, benign
2C25.Y & XH9WD1 Other specified malignant neoplasms of bronchus or lung & Perivascular epithelioid tumour, malignant

Related terminology
Not recommended: sugar tumour; clear cell tumour.

Subtype(s)
PEComa (benign and malignant); PEComatosis

Localization
The tumours usually consist of a solitary, peripheral lung nodule.

Clinical features
Most primary lung PEComas are incidental findings in asymptomatic patients.

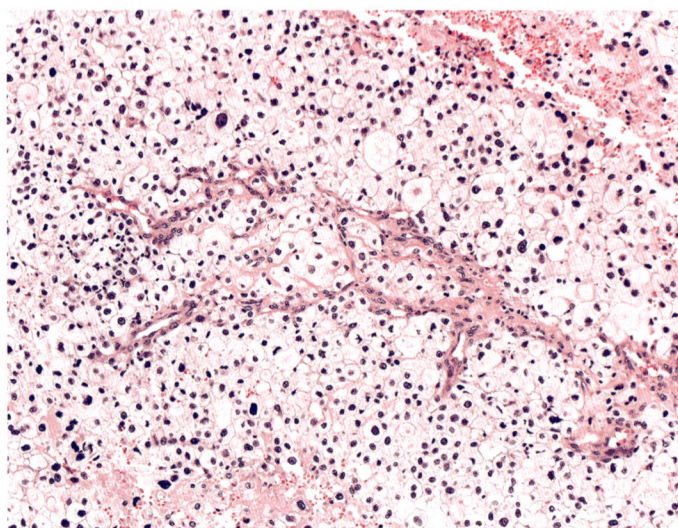

Fig. 1.173 Perivascular epithelioid cell tumour (PEComa). Sheets of epithelioid cells with abundant cytoplasm associated with a prominent thin-walled vascular network.

Epidemiology
The PEComa family includes lymphangioleiomyomatosis, angiomyolipoma, diffuse PEComatosis, and tumours of the lung called PEComas that resemble a group of histologically and immunophenotypically similar tumours arising at a variety of extrapulmonary soft tissue and visceral sites {269}. PEComatous lesions of the lung other than lymphangioleiomyomatosis, such as primary pulmonary PEComas and angiomyolipoma, are rare. Although PEComas are more frequent in females than males overall (M:F ratio: 1:6), primary lung PEComas show a male predilection. There is a wide age range, with a peak in young to middle-aged adults (mean age: 45 years) {849,728}.

Etiology
Most PEComas are sporadic; a small subset of cases are associated with tuberous sclerosis {268,849,728}.

Pathogenesis
Deletion of 16p, the location of the *TSC2* gene, indicates the oncogenetic relationship of PEComas with angiomyolipoma as a *TSC2*-linked neoplasm, and approximately 80% of PEComas show *TSC2* mutations and result in abnormal signalling through the mTOR pathway. *TP53* mutations have been identified in 63% of *TSC2*-mutated PEComas {25}.

A small subset of PEComas harbour *TFE3* gene fusions (and lack *TSC2* mutations / loss of heterozygosity) and show strong nuclear immunoreactivity for TFE3 {99,25,1779}. The most common fusion partner with *TFE3* is *SFPQ* (*PSF*) {25,2432,2984}. Other non-recurrent gene fusions reported include *HTR4-ST3GAL1* and *RASSF1-PDZRN3* {25}. This subtype is very rare in the lung.

Macroscopic appearance
Primary pulmonary PEComas are grossly well circumscribed, with a firm fleshy red-tan cut surface. Tumours usually measure 20–30 mm (range: 1–65 mm) {487,2347}.

Histopathology
PEComa of lung shows a nested or sheet-like architecture and is composed of uniform round/ovoid cells with abundant clear or granular eosinophilic cytoplasm and distinct cell borders. Within the lung, the growth pattern is often predominantly sheet-like. Thin-walled sinusoidal vessels are characteristic. The tumour cells typically show an association with blood vessel walls, with tumour cells arranged radially around thin-walled vessels and showing subendothelial growth, consistent with their perivascular nature. The nuclei are round, with small nucleoli, and usually show at most mild atypia or pleomorphism. Mitotic activity is usually absent or low {487,2347}.

Diffuse PEComatosis shows features overlapping between lymphangioleiomyomatosis and conventional PEComa {1607}. Angiomyolipoma, a member of the PEComa family of tumours, may rarely occur in the lung {1028} and is composed of admixed mature fat and thin and thick-walled blood vessels, along with abnormal spindle to epithelioid smooth muscle cells, similar to its renal counterpart.

Malignant PEComa is characterized by mitotic activity, marked atypia, pleomorphism, and necrosis {207,268,728,849, 431A}. The lung is a common site of metastasis for malignant PEComas of extrapulmonary sites. The presence of multiple nodules, marked atypia, and spindled morphology is suggestive of a metastatic rather than primary lung neoplasm.

Immunohistochemistry

PEComas show myomelanocytic differentiation and therefore typically express melanocytic markers, such as HMB45 (most sensitive), melan-A, and MITF, and muscle markers, such as SMA, desmin, and caldesmon {207,728,1180}. Some tumours lack expression of muscle markers. About 10% of tumours show focal expression of S100 {728}.

Differential diagnosis

PEComas may mimic several different tumour types, depending on their predominant cytomorphology (epithelioid or spindled) and the presence or absence of atypia. Within the lung, the most likely differential diagnostic considerations are metastases, including carcinoma (especially renal cell or hepatocellular), melanoma, alveolar soft part sarcoma, pure smooth muscle tumours, and myoepithelial tumours. The broad differential underscores the role of immunohistochemistry in confirming this diagnosis.

Cytology

There are cohesive clusters of epithelioid cells, with fine vessels sometimes transgressing cell clusters {2369}.

Diagnostic molecular pathology

Approximately 80% of PEComas show *TSC2* mutations, and a small subset show *TFE3* gene rearrangement.

Essential and desirable diagnostic criteria

Essential:
- Epithelioid cells with clear or granular cytoplasm, in sheets or nests, with expression of myoid or melanocytic markers

Desirable:
- Expression of both myoid and melanocytic markers
- *TSC2* mutation

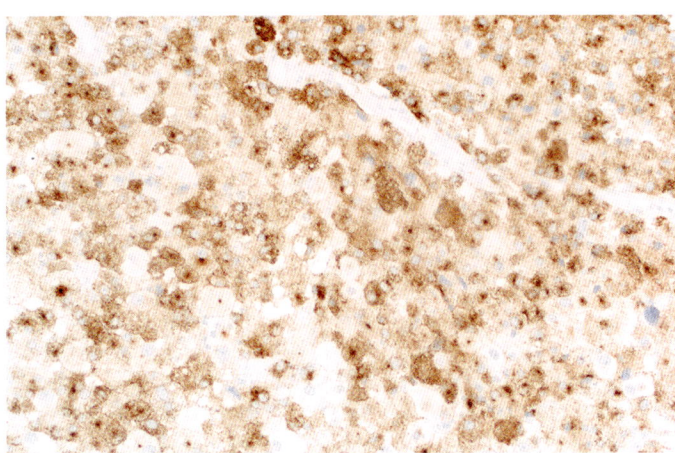

Fig. 1.174 Perivascular epithelioid cell tumour (PEComa). The tumour cells characteristically express a melanocytic marker such as HMB45.

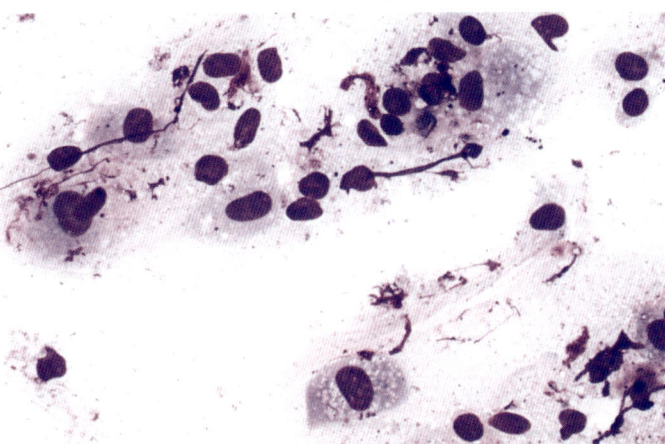

Fig. 1.175 Perivascular epithelioid cell tumour (PEComa). Cytology smears show large polygonal cells with clear and vacuolated cytoplasm (May–Grünwald–Giemsa).

Staging

There is no applicable Union for International Cancer Control (UICC) staging system for PEComa.

Prognosis and prediction

Virtually all primary PEComas of the lung are benign and cured by excision. Diffuse PEComatosis has also been successfully treated with sirolimus {1607}.

Haematolymphoid tumours of the lung: Introduction

Nicholson AG
Dogan A

The lung is commonly involved by haematolymphoid disorders, although primary involvement is rare, with the commonest being extranodal marginal zone lymphoma of mucosa-associated lymphoid tissue (MALT lymphoma) {280}. Secondary involvement by haematolymphoid disease is much more common, often in advanced stages of nodal or systemic disease, and this should always be considered in the differential diagnosis on encountering haematolymphoid diseases in lung tissue. Haematolymphoid neoplasms, in particular lymphomas, often present in hilar nodes, rather than in the parenchyma. Rarely, other primary nodal neoplasms such as follicular dendritic cell sarcoma {3174} can be seen.

Of the many haematolymphoid neoplasms that involve the lung (see Table 1.15), only six types are viewed as primary lung tumours. Although cases of intravascular lymphoma, lymphomatoid granulomatosis, Erdheim–Chester disease, and even Langerhans cell histiocytosis may be systemic, the consensus is that the extent and pattern of primary lung presentation warrants classification as a primary lung tumour. Erdheim–Chester disease and Langerhans cell histiocytosis, historically viewed as reactive entities, are now recognized as neoplasms caused by activating somatic mutations of the MAPK pathway {765,1926, 2228}. In B-cell lymphoproliferative diseases involving the lung, in particular MALT lymphoma and plasmacytoma, some cases may be accompanied by amyloid deposits, light chain deposition disease, or crystal-storing histiocytosis.

Additionally, posttransplant lymphoproliferative disorders may also occur in the lung, although they are not part of the WHO classification of thoracic tumours. Reactive lymphoid proliferations are much more common than primary pulmonary lymphoid neoplasms, and some, such as lymphoid interstitial pneumonia or IgG4-related disease, may mimic neoplastic processes (see Table 1.15). Therefore, diagnosis of haematolymphoid tumours is an area where multidisciplinary review is of particular value: for example, CT features of MALT lymphoma have particular characteristics that may aid in excluding non-MALT lymphomas {484} and reactive disorders such as lymphoid interstitial pneumonia {1460, 1072,2782}. Also, joint review by both thoracic and haematolymphoid pathologists may be of value, because both subspecialties can bring particular expertise to the diagnostic process.

Table 1.15 Classification of lymphoproliferative disease within the lung (types in bold are covered in detail)

Category	Types
Primary pulmonary neoplasms	**Extranodal marginal zone lymphoma of mucosa-associated lymphoid tissue (MALT lymphoma)**
	Diffuse large B-cell lymphoma[a]
	Lymphomatoid granulomatosis
	Classic Hodgkin lymphoma[a]
	Plasmacytoma
	Mast cell tumour
Secondary involvement of the lung	**Intravascular large B-cell lymphoma**
	Classic Hodgkin lymphoma and non-Hodgkin lymphomas
	Myeloid neoplasms (myeloid sarcoma, chronic myeloproliferative disorders)
	Primary mediastinal large B-cell lymphoma
Benign hyperplastic disorders	Reactive pulmonary lymphoid hyperplasia • Lymphoid interstitial pneumonia • Follicular bronchiolitis
	Nodular lymphoid hyperplasia
	Castleman disease, hyaline-vascular and plasma cell subtypes
	IgG4-related disease
Posttransplant lymphoproliferative disorders (PTLDs)	PTLD – early (plasmacytic hyperplasia, infectious mononucleosis–like)
	PTLD – polymorphic
	PTLD – monomorphic (classify according to lymphoma classification)
	Other types (rare; e.g. Hodgkin disease–like lesions, plasmacytoma-like lesion)
Histiocytic neoplasms	**Langerhans cell histiocytosis**
	Erdheim–Chester disease
	Rosai–Dorfman disease

[a]Primary presentations of diffuse large B-cell lymphoma and classic Hodgkin lymphoma of the lung parenchyma are extremely rare if EBV-positive B-cell lymphoproliferative disorders mimicking lymphoma and Hodgkin lymphoma, as well as involvement by primary mediastinal B-cell lymphoma / mediastinal classic Hodgkin lymphoma, are rigorously ruled out.

MALT lymphoma of the lung

Cook JR
Cooper WA
Inagaki H

Definition
Pulmonary extranodal marginal zone lymphoma of mucosa-associated lymphoid tissue (MALT lymphoma) is a low-grade primary extranodal lymphoma recapitulating the morphological features of mucosa-associated lymphoid tissue (MALT).

ICD-O coding
9699/3 MALT lymphoma

ICD-11 coding
2A85.3 & XH3FE9 Extranodal marginal zone B-cell lymphoma, primary site excluding stomach or skin & Mature B-cell lymphomas

Related terminology
Acceptable: bronchus-associated lymphoid tissue (BALT) lymphoma; BALToma; MALToma.
Not recommended: pseudolymphoma (obsolete).

Subtype(s)
None

Localization
There is no zonal or lobar predisposition in the lungs. Some cases extend to and involve the visceral pleura, while rare cases may be predominantly endobronchial {2106,1566,3418,2356}.

Clinical features
Patients may present asymptomatically with lesions identified incidentally on imaging studies. About 55–67% of patients show nonspecific respiratory symptoms such as cough, dyspnoea, or chest pain {2846,2619}. Systemic symptoms, such as fever and night sweats, are uncommon {2356}. Serum monoclonal proteins were reported in 43% of patients {1566}.

Imaging
Chest CT commonly shows one or more nodules or masses, which may be bilateral. Air bronchograms are common. Some patients may show ground-glass opacities or interstitial infiltrates, creating a differential diagnosis with pneumonia or interstitial lung disease {2846,1566,386}.

Epidemiology
MALT lymphomas represent 70–90% of all primary pulmonary lymphomas but < 0.5% of all primary lung neoplasms {2619, 2846,2356}. Patients are middle-aged to elderly, with a median age of 68 years at diagnosis. There is a slight female predominance.

Etiology
A specific infectious agent, analogous to *Helicobacter pylori* in gastric MALT lymphoma, has not been identified in pulmonary

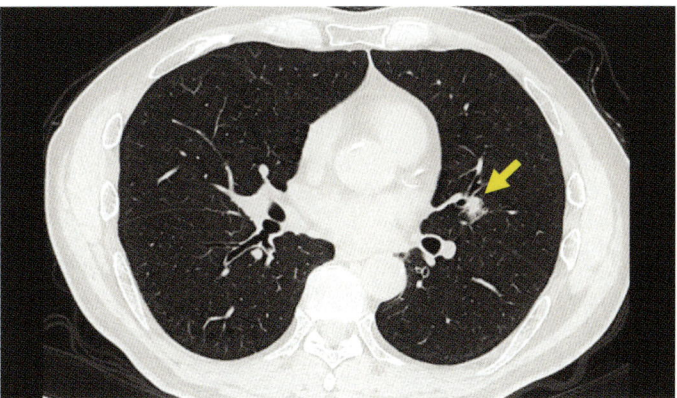

Fig. 1.176 Extranodal marginal zone lymphoma of mucosa-associated lymphoid tissue (MALT lymphoma) of the lung. CT shows an irregularly shaped nodule with marginal ground-glass opacity (arrow).

MALT lymphomas. Underlying autoimmune disorders, especially Sjögren syndrome, have been reported in 10–29% of cases {2356,1566,2846,2619}.

Pathogenesis
MALT is not present in normal lung parenchyma but is acquired in reactive conditions including smoking, infection, and autoimmune disorders. Extranodal MALT lymphomas are thought to arise after long-term antigenic stimulation in the setting of chronic lymphoid hyperplasia. Multiple genetic subsets have been identified, including one group associated with *MALT1* translocations (25–45% of cases) and activation of the NF-κB pathway, and another group associated with increased plasma cells and a plasmacytic gene expression pattern {2176,508, 2466,3349}.

Macroscopic appearance
Grossly, pulmonary MALT lymphomas are consolidated masses with a cut surface that is yellow to cream-coloured.

Histopathology
The lymphomatous infiltrate is heterogeneous, with varying proportions of small lymphocytes, centrocyte-like cells, monocytoid B cells, occasional large transformed cells, and plasma cells {1566,2106,192}. The infiltrate surrounds and, in some cases, colonizes reactive germinal centres. At the periphery of the lesion, the neoplastic cells track bronchovascular bundles, but the centre of the lesion often shows alveolar destruction {2356}. Lymphoepithelial lesions are common. Airways are frequently spared, correlating with the air bronchograms observed on imaging studies. Necrosis is rare and its presence should raise concern for transformation to diffuse large B-cell lymphoma. Amyloidosis, light chain deposition disease, and/or crystal-storing histiocytosis may coexist with MALT lymphoma.

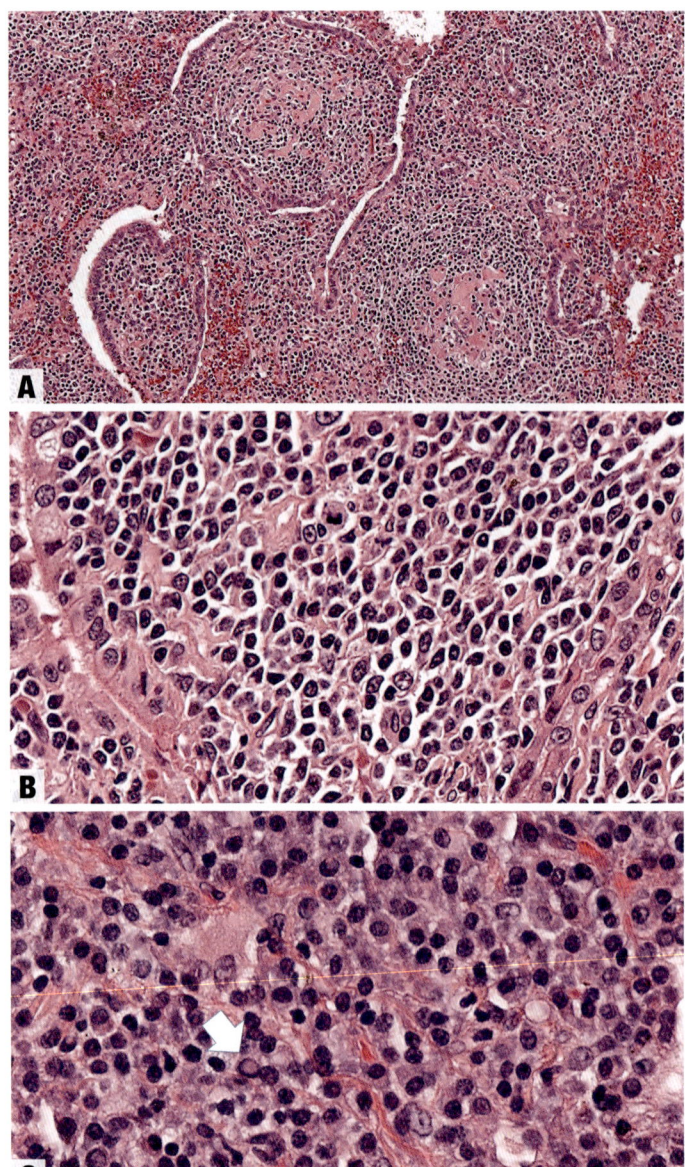

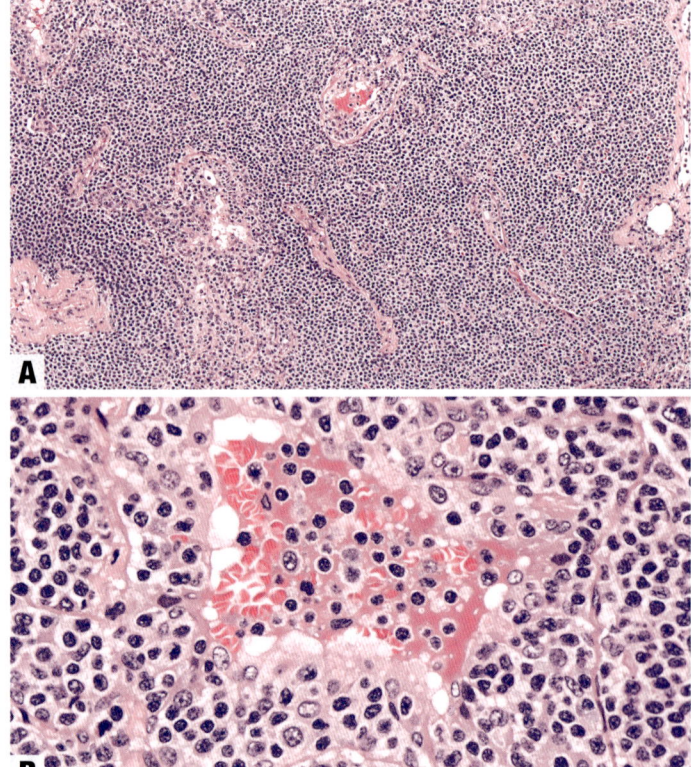

Fig. 1.178 Pulmonary extranodal marginal zone lymphoma of mucosa-associated lymphoid tissue (MALT lymphoma). **A** The lung shows a diffuse and dense infiltrate of small lymphoid cells, which also infiltrate the bronchial and bronchiolar epithelium to form lymphoepithelial lesions. **B** The lymphoid cells are centrocyte-like or monocytoid B cell–like. They show prominent infiltration of the bronchiolar epithelium.

Fig. 1.177 Extranodal marginal zone lymphoma of mucosa-associated lymphoid tissue (MALT lymphoma). **A** The infiltrate shows a nodular appearance, with infiltration of germinal centres by the neoplastic cells. **B** The neoplastic infiltrate includes small lymphocytes, centrocyte-like cells, and rare large cells. **C** This case shows prominent plasmacytic differentiation, with numerous plasma cells and an occasional Dutcher body (arrow).

Immunohistochemistry

The neoplastic B cells express CD20 and CD79a. Flow cytometric studies may show monotypic B cells, although these may in some cases be masked by benign germinal centre cells or other background polytypic B cells. The B cells are negative for CD10, BCL6, and other germinal centre markers. Aberrant CD43 expression has been reported in 30–80% of cases {2356}. Rare cases may express CD5 {1295,3016}. Follicular dendritic cell markers (CD21, CD35) highlight dendritic cell meshworks, which may be disrupted and colonized by the neoplastic cells. The Ki-67 index is typically low (< 20%). Kappa and lambda stains reveal clonal plasma cells or plasmacytoid

cells in a subset of cases {2106,1566,2356}. Keratin stains may be useful to identify lymphoepithelial lesions.

Differential diagnosis

Pulmonary MALT lymphoma must be distinguished from reactive lymphoid proliferations, including nodular lymphoid hyperplasia and lymphocytic interstitial pneumonia. The presence of aberrant CD43 expression on B cells or plasma cells with light chain restriction may be helpful, although each of these findings is present in only a subset of cases. Flow cytometric studies or molecular clonality testing may be helpful to demonstrate the presence of a clonal B-cell population. Other small B-cell neoplasms that may mimic marginal zone lymphoma must also be excluded, using a thorough panel of immunophenotypic markers.

Cytology

FNA smears or bronchoalveolar lavage samples are generally inadequate to establish a definitive diagnosis. Flow cytometry or PCR studies may demonstrate a clonal B-cell population {279,1487}, but distinguishing MALT lymphoma from other small B-cell neoplasms typically requires at least a core biopsy. In cytological preparations, pulmonary MALT lymphomas typically show a heterogeneous mix of small lymphocytes, centrocyte-like cells, plasmacytoid cells, and/or plasma cells {1487}.

Diagnostic molecular pathology

Detection of clonal IG gene arrangements and/or *MALT1*-associated translocations is useful for diagnosis in problematic cases {2466,3349,2176}.

Essential and desirable diagnostic criteria

Essential:

- Destructive infiltrate of small lymphocytes, centrocyte-like cells, monocytoid cells, and/or plasmacytic cells
- B-cell phenotype
- Exclusion of other small B-cell neoplasms

Desirable:

- Neoplastic B cells surround and/or colonize germinal centres
- Lymphoepithelial lesions
- Demonstration of a monoclonal B-cell population

Staging

The American Joint Committee on Cancer (AJCC) staging manual (eighth edition) has adopted the Lugano modification of the Ann Arbor system for the staging of non-Hodgkin lymphomas {75,492}.

Prognosis and prediction

Patients with low-stage disease have achieved prolonged remission with localized therapy, usually surgical resection

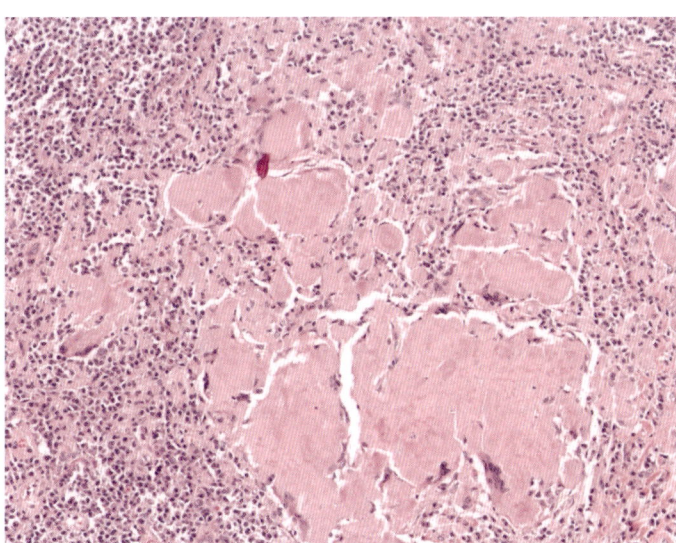

Fig. 1.179 Extranodal marginal zone lymphoma of mucosa-associated lymphoid tissue (MALT lymphoma). Amyloid deposition is present in this MALT lymphoma.

{822,2846,2619}. The 5-year and 10-year overall survival rates are reported at 68–90% and 53–72%, respectively {281,822}. Overall survival is not significantly different between patients presenting at different stages {2846}.

Pulmonary diffuse large B-cell lymphoma

Quintanilla-Martinez L
Guinee DG
Nicholson AG
Takeuchi K

Definition

Primary pulmonary diffuse large B-cell lymphoma (DLBCL) is a non-Hodgkin lymphoma composed of a diffuse proliferation of large B cells with centroblastic or immunoblastic morphology, confined to the lung with or without hilar lymph node involvement at presentation or during the subsequent 3 months.

ICD-O coding

9680/3 Diffuse large B-cell lymphoma, NOS

ICD-11 coding

2A81.Z Diffuse large B-cell lymphoma, NOS

Related terminology

Acceptable: diffuse large B-cell non-Hodgkin lymphoma.
Not recommended: high-grade mucosa-associated lymphoid tissue lymphoma.

Subtype(s)

Diffuse large B-cell lymphoma NOS; EBV-positive diffuse large B-cell lymphoma NOS

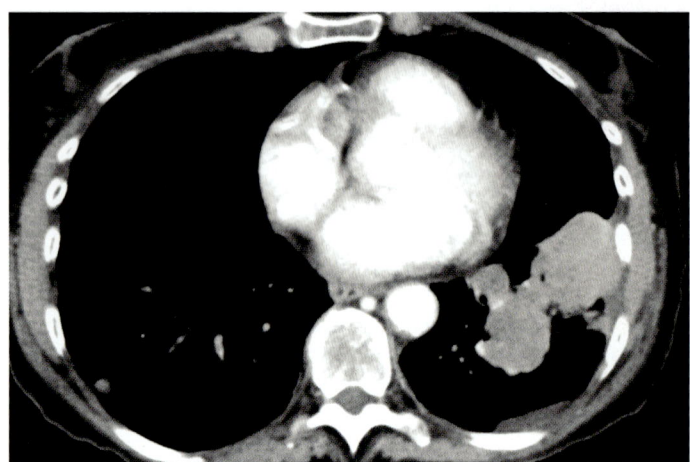

Fig. 1.180 Diffuse large B-cell lymphoma of lung. Chest CT shows a large peripheral mass in the left lower lobe, with sharp borders separating it from the adjacent lung

Localization

Primary pulmonary DLBCL can involve any lobe but is characteristically located peripherally.

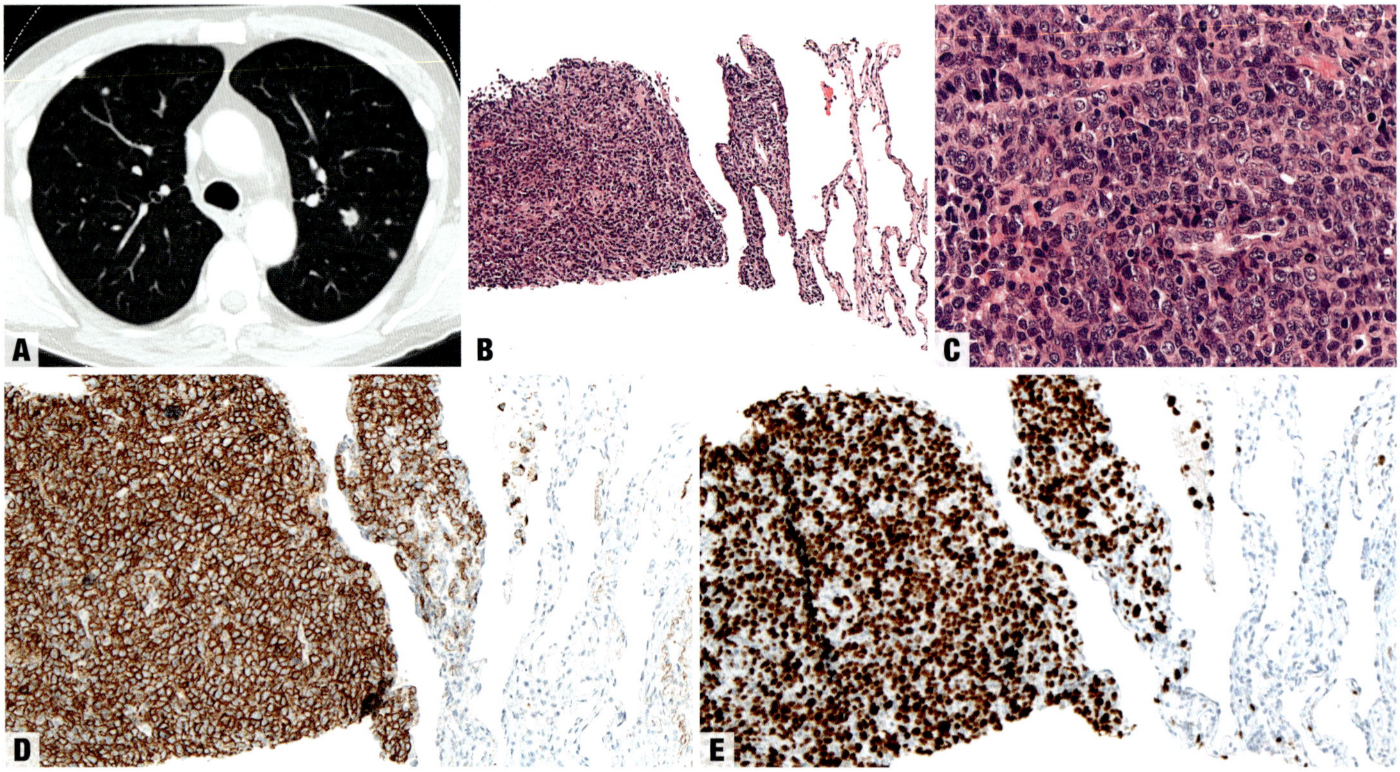

Fig. 1.181 Diffuse large B-cell lymphoma of lung. **A** Chest CT shows bilateral poorly defined nodules. **B** Percutaneous, CT-guided lung biopsy shows residual alveolar spaces and a diffuse infiltration of large lymphoid cells. **C** Diffuse sheets of large lymphoid cells resembling centroblasts. **D** CD20 stain demonstrates the B-cell origin of the lymphoid infiltrate. **E** MIB1 reveals a high proliferation rate of the tumour cells.

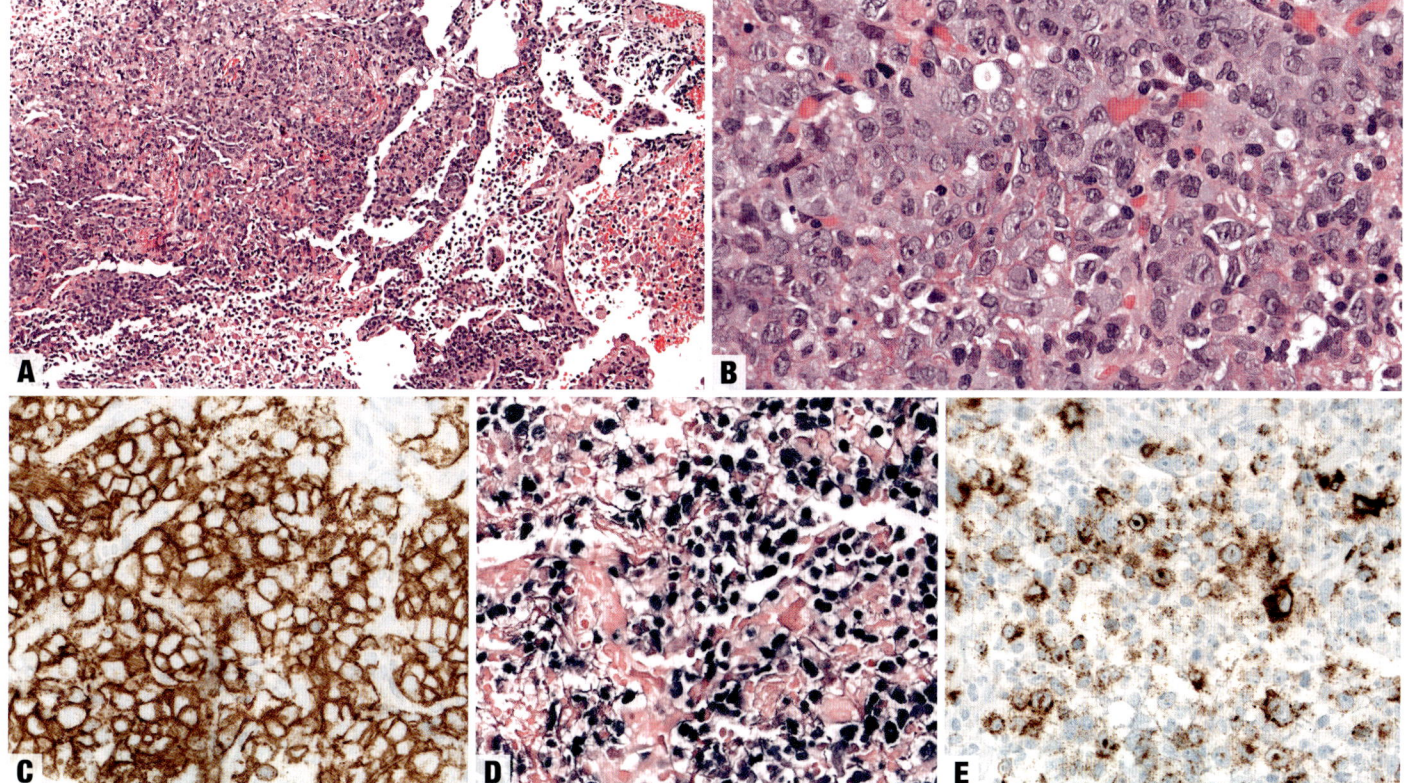

Fig. 1.182 EBV-positive diffuse large B-cell lymphoma NOS. **A** Percutaneous, CT-guided lung biopsy shows a diffuse infiltrate of large lymphoid cells with residual alveolar walls partially infiltrated. Note the tumour necrosis. **B** The infiltrate is characterized by large, pleomorphic lymphoid cells with prominent eosinophilic nucleoli resembling immunoblasts and Reed–Sternberg cells. **C** CD20 staining highlights the diffuse infiltration by neoplastic large B cells. **D** In situ hybridization for EBV-encoded small RNA (EBER) reveals that the majority of the large lymphoid cells are EBER-positive. **E** LMP1 stain is positive in many cells.

Clinical features

Patients are usually symptomatic and present with cough or dyspnoea, or rarely with haemoptysis and systemic B symptoms, which include fever, night sweats, and weight loss {2989, 2356,3313}.

Imaging

Chest CT examination shows consolidation and single or multiple well-defined nodules. CT findings in extranodal marginal zone lymphoma of mucosa-associated lymphoid tissue (MALT lymphoma) and DLBCL can overlap; however, cavitation and/or central necrosis are features more commonly seen in DLBCL {582,1480}. DLBCL can be limited to the lungs or can spread to the mediastinum and other extranodal sites.

Epidemiology

Primary pulmonary DLBCL, although rare, is the second most common type of primary pulmonary lymphoma, accounting for about 5–20% of cases {2107,1666,1446,2086}. The mean age of presentation is 60 years (range: 38–70 years). There is no sex predisposition.

Etiology

The etiology of pulmonary DLBCL is unknown. It occurs in both immunocompetent and immunocompromised patients; however, it occurs often in immunocompromised individuals with underlying inflammatory processes or chronic infections such as HIV infection. DLBCL arising in this setting is often EBV-positive

{2227,1697,2110,1171}. An association between DLBCL and systemic autoimmune disorders has also been described {2107}.

Pathogenesis

Roughly half represent de novo DLBCL, whereas the other half arise from transformation of an underlying MALT lymphoma {1666}.

Macroscopic appearance

Nodules are usually well-circumscribed, cream-coloured, and typically solid, but they may show areas of haemorrhage, central necrosis, and cavitation.

Histopathology

Endobronchial ultrasound–guided transbronchial needle aspiration and percutaneous CT-guided or bronchoscopic biopsy may be sufficient to make a diagnosis in a solid lesion; however, a surgical biopsy may be required {1011,906}. Morphologically, primary pulmonary DLBCL is similar to DLBCL in other sites. The tumour comprises diffuse sheets of large cells that destroy and replace the normal lung parenchyma. The large cells resemble centroblasts and/or immunoblasts and are 2–4 times the size of normal lymphocytes.

The immunophenotype is that of a B cell, with expression of pan–B cell markers (CD20, CD79a). There is variable staining for CD10, BCL6, IRF4 (MUM1), BCL2, and MYC, which is performed to aid in prognostication. Subclassification into germinal-centre B-cell and activated B-cell subtypes should be accomplished through the use of gene expression profiling or immunohistochemical algorithms {2690,1901}. The presence of EBV should be investigated using in situ hybridization for EBV-encoded small RNA (EBER).

The differential diagnoses include undifferentiated carcinoma, anaplastic large cell lymphoma, primary mediastinal large B-cell lymphoma, and rarely germ cell tumours. The most difficult differential diagnosis is between EBV-positive DLBCL-NOS and pulmonary lymphomatoid granulomatosis. The latter shows more reactive T cells, marked angiocentricity, and a greater variability in the number of EBV-positive cells {2813}.

Cytology

Smears show a monotonous population of large atypical cells with blastic chromatin, one or more nucleoli, and fairly abundant cytoplasm. Primary diagnosis of DLBCL in cytological preparations should be made with caution, always in conjunction with ancillary techniques such as immunohistochemistry, flow cytometry, and molecular testing.

Diagnostic molecular pathology

IG genes are clonally rearranged. Little is known about other genetic abnormalities in primary pulmonary DLBCL; however, a molecular classification for DLBCL, in general, has been proposed {456,2666}.

Essential and desirable diagnostic criteria

Essential:
- Large lymphoid cells (tumour cells 2–4 times the size of normal lymphocytes) resembling centroblasts or immunoblasts
- Diffuse infiltration with destruction of lung parenchyma
- Immunophenotyping to confirm B-cell lineage (e.g. CD20, PAX5, CD79a)

Desirable:
- Immunophenotype or gene expression profiling to determine germinal-centre B-cell or activated B-cell subtype
- EBER in situ hybridization and/or LMP1 stain

Staging

The stage of the disease is determined using the Lugano classification, a modification of the Ann Arbor staging system {492}.

Prognosis and prediction

Patients are usually treated with combined immunotherapy and chemotherapy. Surgical resection can be performed in cases with localized tumours. An enhanced International Prognostic Index (IPI) is widely applied as a prognostic guide {2697,3517}. DLBCL in extranodal sites generally has a poorer prognosis than nodal-based disease {405}.

Lymphomatoid granulomatosis of the lung

Pittaluga S
Nicholson AG

Definition

Lymphomatoid granulomatosis is characterized by an angiocentric/angiodestructive polymorphous lymphoid infiltrate composed of EBV-positive B cells admixed with a large number of reactive T cells.

ICD-O coding

9766/1 Lymphomatoid granulomatosis, NOS

ICD-11 coding

2A81.3 Lymphomatoid granulomatosis

Related terminology

Not recommended: angiocentric immunoproliferative lesion (obsolete).

Subtype(s)

None

Localization

Lymphomatoid granulomatosis involves the lung in all cases. Other sites include CNS (40%), skin (34%), kidney (19%), liver (17%), and other organs (e.g. adrenal gland) {2813,465,1397}. Lymph node and/or bone marrow involvement is rare {1522}.

Clinical features

Presenting symptoms are variable (i.e. cough, dyspnoea, and/or chest pain) and may be accompanied by constitutional symptoms. Only one third to two thirds of patients present with overt respiratory symptoms; the rest are identified incidentally by imaging. Other symptoms are related to the site of involvement, such as CNS or skin {1881}.

Imaging

Pulmonary imaging reveals multifocal bilateral nodules or masses, with predilection for the mid-lung to lower-lung fields; occasionally, there is only a solitary lung nodule {2813,465,1397}. Some lesions show evidence of necrosis with central cavitation. In rare instances, more infiltrative interstitial patterns and ground-glass opacities, mimicking interstitial lung disease, are seen {1881}.

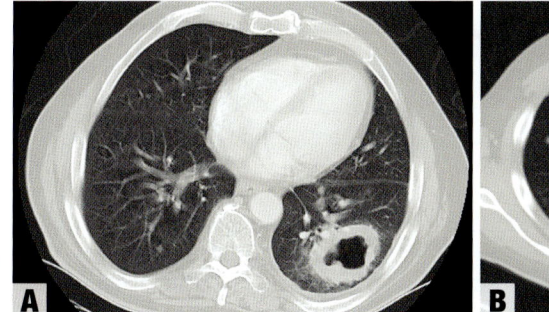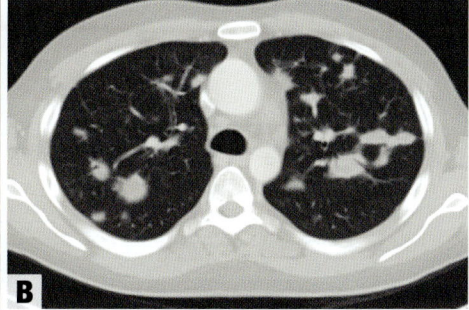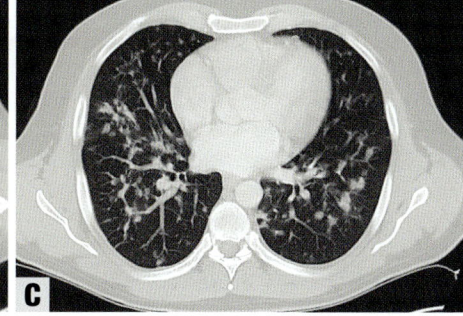

Fig. 1.183 Lymphomatoid granulomatosis. CT of chest shows a nodular cavitary lesion (**A**), multiple bilateral nodular masses affecting mid-lung and lower-lung fields (**B**), and an interstitial pattern of involvement (**C**).

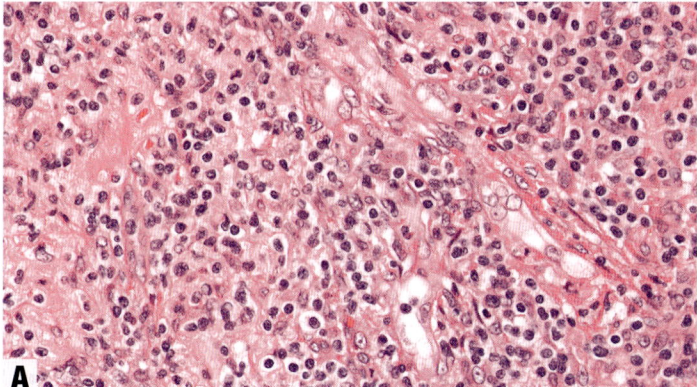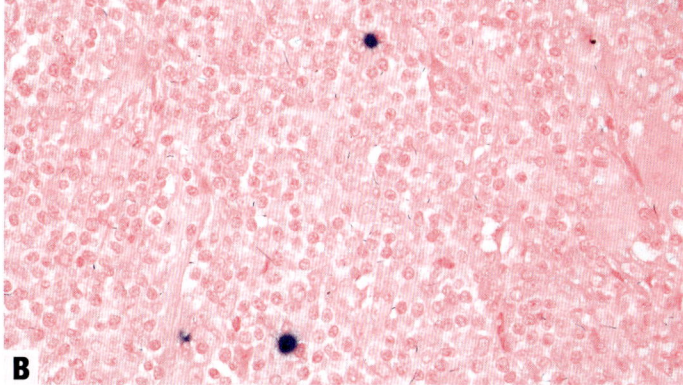

Fig. 1.184 Lymphomatoid granulomatosis, grade 1. **A** There is a polymorphous mixture of inflammatory cells, with large lymphoid cells being inconspicuous. **B** In situ hybridization for EBV-encoded small RNA (EBER) reveals only rare positive medium-sized to large lymphoid cells.

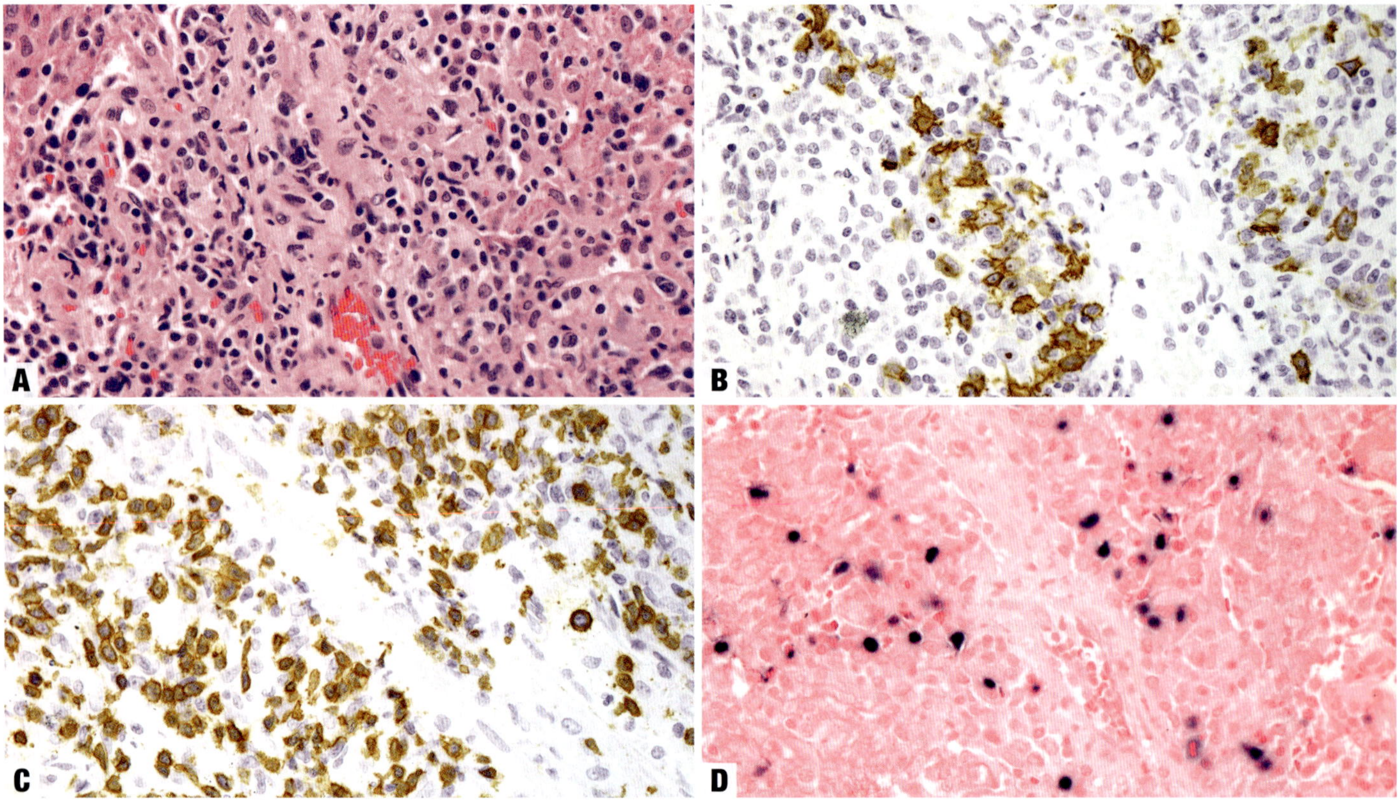

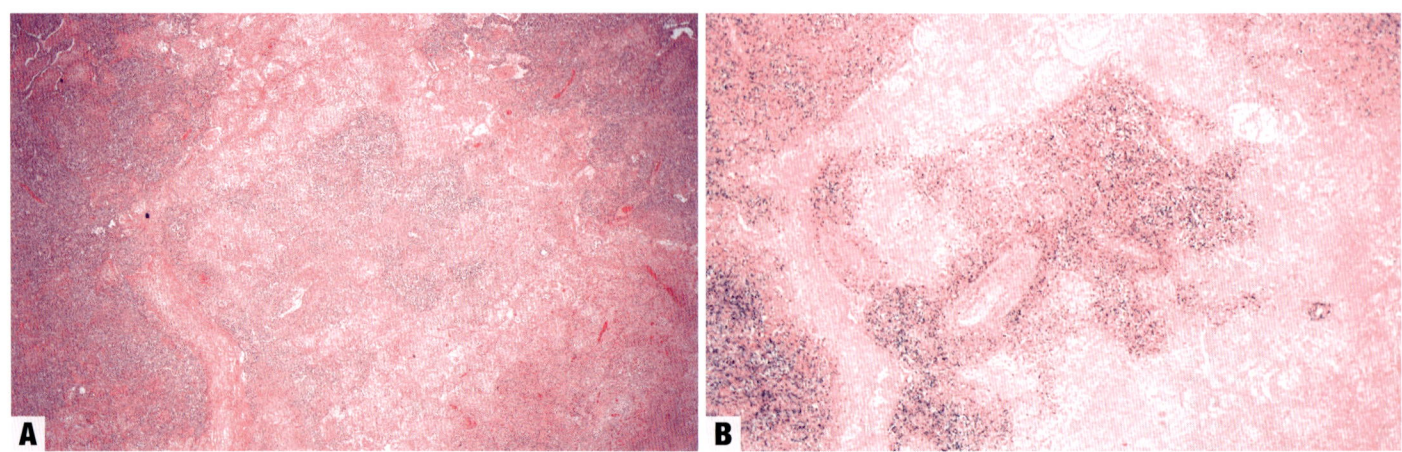

Fig. 1.185 Lymphomatoid granulomatosis, grade 2. **A** Large atypical cells are scattered in a background of lymphoid cells and histiocytes. **B** CD20 immunostaining highlights the large atypical cells. **C** Immunostaining for CD3 highlights the presence of T cells in the background. **D** In situ hybridization for EBV-encoded small RNA (EBER) highlights scattered large atypical cells.

Epidemiology

The disease appears to be more common in North American than in Asian populations {1397,1881}. The incidence also appears to be higher in patients with immunodeficiencies {707, 1066}, but because the disease is rare, reliable data are not available. The median age is in the fourth to sixth decade of life, with 2:1 male predominance.

Etiology

Lymphomatoid granulomatosis is an EBV-associated B-cell lymphoproliferative disorder with a prominent T-cell infiltrate.

Diminished immunity is thought to be an important factor in the development of lymphomatoid granulomatosis.

Pathogenesis

Current hypotheses include defective immune surveillance of EBV and abnormal immune response to EBV, given that previously healthy subjects with lymphomatoid granulomatosis have shown various defects in cell-mediated and/or humoral immunity {2818,3321,3025}. However, if the disease arises in a solid organ transplant recipient, it should be classified as a posttransplant lymphoproliferative disorder.

Fig. 1.186 Lymphomatoid granulomatosis, grade 3. **A** Lung wedge biopsy shows extensive necrosis with an angiocentric lymphoid infiltrate. **B** EBV in situ hybridization, using an EBV-encoded small RNA (EBER) probe, detects numerous EBV-positive cells.

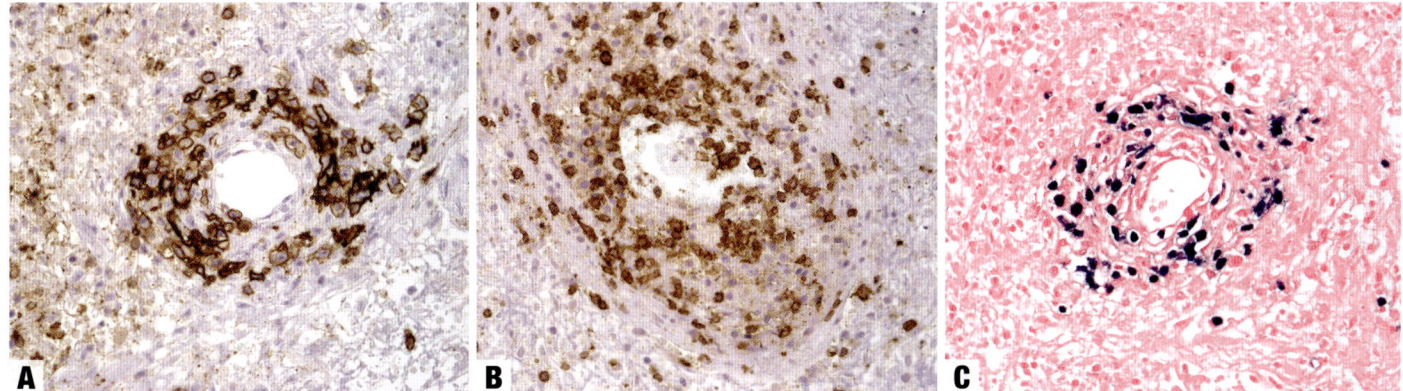

Fig. 1.187 Lymphomatoid granulomatosis, grade 3. **A** Large atypical CD20-positive B cells are present, with a perivascular distribution. **B** CD3-positive T cells within the necrotic area. **C** In situ hybridization shows large atypical perivascular EBV-positive cells.

Macroscopic appearance
The lung shows single or multiple nodules of variable sizes, with or without central necrosis. The nodules are often multiple and bilateral in distribution.

Histopathology
Lymphomatoid granulomatosis is characterized by nodules containing a polymorphous lymphoid infiltrate with an angiocentric distribution. The majority of the cells are small T cells admixed with a variable number of histiocytes, plasma cells, and immunoblasts. Central necrosis is often (although variably) present. The EBV-positive cells vary in size and may show cytological atypia. They may have an appearance of immunoblasts but can rarely resemble Reed–Sternberg cells with multinucleated forms. Despite the name of the lesion, well-formed granulomas are absent. The inflammatory infiltrate affecting the vessels is rich in T cells.

Lymphomatoid granulomatosis is graded by comparing the proportion of EBV-positive B cells and their degree of cytological atypia to the background population of reactive T cells. Three grades are recognized, offering guidance to therapy, notwithstanding issues with reproducibility of the grading system. Grade 1 lesions are composed of a polymorphous lymphoid infiltrate without significant atypia; necrosis may be absent or focal. Large EBV-positive lymphoid cells are rare. In grade 2 lesions, large EBV-positive cells are typically present (40–400/mm²; 5–50/HPF of 0.12 mm²); necrosis is more common. Grade 3 lesions are characterized by a greater number of EBV-positive cells (> 400/mm²; > 50/HPF of 0.12 mm²); necrosis is common and often extensive {2813}. The large atypical cells may occur in clusters. However, if there is a uniform population of large atypical cells beyond the acceptable morphological spectrum of lymphomatoid granulomatosis, a diagnosis of EBV-positive large B-cell lymphoma is more appropriate.

Immunohistochemistry
The large atypical cells are positive for CD20 and EBV by in situ hybridization using EBV-encoded small RNA (EBER) probes. A subset of these positive cells may also stain for EBV LMP1. The cells may be variably positive for CD30 and are negative for CD15. Staining for kappa and lambda light chains is of limited utility, although rare cases may show light chain restriction in the plasma cells. The majority of lymphoid cells in the background are CD3+ T cells, with CD4+ cells outnumbering CD8+ cells {2813}.

Cytology
Tissue biopsy is required for definitive diagnosis.

Diagnostic molecular pathology
Clonal IG gene rearrangements may be identified in most grade 2 and grade 3 lesions. Different clonal rearrangements may be identified in different lesions or from different sites of involvement. B-cell clonality may not be detected in grade 1 lesions, most likely due to the paucity of EBV-positive cells. Clonal TR gene rearrangements are usually not present, although restricted patterns may be observed {1027,2813}.

Essential and desirable diagnostic criteria
Essential:
- Polymorphous lymphoid infiltrate with striking angiocentricity
- Transmural involvement of small to medium-sized arteries by small T lymphocytes
- Presence of variable numbers of large B cells positive for EBV by in situ hybridization

Staging
No staging system applies.

Prognosis and prediction
The prognosis of lymphomatoid granulomatosis is variable. As many as 63% of patients die, with a median overall survival of 14 months. However, as many as 30% undergo spontaneous remission without treatment. Cause of death is related to extensive lung involvement or destruction of other involved organs {1881}.

Intravascular large B-cell lymphoma of the lung

Takeuchi K
Bacon CM
Cooper WA

Definition

Intravascular large B-cell lymphoma (IVLBCL) is an aggressive extranodal non-Hodgkin lymphoma, characterized by the presence of large neoplastic B cells within, if not exclusive to, different-sized vessels, particularly capillaries.

ICD-O coding

9712/3 Intravascular large B-cell lymphoma

ICD-11 coding

2A81.1 Intravascular large B-cell lymphoma

Related terminology

Not recommended (all obsolete): malignant angioendotheliomatosis; neoplastic angioendotheliomatosis; angiotropic lymphoma; intravascular lymphomatosis; angioendotheliotropic lymphoma.

Subtype(s)

Classic, haemophagocytic, and cutaneous subtypes have been proposed.

Localization

IVLBCL involving the lungs generally represents part of systemic disease. However, primary pulmonary cases have been reported {3498}.

Clinical features

IVLBCL is a systemic disorder and thus may show various symptoms according to the involved organs. Haemophagocytic syndrome is observed predominantly in Asian populations (haemophagocytic subtype). IVLBCL may cause pulmonary hypertension, hypoxaemia, and pulmonary embolism. A random skin biopsy and transbronchial lung biopsy are useful to make the diagnosis {775,1838}.

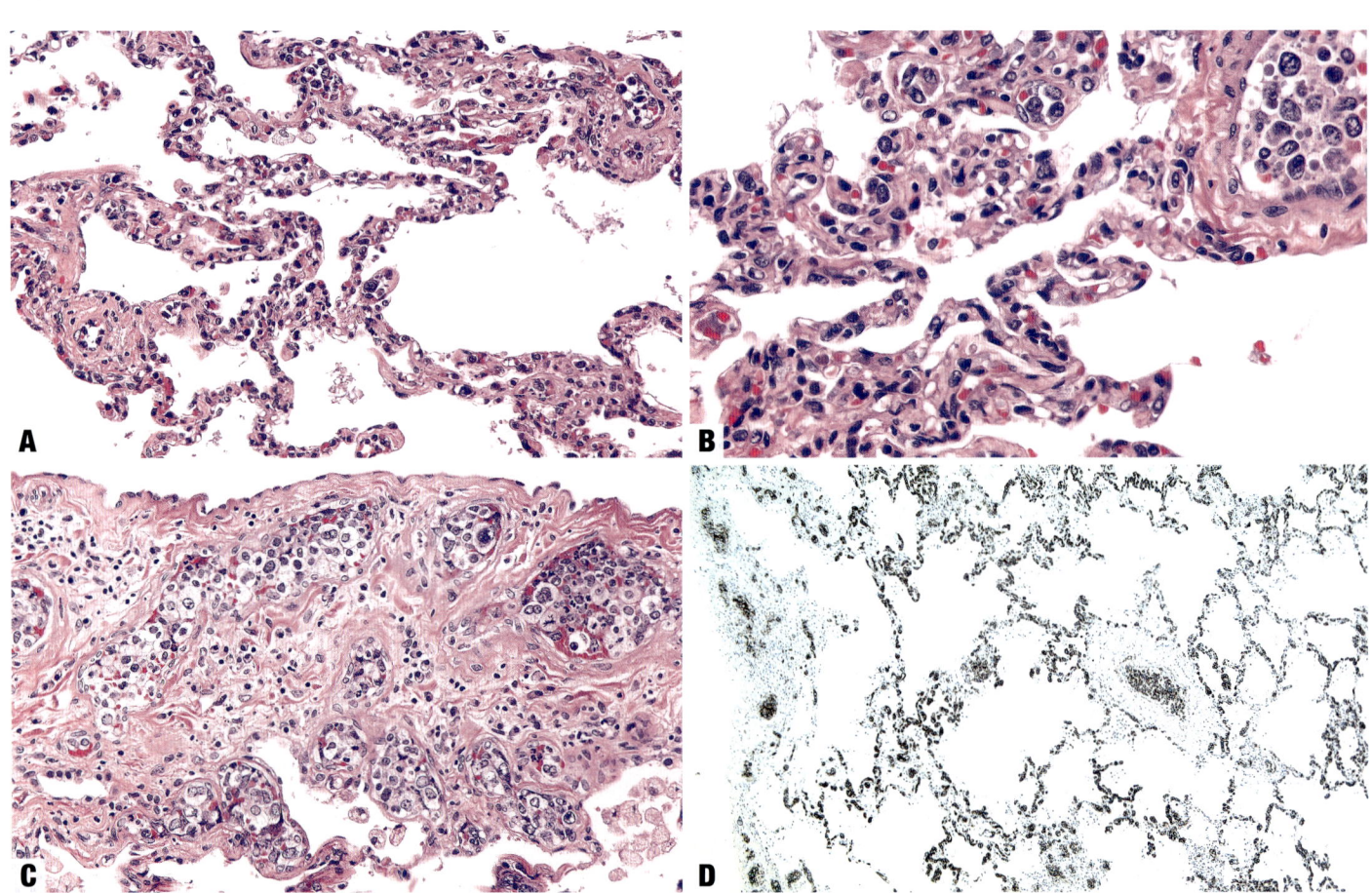

Fig. 1.188 Intravascular large B-cell lymphoma. **A** Large lymphoid cells are observed within the pulmonary capillaries and small vessels. **B** The neoplastic cells show vesicular nuclei. **C** Large anaplastic cells are present in the pleural vessels. **D** Immunohistochemistry for CD20 expressed by the neoplastic cells highlights the vascular network of the affected lung.

Epidemiology
IVLBCL occurs in adults, without sex predisposition.

Etiology
Unknown

Pathogenesis
The neoplastic cells lack adhesion molecules, including CD29 (integrin beta-1) and CD54 (ICAM1) {2372}. *MYD88* p.L265P mutations are reported in about half and *CD79B* p.Y196 mutations in one third to two thirds of cases examined {2676,2890}. Unlike for other lymphoma types, detection of mutations in cell-free DNA by liquid biopsy is more highly sensitive than in tissue-derived DNA {2890}.

Macroscopic appearance
Not relevant

Histopathology
Large lymphoid cells with vesicular nuclei and often showing mitotic figures are observed within small vessels, especially capillaries, sometimes showing minimal extravasation. Rarely, the lymphoid cells can be anaplastic. Mature B-cell markers are expressed, often with CD5 and PDL1 (CD274) expression (20–40%) {1035,2596}. Most cases have a non–germinal-centre B-cell immunophenotype, but approximately 13% are CD10-positive {2032}.

Cytology
Not relevant

Diagnostic molecular pathology
Not clinically relevant

Essential and desirable diagnostic criteria
Essential:
- Large lymphoid cells resembling centroblasts or immunoblasts in blood vessels, especially capillaries
- Mature B-cell markers (e.g. CD20, CD79a, PAX5) are positive

Staging
Staging is according to the Lugano modification of the Ann Arbor staging system.

Prognosis and prediction
IVLBCL is an aggressive lymphoma. The poor prognosis is often caused by delayed diagnosis. Cases with disease limited to the skin (cutaneous form) have a better outcome {823,2746}. Chemotherapy with rituximab has improved the outcomes, with a 3-year overall survival rate of 60–81% {824,825,2746,2747}.

Pulmonary Langerhans cell histiocytosis

Yi ES
Go RS
Weiss LM

Definition

Pulmonary Langerhans cell histiocytosis (PLCH) is a proliferative, usually clonal, disorder of Langerhans cells, with associated interstitial changes in the lung tissue, manifesting as a variable combination of cellular, cystic, and fibrotic lesions.

ICD-O coding

9751/1 Langerhans cell histiocytosis

ICD-11 coding

2B31.2Y & XH51C6 Other specified Langerhans cell histiocytosis & Pulmonary Langerhans cell histiocytosis

Related terminology

Not recommended: pulmonary eosinophilic granuloma; pulmonary Langerhans cell granulomatosis; pulmonary histiocytosis X (obsolete).

Subtype(s)

None

Localization

PLCH mainly involves the upper and middle lung fields, with relative sparing of the lung bases.

Clinical features

PLCH in adults usually occurs in one of three clinical settings: (1) respiratory symptoms (cough and dyspnoea), in about two thirds of patients, with or without constitutional symptoms (fever, malaise, sweats, and weight loss, seen in 15–20% of patients); (2) acute presentation with spontaneous pneumothorax, in 15–20% of cases, which can be bilateral or recurrent; or (3) as an incidental finding on routine chest X-ray, in

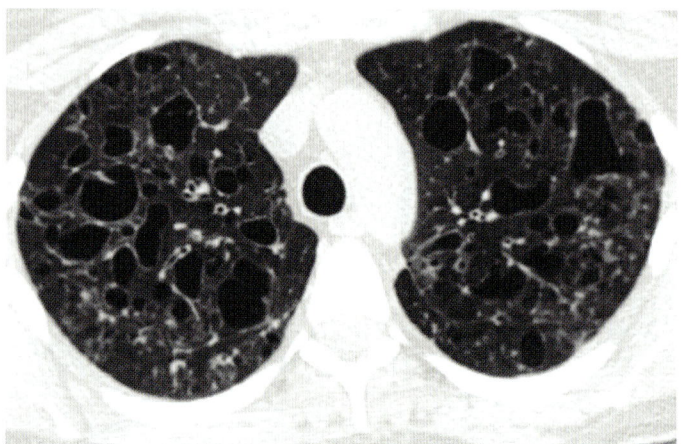

Fig. 1.189 Pulmonary Langerhans cell histiocytosis. Chest CT from a 31-year-old smoker showing many small non-calcified nodules and irregular cysts of varying size, mostly in the upper-lung and mid-lung zones.

5–25% of cases {3155}. Haemoptysis is rare but should raise the possibility of complications or alternative diagnosis (e.g. infection and cancer). Approximately 15% of adults with PLCH have extrapulmonary involvement, including bone involvement, hypothalamic–pituitary axis involvement causing diabetes insipidus, and rarely skin disease {3157}. The systemic form of Langerhans cell histiocytosis (LCH) may have secondary lung involvement {3157}.

Pulmonary function abnormalities vary according to the extent of cystic involvement and disease duration. Reduction of diffusing capacity of the lung for carbon monoxide (D_{LCO}) is observed in 80–90% of cases. Obstructive ventilatory defects are more common than restrictive patterns, and mixed restrictive and obstructive patterns may be seen. The severity of airflow limitation on lung function testing correlates with the extent of cystic lesions on high-resolution CT {3005}.

Imaging

Chest X-ray shows symmetrical bilateral reticulonodular changes predominantly involving the upper and middle lung fields with relative sparing of the lung bases {1578}. High-resolution CT demonstrates a combination of nodules, cavitating nodules measuring 1–10 mm in diameter, and thick-walled or thin-walled cysts. Cysts vary in size and may coalesce to form irregular shapes. In early stages, nodules and cavitating nodules are more numerous than lung cysts, whereas cystic change dominates in later stages. Extensive ground-glass opacities may be present as a result of concomitant smoking-related interstitial lung disease such as desquamative interstitial pneumonia. Pulmonary nodules in PLCH may be hypermetabolic and can be indistinguishable from malignant disease {3156}.

Epidemiology

PLCH is uncommon and estimated as the cause of 3–5% of all adult diffuse lung disease {897}. However, the prevalence of PLCH may be higher, given that it may be asymptomatic, may undergo spontaneous remission, or may be difficult to identify in very advanced forms. PLCH occurs predominantly in young smokers or ex-smokers, with a peak incidence between the ages of 20 and 40 years and equal frequency in men and women {3157}.

Etiology

The majority of patients (> 95%) are current or former cigarette smokers, suggesting cigarette smoke as an etiological agent {3157}.

Pathogenesis

Activating mutation of specific MAPK pathway genes, most commonly *BRAF* p.V600E, have been found in 38–57% of cases {134,2508}. This oncogenic mutation leads to a constitutively

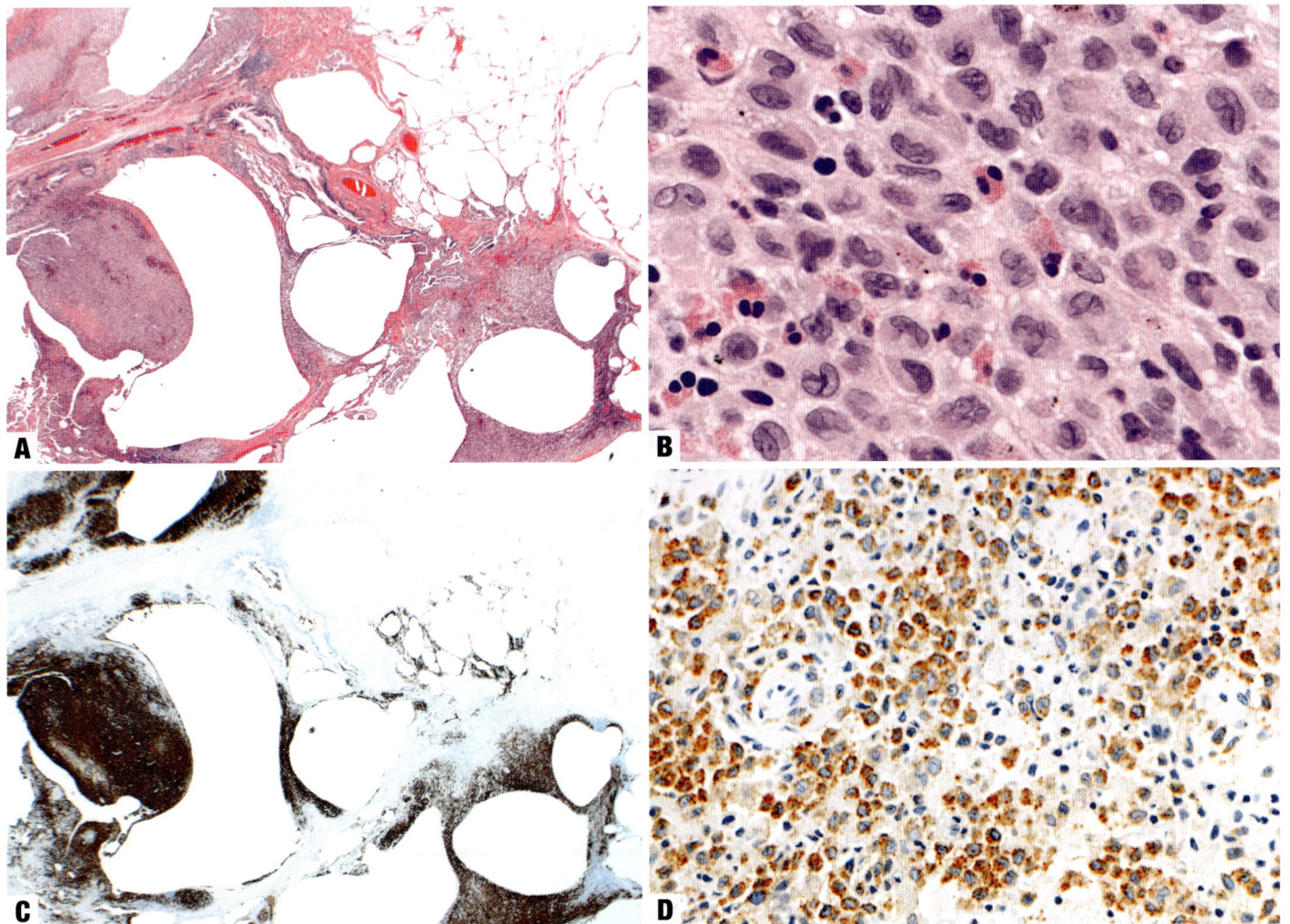

Fig. 1.190 Pulmonary Langerhans cell histiocytosis. **A** Langerhans cell collections with central cavitation and surrounding cystic changes. **B** The Langerhans cells have deeply grooved to contorted nuclei, delicate chromatin, and a moderate amount of lightly eosinophilic cytoplasm. There are some admixed eosinophils. **C** Nodular lesions of Langerhans cells highlighted by CD1a immunostain. **D** BRAF p.V600E immunostain shows granular cytoplasmic positivity in the Langerhans cells.

activated MAPK pathway that promotes cell survival. MAPK pathway activation is also found in PLCH that lacks *BRAF* mutations {432,3155}.

Macroscopic appearance

The lungs may appear cystic, with variable numbers of solid nodules or fibrotic scars depending on the activity and severity of disease.

Histopathology

The histological hallmark of PLCH is accumulation of Langerhans cells forming loose aggregates. The Langerhans cells have convoluted nuclei and pale, lightly eosinophilic cytoplasm. The cellular lesions are mainly present along the bronchioles and alveolar ducts. The aggregates of Langerhans cells may rarely be in the alveolar spaces. Variable numbers of lymphocytes, monocytes/macrophages, and eosinophils are admixed in the cellular lesions. As the lesions enlarge, rounded or stellate nodules develop and the bronchiolocentricity becomes less apparent. The nodules tend to progress from cellular lesions with abundant Langerhans cells to more-fibrotic (often stellate)

scars with sparse to absent Langerhans cells at the end stage. Thus, the diagnosis of healed PLCH may be based on the presence of stellate centrilobular scarring in the appropriate clinical and radiological setting. Cystic changes are prominent in late stages of the disease. Background lung tissue usually shows concomitant features of smoking, including emphysema, respiratory bronchiolitis, smoking-related interstitial fibrosis, and even desquamative interstitial pneumonia in some cases.

Immunohistochemistry

Langerhans cells are positive for S100, CD1a, and langerin. Cellular PLCH shows numerous Langerhans cells, but burnt-out or healed PLCH may not show any identifiable Langerhans cells even on immunohistochemical stains. BRAF p.V600E immunohistochemical stain correlates well with the mutation status of *BRAF* in both PLCH and systemic LCH cases {2508}.

Cytology

Bronchoalveolar lavage may reveal an increased number of CD1a-positive cells in a minority of cases but is rarely useful in the diagnosis of PLCH in adults {612}.

Diagnostic molecular pathology

BRAF p.V600E immunohistochemical stain correlates well with the mutation status of this gene {2508}.

Essential and desirable diagnostic criteria

Essential:
- Langerhans cell aggregates, usually in a centriacinar distribution
- Immunohistochemical confirmation of Langerhans cells (e.g. CD1a, langerin)

Desirable:
- Associated cystic and fibrotic changes may be present
- Background of smoking-related changes
- Assessment of *BRAF* mutation status if targeted therapy contemplated

Staging

There is no staging system for LCH.

Prognosis and prediction

The natural history of PLCH is unpredictable. Some cases may remit or stabilize after smoking cessation. However, approximately 15% of patients develop progressive disease, often associated with airflow limitation and pulmonary vascular dysfunction {256}. Predictors of shorter survival include older age, lower forced expiratory volume in 1 second (FEV1), higher residual volume, lower ratio of FEV1 to forced vital capacity (FVC), and reduced D_{LCO} {3157}. Development of pulmonary hypertension is also associated with higher mortality {1619}.

For treatment of PLCH, smoking cessation is essential, and a prospective multicentre study showed its effectiveness {3004, 544}. Pharmaceutical treatment with corticosteroid or chemotherapeutic agents can be considered for patients with severe or progressive disease despite smoking cessation.

Clinical trials with BRAF inhibitors have shown efficacy in systemic LCH with mutant *BRAF* {699,2262A,1103A}, but the role of BRAF inhibitors in PLCH, if any, remains to be defined because the main morbidities in PLCH are due to complications of the disease rather than Langerhans cell proliferation (which tends to abate with disease course).

Pulmonary Erdheim–Chester disease

Ozkaya N
Emile JF
Go RS

Definition
Erdheim–Chester disease (ECD) is a systemic histiocytic neoplasm characterized by multiorgan accumulation of mature histiocytes in a background of fibrosis.

ICD-O coding
9749/3 Erdheim–Chester disease

ICD-11 coding
2B31.Y & XH1VJ3 Other specified histiocytic or dendritic cell neoplasms & Erdheim–Chester disease

Related terminology
Not recommended: lipogranulomatosis; lipoid granulomatosis; lipid (cholesterol) granulomatosis; polyostotic sclerosing histiocytosis

Subtype(s)
None

Localization
ECD can affect virtually any organ system, including lung and pleura (see Table 1.16) {696,785,555,1000}.

Clinical features
Patients mostly present with non-respiratory symptoms (see Table 1.16). Lung involvement may be asymptomatic or may cause cough and/or progressive dyspnoea {785,1076,107,408, 1000}. Pleural effusion and/or mediastinal infiltration is also common {1000,107}. Pulmonary function studies can show a restrictive pattern or may be normal. ECD can rarely be associated with Langerhans cell histiocytosis and Rosai–Dorfman disease, as well as autoimmune diseases {1136,765,2514,2443}. Myeloid neoplasms can be present in as many as 10% of cases {2263,271,999,998}.

Imaging
CT is helpful to demonstrate the pleural and/or parenchymal involvement, with reticulations and ground-glass opacities being the predominant parenchymal findings.

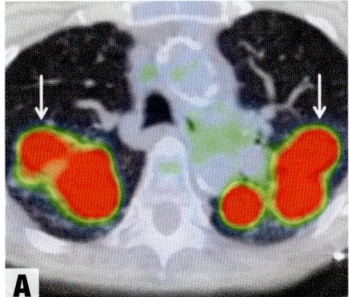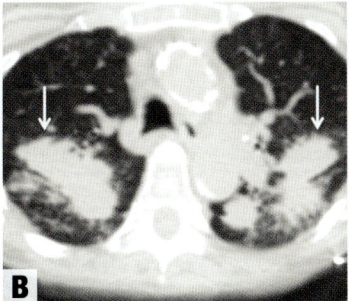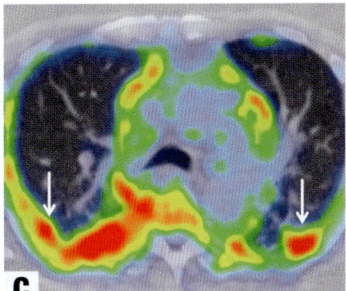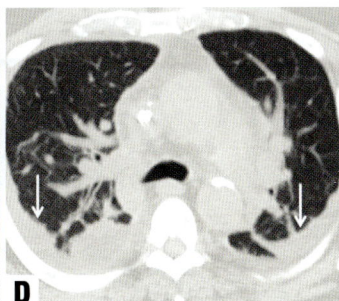

Fig. 1.191 Erdheim–Chester disease. **A** Axial FDG PET-CT of lungs demonstrates bilateral FDG-avid (12.0 maximum standardized uptake value) lung masses (arrows). **B** Corresponding axial CT demonstrates large ill-defined solid masses involving the central bronchovascular architecture (arrows). **C** FDG PET-CT of chest demonstrates FDG-avid (8.9 maximum standardized uptake value) disease involving the pleura bilaterally (arrows). **D** Corresponding axial chest CT elucidates thick confluent soft tissue thickening of the pleura, extending into the interlobular septa (arrows).

Table 1.16 Common sites of involvement by Erdheim–Chester disease

Site	Manifestations
Bones (80–95%)	Bilateral symmetrical long bone involvement at the metadiaphysis
Retroperitoneum (55–65%)	Perinephric infiltration ("hairy kidneys")
Vasculature (50–80%)	Periaortic infiltration of the entire thoracoabdominal aorta ("coated aorta"), supra-aortic trunks, and coronary arteries
Heart (40–70%)	Right atrial pseudotumour; valvular infiltration; pericardial infiltration and effusion
Endocrine system (40–70%)	Diabetes insipidus; anterior pituitary dysfunction; testicular insufficiency; adrenal infiltration
Nervous system (40%)	Brainstem/cerebellum masses; cerebral white matter enhancement; dural and pituitary stalk thickening
Respiratory tract (30–55%)	Mediastinal infiltration; pleural, septal, and maxillary sinus thickening
Orbits (30%)	Orbital masses
Skin (25–30%)	Xanthelasma-like lesions around the eyes, face, neck, and inguinal folds

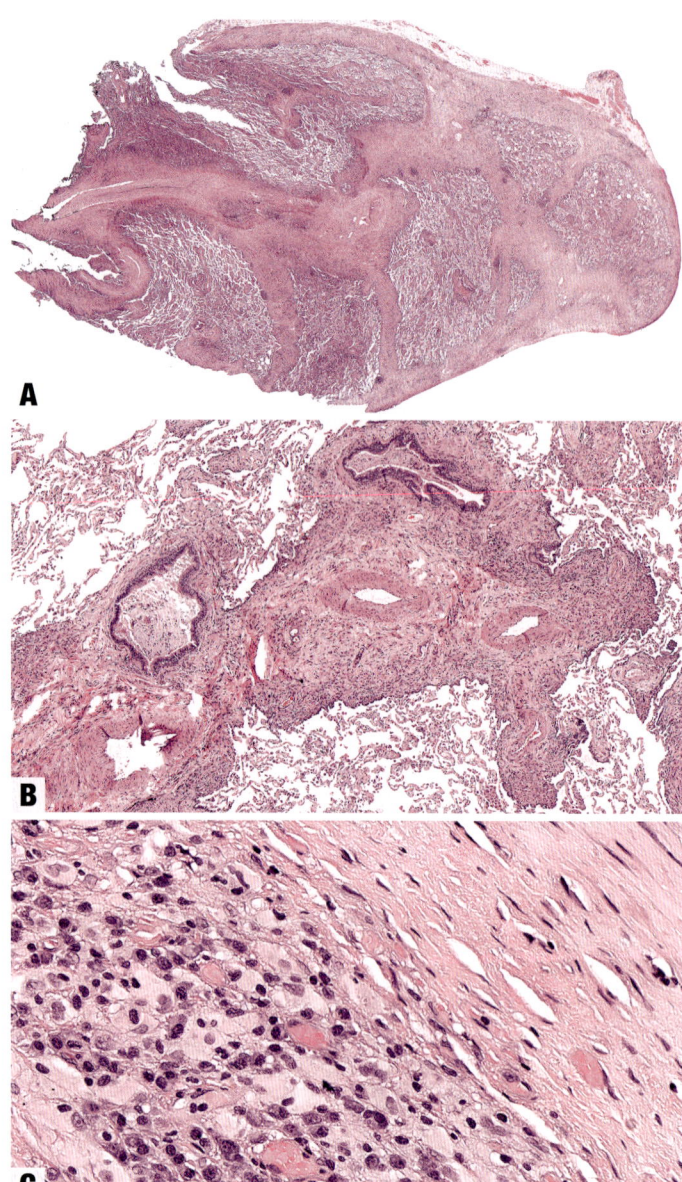

Fig. 1.192 Erdheim–Chester disease. **A** Low-power view of the lung shows thickening of pleura and interlobular septa by a histiocytic infiltrate in a background of fibrosis. **B** Involvement of perivascular and peribronchiolar interstitium is present, with areas of relatively normal alveolar parenchyma. **C** High-power view of the subpleura showing accumulation of histiocytes with round to oval nuclei and abundant eosinophilic cytoplasm interspersed with plasma cells.

Epidemiology

ECD is a rare disease. The age range is 15–80 years, with a male predominance (~70%) {696,785,555,1000}. ECD is extremely rare in children, in whom it is generally associated with Langerhans cell histiocytosis {3060,1451,1065}.

Etiology

ECD is a clonal neoplastic disorder {1075,697,2228}. Unlike in Langerhans cell histiocytosis, no association with cigarette smoking has been shown {2228}.

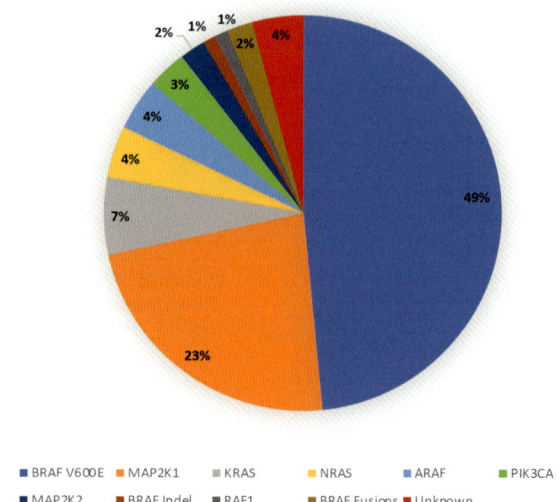

Fig. 1.193 Erdheim–Chester disease. Pie chart showing relative frequencies of activating signalling pathway alterations.

Pathogenesis

Functional studies have shown that some cases derive from haematopoietic/myeloid progenitors {746,1926}. A characteristic cytokine signature responsible for local activation and recruitment of histiocytes has been identified {105,2233}. Gain-of-function alterations activating cell signalling pathways have been identified in nearly all cases {766,1075,745,697}.

Macroscopic appearance

The lung is firm, with pleural and interlobular septa often visible due to thickening.

Histopathology

Lung involvement has a characteristic lymphangitic distribution, along with involvement of the visceral pleura, interlobular septa, and perivascular interstitium as well as lesser involvement of the peribronchiolar areas. The disease typically spares perialveolar spaces {2228}. The lesional histiocytes have foamy and/or eosinophilic cytoplasm, but they can be sparse and may have a distorted shape due to marked fibrosis admixed with chronic inflammatory cells. Eosinophils are rare to absent. Touton giant cells can be seen occasionally.

Immunohistochemistry

The lesional cells are positive for histiocytic markers (CD163, CD68, CD14, CD4, and factor XIIIa) and negative for CD1a and CD207 (langerin). S100 is variably positive. Immunostaining with BRAF p.V600E antibody (VE1) is not an optimal method to demonstrate *BRAF* p.V600E mutation in Erdheim–Chester disease {2228}.

Cytology

Bronchoalveolar lavage may show a nonspecific increase in histiocytes and/or chronic inflammatory cells {107}.

Diagnostic molecular pathology

Demonstration of a corroborating genomic alteration may aid in diagnosis and treatment.

Box 1.09 Diagnostic criteria for lung involvement by Erdheim–Chester disease (ECD) {3332,753,107,696}

For first-time diagnosis of ECD (with pulmonary presentation):

Essential:

- Histiocytic infiltrate with characteristic lymphangitic distribution[a]
- Non-Langerhans cell phenotype
- Characteristic chest CT findings
- Additional systemic findings[b]

Desirable:

- Corroborating genetic alteration

When there is already a well-established diagnosis of ECD involving another site[b]:

Essential[c]:

- Characteristic chest CT findings
- Exclusion of other possible etiologies of interstitial lung disease

Desirable:

- Histiocytic infiltrate with characteristic lymphangitic distribution[a]
- Non-Langerhans cell phenotype
- Corroborating genetic alteration

[a]Transbronchial lung biopsies are often unhelpful in showing the characteristic distribution, but wedge biopsies can exhibit diagnostic features.
[b]The diagnosis of ECD should be made by identifying distinctive histopathological findings from any site in the appropriate clinical and radiological context (see Table 1.16, p. 189).
[c]Diagnosis of pulmonary ECD is highly likely under these circumstances, although a definitive diagnosis always requires histopathological evaluation.

Essential and desirable diagnostic criteria

See Box 1.09.

Staging

Not relevant

Prognosis and prediction

Most patients require systemic therapy. Traditionally, drugs such as peginterferon and cladribine have been used as initial treatments. However, in recent years, *BRAF* mutations have been recognized and tyrosine kinase inhibitors are used more frequently {555,1135,696,997A}. Recent studies reported a 43–100% response rate and almost no disease progression with the use of BRAF and/or MEK inhibitors {698,552,699}. Prognosis depends on site and extent of the involvement. CNS involvement and multisystemic disease are poor prognostic factors {106}. Lung involvement is not an independent poor prognostic factor in recent case series {555,107}.

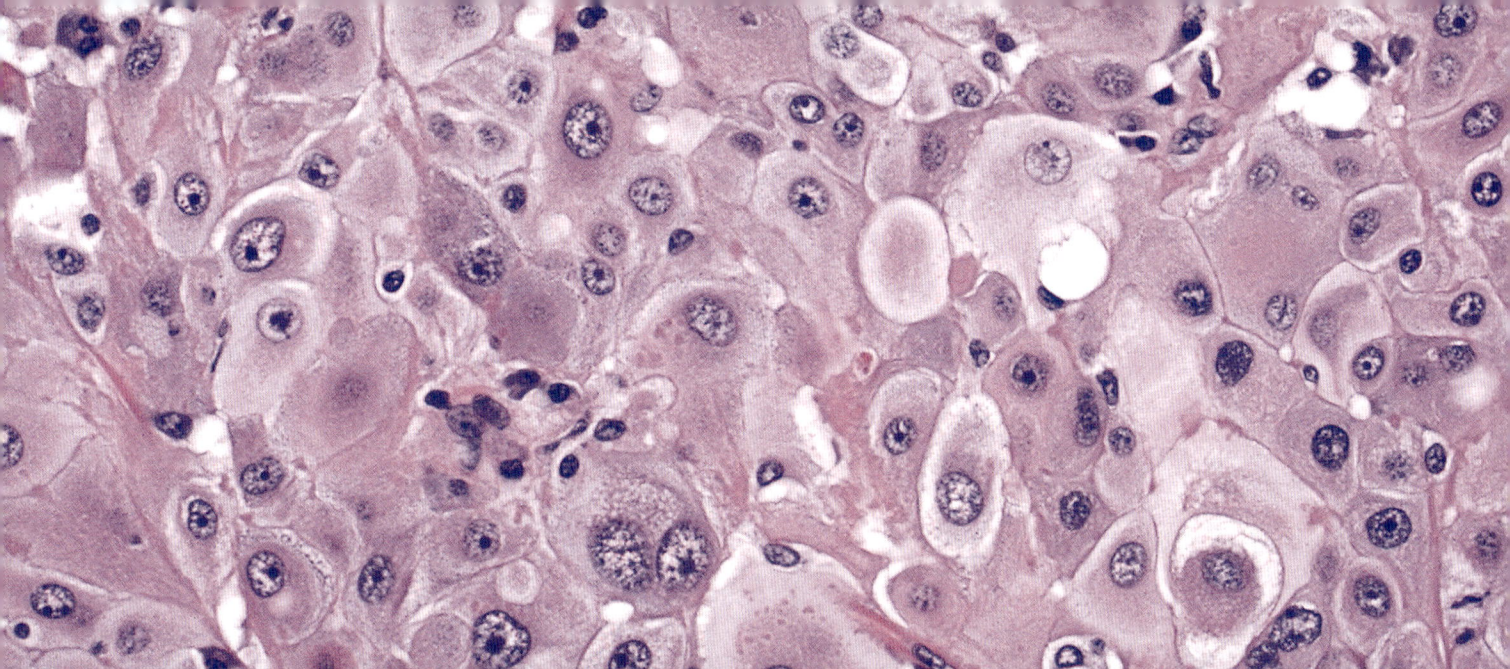

2

Tumours of the pleura and pericardium

Edited by: Chan JKC, Galateau-Salle F, Nicholson AG, Travis WD, Tsao MS

Adenomatoid tumour
Well-differentiated papillary mesothelial tumour
Mesothelioma in situ
Localized mesothelioma
Diffuse mesothelioma
Primary effusion lymphoma
Diffuse large B-cell lymphoma associated with chronic inflammation

Tumours of the pleura and pericardium: Introduction

Nicholson AG
Dacic S
Znaor A

Pleural tumours

The classification of pleural tumours centres primarily on the identification of mesothelioma and its differential diagnoses – namely, metastatic carcinomas (particularly from the lung) and mesenchymal tumours. The three main histological subtypes (epithelioid, sarcomatoid, biphasic) remain the same, although there is increased recognition of architectural patterns, cytological features, and stromal features {2103}. Localized mesothelioma also remains a separate category, because of the better prognosis afforded by complete resection in some cases {1800}. However, since the previous WHO classification, with the understanding of genomics in mesothelioma advancing significantly, this has led to the recognition and establishment of criteria for mesothelioma in situ {533}.

Epidemiology

Pleural mesotheliomas are rare cancers that account for < 2% of all malignancies. In 2018, there were 30 440 estimated new cases and 25 580 estimated mesothelioma (as defined by ICD-10 code C45) deaths worldwide, with the highest incidence observed in high-income countries {309}. According to the observed cancer registry data from the period 2008–2012, the age-standardized incidence rates (World) among males varied from > 4.5 cases per 100 000 person-years in some populations in the United Kingdom, Germany, and Australia to < 0.1 cases per 100 000 person-years in Asia and South America. Incidence rates among females were lower, with highest rates recorded in Eskişehir, Turkey (2.9/100 000) and South Lombardy, Italy (2.2/100 000) {308}. Mesothelioma incidence rates have stabilized in the USA, Australia, France, the United Kingdom, Poland, Finland, and Norway {228,2798,2039,1423, 948}, while still increasing in other countries, such as China {3504}. A recent analysis of age-specific mortality trends (used as a proxy for incidence trends, given the poor survival) in high-income countries reported trends of increasing mortality in older age groups alongside decreases in younger age groups in most countries, probably reflecting lower levels of asbestos exposure in younger cohorts {251}.

Etiology

The majority of mesotheliomas are caused by asbestos, with the strength of the relationship being dependent on fibre type. Commercial amphibole asbestos types, such as amosite and crocidolite, are more carcinogenic than serpentine asbestos (chrysotile) {1220A}. There is also variation in population attributable fractions by sex: in the USA and France, 80–90% of mesotheliomas in men are caused by asbestos, but only 20–40% in women {1120,1577,83}. Other types of mineral fibres may also induce mesothelioma {119}. Where erionite is present naturally, mainly in the Cappadocia region of Turkey, there is a very high incidence of mesothelioma {382,385}. A raised incidence of mesothelioma has also been reported in a rural village in central

Estimated age-standardized incidence rates (World) in 2018, mesothelioma, both sexes, all ages

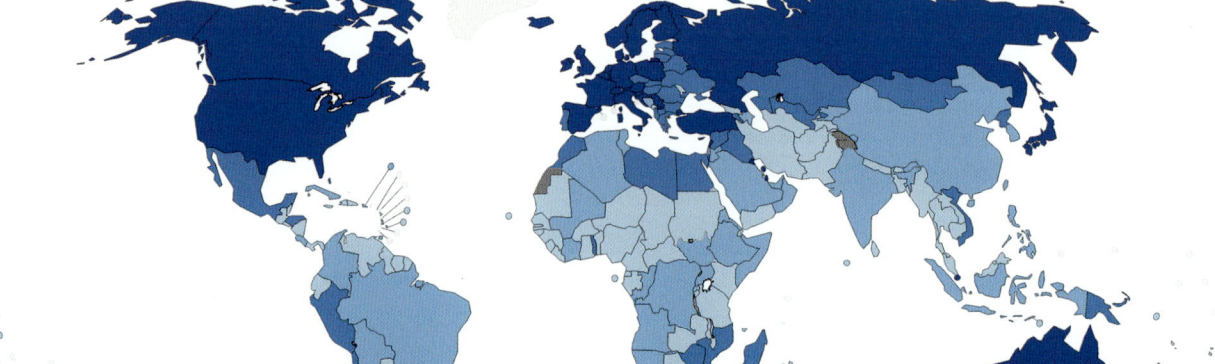

ASR (World) per 100 000

- ≥ 0.44
- 0.16–0.44
- 0.06–0.16
- 0.0–0.06
- Not applicable
- No data

Data source: GLOBOCAN 2018
Graph production: IARC
(http://gco.iarc.fr/today)
World Health Organization

World Health Organization
© International Agency for Research on Cancer 2018

Fig. 2.01 Mesothelioma map. Estimated age-standardized global incidence rates (ASRs; World), per 100 000 person-years, of mesothelioma in 2018.

Mexico {2216} where erionite is present in the soil and rocks. Erionite has also been reported as being used in gravel in the US state of North Dakota {382} and being present in soil in the Southern Nevada region of the US state of Nevada, although it remains uncertain whether these exposures are associated with increased incidence of mesothelioma {177,2358,176}.

Mesothelioma typically develops 20–40 years after exposure {1594}, sometimes after exposure in childhood {2448,610}. Prospectively, rates will probably vary as asbestos bans (or a lack thereof) take effect and both occupational and environmental exposures change {385,949,2473}.

Other established causes of mesothelioma include therapeutic and occupational radiation, with a risk for development of mesothelioma in directly irradiated tissues {801,119}. A high risk for mesothelioma development has been reported in families with *BAP1* tumour predisposition syndrome {3026,383,384, 2156} (see *BAP1 tumour predisposition syndrome*, p. 476).

Mesothelioma in situ

Mesothelioma in situ was originally described in patients who also had invasive mesotheliomas, so proof of in situ disease as opposed to surface spread of the underlying invasive tumour was challenging {3294}. Until recently, the consensus among pathologists had been that it was impossible to recognize mesothelioma in situ based on morphology alone. Recently published studies reintroduced the concept of mesothelioma in situ in patients with recurrent unexplained pleural effusions over a longer period of time and in the absence of gross evidence of disease on imaging or thoracoscopic inspection {534, 1928,533}. In addition to these unique clinical criteria, ancillary studies such as immunohistochemistry for BAP1 and/or MTAP as a surrogate for FISH for *CDKN2A* homozygous deletion are necessary to establish the diagnosis {534,1928,533}. The proposed markers are well-established diagnostic markers for separating benign mesothelial proliferations from mesothelioma {532}. These will be informative in about 60–70% of cases, and it is currently unknown what other markers should be used to establish the diagnosis of mesothelioma in situ. Therefore, the diagnosis of mesothelioma in situ is based on a combination of clinical, imaging, and morphological criteria with loss of BAP1 and/or MTAP and/or *CDKN2A*.

This definition raises several issues for practising pathologists. The pathologist must be aware of the clinical presentation and imaging findings; therefore, communication with the treating/procedure physician and review of the medical records are essential. The diagnosis of mesothelioma in situ cannot be made in small biopsies, cytology, or effusion samples alone, because the presence of invasion cannot be excluded. The diagnosis requires submission of biopsy samples (ideally 100–200 mm²) from different areas of the pleura, in combination with clinical presentation and imaging data.

Biomarker testing

From an assay establishment standpoint, immunohistochemistry for BAP1 and MTAP as well as and FISH for *CDKN2A* homozygous deletion must be rigorously validated and performed in an accredited laboratory. The laboratory may choose which antibody to use on the basis of analytic precision, clinical sensitivity, and clinical specificity in accordance with published standards. The laboratory must perform technical validation of the antibody and platform selected for clinical use and must develop a standard operating procedure for the test to be offered. Similar rules apply to the validation of FISH assays. The number of tests required for a reliable validation usually includes 20 positive and 20 negative samples, with results comparable to published data on specificities and sensitivities. If a laboratory chooses to use alternative fixatives other than buffered formalin, the laboratory is obligated to validate those fixatives' performance against the results of testing of the same samples fixed in buffered formalin {3335}.

Well-differentiated papillary mesothelial tumour

The tumour previously classified as well-differentiated papillary mesothelioma has been renamed to well-differentiated papillary mesothelial tumour. This new term is intended to recognize the relatively indolent clinical behaviour of most well-differentiated papillary mesothelial tumours and to help avoid confusion with the much more clinically aggressive diffuse mesothelioma (see below).

Diffuse and localized pleural mesothelioma

The word "malignant" has been removed from the diagnostic terminology for diffuse and localized pleural mesothelioma, because all mesotheliomas are malignant. Historically, the term "malignant" was preserved to contrast with well-differentiated papillary mesothelioma, which is now called well-differentiated papillary mesothelial tumour.

Pericardial tumours

Pericardial tumours were classified with cardiac tumours in the previous edition, but they are now discussed within the chapters on tumours of the pleura and pericardium (mesothelioma), mesenchymal tumours, and metastases.

Adenomatoid tumour of the pleura

Hiroshima K
Karpathiou G

Definition

Pleural adenomatoid tumour is a benign tumour of mesothelial origin.

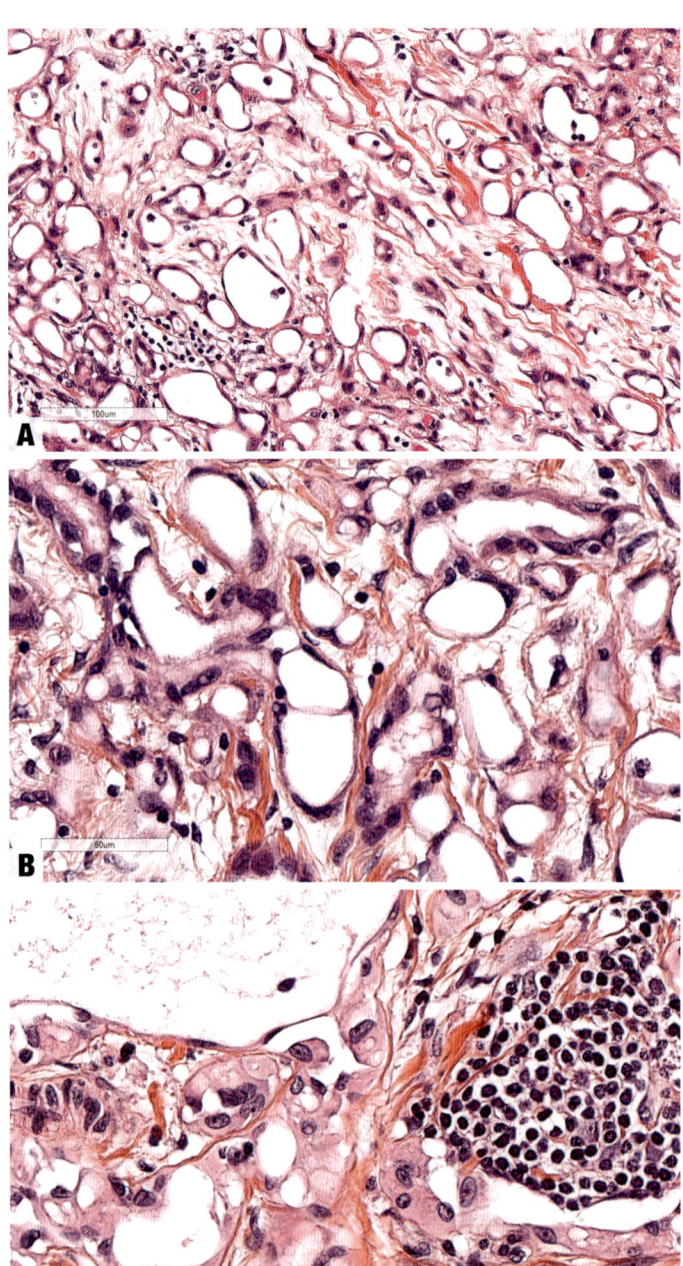

Fig. 2.02 Adenomatoid tumour. **A** Adenomatoid tumour composed of small tubular or gland-like spaces, many of which are dilated. **B** Vacuolated cells contain strands that bridge the lumina of the tubular and slit-like spaces and may form a fine network. **C** Pseudoglandular spaces and a lymphoid aggregate.

ICD-O coding

9054/0 Adenomatoid tumour

ICD-11 coding

2E8Y & XH6BY3 Benign neoplasm of mesothelial tissue, other specified organs & Adenomatoid tumour, NOS

Related terminology

None

Subtype(s)

None

Localization

The tumours can occur on the visceral or parietal pleura {1384, 1930,1063,1237}.

Clinical features

The tumour is usually found incidentally during surgery or at autopsy.

Epidemiology

Adenomatoid tumour is extremely rare in the pleura, with < 20 cases described in the literature to date {1930,1420,1384}. The age range is reported to be 40–70 years. The role of asbestos exposure is unknown.

Etiology

Unknown

Pathogenesis

Adenomatoid tumours of the genital tract harbour somatic missense mutations in the *TRAF7* gene, a member of the family of TNF receptor–associated factors {988}, but this has not yet been identified in thoracic tumours. Adenomatoid tumours in the genital tract do not harbour alterations in *BAP1*, *NF2*, or *CDKN2A* {988,2962}. It is not known why adenomatoid tumours occur more frequently in the genital tract than in the serosal surfaces of the pleura {1384}.

Macroscopic appearance

The tumour is an unencapsulated, relatively circumscribed, firm grey to yellow-tan nodule measuring 5–30 mm in greatest dimension {1384,1063,1237}.

Histopathology

Tumours are circumscribed and nodular, arising on the pleural surfaces. Localized infiltration of surrounding soft tissues adjacent to the tumour may be seen. Combinations of interanastomosing pseudoglands, pseudovascular spaces, tubules, signet-ring–like spaces, and papillae lined by flat to cuboidal cells can be seen {1384,2858}. The tumour cells have scant epithelioid or vacuolated cytoplasm and bland nuclei. Spaces may contain basophilic material. Vacuolated cells contain strands that bridge the lumina of the tubular and slit-like spaces and may form a fine network {1137,2623}. Adenomatoid tumours often harbour lymphoid aggregates {1137,2623}.

Sampling the entire tumour is recommended to rule out epithelioid mesotheliomas with adenomatoid-appearing areas.

Immunohistochemistry
The tumour stains for cytokeratins and mesothelial cell markers, such as calretinin, D2-40, and WT1 {2623,1565,2204,1747, 2684}, with retained BAP1 expression {1328,777} (see *Diffuse pleural mesothelioma*, p. 204).

Differential diagnosis
The most important differential diagnosis is mesothelioma, which typically shows more diffuse pleural involvement and invasive growth as well as malignant histological characteristics such as cytological atypia, necrosis, or sarcomatoid patterns. Entities such as lymphangioma, epithelioid haemangioendothelioma, and metastatic signet-ring cell carcinoma should be excluded by immunohistochemistry.

Cytology
Insufficient data available

Diagnostic molecular pathology
Not relevant

Essential and desirable diagnostic criteria
Essential:
- Focal proliferation of tubular spaces or vacuoles lined by flattened or cuboidal mesothelial cells in a fibrous stroma
- Lack of diffuse or multifocal spread along the pleura and absence of malignant histological features such as invasive growth into the underlying stroma, cytological atypia, necrosis, or sarcomatoid patterns

Desirable:
- Immunohistochemistry for mesothelial markers, if needed
- Staining for L1CAM, a marker of *TRAF7* mutation, may be useful {988}
- BAP1 retained and absence of homozygous deletion of *CDKN2A*

Staging
Not relevant

Prognosis and prediction
Tumours follow a benign clinical course {1384,1063,1930}.

Well-differentiated papillary mesothelial tumour of the pleura

Butnor KJ
Roden AC
Tazelaar HD
Wang J

Definition

Well-differentiated papillary mesothelial tumour (WDPMT) of the pleura is a neoplasm of mesothelial origin composed of papillary stromal formations covered by bland mesothelial cells lacking invasion.

ICD-O coding

9052/1 Well-differentiated papillary mesothelial tumour

ICD-11 coding

2C26.0 & XH85T6 Mesothelioma of pleura & Well-differentiated papillary mesothelioma of the pleura

Related terminology

Not recommended: well-differentiated papillary mesothelioma; benign papillary mesothelioma.

Subtype(s)

None

Localization

WDPMT arises from the visceral and/or parietal pleura.

Clinical features

Patients with WDPMT commonly present with dyspnoea. Unilateral pleural effusion is frequent and often recurrent. Some tumours are discovered incidentally.

Epidemiology

With fewer than 50 cases reported, pleural WDPMT is less common than its counterpart in the peritoneum and far rarer than pleural diffuse mesothelioma. Pleural WDPMT shows no apparent sex predilection and occurs over a wide age range (median age: ~62 years) {357,904,483,2901}.

Etiology

The etiology remains uncertain. Although asbestos exposure has been documented in some patients, the rarity of WDPMT poses challenges to conducting epidemiological studies {357, 904}.

Pathogenesis

Pathogenic mechanisms of WDPMT have not been established. A *BAP1* germline mutation has rarely been detected {2474}. *CDKN2A* homozygous deletion has not been observed in pleural WDPMT {1630,528}.

Macroscopic appearance

Tumours protrude from the pleura as single arborescent masses as large as 50 mm or as multifocal nodules < 10 mm that stud the pleura and impart a granular to velvety appearance {357, 904}.

Histopathology

The tumour arises from the pleural surface as distinct thin to broad papillary formations covered by a single layer of flattened to cuboidal bland mesothelial cells with inconspicuous nucleoli, rare to absent mitoses, and no stromal invasion. The papillae

Table 2.01 Pathological features of well-differentiated papillary mesothelial tumour of the pleura and its differential diagnosis

Feature	Well-differentiated papillary mesothelial tumour	Reactive pleuritis with mesothelial hyperplasia	Diffuse epithelioid mesothelioma with papillary pattern
Macroscopic appearance	Single arborescent mass or small multifocal nodules	Masses/expansile nodules absent; may have accompanying effusion, overlying exudate, and/or adhesions	Diffuse rind-like pleural thickening or coalescent nodular masses
Histological growth pattern	Surface growth	Surface involvement ± overlying fibrin and associated granulation tissue featuring capillaries oriented perpendicular to surface	Surface papillary proliferation with underlying complex/haphazard expansile growth
Papillae	Range from relatively thin to broad with paucicellular myxoid or fibrovascular cores ± foamy macrophages	Uncommon; stubby with simple architecture	Architecturally complex
Mesothelial cell morphology	Bland monotonous monolayer	Reactive atypia ± nucleolar prominence	Cellular stratification/multilayering ± cytological atypia, can be deceptively bland
Inflammation	Rare to absent	Usually present and often prominent	If present, usually at interface of tumour with adipose tissue
Mitoses	Rare to absent	May be abundant (not atypical)	Relatively few, but atypical forms may be seen
Stromal invasion	Absent	Absent	Present and typically deep into submesothelial connective tissue or beyond

consist of paucicellular myxoid or fibrovascular cores devoid of inflammation that infrequently show hyalinization and occasionally contain foamy macrophages. Psammomatous calcifications are rare. Papillae infrequently exhibit compressive crowding, in which back-to-back arrangements simulate invasion, but keratin staining demonstrates maintained papillary architecture {528}.

Immunohistochemistry
WDPMT stains with mesothelial markers {1630} (see *Diffuse pleural mesothelioma*, p. 204).

Differential diagnosis
The diagnosis of WDPMT requires histological examination of the entire tumour to exclude invasion. Principal differential considerations include mesothelial proliferations with the histological appearance of WDPMT that show focal invasion, reactive mesothelial hyperplasia, and diffuse mesothelioma (see Table 2.01). Rarely, mesothelial proliferations with the architecture of WDPMT invade the papillary cores and/or focally invade the submesothelial connective tissue as bland tubules or solid foci of epithelioid or spindle cells {528}. It has not been established whether such lesions, which have been referred to as well-differentiated papillary mesothelioma with invasive foci, are best considered a subtype of WDPMT, represent early diffuse mesothelioma, or are a distinct entity. Nor have invasive size and depth criteria been defined. The mesothelium in reactive pleuritis occasionally forms papillae, but unlike those of WDPMT, the papillae are stubby and have reactive cytological features and accompanying inflammation. Epithelioid diffuse mesothelioma with papillary growth can bear a striking resemblance to WDPMT, but it is distinguished by invasion into the deep pleural connective tissue or beyond.

Cytology
Cytological samples are not relevant to the diagnosis of WDPMT, because invasion cannot be excluded.

Diagnostic molecular pathology
Molecular data are extremely limited. BAP1 is usually retained {1630}.

Essential and desirable diagnostic criteria
Essential:
- Papillary stromal formations covered by bland mesothelium
- No stromal invasion

Desirable:
- Immunohistochemical staining for mesothelial markers
- BAP1 positivity retained

Staging
Not clinically relevant

Prognosis and prediction
Although a minority of cases follow a benign clinical course after complete resection, most WDPMTs are characterized by slow growth of recurrent disease, with extended survival of several years or longer {357,904}. For this reason, and to avoid confusion with diffuse mesothelioma, the designation

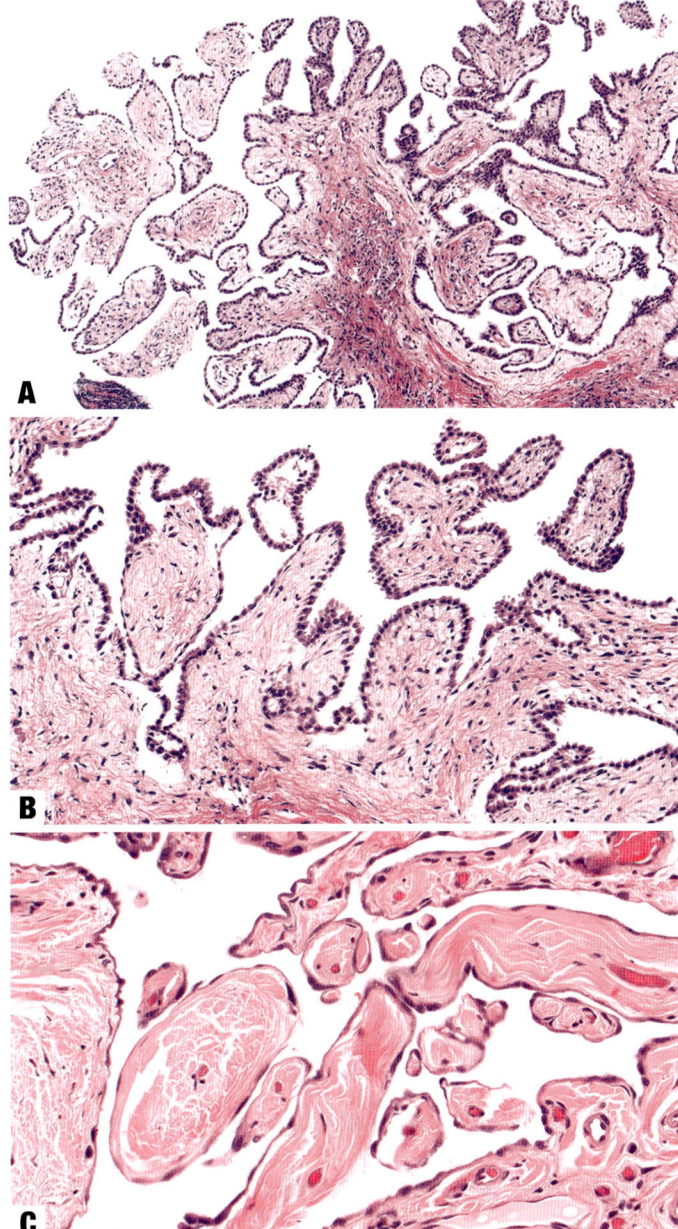

Fig. 2.03 Well-differentiated papillary mesothelial tumour. **A** Low-power examination shows arborescent papillary formations. **B** Papillae are covered by a single layer of bland mesothelial cells. **C** Although typically myxoid or fibrous, the papillary cores are sometimes hyalinized.

"well-differentiated papillary mesothelial tumour", rather than the historical term "well-differentiated papillary mesothelioma", is recommended. Mesothelial proliferations with the appearance of WDPMT that show focal invasion have a propensity for multifocality and recurrence, but they are rarely fatal {528}.

Whether pleural WDPMT is a precursor of diffuse mesothelioma is unresolved {579}. Exceptional cases of pleural WDPMT with concomitant or subsequent diffuse mesothelioma show BAP1 loss in both neoplasms, raising the possibility of a clonal relationship {1630}.

Mesothelioma in situ

Dacic S
de Perrot M
Gill RR
Hiroshima K
Klebe S
Nabeshima K

Definition
Mesothelioma in situ is a preinvasive single-layer surface proliferation of neoplastic mesothelial cells.

ICD-O coding
9050/2 Mesothelioma in situ

ICD-11 coding
None

Related terminology
None

Subtype(s)
None

Localization
Mesothelioma in situ occurs on the serosal surfaces, including pleura (parietal and/or visceral) and peritoneum.

Clinical features
Mesothelioma in situ is clinically suspected in patients presenting with non-resolving pleural effusion(s) in the setting of heavy asbestos exposure, with or without pleural plaques, after irradiation and in patients with familial predisposition {533,2103,2243}. The diagnosis is made on the basis of a combination of clinical, imaging, and pathological features. No mass lesions are identified on imaging or thoracoscopy.

The diagnosis requires submission of sufficient tissue for diagnosis – in most instances, this requires thoracoscopic evaluation with large biopsy samples (ideally 100–200 mm²) of different areas of the pleura in patients with non-resolving effusions. Small biopsy and cytology samples are not appropriate.

Because of the variable and long latency period, no current screening guidelines or imaging strategies are currently in

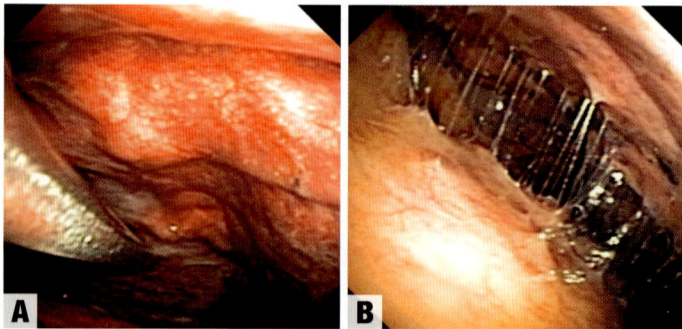

Fig. 2.04 Mesothelioma in situ. **A** Thoracoscopic inspection of pleura with no evidence of nodules or thickening. **B** Thoracoscopic inspection of pleura with no evidence of thickening or nodules. Adhesions are present between the two surfaces.

practice. However, if the pathology is inconclusive, patients are longitudinally followed with regular CT to ensure that an invasive component was not missed during the initial workup. After that, patients can be followed as required within a multidisciplinary setting {955}.

Epidemiology
To date, very few cases of pleural mesothelioma in situ have been reported worldwide, with a male predominance and an age range of 67–79 years {534,533,1928,2395}.

Etiology
See *Tumours of the pleura and pericardium: Introduction* (p. 194).

Pathogenesis
BAP1 inactivation and *CDKN2A* homozygous deletion are considered to be early events in mesothelioma development {1166, 534,533,1928,601A,497A}. In animal models, it has been shown that inactivation of *BAP1* cooperates with loss of either *NF2* or *CDKN2A* to drive development of mesothelioma {1545}.

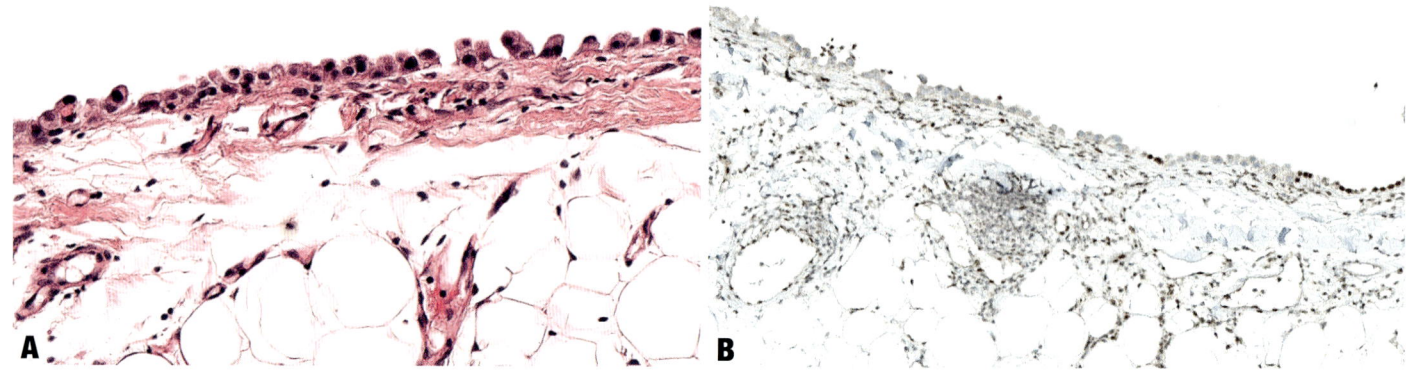

Fig. 2.05 Mesothelioma in situ. **A** Parietal pleura with a single layer of cuboidal mesothelial cells with mild cytological atypia. **B** BAP1 loss is seen within tumoural mesothelial cells, with retention of staining (right) within non-neoplastic mesothelial cells.

Macroscopic appearance

At thoracoscopy, no mass is identified; visually normal pleura, smooth pleural thickening, and tiny nodules are all described {534,533}.

Histopathology

Mesothelioma in situ shows a layer of flat or cuboidal cells with or without minimal cytological atypia, without evidence of invasion {533,534}. The cells have bland nuclear features and may have a prominent nucleolus {533,3294}. Mitoses are typically absent. Other appearances include small papillary projections or small nodules that may show moderate to severe cytological atypia {533,3294,2395}.

Immunohistochemistry

The diagnosis of mesothelioma in situ cannot be made on H&E stains. Loss of BAP1 nuclear expression by immunohistochemistry and/or CDKN2A homozygous deletion identified either by FISH or by MTAP immunohistochemistry (cytoplasmic staining) must be demonstrated using a validated assay with appropriate internal controls and external quality assurance {2103,533, 534}. Loss of these markers in isolation of other data does not exclude malignancy. This workup should be limited to patients with non-resolving pleural effusions or for whom there is clinical suspicion of mesothelioma {2103}.

Differential diagnosis

Reactive mesothelial proliferation can usually be distinguished from mesothelioma in situ by BAP1 and/or MTAP immunohistochemistry and/or FISH for CDKN2A homozygous deletion. These ancillary studies are not helpful in the differential diagnosis of other malignant processes. Surface spread of adjacent invasive mesothelioma can be difficult to distinguish from mesothelioma in situ, and a correlation with imaging studies and intraoperative findings is essential in order to avoid the misinterpretation of a non-representative sample. Well-differentiated papillary mesothelial tumour can be difficult to differentiate from mesothelioma in situ, and thoracoscopy showing a granular pleural surface or multiple millimetre-sized pleural nodules favours the former.

Cytology

Cytological evaluation of pleural fluid, including morphological assessment and ancillary studies for BAP1, MTAP, and/or p16 (CDKN2A), can be an initial screening test for malignant mesothelial proliferation, but it is not diagnostic {3191,214,1961,1465}. Specific diagnosis of mesothelioma in situ cannot be made in

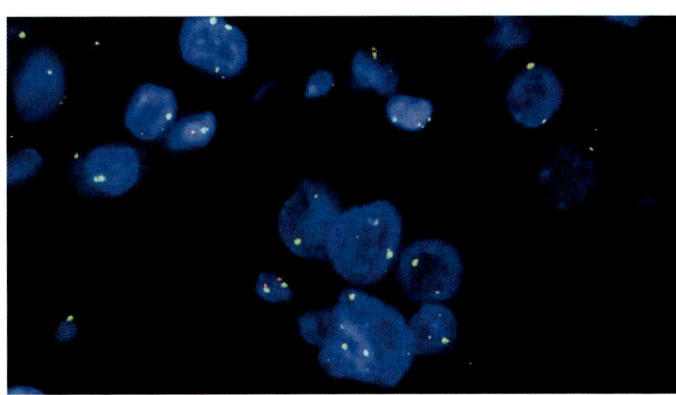

Fig. 2.06 Mesothelioma in situ. *CDKN2A* FISH showing loss of signal (homozygous deletion) in a papillary cluster and flat mesothelial cells.

cytology specimens in isolation of clinical data, because the presence of invasion cannot be excluded.

Diagnostic molecular pathology

Immunohistochemical detection of loss of BAP1 nuclear staining or MTAP cytoplasmic staining as a surrogate for FISH *CDKN2A* homozygous deletion discriminates neoplastic from benign mesothelial proliferations in histological sections or cell blocks {1213,214,452,215}.

Essential and desirable diagnostic criteria

Essential:
- Pleural effusion (non-resolving)
- No thoracoscopic or imaging evidence of tumour
- Single layer of mesothelial cells (with or without atypia) on pleural surface
- No histological features of invasive growth
- Loss of BAP1 and/or MTAP by immunohistochemistry and/or *CDKN2A* homozygous deletion by FISH
- Multidisciplinary discussion of diagnosis

Staging

The clinical TNM staging system does not currently have a category for mesothelioma in situ, and there are currently no data to support assignment of a separate category.

Prognosis and prediction

Mesothelioma in situ may progress to invasive epithelioid mesothelioma {533}. The prognosis is unknown and depends on the risk of progression to invasive mesothelioma, which can reach 70% after a median follow-up of 5 years {533}.

Localized pleural mesothelioma

Khoor A
Bironzo P
Bueno R
Nowak AK
Schmitt F

Definition

Localized mesothelioma is a rare malignant neoplasm of mesothelial cell origin that occurs as a circumscribed mass with no clinical or histological evidence of diffuse serosal spread.

ICD-O coding

9050/3 Localized mesothelioma

ICD-11 coding

2C26.0 Mesothelioma of pleura

Related terminology

Acceptable: localized mesothelioma.
Not recommended: localized malignant mesothelioma; solitary malignant mesothelioma.

Subtype(s)

Epithelioid mesothelioma; sarcomatoid mesothelioma (including desmoplastic); biphasic mesothelioma

Localization

Most cases (82–88%) occur as an intrathoracic mass localized to the pleura, chest wall, lung, or mediastinum {1800}. Extrathoracic sites of origin include the abdominal wall, fallopian tube, gastric serosa, hepatic capsule, tunica albuginea, and broad ligament.

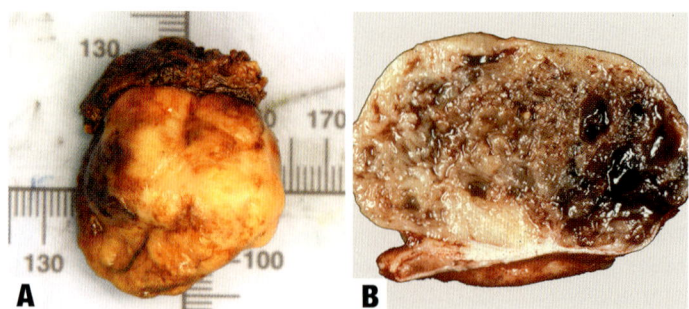

Fig. 2.07 Localized mesothelioma. **A** Macroscopic appearance of a localized tumour on the pleural surface. **B** This mesothelioma consists of a circumscribed pleural-based mass. The cut surface is tan-brown, with focal haemorrhage and cystic changes.

Clinical features

Patients can be asymptomatic or present with chest pain, dyspnoea, or other symptoms related to compression of various structures {1800}. Imaging studies reveal a mass lesion that is clinically suspicious for sarcoma or metastasis to the serosal membranes {3388}.

Epidemiology

The tumour is rare and poorly recognized; approximately 160 cases have been reported {1800}. Men are more often

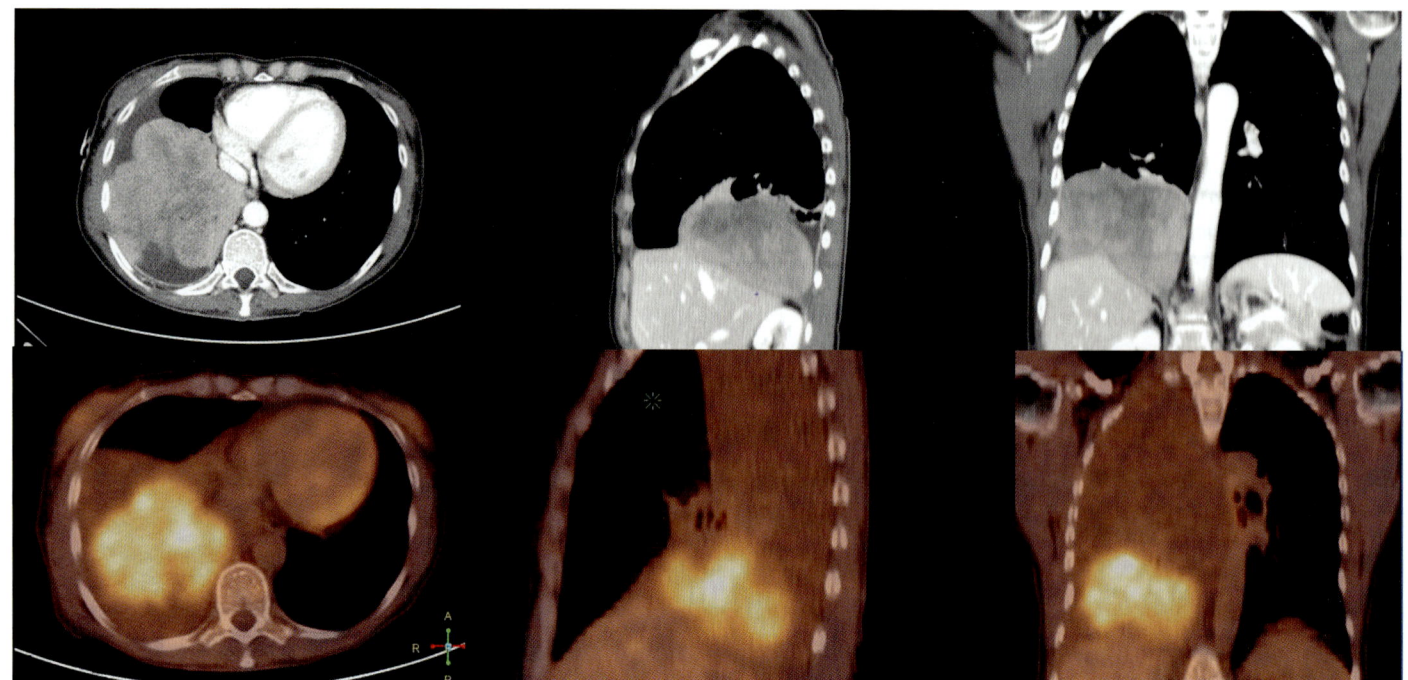

Fig. 2.08 Localized mesothelioma. CT and PET-CT of a 52-year-old woman with a localized epithelioid pleural mesothelioma. An FDG-avid circumscribed tumour is present in the right lower chest abutting the diaphragm.

affected than women (M:F ratio: 2.7:1). Patients range in age from 6 to 82 years, with a mean age of 59 years.

Etiology
Localized mesothelioma appears to show a loose association with exposure to asbestos. Approximately 37% of the reported patients have a history of asbestos exposure, which, in general, is poorly documented with no clear characterization of the fibre type and levels of exposure {1800}.

Pathogenesis
BAP1 mutations, *TRAF7* mutations, and genomic near-haploidization have recently been described as potential pathogenetic pathways in localized mesothelioma {1209}.

Macroscopic appearance
Localized mesothelioma is a solitary, circumscribed mass attached to the pleura or other serosal surfaces {3388}.

Histopathology
The histopathological, ultrastructural, and immunophenotypic features of localized mesothelioma are identical to those of diffuse mesothelioma {594,63,1785,1800}. Approximately 55% of the tumours are epithelioid lesions; others exhibit biphasic or sarcomatoid morphology. Rare epithelioid localized mesotheliomas with pleomorphic, microcystic, and rhabdoid features have also been described. Occasional sarcomatoid tumours showed desmoplastic or lymphohistiocytoid differentiation.

Immunohistochemistry
Immunohistochemistry is the same as in diffuse mesothelioma.

Differential diagnosis
The differential diagnosis includes solitary fibrous tumour (see *Solitary fibrous tumour of the thorax*, p. 284), metastatic carcinoma and sarcoma (see *Metastasis to the pleura*, p. 459), primary pleural and peripherally located pulmonary synovial and other sarcomas (see *Synovial sarcoma of the thorax*, p. 314), and diffuse mesothelioma (see *Diffuse pleural mesothelioma*, p. 204).

Cytology
FNA can be diagnostic of localized mesothelioma, especially the epithelioid subtype, by revealing malignant cells identical to those described in diffuse mesothelioma (see *Diffuse pleural mesothelioma*, p. 204). Pleural fluid cytology should be negative for malignant cells in these patients by definition {1800}.

Diagnostic molecular pathology
Diagnostic molecular pathology is the same as for diffuse mesothelioma (see *Diffuse pleural mesothelioma*, p. 204).

Essential and desirable diagnostic criteria
Essential:
- Presentation as a solitary localized mass by imaging, surgical findings, and histology
- Examination of a surgical resection specimen showing lack of invasion beyond the circumscribed borders of the tumour
- Histological features of diffuse mesothelioma
- Immunohistochemical evidence of mesothelial origin

Desirable:
- Multidisciplinary discussion to confirm the diagnosis

Staging
Staging is the same as for diffuse pleural mesothelioma.

Prognosis and prediction
Patients are usually treated with surgical resection {2060}, which is sometimes supplemented by chemotherapy and/or radiation therapy {1800}. In earlier series, the median survival time of patients with localized mesothelioma reported in the English-language literature ranged from 12 to 36 months, with a pooled median survival time of 29 months {936A}. However, in a more recent study, for 51 localized mesothelioma patients diagnosed by the International Mesothelioma Panel, the median survival time was 134 months {1800}. Patients with complete resection and epithelioid histology have a better prognosis than those with postsurgical residual disease and/or sarcomatoid or biphasic histology.

Diffuse pleural mesothelioma

Sauter JL
Bueno R
Dacic S
Gill RR
Husain AN

Kadota K
Ladanyi M
Nowak AK
Schmitt F

Definition
Diffuse mesothelioma is a tumour of malignant mesothelial cells showing diffuse involvement of the pleura or pericardium.

ICD-O coding
9050/3 Diffuse mesothelioma, NOS

ICD-11 coding
2C26.0 Mesothelioma of pleura
2C28.1 Mesothelioma of pericardium

Related terminology
Not recommended:
Epithelial-type mesothelioma; epithelial mesothelioma.
Sarcomatous mesothelioma.
Mixed mesothelioma; mixed epithelioid and sarcomatoid mesothelioma; mixed epithelioid and sarcomatous mesothelioma.

Subtype(s)
Epithelioid mesothelioma; sarcomatoid mesothelioma (including desmoplastic); biphasic mesothelioma

Localization
There is no significant difference in location between the histological subtypes of pleural mesothelioma. Right-sided involvement is more common than left-sided by a 3:2 ratio. Bilateral involvement at diagnosis is unusual {3394}.

Pericardial mesotheliomas are localized to the pericardium, without a primary lesion in the pleura. Most pericardial mesotheliomas are diffuse mesotheliomas. Localized mesothelial tumours such as well-differentiated papillary mesothelial tumour are exceedingly rare in the pericardium {2000,2621}.

Diffuse mesotheliomas must be differentiated from localized mesotheliomas due to different clinical behaviour.

Clinical features
Presenting symptoms
Pleural mesothelioma: Initial presenting symptoms of diffuse mesothelioma usually include dyspnoea, unilateral chest pain or discomfort, cough, unintended weight loss, low-grade fever, and night sweats {761,1148,2656}. A frequent initial manifestation is symptomatic unilateral pleural effusion, with dyspnoea and a cough, which can resolve on effusion drainage. Less commonly, pleural effusion or thickening may be identified incidentally or during screening after known asbestos exposure. Patients presenting with pleural effusion only, or on screening, may have a more indolent clinical course. As pleural thickening advances, chest wall contraction occurs, and chest pain can be prominent, often including neuropathic characteristics from involvement of adjacent intercostal nerves, and bone pain from rib invasion or pathological fractures. Reduced ipsilateral chest expansion on examination is common, as is dullness to percussion and

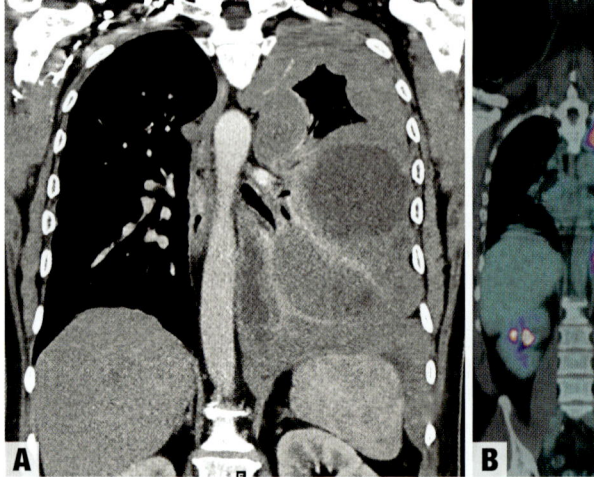

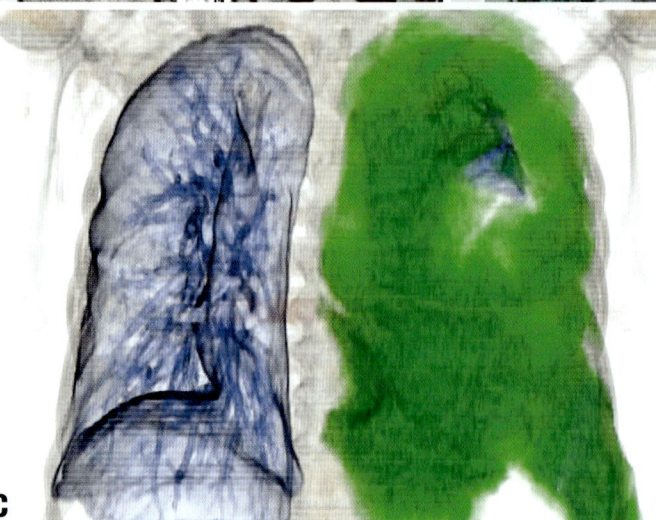

Fig. 2.09 Radiology of diffuse malignant pleural mesothelioma. **A** Coronal CT showing diffuse circumferential pleural thickening surrounding the left pleural space and a moderate loculated effusion and complete atelectasis of the left lower lobe, as well as partial atelectasis in the left upper lobe. **B** Coronal fused FDG PET-CT showing moderate avidity within the pleural tumour. **C** Volume-rendered radiology image showing the circumferential pleural tumour (green) encasing the left lung.

reduced volume breath sounds, even when pleural effusion is not present. Neuropathic arm pain, occasionally with sensory or motor deficits, can occur from apical disease involving the brachial plexus, and palpable cervical lymphadenopathy may be seen. Later findings include externally palpable chest wall masses, abdominal pain and distension from peritoneal involvement leading to ascites or intra-abdominal masses, and symptoms of pericardial effusion. However, all these findings can be present at diagnosis. Some patients present with acute pleuritic chest pain and small effusion, and initial investigations may fail to provide a diagnosis. Patients may remain symptom-free for

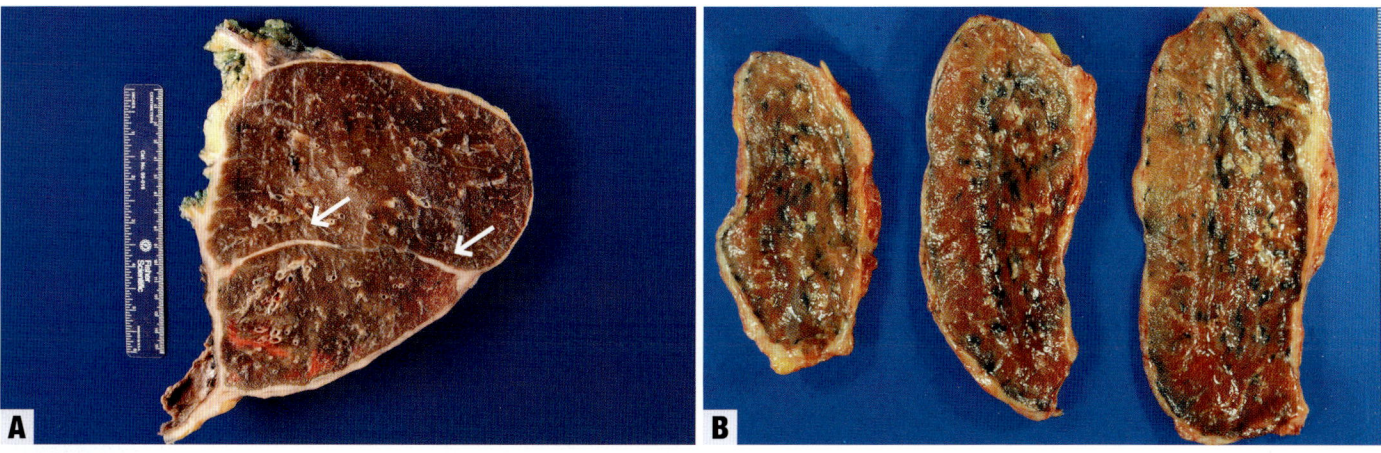

Fig. 2.10 A Diffuse mesothelioma. The tumour encases the lung as a rind and grows along the interlobar septa (arrows), compressing the lung parenchyma. **B** Pseudomesotheliomatous adenocarcinoma. The tumour encases the lung, mimicking a mesothelioma.

months until recurrence of fluid or development of chest pain leads to further investigation. Unusual misleading presentations include recurrent pneumothoraces {2641} and diffuse intrapulmonary mesothelioma masquerading as interstitial lung disease {1597}. Mesothelioma can occur as a distant metastasis.

Pericardial mesothelioma: Patients with primary pericardial mesotheliomas may present with symptoms related to a mass in the pericardium, which may cause compression of the heart. Pericardial effusion is often asymptomatic, with tamponade as disease progresses.

Imaging

Pleural mesothelioma: Imaging of diffuse pleural mesothelioma is complex because of its rind-like circumferential growth, usually arising from diaphragmatic surface of pleura and extending along pleural reflections with propensity to invade multiple structures simultaneously {952}. Radiographic assessment includes characterization of pleural involvement and determination of extent of disease and invasion of adjacent structures to determine resectability, clinical staging, and response to therapy {953,956,1109}. The imaging appearance of diffuse pleural mesothelioma most often consists of a circumferential rind of nodular pleura, usually associated with ipsilateral effusion. Less commonly, a pleural effusion without obvious pleural nodularity is seen. Rarely, an isolated nodular pleural density is seen, with or without an effusion. Pleural plaques are present in 20% of mesothelioma on CT {2243}. CT-derived tumour volume and maximum standardized uptake value > 10 on FDG PET-CT have been shown to be prognostic {957,954,2571,940}.

Pericardial mesothelioma: Echocardiography and CT of pericardial mesothelioma show cardiac enlargement, with pericardium thickened by tumour nodules and associated effusion {2627}.

Tumour spread

Pleural mesothelioma: Disease progression is variable. Growth is often characterized by diffuse pleural thickening, with areas of nodularity, ranging from subtle nodularity within diffuse thickening throughout to large pleural masses. Spread generally occurs along interlobar fissures, extending into lung, diaphragm, and/or chest wall. Mediastinal involvement, with direct invasion of pericardium and other mediastinal structures, is common. Progression of disease more often occurs by local extension into chest wall and lung than by haematogenous spread. However, lymphangitic involvement is more common in the epithelioid type, particularly with micropapillary pattern {1344}. Mediastinal lymphadenopathy develops, and it may occur without hilar lymphadenopathy. Pericardial, peridiaphragmatic, internal mammary, supraclavicular, abdominal, and intercostal lymph node involvement is frequent during progression {2476}. Although development of early symptomatic systemic metastases is unusual, tumour involvement of extrathoracic sites is common in end-stage disease. More than 85% of patients in postmortem series have disease beyond the ipsilateral hemithorax {838}. Disease dissemination is most commonly via invasion of contiguous structures, with transdiaphragmatic spread, invasion of liver or spleen, pericardial invasion, and involvement of contralateral pleural space. Haematologically disseminated metastases to lung, bone, liver, and brain also occur. The clinical symptoms and imaging findings described above are not specific and may be seen in other pleural tumours, including metastases.

Pericardial mesothelioma: Pericardial mesotheliomas are locally aggressive and may extend to pleura, encase heart and great vessels, and invade the mediastinum {2450}. Distant metastasis has not been reported.

Epidemiology

See *Tumours of the pleura and pericardium: Introduction* (p. 194).

Etiology

See *Tumours of the pleura and pericardium: Introduction* (p. 194).

Pathogenesis

The pathogenesis of mesothelioma is complex. Mechanisms include chronic inflammation, deregulation of cell death, and genomic copy-number losses and some gains. Asbestos causes genotoxic effects (mutagenic and clastogenic) and nongenotoxic effects.

Somatic mutation burden in mesothelioma is low, usually < 2 non-synonymous mutations per megabase, and with no difference between the histological subtypes {330}.

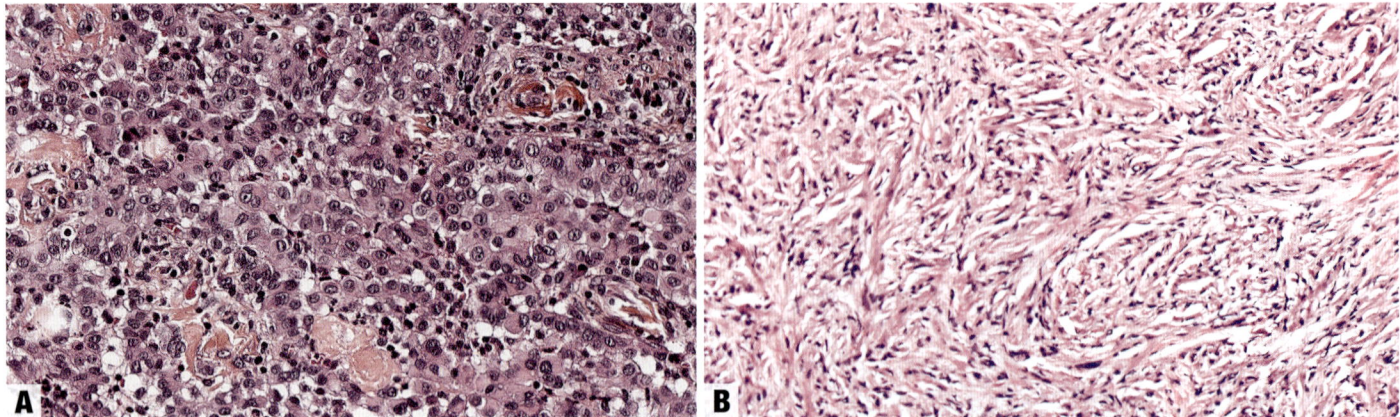

Fig. 2.11 Diffuse mesothelioma. **A** Epithelioid mesothelioma characterized by rounded cells with eosinophilic cytoplasm and round nuclei with small nucleoli. The tumour shown here demonstrates the solid pattern of epithelioid mesothelioma. **B** Sarcomatoid mesothelioma characterized by malignant spindle-shaped cells within a fibrous stroma.

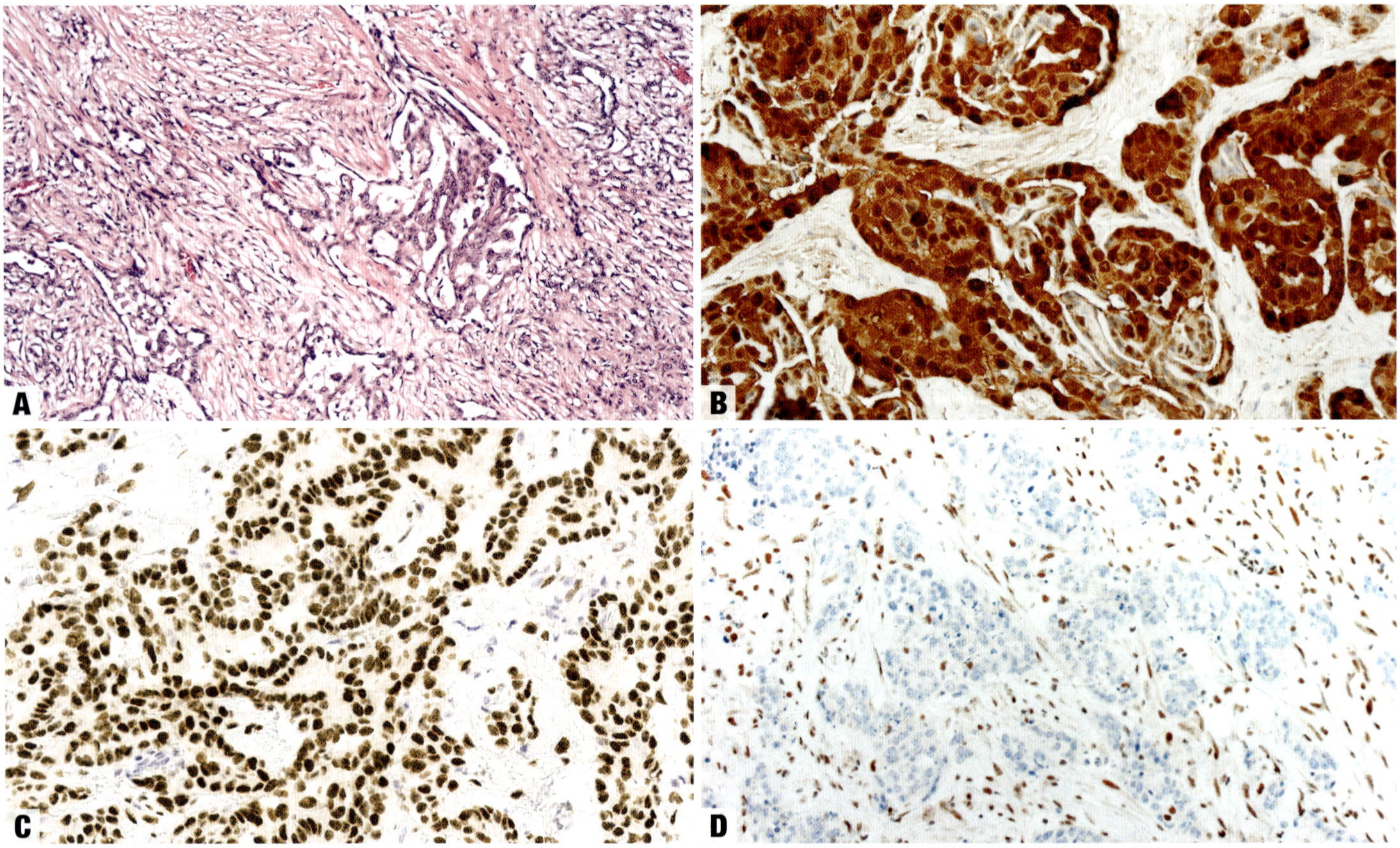

Fig. 2.12 Diffuse biphasic mesothelioma. **A** Biphasic mesothelioma shows both epithelioid and sarcomatoid malignant areas. **B–D** Immunohistochemistry shows positive cytoplasmic and nuclear staining for calretinin (**B**), positive nuclear staining for WT1 (**C**), and loss of BAP1 (**D**). The BAP1 stains the nuclei of benign stromal cells as a positive internal control.

Comprehensive genomic analyses have demonstrated that the most frequently mutated genes include *BAP1*, *NF2*, *TP53*, *SETD2*, *DDX3X*, *ULK2*, *RYR2*, *CFAP45*, *SETDB1*, and *DDX51*. In patients with germline mutations (including in *BAP1*; see *BAP1 tumour predisposition syndrome*, p. 476), exposure to even small amounts of asbestos increases risk of mesothelioma {2763}.

Most pleural mesotheliomas with inactivating mutations in *BAP1* also have concurrent loss of heterozygosity on chromosome 3p21. A recent study suggests that loss of BAP1 may serve as a predictive biomarker for immunotherapy in peritoneal mesothelioma {2763}. Similarly, The Cancer Genome Atlas (TCGA) data in pleural mesothelioma found that BAP1-altered pleural mesotheliomas have an mRNA signature of activated dendritic cells and tend to show higher expression of PDL1 (CD274) {1581}. RNA sequencing data from 216 pleural mesotheliomas found mostly sarcomatoid mesotheliomas to be positive for PDL1 (CD274) {330}. The same study showed

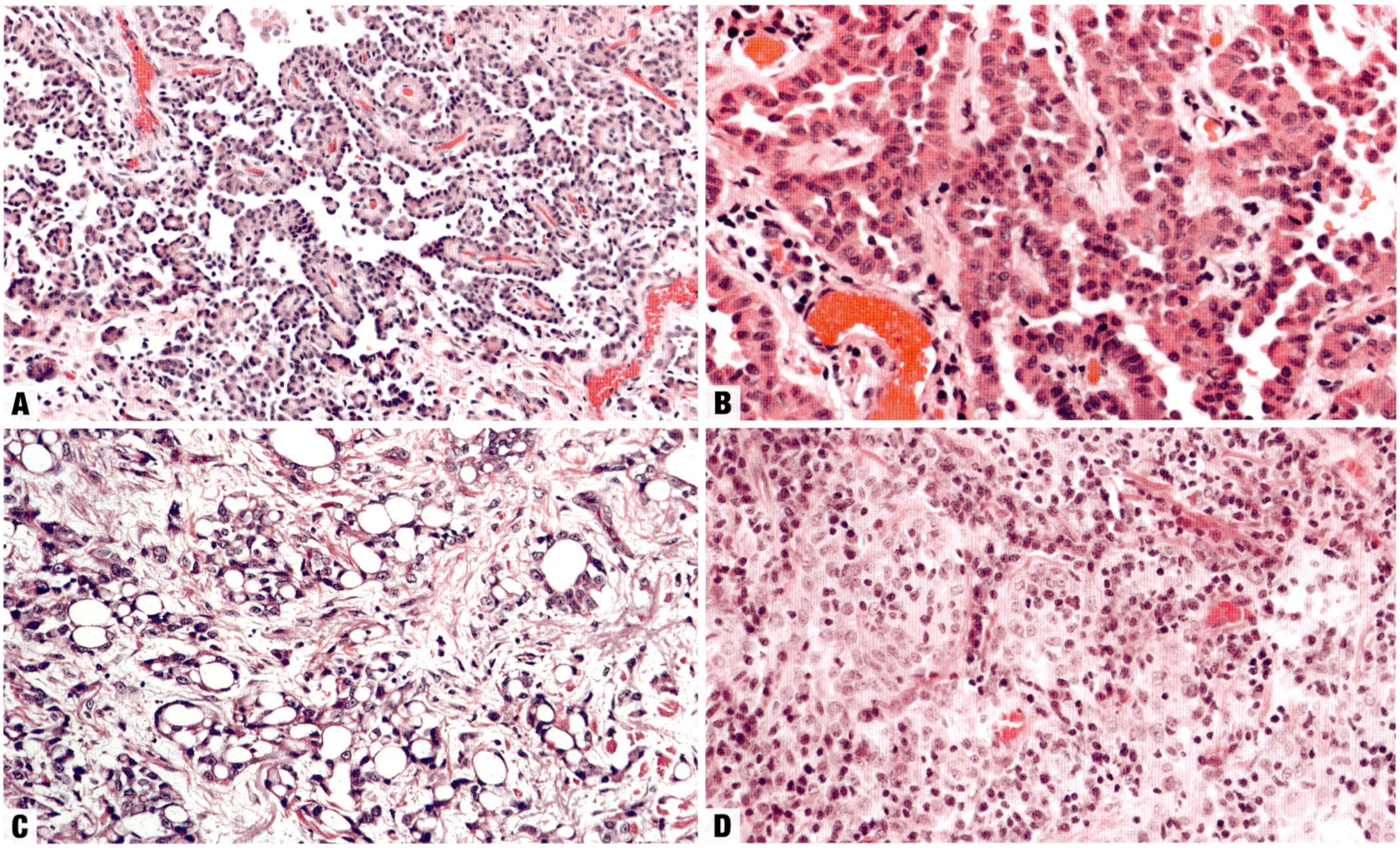

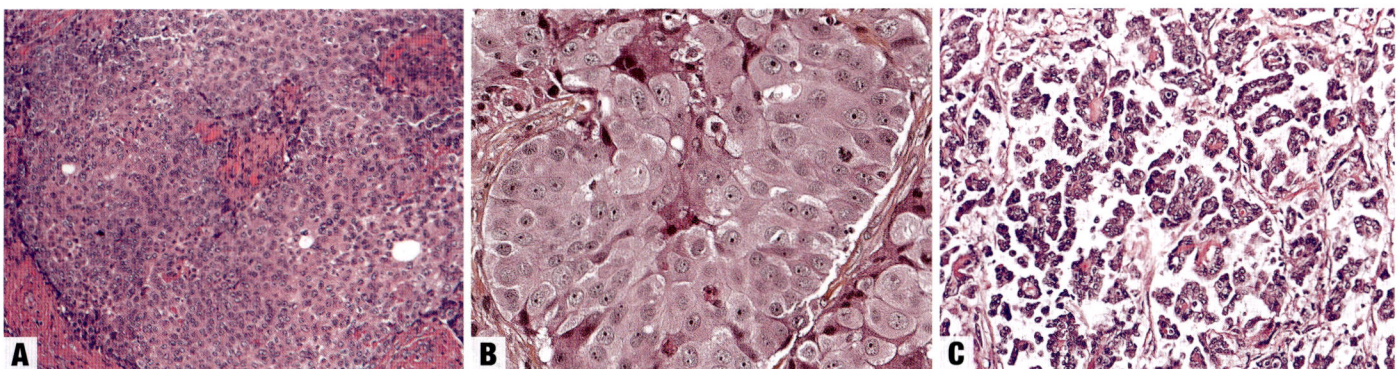

Fig. 2.13 Histological patterns considered favourable in diffuse epithelioid mesothelioma. **A** Tubulopapillary pattern, a combination of tubular and papillary patterns, which is commonly seen in epithelioid mesothelioma. **B** Trabecular pattern, characterized by interconnected linear arrangements of single or dual layers of malignant epithelioid cells. **C** Adenomatoid pattern, composed of gland-like structures lined by flat to cuboidal malignant epithelioid cells resembling adenomatoid tumour. **D** Lymphohistiocytoid pattern with prominent stromal lymphocytes.

that somatic alterations in significantly mutated genes such as *BAP1*, *NF2*, and *TP53* resulted in multiple neoepitopes predicted to be immunogenic {330}. Among all tumour types analysed by TCGA, neoplastic cells of epithelioid pleural mesotheliomas have the highest expression of *VSIR* (*VISTA*), an immune checkpoint gene that inhibits anti-tumour immune responses {1166,51}. In contrast, PDL1 is expressed in approximately 30% of epithelioid mesotheliomas, which in part may explain lack of response to anti-PD(L)1/CTLA-4 therapies {2023,1899,412, 567}. Sarcomatoid mesotheliomas show the opposite, with high

PDL1 expression and infrequent VISTA expression by immunohistochemistry {2023}.

Through exome analysis, the tumour suppressor *TP53* was found to be mutated in 8% of mesotheliomas and was associated with aggressive clinical behaviour {330}. In the TCGA cohort, a subset of mesotheliomas with *TP53* and *SETDB1* co-mutations associated with genome-wide loss of heterozygosity that affects > 80% of the genome ("genomic near-haploidization") was identified mostly in young female patients (M:F ratio: 1:4) {1166}.

Fig. 2.14 Histological patterns considered unfavourable in diffuse epithelioid mesothelioma are solid pattern (**A,B**) (mesothelioma consisting of continuous sheets of malignant epithelioid cells) and micropapillary pattern (**C**), which shows small groups of epithelioid cells forming papillary structures but lacking true fibrovascular cores.

Table 2.02 Histological classification of diffuse pleural mesothelioma {2103}

Type	Description	Patterns/features	Favourable	Unfavourable	Reporting
Epithelioid mesothelioma	Composed of round, epithelioid cells, usually with cohesive architecture, but single cells within a fibrous stroma may also be seen	Architectural patterns: Tubulopapillary Trabecular Adenomatoid Solid Micropapillary	Architectural patterns: Tubulopapillary Trabecular Adenomatoid	Architectural patterns: Solid (≥ 50%) Micropapillary	Grade (high or low), architectural patterns present (and in definitive resection specimens such as EPD and EPP, percentages of each pattern; for all other specimens, indicate "with ... patterns/features")
		Cytological features: Rhabdoid Deciduoid[a] Small cell[a] Clear cell[a] Signet ring[a] Lymphohistiocytoid Pleomorphic	Cytological features: Lymphohistiocytoid Low nuclear grade[b]	Cytological features: Rhabdoid Pleomorphic High nuclear grade[b]	
		Stromal features: Myxoid	Stromal features: Myxoid (if predominant, i.e. when ≥ 50% of tumour with < 50% solid pattern contains myxoid stroma)	Necrosis (included in grading)	
Sarcomatoid mesothelioma, including desmoplastic pattern	Composed of elongated/spindle cells (> 2 times longer than wide) arranged in solid sheets or within a fibrous stroma	Cytological features: Lymphohistiocytoid Transitional Pleomorphic	Cytological features: Lymphohistiocytoid	Cytological features: Transitional	
		Stromal features: Desmoplastic With heterologous differentiation			
Biphasic mesothelioma	Showing both epithelioid and sarcomatoid components (in definitive resection specimens, namely EPD and EPP, ≥ 10% of each component is required for diagnosis); for smaller samples, including biopsy and cytology specimens, the diagnosis of biphasic mesothelioma can be rendered regardless of percentages of each component present				Percentage of each component should be reported regardless of specimen type

EPD, extended pleurectomy/decortication; EPP, extrapleural pneumonectomy.
[a]These cytological features carry no prognostic significance but are important to recognize to avoid misdiagnosis with other entities in the differential diagnosis.
[b]See Box 2.01 (p. 210) for nuclear grading.

Somatic copy-number alterations in mesothelioma include frequent recurring focal or arm-level deletions, but no amplifications. Homozygous deletion of *CDKN2A* ranges between 67% and 83% in epithelioid and biphasic mesotheliomas, with rates approaching 100% in the sarcomatoid subtype. *CDKN2A* is frequently co-deleted with *MTAP*, the adjacent gene on 9p21, which encodes the protein MTAP whose deficiency may increase sensitivity to PRMT inhibitors {1851,805}. Loss of *CDKN2A* is strongly associated with shorter overall survival. *NF2* deletions and losses occur in about 30–40% of pleural mesotheliomas. *NF2* inactivation has not been associated with a specific histological subtype of mesothelioma or prognosis. Recurrent copy losses that include the genes *LATS1* and *LATS2*, key members of the Hippo signalling pathway, have also been reported {330, 1943,3061}.

RNA sequencing data for gene fusions are somewhat inconsistent. Recurrent fusions involving *NF2*, *BAP1*, *SETD2*, *PBRM1*, and *PTEN* have been reported {330}. *ALK* fusions were reported in rare cases of peritoneal mesothelioma in children and young adults {1210,1905,1620A}. *EWSR1* fusions have been found in rare cases of epithelioid pleural and peritoneal mesotheliomas occurring in younger patients without history of asbestos exposure {675,2254}. No gene fusions were identified in the TCGA cohort of 73 pleural mesotheliomas {1166}.

Unlike with pleural mesothelioma, the link between asbestos exposure and pericardial mesothelioma is weak, with one review reporting only 14% of patients with documented asbestos exposure {1091,1888,2285,2516,3034}. Radiation-associated mesothelioma following radiation treatment for other malignancies is another etiopathogenic mechanism of both pleural and pericardial mesotheliomas {505,2042}.

Macroscopic appearance

Pleural mesothelioma: Once invasive, early diffuse pleural mesothelioma appears macroscopically as multiple small nodules scattered in parietal pleura, less frequently in visceral pleura, or as a pleural-based mass, usually with limited spread into the lung parenchyma. As disease progresses, nodules coalesce, forming a rind encasing underlying lung. Growth typically occurs along interlobar fissures and can invade lung parenchyma, chest wall skeletal muscle, or skin. Grossly, the tumour is grey-white, soft, and with or without cystic areas containing mucoid-like material.

Pericardial mesothelioma: This typically involves the pericardium diffusely, forming multiple nodules along its surface. Involvement of great vessels is common. Infiltration into myocardium is uncommon {1155}.

Histopathology

Mesotheliomas are classified as epithelioid, sarcomatoid (including desmoplastic), and biphasic subtypes. Several architectural patterns, cytological features, and stromal features need to be recognized – some because they have prognostic value and others in order to avoid misdiagnosis. The histological classification of diffuse pleural mesothelioma is summarized in Table 2.02.

Epithelioid mesothelioma

Epithelioid mesothelioma is often cytologically bland, but marked cytological atypia can occur {2210,1344,310,530}. Cells typically display eosinophilic cytoplasm, round nuclei with vesicular chromatin, small nucleoli, and infrequent mitoses, but coarse chromatin, prominent nucleoli, and high mitotic count can be seen in poorly differentiated tumours {1213}.

Architectural patterns: There are a wide range of architectural patterns, and several are often observed in the same tumour. Common patterns include tubulopapillary, trabecular, micropapillary, and solid, while adenomatoid is less common. The solid pattern is composed of solid sheets of cohesive tumour cells. The tubulopapillary pattern exhibits varying combinations of tubules and papillae, with connective tissue cores and/or clefts lined by a range of relatively bland cuboidal cells to larger more atypical cells. The trabecular pattern consists of relatively small, uniform cells forming thin cords, or sometimes a single-file arrangement. The adenomatoid pattern shows microcystic structures with lace-lake or signet-ring appearance. The micropapillary pattern consists of papillary structures lacking fibrovascular cores. Psammoma bodies may be seen.

Cytological features: Clear cell features show large cells with clear cytoplasm and round central nuclei mimicking renal cell carcinoma or another clear cell carcinoma. Rhabdoid features are tumour cells with cytoplasmic eosinophilic globules that express cytokeratins and not muscle markers, resembling rhabdomyoblastic tumours {2207}. Cells with abundant eosinophilic cytoplasm, resembling deciduoid cells of pregnancy, can be observed in epithelioid mesothelioma (so-called deciduoid mesothelioma) {2205,2206,1197,2716}. Small tumour cells mimicking small cell carcinoma can be observed in rare cases; however, the term "small cell mesothelioma" is discouraged in diagnostic reports, to avoid confusion with small cell carcinoma {1852,2208}. Signet-ring features are the result of optically clear cytoplasmic vacuoles pushing the nucleus to one side within tumour cells. This is rarely seen and is important to recognize so as not to misdiagnose adenocarcinoma {2207A}. Pleomorphic features are characterized by tumour cells with prominent anaplastic nuclei, as well as bizarre nuclei often also containing

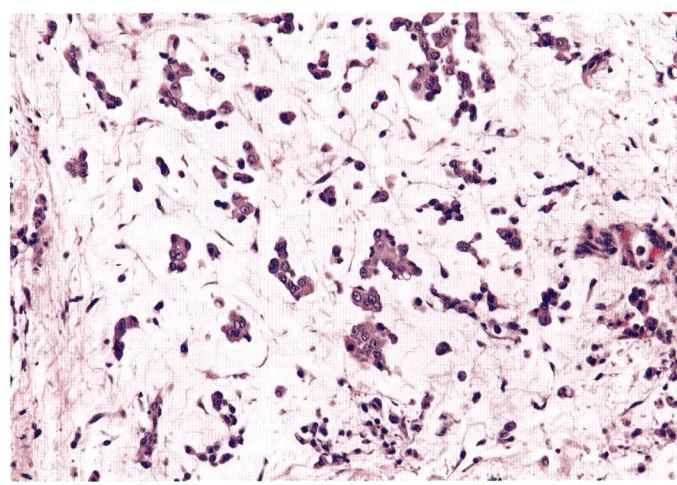

Fig. 2.15 Diffuse epithelioid mesothelioma. Stromal features seen in epithelioid mesothelioma include myxoid features; tumour cells lie within a pale haematoxyphilic mucoid stroma. This feature should be noted when ≥ 50% of a tumour with < 50% solid pattern shows this feature, which is prognostically favourable in this context.

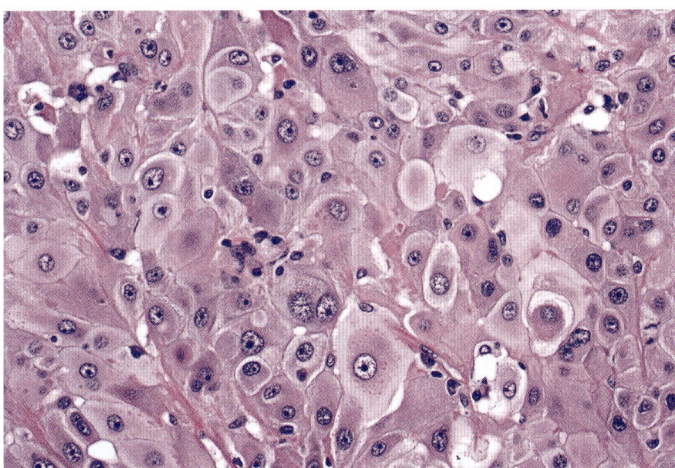

Fig. 2.16 Diffuse epithelioid mesothelioma. Deciduoid features consist of malignant epithelioid tumour cells that contain abundant richly eosinophilic cytoplasm, resembling decidua from the placenta.

multinucleated tumour giant cells. Recent studies have shown similar survival in patients with epithelioid mesotheliomas with pleomorphic features as in patients with sarcomatoid mesothelioma {1344,2210}. Therefore, reporting the presence of a pleomorphic component in epithelioid mesothelioma is important because of its aggressiveness. Lymphohistiocytoid features can mimic lymphoma or lymphoepithelial carcinoma and are characterized by marked lymphoid infiltrates composed of mainly CD8+ T lymphocytes obscuring polygonal malignant mesothelial cells that show histiocytoid morphology. Lymphohistiocytoid features do not simply represent prominent lymphocytic infiltration in an epithelioid mesothelioma {903,1408,3386, 1117}. Mesothelioma showing pleomorphic or lymphohistiocytoid features should be subtyped as epithelioid, biphasic, or sarcomatoid on the basis of the tumour cell morphology {3386}.

Stromal features: Fibrous stroma can vary from scant to prominent, showing varying degrees of cellularity from hyalinized acellular to highly cellular, which may make distinguishing a true sarcomatoid component difficult, and such tumours may be confused with biphasic mesothelioma. Myxoid change may be seen in a minority of cases, with single or nests of cytologically bland, often vacuolated epithelioid cells floating in a matrix of hyaluronate that shows hyaluronidase-sensitive staining with Alcian blue {52,2734}. Mesotheliomas are generally negative for neutral mucin using PASD or mucicarmine stains, but exceptions occur, limiting the diagnostic utility of these stains.

Grading of epithelioid mesothelioma: Although grading has not hitherto been performed in mesothelioma, a two-tiered system (low and high grade), combining nuclear grade (mitotic count and nuclear atypia) and presence of necrosis, has been proposed (see Box 2.01), because these features have been demonstrated to be strongly predictive of survival in patients with epithelioid mesothelioma {1343,2532,2103,3499}. Areas showing the highest-grade features should be used to assign tumours to low grade (any nuclear grade I and nuclear grade II without necrosis) or high grade (nuclear grade II with necrosis and any nuclear grade III). Grade should be routinely reported in both biopsy and resection specimens of diffuse epithelioid mesothelioma to help identify tumours that may behave more aggressively.

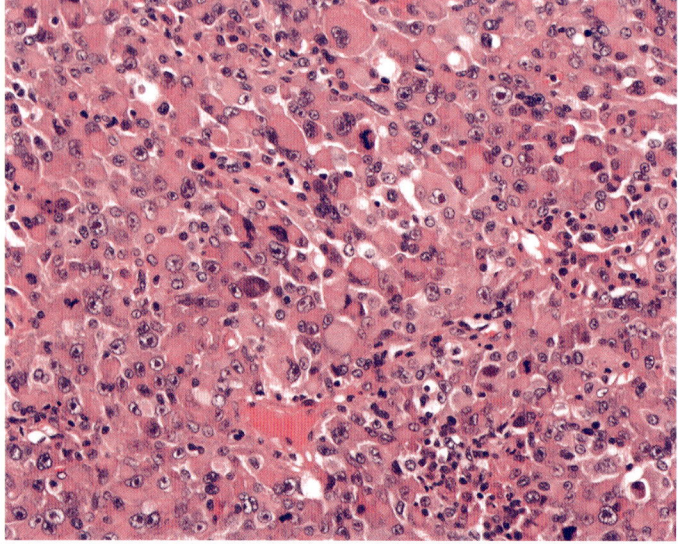

Fig. 2.17 Diffuse epithelioid mesothelioma. Rhabdoid features consist of tumour cells that resemble the rhabdoid cells seen in rhabdomyoblastic tumours, typically with a cytokeratin-positive eosinophilic cytoplasmic globule and usually negative for muscle markers. This is an unfavourable cytological feature when seen in epithelioid mesothelioma.

Sarcomatoid mesothelioma

Sarcomatoid mesothelioma is characterized by a proliferation of spindle cells arranged in fascicles or in haphazard patterns invading adipose tissue and/or lung parenchyma. Sarcomatoid mesothelioma may show a wide range of morphologies. Spindle cells are elongated (> 2 times as long as wide) and tapered, with nuclei that range from relatively bland to highly atypical/pleomorphic. Nucleoli may be prominent and multiple, with variable mitoses. Necrosis is frequent.

Cytological features: Transitional features are signified by elongated yet plump cells appearing intermediate between epithelioid and sarcomatoid in morphology, arranged in a sheet-like pattern, containing moderate cytoplasm and prominent nucleoli. These cells appear more round than sarcomatoid cells but more discohesive than epithelioid cells, and like in sarcomatoid mesotheliomas, reticulin stain highlights single cells. Recent studies have shown the presence of transitional features to be associated with worse prognosis {601,535,580}. In light of these data, a mesothelioma with transitional features is now classified under sarcomatoid mesothelioma. Sarcomatoid mesotheliomas with pleomorphic features show areas of large, pleomorphic, and atypical giant cells with multinucleation, marked atypia, hyperchromatic nuclei, and many mitoses (including bizarre mitoses) {1344}. See the *Epithelioid mesothelioma* subsection above for discussion of both pleomorphic and lymphohistiocytoid cytological features, which can both be seen in sarcomatoid as well as epithelioid mesothelioma.

Occasionally, heterologous elements, such as rhabdomyosarcoma, osteosarcoma, or chondrosarcoma, are present, and the term "with heterologous elements" is applied {1476}. These elements must be differentiated from osteoid and chondroid metaplasia. Any of these patterns may sometimes contain benign osteoclast-type giant cells.

Desmoplastic mesothelioma

Desmoplastic mesothelioma is a pattern of sarcomatoid mesothelioma characterized by spindle cells with minimal atypia arranged haphazardly in a so-called patternless pattern within a dense, hyalinized stroma {1782,561,1087}. Desmoplastic mesothelioma can be diagnosed in definitive resection specimens (extended pleurectomy/decortication [EPD] / extrapleural pneumonectomy [EPP]) if ≥ 50% of the tumour shows desmoplastic features. In small biopsy specimens, the term "with desmoplastic features" should be used {2103}.

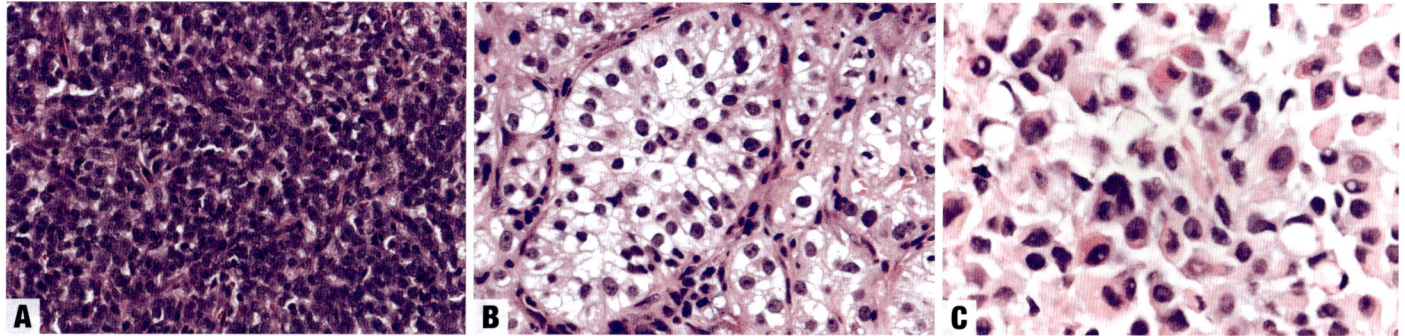

Fig. 2.18 Features seen in epithelioid mesothelioma that do not carry prognostic significance but are important to recognize to avoid misdiagnosis. **A** Small cell features. Some mesotheliomas are composed of small hyperchromatic tumour cells that morphologically resemble small cell carcinoma but demonstrate a mesothelial immunophenotype. **B** Some epithelioid mesotheliomas contain tumour cells with clear cytoplasm showing a mesothelial immunophenotype. **C** Signet-ring features. Rarely, epithelioid mesotheliomas contain tumour cells with intracytoplasmic vacuoles that push nuclei to the side and resemble a signet ring. It is important to recognize that signet-ring features can occur in mesotheliomas and to distinguish these tumours from signet-ring carcinomas from other sites by immunohistochemistry.

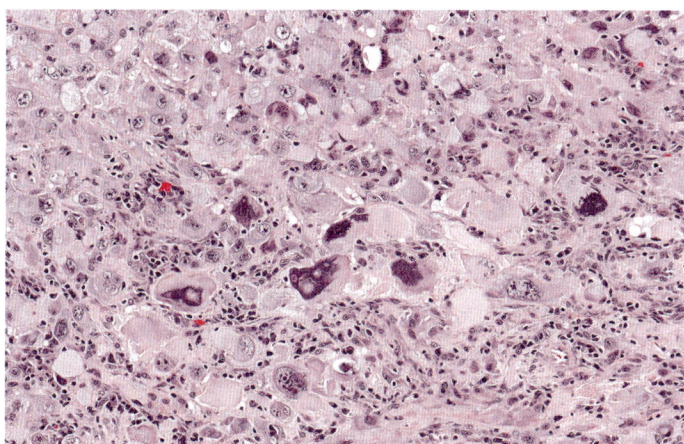

Fig. 2.19 Epithelioid mesothelioma with pleomorphic features. The tumour consists of malignant epithelioid cells with abundant cytoplasm. Some tumour cells are markedly enlarged, with highly atypical hyperchromatic nuclei.

Biphasic mesothelioma

Biphasic mesotheliomas are composed of both epithelioid and sarcomatoid morphology. In definitive resection specimens (EPD/EPP), by consensus, ≥ 10% of each component must be present. However, any tumour can be diagnosed as biphasic mesothelioma regardless of percentages of each component in small biopsy specimens {2103}. In all specimen types, reporting the percentage of sarcomatoid component is recommended because of potential implications for prognosis and therapeutic management. When transitional features are observed in an otherwise epithelioid mesothelioma, the tumour should be classified as biphasic mesothelioma.

Pericardial mesothelioma

Pericardial mesotheliomas are also subtyped as epithelioid, biphasic, or sarcomatoid {1148,3018}. One deciduoid tumour and one case of desmoplastic mesothelioma have also been reported in the pericardium {2450,2111}.

Immunohistochemistry of epithelioid mesothelioma

Distinguishing epithelioid mesotheliomas from other tumours involving pleura, most commonly metastatic carcinoma, can be facilitated by use of a minimum of two mesothelial and two carcinoma markers. On the basis of specificity and sensitivity,

calretinin, WT1, D2-40, and CK5/6 are recommended mesothelial markers, whereas claudin-4, BerEP4 or MOC31, B72.3, CEA, CD15 (LeuM1), and BG8 are commonly used carcinoma markers {3395,1213,2203}. Claudin-4 immunohistochemistry for the diagnosis of carcinoma performed with a higher sensitivity and specificity than conventional carcinoma markers {2282}. Site-specific markers can help in determining tumour origin (see *Metastasis to the pleura*, p. 459).

Pancytokeratins are also useful, because a negative result suggests the possibility of other tumours. Several non-epithelial tumours (including epithelioid haemangioendothelioma, angiosarcoma, melanoma, and large cell lymphoma) can mimic epithelioid mesothelioma (see *Metastasis to the pleura*, p. 459). Keratins can occasionally be positive in epithelioid vascular tumours, although usually only focally.

Immunohistochemistry of sarcomatoid and desmoplastic mesothelioma

Sarcomatoid mesotheliomas are generally at least focally positive with pancytokeratin antibodies including AE1/AE3, OSCAR, and KL1, as well as CAM5.2, which reacts with CK8 and CK18 {506,1213,2967}. CK18 alone may be positive in tumours in which other keratins are negative. However, sarcomatoid mesotheliomas can be keratin-negative {1476}.

About 30% of sarcomatoid mesotheliomas express calretinin {120,1149,1475}, but are more often positive for D2-40 {506, 1149,2238}. Other mesothelial markers, including CK5/6 and WT1, are relatively insensitive {1213}. Sarcomatoid mesotheliomas are often vimentin-positive, whereas epithelioid mesotheliomas are often negative for vimentin. Occasionally, sarcomatoid mesotheliomas express actin, desmin, or S100. TTF1 (clone 8G7G3/1) and/or p40 expression supports a diagnosis of sarcomatoid carcinoma.

Ancillary studies for distinguishing mesothelioma from benign mesothelial proliferations

Ancillary studies can aid in distinguishing diffuse pleural mesothelioma from reactive mesothelial proliferations. Loss of BAP1 expression by immunohistochemistry and homozygous deletion of *CDKN2A* (9p21; encoding p16) by FISH and/or cytoplasmic loss of MTAP expression by immunohistochemistry to identify *CDKN2A* homozygous deletion can distinguish mesothelioma from benign proliferations {215,1141,1466,1465,1218}. Loss of

Table 2.03 Immunohistochemistry to aid in distinguishing mesothelioma from reactive mesothelial proliferations {215,1141,1466,1620}

	Mesothelioma	
Markers	**Sensitivity**	**Specificity vs reactive mesothelial hyperplasia**
BAP1	42–65%	100%
MTAP	42–48%	100%

BAP1 nuclear expression is seen more commonly in epithelioid mesotheliomas, whereas homozygous deletion in the region of 9p21 is seen in > 80% of sarcomatoid pleural mesotheliomas {1862}. High expression of EZH2 by immunohistochemistry may also be useful {3431,83A,2753A}. Immunohistochemistry to aid in distinguishing mesothelioma from reactive mesothelial proliferations is summarized in Table 2.03. Note that these ancillary studies can be useful for distinguishing mesothelioma from benign mesothelial proliferations but are not appropriate for distinguishing mesothelioma from other malignant tumours.

Keratins can also be useful for highlighting tumour cells and invasion into adjacent soft tissues (in particular adipose tissue), because in some cases sarcomatoid or desmoplastic malignant mesothelial cells can be difficult to distinguish from reactive fibrous pleuritis by histology alone. Careful quality assurance and validation of methods for immunohistochemistry and FISH are critical, including examination of proper controls to avoid false negative results.

Differential diagnosis of epithelioid mesothelioma

Epithelioid mesothelioma must be distinguished from carcinomas and other epithelioid malignancies that can show diffuse pleural (pseudomesotheliomatous) spread. Immunohistochemistry is essential in establishing the diagnosis, and the choice of antibodies, particularly carcinoma markers, depends on morphology (see *Metastasis to the pleura*, p. 459). The most common carcinomas in the differential diagnosis include lung adenocarcinoma and squamous cell carcinoma, but metastases from breast, kidney, ovary, prostate, pancreas, and gastrointestinal tract could potentially be confused with epithelioid mesotheliomas. Epithelioid mesothelioma with clear cell features must be distinguished from clear cell renal cell carcinoma, melanoma, and other metastatic clear cell tumours. Mesotheliomas with small cell features should be distinguished from small cell carcinomas of lung, desmoplastic small round cell tumours, lymphomas, and other tumours with small blue cell morphology {2208}.

Proximal epithelioid sarcoma and SMARCA4-deficient undifferentiated thoracic tumours (see *Thoracic SMARCA4-deficient undifferentiated tumour*, p. 111) can be mistaken for epithelioid mesotheliomas with rhabdoid features {2324,2460,2643, 3421,1617,1086}. Focal or negative keratin staining and loss of SMARCB1 (INI1/BAF47) or SMARCA4 (BRG1) expression by immunohistochemistry, respectively, or detection of either of these mutations by next-generation sequencing, in addition to mesothelial markers, should help to establish a correct diagnosis.

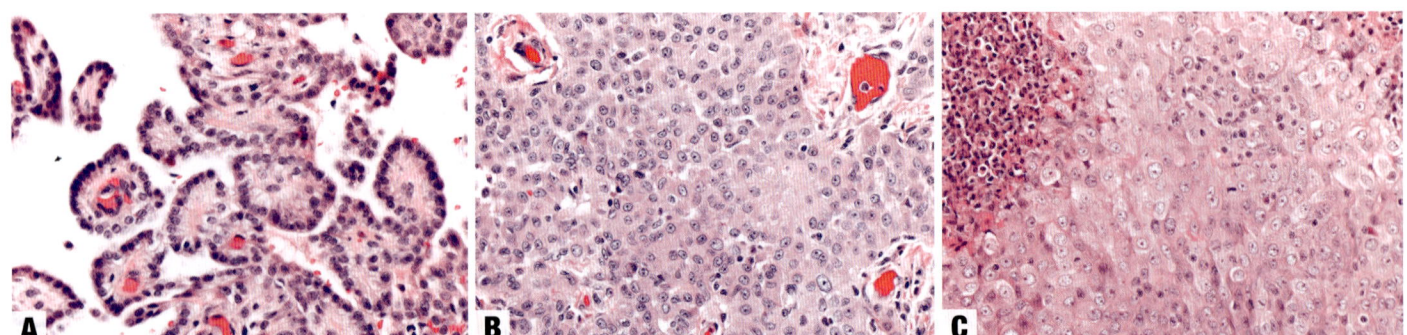

Fig. 2.20 Diffuse epithelioid mesothelioma. Nuclear grading of epithelioid mesothelioma includes nuclear atypia and mitoses. **A** Nuclear atypia score of 1 (mild) shows small, uniform, and round nuclei with inconspicuous nucleoli and finely granular chromatin. **B** Nuclear atypia score of 2 (moderate) shows nuclei that are intermediate in size with limited anisonucleosis and pleomorphism, coarser chromatin, and more conspicuous nucleoli. **C** Nuclear atypia score of 3 (severe) shows large nuclei with anisonucleosis, pleomorphism, coarse chromatin, and prominent nucleoli. Necrosis and a mitotic figure are present.

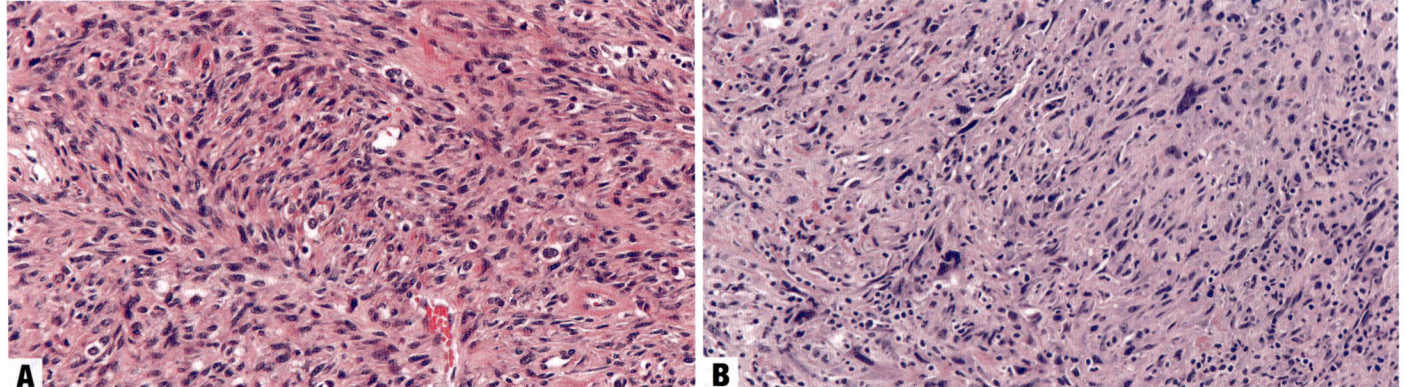

Fig. 2.21 Diffuse sarcomatoid mesothelioma. **A** The tumour cells are spindled, with fascicular arrangement. **B** The tumour nuclei show varying degrees of pleomorphism, with some nuclei being small and others large, hyperchromatic, and irregular.

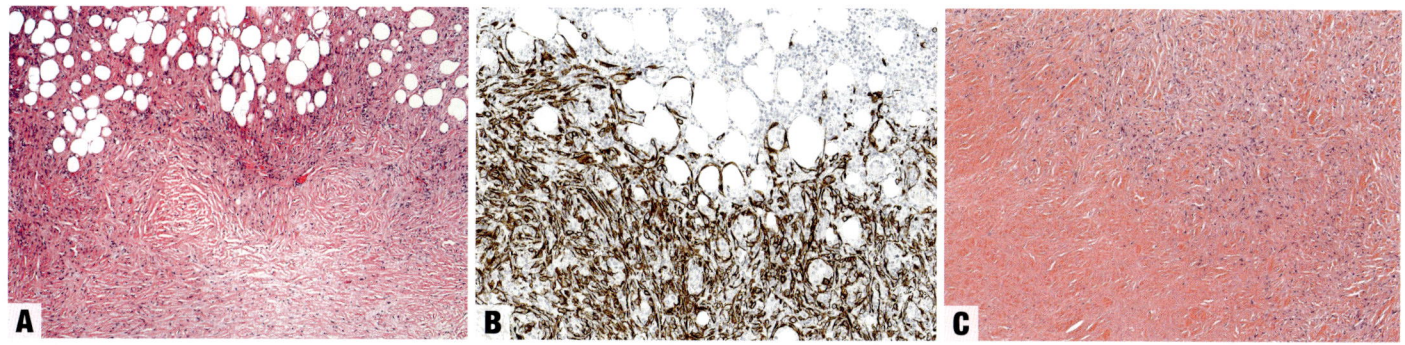

Fig. 2.22 Diffuse desmoplastic mesothelioma. **A** This desmoplastic mesothelioma shows pleural thickening by nodules of paucicellular tumour characterized by haphazard slit-like spaces. There is extensive invasion into the adjacent parietal pleural fat. **B** Invasion is highlighted by cytokeratin-positive cells between adipocytes. **C** Diffuse desmoplastic mesothelioma with a paucicellular spindle cell area and bland necrosis.

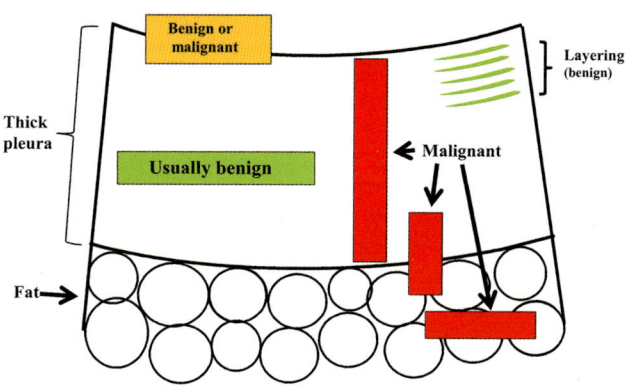

Fig. 2.23 Benign mesothelial proliferations versus mesothelioma. Schematic diagram showing benign versus malignant processes as a function of the distribution of mesothelial cells in a thickened pleura.

Other epithelioid tumours that can demonstrate a pseudomesotheliomatous appearance include epithelioid haemangioendothelioma, angiosarcoma, intrapleural thymomas, melanoma, lymphoma, and monophasic synovial sarcomas.

CAMTA1-WWTR1 and YAP1-TFE3 gene fusions are characteristic of epithelioid haemangioendothelioma. FISH or molecular testing for t(X;18) to confirm a diagnosis of synovial sarcoma in the pleura is preferred, because TLE1 immunohistochemistry may not discriminate between mesothelioma and synovial sarcoma {1477,3250,1844}. Melanoma markers such as HMB45 or SOX10 and the presence of BRAF p.V600E mutation are very helpful in the separation of melanoma from mesothelioma. Concurrent mesothelioma and adenocarcinoma in an asbestos-exposed patient is a rare event that can be identified using a panel of mesothelial and specific organ markers by immunohistochemistry, as discussed above {360}.

Separation of benign processes and malignant mesothelial proliferation

Reactive mesothelial hyperplasia may be extremely florid and atypical and mimic epithelioid mesothelioma, particularly in the context of infection, collagen vascular disease, pulmonary embolism, or pulmonary infarction. The presence of unequivocal invasion of chest wall, soft tissue, or underlying lung parenchyma by mesothelial cells is a robust criterion for malignancy. Ancillary studies may be useful, particularly in small biopsy or cytology specimens (see the *Immunohistochemistry* subsection above). Hyperplastic mesothelial cells may transit into draining lymph nodes from reactive mesothelial lesions without evidence

Table 2.04 Reactive atypical mesothelial hyperplasia versus mesothelioma {531}

Histological features	Atypical mesothelial hyperplasia	Mesothelioma
Major criteria		
Stromal invasion	Absent	Present (the deeper, the more definitive)
Cellularity	Confined to the pleural surface	Dense, with stromal reaction
Papillae	Simple, lined by single-cell layer	Complex, with cellular stratification
Growth pattern	Surface growth	Expansile nodules, complex and disorganized pattern
Zonation	Process becomes less cellular towards chest wall	No zonation of process, often more cellular away from effusion
Vascularity	Capillaries are perpendicular to the surface	Irregular and haphazard
Inflammation	Often present	Uncommon
Minor criteria		
Cytological atypia	Confined to areas of organizing effusion	Present in any area, but many cells are deceptively bland and relatively monotonous
Necrosis	Rare (necrosis may be within pleural exudate)	Necrosis of tumour area is usually a sign of malignancy
Mitoses	Mitoses may be plentiful	Many mesotheliomas show very few mitoses (but atypical mitoses favour malignancy)

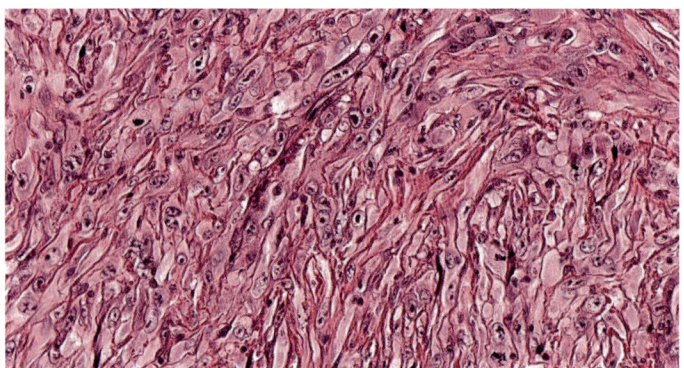

Fig. 2.24 Epithelioid mesothelioma. Unfavourable cytological features seen in epithelioid mesothelioma include transitional features, which comprise tumour cells with features intermediate between epithelioid and sarcomatoid morphology.

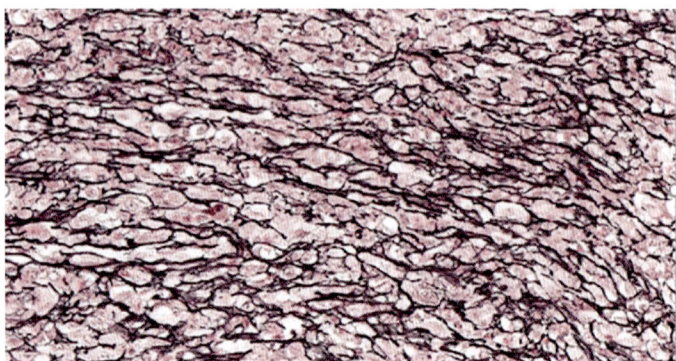

Fig. 2.25 Diffuse mesothelioma. Reticulin stain in a tumour with a transitional appearance.

of mesothelioma, typically involving subcapsular sinuses without destruction of lymph node architecture {101,559}.

Pleural nodular histiocytic/mesothelial hyperplasia (BAP1 retained) is a nodular histiocytic/mesothelial proliferation, rarely observed in the pleural cavity, due to irritation of the pleura, that should be distinguished from mesothelioma showing a large number of histiocytes {359}. Pleural exudates with necrotic cells should not be called malignant in the absence of viable malignant cells either forming tumour nodules or showing invasive growth.

Fake fat phenomenon in organizing pleuritis can be a pitfall; S100 immunohistochemistry can aid in distinguishing fat-like spaces in pleuritis from true adipose tissue {529}. Desmoid fibromatosis arising from the pleura can mimic desmoplastic mesothelioma. The lack of cytokeratin expression, β-catenin nuclear staining, and *CTNNB1* mutation support desmoid fibromatosis {565,1616,3170A,2319A}.

The histological features of reactive atypical mesothelial hyperplasia versus mesothelioma are summarized in Table 2.04 (p. 213).

Differential diagnosis of sarcomatoid mesothelioma

Sarcomatoid mesothelioma should be distinguished from metastatic sarcomatoid carcinomas from lung and other sites, particularly renal cell carcinomas. Distinction between sarcomatoid carcinoma and sarcomatoid mesothelioma can be challenging, because expression of markers of specific differentiation can be negative in both, and both tumours may be weakly or focally positive for mesothelial markers (WT1, calretinin, D2-40) {1801}. Expression of carcinoma markers (see the *Immunohistochemistry* subsection above), even weak and focal, supports sarcomatoid carcinoma, and strong and diffuse GATA3 favours sarcomatoid/desmoplastic mesothelioma {213,1913}, except for urothelial and breast carcinoma (see *Metastasis to the pleura*, p. 459). Molecular testing can be helpful in difficult cases, because sarcomatoid carcinomas of lung are frequently associated with *MET* exon 14 splice-site mutations {1714,2679}. When immunohistochemical and/or molecular results are not definitive, the final diagnosis may rest on clinical and radiological correlation, where diffuse pleural thickening would favour mesothelioma, and a localized mass would favour carcinoma.

Primary chest wall and metastatic sarcomas are important in the differential diagnosis of sarcomatoid mesothelioma. Focal cytokeratin positivity can be seen in many different types of sarcomas, including primary angiosarcoma of the pleura and monophasic synovial sarcoma. Calretinin, and/or D2-40 expression alone in the absence of keratin expression should not be interpreted as evidence of mesothelial differentiation, because these markers can be variably positive in sarcomas. Many different sarcoma types may be considered (angiosarcoma, synovial sarcoma, liposarcoma, myogenic sarcomas, and

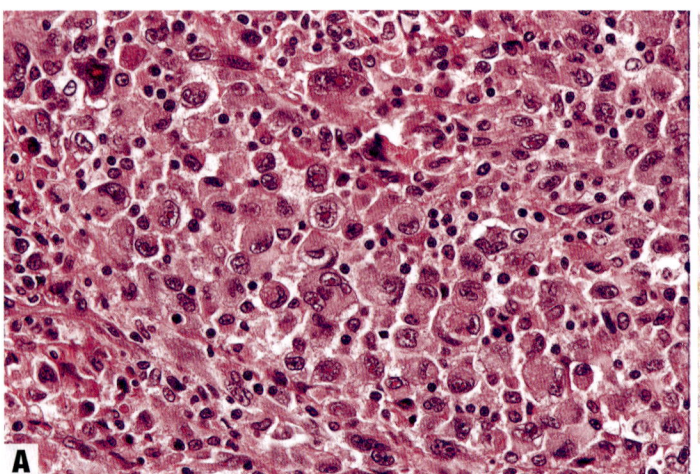
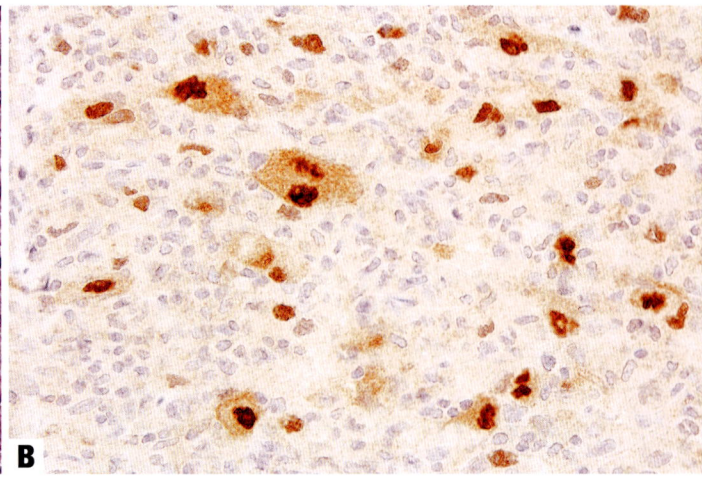

Fig. 2.26 Sarcomatoid malignant mesothelioma with rhabdomyosarcoma differentiation. **A** This mesothelioma shows some pleomorphic tumour cells with abundant eosinophilic cytoplasm, which suggests the possibility of rhabdomyosarcoma. **B** Scattered tumour cells show positive staining for myogenin.

Table 2.05 Immunochemistry and molecular findings in the differential diagnosis between sarcomatoid mesothelioma and selected other neoplasms {213,1714,2679,1801,1485,3250}

Neoplasm	Immunohistochemistry	Molecular findings
Sarcomatoid mesothelioma	Keratin positive Low expression of mesothelial markers GATA3 often positive (high expression)	Not usually applicable
Sarcomatoid carcinoma	Keratin positive TTF1 or p63/p40 positive Carcinoma markers positive (see *Metastasis to the pleura*, p. 459)	*MET* exon 14 splice-site mutations *EGFR* mutations (rare)
Monophasic synovial sarcoma	Keratin usually weak and/or focal	Translocation t(X;18)(p11.2;q11.2) *SS18* (*SYT*)-SSX fusion
Solitary fibrous tumour	Keratin usually negative; rarely focally positive STAT6 positive	Translocation *NAB2-STAT6*
Angiosarcoma	Keratin usually negative; can be focal/weak; rarely strong CD31 and CD34 positive ERG and FLI1 positive	

undifferentiated pleomorphic sarcoma. Immunohistochemical and molecular workup should be performed accordingly. Negative STAT6 immunohistochemistry would suggest a tumour other than malignant solitary fibrous tumour. Primary pleural tumours causing diffuse pleural thickening with osteosarcomatous or chondrosarcomatous differentiation, even in the absence of keratin or mesothelial marker expression, are probably all mesotheliomas, although osteosarcomas and chondrosarcomas mimicking mesothelioma growth patterns have been reported {944,1390}. *IDH1/2* mutation can differentiate chondrosarcoma from mesothelioma with a heterologous element. Mesothelioma with heterologous elements is also applied to rhabdomyosarcomatous differentiation with positive expression of desmin, myogenin, and/or MYOD1 {3065A,1476}.

Sarcomatoid and desmoplastic mesotheliomas must be distinguished from organizing pleuritis {531,1782}. Morphological features such as a lack of zonation, inconspicuous capillaries, cellular stromal nodules, and chest wall invasion are seen in desmoplastic mesotheliomas. Invasion of adjacent tissues, particularly adipose tissue, is the most reliable criterion for distinguishing desmoplastic mesothelioma from pleuritis. Bland

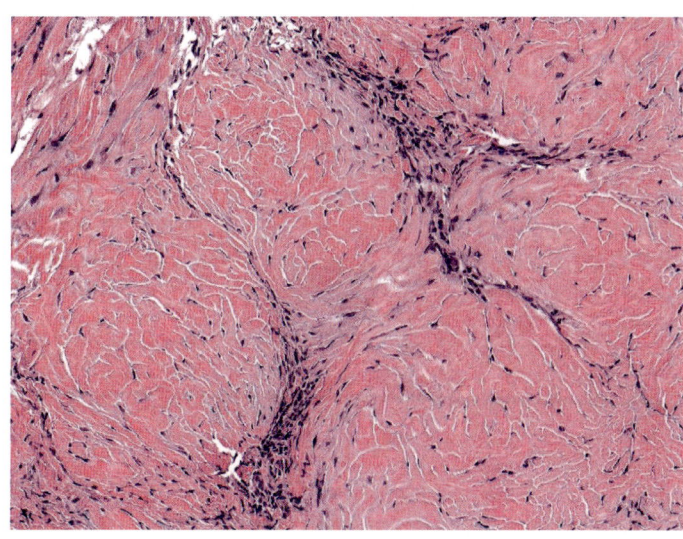

Fig. 2.27 Diffuse sarcomatoid mesothelioma, desmoplastic pattern. Proliferation nodules and desmoplastic round nodules are a feature occasionally seen in the desmoplastic pattern of mesothelioma.

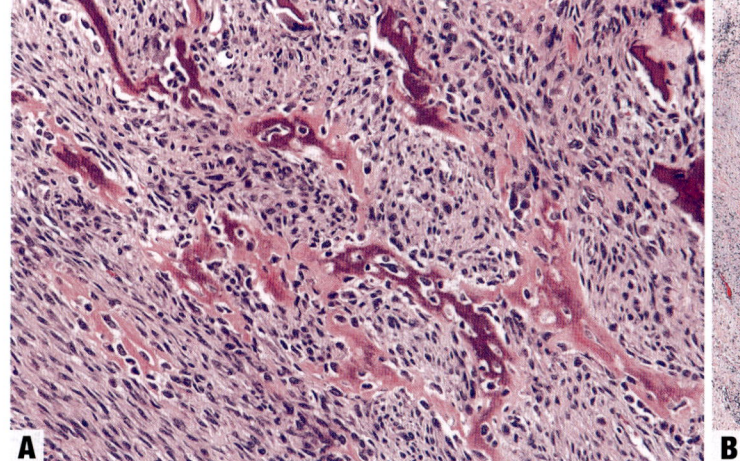

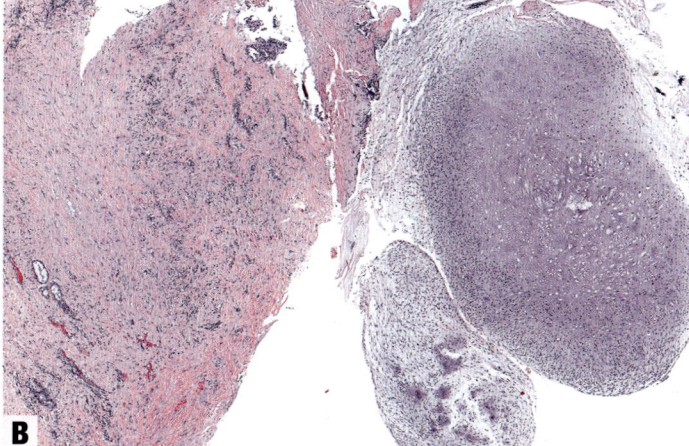

Fig. 2.28 Sarcomatoid mesothelioma with heterologous elements. **A** Osteosarcoma. **B** This mesothelioma shows an epithelioid and sarcomatous component (left) and nodules of chondrosarcoma (right).

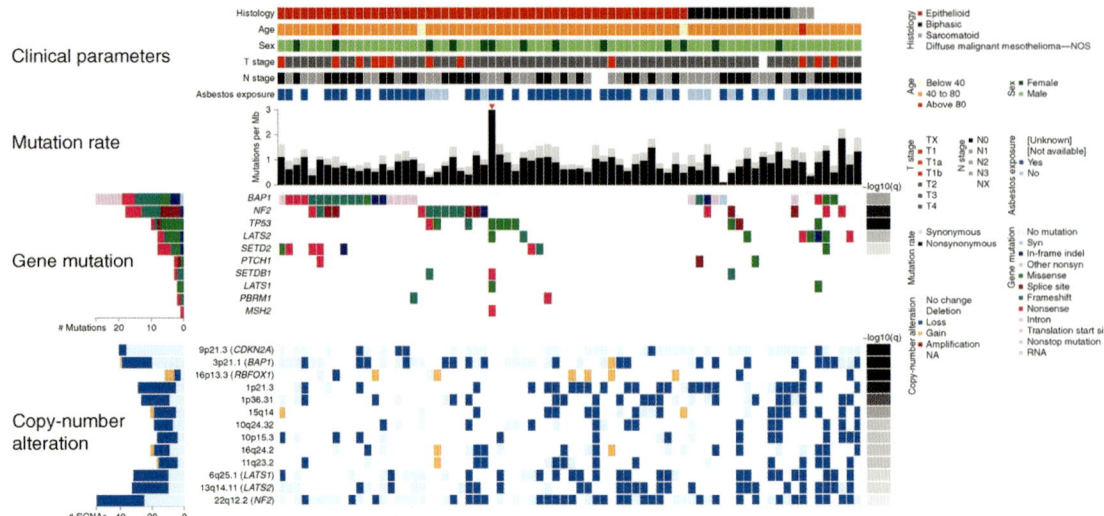

Fig. 2.29 Malignant pleural mesothelioma (MPM). iCoMut plot describing clinical and molecular features of The Cancer Genome Atlas (TCGA) MPM cohort. Each column represents an individual case; rows represent clinical and molecular features. Samples are grouped by MPM histological type. The red arrowhead indicates the hypermutated case. Copy-number alterations are defined as follows: "deletion" is a deep loss, possibly a homozygous deletion; "loss" is a shallow loss (possibly heterozygous deletion); "gain" indicates a low-level gain; "amplification" is a high-level amplification. The individual genes shown include significantly mutated genes and selected additional genes of interest.

necrosis, stromal nodules sometimes referred to as "proliferation nodules", and adjacent areas of definitive epithelioid or sarcomatoid mesothelioma are also useful diagnostic features. In difficult cases and in limited biopsy material, ancillary tests may help in confirming malignancy (see the *Immunohistochemistry* subsection above).

Biphasic mesothelioma must be distinguished from pleomorphic carcinomas and synovial sarcomas. Pleomorphic carcinomas usually form a peripheral lung mass that can invade the chest wall, and they usually show areas of conventional non-small cell carcinoma. Biphasic synovial sarcomas show t(X;18) translocation {1485,3250}.

Immunohistochemistry and molecular findings in the differential diagnosis between sarcomatoid mesothelioma and selected other neoplasms are summarized in Table 2.05 (p. 215).

Differential diagnosis of pericardial mesothelioma
Pleural mesotheliomas extending to the pericardium are far more common than primary pericardial mesotheliomas, and this possibility must be excluded before the diagnosis can be made. Other tumours in the differential diagnosis include metastatic carcinomas, especially lung adenocarcinomas, angiosarcomas, synovial sarcomas, malignant solitary fibrous tumours, and rarely germ cell tumours.

Cytology
In industrialized countries, < 10% of malignant pleural effusions are caused by diffuse mesothelioma {108,414}. Malignant mesothelial cells in effusions are nearly always epithelioid morphologically, because sarcomatoid mesotheliomas seldom shed cells into effusions. Mesothelioma cells in effusions may be arranged in sheets, clusters, morules, or papillae, with a range of cytological atypia, from bland to pleomorphic {2906}. Psammoma bodies may be present but can also be seen in malignant effusions from carcinomas. Reactive benign mesothelial cells may exhibit features often associated with malignancy, such as increased cellularity, nuclear pleomorphism, and mitotic activity. Therefore, differentiation of mesothelioma from benign

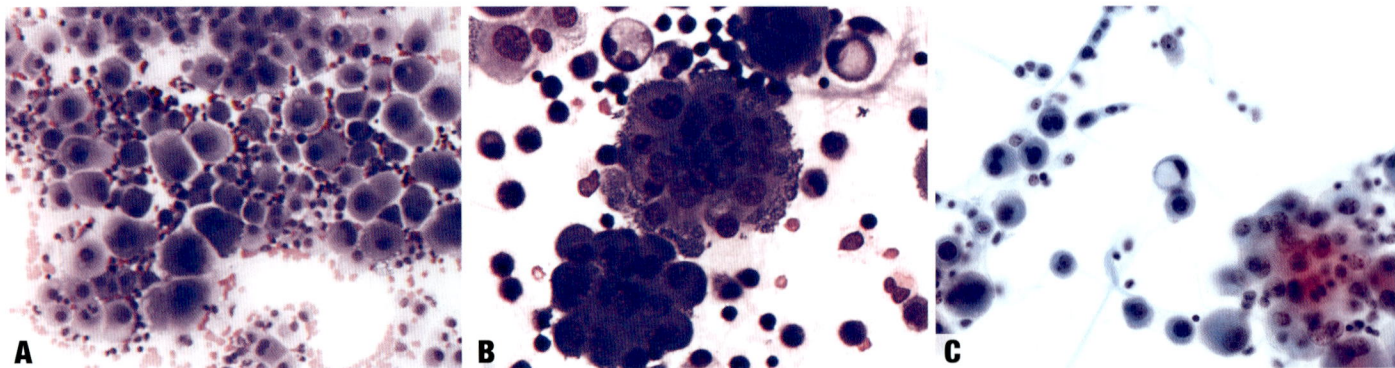

Fig. 2.30 Epithelioid mesothelioma, cytology. **A** This specimen shows high cellularity composed of diffuse mesothelial neoplastic cells of various sizes. **B** This specimen shows a 3D morula composed of atypical mesothelial cells with round nuclei and prominent nucleoli mixed with inflammatory cells. **C** Diffuse epithelioid mesothelioma with signet-ring features. Rarely, epithelioid mesotheliomas contain tumour cells with intracytoplasmic vacuoles that push nuclei to the side and resemble a signet ring. It is important to recognize that signet-ring features can occur in mesotheliomas and to distinguish these tumours from signet-ring carcinomas from other sites by immunohistochemistry.

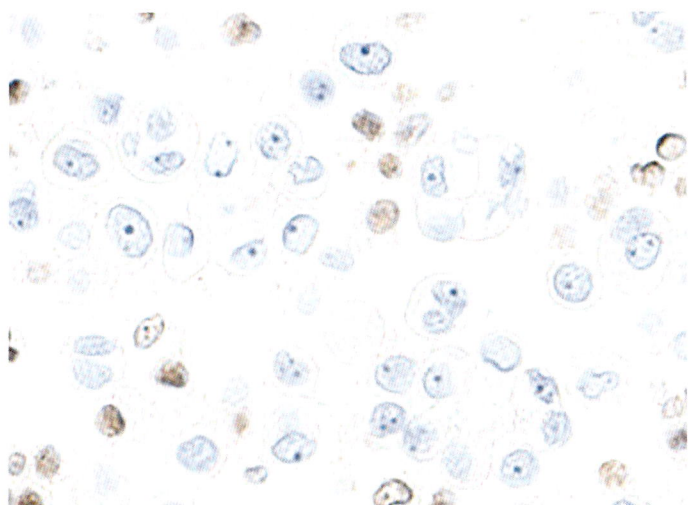

Fig. 2.31 Mesothelioma. Pleural fluid cytology shows malignant mesothelial cells with prominent nucleoli and BAP1 loss mixed with reactive mesothelial cells and inflammatory cells showing retained BAP1.

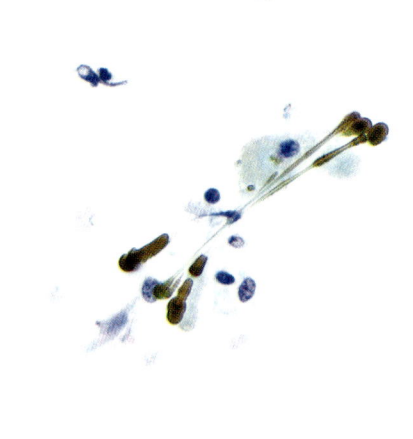

Fig. 2.33 Asbestos bodies. Fibres with thin transparent cores and iron-rich deposits on their surfaces.

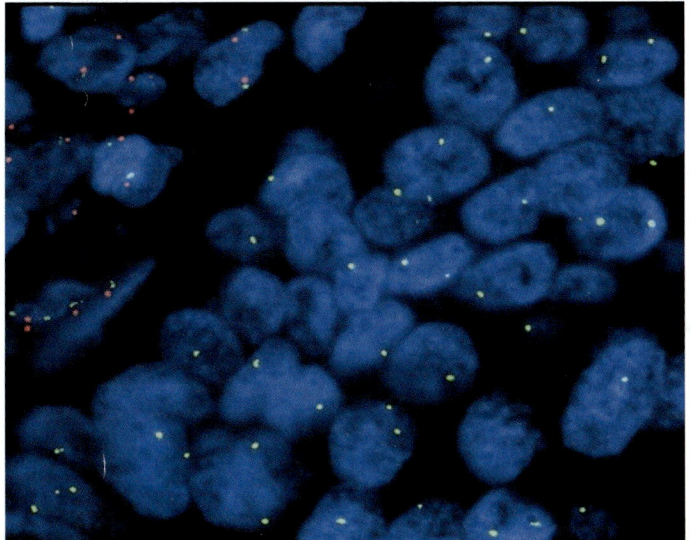

Fig. 2.32 Epithelioid mesothelioma. 9p21 (*CDKN2A*) FISH; malignant mesothelial cells with homozygous deletion of 9p21 show centromere of chromosome 9 only (green signal) and lack the *CDKN2A* gene (red signal). Normal cells (as a positive control) show both red and green signals.

mesothelial reactions may be difficult or even impossible in cytological specimens. Similarly, tissue invasion (an important histological feature of malignancy) cannot be evaluated in effusion specimens. However, ancillary studies may aid in differentiating mesothelioma from benign effusions (see the *Immunohistochemistry* subsection above), and the use of cell block material can be helpful. It should be noted that fixation differences may cause differences in immunocytochemistry results (in particular, issues with false negative staining) {336,2643A}. BAP1 and MTAP immunostains must only be interpreted in the presence of a positive internal control.

Mesothelioma in effusion specimens can be distinguished from metastatic tumours, in particular carcinomas, morphologically by the absence of a "second" population of cells. However, the use of immunocytochemistry to determine cell of origin is recommended (see *Metastasis to the pleura*, p. 459).

In FNA specimens, sarcomatoid mesotheliomas may demonstrate features similar to those of other soft tissue sarcomas or sarcomatoid carcinoma, with spindle morphology and varying degrees of atypical nuclear features.

Diagnostic molecular pathology

Blood-based biomarkers such as SMRP, HMGB1, fibulin-3, and calretinin are still under evaluation and currently not recommended for clinical use because the sensitivities and specificities are still inadequate for monitoring response to treatment or for predicting outcome {1459,3093,2279,2436,2073,1320,351,596}.

Essential and desirable diagnostic criteria

Essential:
- Diffuse pleural thickening by a malignant neoplasm with epithelioid, sarcomatoid, or biphasic histology
- Invasion of adjacent structures (i.e. adipose tissue, skeletal muscle, and/or lung parenchyma), tumour necrosis, or formation of unequivocal malignant tumour nodules
- Desmoplastic mesothelioma is characterized by dense collagenized tissue separated by malignant mesothelial cells arranged in a storiform or so-called patternless pattern, which must be present in ≥ 50% of the tumour in definitive resection specimens
- Biphasic mesothelioma is mesothelioma showing ≥ 10% each of epithelioid and sarcomatoid patterns in definitive resection specimens, or any percentage of each component in smaller biopsy and cytology specimens
- Immunohistochemistry confirming mesothelial origin

Desirable:
- Loss of BAP1 and/or CDKN2A and/or MTAP by immunohistochemistry
- *BAP1* or *CDKN2A* loss demonstrated by FISH or next-generation sequencing

Box 2.02 Examples of pathology reporting of diffuse pleural mesothelioma in biopsy and resection specimens (EPD/EPP) {2103}

Resection specimens (EPD/EPP):

Tumour site, specimen type:

Histological type (epithelioid, biphasic[a], or sarcomatoid/desmoplastic)

High/low grade (use only for epithelioid)

List all architectural patterns present (give predominant pattern and percentages for each pattern listed) and any cytological and/or stromal features present

> Example of a pathology report for a resection specimen:
>
> Extended pleurectomy: Epithelioid mesothelioma, high grade. Predominantly tubulopapillary pattern (80%), also with micropapillary pattern (20%) and pleomorphic features (20%).

Biopsy specimens:

Tumour site, specimen type:

Histological type (epithelioid, biphasic[a], or sarcomatoid; if desmoplastic features are present, include "with desmoplastic features")

High/low grade (use only for epithelioid)

List all architectural patterns present (do not give a percentage) and any cytological and/or stromal features present (do not give a percentage)

> Example of a pathology report for a biopsy specimen:
>
> Pleura (biopsy): Epithelioid mesothelioma, high grade. Solid pattern and with rhabdoid cytological features

EPD, extended pleurectomy/decortication; EPP, extrapleural pneumonectomy.
[a]When a diagnosis of biphasic mesothelioma is made, a comment should be included to indicate the percentages of each component present.

Staging

Current staging, the eighth edition of TNM, adopted by the American Joint Committee on Cancer (AJCC) and the Union for International Cancer Control (UICC), is based on retrospective analysis of a large series of patients accumulated by the International Association for the Study of Lung Cancer (IASLC) {2278,2476,2145,2570} and applies to both clinical and pathological staging {75}. Changes from the previous edition include collapsing T1a and T1b and N1 and N2 into single T1 and N1 categories, respectively. Accordingly, T1N0, T2–3N0, T1–2N1, T3N1, and any T4 or N2 now constitute stages IA, IB, II, IIIA, and IIIB, respectively, while any M1 remains stage IV.

Definitive resection specimens (EPD/EPP) should be pathologically staged, with smaller specimens being clinically staged via multidisciplinary review. It is recommended to discuss intraoperative findings with the surgeon before completion of pathological staging.

Clinical staging is inaccurate for early stages, due to low accuracy of CT and MRI {2103}. Integrated FDG PET-CT may improve accuracy {2365}. In clinical series, patients most commonly presented with locally advanced disease (stage III, 40%), followed by advanced (stage IV, 35%) and local (stage I–II, 25%) disease.

Current T descriptors are qualitative and applicable for invasive staging procedures, as well as T1, which requires thoracoscopic assessment of pleural cavity. They account insufficiently for invasion, extent, thickness, and volume of the circumferential pleural rind. The regional lymph node map and nomenclature are the same as those used for lung cancer, with the addition of lymph nodes in the anterior peridiaphragmatic region and around the internal mammary artery as N2 nodes. This empirical assumption discounts the possible prognostic role of lymph nodes in the extrapleural space and pericardial fat, and it associates better prognosis with intrapulmonary nodes. It may not be possible to perform a thorough N classification, particularly in unresectable tumours.

The IASLC has also created a prospective database, including a broader patient population by expanding to include clinical staging data for patients who did not undergo surgery, to obtain more-meaningful long-term data for future staging classifications {2573,2278}.

Prognosis and prediction

Although histological classification of pleural mesotheliomas is prognostically valid, there is variability in clinical behaviour and outcomes within subtypes. Comprehensive genomic analyses have been shown to improve prognostic classification and suggest that histological and molecular classifications may be discordant {1166,330,51}. On the basis of transcriptome data, four different prognostic molecular clusters were identified that correlated with survival and the degree of epithelial–mesenchymal transition {330}: sarcomatoid, epithelioid, biphasic-epithelioid, and biphasic-sarcomatoid {330}. Similarly, the TCGA cohort study identified four distinct subtypes of pleural mesothelioma based on integrated genomic, transcriptomic, and epigenomic data {1166}. The poor prognostic cluster has a high score of epithelial–mesenchymal transition, low mRNA expression of mesothelin, a higher score for the T helper 2 (Th2) cell signature, and enrichment for *LATS2* mutations and *CDKN2A* homozygous deletions {1166}. Recently, reanalysis of these two large cohorts of pleural mesotheliomas showed that a continuous classification of pleural mesothelioma explains prognosis better than any discrete model {51,245}, and these differences in prognosis are mainly driven by an interaction of the immune and vascular pathways with major differences in expression of immune checkpoint and proangiogenic genes {51}.

Long-term survival in patients with mesothelioma is poor, with median survival times of 19, 13, and 8 months in patients with epithelioid, biphasic, and sarcomatoid tumours, respectively {2573,2574,3141}. Younger age, epithelioid type (vs sarcomatoid or biphasic type), and early TNM staging are indicators of longer median survival and strongly influence therapeutic strategy {845,2569,2572,2573}. Although evidence is sparse, multimodality therapy is indicated in patients with good performance status and early-stage disease {3144}. Some histological features of epithelioid mesothelioma (i.e. abundant myxoid changes {52}) are more prognostically favourable, whereas the presence of micropapillary pattern, pleomorphic features, transitional features, or solid pattern strongly predict poor survival {2103,1344,2210,902,902A}. A histological grading system has been proposed for epithelioid mesothelioma, with high nuclear grade (including nuclear atypia and a high mitotic count) found to be an independent poor prognostic factor {3499,580}.

Reporting of histological patterns and features in diffuse epithelioid mesothelioma: Solid (≥ 50%) {2532}, pleomorphic {1344,2210}, and rhabdoid {2207} features have been shown to be associated with poor prognosis, whereas lymphohistiocytoid features {903,1408} and myxoid stroma (when ≥ 50% in tumours with < 50% solid pattern) {52} have been shown to be associated with better prognosis. Favourable/unfavourable histological characteristics (architectural patterns, cytological features, and stromal features) should be routinely reported {2103}. However, specific terminology and classification criteria differ between small biopsy/cytology and definitive resection (namely, EPD and EPP) specimens {2103}. Templates for pathology reporting of diffuse pleural mesothelioma in biopsy and resection specimens (EPD/EPP) are presented in Box 2.02.

The treatment of choice for localized pericardial mesothelioma is surgical resection, but most patients present with diffuse disease. Even with therapy, the median survival time from onset of symptoms is only about 6 months {1399,2512A}. However, new chemotherapeutic regimens have been attempted with longer survival {1419}.

Haematolymphoid tumours of the pleura and pericardium: Introduction

Chan JKC
Cooper WA

Overview

Lymphomatous involvement of the pleural and pericardial cavities in disseminated lymphoma or in association with an underlying pulmonary lymphoma is not uncommon {614,3163}. However, primary pleural or pericardial lymphoma is rare.

Two distinct types of lymphoma characteristically involve the pleura and/or pericardium. Primary effusion lymphoma (PEL), which is invariably associated with HHV8 and frequently associated with EBV, may involve the pleural or pericardial cavity, and manifests as effusion without formation of a solid tumour mass. Diffuse large B-cell lymphoma associated with chronic inflammation (pyothorax-associated lymphoma being the prototype) is a mass-forming lymphoma involving the pleura and consistently associated with EBV.

Other types of lymphoma, such as follicular lymphoma {2172,2852,3163}, extranodal marginal zone lymphoma {1934, 1406,156,2013}, and anaplastic large cell lymphoma {439}, may also exceptionally occur as a primary pleural or pericardial tumour, in the form of a serous effusion or plaque-like mass lesion. Details of these lymphoma types are available in the 2017 volume on tumours of haematopoietic and lymphoid tissues {2941}.

So-called PEL-like lymphoma

An unresolved issue is whether diffuse large B-cell lymphoma occurring primarily as pleural or pericardial effusion, also known as PEL-like lymphoma or HHV8-unrelated PEL-like lymphoma, represents a distinct entity or merely conventional high-grade B-cell lymphoma involving the pleural/pericardial cavity {3346, 381,1493}. In contrast to PEL, the lymphoma uncommonly occurs in the setting of HIV-associated immunodeficiency, HHV8 is by definition negative, EBV association is present in only a proportion of cases (< 30%), and the neoplastic cells often exhibit a mature peripheral B-cell phenotype (CD20+) instead of a plasmablastic phenotype {2052,1493,3346,1225, 56}. Some studies have shown the lymphoma to be associated with HCV infection and with fluid overload states in a proportion of cases {1225,3346,56}. The lymphoma appears to have a more favourable prognosis than PEL {3366,1225,3020,56}.

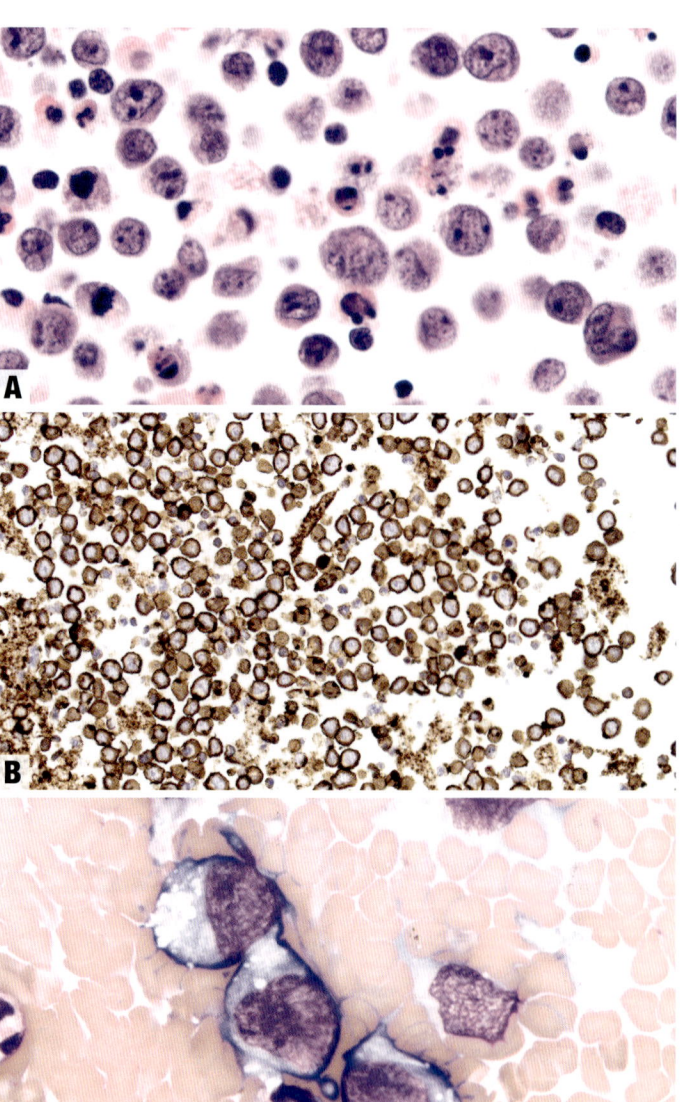

Fig. 2.34 Primary pericardial HHV8-unrelated diffuse large B-cell lymphoma occurring as pericardial effusion (so-called PEL-like lymphoma). **A** Cell block preparation of pericardial fluid shows non-cohesive large cells with variably sized nuclei that often show irregular foldings. Nucleoli are distinct. **B** Immunostaining performed on a histological section cut from the cell block shows CD20 staining of the lymphoma cells (which contrasts with the usually negative staining in PEL). **C** Giemsa-stained smear of pericardial fluid shows large atypical lymphoid cells with abundant lightly basophilic cytoplasm.

Primary effusion lymphoma

Said JW
Bacon CM
Cesarman E

Definition

Primary effusion lymphoma (PEL) is a large B-cell lymphoma of terminally differentiated B cells, consistently associated with HHV8 (Kaposi sarcoma–associated herpesvirus) and often co-infected with EBV, occurring as a serous effusion in the absence of lymph node involvement or a tumour mass.

ICD-O coding

9678/3 Primary effusion lymphoma

ICD-11 coding

2A81.9 Primary effusion lymphoma

Related terminology

Not recommended: body cavity–based lymphoma.

Subtype(s)

Extracavitary (solid) PEL

Localization

PEL affects the major body cavities, including the pleura, peritoneum, and pericardium.

Clinical features

PEL manifests with lymphomatous effusions involving serous cavities {419}. The majority of patients are HIV-positive men in the fifth decade of life, with low CD4 cell counts ($\leq 200 \times 106/L$) {1021}. Other features of HHV8 infection, including Kaposi sarcoma and multicentric Castleman disease, are present in as many as 50% of patients at presentation. Extracavitary PEL occurs as solid tumours in sites such as the lung, gastrointestinal

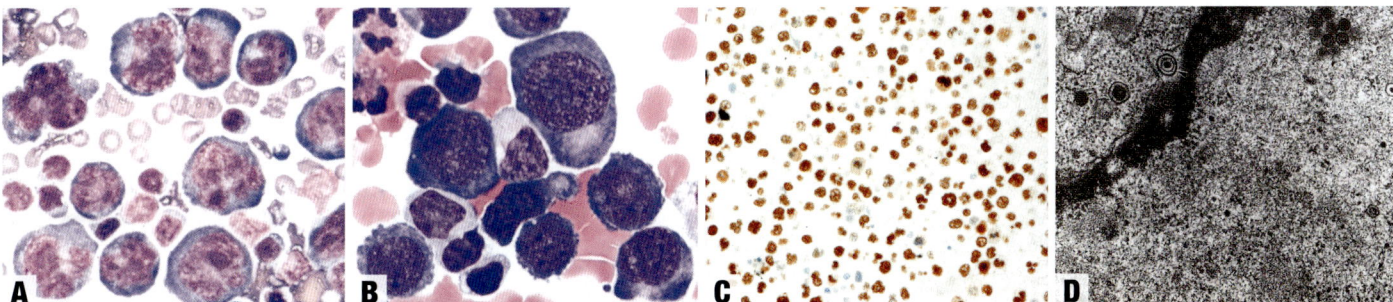

Fig. 2.35 Primary effusion lymphoma. **A** Cytological preparation from a patient with a serous pleural effusion. The cells are large and pleomorphic with lobated nuclei and prominent nucleoli (Giemsa). **B** Cytology. In this effusion, the cells have a plasmacytoid appearance with a prominent Golgi zone or hof. There is marked variation in size and shape of the malignant cells (Giemsa). **C** Cytological preparation from a patient with primary effusion lymphoma stained for HHV8 latency-associated nuclear antigen (LANA) by immunohistochemistry. There is granular brown nuclear staining in all the malignant cells infected with HHV8 (Kaposi sarcoma–associated herpesvirus). **D** Electron photomicrograph shows herpesvirus particles in the nucleus and packaged in the cytoplasm before shedding from the cell surface.

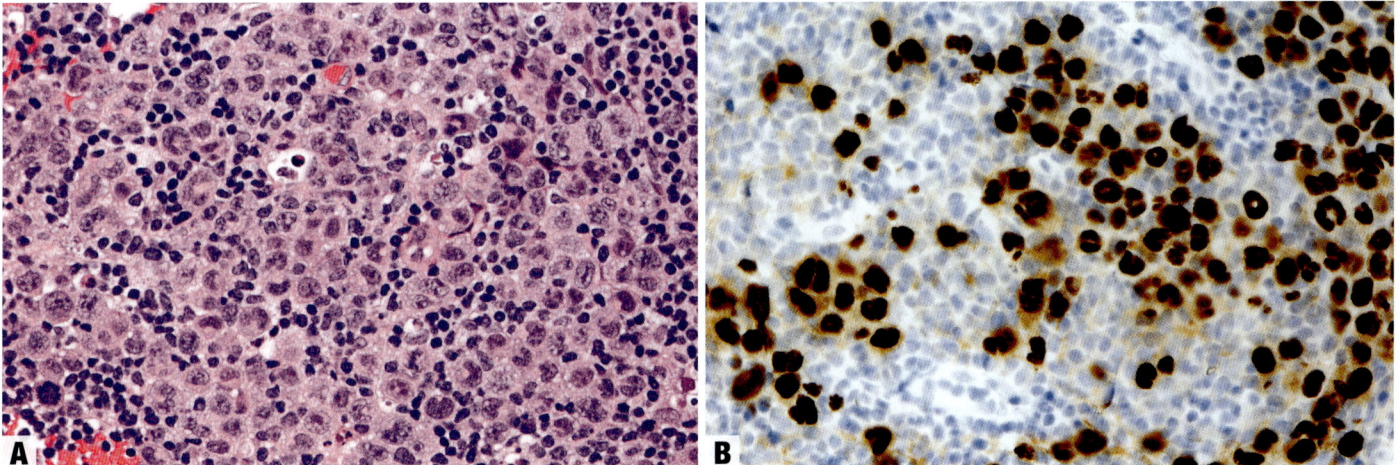

Fig. 2.36 Extracavitary primary effusion lymphoma. **A** Extracavitary primary effusion lymphoma from a patient with a thoracic mass without pleural effusion. The cells are large and pleomorphic with prominent nucleoli, many resembling the hallmark cells seen in anaplastic large cell lymphoma. **B** Extracavitary primary effusion lymphoma stained for HHV8 latency-associated nuclear antigen (LANA) using an immunohistochemical technique. All the large malignant cells show nuclear staining, emphasizing the markedly pleomorphic nature of the nuclei. The adjacent non-infected nuclei are unstained.

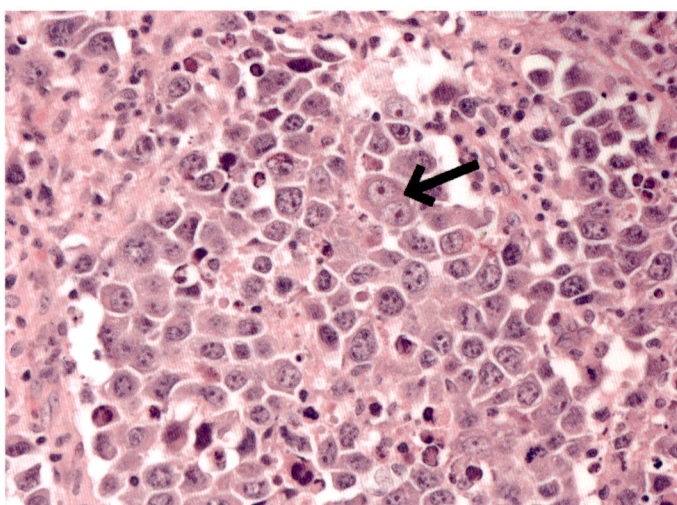

Fig. 2.37 Extracavitary primary effusion lymphoma. Sheets of large malignant cells including multinucleated forms resembling Hodgkin or Reed–Sternberg cells (arrow). There are frequent apoptotic cells.

tract, skin, and CNS {1536}. It is usually associated with HIV, but most patients are less immunosuppressed than in classic PEL.

Epidemiology
PEL usually occurs in immunosuppressed patients, particularly those with HIV, as well as in the posttransplantation setting. In HHV8-endemic areas, PEL is also reported in elderly patients without other known risk factors. PEL represents about 4% of HIV-related lymphomas and < 1% in the non–HIV-infected population {818}. Although there has been a decrease in diffuse large B-cell lymphoma among HIV-infected patients with antiretroviral therapy, the incidence of PEL may be increasing {2419}.

Etiology
PEL is thought to be caused by infection of post–germinal-centre B cells by HHV8, with or without co-infection by EBV.

Pathogenesis
PEL cells are infected with HHV8, with persistence of naked viral episomes and expression of latent viral gene products including the latency-associated nuclear antigen (LANA) LANA1, viral cyclin, vFLIP, vIRF3/LANA2, and kaposins {420}. All of these viral proteins have oncogenic functions, such as activation of NF-κB by vFLIP through binding to IKKγ, effects on cell cycle and prevention of RB1-mediated cell-cycle arrest by viral cyclin, and inhibition of p53 and RB1 by LANA. Virus is replicated and encapsidated in the nuclei of the malignant cells and then enveloped in cytoplasmic and plasma membranes for shedding. Viral lytic gene transcription leads to virion formation. EBV is not required for the pathogenesis of PEL, but EBNA1 enhances the maintenance of HHV8 genomes and LANA expression {231}. The HHV8-encoded homolog of human IL-6, viral IL-6, is produced and secreted by a subset of PEL cells; both IL-6 and IL-10 levels contribute to the natural history of PEL and may be associated with inferior survival {1750}.

PELs are monoclonal lymphomas with somatic hypermutation of IGH variable region genes, resembling post–germinal-centre B cells {428}. They lack translocations involving *MYC*, *BCL6*,

and *BCL2* but may have deregulated expression of MYC protein. Cytogenetic studies reveal a complex karyotype and recurrent alterations that include trisomy 7, trisomy 12, and aberrations of the proximal region of 1q {1750,3318}.

Macroscopic appearance
PEL occurs as a serous effusion. Extracavitary PEL occurs as a mass.

Histopathology
Diagnosis is usually made in cytological preparations (see *Cytology*, below). In extracavitary PEL, the infiltrate comprises sheets of large malignant cells with plasmablastic, pleomorphic, or anaplastic nuclei; prominent nucleoli; and basophilic cytoplasm. Some cells may resemble Reed–Sternberg cells. The cells are usually cohesive with few infiltrating lymphocytes. There may be apoptotic cells or necrosis. A sinusoidal pattern of infiltration mimicking other malignant tumours, such as anaplastic large cell lymphoma or carcinoma, can occur.

Immunohistochemistry
PEL cells are terminally differentiated B cells, but in contrast to other post–germinal-centre B cells and plasma cells, they usually lack surface and cytoplasmic immunoglobulins. They generally lack CD45 (LCA) and can express cytokeratins, causing confusion with other tumours {3365}. They also lack B-cell markers, including CD19, CD20, PAX5, OCT2, BOB1, and CD79a. They most often express non-lineage activation and plasma cell markers, including HLA-DR, CD38, VS38c, CD138, and EMA, as well as CD30 and PDL1 {469}. The cells usually lack T-cell or NK-cell antigens, but aberrant expression of T-cell markers such as CD4 and CD7 can occur in as many as 30% of cases {295,2592,1021}. Demonstration of HHV8, usually by immunostaining for LANA, is required for diagnosis. Most (if not all) cases in HIV-positive patients are positive for EBV-encoded small RNA (EBER) by in situ hybridization, but latent membrane protein LMP1 and EBNA2 are absent (type I latency). Extracavitary PELs express B cell–associated antigens, CD45, and immunoglobulins slightly more often than classic PEL, and they more often have aberrant expression of T-cell markers {428}.

Differential diagnosis
Lymphomas other than PEL may also occur as pleural effusions. Effusion-based large B-cell lymphomas occur in older immunocompetent individuals, in association with fluid overload states usually related to cirrhosis or congestive cardiac failure {56}. These HHV8-negative B-cell lymphomas are not related to PEL and have a relatively favourable prognosis.

Pyothorax-associated lymphomas arise in the pleural cavity after longstanding inflammation, usually due to tuberculosis or chronic pneumothorax. These B-cell lymphomas do not exhibit a plasmablastic immunophenotype, and they are associated with EBV but not HHV8 {422}.

Primary mediastinal (thymic) large B-cell lymphoma may also involve the pleura or pericardium {3087}, but it is a B-cell lymphoma lacking a plasmablastic immunophenotype and HHV8.

HHV8-positive diffuse large B-cell lymphomas associated with multicentric Castleman disease may be difficult to differentiate from extracavitary PEL. These usually involve lymph nodes, are negative for EBER and CD138, and express IgM.

PELs may resemble anaplastic large cell lymphomas, which are T-cell lymphomas negative for HHV8.

ALK-positive large B-cell lymphomas have immunoblastic or plasmablastic morphology and characteristically express plasma cell but not B-cell antigens. They are ALK-positive, usually express immunoglobulin, and are negative for HHV8 and EBV.

Cytology
The cells exhibit a range of appearance, from large immunoblastic or plasmablastic cells to cells with pleomorphic or anaplastic nuclei. Nucleoli are prominent and a perinuclear hof may be seen. The cytoplasm is abundant and basophilic or amphophilic, with occasional vacuoles. Some cells resemble Reed–Sternberg cells. The cytoplasmic characteristics are best appreciated in Giemsa-stained preparations and may appear more uniform in histological sections of cell blocks.

Diagnostic molecular pathology
Demonstration of HHV8 with or without EBV is required for the diagnosis.

Essential and desirable diagnostic criteria
Essential:
- Large pleomorphic malignant cells with plasmablastic immunophenotype (but immunoglobulin is often negative)
- HHV8 is positive (usually by LANA immunohistochemistry)

Desirable:
- The presence of EBV, although neither necessary nor sufficient, is supportive of the diagnosis

Staging
PELs are characterized by diffuse involvement of body cavities without associated nodal involvement, and they are therefore stage IV. Most cases of extracavitary PEL involve a single extralymphatic site in the absence of nodal involvement (stage IE).

Prognosis and prediction
PEL is an aggressive lymphoma with a relatively poor prognosis {1021}. Patients treated with modified EPOCH (etoposide, vincristine, doxorubicin, cyclophosphamide, prednisone) had

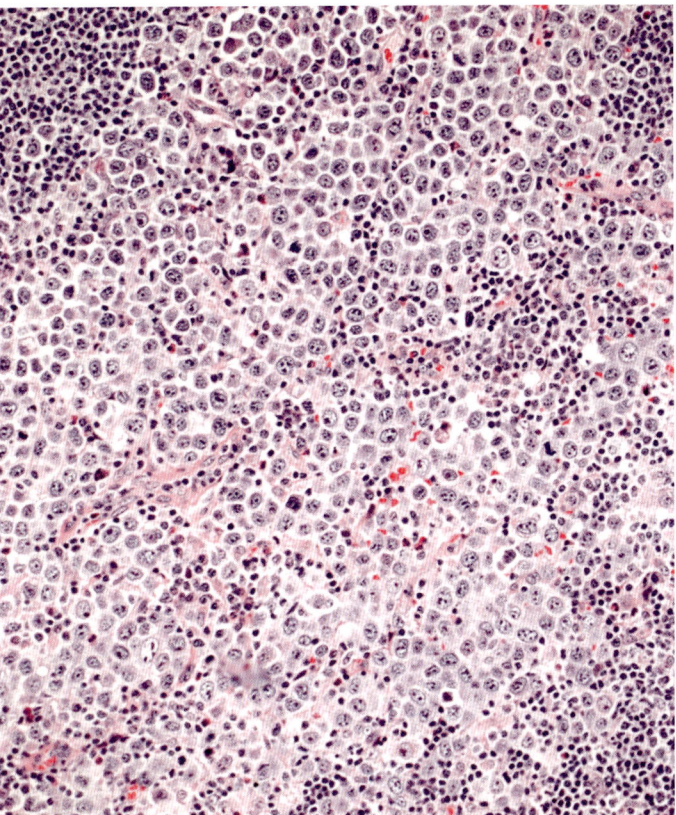

Fig. 2.38 Extracavitary primary effusion lymphoma with extension to regional nodes. Extracavitary primary effusion lymphoma showing sheets of large malignant cells including multinucleated forms and apoptotic cells. There is intrasinusoidal involvement mimicking anaplastic large cell lymphoma or metastatic carcinoma.

an overall survival of 22 months, with a plateau after 2 years, and a 3-year cancer-specific survival rate of 47%. Prolonged survival has been reported in patients who maintain a remission on chemotherapy and antiretroviral therapy {709,2492}. EBV-positive tumours are associated with better survival, whereas patients with elevated IL-6 fare worse {1750}. The prognosis of extracavitary PEL is somewhat better than that of PEL, with fewer relapses after complete remission {428,1021}.

Diffuse large B-cell lymphoma associated with chronic inflammation of the pleura

Chan JKC
Aozasa K
Gaulard P

Definition

Diffuse large B-cell lymphoma (DLBCL) associated with chronic inflammation is an EBV-associated mature B-cell neoplasm occurring in the context of longstanding chronic inflammation, usually in confined anatomical sites.

ICD-O coding

9680/3 Diffuse large B-cell lymphoma associated with chronic inflammation

ICD-11 coding

2A81.7 Diffuse large B-cell lymphoma associated with chronic inflammation

Related terminology

None

Subtype(s)

None

Localization

The commonest site of involvement is the pleural cavity (pyothorax-associated lymphoma [PAL]). Lymphoma occurring in other sites (e.g. bone, joint, and periarticular soft tissue) is not discussed in this section {572,493}. Fibrin-associated DLBCL was previously considered a subtype of DLBCL associated with chronic inflammation, but it is now considered a separate, distinct entity (see *Cardiac fibrin-associated diffuse large B-cell lymphoma*, p. 269).

In PAL, there is direct invasion of adjacent structures, but the tumour is often confined to the thoracic cavity at the time of diagnosis, with about 70% of patients presenting with clinical stage I/II disease {94,2066}.

Clinical features

PAL is the prototypical form, developing in the pleural cavity of patients with longstanding pyothorax. Patients present with chest pain, back pain, fever, or tumorous swelling in the chest wall, or with respiratory symptoms such as productive cough, haemoptysis, or dyspnoea. The serum LDH level is commonly elevated {2066,2332}.

Imaging

Radiological examination reveals a tumour mass in the pleura (80%), pleura and lung (10%), and lung near the pleura (7%).

Epidemiology

PAL develops in patients with a 20- to 64-year (median: 37-year) history of pyothorax resulting from artificial pneumothorax for treatment of pulmonary or pleural tuberculosis {94,1273,2066, 2332,2075}. Patient age at diagnosis ranges from the fifth to eighth decade of life, with a median age of 65–70 years {2066,

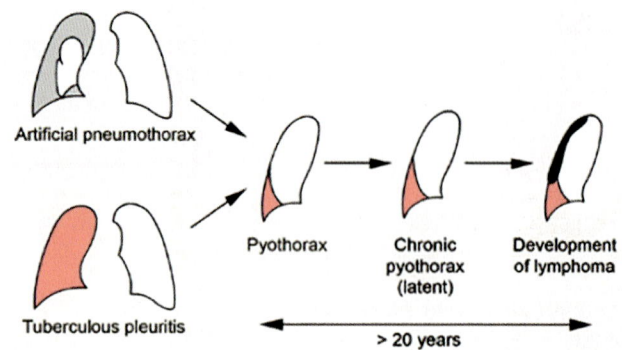

Fig. 2.39 Pyothorax-associated lymphoma. Development of pyothorax-associated lymphoma.

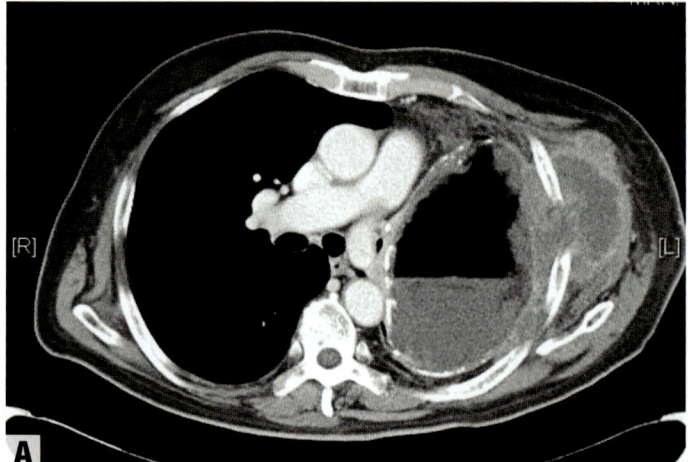

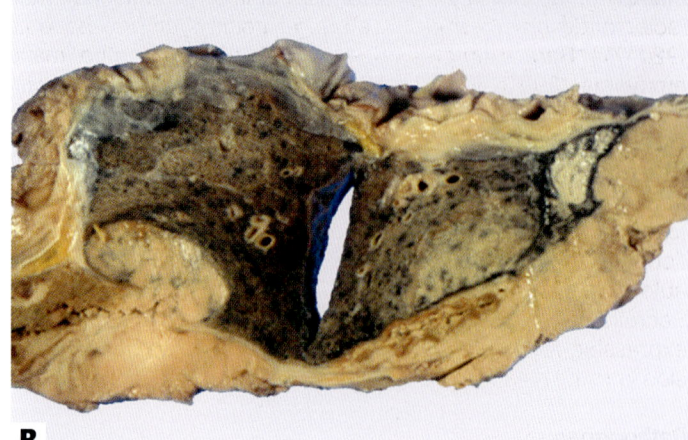

Fig. 2.40 A Pyothorax-associated lymphoma. CT of the thorax shows a destructive tumour mass in the pleura, with invasion into the chest wall tissues. Pleural effusion is also evident. **B** Diffuse large B-cell lymphoma with chronic inflammation. At autopsy, a dense, tan-coloured mass surrounds and compresses the adjacent lung.

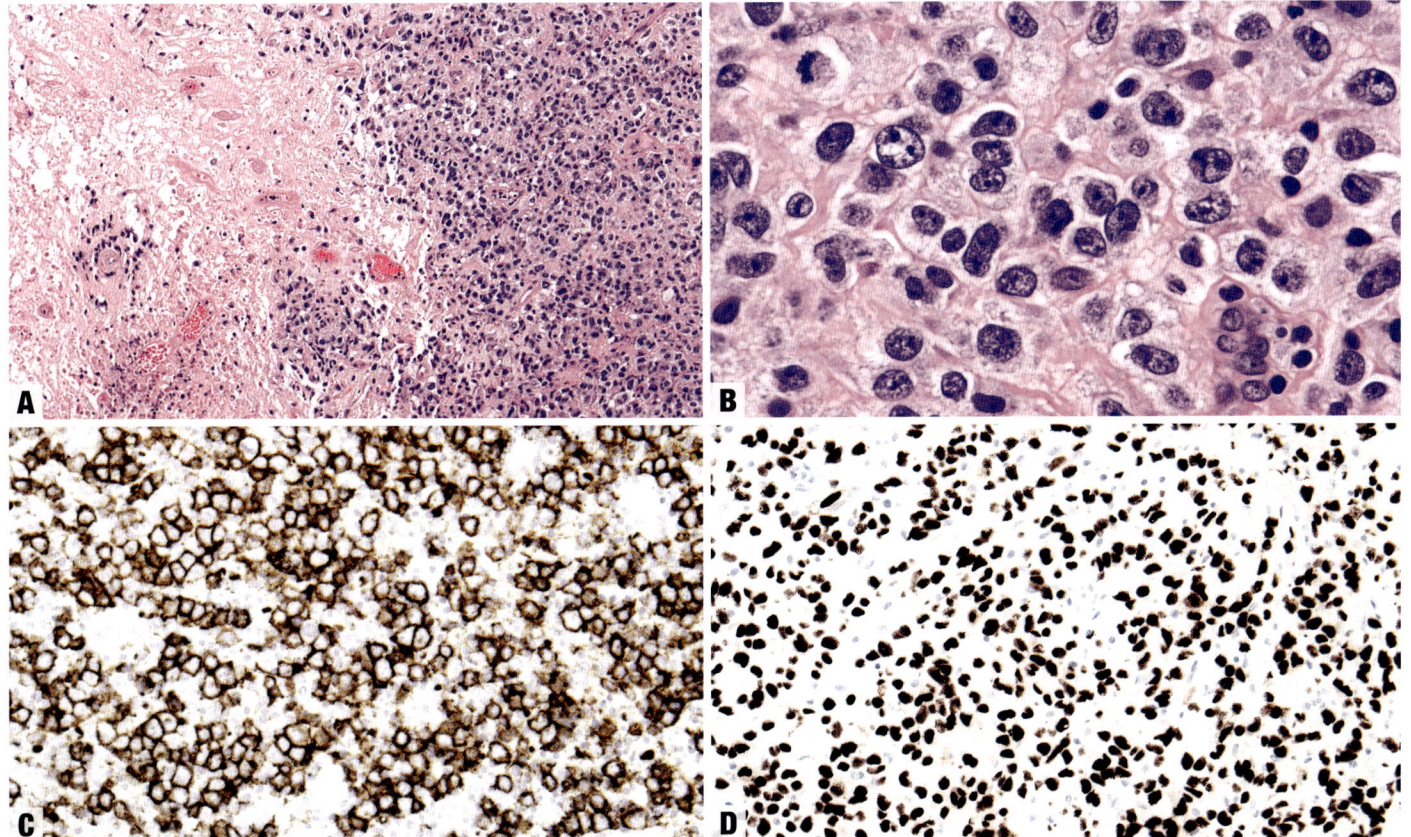

Fig. 2.41 Pyothorax-associated lymphoma. **A** The tumour shows a diffuse dense infiltrate of large lymphoma cells, with areas of coagulative necrosis. **B** The lymphoma cells are large and show distinct nucleoli and voluminous cytoplasm. **C** Positive immunostaining for CD20. **D** Positive immunostaining for EBNA2, indicating type III EBV latency.

2075}. The M:F ratio is 12:3, versus near equality for chronic pyothorax, suggesting that men are more susceptible to this type of lymphoma {1273,2066}. Although most cases of PAL have been reported in Japan, this lymphoma has also been described in Europe {2332,115}.

Etiology

Artificial pneumothorax, used in the past as a form of surgical therapy for pulmonary tuberculosis, is the most significant risk factor for development of PAL among chronic pyothorax patients {92,1177}. Rare examples arise in the setting of posttraumatic empyema {2991}. PAL is strongly associated with EBV, with expression of EBNA2 and/or LMP1 together with EBNA1 {2165, 2955,1177,2635}, i.e. usually type III EBV latency {2954,2332}. Chronic inflammation at the local site probably plays a role in the proliferation of EBV-transformed B cells by enabling them to escape from the host immune surveillance through production of IL-10 (an immunosuppressive cytokine) and by providing autocrine to paracrine growth via IL-6 and IL-6R {1371,1374}. Secretion of CCL17 and CCL22 (chemokines that attract CCR4-expressing regulatory T cells) may play a role in immune evasion in PAL {1145}.

Pathogenesis

IG genes are clonally rearranged and hypermutated but lack ongoing mutations {1939,2956}. *TP53* mutations occur in about 70% of cases, usually involving dipyrimidine sites, which are known to be susceptible to mutagenesis induced by ionizing

radiation {1177}. *MYC* gene amplification is common {3368}, and *TNFAIP3* (*A20*) is deleted in a proportion of cases {80}. Cytogenetic studies show complex karyotypes with numerous numerical and structural abnormalities {2955}. The gene expression profile of PAL is distinct from that of nodal DLBCL {2119}. One of the most differentially expressed genes is *IFI27*, which is known to be induced in B lymphocytes by stimulation of interferon-α, in keeping with the role of chronic inflammation in this condition. Downregulation of HLA class I expression, which is essential for efficient induction of host cytotoxic T lymphocytes (CTLs), and mutations of CTL epitopes in EBNA3B, an immunodominant antigen for CTL responses, might also contribute to escape of PAL cells from host CTLs {1372,1373}.

Macroscopic appearance

The fleshy tumour mass is > 100 mm in more than half of the cases.

Histopathology

The morphological features are the same as those of DLBCL-NOS. Most cases show centroblastic/immunoblastic morphology, with round nuclei and large single or multiple nucleoli. Massive necrosis and angiocentric growth may be present.

Immunohistochemistry

Most cases express CD20 and CD79a. However, a proportion of cases may show plasmacytic differentiation, with loss of CD20 and/or CD79a and expression of IRF4 (MUM1) and CD138. The lymphoma exhibits an activated B-cell / non–germinal-centre B-cell phenotype. CD30 can be expressed. Occasional cases may express in addition one or more T-cell markers (CD2, CD3, CD4, and/or CD7), causing problems in lineage assignment {572,2066,2332,3047}.

In situ hybridization for EBV-encoded small RNA (EBER) shows positive labelling of the lymphoma cells. Type III EBV latency is characteristic (LMP1+, EBNA2+) {2332,880}. HHV8 is negative.

Differential diagnosis
PAL is distinguished from primary effusion lymphoma in that a solid tumour mass is formed, the lymphoma cells often express B-lineage markers, and HHV8 is negative.

Cytology
Unknown

Diagnostic molecular pathology
EBER may be helpful, as described above.

Essential and desirable diagnostic criteria
Essential:
- Mass-forming tumour involving the pleura
- Large cell lymphoma with expression of B-lineage markers
- EBV positivity
- History of longstanding chronic inflammation

Staging
Not clinically relevant

Prognosis and prediction
DLBCL associated with chronic inflammation is an aggressive lymphoma. For PAL patients, the 5-year overall survival rate is 20–35% {2066,2075}. For patients achieving complete remission with chemotherapy and/or radiotherapy, the 5-year survival rate is 50% {2066}. Complete tumour resection (pleuropneumonectomy with or without resection of adjacent involved tissues) or chemotherapy plus rituximab has been reported to give good results {2051,3200}. Poor performance status; high serum levels of LDH, alanine transaminase, or urea; and high clinical stage are unfavourable prognostic factors {93,2075}.

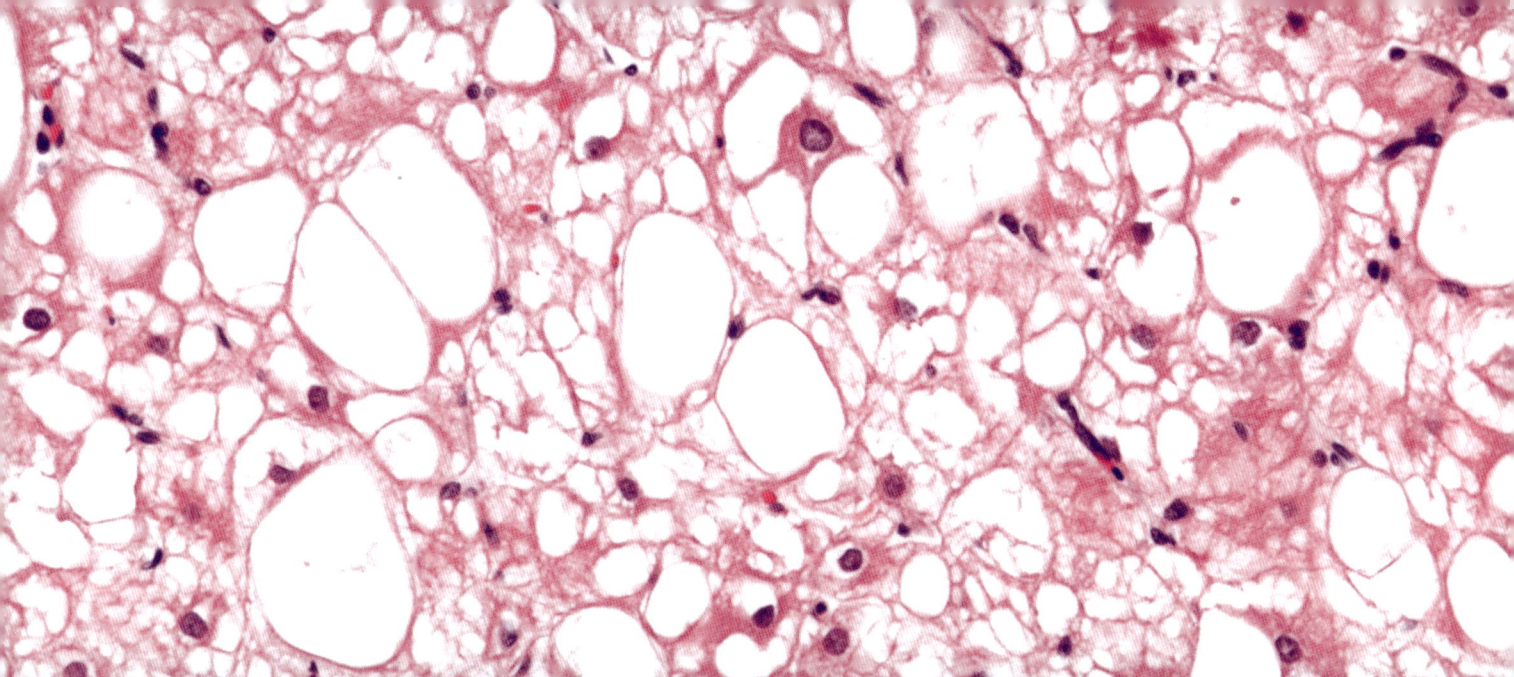

3

Tumours of the heart

Edited by: Chan JKC, Cooper WA, Jain D, Lazar AJ, Maleszewski JJ

Papillary fibroelastoma
Cardiac myxoma
Cardiac fibroma
Cardiac rhabdomyoma
Adult cellular rhabdomyoma
Cardiac lipoma and lipomatous hypertrophy of the atrial septum
Lipomatous hamartoma of the atrioventricular valve
Hamartoma of mature cardiac myocytes
Mesenchymal cardiac hamartoma
Cardiac haemangiomas
Conduction system hamartoma
Cystic tumour of the atrioventricular node
Cardiac angiosarcoma
Cardiac leiomyosarcoma
Cardiac undifferentiated pleomorphic sarcoma
Other sarcomas that may involve the heart
Cardiac diffuse large B-cell lymphoma
Cardiac fibrin-associated diffuse large B-cell lymphoma

Tumours of the heart: Introduction

Maleszewski JJ

Overview

Primary cardiac tumours have long been held to be rare. However, advances in molecular techniques and imaging have improved our understanding of these tumours, as well as our ability to recognize them. They are still considered uncommon, but their prompt identification and management is paramount, given the relatively high morbidity and mortality associated with them.

Unlike tumours in many other organs, those that involve the heart can have devastating consequences, irrespective of histological benignity. Cardiac tumours may interfere with the heart's mechanical or electrical function and cause dramatic presentation or even sudden death.

Etiology and epidemiology

Cardiac tumours can be broadly dichotomized into metastatic and primary forms. Metastasis to the heart is about 20-fold to 30-fold more common than primary cardiac tumours {1775}. In fact, cardiac involvement is found in upwards of 9–14% of autopsies of patients with underlying malignancy {325,3461,64, 2471,352}. Although nearly any malignancy has the potential to metastasize to the heart, thoracic malignancies, along with melanoma, extracardiac sarcomas, and renal cell carcinoma, account for the majority of cases {1774}.

Primary cardiac tumours can be either benign or malignant, with the former outnumbering the latter by about 10:1. The most common primary cardiac tumour is the papillary fibroelastoma, which typically arises on one of the left-sided valves. Cardiac myxoma, perhaps the most well-studied, is the second most common cardiac tumour in adults. In children, cardiac rhabdomyoma is the most common cardiac tumour, often arising in the setting of tuberous sclerosis due to mutations in the underlying TSC1 and TSC2 genes {1775}.

Rhabdomyoma is not the only cardiac tumour to occur in a syndromic context. Approximately 5% of cardiac myxomas arise in association with Carney complex, an autosomal dominant condition caused by mutations in PRKAR1A {1777}. Likewise, cardiac fibromas may be associated with Gorlin syndrome (naevoid basal cell carcinoma syndrome), resulting from mutation in the PTCH1 gene {3159}. Recently, some subsets of cardiac angiosarcoma have been noted to occur in kindreds with Li–Fraumeni–like syndrome and POT1 mutation {364}. Therefore, the possibility of a syndromic condition should be investigated in many cases when a cardiac tumour has been diagnosed.

Cardiac tumours have been reported across the entire human age spectrum, including in fetuses and in people aged > 100 years. They do, however, exhibit age-related trends by tumour type. Cardiac rhabdomyoma, cardiac fibroma, and cardiac haemangioma are identified (in order of decreasing frequency) disproportionately in children {2993}. Most other cardiac tumours are seen more commonly in adults. Nearly all malignant diseases of the heart, both primary and metastatic, are encountered far more frequently in adults as well.

Clinical features

Clinical features of cardiac tumours, both benign and malignant, are wide-ranging and often nonspecific, delaying diagnosis and management. Many cardiac tumours are asymptomatic and are incidental findings on imaging or routine examination. When symptoms are present, they may relate to involvement of the heart itself, producing valvular dysfunction, arrhythmia, or obstruction. Additionally, embolization resulting from either the tumour or a surface thrombus may result in any number of systemic effects. Finally, constitutional symptoms such as fever, malaise, and weight loss may occur as a result of elaboration of substances by the tumour.

A multitude of factors drive the presentation of cardiac tumours, including size, location, site, and type. Large masses, such as rhabdomyomas, often have a propensity to interfere with the normal flow of blood throughout the heart. Alternatively, some small masses, such as cystic tumours of the atrioventricular node (a lesion not usually visible to the naked eye), may have calamitous consequences owing to the extreme sensitivity of the cardiac conduction system, which they involve. Lesions that more commonly involve the left side of the heart, such as papillary fibroelastoma or cardiac myxoma, are obviously much more likely to occur with embolic phenomenon {1288,3127}.

Technical considerations

Most cardiac tumours can be processed in a similar fashion to tumours excised from elsewhere in the body. As is true with all specimens, careful gross examination can be very helpful in narrowing the differential diagnosis. Papillary fibroelastomas, for instance, may have a somewhat mucoid appearance (mimicking cardiac myxoma) when they are not in solution. However, when they are placed in an aqueous medium, their papillary nature becomes readily apparent. Careful sampling and routine processing are also important, as with other tumours.

Changes from the prior edition

Advances in molecular techniques have allowed for a deepened understanding of certain tumours. Papillary fibroelastomas, for instance, have been shown to demonstrate KRAS driver mutations in a subset of cases – indicating they are probably neoplastic in nature {3333,257}. Similarly, cases of lipomatous hypertrophy of the atrial septum have been shown to harbour molecular genetic alterations similar to those seen in lipomas, debunking the notion that all of these cases are simply due to displaced fat during embryogenesis {255}.

New ancillary tools have become available that allow for screening for underlying and associated syndromes, such as for Carney complex in patients with cardiac myxomas {1777}.

These techniques allow for rapid and reliable screening that enables the treating team to react and follow up in accordance with newer guidelines. Molecular advances continue to drive sarcoma research, with the promise of identifying targeted and personalized therapeutics.

Several entities are new to the classification, including hamartomatous lesions such as lipomatous hamartoma of the atrioventricular valve and mesenchymal cardiac hamartoma. These newly described entities expand the spectrum of recognized tumours that arise in the heart.

Finally, legacy terms have been carefully evaluated and changed where appropriate. The term "conduction system hamartoma" was coined to refer to the lesion formerly known as histiocytoid cardiomyopathy, after careful consideration of the underlying molecular biology and presentation of this entity; because this lesion is not generally a diffuse primary muscular disease of the heart, calling it a cardiomyopathy resulted in confusion. The nodular proliferation of Purkinje cells that tracks along the cardiac conduction system is far better represented by the new name.

Papillary fibroelastoma

Buettner R
Maleszewski JJ

Definition
Papillary fibroelastoma is a benign endocardial neoplasm, consisting of endothelium overlying avascular fibroelastic fronds.

ICD-O coding
8820/0 Papillary fibroelastoma

ICD-11 coding
2F01 Benign neoplasm of intrathoracic organs

Related terminology
Not recommended: fibroelastic papilloma; cardiac papilloma; giant Lambl excrescence.

Subtype(s)
None

Localization
By definition, papillary fibroelastomas arise on endocardial surfaces, mostly on the valves. In surgical series, the left-sided

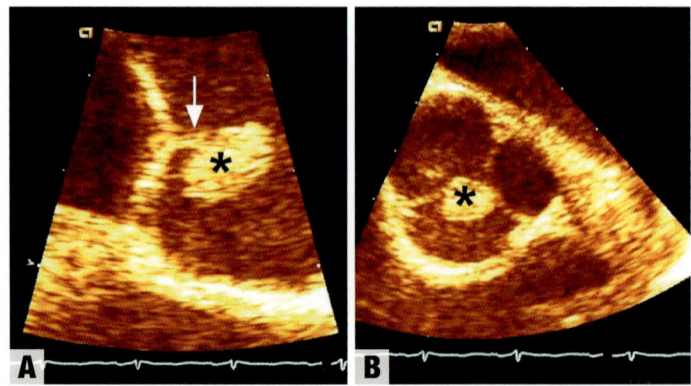

Fig. 3.01 Papillary fibroelastoma. Transoesophageal echocardiographs showing a papillary fibroelastoma (asterisks) arising from the aortic valve. A short stalk (arrow) can be seen (**A**), as can the relationship to the closed tricuspid aortic valve (**B**).

valves are most commonly involved, with the aortic valve being the usual site. Papillary fibroelastomas often arise on the surface of diseased valves (e.g. in degenerative fibrocalcific disease or

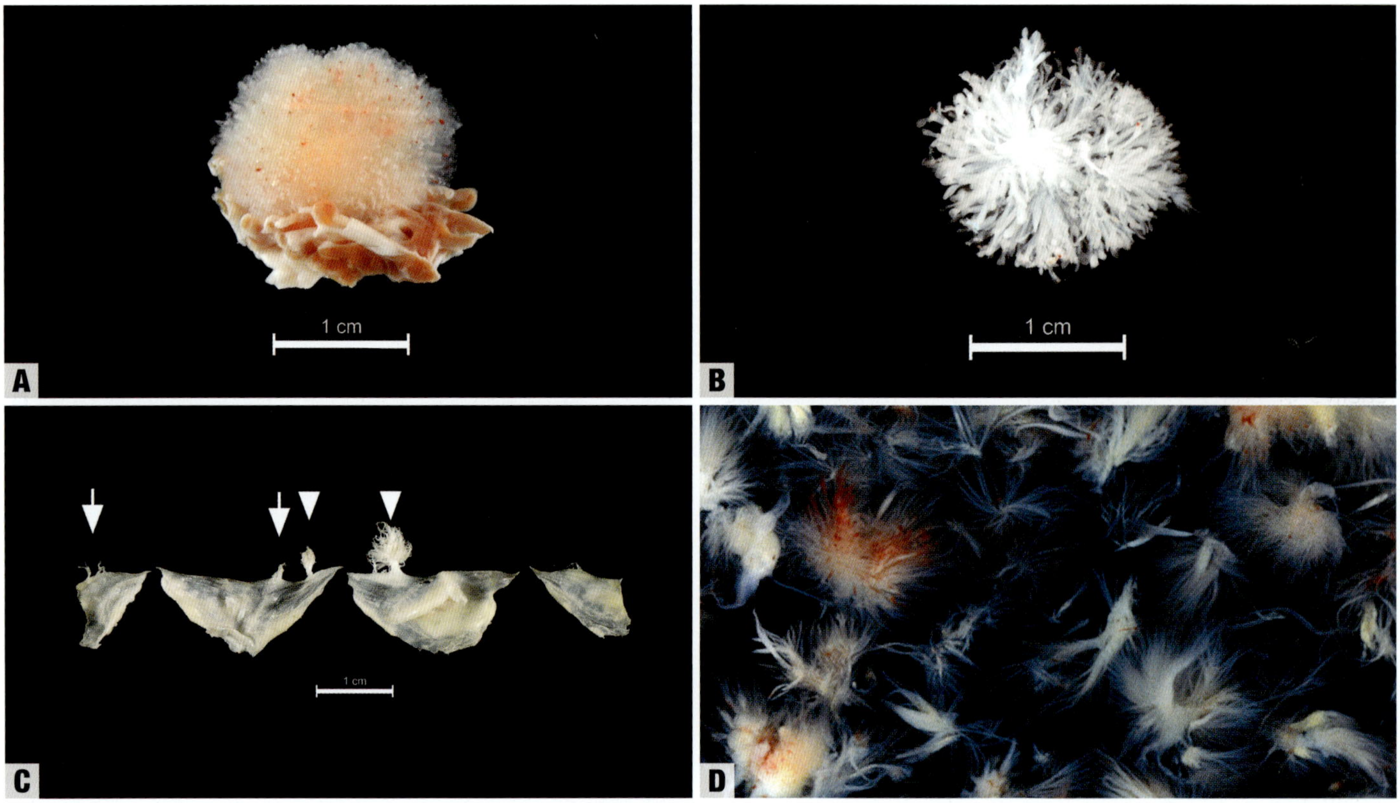

Fig. 3.02 Papillary fibroelastoma. **A** Papillary fibroelastoma arising from the left ventricle; the sea anemone–like quality of the tumour can be clearly seen. **B** Multiple fronds are visible, with complex branching. **C** Two papillary fibroelastomas arise from the free edge of two aortic valve cusps (arrowheads); small Lambl excrescences (arrows) that consist of simple, singular fronds also arise from the free edge of the cusps. **D** Multiple (> 40) papillary fibroelastomas resected from the left ventricular outflow tract, 17 years after subaortic septal myectomy for hypertrophic obstructive cardiomyopathy.

chronic rheumatic valvulopathy). Less common sites of involvement include the right-sided valves, cardiac chambers, papillary muscles, and (rarely) the aortic sinus {1567,47}.

Papillary fibroelastomas may occur singly or as multifocal lesions (which are particularly common in iatrogenic settings and rheumatic valve disease). Individual patients with > 40 discrete synchronous papillary fibroelastomas have been reported {2091}.

Clinical features
The clinical presentation of papillary fibroelastomas varies greatly, from asymptomatic incidental findings on echocardiography to symptoms of heart failure, syncope, embolic phenomena, or sudden death {171}. As is the case with most cardiac tumours, the clinical symptoms depend primarily on the size and location of the mass. Tumours arising from the aortic valve may obstruct blood flow, causing chest pain or dyspnoea {537}. Embolic symptoms such as transient ischaemic attacks or stroke have been reported in as many as 33% of patients with papillary fibroelastomas found on imaging {2980}. Such embolic phenomena may be related to embolization of the tumour itself or adherent surface thrombus {997,2980}.

Imaging
Transoesophageal echocardiography is the preferred imaging modality for visualization of papillary fibroelastomas, which typically manifest as small mobile masses attached to an endocardial surface, with independent motion and a contour that is either stippled or shimmering {568}.

Epidemiology
Papillary fibroelastoma is the most common primary cardiac neoplasm. Due to improved recognition through higher-resolution imaging techniques, they are increasingly encountered {171}. Patients are typically 60–70 years old, with a recently published series reporting an age range of 42–80 years {3333}, but lesions have been reported in individuals from the neonatal period up to 92 years of age. Papillary fibroelastomas have no clear sex predilection {997,2980}.

Etiology
Although papillary fibroelastoma was initially considered a reactive or hamartomatous lesion, recent studies have provided evidence that a subset of papillary fibroelastomas harbour canonical oncogenic driver mutations in *KRAS* exon 2 or 3, which impair the protein's GTPase activity {3333,257}. Thus, papillary fibroelastomas must be considered benign neoplasms with limited growth capacity resulting from constitutive activation of the RAS/MAPK signalling pathway. However, this finding does not exclude the possibility that endothelial injury may be a contributing factor, because these tumours clearly occur more commonly in a variety of conditions associated with damaged endocardium (e.g. rheumatic valvulopathy, hypertrophic cardiomyopathy, and congenital heart disease) {2732,1547}. Their benign neoplastic nature is further supported by the fact that these neoplasms frequently arise on areas of damaged endothelium or haemodynamic trauma (e.g. in structural heart disease or at sites of prior surgery, instrumentation, or irradiation) {1567}.

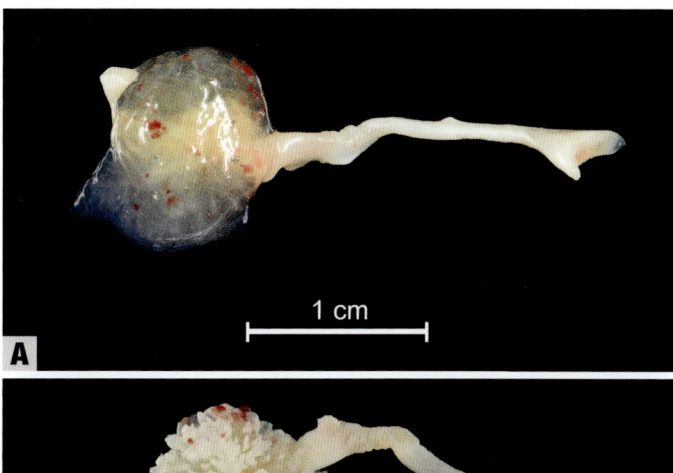
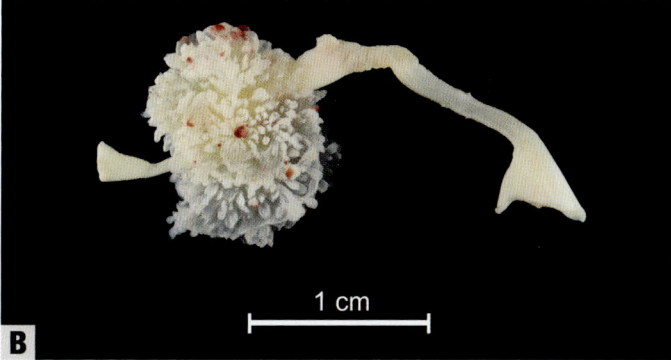

Fig. 3.03 Papillary fibroelastoma. **A** The myxoid appearance of a surgically resected papillary fibroelastoma arising from a left ventricular pseudotendon can closely mimic that of a myxoma. **B** Placing the tumour in an aqueous medium reveals its papillary architecture.

Pathogenesis
The genetic hallmark of papillary fibroelastoma is an oncogenic *KRAS* mutation found in as many as 80% of cases {3333}. Two cases have been cytogenetically studied, showing heterogeneous translocations involving chromosomes 5, 21, and 15 in one case and nullisomy Y with trisomies 12 and 20 in the other {3237,2828}. However, these inconsistent genomic aberrations may result from oncogenic stress induced by constitutive KRAS/MAPK activation.

Macroscopic appearance
Grossly, excised papillary fibroelastomas often have a round, whitish appearance and a soft consistency. When placed into solution, multiple delicate fronds unfurl, giving the tumour what has been described as a sea anemone–like appearance. The tumours range in size from 2 to 50 mm and are usually attached to the endocardium by a single stalk. Occasionally, the stalk and fronds can be matted together with thrombus, fibrosis, or calcification {171,836}.

Histopathology
Papillary fibroelastomas consist of narrow avascular papillary fronds that often exhibit complex branching patterns. Histologically, the collagen and elastic fibre arrangements are reminiscent of the tendinous cords of the atrioventricular valves. An elastic stain is helpful to delineate the fibroelastic core, and a Movat pentachrome stain can highlight the rich mucopolysaccharide and proteoglycan matrix. The elastic fibres may be sparse or absent at the tips of the lesion. Occasionally, the fronds can fibrotically fuse together, but the fibroelastic fronds

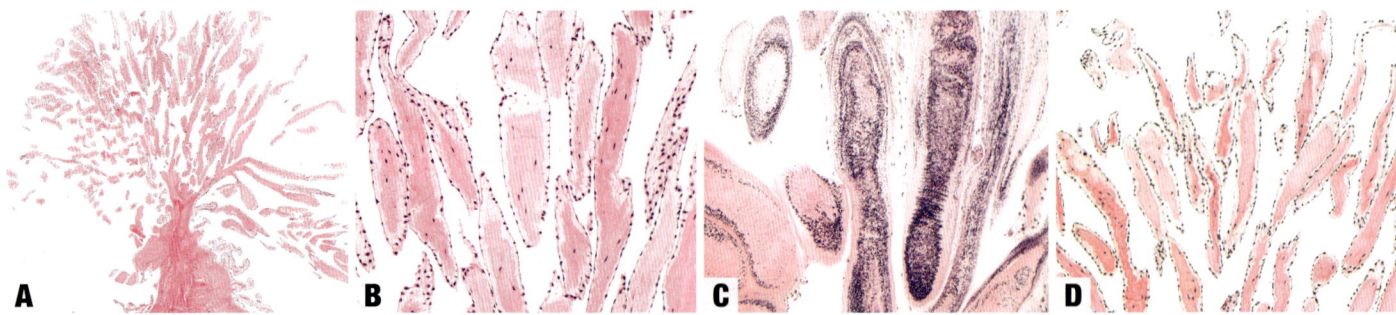

Fig. 3.04 Papillary fibroelastoma. **A** At low power; numerous arborizing fronds arise from a common central stalk. **B** At high power; avascular fronds, coated by bland endothelium, are prototypical of the lesion. **C** An elastic stain highlights the fibroelastic nature of the fronds. **D** Elastic fibres may be sparse or absent in the fronds, particularly at the tips.

can still be visualized histologically. A single layer of endothelial cells coats the fronds and may have adherent surface thrombus.

Immunohistochemistry

Surface endothelial cells express factor VIII, CD34, CD31, and S100 {2561}. Some spindle cells within deeper layers may express S100, possibly representing dendritic cells.

Differential diagnosis

The differential diagnosis of papillary fibroelastoma includes cardiac myxoma, vegetations (infected or sterile), valvular strands, calcification (mural or valvular), and Lambl excrescences. Cardiac myxoma, particularly the villiform variety, can mimic a papillary fibroelastoma on imaging or gross evaluation. However, it is most unusual for a myxoma to arise in a valvular location. Additionally, papillary fibroelastomas do not contain myxoma cells {20}, and they have a characteristic fibroelastic core.

There is significant histological overlap between Lambl excrescences and papillary fibroelastomas, and it has been postulated that these entities may represent a spectrum of the same process. The term "Lambl excrescence" should be applied only to simple fronds (without branching) that are found on the closing surface of the valves (usually the aortic). Papillary fibroelastomas exhibit more-complex branching patterns and may arise on any endothelial surface.

Cytology

Not clinically relevant

Diagnostic molecular pathology

Not clinically relevant

Essential and desirable diagnostic criteria

Essential:
- Avascular fibroblastic fronds lined by endocardium

Desirable:
- Papillary architecture (may be obscured by fibrotic matting)

Staging

Not clinically relevant

Prognosis and prediction

Despite their benign histology and limited growth, papillary fibroelastomas may have potentially devastating clinical sequelae, usually resulting from their thromboembolic potential. Consequently, resection is recommended (particularly for left-sided lesions), and it can often be done sparing the underlying cardiac structures, obviating the need for a valve replacement. Anticoagulation may also be used, if thromboembolic symptoms are present. Surgery provides excellent short- and long-term outcomes without significant recurrence, even when resection is incomplete {997,989,3375}. Regardless, follow-up echocardiography is recommended after surgery.

Cardiac myxoma

Maleszewski JJ
Castonguay MC

Definition
Cardiac myxoma is a benign neoplasm consisting of stellate, ovoid, or plump spindle cells within a vascular myxoid matrix.

ICD-O coding
8840/0 Myxoma, NOS

ICD-11 coding
2F01 & XH6Q84 Benign neoplasm of intrathoracic organs & Myxoma, NOS

Related terminology
Not recommended: left atrial myxoma; atrial myxoma.

Subtype(s)
None

Localization
Cardiac myxomas are intracavitary endocardial lesions, most often arising in the left atrium (in 80–90% of cases) in the region of the fossa ovalis {1777,3453}. The tumours have also been reported in all other cardiac chambers, and very rare examples of valvular myxomas have been described {813,2637,3428}. About half of the cardiac myxomas that arise in the setting of Carney complex occur outside of the left atrium, whereas < 20% occur outside of the left atrium in non-syndromic circumstances {1777}. Thus, a myxoma occurring in a non-left atrial site should raise suspicion for underlying Carney complex. The tumours can be multicentric, raising further suspicion for Carney complex {3057}.

Clinical features
Signs and symptoms
The clinical presentation of cardiac myxoma is diverse and (as is the case with most cardiac tumours) primarily dependent on tumour location, size, shape, mobility, and rate of growth. Patients with cardiac myxomas may be entirely asymptomatic (10–20%), have symptoms of heart failure, or rarely present with sudden death {1562}.

Cardiac symptoms
Cardiac myxomas can produce several cardiac symptoms, including syncope, dyspnoea, chest pain, and palpitations {2707}. Most cardiac symptoms are related to tumoural obstruction of blood flow through the heart. Occasionally, atrial myxomas may obstruct the atrioventricular valve orifice, causing a diastolic tumour plop on auscultation. Some authors have noted an association between septal tumour location and heart failure, and between extraseptal location and neurological events {2940}.

Embolism
Villiform tumours and tumours with abundant myxoid stroma are more likely to be associated with embolization. Tumour degeneration by overexpression of matrix metalloproteinases may hasten embolization {2214}. Embolization of associated surface thrombi can also occur {1326}. Embolization can result in pulmonary embolism, acute myocardial ischaemia, or stroke {1513, 3122}.

Constitutional symptoms
Constitutional symptoms, which can include fever, weight loss, and arthralgias, are frequently associated with large or multiple tumours {768}. Clinical signs such as anaemia, leukocytosis, and elevated erythrocyte sedimentation rate may also be observed. Many of the phenomena are believed to be related to cytokine elaboration by the tumours themselves, including of IL-6, IL-4, IL-12, interferon-γ, and TNF {2792}. A wide range of paraneoplastic syndromes (e.g. vasculitis/vasculopathy,

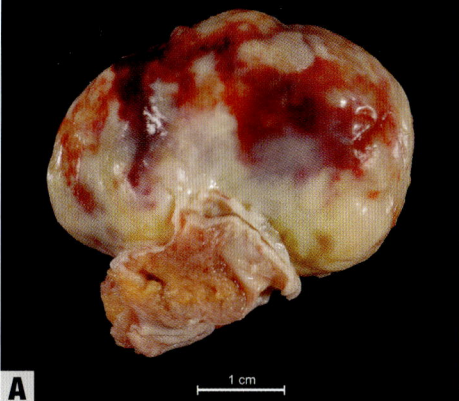
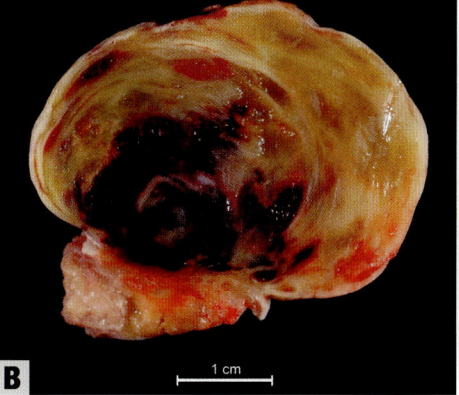
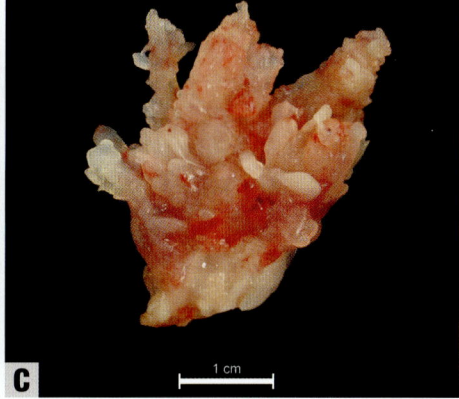

Fig. 3.05 Cardiac myxoma. **A** Gross photo of a globular, smooth-surfaced myxoma that was surgically resected from the left atrium. **B** Gross photo of the cut surface of a globular myxoma. The cut surface is variegated, with areas of intratumoural haemorrhage. **C** Gross photo of a villiform myxoma that was surgically resected from the left atrium.

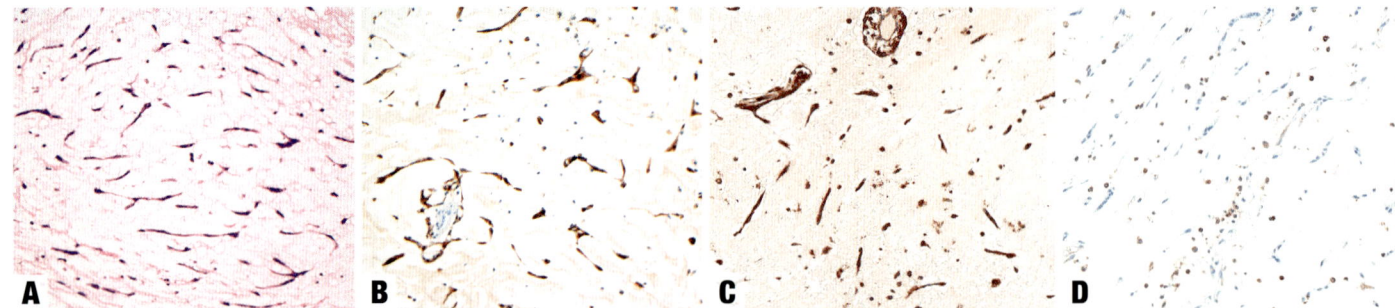

Fig. 3.06 Cardiac myxoma. **A** Photomicrograph showing bland, spindle (myxoma) cells occurring singly and in small cords residing in a myxoid background. **B** Myxoma cells are typically reactive with antibodies directed against calretinin. **C** A non-syndromic cardiac myxoma exhibiting retained expression of PRKAR1A within both the neoplastic cells and the background inflammatory cells. **D** Syndromic cardiac myxoma, arising in the setting of Carney complex, showing lost expression of PRKAR1A within the myxoma cells. Note that the background inflammatory cells have retained expression.

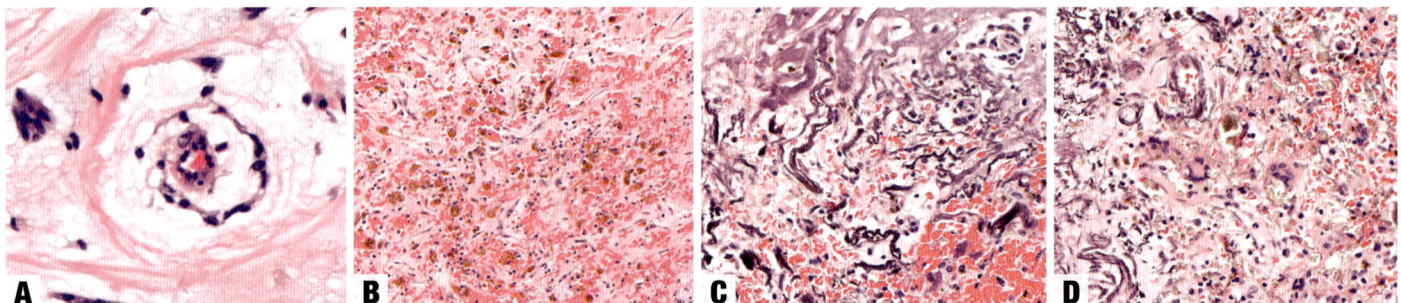

Fig. 3.07 Cardiac myxoma. **A** Perivascular ring structures composed of myxoma cells growing around small intratumoural blood vessels. **B** Prominent haemosiderosis, a consequence of intratumoural haemorrhage. **C** Gamna–Gandy bodies within a cardiac myxoma. **D** Intratumoural giant cells within a cardiac myxoma.

pancreatitis, demyelinating neuropathy, and epistaxis) have been reported {2286,2625,2792}.

Carney complex

Less than 10% of cardiac myxomas arise in the setting of Carney complex, an autosomal dominant disorder characterized by the constellation of myxomas (cardiac or otherwise), endocrinopathy (Cushing syndrome and acromegaly), and spotty skin pigmentation. See *Carney complex* (p. 478) for more detailed information on this syndrome.

Imaging

Transthoracic echocardiography is the diagnostic imaging modality of choice {332}. Echocardiographically, a cardiac myxoma usually appears as a mobile endocardial mass of irregular shape, most often arising in the left atrium in the region of the fossa ovalis. Areas of variable echogenicity and calcification may be seen. More advanced echocardiographical modalities, such as contrast and 3D echocardiography, may help provide a more complete characterization of the tumour appearance, size, and location {1787,2190,3046}.

If a definitive tumour stalk is not visible, cardiac MRI and CT may help to exclude the myocardial infiltration seen in malignant processes {966}. Most frequently, myxomas are T1-isointense and T2-hyperintense, owing to their gelatinous nature and high extracellular water content {562}. Myxomas usually show no or weak contrast enhancement on CT {562}.

Tumour spread

Myxomas can recur locally, a phenomenon that is usually explained by incomplete resection {1777,2437}. They can also spread to distant sites through embolization, after which they can infiltrate the arterial wall and produce histologically identical tumours at the embolization site. Myxoma cell infiltration can result in arterial wall weakening and aneurysm formation, even years after resection of the primary tumour {1296,3170,2626}.

Epidemiology

Cardiac myxoma is the second most common primary cardiac neoplasm of adults, after papillary fibroelastoma. It occurs in all age groups (having been described prenatally through the age of 97 years), but it manifests most commonly between the fourth and seventh decades of life {1562,1590,2491}. Cardiac myxomas occur, on average, twice as commonly in women as in men {3414}, but this female predominance is less pronounced in patients aged > 65 years {276}.

More than 90% of cardiac myxomas arise in an isolated fashion. The remaining cases arise in association with Carney complex. Syndromic tumours generally occur in younger patients, with no sex predominance {991}.

Etiology

The histogenesis of cardiac myxomas has been controversial since they were first described. Initially, they were thought to be reactive lesions or organizing thrombi; however, their locations within the heart, their genetics, and their overall histology are more characteristic of a neoplastic process. The origin of the myxoma cell (or lepidic cell) has also proved enigmatic.

Pathogenesis

Recent molecular characterization studies have revealed protein expression profiles similar to those seen in

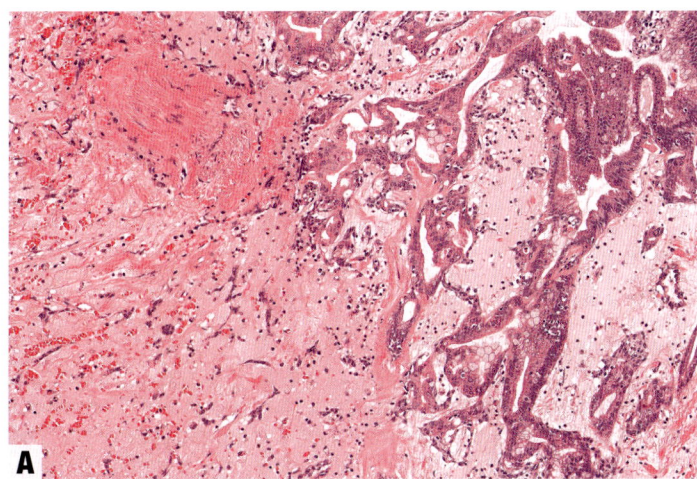 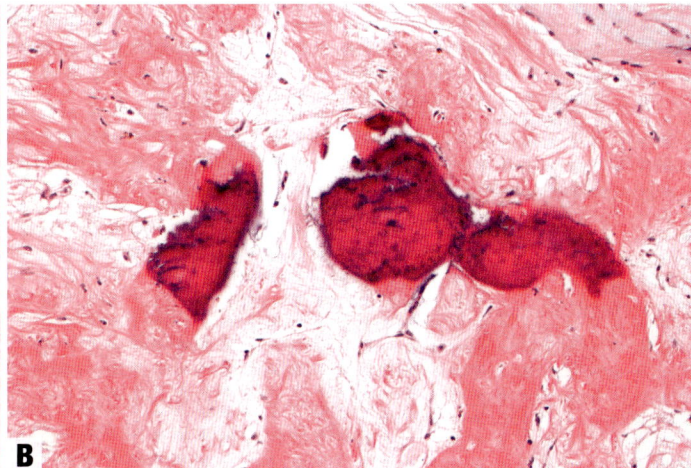

Fig. 3.08 Cardiac myxoma. **A** Heterotopic glands arising within a myxoma. **B** Heterotopic bone formation within a cardiac myxoma.

endocardial–mesenchymal transformation of the endocardial cushion {1495,2213,715}. Whether these cells ultimately derive from developmental remnants or from redifferentiation of a terminally differentiated cardiac cell is not yet clear.

Although initially thought to play a role only in syndromic tumour formation {1753,1790}, *PRKAR1A*, encoding the cAMP-dependent protein kinase type Iα regulatory subunit, has also been implicated in a subset of patients without Carney complex {1777,3169}. Cytogenetic data on myxoma are limited, but 15 previously analysed myxomas contained clonal numerical or non-clonal structural abnormalities. Cytogenetic analyses of 3 cases of Carney complex revealed similar chromosomal patterns as in non-syndromic cases {705,1017}.

Macroscopic appearance

The gross appearance of cardiac myxomas is quite variable. The tumours can measure < 10 mm or > 150 mm {512,2357, 2518,3491}. They may be either sessile and broad-based or pedunculated – arising from a stalk. Tumour stalks may occasionally be long, resulting in free mobility of the tumour within the chamber or through a valvular orifice. Two basic gross appearances have been described: solid and villiform. Tumours of the solid type may be globular or elongated, with a smooth, shiny, and sometimes undulant surface. Tumours of the villiform type (as the name would imply) have irregular, often friable, extensions. The cut surface is variegated, usually owing to the myxoid tissue and areas of intratumoural haemorrhage, which is common. Areas of necrosis, cystic change, fibrosis, and calcification can also be seen {13,2271}. Rarely, cardiac myxomas show extensive calcifications with a stone-like appearance – the so-called lithomyxoma {169}.

Histopathology

Cardiac myxomas exhibit considerable histological variability, sometimes even in different regions of the same tumour. The one defining characteristic is the presence of the so-called myxoma cell (or lepidic cell), a cytologically bland cell with eosinophilic cytoplasm and an oval or round nucleus. These stellate, ovoid, or plump spindle cells may occur singly or in groups. When in groups, the cells can form cords, nests, or rings. Rings frequently occur around capillaries or small vessels and have been termed perivascular rings.

The cells reside in a myxoid matrix that is rich in mucopoly-saccharides, with variable amounts of proteoglycan, collagen, and elastin {1285}. The matrix shows strong reactivity with Alcian blue, is resistant to hyaluronidase, and shows patchy positivity with mucicarmine and PAS stains. The background may also contain variable numbers of inflammatory cells and (rarely) multinucleated giant cells {346,1116}.

Larger, thick-walled vessels are often present near the stalk or base of the lesion, while smaller vessels are present throughout {2213}. Haemorrhage, both recent and remote, is frequently encountered and is probably a product of the vascularity and trauma throughout the cardiac cycle. Remote haemorrhage can manifest as haemosiderin-laden macrophages and/or iron encrustation of intratumoural elastic fibres (Gamna–Gandy bodies). Secondary degenerative changes such as fibrosis, cystic change, necrosis, thrombosis, calcification, and metaplastic bone formation can also be present {169}.

Glandular elements are very rare – identified in < 3% of all myxomas {3489}. The glands are predominantly located at the base of the tumour, without local infiltration. Similarly, diffuse large B-cell lymphomas, some associated with EBV, have been described in the background of otherwise classic cardiac myxomas (see *Cardiac fibrin-associated diffuse large B-cell lymphoma*, p. 269) {2936,2269}.

Foci of extramedullary haematopoiesis may be seen in 7% of myxomas {1626}. Thymic rests and cellular thymoma-like elements have been observed {1923}. There have also been rare reports of gastric heterotopia, chondroid differentiation, and prominent oncocytic change {197,380,2397,3317}.

Immunohistochemistry

Myxoma cells exhibit reactivity with antibodies directed against calretinin in nearly all cases, while variable reactivity has been observed with antibodies directed against NSE, S100, synaptophysin, SMA, and desmin {11}. Endothelial markers (e.g. CD31, CD34, thrombomodulin, and endothelin) are, as expected, positive in endothelium, with variable reactivity reported in myxoma cells {2600}.

Demonstration of lost PRKAR1A expression within the myxoma cells raises the possibility of underlying Carney complex, which should prompt clinical consideration of the syndrome (possibly including germline genetic testing) {1777}.

Differential diagnosis

The primary differential diagnoses of cardiac myxoma include organizing thrombus, so-called calcified amorphous tumour (when calcification is present), papillary fibroelastoma (particularly with villiform myxomas), and other rare entities. When heterologous glands are identified, differentiation from metastatic adenocarcinoma is paramount, and this can usually be achieved with clinical history, imaging, and ancillary studies.

Cytology

Cytological descriptions are scarce, with < 15 cases reported in the literature {1275,1876}. The characteristic features are polyhedral or stellate tumour cells in a myxoid or mucinous background. Interspersed inflammatory cells, haemosiderin-laden macrophages, and Gamna–Gandy bodies may also be seen {1316}.

Diagnostic molecular pathology

Not relevant

Essential and desirable diagnostic criteria

Essential:
- Myxoma cells within a myxoid stroma
- Appropriate location

Desirable:
- Calretinin reactivity within the myxoma cells
- Perivascular rings

Staging

Not relevant

Prognosis and prediction

Non-syndromic and familial myxomas differ not only in their clinical features and etiology, but also in their prognosis. The tumour recurrence rate is relatively low in non-syndromic patients (< 5%), but it approaches 10–20% in Carney complex patients. Patients with Carney complex may also develop multiple tumours (in a synchronous or metachronous fashion), and they are more likely to have atypical cardiac locations {235,2730}.

Cardiac fibroma

Sheppard MN
Glass C

Definition
Cardiac fibroma is a benign mesenchymal tumour, composed of bland fibroblasts in a variably collagenized stroma.

ICD-O coding
8810/0 Fibroma, NOS

ICD-11 coding
2F01 & XH8E66 Benign neoplasm of intrathoracic organs & Fibroma, NOS

Related terminology
Not recommended: cardiac fibromatosis; fibrous hamartoma; fibroelastic hamartoma.

Subtype(s)
None

Localization
Nearly all cardiac fibromas arise in the ventricular septum; for the remaining cases, the most common site is the ventricular free wall (localization in the left ventricle is 5 times as common as in the right ventricle), followed by the right and left atria {2993}.

Clinical features
Due to the predilection of cardiac fibroma for the ventricular septum, one third of patients present with arrhythmias {185,1260}. Cardiac fibromas may cause obstruction or abnormal valvular function, leading to heart failure. Patients with asymptomatic tumours may present with a heart murmur, or the tumour may be identified incidentally on imaging.

Epidemiology
Most cardiac fibromas (90%) occur in children, and they are the second most common cardiac tumour of childhood after rhabdomyoma. One third arise before the age of 1 year, without sex predilection {3126}.

Etiology
The *PTCH1* gene appears to play a role in at least a subset of cardiac fibromas. Mutations may be somatic, resulting in sporadic tumour formation, or within a syndromic context, associated with Gorlin syndrome (naevoid basal cell carcinoma syndrome). Gorlin syndrome is an autosomal dominant disorder caused by germline *PTCH1* mutation, characterized by multiple basal cell carcinomas, skeletal anomalies, distinct facies, and intracranial calcifications.

Pathogenesis
Unknown

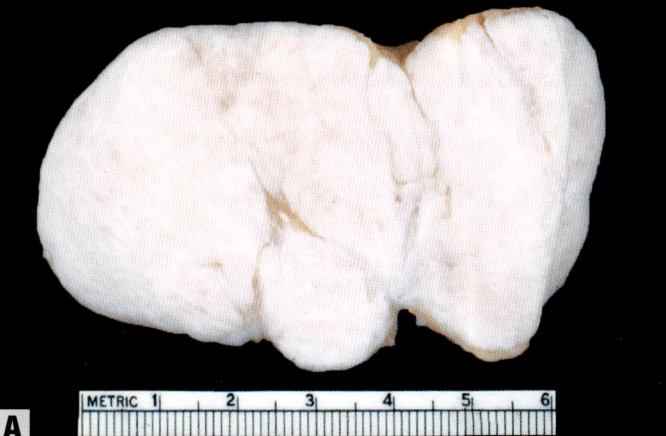

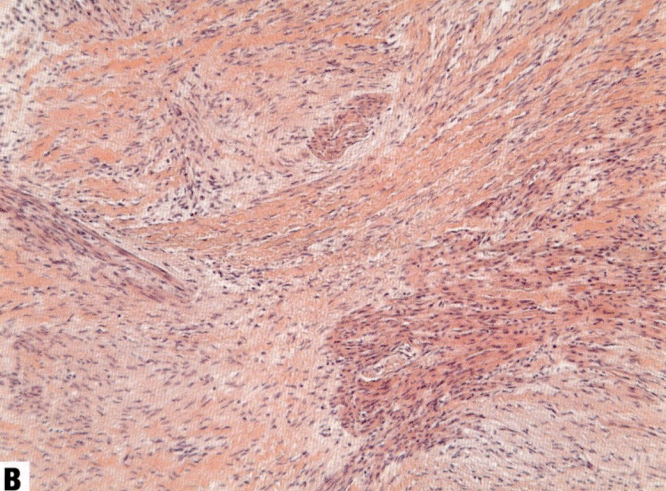

Fig. 3.09 Cardiac fibroma. **A** Cross-section of a resected cardiac fibroma, exhibiting the white, whorled surface. **B** Spindle cell fibroma infiltrating the surrounding pinker-appearing cardiac myocytes.

Macroscopic appearance
Cardiac fibromas are often large (mean: 50 mm), well-circumscribed, solitary tumours with a white whorled appearance. Although rare, multiple tumours have been reported. Calcification is common in this tumour and helps distinguish it from rhabdomyoma, particularly on imaging {2807}.

Histopathology
Cardiac fibromas consist of benign fibroblasts within a variably collagenous background. Although the tumours are well circumscribed grossly, fibroblasts and collagen may infiltrate adjacent cardiac muscle histologically, but this does not correlate with recurrence risk. Cellularity frequently decreases with age of the patient, and the amount of collagen increases {2284}. Microcalcifications and elastic fibres are variably present in patients of any age.

The lesional cells exhibit myofibroblastic differentiation and are reactive with antibodies directed against SMA.

Cytology
Not clinically relevant

Diagnostic molecular pathology
Demonstration of germline *PTCH1* mutation in Gorlin syndrome may be helpful in some cases {286}.

Essential and desirable diagnostic criteria
Essential:
- Nodular collection of fibroblasts within a fibrotic stroma

Desirable:
- Microcalcifications
- Ventricular involvement

Staging
Not relevant

Prognosis and prediction
Surgical excision is the treatment of choice for large tumours, and the recurrence rate is low, with excellent outcome. In asymptomatic patients, spontaneous regression is rare but has been reported {930,345,511}.

Cardiac rhabdomyoma

Basso C
Bois MC

Definition
Rhabdomyoma is a benign tumour of striated cardiac myocytes.

ICD-O coding
8900/0 Rhabdomyoma, NOS

ICD-11 coding
2F01 & XH8WG9 Benign tumour of intrathoracic organs & Rhabdomyoma, NOS
2F01 & XH4729 Benign tumour of intrathoracic organs & Fetal rhabdomyoma

Related terminology
Not recommended: congenital glycogenic tumour.

Subtype(s)
None

Localization
The most frequent location is the ventricular myocardium, but cardiac rhabdomyomas may also occur in the atria. Although mostly intramural, they may also appear as intracavitary pedunculated or sessile masses {2713,1173,189}.

Clinical features
The clinical features depend on the localization, number, and dimensions of the tumour(s). Prenatal detection is increasing dramatically in frequency and usually occurs when arrhythmias, hydrops, delayed fetal growth, or family history of tuberous sclerosis is reported {1173,1150}. Children may be asymptomatic or mildly symptomatic, presenting with a cardiac murmur {185,189, 863}. Haemodynamic impairment can occur either due to intracavitary protrusion of a large mass causing outflow obstruction

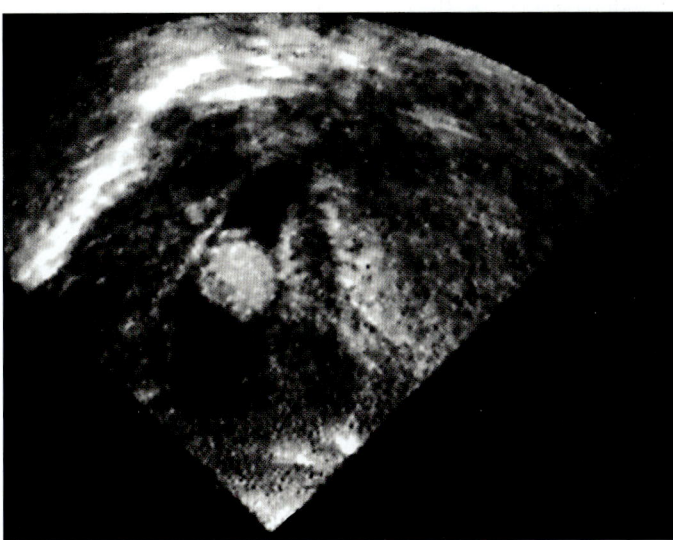

Fig. 3.10 Rhabdomyoma. 2D echocardiography showing an intracavitary rhabdomyoma of the right ventricular outflow tract.

and valve impairment or in the setting of extensive intramural growth with systolic and diastolic dysfunction {2114,2234,2235}. Both atrial and ventricular arrhythmias have been described, as well as conduction abnormalities due to direct compression of the specialized conduction system {1227}. When located in the atrioventricular junction, the tumour may serve as an accessory pathway, resulting in pre-excitation {1820}.

Imaging
2D echocardiography remains the main diagnostic tool, and rhabdomyomas show a homogeneous echogenicity different from that of other cardiac masses. By cardiac MRI, the signal

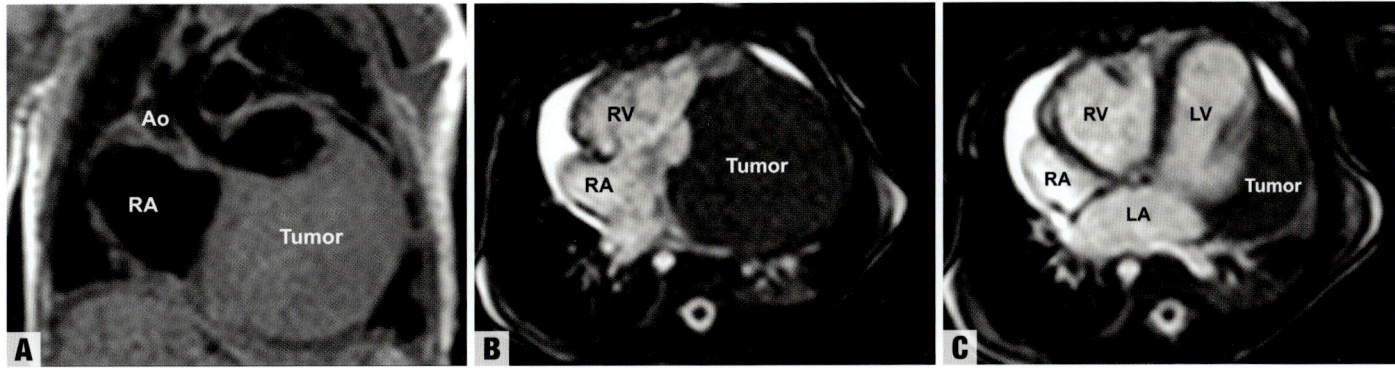

Fig. 3.11 Cardiac rhabdomyoma of the left ventricle. **A** Electrocardiography-triggered breath-hold proton density T1-weighted fast spin-echo in coronal plane, showing a large homogeneous isointense mass involving the left ventricular wall. **B** Electrocardiography-triggered breath-hold cine steady-state free precession in axial plane, showing the cardiac mass involving the interventricular septum. **C** Electrocardiography-triggered breath-hold cine steady-state free precession in four-chamber view, showing no intracardiac obstruction. Ao, aorta; LA, left atrium; LV, left ventricle; RA, right atrium; RV, right ventricle.

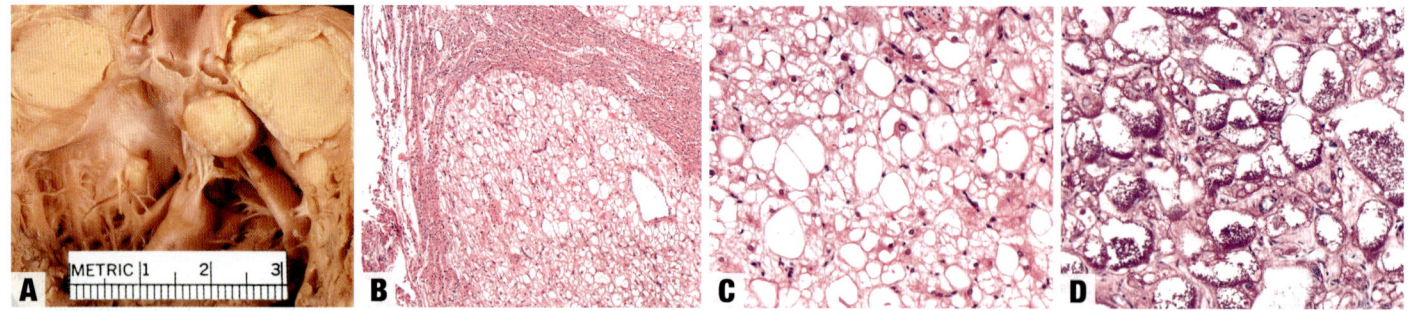

Fig. 3.12 Rhabdomyoma. **A** Autopsy specimen demonstrating multiple cardiac rhabdomyomas involving the left ventricle. The masses can be seen obstructing the ventricular outflow tract. **B** Panoramic view showing the border between tumour and normal cardiac myocytes. **C** At high magnification, enlarged swollen myocytes with clear cytoplasm are visible. Strands of cytoplasm are connected to the peripheral cell membrane. **D** The swollen cardiac myocytes are full of glycogen, shown on PAS stain.

characteristics are almost identical to those of the normal myocardium {863,168}.

Epidemiology

Rhabdomyoma is the most common heart neoplasm in children, accounting for > 60% of cardiac tumours {185,189,863}. It is also the most common heart tumour diagnosed prenatally {1173}. Although its prevalence in surgical series is lower because it does not necessarily represent an indication for resection, in a multicentre surgical series of paediatric cardiac tumours, rhabdomyoma was the most frequent (36%) {2235}. As many as 70–90% of cardiac rhabdomyomas have been reported in association with tuberous sclerosis {283,1070,2713,1150}, and > 50% of children with tuberous sclerosis are diagnosed with a cardiac rhabdomyoma by echocardiography {3239}. However, the true incidence in tuberous sclerosis patients probably remains underestimated.

Etiology

Two genes have been identified in tuberous sclerosis (an autosomal dominant disease with variable penetrance and expression): *TSC1* (9q34), which encodes the protein hamartin, and *TSC2* (16p13.3), which encodes the protein tuberin {1150}. These two proteins normally combine to suppress the growth-promoting mTORC1. Consequently, dysregulation of the *TSC1-TSC2* complex is a molecular driver of tumorigenesis.

Pathogenesis

Rhabdomyoma is a lesion of striated muscle without proliferative activity, and as such it is considered to be a hamartoma of developing cardiac myocytes (i.e. embryonic cardiac myoblasts) {2912}.

Macroscopic appearance

Rhabdomyomas are well-defined, unencapsulated, typically multiple, white-yellow masses, of variable size {1150}.

Histopathology

The tumours consist of well-demarcated but unencapsulated nodules, easily distinguished from the surrounding myocardium, with enlarged vacuolated cells. Abundant glycogen accounts for the clear sarcoplasm of the myocytes, and the characteristic spider-cell feature is the consequence of radial sarcoplasmic extensions emanating from the centrally located nucleus to the sarcoplasmic membrane {1150,2912}. Transmission electron microscopy shows myocytes with abundant glycogen, rare mitochondria, and peripherally distributed intercalated discs {809}. Positive expression of markers of striated muscle cells (myoglobin, desmin, actin, and vimentin) is detected by immunohistochemistry {2085}.

Cytology

Not relevant

Diagnostic molecular pathology

Not clinically relevant

Essential and desirable diagnostic criteria

Essential:
- Collection of vacuolated cells with radial sarcoplasmic extensions extending from the nucleus to the sarcoplasmic membrane

Desirable:
- Tuberous sclerosis

Staging

Not relevant

Prognosis and prediction

The most common symptoms necessitating intervention are ventricular arrhythmia and obstruction. Despite what can be considered rather dramatic presentations, cardiac rhabdomyomas are peculiar in that they have a propensity to resolve spontaneously with age. For this reason, a conservative approach is typically warranted unless the patient is symptomatic and refractory to medical therapy. Partial resection, aimed at preserving adjacent vital cardiac structures, can still be successful owing to this time-based regression {2235}. mTOR pathway inhibitors (e.g. everolimus) have been used with success to hasten tumour regression {654}.

Adult cellular rhabdomyoma

Burke AP
Jain D

Definition
Adult cellular rhabdomyoma is a benign neoplasm with striated muscle differentiation that occurs in the heart. It is the cardiac counterpart of extracardiac rhabdomyoma, adult type, which usually occurs in the head and neck region of adults aged > 40 years.

ICD-O coding
8904/0 Adult cellular rhabdomyoma

ICD-11 coding
2F01 & XH4BG5 Benign tumour of intrathoracic organs & Adult rhabdomyoma

Related terminology
Acceptable: adult intracardiac rhabdomyoma resembling the extracardiac tumour; adult rhabdomyoma.

Subtype(s)
None

Localization
Cellular rhabdomyomas have been reported in the right atrium, tricuspid valve, atrial septum, right ventricle, and left ventricle {41,293,343,499,712,3448}.

Clinical features
Clinical symptoms vary depending on intracardiac location. Patients with tumours in the atria present with supraventricular tachycardia and palpitations. Right ventricular tumours may be incidental findings or result in right bundle branch block. A left ventricular tumour caused dyspnoea on exertion and palpitations {499}.

Epidemiology
Adult extracardiac rhabdomyoma is a rare soft tissue tumour, accounting for < 2% of soft tissue neoplasms. There are < 10 reports of adult cellular rhabdomyoma involving the heart. The reported patient age range is 23–62 years. There is no sex predilection among the few reported cases.

Etiology
The etiology is unknown. There is no association with tuberous sclerosis or any syndrome. Adult cellular rhabdomyoma is not related to cardiac rhabdomyoma.

Pathogenesis
Reciprocal translocation of chromosomes 15 and 17 and abnormalities in the long arm of chromosome 10 have been described in a parapharyngeal rhabdomyoma {945}, but the pathogenesis of cardiac adult cellular rhabdomyoma is unknown.

Macroscopic appearance
Cellular rhabdomyomas are homogeneous, circumscribed fleshy tan masses that may be pedunculated and protrude into the atrium or ventricle or that are situated within the atrial septum. They are usually smooth, but a lobulated surface has also been described {499}.

Histopathology
Adult cellular rhabdomyomas are similar in appearance to adult extracardiac rhabdomyoma {343,3448}. The tumours are composed of small round, ovoid, or spindled cells that form sheets, with prominent vascularity. Sarcoplasmic vacuolization is usually prominent. Cross-striations may be seen. Tumour cells express skeletal muscle markers such as myogenin immunohistochemically, in addition to desmin. Occasionally, perinuclear haloes and multinucleation occur, resulting in cells resembling

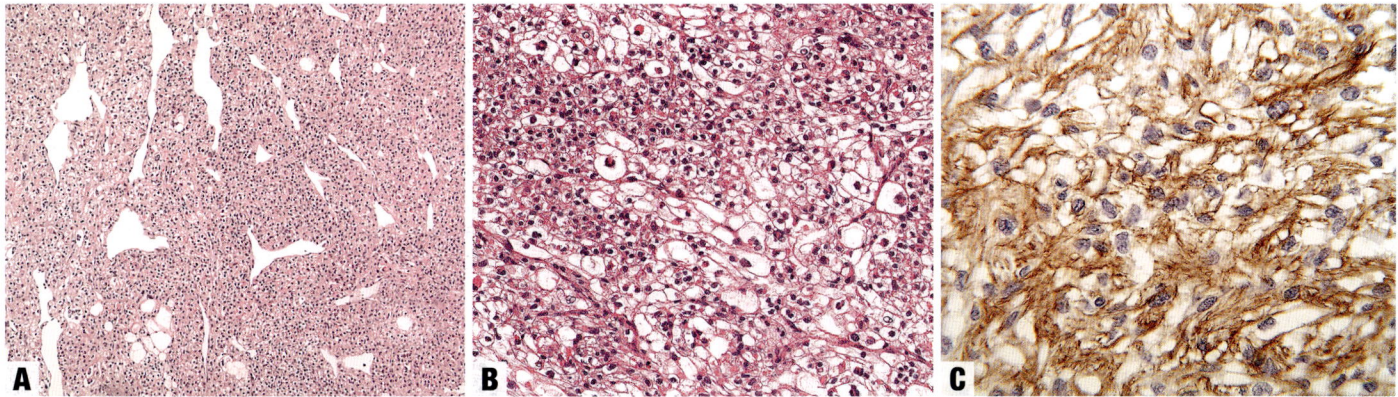

Fig. 3.13 Adult cellular rhabdomyoma. **A** Low magnification demonstrates a cellular tumour with prominent vascularity. **B** A high-magnification view demonstrates a solid pavement-like growth pattern. There is prominent sarcoplasmic clearing. Scattered cells are reminiscent of the spider cells of cardiac rhabdomyoma, but the cytological enlargement and radial sarcoplasmic strands are absent. **C** Immunohistochemical stain for desmin shows sarcoplasmic reactivity.

the spider cells seen in cardiac rhabdomyoma. However, classic spider cells are absent. There is a low but significant proliferation index by immunostaining for Ki-67, unlike in cardiac rhabdomyoma, which is non-reactive {343}.

Cytology

Cytological diagnosis of adult cellular rhabdomyoma has not been described. Aspirates of extracardiac rhabdomyoma of the adult type show clusters and isolated polygonal cells with abundant granular cytoplasm and small peripherally located nuclei {241,669}.

Diagnostic molecular pathology

The diagnostic molecular pathology has not been described. Unlike in cardiac rhabdomyoma, there are no alterations in *TSC1* or *TSC2*.

Essential and desirable diagnostic criteria

Essential:
- Cellular neoplasm expressing skeletal muscle markers
- Age > 20 years
- Absence of signs of tuberous sclerosis
- Absence of pleomorphism, mitotic activity, or necrosis

Desirable:
- Ki-67 proliferation index > 1% and < 20%

Staging

Not clinically relevant

Prognosis and prediction

No patient has been described with recurrence to date. Extracardiac rhabdomyomas of the adult type recur uncommonly.

Cardiac lipoma and lipomatous hypertrophy of the atrial septum

Basso C
Fritchie KJ

Definition
Cardiac lipoma is a benign mesenchymal tumour of mature adipocytes. Lipomatous hypertrophy of the atrial septum (LHAS) is a collection of immature (brown) fat, mature (yellow) fat, and atrial myocytes, expanding the atrial septum.

ICD-O coding
8850/0 Lipoma, NOS

ICD-11 coding
2F01 & XH1PL8 Benign neoplasm of intrathoracic organs & Lipoma, NOS

Related terminology
Not recommended: fibrolipoma; sclerosed lipoma.

Subtype(s)
None

Localization
Lipomas are most often epicardial but may be endocardial, intracavitary, or pericardial. They can be also intramyocardial, although less commonly {798,3220,19}. LHAS is a collection of fatty tissue located within the atrial septum.

Clinical features
The majority of cardiac lipomas are solitary asymptomatic masses discovered incidentally on imaging or autopsy, but rare cases may be associated with arrhythmias, chest pain, syncope, or sudden death {255,138,3164,2502}. There is variable echogenicity by echocardiogram, and MRI/CT should facilitate diagnosis {2416,3164,3107,126,168}.

LHAS is generally asymptomatic and discovered incidentally. Occasionally, atrial arrhythmias have been attributed to lipomatous hypertrophy {2148}. Rarely, the hypertrophy can become large enough to cause obstruction of blood flow within the heart.

Epidemiology
Lipomas of the heart are rare, representing 0.5–3% of excised cardiac tumours, although surgical prevalence is probably an underestimation because cardiac lipomas do not usually require resection {759,148,285,1365,2149,3032,1003}. All ages are affected, and there is no sex predilection.

Etiology
Little is known about the etiology of cardiac lipomas. It is hypothesized that, similar to in extracardiac lipomas, reactivated expression of the high-mobility group AT-hook 2 (HMGA2) protein plays a role. This hypothesis is supported by the finding of *HMGA2* rearrangement in a cardiac lipoma {102,1678,255} and in a case of LHAS, raising the possibility that a subset of LHAS cases may represent a clonal adipocytic process, or

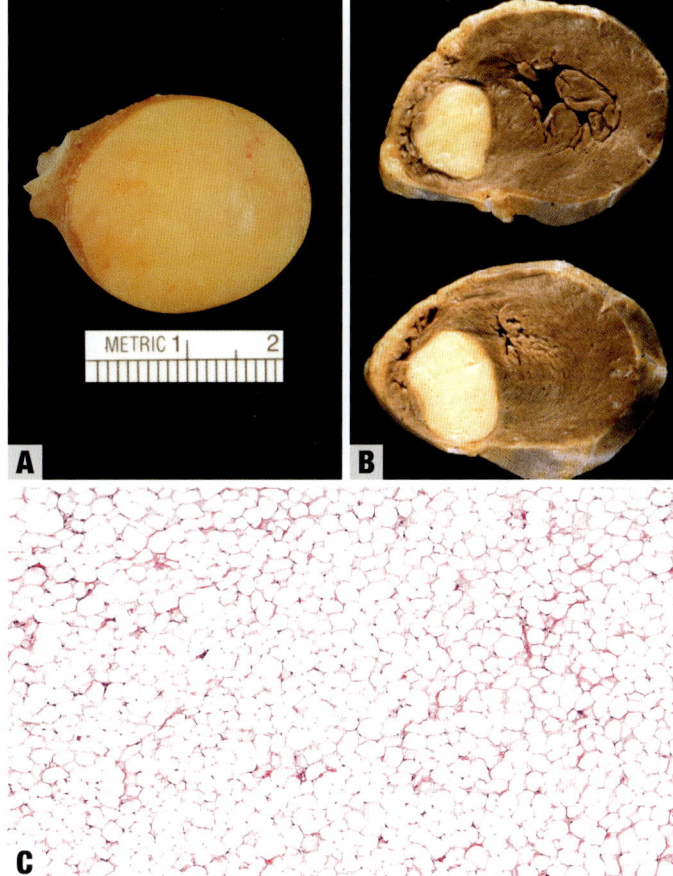

Fig. 3.14 Cardiac lipoma. **A** Gross appearance of a resected cardiac lipoma; note the rim of cardiac muscle at the left. **B** At autopsy there was a round homogeneous fatty tumour within the myocardium. **C** There is a proliferation of mature adipocytes with a delicate intermixed vasculature.

(less probably) lipomas may rarely arise within LHAS {255}. A large epicardial lipoma with a novel t(2;19)(p13;p13.2) has also been reported, and there is a single case report of a right atrial lipoma arising in a patient with Cowden syndrome {3160,416}.

Pathogenesis
Unknown

Macroscopic appearance
Lipomas are encapsulated, yellow, smooth, soft masses with a yellow glistening cut surface. LHAS is a somewhat related entity involving the atrial septum, with a similar gross appearance otherwise. It often imparts a dumbbell appearance to the septum.

Histopathology
Histological examination of cardiac lipoma reveals a proliferation of mature adipocytes with a fibrous capsule and variable

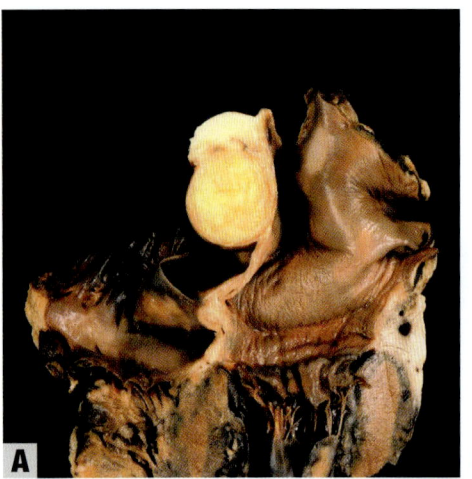 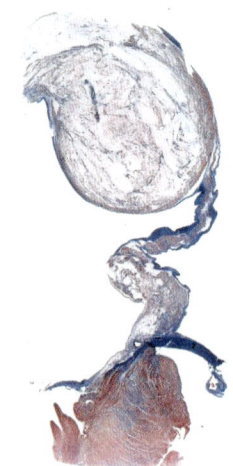 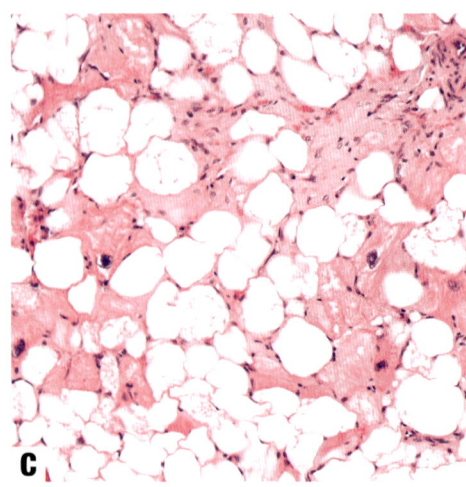

Fig. 3.15 Lipomatous hypertrophy of the atrial septum. **A** This 30 × 20 mm mass was found incidentally at autopsy. **B** By histology, the unencapsulated mass contained mature adipocytes with intermingled myocytes and mild interstitial fibrosis (trichrome stain). **C** Histological sections show a mixture of mature adipocytes, brown fat, and hypertrophied myocytes.

septa. Rare entrapped myocytes may be seen at the periphery of the lesion. LHAS is characterized by an unencapsulated collection of brown fat, mature fat, and atrial myocytes located within the limbus of the fossa ovalis {167}.

Cytology
Not clinically relevant

Diagnostic molecular pathology
Diagnostic molecular pathology is not usually required. *MDM2* amplification studies can be performed if there is concern for well-differentiated liposarcoma.

Essential and desirable diagnostic criteria
Lipoma
Essential:
- Encapsulated mass composed of mature adipocytes

LHAS
Essential:
- Collection of immature (brown) fat, mature (yellow) fat, and atrial myocytes within the atrial septum

Desirable:
- ≥ 15 mm in thickness

Staging
Not clinically relevant

Prognosis and prediction
Lipomas and LHAS typically do not require surgery unless the patient is symptomatic. Tumours requiring surgical intervention can usually be completely excised without complications {3167, 2447,2033,2502}.

Lipomatous hamartoma
of the atrioventricular valve

Bois MC
Singaravel S

Definition

Lipomatous hamartoma of the atrioventricular valve (LHAV) is a benign valvular mass composed of unencapsulated mature adipocytes, small capillaries, and fibrous connective tissue.

ICD-O coding

None

ICD-11 coding

2F01 Benign neoplasm of intrathoracic organs

Related terminology

Acceptable: primary valvular lipomatous hamartoma.
Not recommended: cardiac valve lipomatosis.

Subtype(s)

None

Localization

As the name implies, these lesions are found in atrioventricular valves. Right-sided LHAVs are generally associated with the septal leaflet of the tricuspid valve, whereas LHAVs of both the anterior and posterior mitral valve leaflets have been observed {224}.

Clinical features

Clinical features vary based on lesional location or may be entirely absent. In the few cases reported, flow murmurs with valvular insufficiency were the most common presenting findings {1386}. Owing to their anatomical location, right-sided LHAVs have been associated with dyspnoea, whereas left-sided lesions may be associated with thromboembolic phenomena {858}.

Epidemiology

LHAV is exceedingly rare, with < 15 reported cases in the literature. The lesion has been documented in a wide age range (2–76 years). There is no sex predilection {1386}.

Etiology

Hamartomatous lesions, such as LHAV, are thought to be congenital in nature. There are no known genetic predispositions or associated causes.

Pathogenesis

Although probably present at birth, the lesion may slowly enlarge (stretch) over time as the structurally dysplastic leaflet is subjected to ventricular systolic pressures {593}.

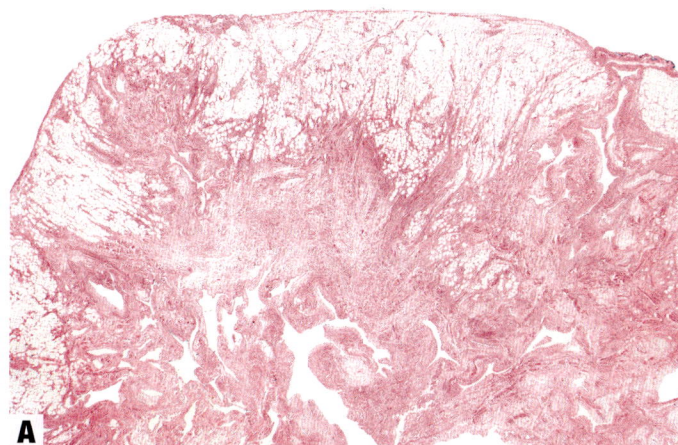
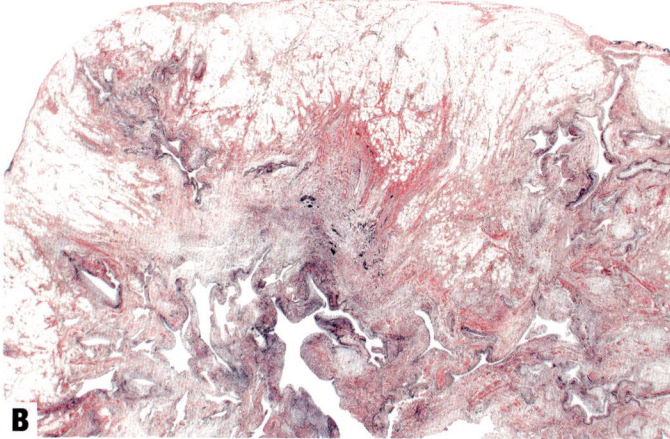
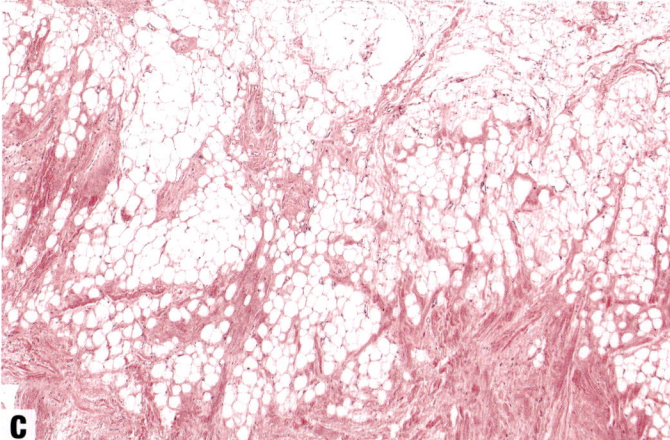

Fig. 3.16 Lipomatous hamartoma of the atrioventricular valve. **A** This lesion shows diffuse involvement of the leaflet by unencapsulated mature adipocytes and fibroconnective tissue. **B** There is diffuse involvement of a leaflet by unencapsulated mature adipocytes and fibroconnective tissue (Verhoeff–Van Gieson stain). **C** Higher magnification shows involvement of a leaflet by disorganized mesenchymal tissue native to the anatomical site.

Macroscopic appearance

The valve may appear thickened with a billowing contour, or it may show a nodular protuberance on either the ventricular or the atrial aspect of the leaflet {593,1386}.

Histopathology

LHAV is composed of mature adipocytes admixed with mesenchymal elements native to the atrioventricular valve, such as fibroconnective tissue and thin-walled vasculature. Importantly, LHAV shows no features of fibrous encapsulation, distinguishing it from entities in the differential diagnosis, such as lipoma {224}.

Cytology

Not described

Diagnostic molecular pathology

Not clinically relevant

Essential and desirable diagnostic criteria

Essential:
- Unencapsulated collection of fat within the atrioventricular valve

Desirable:
- Grossly mass-forming

Staging

Not relevant

Prognosis and prediction

Although LHAV is histopathologically benign, it may have haemodynamic consequences secondary to its anatomical localization. Significant valvular regurgitation, premature ventricular contractions, presyncope, (thrombo)embolism, and sudden death have all been reported or are theoretical risks.

Hamartoma of mature cardiac myocytes

Miller DV
Jain D

Definition
Hamartoma of mature cardiac myocytes is a benign growth of differentiated mature striated cardiac myocytes.

ICD-O coding
None

ICD-11 coding
2F01 Benign neoplasm of intrathoracic organs

Related terminology
Not recommended: hamartoma of adult cardiac myocytes; cardiac hamartoma.

Subtype(s)
None

Localization
Usually arising in the ventricles, hamartomas of mature cardiac myocytes have also been reported in the atria {2019,3516}. They may be multiple or (more commonly) solitary lesions {804}.

Clinical features
Most cases are asymptomatic and incidental at the time of autopsy or imaging (echocardiography, CT, MRI, and PET) {959,874}. In symptomatic cases, the clinical features are often related to arrhythmia (palpitations, syncope, chest pain, and sudden death) {649}. Variable electrocardiographic abnormalities have been reported {804}.

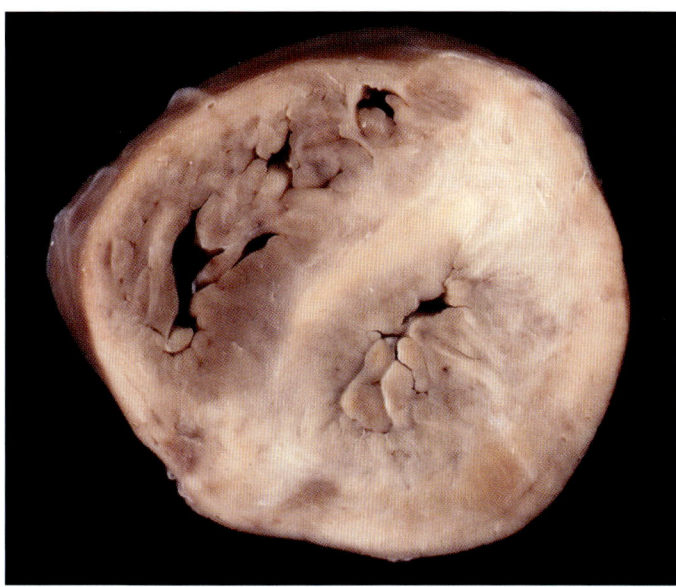

Fig. 3.17 Hamartoma of mature cardiac myocytes. A poorly defined, vaguely circular pale area can be seen in the anteroseptal region of this mid-ventricular, short-axis specimen.

Epidemiology
Fewer than 50 cases have been reported in the literature, with patient ages spanning 6 months to 76 years. Hamartoma of mature cardiac myocytes is most common in younger patients (median age: 24 years), and two thirds arise in men {524,804}.

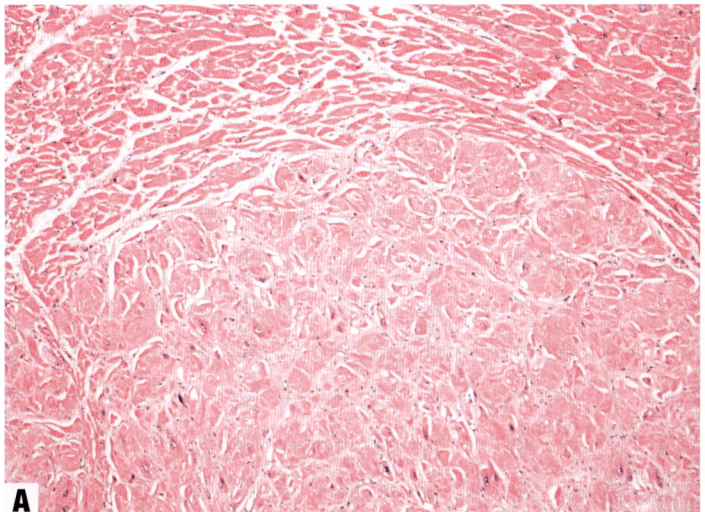
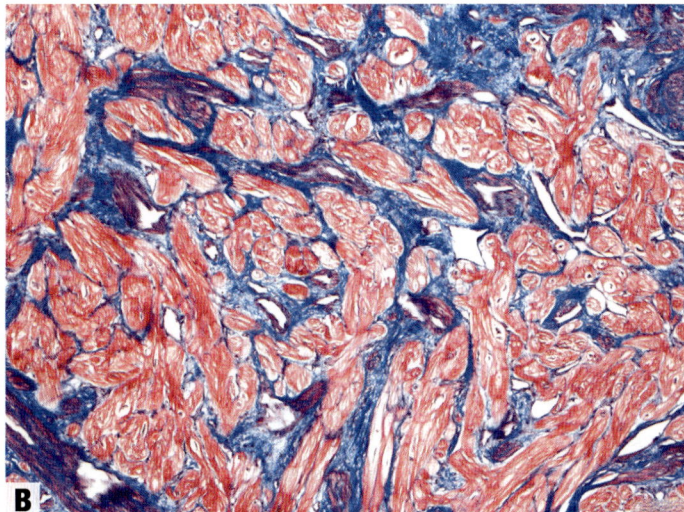

Fig. 3.18 Hamartoma of mature cardiac myocytes. **A** Enlarged and disorganized myocytes are seen in this photomicrograph, forming a distinct border with the adjacent normal myocardium. **B** A Masson trichrome stain highlights the degree of myocyte disorganization within the tumour, as well as the fibrosis interspersed throughout.

Etiology
Unknown

Pathogenesis
Unknown

Macroscopic appearance
Grossly, lesions consist of firm, poorly defined areas of pale-grey tissue that look somewhat fibrotic. The lesions are usually < 50 mm, although a 90 mm tumour has been reported {804}. Tissue interdigitation makes complete surgical excision difficult {2411}.

Histopathology
The lesions are composed of enlarged, disorganized, striated cardiac myocytes with sarcoplasmic vacuolization and bizarre nuclei. They are associated with interstitial fibrosis and may be arranged in disorganized whorls or a herringbone pattern {344}. Fat and nerves may be intermixed. The tumours express muscle markers such as desmin, troponin, actin, and myosin. Ki-67 studies have shown the lesions to be non-proliferative {344}.

The differential diagnoses include cardiac rhabdomyoma (but hamartoma of mature cardiac myocytes lacks spider cells) and cardiac fibroma (which lacks myocytes). The appearance actually closely resembles that of hypertrophic cardiomyopathy, but hamartomas of mature cardiac myocytes are discrete and localized.

The term "mesenchymal hamartoma" is used to describe lesions composed of blood vessels, smooth muscle, fat, and nerves within myocardium {298}.

Cytology
Not described

Diagnostic molecular pathology
Not clinically relevant

Essential and desirable diagnostic criteria
Essential:
- Discrete, nodular collections of enlarged, disorganized cardiac myocytes forming a myocardial mass

Desirable:
- Admixed adipose tissue and nerves

Staging
Not clinically relevant

Prognosis and prediction
Although histopathologically benign, these tumours can cause death from intractable arrhythmias or sudden death {804}. Surgical excision (even when incomplete) has proved effective for tumours causing arrhythmia and/or obstruction {649,2411}.

Mesenchymal cardiac hamartoma

Veinot JP
Bois MC
Singaravel S

Definition
Mesenchymal cardiac hamartoma is a myocardial collection of mature, irregularly arranged mesenchymal tissues normally found within the heart.

ICD-O coding
None

ICD-11 coding
2F01 Benign neoplasm of intrathoracic organs

Related terminology
Not recommended: cardiac hamartoma.

Subtype(s)
None

Localization
Mesenchymal cardiac hamartomas occur in both the septum and the free walls of the ventricles.

Clinical features
Mesenchymal cardiac hamartomas may be associated with dyspnoea, fatigue, or syncope. Ventricular arrhythmias and sudden death have been reported.

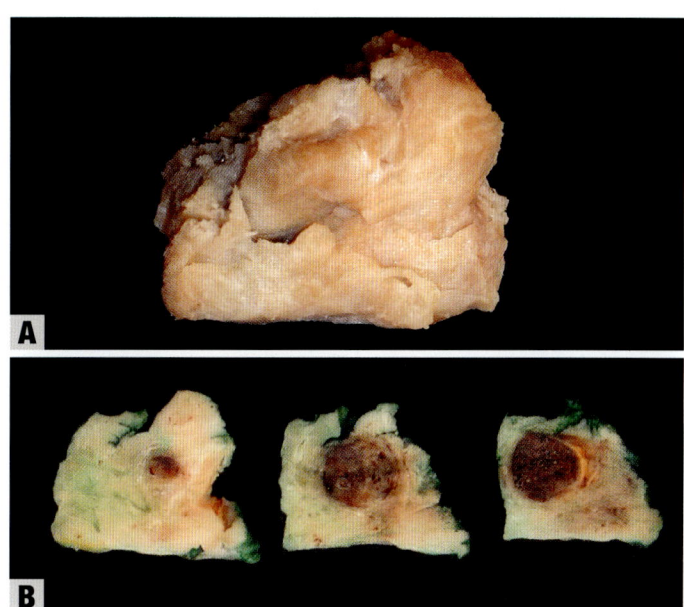

Fig. 3.19 Mesenchymal cardiac hamartoma. **A** External view of a tan fleshy ventricular mass. **B** Cut sections showing tan fleshy tissue with a round vascular area.

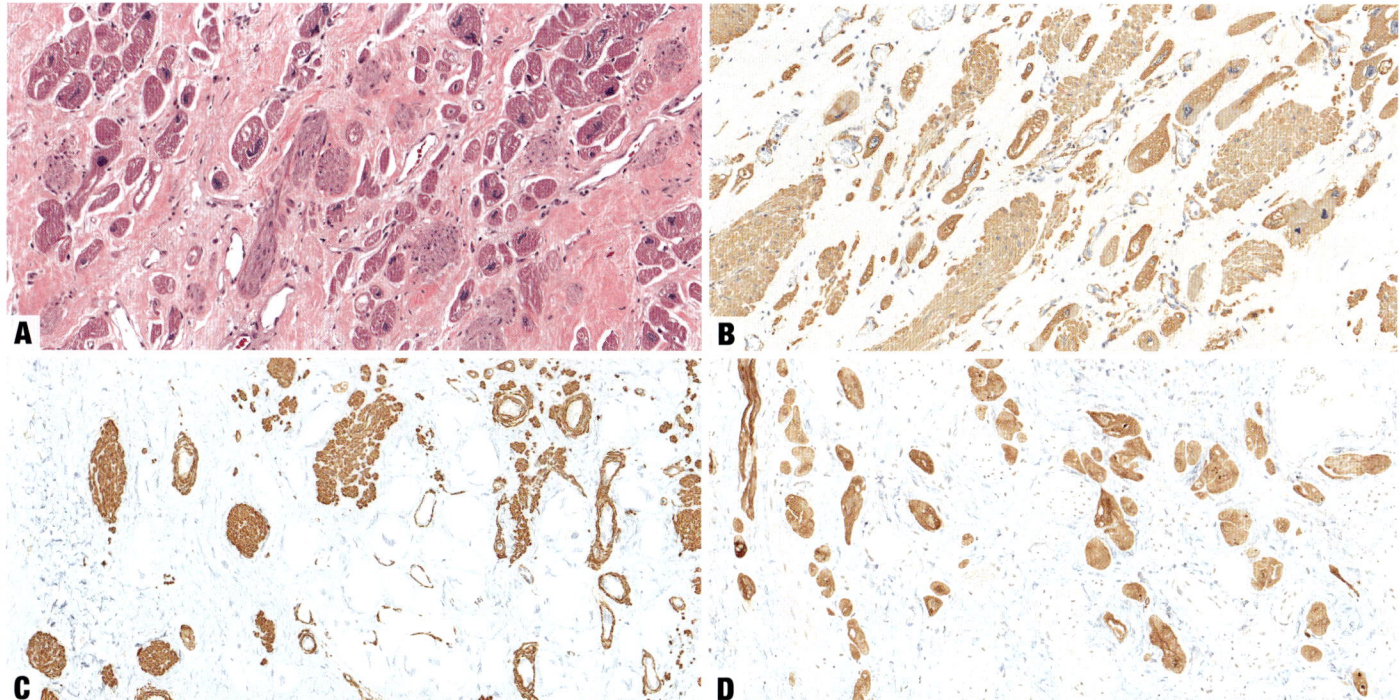

Fig. 3.20 Mesenchymal cardiac hamartoma. **A** Admixed smooth muscle, cardiac muscle, and blood vessels are the main components of the mass. **B** Immunohistochemistry for MSA stains both muscle types and the smooth muscle of the blood vessels. **C** Immunohistochemistry for SMA stains smooth muscle fascicles and blood vessel smooth muscle, leaving the cardiomyocytes unstained. **D** Immunohistochemistry for troponin stains the cardiac myocytes, leaving the smooth muscle fascicles and cells unstained.

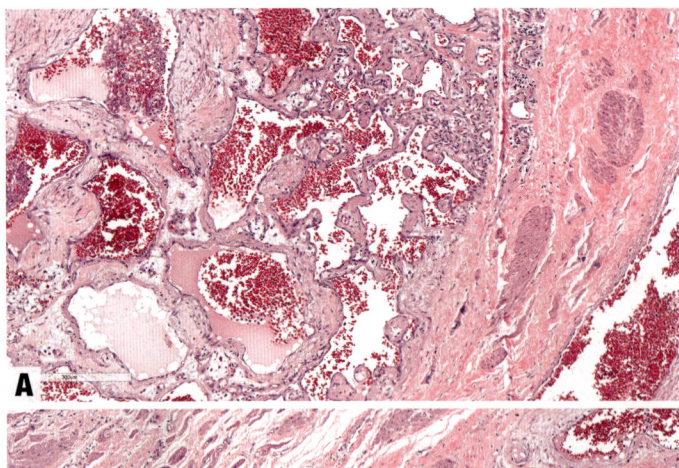
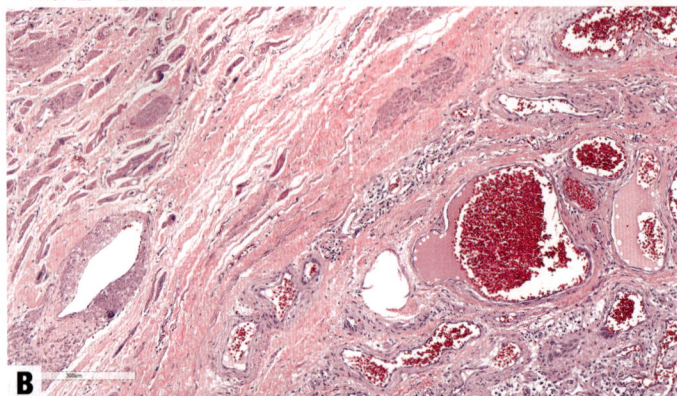
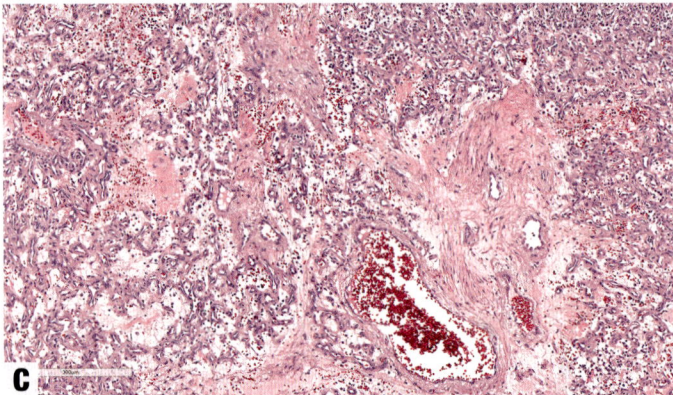

Fig. 3.21 Mesenchymal cardiac hamartoma. **A–C** Microscopy of a vascular region of a mass with variably sized blood vessels, including areas resembling a haemangioma. The surrounding tissues show muscle cells, blood vessels, and collagen.

Epidemiology
Cases in adult men and women have been reported.

Etiology
The etiology is unknown. Although few data exist, the lesion is probably congenital in origin.

Pathogenesis
No genetic or syndromic predispositions have been identified.

Macroscopic appearance
The lesion appears as a soft tissue mass involving the endocardium, myocardium, or epicardium. It may protrude into the cardiac chamber. Grossly, mesenchymal hamartomas are tan or pink in colour and may shell out easily, but the lesion has infiltrative borders that extend irregularly into the adjacent myocardium on microscopy. Neither gross necrosis nor calcifications are typically present {298}.

Histopathology
The lesion contains an admixture of mature tissues including irregularly arranged cardiomyocytes, smooth muscle cells, fibroblasts, blood vessels (veins, arteries, arterioles, venules, and capillaries), nerves, fibrous tissue, and adipose tissue. Scattered inflammatory cells, such as lymphocytes and macrophages, may be seen. The low mitotic activity, as well as the lack of necrosis and cytological atypia, is consistent with the benign nature of these lesions. The cardiac myocytes may have nuclear hypertrophy, sarcoplasmic degenerative changes (myocytolysis), and haphazard arrangement. The vessels may have intimal myxoid narrowing and be inflamed.

Immunohistochemistry shows variable reactivity with desmin and MSA (smooth and cardiac muscle), SMA (smooth muscle), troponin (cardiac muscle), S100 (fat and nerves), CD31 and factor VIII (vascular endothelium), cytokeratin AE1/AE3 (focal endothelial cells), and lymphoid and macrophage markers in areas of inflammation (CD3, CD20, CD68, and others) {1710}. The differential diagnosis includes fibroma, rhabdomyoma, hamartoma of mature cardiac myocytes, mature teratoma, lipoma, and vascular hamartoma.

Cytology
Not described

Diagnostic molecular pathology
Not relevant

Essential and desirable diagnostic criteria
Essential:
- Discrete collection of mature mesenchymal tissues in the heart

Desirable:
- Ventricular involvement

Staging
Not clinically relevant

Prognosis and prediction
The prognosis is not definitively known, owing to the rarity of the lesion and its relatively new description. Mesenchymal cardiac hamartomas may be surgically excised. Although the margins may seem clear grossly, they are seldom clear histologically; however, the implication of this for recurrence is not yet known.

Cardiac haemangiomas

Tavora F
Calonje JE

Definition
Cardiac haemangiomas are a family of benign vascular tumours arising in the heart and are broadly divided morphologically as capillary, cavernous, and arteriovenous types.

ICD-O coding
9120/0 Haemangioma, NOS
9122/0 Venous haemangioma
9131/0 Capillary haemangioma
9123/0 Arteriovenous haemangioma
9121/0 Cavernous haemangioma

ICD-11 coding
2F01 & XH3U29 Benign neoplasm of intrathoracic organs & Capillary haemangioma
2F01 & XH1GU2 Benign neoplasm of intrathoracic organs & Cavernous haemangioma
2F01 & XH5AW4 Benign neoplasm of intrathoracic organs & Haemangioma, NOS

Related terminology
Not recommended: cardiac angioma; cardiac vascular malformation.

Subtype(s)
None

Localization
Haemangiomas may arise from the endocardium, myocardium, or pericardium. The ventricular free walls are the most common sites of involvement. Congenital haemangiomas most frequently involve the right atrium {147,1757,3340}.

Clinical features
Most cardiac haemangiomas are asymptomatic and incidental. Symptomatic patients may present with dyspnoea, palpitations, murmur, or (unusually) thromboembolic events. Arrhythmia and conduction disturbances may be related to an intramyocardial location. Pericardial involvement may lead to effusion, haemopericardium, or potentially tamponade {648,2648}. Congenital

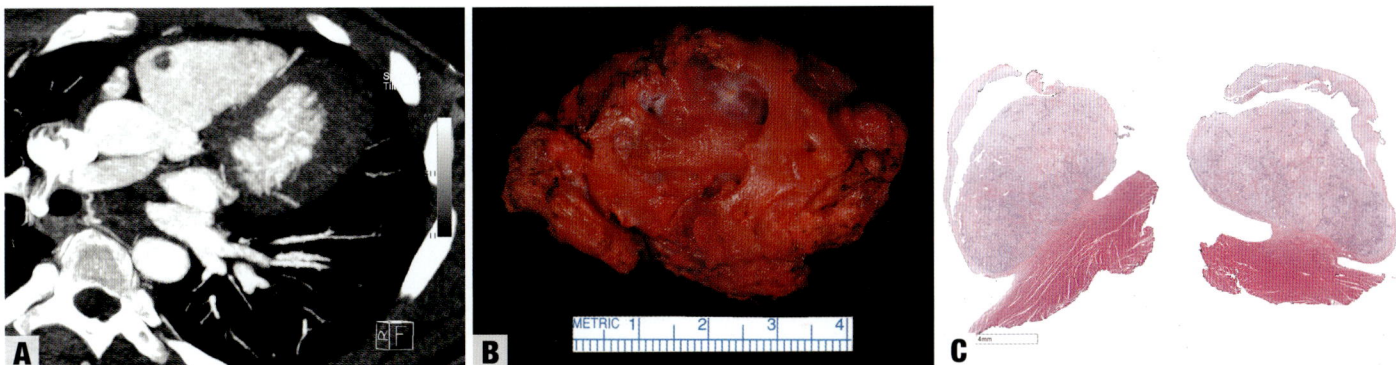

Fig. 3.22 Cardiac haemangioma. **A** CT appearance of cardiac haemangioma; note the filling defect due to the endocardial-based pedunculated mass in the anterior wall. **B** Gross photo of a cardiac haemangioma, surgically excised from the right ventricle. This red lobulated mass exhibited primarily intramyocardial growth, with extension into the ventricular chamber. **C** Low-magnification view of a resected endocardial haemangioma, capillary type.

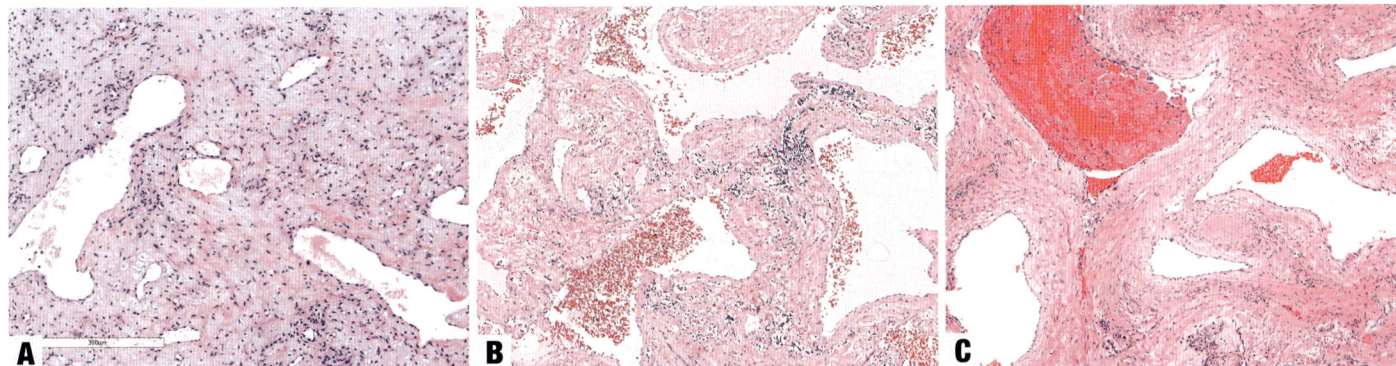

Fig. 3.23 Cardiac haemangioma. **A** Capillary type, with a grouping of capillary-sized vessels in a myxoid background. **B** Cavernous type, consisting of large dilated vessels and thick fibrous septa. **C** Arteriovenous type, consisting of a mixture of thin- and thick-walled vessels, some of which may be thrombosed.

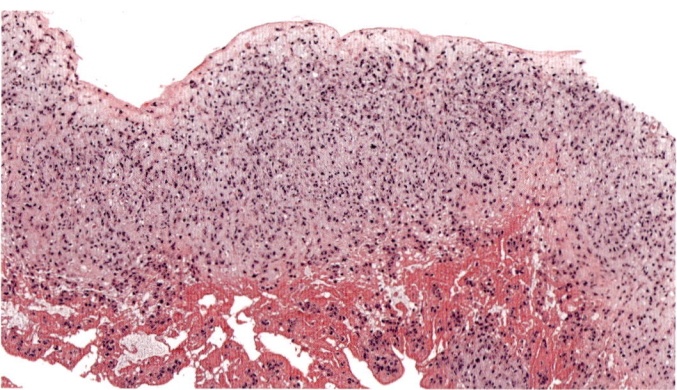

Fig. 3.24 Cardiac haemangioma, capillary type. The vascular proliferation is present in a myxoid background, with overlying fibrin deposition.

haemangiomas, frequently associated with pericardial effusion, may be diagnosed in utero {306,2908,2648}. The malformation type of cardiac haemangioma has been rarely reported with in Klippel–Trénaunay syndrome {2025}.

Epidemiology

Age at presentation ranges widely, from the neonatal period to old age. Approximately 10% of cases occur in children, and 10% are diagnosed in utero or in infancy {147}. There is a slight male predominance.

Etiology

The clinical evolution and clinicopathological features suggest that these lesions represent vascular malformations.

Pathogenesis

Unknown

Macroscopic appearance

Tumours are usually single and nodular. Intramyocardial lesions often merge with the adjacent tissue, whereas endoluminal lesions (80% of the cases) can be sessile or polypoid {340,2425}.

Histopathology

The histological patterns, which overlap, are capillary, cavernous, and arteriovenous. The most frequent type is cavernous, followed by mixed cavernous-capillary and capillary. Cardiac haemangiomas with adipocytes similar to intramuscular haemangiomas are very rare. Atrial haemangiomas may be diagnostically challenging because of the trabeculations of the atrial wall.

Capillary haemangiomas consist of small, thin-walled vessels arising from and clustered around a larger "feeder" vessel. Small capillary lumina may be difficult to immediately appreciate in cellular lesions. The intervening stroma may have a myxoid character, and scattered pericytes and fibroblasts may be seen. So-called infantile haemangiomas, which are considered a type of capillary haemangioma, contain back-to-back capillaries and no intervening fibrous tissue {1757}. In this later type, mitoses may be numerous at the proliferative stage and immunohistochemical expression of GLUT1 is characteristic {1757}.

Cavernous types exhibit large, dilated vascular spaces, often situated within the myocardium itself. The vessels may be thin- or thick-walled, and pools of blood may be present throughout.

The arteriovenous types are characterized by arterial and venous structures, the latter of which often exhibit remodelling and arterialization owing to complex arterial anastomoses and exposure to systemic pressures. Similar to in the extracardiac variety, adipose tissue and collagen may be admixed.

Cytology

Not clinically relevant

Diagnostic molecular pathology

Not clinically relevant

Essential and desirable diagnostic criteria

Essential:
- Benign tumour composed of thin-walled vascular spaces, without atypia

Desirable:
- Expression of CD31, CD34, and ERG

Staging

Not clinically relevant

Prognosis and prediction

Surgical excision of haemangioma is generally successful, with rare postsurgical events {340}.

Conduction system hamartoma

Shehata BM
Basso C

Definition
Conduction system hamartoma (CSH) is a hamartomatous lesion consisting of a multifocal proliferation of Purkinje or Purkinje-like cells throughout the endocardium, with a predilection for the cardiac conduction system (including the sinoatrial node, atrioventricular node, bundle of His, and Purkinje fibres).

ICD-O coding
None

ICD-11 coding
2F01 Benign neoplasm of intrathoracic organs

Related terminology
Acceptable: Purkinje cell hamartoma.

Not recommended: histiocytoid cardiomyopathy; arachnocytosis of the myocardium; infantile cardiomyopathy; infantile xanthomatous cardiomyopathy; oncocytic cardiomyopathy; focal lipid cardiomyopathy; isolated cardiac lipidosis; foamy myocardial transformation; congenital cardiomyopathy.

Subtype(s)
None

Localization
The lesions are multifocal and appear predominantly in the subendocardial distribution of the conduction system. However, they can appear in the middle of the myocardium and, rarely, in the subepicardium. Additionally, the lesions have a tendency to involve the cardiac valve cusps, which is a major differentiating characteristic from rhabdomyoma.

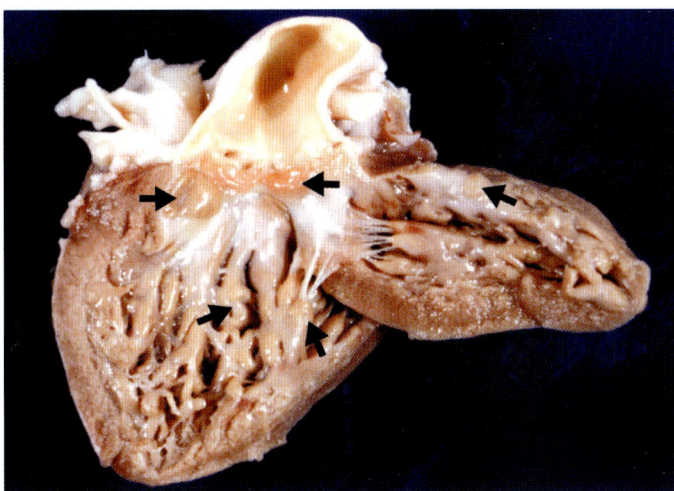

Fig. 3.25 Conduction system hamartoma. Gross view of the heart, showing multiple lesional nodules (arrows) in the aortic valve leaflets, endocardium, and papillary muscles.

Clinical features
CSH is a distinct arrhythmogenic disorder that has a spectrum of clinical presentations in 70% of patients {3526}. Aside from arrhythmic presentation, patients may present with sudden death. Approximately 20% of cases are mistaken for sudden infant death syndrome (SIDS), which may be preceded by a short-duration coryzal illness {2723}.

Epidemiology
In the USA, CSH most commonly affects white people (> 80% of the cases), followed by African-Americans (15%) and others (5%) {2723}. More than 60% of CSH cases are diagnosed in the

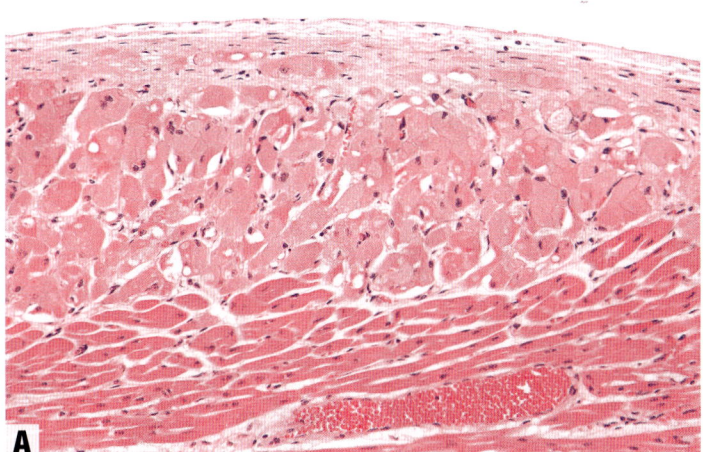

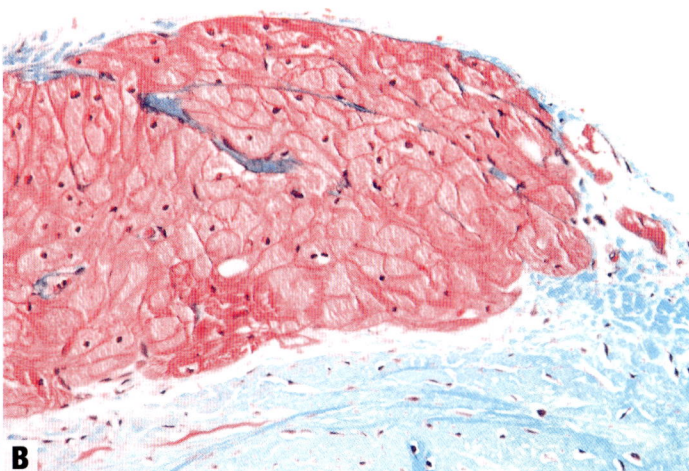

Fig. 3.26 Conduction system hamartoma nodule. **A** Subendocardial nodule. Note the poorly defined border with the underlying normal myocardial fibres. **B** This nodule was located on the edge of a heart valve leaflet (trichrome stain).

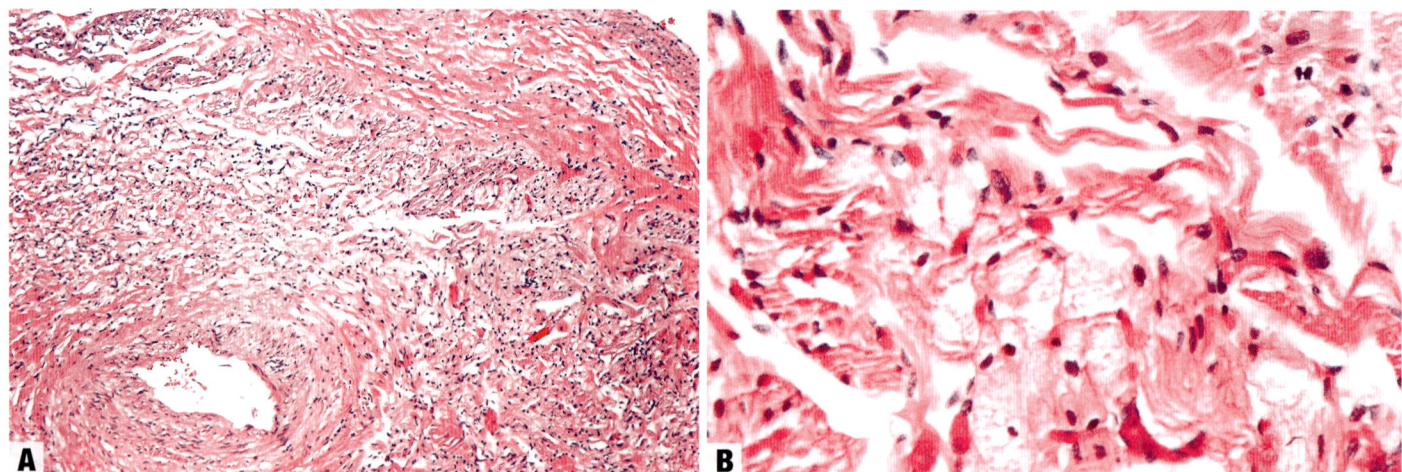

Fig. 3.27 Conduction system hamartoma. **A** The artery to the sinoatrial node is surrounded by wavy conduction system fibres. **B** Higher magnification. Large polygonal cells infiltrate between the wavy sinoatrial node fibres.

first year of life, and it is extremely rare after the age of 2 years. CSH has a predilection for girls (M:F ratio: 1:3), and it can be associated with cardiac malformations (16%) and extracardiac malformations (17%) {2723}. Recently, CSH has been diagnosed in infants with long QT syndrome. An interesting association has been reported with microphthalmia with linear skin defects syndrome {234}.

Etiology
Nonsense mutations involving the *NDUFB11* gene, encoding for complex I of the electron transport chain, have been described {2722}.

Pathogenesis
Several members of the NDUF gene family, all of which encode for proteins involved in the oxidative phosphorylation pathway, are now potential candidate genes in the pathogenesis of CSH {2444}.

Macroscopic appearance
Cardiomegaly is observed in > 95% of cases. The lesions are usually visible grossly and form yellow-tan endocardial and subendocardial nodules as large as 3 mm, which can be seen in both the right and left ventricular endocardium. Additionally, nodules can be seen in the papillary muscles, the tendinous cords, and the atrioventricular valves.

Histopathology
The lesional nodules are composed of large polygonal cells mimicking histiocytes, measuring 30–40 μm in diameter. The lesional cells show granular eosinophilic sarcoplasm, containing variable amounts of glycogen and lipids. The nucleus is oval in shape, with occasional prominent nucleoli. Sections of sinoatrial and atrioventricular nodes usually show lesional cells interspersed between the conduction system fibres.

By electron microscopy, these cells show poorly defined intercellular junctions. Abundant (often swollen and abnormal) mitochondria push the myofibrils peripherally. Mitochondria show disorganized cristae and contain dense membrane-bound granules. Scattered lipid droplets may also be seen.

The immunohistochemistry panel shows reactivity with antibodies directed against myosin, desmin, MSA, and myoglobin. Histiocyte and macrophage markers (CD68, CD163, MAC387, LN3, and HAM56) are all negative. The lesional cells show variable reactivity with antibodies directed against S100.

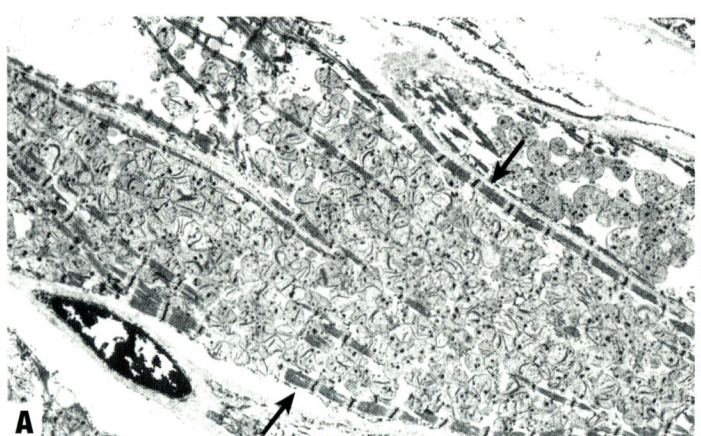
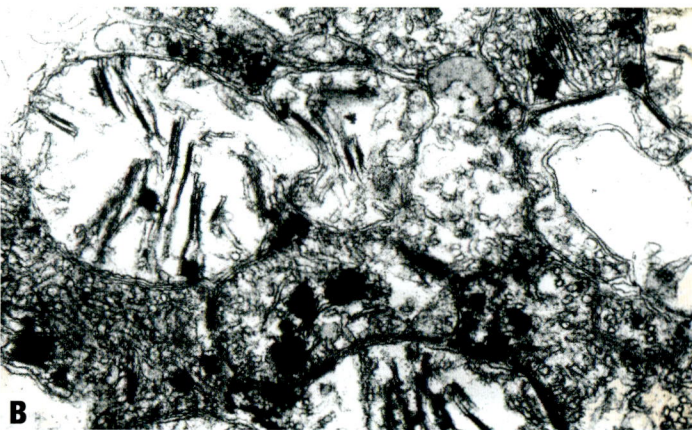

Fig. 3.28 Conduction system hamartoma. **A** Electron microscopy shows conduction system hamartoma cells packed with mitochondria; the diminished myofibrils are displaced to the periphery of the cell (arrows). **B** Higher power electron microscopy shows swollen mitochondria with disorganized cristae and dense membrane-bound granules.

Cytology
Not relevant

Diagnostic molecular pathology
A mutation in *NDUFB11* or another NDUF-family gene can be helpful in supporting the diagnosis, although this is not widely used clinically.

Essential and desirable diagnostic criteria
Essential:
- Collections of pale, eosinophilic Purkinje cells distributed along the endocardium

Desirable:
- Demonstration of a mutation in one of the NDUF-family genes

Staging
Not relevant

Prognosis and prediction
Historically, the condition was universally fatal; however, successful surgical excision targeting the arrhythmogenic focus has been achieved {1415}. Treatment may also include antiarrhythmic medication and/or ablation of the arrhythmogenic foci after electrophysiological mapping. Cardiac transplantation has also been successful {3471}.

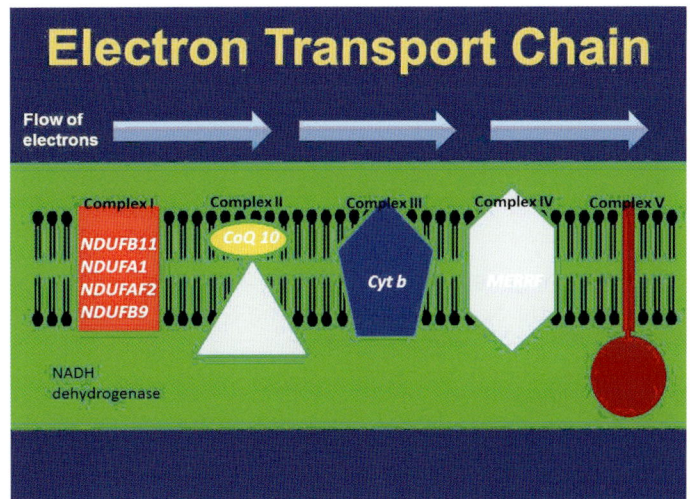

Fig. 3.29 Electron transport chain. NDUF family members' role in respiratory complex I.

Cystic tumour of the atrioventricular node

Singaravel S
Cohle SD

Definition

Cystic tumour of the atrioventricular node (CTAVN) is a benign endodermal developmental rest forming a mass lesion in the region of the atrioventricular node.

ICD-O coding

8454/0 Cystic tumour of atrioventricular node

ICD-11 coding

2F01 & XH55F1 Benign neoplasm of intrathoracic organs & Cystic tumour of atrioventricular node

Related terminology

Acceptable: endodermal heterotopia.
Not recommended: mesothelioma of the atrioventricular node.

Subtype(s)

None

Localization

CTAVN occurs in the triangle of Koch, within the atrioventricular septum.

Clinical features

Initially asymptomatic tumours may manifest later in life as the tumours enlarge due to glandular secretions. Symptoms may range from none to palpitations, dyspnoea, syncope, dizziness, partial or complete heart block, and sudden cardiac death.

Epidemiology

CTAVN accounts for about 2.7% of cardiac tumours at autopsy {1746}. The mean age at diagnosis is about 38 years (range: 0–95 years). Women are affected more often than men. No racial or ethnic predilection has been noted.

Etiology

CTAVN is thought to be congenital in nature, although its precise etiology is unknown.

Pathogenesis

This endodermal rest is believed to occur due to abnormal migration during embryogenesis. About 10% of individuals with CTAVN also have midline developmental defects suggestive of a genetic defect affecting migration of embryological tissues.

Macroscopic appearance

A CTAVN may be apparent as a small bulge or swelling within the atrioventricular septum. The cysts may or may not be apparent grossly and may contain fluid or pultaceous debris.

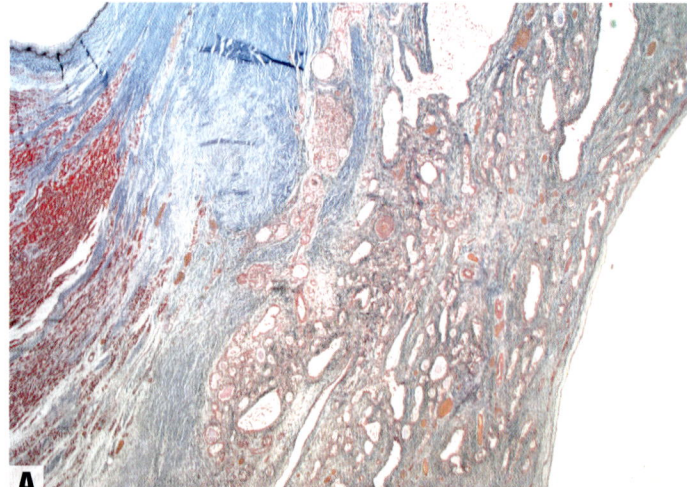

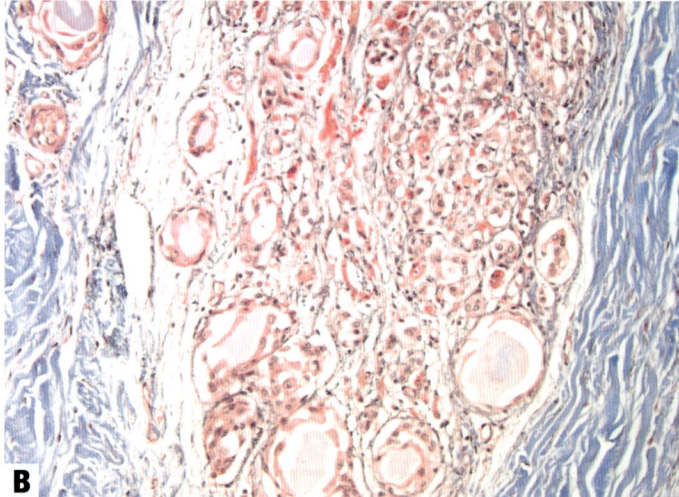

Fig. 3.30 Cystic tumour of the atrioventricular node. **A** Low-power view showing replacement of the nodal tissue by a cystic tumour of the atrioventricular node (Masson trichrome stain). **B** Higher-power view of the lesion showing solid nests of cells, as well as glands, some of which have intraluminal secretions (Masson trichrome stain).

Histopathology

The cysts are lined by columnar, transitional, or squamous cells. Goblet cells and sebaceous cells have also been described. No cellular atypia is present and mitotic figures are rare.

CTAVN stains with Alcian blue and PAS, exhibiting resistance to both hyaluronidase and diastase digestion. There is positive staining for cytokeratin AE1/AE3, CK5, and CEA. Scattered cells may be positive for serotonin, chromogranin, and calcitonin. Mesothelial, endothelial, and lymphatic markers are negative {556}.

On electron microscopy, the cells form solid nests with a basement membranes. Cytoplasmic tonofilaments, desmosomes, electron-dense material, and short microvilli are seen.

Differential diagnoses include simple cysts or bronchogenic cysts and intracardiac teratoma.

Cytology
Not described

Diagnostic molecular pathology
Not clinically relevant

Essential and desirable diagnostic criteria
Essential:
- Endodermal inclusion forming a cystic lesion within the atrio-ventricular septum

Staging
Not clinically relevant

Prognosis and prediction
The tumours are usually apparent only at autopsy. Rare cases have been surgically excised. Fatal arrhythmias may occur despite pacemaker placement. There is no correlation between tumour size and occurrence of arrhythmia.

Cardiac angiosarcoma

Leduc C
Thway K

Definition

Cardiac angiosarcoma is a primary cardiac malignant mesenchymal neoplasm with endothelial differentiation by morphology and/or immunohistochemistry.

ICD-O coding

9120/3 Angiosarcoma

ICD-11 coding

2B56.0 Angiosarcoma of heart

Related terminology

Not recommended: haemangiosarcoma; lymphangiosarcoma; malignant haemangioendothelioma; malignant angioendothelioma.

Subtype(s)

None

Localization

Angiosarcomas can occur anywhere in the heart and pericardium; however, the vast majority originate in the right atrium within the atrioventricular groove. Extension to adjacent chambers and pericardium is common {356,1132,1291,1671,3451}. Tumour spread is generally by direct extension or haematogenous dissemination, most commonly to lung, liver, brain, and bone. Lymph node metastases occur in a minority of cases {3481,1291,802,1438}. See *Angiosarcoma of the thorax* (p. 299).

Clinical features

Dyspnoea, chest pain, and syncope are the most common symptoms. Clinical signs include haemopericardium (with or without tamponade), arrhythmias, and signs of right heart failure {356,1291,929,802,1731,1671}.

Imaging

Echocardiographic findings are nonspecific {2166}. Tumours are hypermetabolic on PET, with heterogeneous attenuation on CT and MRI {1671,40,3355,563,1442}.

Epidemiology

Cardiac angiosarcoma is the most common differentiated cardiac sarcoma, representing approximately one third of all primary cardiac sarcomas {2777,2429,480}. It occurs most commonly between the fourth and sixth decades of life, with a wide age range (8–90 years). It is more frequent in men and in white people {3481,356,1132,1291}.

Etiology

The etiology of most cases is unknown; however, cases secondary to chest irradiation and cases within Li–Fraumeni–like families have been reported {2718,1435,364,401,1416,363}.

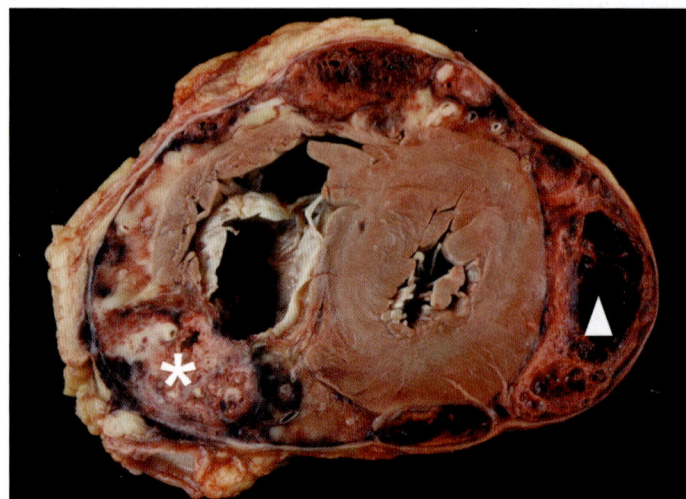

Fig. 3.31 Cardiac angiosarcoma. This autopsy specimen exhibits a high mid-ventricular short-axis section exhibiting a variegated mass growing along the right atrioventricular groove (asterisk), infiltrating the right ventricular myocardium, with associated haemopericardium (arrowhead).

Pathogenesis

Upregulation of genes in the VEGF pathway (including *KDR* and *VEGFA*) appears to play a role {363,1269}. Cardiac angiosarcomas have complex karyotypes, with trisomy 8, trisomy 17, and gain of 1q being the most common anomalies {1622,1553, 3527}. Point mutations have been identified in a variety of genes, including *TP53*, *KRAS*, *KDR*, *PLCG1*, KMT2 (*MLL2*), and *KMT2D* {1553,3527,3518,2047,912}. Recurrent *POT1* mutations have been identified in cardiac angiosarcomas in Li–Fraumeni–like families {364}.

Macroscopic appearance

Tumours have a broad infiltrative endocardial base with lobules protruding into and occasionally filling the involved chamber. Haemorrhage and necrosis are common. With pericardial involvement, there is extensive and often circumferential filling of the pericardial space by haemorrhage and tumour {356,1671}. Tumour size ranges from 20 to 130 mm, with most tumours being ≥ 50 mm {3481,356,1132,1291,929}.

Histopathology

Histologically, conventional angiosarcoma is typically vasoformative, consisting of anastomosing thin-walled vascular channels filled with erythrocytes and lined by moderately pleomorphic hyperchromatic round to spindle-shaped cells with distinct nucleoli. Vascular spaces can be slit-like and inapparent, resulting in a sheet-like proliferation of spindle cells. The epithelioid pattern has plump polygonal tumour cells with prominent nucleoli, arranged in cords, nests, or papillae. Haemorrhage and necrosis are common. Biphasic morphology, with both

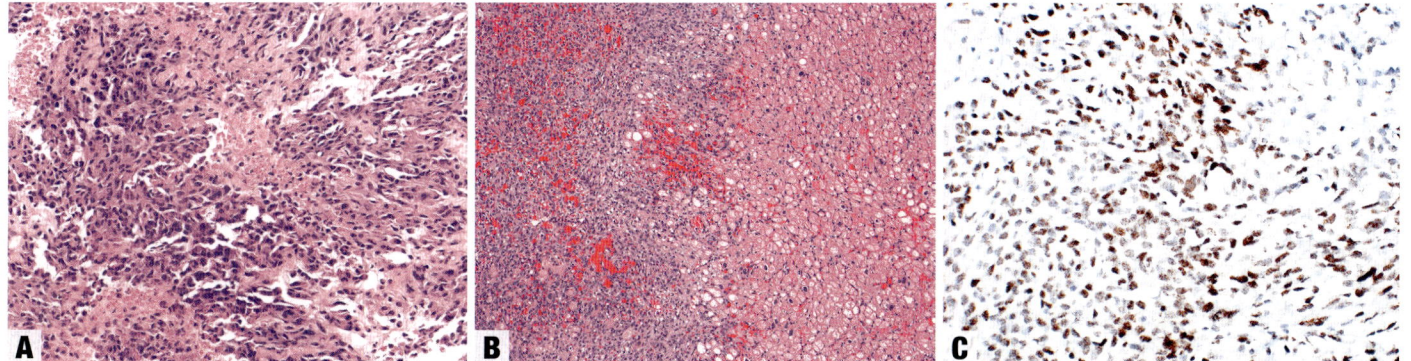

Fig. 3.32 Cardiac angiosarcoma, conventional pattern. **A** Round to oval tumour cells with vasoformative and papillary architecture and associated haemorrhage and necrosis. **B** Highly cellular, vasoformative tumour (left) infiltrating cardiac myocytes (right). **C** Diffuse nuclear immunoreactivity for FLI1.

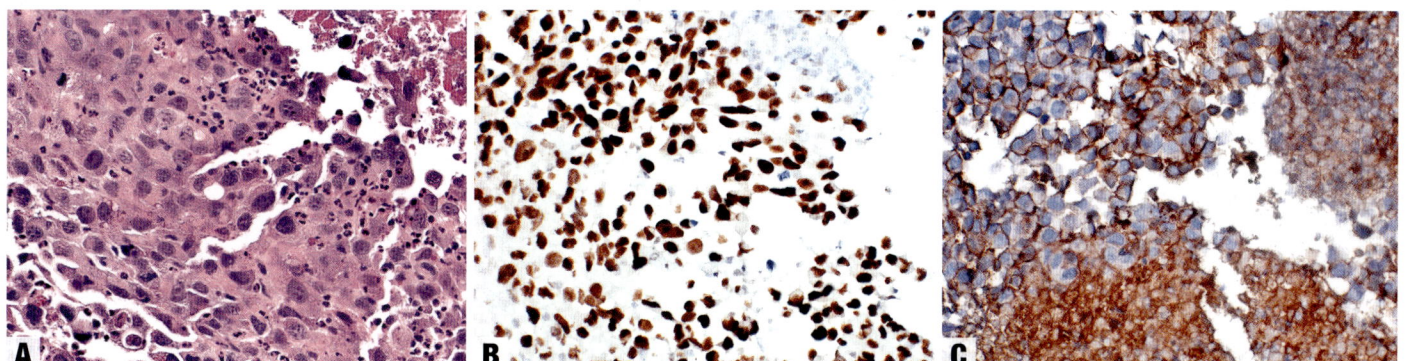

Fig. 3.33 Cardiac angiosarcoma, epithelioid pattern. **A** Large mitotically active epithelioid tumour cells forming abortive lumina with associated necrosis. **B** Diffuse nuclear immunoreactivity for ERG. **C** Diffuse membranous immunoreactivity for CD31 in viable tumour cells.

conventional and epithelioid components, has been reported {1731,1622}. Grading is according to the French Fédération Nationale des Centres de Lutte Contre le Cancer (FNCLCC) system, with a tumour differentiation score of 2 for conventional angiosarcoma and 3 for epithelioid angiosarcoma {1024,558}.

Immunohistochemically, ERG is the most sensitive and specific antibody for confirming endothelial differentiation, with most tumours also being reactive with other endothelial markers such as FLI1, CD31, and CD34 {1622,2288}. Cytokeratin reactivity is common in epithelioid angiosarcoma, as well as in a minority of conventional cardiac angiosarcomas {1622,485}.

Cardiac angiosarcoma can be distinguished from benign vascular proliferations by the presence of extensively infiltrative borders, readily apparent cytological atypia, and an elevated proliferation index (Ki-67 generally ≥ 10%) {929,1878}. Exclusion of metastatic carcinoma, mesothelioma, and non-endothelial sarcomas is achieved by confirming vascular differentiation by immunohistochemistry. Epithelioid cases should be distinguished from epithelioid haemangioendothelioma, which is characterized morphologically by cytoplasmic vacuoles, nuclear inclusions, and chondroid/myxoid stroma and typically harbours the pathognomonic *CAMTA1-WWTR1* fusion {78}.

Cytology
On cytological preparations, tumour cells tend to occur individually; however, 3D clusters and/or papillary structures can be observed. Other cytological features commonly present include frequent mitoses, nuclear grooves, and readily apparent nucleoli {936,1549}.

Diagnostic molecular pathology
Not clinically relevant

Essential and desirable diagnostic criteria
Essential:
- Malignant cells with vascular differentiation (morphologically or immunophenotypically)

Desirable:
- Vascular structures or intracytoplasmic lumina

Staging
While the American Joint Committee on Cancer (AJCC) has included angiosarcoma in the staging of soft tissue sarcomas of the thoracic visceral organs, the Union for International Cancer Control (UICC) has not.

Prognosis and prediction
The prognosis is worse than that of other cardiac sarcomas and non-cardiac angiosarcoma, probably because of the high likelihood of developing cardiac tamponade {2777,480,1717}. The majority of cases are of advanced stage at diagnosis, and the 5-year overall survival rate is approximately 10% {3481,356, 1731}. Poor prognostic factors include age ≥ 45 years; tumour size > 50 mm; and spread to adjacent organs, regional lymph nodes, or distant organs. Tumour grade does not seem to have a significant impact on survival {3481}. For surgically amenable tumours, complete resection is the treatment of choice and has been shown to improve overall survival {3481,1696,2424,2780}.

Cardiac leiomyosarcoma

Basso C
Dry SM

Definition

Cardiac leiomyosarcoma is a malignant mesenchymal tumour arising in the heart showing smooth muscle cell differentiation.

ICD-O coding

8890/3 Leiomyosarcoma, NOS

ICD-11 coding

2B58.Y & XH7ED4 Leiomyosarcoma, other specified primary site & Leiomyosarcoma, NOS
2B58.Z & XH7ED4 Leiomyosarcoma, unspecified primary site & Leiomyosarcoma, NOS

Related terminology

None

Subtype(s)

None

Localization

The left atrium is the most common location, followed by the right atrium and the ventricular chambers, with the tumours being either intracavitary or infiltrating. When in the atria, cardiac leiomyosarcomas usually arise from the free wall and rarely have a stalk {3208,1853,931,2327}.

Clinical features

Clinical presentation for left atrial tumours is often dyspnoea, haemoptysis, or atrial fibrillation, and for right-sided tumours is peripheral oedema and ascites. The median age is 48 years (range: 6 months to 86 years), and there is no sex predominance {3208}.

Epidemiology

Leiomyosarcoma accounts for < 20% of primary cardiac sarcomas in published series {170,3003}.

Etiology

Etiology has not been reported specifically for primary cardiac leiomyosarcomas.

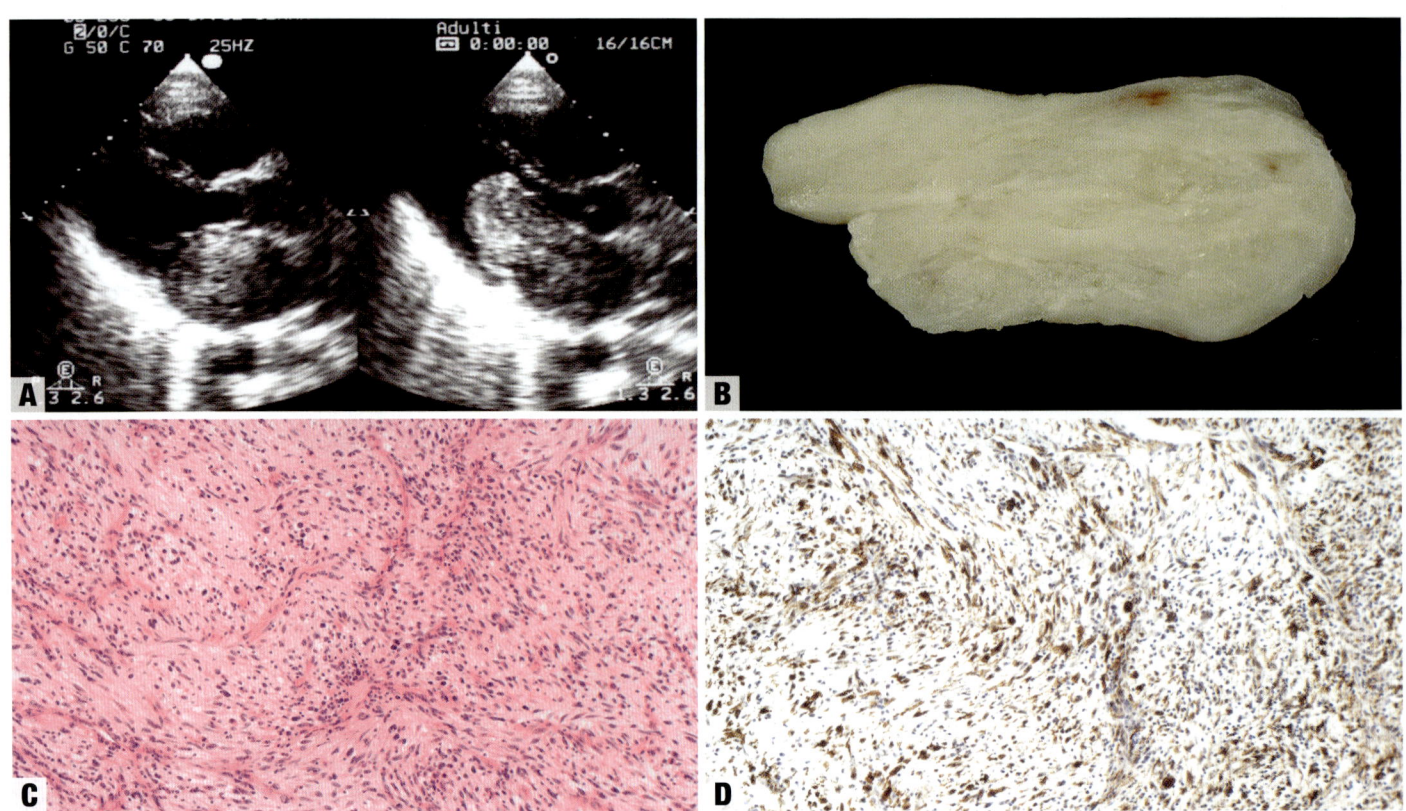

Fig. 3.34 Leiomyosarcoma. **A** Preoperative transthoracic echocardiography. The left atrial mass (**left**) is moving towards the left ventricular cavity during diastole (**right**) through the mitral valve. **B** The mass appears firm, whitish, and ovoid on gross examination. **C** Storiform proliferation with pleomorphic cells enmeshed in a myxoid extracellular matrix with a high mitotic count. **D** At immunohistochemistry, the neoplastic cells appeared positive for α-SMA (shown here) and desmin.

Pathogenesis

Pathogenesis has not been reported specifically for cardiac leiomyosarcomas. For information on general pathogenesis of leiomyosarcoma, see the *Soft tissue and bone tumours* volume of this series {3298}.

Macroscopic appearance

Leiomyosarcomas are homogeneous, firm, grey to white to tan masses, often multilobular. A whorled appearance may be evident. Variable necrosis can be present.

Histopathology

The majority of leiomyosarcomas are high-grade. They show spindle-shaped cells with plump, blunt-ended nuclei and moderate to abundant, pale to brightly eosinophilic fibrillary cytoplasm. The cells are set in long intersecting fascicles parallel and perpendicular to the plane of section; some tumours show areas with storiform or palisade patterns. Moderate nuclear pleomorphism is usually present. Mitotic figures, including atypical ones, are easy to find. Usually there is diffuse hypercellularity, although focal fibrosis, myxoid change, and hyalinized hypocellular areas can be present. There is often necrosis in larger tumours. By immunohistochemistry, SMA and desmin are typically positive {3208,662}.

Cytology

Not clinically relevant

Diagnostic molecular pathology

Not clinically relevant

Essential and desirable diagnostic criteria

Essential:
- Fascicles of eosinophilic spindled cells with blunt-ended nuclei showing variable pleomorphism
- Immunolabelling for SMA, desmin, and/or caldesmon

Staging

Not clinically relevant

Prognosis and prediction

Cardiac leiomyosarcomas are generally clinically aggressive neoplasms with frequent local recurrences and distant metastases. Adjuvant chemotherapy and radiation therapy is of unclear benefit in primary cardiac sarcomas. The completeness of excision in general affects survival. In a recent review of published cases, the 5-year overall survival rate and the local and metastatic recurrence-free survival rate were 25.4% and 14.7%, respectively {3208}.

Cardiac undifferentiated pleomorphic sarcoma

Burke AP

Definition

Undifferentiated pleomorphic sarcoma is a high-grade sarcoma composed of pleomorphic spindled or epithelioid cells with no areas of differentiation that would indicate a specific subset of sarcoma.

ICD-O coding

8802/3 Pleomorphic sarcoma

ICD-11 coding

2B54.Y Unclassified pleomorphic sarcoma, primary site, other specified site

Related terminology

Not recommended: intimal sarcoma; undifferentiated sarcoma; undifferentiated spindle cell sarcoma.

Subtype(s)

None

Localization

Undifferentiated pleomorphic sarcoma most commonly occurs in the left atrium. The site of attachment is usually the posterior or lateral wall, although the attachment site may be the atrial appendage or mitral valve. In rare instances, the attachment site is the atrial septum, mimicking cardiac myxoma. Occasionally, tumours can fill the entire atrial cavity {2825}. Multiple tumours studding the endocardium have been reported {1175}.

Pulmonary intimal sarcomas with histological features of undifferentiated sarcoma may extend retrograde from the pulmonary valve or trunk into the right ventricle and atrium and are best considered to be of pulmonary artery origin.

Clinical features

The majority of patients present with symptoms related to a left atrial mass, especially respiratory symptoms related to mitral stenosis, cardiac arrhythmias, and heart failure. In some patients, fever and constitutional symptoms are prominent {1815}. In rare examples, patients present with metastatic disease {589}. A wide variety of metastatic sites have been reported, including soft tissue, bone, gastrointestinal tract, and CNS. There is no sex predilection. The mean age at presentation is 50–55 years {3129,3240,1156,392,1441,32,1142,200}.

Epidemiology

Cardiac undifferentiated pleomorphic sarcoma accounts for approximately one third of cardiac sarcomas. Primary cardiac sarcoma is rare, accounting for just under 1% of sarcomas in the US population {1056}.

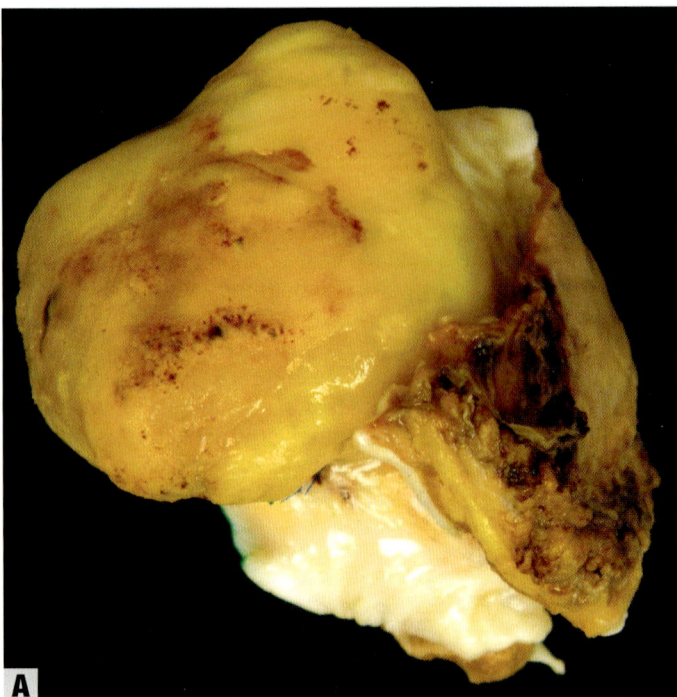

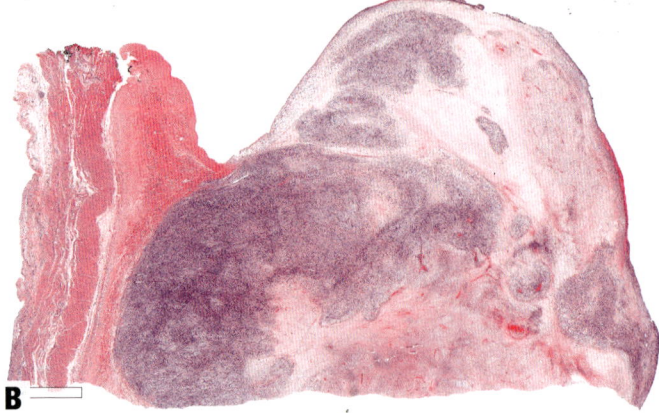

Fig. 3.35 Undifferentiated pleomorphic sarcoma. **A** Gross photo of a resected left atrial tumour that is polypoid and exophytic. **B** The histological section demonstrates a polypoid highly cellular mass, with lighter areas representing necrosis. There was little invasion into the left atrial wall at the left of the figure.

Etiology

The etiology of undifferentiated pleomorphic sarcoma of the heart is unknown.

Pathogenesis

MDM2 amplification using FISH, PCR, and array comparative genomic hybridization has been observed in about 30% of cardiac undifferentiated pleomorphic sarcomas, a lower rate than

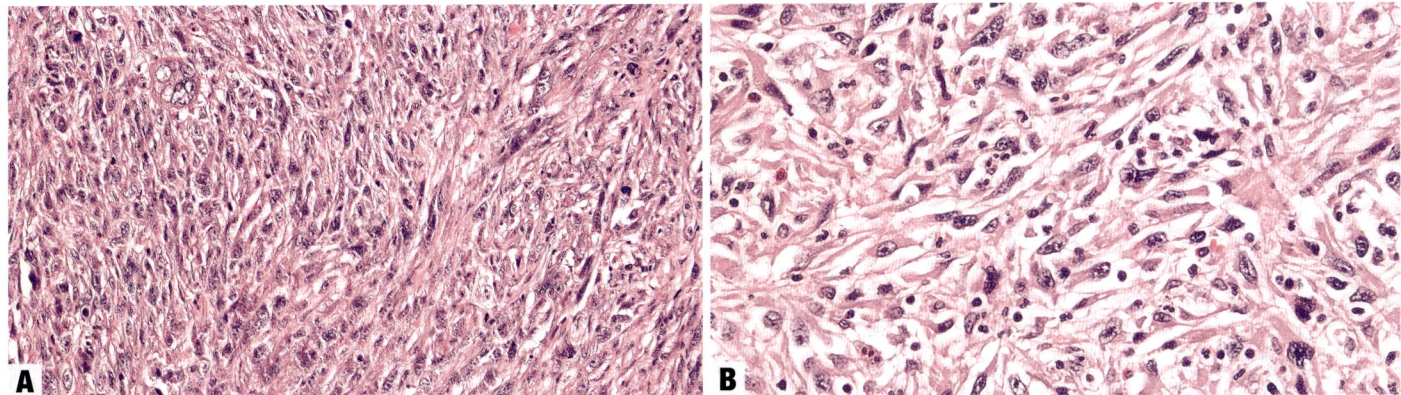

Fig. 3.36 Undifferentiated pleomorphic sarcoma with predominant spindled component. **A** The spindle cells are highly atypical and pleomorphic, without significant amounts of stroma. **B** A different example at higher magnification shows similar features.

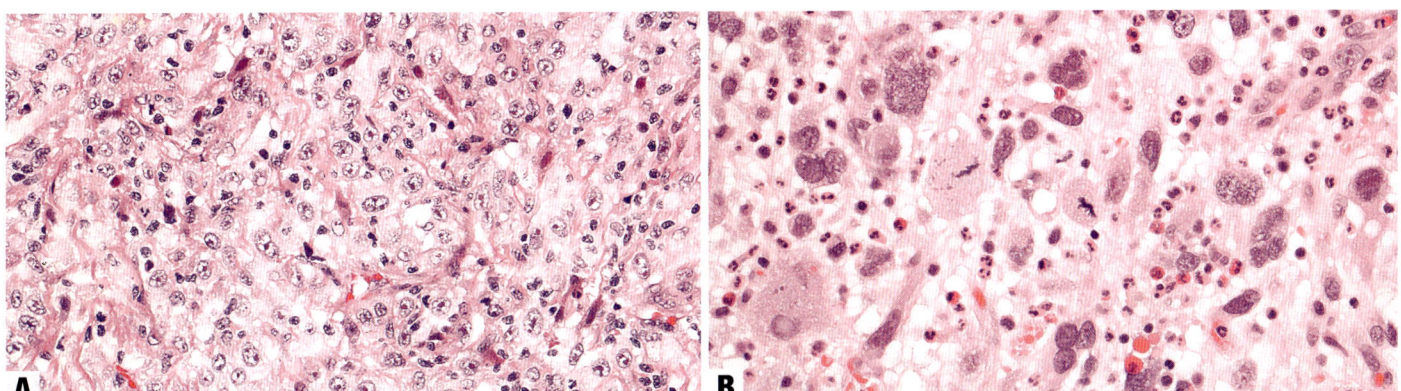

Fig. 3.37 Undifferentiated pleomorphic sarcoma. **A** Undifferentiated pleomorphic sarcoma with predominant epithelioid component. There is no significant spindling; the cells are epithelioid and pleomorphic. **B** Undifferentiated pleomorphic sarcoma, epithelioid, with extreme pleomorphism. There are numerous mitotic figures and pronounced variation in cell size.

in better-differentiated intimal sarcomas {2089}. Immunohisto-chemical overexpression of the protein product and amplification of *PDGFRA* and *KIT* (CD117) are frequently seen in these cases {589,3240,32,7,10,873,1272}.

Macroscopic appearance

Cardiac undifferentiated sarcomas are similar in gross appearance to intimal sarcomas, and they typically project into the left atrial lumen as polypoid masses, with little invasion into the muscle early in the course of disease. A lobulated appearance can sometimes mimic myxoma {3240}. Tumours tend to be large (50–100 mm). A 5 mm cardiac pleomorphic sarcoma that caused symptoms because of location on the mitral valve was completely excised and yet metastasized within 6 months {32}.

Histopathology

Undifferentiated pleomorphic sarcomas are composed of atypical, pleomorphic spindle cells and epithelioid cells. Mitotic figures are usually numerous, and necrosis is common. Some tumours have areas that may mimic myxofibrosarcoma, with curvilinear vessels and a myxoid background {2027,2434}. Foci of malignant bone matrix, in the form of chondrosarcoma or osteosarcoma, are occasionally seen {1223}. There is often an eroded surface lined by fibrin {3129}.

As more cardiac undifferentiated pleomorphic sarcomas with molecular alterations typical of intimal sarcoma are being

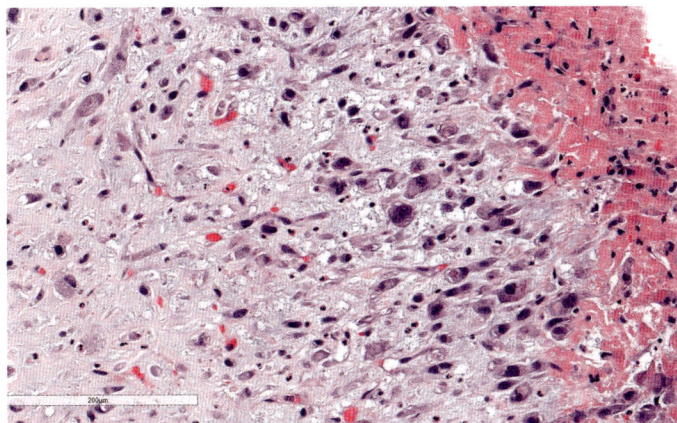

Fig. 3.38 Undifferentiated pleomorphic sarcoma with predominant epithelioid component and surface fibrin. Organizing fibrin layers are common on the surface of intimal sarcomas, such as this example in the left atrium.

described, the two entities are becoming merged into a single spectrum. Also, there are tumours that have histological features of both, with some areas typical of myxofibrosarcoma and others that are undifferentiated. Many primary cardiac sarcomas with histological features of undifferentiated pleomorphic sarcoma are currently being reported as intimal sarcoma, especially if there is MDM2 expression.

Cytology

Aspirates of undifferentiated pleomorphic sarcoma show pleomorphic tumour cells with large vesicular nuclei and prominent nucleoli, with a high mitotic count.

Diagnostic molecular pathology

Not clinically relevant

Essential and desirable diagnostic criteria

Essential:
- Histological features of pleomorphic spindled or epithelioid cells (or both) in the majority of the tumour
- Absence of histological or molecular evidence of leiomyosarcoma or synovial sarcoma

Desirable:
- Location in the left atrium as a polypoid mass
- Minimal or no myxoid or fibrotic stroma

Staging

There is currently no clinically relevant staging system for these tumours.

Prognosis and prediction

The prognosis of cardiac undifferentiated pleomorphic sarcoma is poor, with survival typically being weeks to months. Some patients survive as long as 2 years {1156}. No correlation has been demonstrated between histological features and survival.

Other sarcomas that may involve the heart

Fritchie KJ
Leduc C

In addition to angiosarcoma and leiomyosarcoma, a variety of other sarcomas can also be primary to the heart. Of these, myxofibrosarcoma and synovial sarcoma are the most common and are covered elsewhere (see *Myxofibrosarcoma of the thorax*, p. 290, and *Synovial sarcoma of the thorax*, p. 314). Others include rhabdomyosarcoma (embryonal and pleomorphic subtypes), osteosarcoma, dedifferentiated liposarcoma, malignant peripheral nerve sheath tumour, and Ewing sarcoma {3472, 1104, 16, 339, 3492, 342, 1854, 2805, 1456, 406, 2043, 2662, 861, 1051, 3171, 1681, 26, 3382, 58, 3111, 1206, 480, 2424, 3211, 2429, 1438, 2617, 2781, 2726}. Although data are scarce, these sarcomas do not seem to show a predilection for the pericardium or particular cardiac chambers, and prognosis is generally poor. Intimal sarcoma is considered a sarcoma of vascular intima (not endocardium) and is covered elsewhere (see *Pulmonary artery intimal sarcoma*, p. 164). Cardiac sarcomas without morphological, immunohistochemical, or molecular differentiation are now considered to represent undifferentiated pleomorphic sarcoma (see *Cardiac undifferentiated pleomorphic sarcoma*, p. 262).

Haematolymphoid tumours of the heart: Introduction

Cooper WA
Chan JKC
Maleszewski JJ

Overview

Tumours of the heart are rare, and haematolymphoid tumours make up only about 1% of neoplasms at this site {996,355}. Primary lymphomas of the heart are rare and account for only about 0.5% of all extranodal lymphomas {996,391}. By definition, primary cardiac lymphomas show involvement of the heart and/or pericardium only, with no or minimal extracardiac disease {187}. In contrast, secondary involvement of the heart by disseminated lymphoma is not uncommon, occurring in approximately 20–25% of lymphoma patients {996,1306}.

Primary cardiac lymphomas occur in immunocompetent and, disproportionately, immunodeficient patients (especially HIV-positive patients and transplant recipients) {502,1172}. The clinical presentation is variable, depending on the exact tumour location, but imaging evidence of a cardiac mass or an unexplained pericardial effusion are clues to possible lymphoma or other tumours {996}. Other, less specific presentations include cardiac failure, tamponade, and arrhythmias {502,2333}. Cytological assessment of pericardial fluid can be diagnostic in a large proportion of cases, but a histological biopsy may be required for diagnosis {417}. Because of their critical location and potential delays in diagnosis, the prognosis of primary cardiac lymphomas is generally poor, with chemotherapy being the mainstay of treatment {502}.

Classification of primary cardiac lymphoma

Primary cardiac lymphomas are non-Hodgkin lymphomas, most commonly diffuse large B-cell lymphoma, which accounts for ≥ 80% of cases {996,2333}. Other types of B-cell and T-cell lymphomas, such as Burkitt lymphoma, have also been reported but are extremely rare {2333}.

Although rare, fibrin-associated diffuse large B-cell lymphoma is a unique type of diffuse large B-cell lymphoma that can occur in the heart, in addition to other sites of chronic fibrin deposition {1733,1461}. This is newly listed as a distinct entity in the fifth edition of the WHO classification of thoracic tumours.

Primary effusion lymphoma is another rare but distinct lymphoma type that can occur in the pericardial cavity. This entity is covered in the section *Primary effusion lymphoma* (p. 221).

Cardiac diffuse large B-cell lymphoma

Miller DV
Quintanilla-Martinez L

Definition
Primary cardiac (extranodal) diffuse large B-cell lymphoma (DLBCL) arises in the heart, although it may extend to adjacent tissues.

ICD-O coding
9680/3 Diffuse large B-cell lymphoma, NOS

ICD-11 coding
2A81.Z Diffuse large B-cell lymphoma, NOS

Related terminology
None

Subtype(s)
None

Localization
The right atrium is the most common site. Roughly one third of all cases involve the pericardium {2333}. Valvular involvement is rare {3524}.

Clinical features
Symptoms vary with the size and location of involvement. Dyspnoea, chest pain, and heart failure are frequent {2333}. Pulmonary embolism has also been reported {516,2786}. Arrhythmias and sudden cardiac death may also occur {1486,503}.

Imaging
On echocardiography, cardiac lymphoma usually manifests as hypoechogenic infiltration of the myocardium, often with pericardial effusion {1306}. CT and MRI can provide additional detail. Endomyocardial biopsy may lead to histological diagnosis (and treatment) without thoracotomy {1628}.

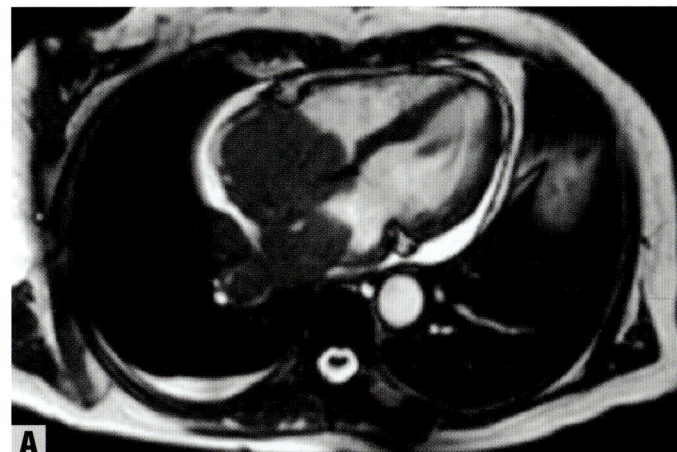

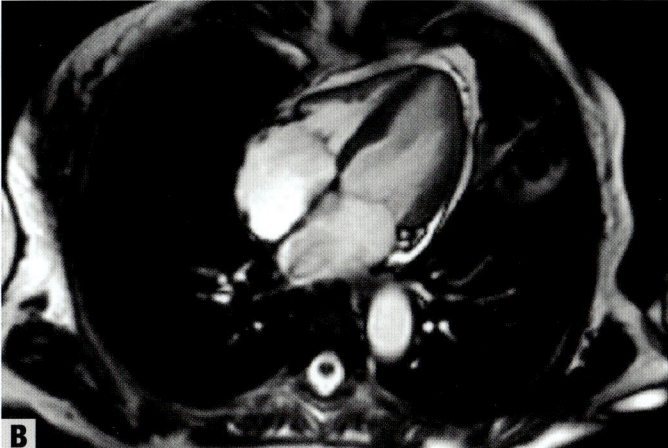

Fig. 3.39 Cardiac lymphoma. **A** A mass occupies both atria, extending to the pulmonary veins. **B** At last follow-up, 2 years later (after R-CHOP chemotherapy), there is complete remission.

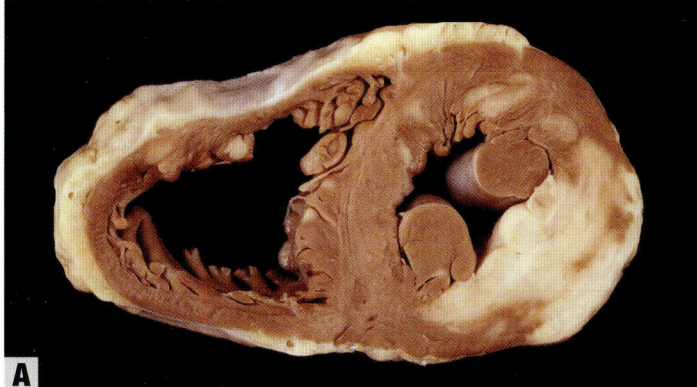

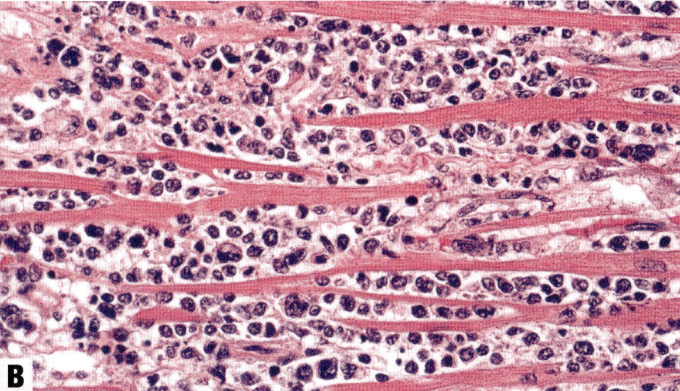

Fig. 3.40 Primary cardiac lymphoma. **A** An infiltrative mass is noted primarily along the inferolateral left ventricle, with smaller satellite foci along the anterior aspect of the ventricle; the tumour involves the epicardium, myocardium, and endocardium. **B** This proliferation of atypical, malignant B lymphocytes exhibits extensive interstitial infiltration with both atrophic and damaged cardiac myocytes.

Epidemiology

Primary cardiac lymphomas (the majority of which are DLBCL) account for < 2% of primary cardiac neoplasms in surgical series {1307,2333}, with an M:F ratio of 2:1 {2333}. The median age is 63 years, but occurrence in a 9-year-old has been reported {433}.

Etiology

Unknown

Pathogenesis

Perhaps the most notable feature of cardiac DLBCL is the high frequency of lymphoma types associated with impaired immunity. These types include EBV-associated DLBCL, DLBCL associated with chronic inflammation {137,1922,272}, and fibrin-associated large B-cell lymphoma {1012,1922}. Primary cardiac low-grade B-cell lymphomas also occur {951,1649,2192}.

Macroscopic appearance

Grossly, primary cardiac lymphomas are multinodular grey-white coalescing masses that can involve any or all tissue layer(s). They may also extend to the great arteries.

Histopathology

Cellular monotony, dyscohesion, and large cell size are hallmarks of DLBCL. Immunophenotyping is critical, especially to characterize the cell of origin (germinal-centre B cell vs activated B cell), MYC/BCL2 coexpression, and EBV status.

Cytology

Cytological evaluation, particularly in cases with pericardial effusion, can be diagnostic {2519}.

Diagnostic molecular pathology

MYC and *BCL2* FISH and EBV in situ studies assist in classification. A molecular classification for DLBCL, based on whole-exome sequencing, has been proposed {456,2666}.

Essential and desirable diagnostic criteria

Essential:

- Large B-cell lymphoma involving the heart/pericardium with no or minor extracardiac component
- Mature B-cell immunophenotype (as described above)

Staging

Staging is according to the Lugano classification, a modification of the Ann Arbor staging system {492}.

Prognosis and prediction

The prognosis is typically poor, especially if myocardial rupture occurs {1953}. Response to chemotherapy is generally on par with that of DLBCL at extracardiac sites {2333}.

Cardiac fibrin-associated diffuse large B-cell lymphoma

Boyer DF
Cheuk W
Maleszewski JJ

Definition

Fibrin-associated diffuse large B-cell lymphoma (FA-DLBCL) is a microscopic proliferation of large B cells found incidentally within fibrin exudate in confined anatomical spaces. The neoplastic cells of FA-DLBCL do not exert a mass effect or infiltrate normal tissues, which distinguishes this entity from EBV-positive diffuse large B-cell lymphoma (DLBCL) and DLBCL associated with chronic inflammation.

ICD-O coding

9680/3 Fibrin-associated diffuse large B-cell lymphoma

ICD-11 coding

2A81.Y Other specified diffuse large B-cell lymphomas

Related terminology

Not recommended: fibrin-associated EBV-positive large B-cell lymphoma; microscopic/incidental DLBCL associated with chronic inflammation; EBV-positive large B-cell lymphoma arising in atrial myxoma; microscopic DLBCL occurring in pseudocyst.

Subtype(s)

None

Localization

FA-DLBCL arises in sites of chronic fibrin deposition, including cysts and pseudocyst cavities {282}, chronic haematomas {3470}, and intravascular or intracardiac locations with chronic perturbation of blood flow (e.g. the surface of atrial myxomas {3372}, endovascular grafts, and prosthetic cardiac valves {1922}). Embolism of fibrinous material from sites involved by FA-DLBCL can carry the lymphoma cells along with the embolus {296}, but dissemination of lymphoma into distant tissues via embolism has not been demonstrated.

Clinical features

The clinical presentation depends on the underlying anatomical lesion that is incidentally involved by FA-DLBCL. Some patients with FA-DLBCL associated with atrial myxoma or endovascular grafts have presented with thromboembolic events, but it is unknown whether the risk of thromboembolism differs from that associated with similar vascular grafts or atrial myxomas without FA-DLBCL. Table 3.01 displays clinical features of reported cases.

Epidemiology

This is a relatively recently described entity, and the overall incidence is unknown. The diagnosis depends on recognition of small aggregates of atypical lymphocytes when evaluating

Table 3.01 Localization and clinical characteristics of reported cases of fibrin-associated diffuse large B-cell lymphoma

Site	Number of reported cases	Median age (range), in years	M:F ratio	Foreign body cases per reported cases	Persistent/recurrent cases per reported cases with follow-up
Cardiac					
Atrial myxoma	14	54 (46–70)	2:5	0/14	1/14
Atrial thrombus	2	42.5 (29–56)	2:0	0/2	0/2
Cardiac valve	5	66 (50–80)	3:2	4/5	0/5
Cyst/pseudocyst					
Adrenal	5	70 (48–71)	3:2	0/5	0/5
Kidney	2	53.5 (46–61)	2:0	0/2	0/1
Spleen	2	33 (29–37)	1:1	0/2	0/2
Retroperitoneum	2	58.5 (44–73)	2:0	0/2	0/2
Ovary	2	56.5 (56–57)	0:2	0/2	0/2
Testis	2	57.5 (27–88)	2:0	0/2	0/1
Breast implant capsule	1	69	0:1	1/1	0/1
Haematoma/thrombus					
Endovascular graft	6	62 (48–79)	5:1	6/6	3/5
Intracranial	4	70.5 (25–81)	3:1	1/4	0/3
Large artery aneurysm	2	82.5 (74–91)	5:1	1/2	0/2
Testicular haematoma	1	79	1:0	0/1	0/1

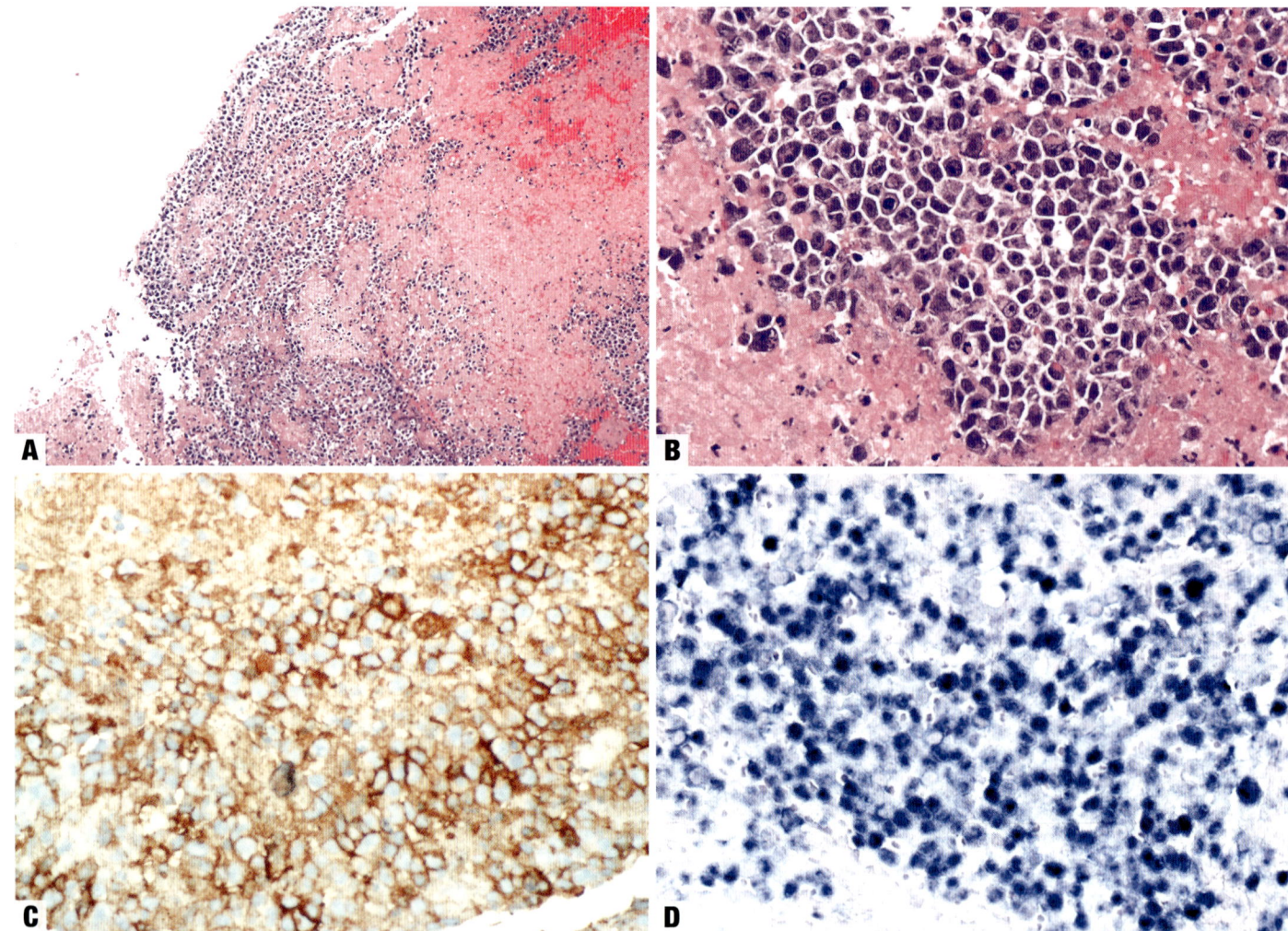

Fig. 3.41 Fibrin-associated diffuse large B-cell lymphoma. **A** Loose aggregates of large lymphocytes on the surface of a fibrin thrombus removed from an abdominal aortic aneurysm. **B** High magnification of the lymphoid aggregates shows immunoblastic cytomorphology with frequent mitotic figures and apoptotic bodies. **C** The large lymphocytes are positive for CD20 (brown). **D** The large lymphocytes are positive for EBV-encoded small RNA (EBER) (blue).

specimens that have been excised or biopsied for other reasons. FA-DLBCL has been diagnosed in adults with a wide age range (25–91 years; median age: 56.5 years). It has been reported in more men than women (M:F ratio: 3:2); however, sex bias is related to the underlying lesions that create a permissive microenvironment for FA-DLBCL (see Table 3.01, p. 269).

Etiology

FA-DLBCL is strongly associated with infection of lesional B cells by EBV, usually with type III latency. Rare EBV-negative lymphoproliferations with features similar to those of typical FA-DLBCL have also been described {1461}. Despite the type III latency profile, patients rarely have evidence of immunosuppression, and the EBV-positive B cells appear to be protected from immune surveillance by the local microenvironment {1733}. Some cases of FA-DLBCL arise in association with foreign bodies/implants, most commonly endovascular grafts.

Pathogenesis

FA-DLBCL is an incidental lymphoproliferative disorder. It is unknown whether the presence of FA-DLBCL modifies the natural history of the underlying anatomical lesions with which it is associated.

Macroscopic appearance

FA-DLBCL is a microscopic, non–mass-forming lymphoproliferation.

Histopathology

Loose aggregates of large lymphoid cells are surrounded by fibrin and cellular debris. There may be focal infiltration of abnormal tissue, such as myxomatous stroma or fibrous capsule, but there is no infiltration into histologically normal tissue. The lymphoma cells often have atypical immunoblastic cytomorphology, with irregular nuclei, coarse chromatin, prominent nucleoli, and amphophilic cytoplasm. Mitotic figures and apoptotic changes are frequent. Associated inflammation is usually sparse and comprises macrophages and small lymphocytes; however, some specimens have a prominent lymphoplasmacytic infiltrate near the lymphoma cells {296}.

The immunophenotype is typical of activated B cells or B immunoblasts: CD20+, CD79a+, PAX5+, CD45+, IRF4 (MUM1)+, BCL2+/–, BCL6+/–, CD30+/–. Rare cases with positivity for CD10 have been reported {3372}. Ki-67 staining shows a high proliferation index, usually > 90%. Some cases overexpress MYC protein by immunohistochemistry but are negative for *MYC* gene rearrangement. In situ hybridization for EBV-encoded small RNA (EBER) is nearly always positive, and the vast majority of cases show evidence of type III latency, signified by positivity for LMP1 and EBNA2 and negativity for BZLF1 {296}. HHV8 latency-associated nuclear antigen (LANA) is negative.

Cytology

The lymphoma cells often have atypical immunoblastic cytomorphology, with irregular nuclei, coarse chromatin, prominent nucleoli, and amphophilic cytoplasm.

Diagnostic molecular pathology

No specific genetic abnormalities have been associated with FA-DLBCL. Cases tested for rearrangements of the *MYC* and *BCL2* genes have been negative. Rare cases with detection of *BCL6* gene rearrangement by FISH have been reported {3372}. Clonal rearrangement of IGH is usually present, but demonstration of clonality is not required for the diagnosis of FA-DLBCL.

Essential and desirable diagnostic criteria

Essential:
- Abnormal lymphoid population associated with fibrin/thrombus with the aforementioned immunophenotype

Desirable:
- EBV reactivity

Staging

All reported cases have been localized to a single extranodal site, consistent with stage IE of the Lugano classification for lymphoma staging.

Prognosis and prediction

No deaths directly attributable to lymphoma have been reported, with some patients being followed for several years {296,3470, 3372}. Retrospective reports show no difference in outcomes for patients treated with chemotherapy, chemoimmunotherapy, or surgical excision {296}. When the underlying lesion cannot be completed excised, persistence or local regrowth of FA-DLBCL has been reported {296,272}. One report described a patient with EBV-positive DLBCL in the brain with an adjacent area of chronic subdural haemorrhage containing aggregates resembling FA-DLBCL, raising concern that FA-DLBCL may have the potential to progress to invasive DLBCL {1362}.

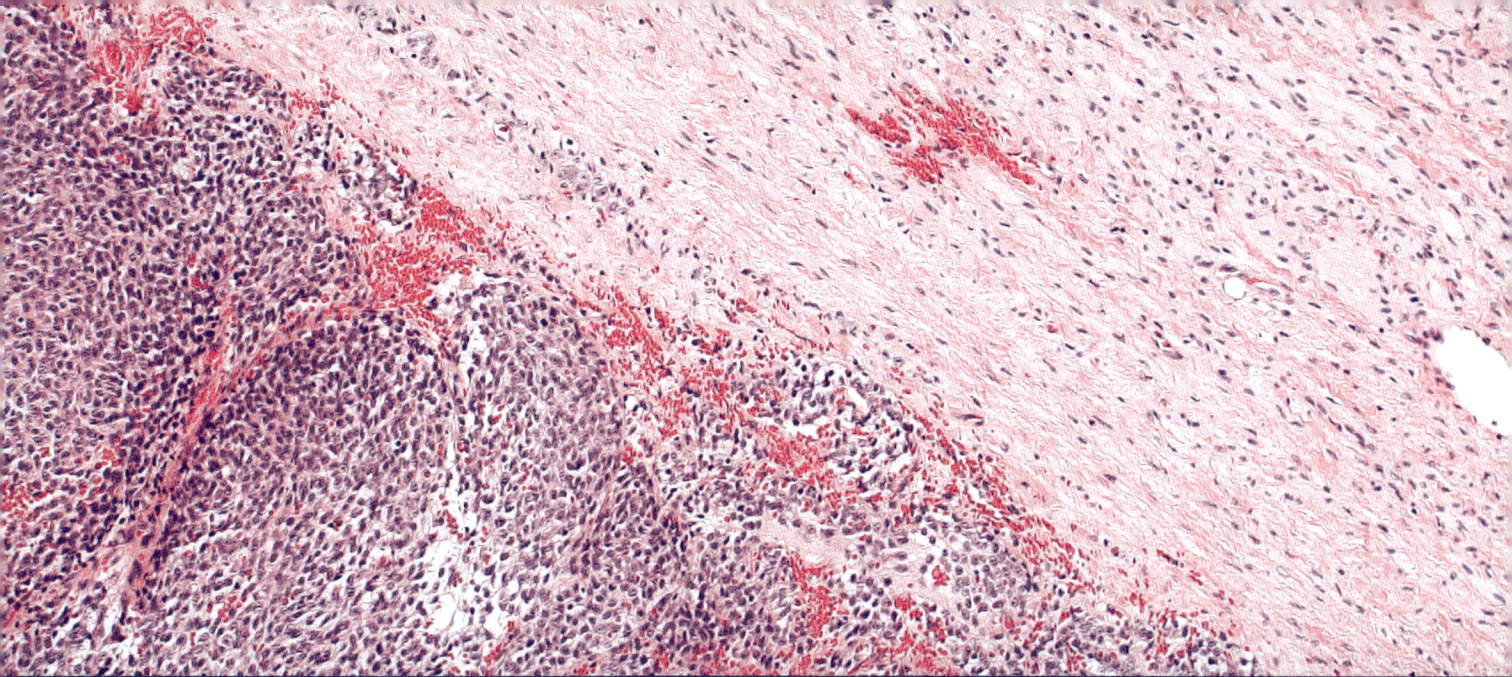

4

Mesenchymal tumours of the thorax

Edited by: Dacic S, Jain D, Lazar AJ, Maleszewski JJ, Noguchi M

Lipoma
Thymolipoma
Liposarcoma
Desmoid fibromatosis
Solitary fibrous tumour
Calcifying fibrous tumour
Inflammatory myofibroblastic tumour
Myxofibrosarcoma
Haemangioma
Lymphangioma
Epithelioid haemangioendothelioma
Angiosarcoma
Rhabdomyosarcoma
Paraganglioma
Granular cell tumour
Schwannoma
Malignant peripheral nerve sheath tumour
Peripheral neuroblastic tumours
Synovial sarcoma
Undifferentiated small round cell sarcomas

Mesenchymal tumours of the thorax: Introduction

Dacic S
Noguchi M

Although this chapter on mesenchymal tumours focuses on the entities most frequently encountered in the thorax (including lung, pleura, chest wall, and mediastinum), a more general introduction to soft tissue pathology is presented here, given that virtually any soft tissue tumour can arise at almost any site on at least rare occasions.

Incidence

The incidence of soft tissue sarcomas is fairly consistent, at 30–50 cases per 1 million person-years {921,1046,1826,811}. Benign soft tissue neoplasms as a group show an incidence at least 100-fold higher in aggregate. Individual benign mesenchymal entities range from frequent (e.g. lipoma) to rare (e.g. spindle cell haemangioma) {2040}. Sarcomas are a rare subset of thoracic tumours, far outnumbered by carcinomas and benign mesenchymal tumours.

The most common benign mesenchymal tumour of the lung is pulmonary hamartoma, accounting for 8% of radiographically detected coin lesions {3052}. Hamartomas have a male predominance, with peak incidence in the sixth decade of life, and they rarely occur in children {3138,578}.

Most hamartomas are peripheral and asymptomatic, with approximately 10% located centrally in a bronchus. Other benign mesenchymal neoplasms encountered in the thorax are not site specific and occur in other anatomical locations. For example, inflammatory myofibroblastic tumour most frequently occurs in the lung and accounts for as many as 1% of all lung tumours {2610}. In children, inflammatory myofibroblastic tumours represent 50% of all benign pulmonary neoplasms {2281,2909}. Most intrathoracic solitary fibrous tumours (SFTs) arise from the visceral pleura, representing < 5% of primary pleural neoplasms. However, SFTs can occur at any cardiopulmonary site, including within the lung parenchyma and pericardium {2431}. Occurrence in the mediastinum is rare. Recurrence occurs in 10–25% of thoracic SFTs and is associated with incomplete surgical resection {230,772,1721,2431,889}. Recurrent SFTs can show more aggressive behaviour {1254,2009}. Other mesenchymal tumour types of the soft tissue can also be seen, with those most frequently and/or characteristically encountered discussed in this volume. The full breadth of soft tissue tumours is covered in the *Soft tissue and bone tumours* volume of this series {3298}. Bronchopulmonary sarcomas are rare and generally affect the middle-aged and elderly. Many types are described, all of which resemble, morphologically and genetically, their counterparts elsewhere in the body. They should be classified according to the current criteria for soft tissue tumours, independent of their thoracic origin.

Etiology and pathogenesis

Most soft tissue neoplasms arise spontaneously, with an unknown pathogenesis, but for some cases a clear etiology can be discerned. Viruses associated with soft tissue tumours include EBV (associated with some smooth muscle tumours in immunosuppressed patients, particularly transplant patients) {692,2883} and HHV8 (associated with Kaposi sarcoma) {421}. Sarcomas such as angiosarcoma and undifferentiated sarcomas can also arise in fields of prior therapeutic irradiation {1435,1640,968}.

Soft tissue tumours (both benign and malignant) in the thorax can also be associated with inherited syndromes, such as *DICER1* syndrome (pleuropulmonary blastoma), Li–Fraumeni syndrome (embryonal rhabdomyosarcoma) {1220}, and tuberous sclerosis (PEComatous tumours, lymphangioleiomyomatosis, and cardiac rhabdomyoma) {1146,3450,1124,1587}. It is uncertain what proportion of patients with intrapulmonary nerve sheath tumours have neurofibromatosis. Hereditary paraganglioma-phaeochromocytoma syndromes occur secondary to germline SDH mutations {179}. Patients with the autosomal dominant Carney–Stratakis syndrome have germline SDH mutations and develop paragangliomas and gastrointestinal stromal tumour {2869}. Paragangliomas, gastrointestinal stromal tumour, and pulmonary chondroma are features of Carney triad; however, Carney triad is non-familial; tumours in affected patients have *SDHC* promoter hypermethylation {1054,389,2869}. These syndromes are discussed in more detail in the *Soft tissue and bone tumours* volume of this series {3298}. The cell of origin of most sarcomas is unknown, and precursor or in situ lesions are not recognized. It remains uncertain whether some postradiation atypical vascular lesions represent precursors to (or a risk factor for) cutaneous angiosarcoma {846}. Somatic genetic factors such as recurrent chromosomal translocations drive the pathogenesis of some sarcomas, but how and in what cell these somatic genetic factors arise remains largely unknown.

Clinical features

Benign and malignant soft tissue tumours typically occur as painless masses, and their growth rates vary. The presentation of mesenchymal tumours of the thorax largely depends on the anatomical location. Pulmonary tumours may occur as solitary or multiple nodules, and patients can range from asymptomatic to presenting with pain, cough, dyspnoea, haemoptysis, or systemic symptoms. Pleural involvement may cause diffuse pleural thickening, with effusion and pleuritic pain. Pulmonary artery intimal sarcomas mimic acute or chronic thromboembolism and pulmonary hypertension.

Histopathology

Malignant soft tissue neoplasms often exhibit nuclear pleomorphism, mitotic activity, and necrosis, although the significance of nuclear atypia should be assessed in the context of the tumour type. For example, nuclear atypia can be seen in schwannoma with ancient change and does not affect behaviour, whereas in other entities (e.g. SFT), increased cellularity, nuclear pleomorphism, elevated mitotic activity, and necrosis can be associated with aggressive behaviour {772,2994,2995, 2449,652}. Aggressive thoracic malignant neoplasms with SMARCA4 deficiency and undifferentiated round cell or rhabdoid morphology were originally proposed to represent thoracic sarcomas {1617}. However, a recent study suggested that these malignant tumours represent smoking-associated undifferentiated/dedifferentiated carcinomas, and they are currently classified under epithelial tumours of lung as thoracic SMARCA4-deficient undifferentiated tumour {2460}.

Genetics

Benign soft tissue tumours feature simple genetic properties, with diploid karyotypes or a single characteristic chromosomal rearrangement. As an intermediate tumour that locally recurs but does not metastasize, desmoid fibromatosis is generally associated with a single activating somatic mutation in *CTNNB1* and much less commonly with loss of function in *APC* {718, 583,219,1042}. In soft tissue malignancies, two broad genetic classes exist: simple-karyotype sarcomas (e.g. synovial sarcoma), associated with a recurrent mutation or translocation, and complex-karyotype sarcomas (e.g. leiomyosarcoma), with numerous chromosomal aberrations but generally lacking recurrent mutations other than loss-of-function mutations in genes such as *TP53*, *RB1*, and *ATRX*, depending on the tumour type {277,371}.

Diagnostic procedures

Investigation includes clinical assessment of the size and anatomical extent of the tumour, the use of imaging modalities (CT, MRI), and biopsy. Imaging can be used to assess the extent of a primary tumour, to determine its relationship to anatomical structures, and to identify metastases. FNA and core needle biopsy (often image-guided) can provide diagnostic information on malignancy, subtype, and grade.

Tumour behaviour

The WHO classification of tumours of soft tissue and bone recognizes four tumour behavioural categories: benign, intermediate (locally aggressive), intermediate (rarely metastasizing), and malignant {3298}. Benign tumours are usually cured by local excision. Intermediate tumours can be either locally aggressive (e.g. desmoid fibromatosis, which locally infiltrates surrounding tissues) or rarely metastasizing (i.e. tumours with a very low [< 2%] but definite risk of metastasis; e.g. inflammatory myofibroblastic tumour). Malignant tumours such as synovial sarcoma can recur locally and metastasize.

Grading

Grading is an attempt to predict clinical behaviour on the basis of histological variables, but it can only be performed using material from primary untreated neoplasms. It is not applicable to all sarcomas; for example, angiosarcomas and undifferentiated sarcomas are always considered to be high-grade. The most widely used system for grading soft tissue sarcomas is the three-tiered system developed by the French Fédération Nationale des Centres de Lutte Contre le Cancer (FNCLCC) {558,2088}. It uses a combination of tumour differentiation, mitotic activity, and necrosis to categorize tumours as being of low, intermediate, or high grade. More-broadly applicable molecular approaches are currently in development {500,1656}.

Staging

The American Joint Committee on Cancer (AJCC) and Union for International Cancer Control (UICC) TNM staging systems are used {75,315}. Sarcoma staging incorporates histological grading and site of involvement along with histological type, tumour size, extent of lymph node involvement, and presence or absence of distant metastasis. Alternative staging and risk assessment approaches incorporating non-anatomical variables such as age and sex are also under consideration {311, 2440}.

Prognosis and predictive factors

Complete excision is the most important factor in preventing local recurrence {744,2799,2731}. Some sarcomas (notably epithelioid sarcoma) are relentlessly recurrent, often with late metastases {2607,2831}. Factors generally associated with a greater risk of metastasis are larger tumour size and higher grade.

Lipoma of the thorax

Creytens D
Fritchie KJ

Definition
Lipoma is a benign neoplasm of mature adipose tissue.

ICD-O coding
8850/0 Lipoma, NOS

ICD-11 coding
2E80.0 & XH1PL8 Lipoma & Lipoma, NOS

Related terminology
None

Subtype(s)
None

Localization
Intrathoracic lipomas may be located in any compartment of the mediastinum {658}, diaphragm {2704,2259}, bronchus {2370, 261,2031,1985}, lung {776}, or chest wall {3315,2611}.

Clinical features
Although most intrathoracic lipomas are asymptomatic, patients may occasionally present with cough, dyspnoea, heart failure, or even death {2611}.

Epidemiology
Intrathoracic lipomas are rare, most frequently reported in the mediastinum as thymolipomas (see *Thymolipoma*, p. 278) and chest wall; they account for 1–9% of primary thymic masses {658}.

Etiology
Unknown

Pathogenesis
Translocations involving 12q13-q15, resulting in fusion of *HMGA2* with a variety of gene partners, are the most common alterations and drive the pathogenesis of lipomas. Other reported chromosomal abnormalities include 6p and 13q rearrangements {3312, 261}.

Macroscopic appearance
Lipomas are well-circumscribed tumours with a uniform glistening yellow to pale-tan cut surface.

Histopathology
The majority of intrathoracic lipomas are composed predominantly of mature adipose tissue, with limited variability in adipocyte size. Occasionally, myxoid change or areas of fibrosis are present. Scattered atypical spindled or multinucleated cells can be appreciated in endobronchial lipomas, but evidence suggests that these tumours share molecular characteristics with lipomas at other sites {2370,1832,261}.

Cytology
Aspiration specimens show adipocytes containing a single large lipid droplet with a compressed rim of cytoplasm and a flattened inconspicuous nucleus.

Diagnostic molecular pathology
Diagnostic molecular pathology is not usually required. In large tumours (> 100 mm) and/or tumours with cytological atypia, exclusion of *MDM2* amplification may be helpful to exclude well-differentiated liposarcoma {2783,3243,540,233}.

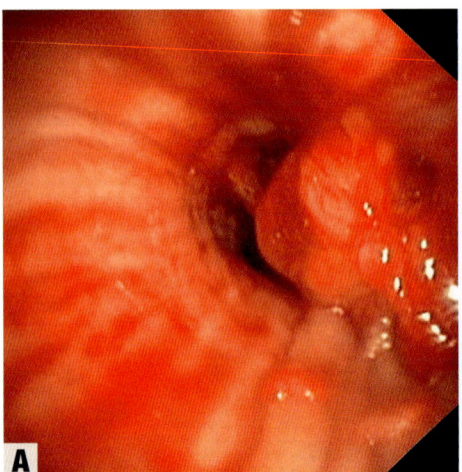 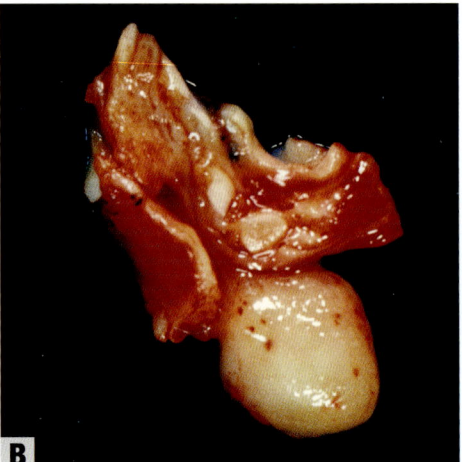 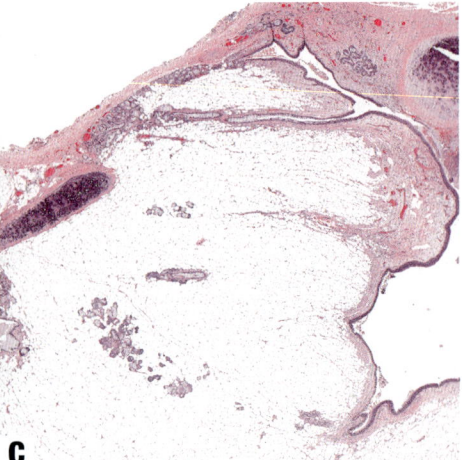

Fig. 4.01 Endobronchial lipoma. **A** Bronchoscopy image of an endobronchial lipoma. **B** Gross image of an endobronchial lipoma. **C** Endobronchial lipoma showing mature adipose tissue forming an endobronchial polypoid mass.

Essential and desirable diagnostic criteria

Essential:

- Mature uniform adipocytes without cytological atypia

Desirable:

- Absence of *MDM2* amplification in large tumours and/or cases with cytological atypia

Staging

Not clinically relevant

Prognosis and prediction

Intrathoracic lipomas are benign, with recurrence rates of < 5% {2611,261}.

Thymolipoma

Rieker RJ

Definition
Thymolipoma is an encapsulated tumour that consists of mature adipose tissue with interspersed non-neoplastic thymic tissue.

ICD-O coding
8850/0 Thymolipoma

ICD-11 coding
2E80.Y & XH4G31 Other specified benign lipomatous neoplasm & XH4G31 Thymolipoma

Related terminology
Not recommended: thymolipomatous hamartoma.

Subtype(s)
None

Localization
Thymolipomas occur mostly in the anterior (prevascular) mediastinum.

Clinical features
Most thymolipomas are detected incidentally; others are found as a result of local symptoms (e.g. cough, dyspnoea, chest pain, hoarseness, and cyanosis) or paraneoplastic syndromes. Myasthenia gravis is the most common paraneoplastic syndrome {2251,2526,3098}; aplastic anaemia, Graves disease, and hypogammaglobulinaemia are rare {611,2223}.

Epidemiology
Thymolipomas are rare tumours of the anterior (prevascular) mediastinum, accounting for 2–9% of all thymic neoplasms. The tumours can occur at any age, with no sex predominance {1969,2482}.

Etiology
Theories postulated for the development of thymolipoma include a benign tumour of specialized thymic stroma (fat) arising in relation with the thymic epithelium, an aberrant development of the third pharyngeal pouch, and fatty regression of a hyperplastic thymus or thymoma {2482,1099,1204}.

Pathogenesis
In one case, translocation involving the *HMGA2* gene on chromosome 12q15 was found {1204}.

Macroscopic appearance
Thymolipomas are encapsulated tumours. They range in size from 30 to > 300 mm {2482,3161,2295}. The tumours are fairly well circumscribed, soft, and yellow on cut surface. Scattered

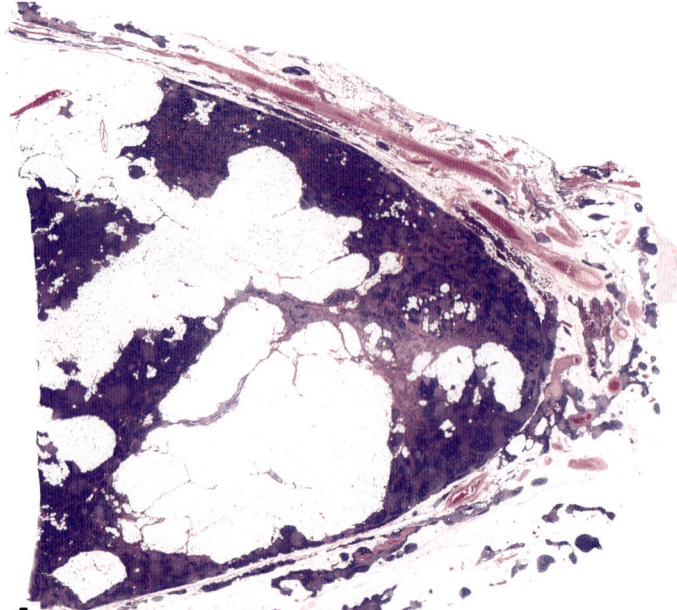

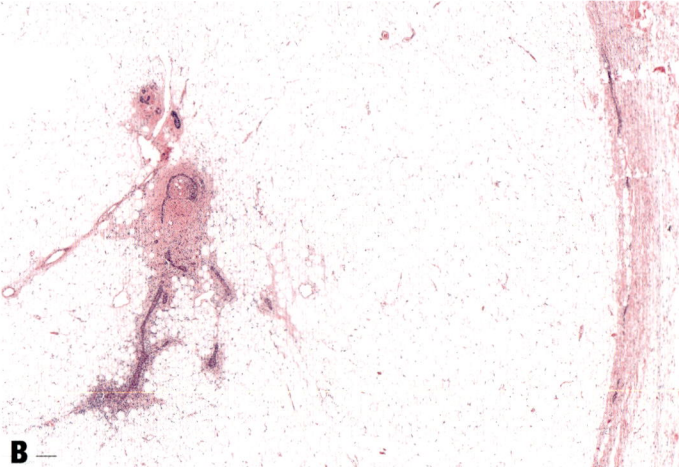

Fig. 4.02 Thymolipoma. **A** Low power showing a well-circumscribed tumour comprising an admixture of mature adipose tissue and thymic tissue. **B** Well-circumscribed tumour comprising mature adipose tissue interspersed with occasional strands of atrophic thymic tissue.

streaks or solid areas representing entrapped thymic tissue may be evident on gross inspection.

Histopathology
Histologically, the tumours consist of mature adipose tissue with strands or even large areas of thymic tissue that is mostly atrophic but may contain lymphoid follicles and Hassall

corpuscles. Atypia and mitotic activity are absent. Thymolipomas may rarely contain thymomas or neuroendocrine tumours (NETs) {1026,2847,3462}. Immunohistochemistry is usually not necessary.

Cytology
Cytological smears or FNA specimens show few if any lymphocytes and scattered epithelial cells {1041}.

Diagnostic molecular pathology
Not clinically relevant

Essential and desirable diagnostic criteria
Essential:
- An encapsulated tumour consisting of mature fat and thymic tissue, usually atrophic

Staging
Not clinically relevant

Prognosis and prediction
Complete resection is curative. No metastases, recurrences, or tumour-related deaths have been reported.

Liposarcoma of the thorax

Creytens D
Folpe AL

Definition

Liposarcoma is a heterogeneous group of mesenchymal neoplasms with adipocytic differentiation and varying biological behaviour, ranging from locally aggressive to metastasizing.

ICD-O coding

8850/3 Liposarcoma, NOS
8851/3 Liposarcoma, well differentiated
8852/3 Myxoid liposarcoma
8854/3 Pleomorphic liposarcoma
8858/3 Dedifferentiated liposarcoma

ICD-11 coding

2B5H & XH7Y61 Well-differentiated lipomatous tumour, primary site & Liposarcoma, well-differentiated
2B59 & XH2J05 Liposarcoma, primary site & Liposarcoma, NOS
2B59 & XH1C03 Liposarcoma, primary site & Dedifferentiated liposarcoma
2B59 & XH3EL0 Liposarcoma, primary site & Myxoid liposarcoma
2B59 & XH25R1 Liposarcoma, primary site & Pleomorphic liposarcoma

Related terminology

Refer to the *Soft tissue and bone tumours* volume of this series {3298}.

Subtype(s)

Well-differentiated liposarcoma: sclerosing; inflammatory

Localization

Liposarcoma occurs in all mediastinal compartments, particularly in the anterior (prevascular) and posterior (paravertebral) mediastinum {658}. An origin from thymic tissue has been shown in a minority of cases (called thymoliposarcoma) {658, 1481}.

Clinical features

Intrathoracic liposarcomas may remain asymptomatic for long periods. Shortness of breath, cough, and pain are the most common symptoms. Despite the tumours' large size, vena cava syndrome has only rarely been reported {658}.

Epidemiology

Primary liposarcomas of the mediastinum are rare, accounting for 0.1–0.75% of all mediastinal tumours {477}. Pleural and pulmonary liposarcomas are rarer yet {477,877}. Most liposarcomas in these anatomical locations represent metastases or direct extension from retroperitoneal tumours {260}. Primary mediastinal liposarcomas have been estimated to account for only 1–2%

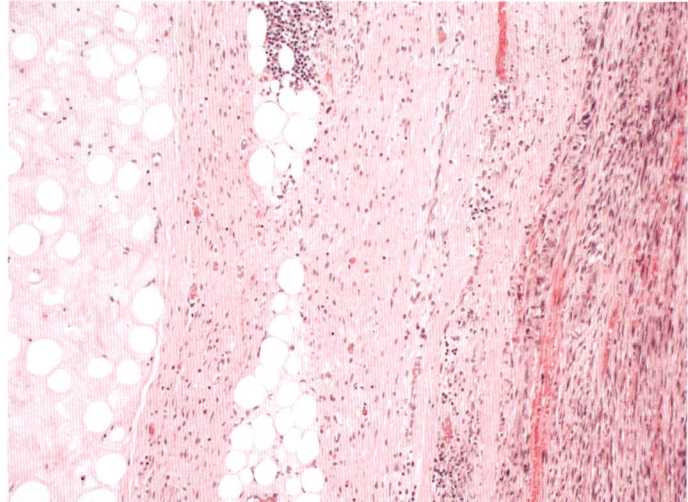

Fig. 4.03 Dedifferentiated liposarcoma. Abrupt transition of a well-differentiated liposarcoma to a high-grade non-lipogenic sarcoma.

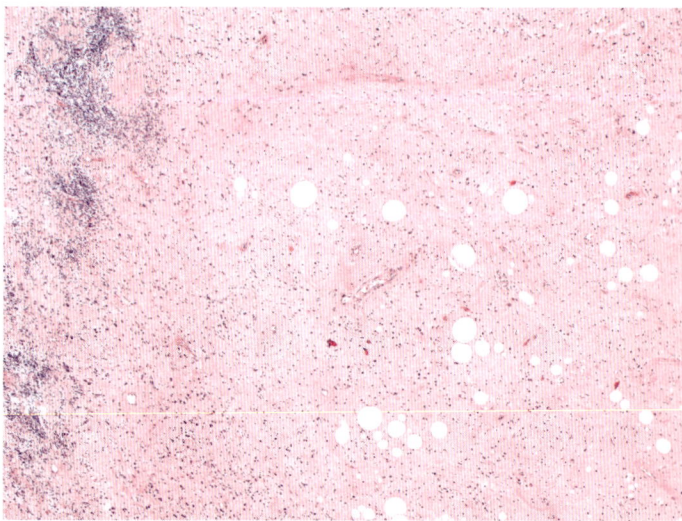

Fig. 4.04 Well-differentiated liposarcoma, inflammatory subtype. Dense chronic inflammatory infiltrate in inflammatory well-differentiated liposarcoma.

of all liposarcomas {658}. However, liposarcoma is by far the most common primary sarcoma of the mediastinum, in particular the anterior (prevascular) mediastinum {2264}. The age range is wide, but liposarcoma usually occurs in adults aged > 40 years {3238}. Paediatric cases have been reported {43}.

Etiology

Unknown

Pathogenesis

Refer to the *Soft tissue and bone tumours* volume of this series {3298}.

Macroscopic appearance

Mediastinal liposarcoma is usually a large, well-circumscribed, multinodular mass with a mixture of lipomatous and myxoid areas.

Histopathology

All types of liposarcoma have been reported in the mediastinum. Well-differentiated and dedifferentiated liposarcomas are most common {1050,1937}. The histopathological findings are identical to those of liposarcomas elsewhere. However, the proportions of liposarcoma types in the mediastinum differ from those in other sites. In particular, pleomorphic liposarcoma is considerably more common in the mediastinum {658,260}. Mediastinal liposarcomas frequently contain myxoid areas {658, 1050,2215,260}. Myxoid pleomorphic liposarcoma has a particular predilection for the mediastinum of young patients {43, 260,587,585,658}. Other unusual types of liposarcoma that have been described in the mediastinum contain elements of smooth muscle (lipoleiomyosarcoma) or skeletal muscle {850, 3265}.

Cytology

Not clinically relevant

Diagnostic molecular pathology

The molecular pathology of intrathoracic liposarcomas corresponds to that of liposarcomas elsewhere (see the *Soft tissue and bone tumours* volume of this series {3298}).

Essential and desirable diagnostic criteria

Well-differentiated liposarcoma

Essential:
- Variation in adipocytic size associated with nuclear atypia in stromal and/or adipocytic cells
- Fibrillary sclerotic background (sclerosing subtype)
- Chronic inflammatory background (inflammatory subtype)
- Lipoblasts are not required for diagnosis

Desirable:
- MDM2 and/or CDK4 nuclear expression or evidence of *MDM2* and/or *CDK4* gene amplification

Dedifferentiated liposarcoma

Essential:
- Abrupt transition to high-grade sarcoma
- Exclusion of metastasis from other (soft tissue) sites

Desirable:
- MDM2 and/or CDK4 nuclear expression or evidence of *MDM2* and/or *CDK4* gene amplification

Myxoid liposarcoma

Essential:
- A mixture of non-lipogenic spindle cells, lipoblasts, myxoid stroma, and thin-walled branched vasculature
- Hypercellularity, diminished myxoid matrix, and elevated nuclear grade (high-grade)
- Exclusion of metastasis from other (soft tissue) sites

Desirable:
- Confirmation of *DDIT3* gene rearrangement or detection of specific *FUS-DDIT3* or *EWSR1-DDIT3* gene fusion

Pleomorphic liposarcoma

Essential:
- Presence of multivacuolated pleomorphic lipoblasts in a high-grade sarcoma
- Exclusion of metastasis from other (soft tissue) sites

Staging

Staging is according to the Union for International Cancer Control (UICC) TNM classification.

Prognosis and prediction

The prognosis for all mediastinal liposarcomas is poor and correlates with tumour type; rapid tumour recurrence and metastatic disease are more common in patients with dedifferentiated, myxoid, and pleomorphic types {1050,260,2215,2264}. Curative surgical resection is the treatment of choice. Local recurrences are common, related to the difficulties in achieving total resection in the mediastinum. The mortality rate associated with mediastinal liposarcomas is 30–50% {658}.

Desmoid fibromatosis of the thorax

Fritchie KJ

Definition
Desmoid fibromatosis is a locally aggressive but non-metastasizing (myo)fibroblastic neoplasm with infiltrative growth and propensity for local recurrence.

ICD-O coding
8821/1 Desmoid-type fibromatosis

ICD-11 coding
2F7C & XH13Z3 Neoplasms of uncertain behaviour of connective or other soft tissue & Desmoid-type fibromatosis (aggressive fibromatosis)

Related terminology
Acceptable: aggressive fibromatosis; desmoid tumour.

Subtype(s)
None

Localization
The majority of intrathoracic desmoid fibromatoses arise from the chest wall; however, cases originating from the pleura, pulmonary parenchyma, and mediastinum have been reported {617,79,1764, 3319,1383,3045,1637,3351,722,2976}.

Clinical features
Intrathoracic desmoid fibromatosis may cause pain, dyspnoea, and kyphoscoliosis or may be detected as an incidental radiological finding {617,2968}. Cases after trauma/surgery have also been reported {2822,1996}.

Imaging
The imaging findings are non-distinct, but MRI often shows mixed hyperintense and isointense signals {3148,2905}.

Epidemiology
Intrathoracic desmoids most often arise in adulthood and show an equal sex distribution {617,2968}.

Etiology
The etiology of desmoid fibromatosis includes genetic factors, and (as at other sites) some cases may be associated with prior trauma.

Pathogenesis
The majority of cases (as many as 95%) are sporadic, resulting from somatic mutations in *CTNNB1*; a smaller subset occur in patients harbouring germline *APC* mutations (Gardner syndrome) {718,583,219,1042}. Both genetic events lead to increased activation of the WNT/β-catenin pathway {159,2146, 1525}.

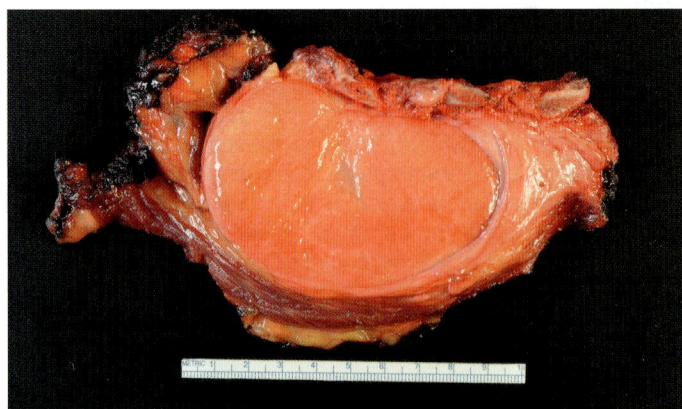

Fig. 4.05 Desmoid fibromatosis. Gross image of desmoid fibromatosis arising in the chest wall.

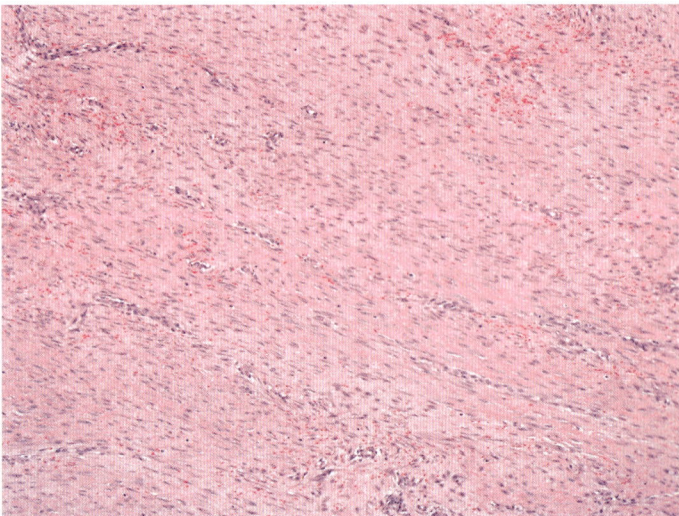

Fig. 4.06 Desmoid fibromatosis. Desmoid fibromatosis shows long sweeping fascicles of uniform fibroblasts and myofibroblasts.

Macroscopic appearance
Gross examination reveals a poorly circumscribed solid mass with a firm, white-tan whorled or trabecular cut surface.

Histopathology
Histological examination reveals long sweeping fascicles of fibroblasts and myofibroblasts, without cytological atypia, that infiltrate into surrounding soft tissue. Lymphoid aggregates are frequently appreciated at the periphery of the lesion. Mitoses may be seen, but atypical mitotic figures are absent. A subset of cases may show myxoid change or keloidal-type collagen deposition. The lesional cells express SMA and MSA

in a tram-track pattern, with variable desmin staining. Nuclear β-catenin expression is present in approximately 80% of cases {388}.

Cytology
FNA specimens may contain fibroblasts/myofibroblasts without atypia or nuclear hyperchromasia; however, the nonspecific cytological features make diagnosis by FNA challenging {2408}.

Diagnostic molecular pathology
CTNNB1 mutation studies may be used to confirm the diagnosis on limited biopsy specimens in the absence of diagnostic morphological features and equivocal β-catenin immunostaining {565,1616}.

Essential and desirable diagnostic criteria
Essential:
- Long fascicles of (myo)fibroblasts lacking atypia with an infiltrative growth pattern

Desirable:
- Nuclear β-catenin expression by immunohistochemistry
- *CTNNB1* mutation studies may be useful to confirm the diagnosis on small specimens

Staging
Not clinically relevant

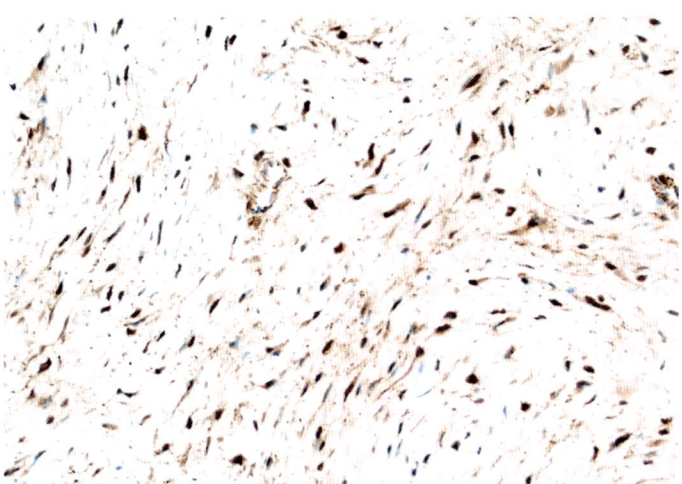

Fig. 4.07 Desmoid fibromatosis. The majority of desmoids show nuclear expression of β-catenin.

Prognosis and prediction
The clinical behaviour of desmoid fibromatosis is unpredictable, with recurrence rates as high as 33%. However, margin status does not consistently correlate with recurrence risk, and an initial watchful waiting approach for asymptomatic patients has been advocated {1392}. *CTNNB1* p.S45F mutations may correlate with increased recurrence risk {246,566,718,1609}.

Solitary fibrous tumour of the thorax

Tavora F
Calabrese F
Demicco EG

Definition
Solitary fibrous tumour (SFT) is a fibroblastic neoplasm with a characteristic histological appearance, immunohistochemical profile, and *NAB2-STAT6* gene rearrangement.

ICD-O coding
8815/1 Solitary fibrous tumour, NOS

ICD-11 coding
2F7C & XH7E62 Neoplasms of uncertain behaviour of connective or other soft tissue & Solitary fibrous tumour, NOS
2B5Y & XH1HP3 Other specified malignant mesenchymal neoplasms & Solitary fibrous tumour, malignant

Related terminology
Not recommended: localized fibrous tumour; pleural fibroma; fibrous mesothelioma; haemangiopericytoma; giant cell angiofibroma.

Subtype(s)
None

Localization
Most intrathoracic SFTs arise from the visceral pleura, but they may occur at any site, including within the lung parenchyma and pericardium {2431}. They rarely occur in the mediastinum.

Clinical features
A great percentage of SFTs are asymptomatic and discovered incidentally. These are slow-growing, relatively benign neoplasms, but as many as 10% behave aggressively. Larger tumours cause symptoms of cough, dyspnoea, or chest pain. Occasionally, patients become hypoglycaemic as a result of tumour production of IGF {139,633,1052}.

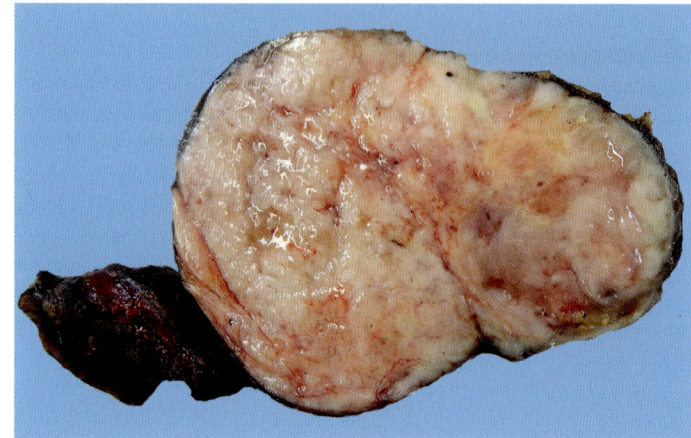

Fig. 4.08 Solitary fibrous tumour, malignant. The cut surface is tan, multinodular, and firm. There is a delicate fibrous capsule.

Imaging
On imaging, SFTs are usually sharply demarcated pleural-based soft tissue masses with no chest wall abnormality. PET usually shows increased avidity in malignant tumours, although there is overlap {1720,1723}. Intracardiac and pericardial tumours have been reported to cause arrhythmias, tamponade, embolism, and heart failure {230}.

Epidemiology
Thoracic SFTs occur most frequently in adults in the sixth decade of life but have been reported in patients from their teens to their nineties {772}. There is no sex predilection. SFTs represent < 5% of primary pleural neoplasms. Intrapulmonary and pericardial SFTs are rare {574,2717,2431}.

Etiology
Unknown

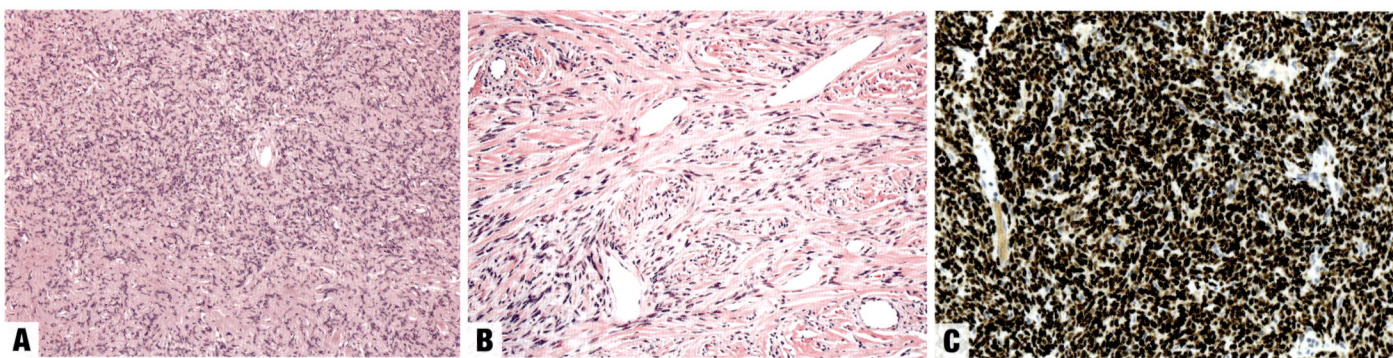

Fig. 4.09 Solitary fibrous tumour. **A** Typical storiform appearance with hypercellular and hypocellular areas. Cytological atypia is minimal. **B** Uniform spindle fibroblastic cells, focal stromal hyalinization, and branching staghorn vessels. **C** The tumour cells show diffuse nuclear positivity for STAT6.

Table 4.01 Three-variable and modified four-variable risk models for the prediction of metastatic risk in solitary fibrous tumours {652,653}

Risk factor	Cut-off value	Points assigned	
		3-variable model	4-variable model
Patient age in years	< 55	0	0
	≥ 55	1	1
Mitoses/mm²	0	0	0
	0.5–1.5	1	1
	≥ 2	2	2
Tumour size in mm	0–49	0	0
	50–99	1	1
	100–149	2	2
	≥ 150	3	3
Tumour necrosis	< 10%	n/a	0
	≥ 10%	n/a	1
Risk	Low	0–2 points	0–3 points
	Intermediate	3–4 points	4–5 points
	High	5–6 points	6–7 points

n/a, not applicable.

Pathogenesis

The genetic hallmark of the tumours is the fusion of the *NAB2* and *STAT6* genes, both located on 12q13.3, with the *NAB2* exon 4–*STAT6* exon 2/3 fusion types being most commonly associated with pleuropulmonary SFTs {139,479,507,651,2501}. *TERT* promoter mutations are present in subsets of SFTs and are associated with aggressive behaviour {139}.

Macroscopic appearance

SFTs are well-circumscribed, solid, tan to grey homogeneous masses, frequently pedunculated and often large (> 100 mm). Cystic necrosis, haemorrhage, and calcification are occasionally present. In 3% of cases, no pleural attachment can be identified, and the tumour is surrounded by lung parenchyma {2431}. Tumours are uncommonly found to involve the pericardium {288, 591,3507}.

Histopathology

SFTs have a distinctive morphology, with uniform fibroblastic spindle cells, varying cellularity, a patternless architecture, fibrosis, and branching staghorn vessels. There is a wide histological spectrum, ranging from paucicellular lesions with abundant stromal keloidal-type collagen to highly cellular tumours consisting of closely spaced cells with little or no intervening stroma. Myxoid change may be present {674}. Most SFTs are circumscribed, but a small portion of tumours may have infiltrative borders and invade the lung parenchyma. Usually there are few mitoses (< 3 mitoses/2 mm²), limited cytological atypia, and infrequent necrosis. More-aggressive tumours show increased mitotic activity and are frequently hypercellular with coagulative necrosis. Rarely, tumours may dedifferentiate

into undifferentiated sarcoma, and a dedifferentiated SFT with heterologous elements has been described. Rather than classifying SFT as benign, malignant, or of uncertain malignant potential, reporting the risk according to the proposed models in Table 4.01 is recommended.

By immunohistochemistry, SFTs are typically positive for CD34 and nuclear STAT6 {507,2501}. Expression may be lost in dedifferentiated SFTs.

Cytology

Cytological examination reveals oval, elongated, or rounded cells with wispy cytoplasm and eosinophilic collagenous stroma {2990}.

Diagnostic molecular pathology

NAB2-STAT6 gene fusions are diagnostic of SFTs. However, because *NAB2* and *STAT6* are in close proximity on chromosome 12q, detection of their fusion is difficult by conventional cytogenetic methods, and the diversity of breakpoints occurring in both exons and introns makes PCR-based detection of fusion variants difficult without multiplexed sequencing assays. STAT6 immunohistochemistry is a sensitive and specific surrogate for all fusions {729,1496,2687}.

Essential and desirable diagnostic criteria

Essential:
- Well-circumscribed mass
- Spindled to ovoid cells arranged around a branching and hyalinized vasculature
- Variable stromal collagen deposition
- CD34 and/or STAT6 expression by immunohistochemistry

Desirable (in selected cases):
- Demonstration of *NAB2-STAT6* gene fusion

Staging

Risk-stratification models are preferred over anatomical staging.

Prognosis and prediction

Recurrence occurs in 10–25% of thoracic SFTs and is associated with incomplete resection {230,772,1721,2431,889}. Recurrent tumours may show more-aggressive behaviour {1254,2009}.

Tumours with > 2 mitoses/mm² in variable association with increased cellularity, atypia, necrosis, or infiltrative growth have a greater rate of recurrence and metastases {772}. Two risk-stratification models incorporating mitotic activity, necrosis, and tumour size have been validated for thoracic SFTs (see Table 4.01); one model also includes patient age (≥ 55 years) and is also applicable to extrathoracic SFTs {2994,2995,652}, while the other includes hypercellularity, haemorrhage, site, and sessile growth as additional criteria {2449}. Both of these models outperform older criteria for the prediction of aggressive behaviour in thoracic SFTs {2449}. It has been suggested that the prognosis of mediastinal and thymic SFTs is worse than that of their pleural counterparts {3330}. See also the *Soft tissue and bone tumours* volume of this series {3298}.

Calcifying fibrous tumour of the thorax

Mehrad M
Hornick JL

Definition
Calcifying fibrous tumour is a rare, benign tumour occurring in visceral pleura, composed of paucicellular collagenized fibrous tissue with associated chronic inflammation and psammomatous and/or dystrophic calcification.

ICD-O coding
8817/0 Calcifying fibrous tumour

ICD-11 coding
2F01 & XH7TH6 Benign neoplasm of intrathoracic organs & Calcifying fibrous tumour

Related terminology
Not recommended: calcifying fibrous pseudotumour; childhood fibrous tumour with psammoma bodies.

Subtype(s)
None

Localization
Calcifying fibrous tumour is typically limited to the pleura, although cases arising within lung parenchyma occur rarely {2294}.

Clinical features
Patients may be asymptomatic or may present with chest pain or non-productive cough.

Imaging
Imaging studies show either a solitary or multiple pleural-based nodular masses. CT shows a well-defined pleural-based tumour (or tumours) with central areas of increased attenuation due to calcification. So-called disseminated (more likely multiple/multicentric) bilateral pleural lesions have been reported {2894,1310, 1825}.

Epidemiology
Pleural calcifying fibrous tumours occur mainly in women, with a median age of 39 years (range: 23–54 years) {1935,2359,2894, 1872}.

Etiology
Unknown

Pathogenesis
Deleterious mutations in *ZNF717*, *FRG1*, and *CDC27*, as well as tumour-specific copy-number losses, including a large (302 kb) loss at 6p22.2 – comprising 32 genes of the histone cluster 1 family and the hemochromatosis gene (*HFE*) – have been reported {1872}, which may contribute to tumorigenesis. Rare familial cases have also been reported {475}.

Macroscopic appearance
The tumours are well circumscribed, unencapsulated, solid, and firm, with a gritty texture. The average size is 50 mm (range: 15–125 mm).

Histopathology
These lesions are hypocellular, consisting of bland fibroblasts in a prominent collagenous stroma with a sparse lymphoplasmacytic infiltrate. There are usually dystrophic or psammomatous calcifications {2359,2894,1872,1262}. By immunohistochemistry, the lesional cells may be CD34-positive, while BCL2, STAT6, β-catenin, and ALK are negative. In the differential diagnosis, both inflammatory myofibroblastic tumour and solitary fibrous tumour are more cellular, the former being fascicular and the latter being patternless with branching, thin-walled vessels. Desmoid fibromatosis has ill-defined borders and lacks the characteristic dystrophic/psammomatous calcifications.

Cytology
Not clinically relevant

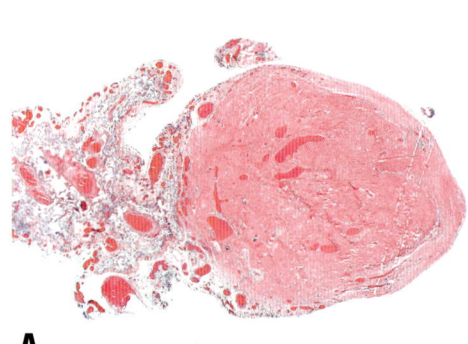 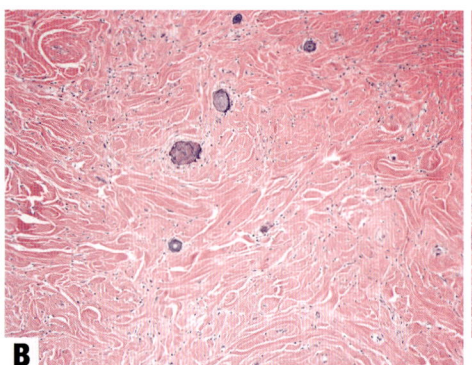 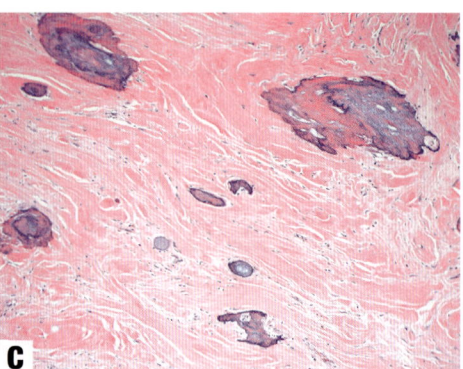

Fig. 4.10 Calcifying fibrous tumour. **A** The tumour is pleural-based and well defined. **B** Note the scattered chronic inflammatory cells and calcospherites. **C** Occasionally, the tumours demonstrate dystrophic calcifications.

Diagnostic molecular pathology
Not clinically relevant

Essential and desirable diagnostic criteria
Essential:

- A well-defined, paucicellular, and collagenized pleural-based mass with associated psammomatous and/or dystrophic calcification

Staging
Not clinically relevant

Prognosis and prediction
Approximately 10–15% of lesions recur locally but not destructively. Local recurrence is not predictable on morphological grounds and is mainly due to incomplete resection. There is no potential for metastasis.

Inflammatory myofibroblastic tumour of the thorax

Tavora F
Glass C
Hornick JL
Jain D
Sheppard MN
Yi ES

Definition

Inflammatory myofibroblastic tumour (IMT) is a distinctive, rarely metastasizing neoplasm composed of myofibroblastic and fibroblastic spindle cells, usually accompanied by a stromal inflammatory infiltrate of plasma cells and lymphocytes.

ICD-O coding

8825/1 Inflammatory myofibroblastic tumour

ICD-11 coding

2B53.Y & XH66Z0 Other specified fibroblastic or myofibroblastic tumour, primary site & Myofibroblastic tumour, NOS

Related terminology

Not recommended: plasma cell granuloma; inflammatory pseudotumour; inflammatory myofibrohistiocytic proliferation; inflammatory fibrosarcoma; pulmonary nodular lymphoid hyperplasia; invasive fibrous tumour of the tracheobronchial tree.

Subtype(s)

Epithelioid inflammatory myofibroblastic tumour

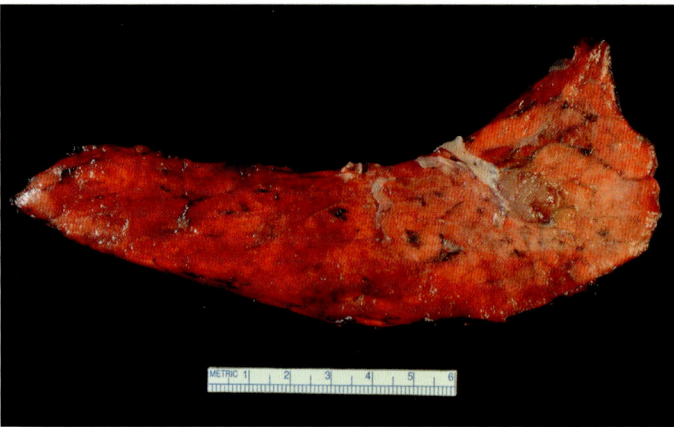

Fig. 4.11 Inflammatory myofibroblastic tumour. Gross appearance showing a well-demarcated tumour with a homogeneous and glistening cut surface within the lung parenchyma.

Localization

IMT shows a wide anatomical distribution and can arise in the lung, tracheobronchial tree, pleura, chest wall, and mediastinum.

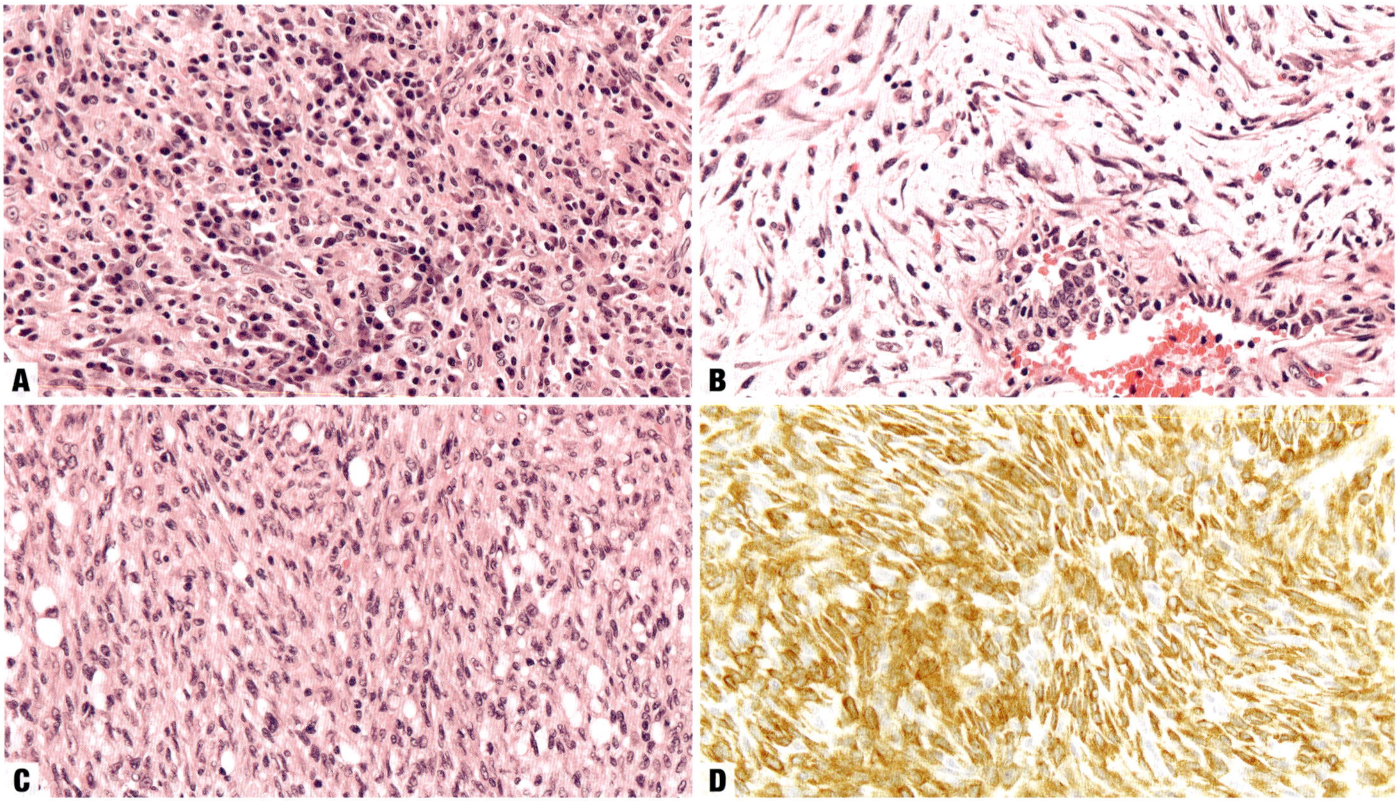

Fig. 4.12 Inflammatory myofibroblastic tumour. **A** Round and spindle cells with vesicular chromatin and small nucleoli admixed with plasma cells and lymphocytes. **B** An example with prominent myxoid stroma. Note the elongated spindle cells with vesicular chromatin and eosinophilic cytoplasm. **C** Some cellular examples contain fewer inflammatory cells and may mimic spindle cell sarcomas. **D** Immunoreactivity for ALK reflects an underlying *ALK* gene rearrangement. A diffuse cytoplasmic staining pattern is most common.

Clinical features

Most patients are asymptomatic, but as many as 25% present with a systemic inflammatory response, which may include fever, weight loss, anaemia, thrombocytosis, elevated erythrocyte sedimentation rate, hypergammaglobulinaemia, and elevated C-reactive protein {418,526,549,2988}. Primary tracheobronchial IMTs are rare and are seen more commonly in children and young adults. This form may occur as well-defined endoluminal masses with an exophytic component {81,335,2115}.

Epidemiology

The lung is the site most frequently affected by IMT, which accounts for as many as 1% of all lung tumours {2610}. In children, IMTs represent 50% of all benign or intermediate pulmonary neoplasms {2281,2909}. The M:F ratio is about 1:1 {2829}.

Etiology

Unknown

Pathogenesis

In about two thirds of cases of IMT in children and young adults, the tumours have clonal rearrangements in chromosome band 2p23 and the 3′ kinase region of the *ALK* gene with various partner genes, including *TPM3*, *TPM4*, *CLTC*, *CARS1* (*CARS*), *ATIC*, *SEC31A* (*SEC31L1*), *PPFIBP1*, *DCTN1*, *EML4*, *PRKAR1A*, *LMNA*, *TFG*, *FN1*, *HNRNPA1*, *RANBP2*, and others {46,2182, 2928,2970}. *ALK* rearrangement is uncommon in IMTs diagnosed in older adults. *ROS1* or *NTRK3* gene rearrangements are each found in about 5% of IMTs {1741,89,3362,46,445}, with *RET* gene rearrangements being less frequent. See also the *Soft tissue and bone tumours* volume of this series {3298}.

Macroscopic appearance

IMTs are lobulated and circumscribed fleshy masses, varying in size from < 10 mm up to 150 mm. Most tumours are solitary. About one fifth may show extraparenchymal involvement including mediastinal or airway invasion. These invasive lesions are more commonly localized to the lower lung lobes and may show associated atelectasis and/or pleural effusions {2909}.

Histopathology

The neoplastic cells of IMT are plump and spindle-shaped with indistinct cell borders, growing in a fascicular pattern {549}. Nuclear atypia is generally absent or only minimal. The morphology can be variable, with myxoid, hypercellular or hypocellular fibrous patterns. The spindle cell component may be obscured by a mixed chronic inflammatory infiltrate (typically rich in plasma cells) and a variable number of lymphocytes, eosinophils, and/or neutrophils {549,2720}. Necrosis is uncommon and mitotic activity is generally low. Secondary changes such as collagen deposition, myxoid change, and oedema may occur. Dystrophic calcifications are seen more frequently in children {2290,2281}.

Spindle cells are positive for SMA, with variable staining for calponin, MSA, and desmin, in keeping with a myofibroblastic immunophenotype. Focal low-molecular-weight keratin immunoreactivity can be seen in as many as 30% of cases. Immunoreactivity for ALK is detectable in 50–60% of cases and is more common in young patients. ALK expression correlates well with the presence of *ALK* gene rearrangement {423,549}. The staining pattern may vary depending on the fusion partner: *RANBP2-ALK* is associated with nuclear membranous staining, *RRBP1-ALK* with a cytoplasmic pattern with paranuclear accentuation, and *CLTC-ALK* with a granular cytoplasmic pattern {1636}. Highly sensitive ALK antibody clones (5A4, D5F3) may improve detection of the ALK protein in IMT {2970,3362}. *ROS1*-rearranged IMT typically shows a cytoplasmic expression of ROS1.

Differential diagnosis

The differential diagnosis of IMT is broad. Several non-neoplastic processes should be considered, including organizing pneumonia, mycobacterial spindle cell tumour, pulmonary hyalinizing granuloma, and IgG4-related disease {3001,223}. Neoplastic processes to be considered, particularly in ALK-negative cases, include sclerosing pneumocytoma, lymphoma, spindle cell carcinoma, and sarcomas.

Cytology

FNA samples usually show spindled fibroblastic to epithelioid myofibroblasts, with a delicate vascular network and admixed plasma cells and lymphocytes. Nuclei are round to oval, with slight hyperchromasia, and nucleoli are inconspicuous {941, 1183,2720,3040}.

Diagnostic molecular pathology

In addition to the detection of ALK by immunohistochemistry, molecular assays for *ALK* can be used to confirm the diagnosis; if such testing is negative, immunohistochemistry for ROS1 or tests for non-*ALK* gene fusions may be useful {46}.

Essential and desirable diagnostic criteria

Essential:
- Loose or compact fascicles of myofibroblastic cells with a prominent inflammatory infiltrate and a variable fibrous or myxoid stroma

Desirable:
- Myofibroblastic differentiation by immunohistochemistry
- Expression of ALK (seen in as many as 60% of cases)
- *ALK* or other gene rearrangements (in selected cases)

Staging

Not clinically relevant

Prognosis and prediction

Most cases of IMT can be cured by complete surgical excision, but approximately 20% recur or show locally aggressive behaviour {418}. Distant metastases are rare {549,2909,2928}.

Myxofibrosarcoma of the thorax

Billings SD
Bois MC
Hornick JL

Definition
Myxofibrosarcoma is a malignant fibroblastic neoplasm with variably myxoid stroma, pleomorphism, and a distinctive curvilinear vascular pattern.

ICD-O coding
8811/3 Myxofibrosarcoma

ICD-11 coding
2B53.0 Myxofibrosarcoma, primary site

Related terminology
Not recommended: myxoid malignant fibrous histiocytoma.

Subtype(s)
Epithelioid myxofibrosarcoma

Localization
Myxofibrosarcoma accounts for approximately 11% of chest wall sarcomas {1866}. About 60% involve superficial soft tissues; the remainder are subfascial/intramuscular. There are case reports of cardiac myxofibrosarcoma, but it is unclear whether these are true myxofibrosarcomas {2898}.

Clinical features
This is a slow-growing mass, with or without pain.

Epidemiology
There is a slight male predominance, with tumours occurring mainly in the sixth to eighth decades of life. It is rare in patients aged < 30 years {1890,2622,1625}.

Etiology
Unknown

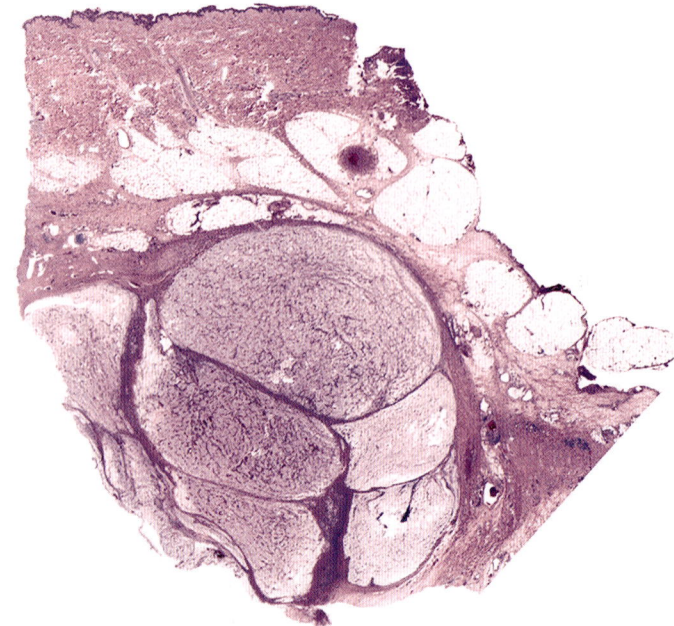

Fig. 4.13 Myxofibrosarcoma. This chest wall tumour shows the characteristic lobulated growth pattern. Note the myxoid nodules demarcated by thin fibrous septa.

Pathogenesis
Myxofibrosarcomas have complex karyotypes {1890}. Progression in grade, seen in recurrences, is accompanied by increased cytogenetic aberrations {3311}. Gains of chromosome 5 are common {1664,1663,1112,2179}. Aberrations in p53 signalling and the cell-cycle G1/S checkpoint play a pathogenetic role in half of myxofibrosarcomas {2154}. For additional information, see the *Soft tissue and bone tumours* volume of this series {3298}.

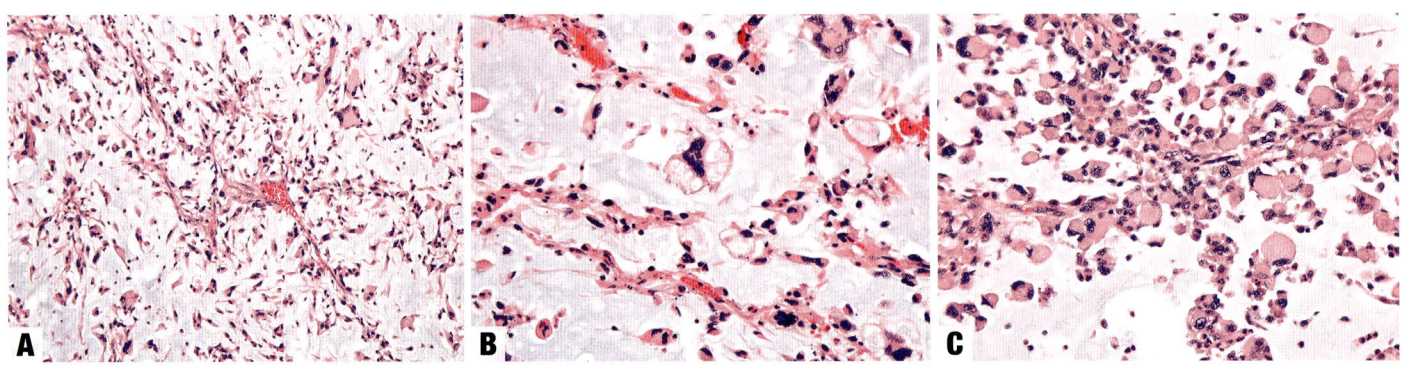

Fig. 4.14 Myxofibrosarcoma. **A** The tumour cells are variably spindled and pleomorphic with hyperchromatic nuclei. Note the thin-walled blood vessels. **B** Matrix-containing vacuolated tumour cells are referred to as pseudolipoblasts. **C** The epithelioid subtype is dominated by polygonal cells with abundant eosinophilic cytoplasm. Such tumours may closely mimic metastatic melanoma or metastatic carcinoma.

Macroscopic appearance

These tumours are infiltrative, with a multinodular, gelatinous to fleshy appearance. Necrosis is often present in high-grade tumours.

Histopathology

Myxofibrosarcomas have a multinodular growth pattern, with myxoid stroma, incomplete fibrous septa, curvilinear vessels, and variably pleomorphic spindled cells {1890,1198}. Low-grade tumours are relatively hypocellular with low mitotic counts. Tumour cells often condense around vessels. Pseudolipoblasts containing cytoplasmic mucin are common. Higher-grade tumours are less myxoid with more solid areas and a greater degree of pleomorphism, and they may have necrosis. Higher-grade tumours often contain areas resembling low-grade tumour.

The epithelioid subtype is composed predominantly of atypical epithelioid tumour cells and may mimic carcinoma or melanoma {2076}. Myxofibrosarcoma may be positive for CD34 and SMA, but it is negative for desmin and S100 {2794}.

In the mediastinum, the differential diagnosis is nearly always with dedifferentiated liposarcoma {2779}. Reported cardiac cases are probably undifferentiated sarcomas or intimal sarcomas (with *MDM2* amplification) {2089}.

Cytology

Not clinically relevant

Diagnostic molecular pathology

Not relevant

Essential and desirable diagnostic criteria

Essential:
- Infiltrative tumour with multinodular architecture, myxoid stroma, variably prominent pleomorphic cells, and distinctive curvilinear vessels
- Higher-grade tumours are more cellular and may have necrosis

Staging

Staging is according to the Union for International Cancer Control (UICC) or American Joint Committee on Cancer (AJCC) TNM system.

Prognosis and prediction

There is frequent local recurrence (30–40%) irrespective of grade. Metastases and mortality are closely related to tumour grade. The overall 5-year mortality rate is 30–35%. In addition to pulmonary and osseous metastases, lymph node metastases are sometimes seen {1198,2622,1625}. The epithelioid subtype of myxofibrosarcoma is more aggressive {2076}.

Haemangioma of the thorax

Thway K
Calonje JE

Definition
Haemangiomas are a family of benign vascular tumours.

ICD-O coding
9120/0 Haemangioma, NOS
9121/0 Cavernous haemangioma
9122/0 Venous haemangioma
9132/0 Intramuscular haemangioma
9123/0 Arteriovenous haemangioma

ICD-11 coding
2F01 & XH3U29 Benign neoplasm of intrathoracic organs &
  Capillary haemangioma
2F01 & XH1GU2 Benign neoplasm of intrathoracic organs &
  Cavernous haemangioma
2F01 & XH5AW4 Benign neoplasm of intrathoracic organs &
  Haemangioma, NOS

Related terminology
Acceptable: angioma; capillary haemangioma; cavernous
haemangioma; venous malformation; arteriovenous malformation; venous or vascular ectasia; haemangiolymphangioma.

Subtype(s)
None

Localization
Haemangiomas can occur at any thoracic site, including the
thoracic vertebrae, chest wall, mediastinum (slightly more frequent in anterior [prevascular] than posterior [paravertebral]),
thymus, lungs, and pleura {1973,837}.

Clinical features
As many as 50% of patients are asymptomatic. Others can
present with nonspecific symptoms, including cough, chest
pain, fever, or dyspnoea (due to compression/adhesion to
adjacent structures) {1973,646}. Rare complications include
dysphagia, superior vena cava syndrome, and neurological
symptoms from intraspinal tumour extension {3245,1129} and
spontaneous haemothorax from rupture {1176}. Haemangiomas
can invade contiguous mediastinal/thoracic structures (e.g.
the aorta, main pulmonary artery, venae cavae, phrenic/vagus
nerves, and carotid artery), precluding complete excision {550}.

Epidemiology
Age ranges from congenital/newborn to the eighth decade of
life.

Etiology
Many lesions previously described as cavernous or venous
haemangiomas are now considered to be venous malformations,

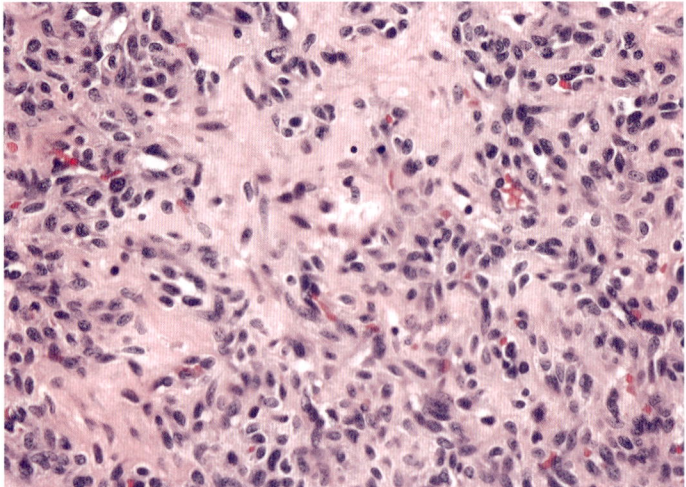

Fig. 4.15 Lobular capillary haemangioma. There are abundant collections of well-formed, often compressed, tightly packed small vessels, giving a somewhat solid appearance.

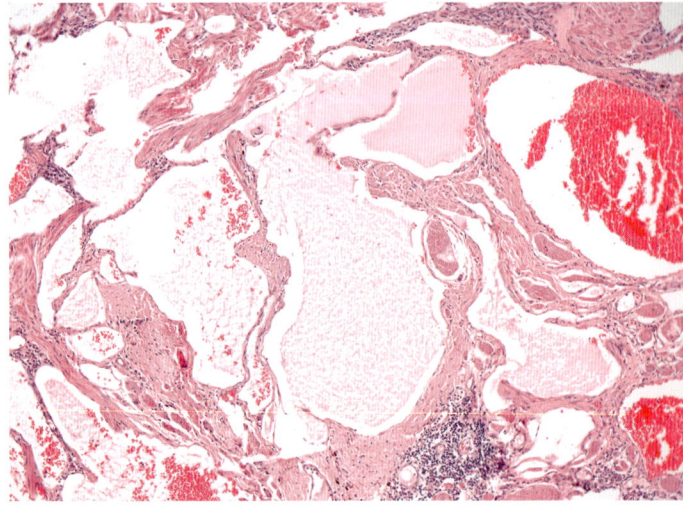

Fig. 4.16 Cavernous haemangioma. This haemangioma shows predominant dilated, cavernous vessels lined by bland, single endothelial layers. Ectatic vessels contain either blood or lymph.

as defined by the International Society for the Study of Vascular
Anomalies classification {3231}.

Pathogenesis
Unknown

Macroscopic appearance
These are typically circumscribed, cystic, haemorrhagic lesions
ranging from 20 to 200 mm {1973}. Appearances depend on

type and anatomical site; lesions can be well or poorly defined or infiltrative with invasion of surrounding structures. They are typically reddish-purple and spongy or are firmer with thrombi/phleboliths.

Histopathology

This is a heterogeneous group, comprising proliferations of lymphatics, capillaries, or veins (with any predominating). Capillary haemangiomas are proliferations of small, thin-walled vessels with lobular and solid growth patterns, with dilated small vessels and more solid endothelial cell proliferations. Cavernous haemangiomas are relatively circumscribed proliferations of large, often dilated, thin-walled vessels or blood-filled sinuses lined by single endothelial layers. There may be fibrosis, interstitial inflammation, smooth muscle proliferation, and thrombosis {1973,550}, and sometimes regressive changes (e.g. hyalinization, dystrophic ossification, cystic and perivascular myxoid changes, and fatty overgrowth) {1973}.

Cytology

Not clinically relevant

Diagnostic molecular pathology

Not clinically relevant

Essential and desirable diagnostic criteria

Essential:
- Morphology dependent on type, with different types and calibres of essentially well-formed vessels lacking atypia

Desirable:
- Immunohistochemical evidence of endothelial differentiation

Staging

Not clinically relevant

Prognosis and prediction

Although these are benign neoplasms treated by surgical excision, they may behave aggressively, with destruction of neighbouring structures. Tumours that cannot be completely excised due to invasion of mediastinal structures have not shown evidence of progression, typically remaining stable without continued local invasion or aggressive recurrence {550}.

Lymphangioma of the thorax

Thway K
Calonje JE

Definition
Lymphangioma is a benign vascular lesion composed of a localized collection of dilated lymphatic channels.

ICD-O coding
9170/0 Lymphangioma, NOS
9173/0 Cystic lymphangioma

ICD-11 coding
LA90.12 & XH9MR8 Lymphatic malformations of certain specified sites & Lymphangioma

Related terminology
Acceptable: cystic hygroma/lymphangioma; lymphatic malformation; cavernous lymphangioma; haemangiolymphangioma.

Subtype(s)
None

Localization
Lymphangiomas may occur on the chest wall or axilla, and they are relatively rare in the thoracic cavity or lung. Lesions on the face and neck area may extend into the thoracic cavity {1550}. Lesions can arise in the anterior (prevascular), superior, and posterior (paravertebral) mediastinum {323} and the paratracheal, subcarinal, and aortopulmonary window areas {458}; < 1% of lymphangiomas are purely mediastinal {2560}.

Clinical features
Symptoms relate to size and site. Some patients are asymptomatic; others may present with pleural effusion and even respiratory distress.

Epidemiology
The age range is wide, but lymphangiomas are usually seen in children and young adults, mainly at birth or during early life {66,2973,2481,2007}, with a slight male predominance. Some are associated with Turner syndrome or other malformative syndromes {201,358,491}.

Etiology
Congenital or early lesions favour developmental malformations, with genetic abnormalities playing an additional role {3307}. Somatic mutations in *PIK3CA* have been reported {1748}.

Pathogenesis
Lymphangiomas are postulated to occur as a result of abnormal lymphatic system development due to mutations in *PIK3CA* and other genes involving endothelial growth factor receptor pathways {1748,2949}.

Macroscopic appearance
Lymphangiomas are multicystic and spongy, and the cavities contain milky or watery chylous fluid.

Histopathology
Most are cystic/cavernous, with variably sized thin-walled, dilated lymphatic vessels lined by flattened endothelium and with frequent peripheral lymphocytic aggregates. Lumina may be empty or may contain proteinaceous fluid or lymphocytes. Larger vessels can be surrounded by a smooth muscle layer. Longstanding lesions may show interstitial fibrosis, stromal inflammation, and/or haemosiderin deposition.

Cytology
Not clinically relevant

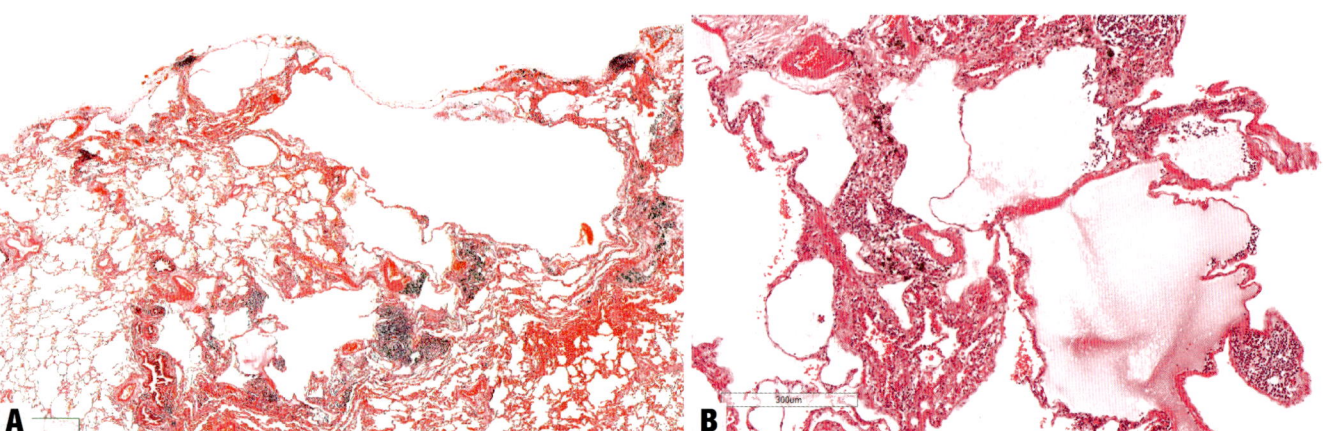

Fig. 4.17 Lymphangioma. **A** Cystic spaces within the lung show focal lymph in their lumina. **B** Lining cells are attenuated and cytologically bland. Staining for D2-40 was positive.

Diagnostic molecular pathology

Not clinically relevant

Essential and desirable diagnostic criteria

Essential:
- Tumour composed of thin-walled vascular spaces

Desirable:
- Expression of CD31, ERG, and D2-40
- Variable CD34 positivity

Staging

Not clinically relevant

Prognosis and prediction

Lymphangiomas are benign, but they may be complex in the thoracic cavity, requiring debulking, repeated drainage, and/or sclerosing procedures {1484}. Surgical excision can be difficult because of lesional size and extension, with infiltration of mediastinal planes, envelopment of great vessels, and displacement of mediastinal organs {623}. Recurrence rates depend on lesion size and depth.

Epithelioid haemangioendothelioma of the thorax

Thway K
Doyle LA

Definition

Epithelioid haemangioendothelioma (EHE) is a malignant vascular neoplasm composed of epithelioid endothelial cells within a distinctive myxohyaline stroma.

ICD-O coding

9133/3 Epithelioid haemangioendothelioma

ICD-11 coding

2B5Y & XH9GF8 Other specified malignant mesenchymal neoplasms & Epithelioid haemangioendothelioma

Related terminology

Not recommended: malignant epithelioid haemangioendothelioma; intravascular bronchioloalveolar tumour.

Subtype(s)

EHE with *WWTR1-CAMTA1* fusion; EHE with *YAP1-TFE3* fusion

Localization

Pulmonary tumours are intraparenchymal and may be multiple (most commonly) or solitary {604}. Pleural tumours may be localized or diffuse {592}. Mediastinal EHEs are rare. Metastatic disease at presentation is common, and lung tumours may be primary or secondary.

Clinical features

In > 60% of cases, parenchymal lung disease is bilateral, occurring as multiple nodules. Symptoms include pain, cough, dyspnoea, haemoptysis, and systemic symptoms {1602}.

Approximately 20% of patients are asymptomatic, with incidentally detected disease.

Imaging

CT of the lung may show well-defined or poorly defined nodules that can mimic metastatic or granulomatous disease or show rare cavitation or calcification. Pleural involvement may cause diffuse pleural thickening with effusion and pleuritic pain. Concurrent lung involvement may be present. Imaging may show pleural nodules or diffuse pleural thickening, mimicking mesothelioma {592}.

Epidemiology

Lung is one of the commonest sites, affected alone or with liver, bone, or soft tissue involvement. EHE of lung and pleura typically affects adults, with a wide age range (median for pulmonary EHE: 38 years; range: 7–81 years). Most patients with pulmonary EHE are female, whereas pleural disease has a marked male predominance {604,592}. Patients with *YAP1-TFE3* fusion tumours tend to be younger {87}.

Etiology

Unknown

Pathogenesis

EHE has a recurrent t(1;3)(p36;q23-q25) translocation resulting in fusion of *WWTR1* (3q23-q24) to *CAMTA1* (1p36) in at least 90% of cases {780,1884,2987}. This is absent in other vascular tumours. Three fusion transcript variants are described, with exon 3 or 4 of *WWTR1* fused to exon 8 or 9 of *CAMTA1*. *WWTR1*

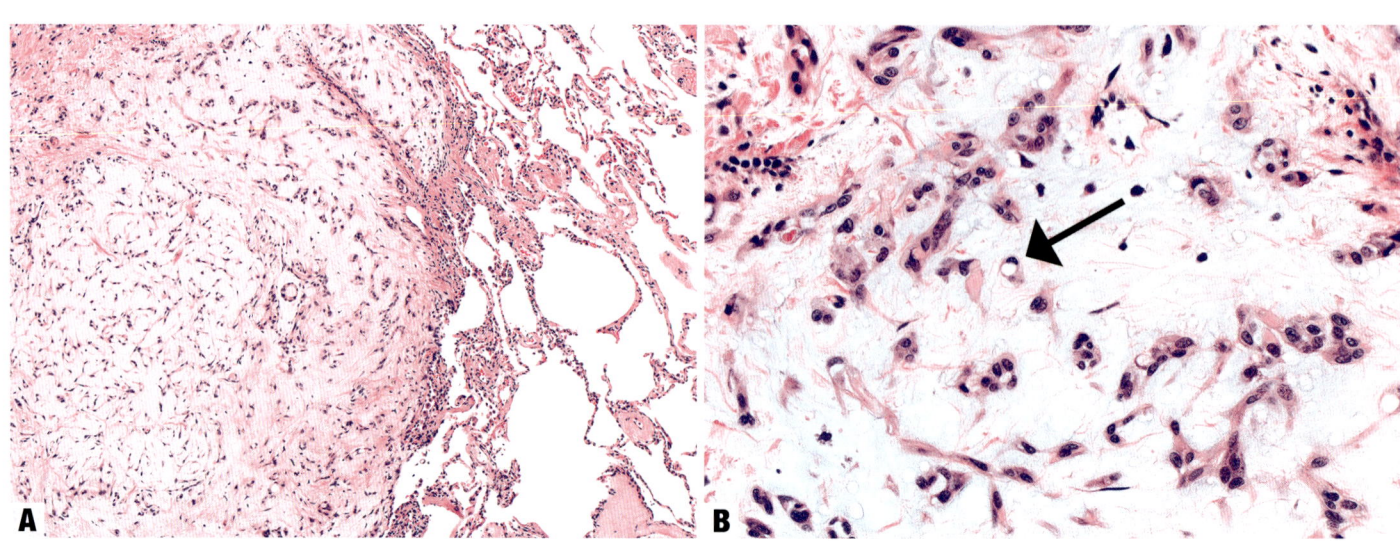

Fig. 4.18 Epithelioid haemangioendothelioma of lung. **A** This tumour is usually reasonably well circumscribed and has a distinct myxoid or myxohyaline stroma, within which cords and single epithelioid cells are embedded. **B** The tumour cells have oval or round nuclei and variable amounts of eosinophilic cytoplasm, imparting an epithelioid appearance; the presence of intracytoplasmic vacuoles (arrow) is a clue to their endothelial nature. Note also the abundant myxohyaline stroma.

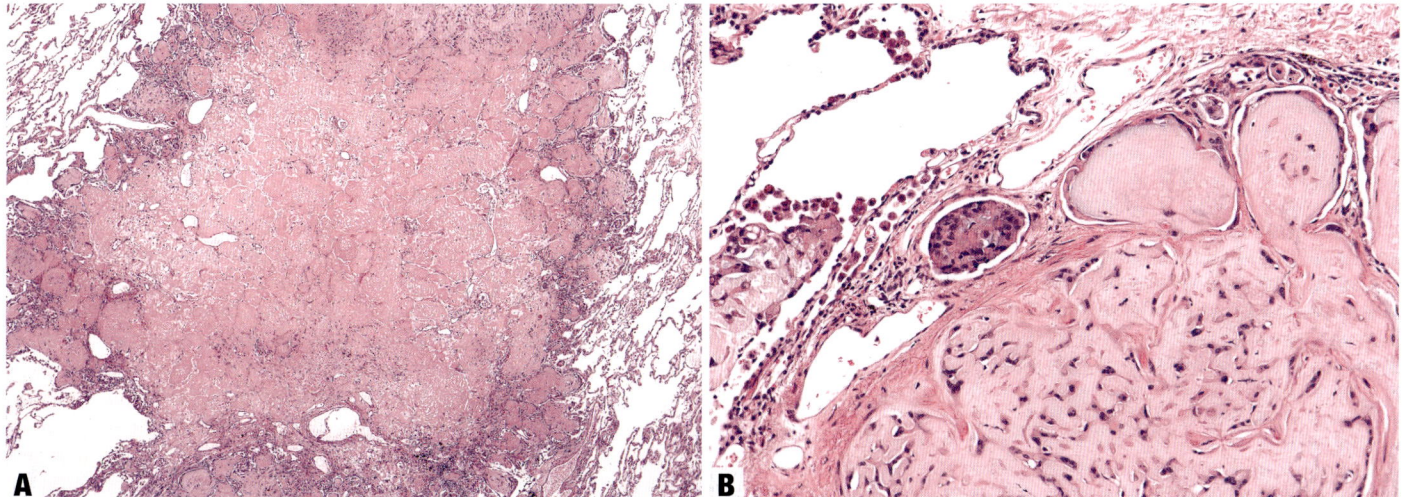

Fig. 4.19 Epithelioid haemangioendothelioma. **A** Low-power magnification of pulmonary epithelioid haemangioendothelioma showing central hypocellular, hyaline stroma and hypercellular periphery. **B** Papillary fronds, covered by tumour cells, project into the adjacent alveoli.

encodes a transcriptional coactivator highly expressed in endothelial cells; CAMTA1 is a DNA-binding transcriptional regulatory protein normally expressed during brain development {1085}. The gene fusions result in dysregulation of the Hippo pathway, driving oncogenic transformation {2986}. Approximately 5% of cases harbour a *YAP1-TFE3* fusion gene and show distinct morphology {87}. TFE3 is a known oncogenic transcription factor involved in translocations in other soft tissue tumours, and it appears likely that EHE with fusion of *YAP1* to *TFE3* has an oncogenic mechanism similar to that of EHE with *WWTR1-CAMTA1* fusions. The monoclonal origin of multifocal EHEs has been established using *WWTR1-CAMTA1* breakpoint analysis, showing that multiple concurrent lesions usually arise from local or metastatic spread from a single primary rather than multiple independent primaries {779}.

Macroscopic appearance

Pulmonary EHEs are circumscribed nodules typically < 20 mm, often distributed perivascularly. Occasional solitary nodules are > 50 mm. The cut surface is grey-white. Pleural tumours are often more infiltrative and poorly defined, and they may mimic mesothelioma.

Histopathology

EHE is often associated with arterioles, venules, or lymphatic vessels and frequently shows an intra-alveolar growth pattern. At low-power magnification, EHE forms round to oval nodules with increased cellularity at the periphery and an abundant hypocellular, eosinophilic sclerotic centre. It is composed of infiltrative cords, strands, and nests of epithelioid cells within a variably myxoid and hyaline stroma. Tumour cells have moderate amounts of glassy eosinophilic cytoplasm, uniform round or ovoid nuclei, and inconspicuous nucleoli. Intracytoplasmic vacuoles are common and may contain erythrocytes {3255}. Intracytoplasmic vacuoles may create a signet-ring appearance. Most cases show only minimal atypia, with a very low mitotic count. Angiocentric tumours expand the vessel wall, may obliterate the lumen, and spread centrifugally into surrounding tissue. Cystic degeneration, haemorrhage, and metaplastic ossification may occur {1889,2925}, with haemorrhage and

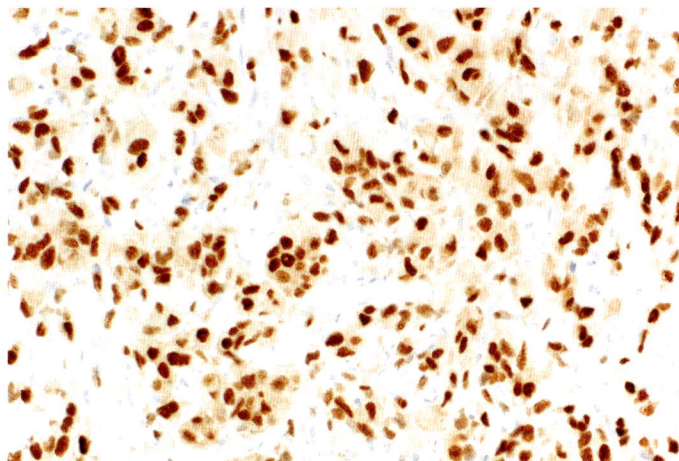

Fig. 4.20 Epithelioid haemangioendothelioma. There is diffuse strong nuclear expression of CAMTA1, reflecting the presence of *WWTR1-CAMTA1* fusion.

sclerosis sometimes obscuring tumour. They may be low-grade or intermediate-grade, with intermediate-grade tumours showing necrosis, increased mitotic activity, and nuclear atypia {78}.

A small subset of cases (< 10%) show atypical histological features (nuclear pleomorphism, increased mitoses, solid sheet-like growth, and necrosis) {694,1889}, with some tumours resembling epithelioid angiosarcoma; areas of conventional EHE or nuclear CAMTA1 expression aid diagnosis. Previously, this group was sometimes labelled as "malignant epithelioid haemangioendothelioma", but EHE is now designated as a malignant neoplasm, so this nomenclature is obsolete. However, the presence of these features should be noted, because there is a tendency for such tumours to have a more aggressive course. EHE with *YAP1-TFE3* fusion shows distinctive features, more frequently showing solid growth, often formation of vascular spaces (generally absent in other EHEs), and cells with brightly eosinophilic cytoplasm {87}.

EHEs express the endothelial markers CD31, ERG, and CD34, although with significant variability in expression {848, 2548,1915}. Keratin (CK7, CK8, CK18, pankeratin) expression is present in as many as 40% of cases, but EMA positivity is unusual {1889,1910}. EHE with *WWTR1-CAMTA1* typically shows diffuse strong nuclear CAMTA1 expression {727}. Tumours with *YAP1-TFE3* fusion show nuclear TFE3 expression {87}, although this is less specific, because TFE3 expression can also be seen in tumours harbouring *WWTR1-CAMTA1* fusion {727,847}.

Histological mimics of EHE, all of which variably express keratins, include epithelioid angiosarcoma and epithelioid haemangioma, other epithelioid mesenchymal neoplasms (e.g. epithelioid sarcoma and myoepithelial tumours), and carcinoma. Epithelioid angiosarcoma may show vasoformation or solid sheet-like growth (both rare in EHE) and shows atypia and endothelial multilayering. CAMTA1 expression is helpful in distinguishing EHE from other epithelioid vascular tumours, whereas ERG and other endothelial markers distinguish EHE from carcinoma and most other sarcomas.

Cytology
Not clinically relevant

Diagnostic molecular pathology
Identification of *WWTR1-CAMTA1* or *YAP1-TFE3* fusion transcripts helps distinguish EHE from histological mimics.

Essential and desirable diagnostic criteria
Essential:
- Classic EHE comprises cords or nests of epithelioid cells with cytoplasmic vacuolization within myxochondroid or hyaline stroma
- EHE with *YAP1-TFE3* fusion shows solid growth or variably formed vascular channels lined by epithelioid endothelial cells with moderate nuclear atypia and abundant pale cytoplasm
- Immunohistochemistry for vascular markers

Desirable (in selected cases):
- CAMTA1 expression by immunohistochemistry and/or *WWTR1-CAMTA1* fusion
- TFE3 overexpression by immunohistochemistry and/or *TFE3* gene rearrangement (*YAP1-TFE3* gene fusion)

Staging
For tumours within the lung or thoracic cavity, American Joint Committee on Cancer (AJCC) eighth-edition staging is not applicable. Instead, it is recommended that the size of the largest lesion be recorded, if possible.

Prognosis and prediction
EHE arising in lung has a worse prognosis than tumours of somatic soft tissue, and patients often present with metastatic disease {2735,78,1771,1602}. Pleural EHE is typically very aggressive, with most patients dying of disease within 1 year {592}. Patients with both lung and pleural involvement have a worse prognosis than those with lung-only disease {78}. Risk stratification (based on data from tumours at various sites) into high-risk and low-risk groups on the basis of a combination of mitotic activity and size (> 30 mm) shows a worse prognosis for patients with both features than for those with neither feature (59% vs 100% 5-year disease-specific survival rate) {694}. The metastatic rate for *YAP1-TFE3* fusion tumours may be higher, with metastases reported in 50% of cases in the original study {87}.

Angiosarcoma of the thorax

Thway K
Billings SD

Definition
Angiosarcoma is a malignant vascular neoplasm with endothelial differentiation.

ICD-O coding
9120/3 Angiosarcoma

ICD-11 coding
2B56.Y & XH6264 Angiosarcoma, other specified primary site & Haemangiosarcoma

Related terminology
Not recommended: haemangiosarcoma; lymphangiosarcoma; malignant haemangioendothelioma; malignant angioendothelioma.

Subtype(s)
None

Localization
These tumours can arise in all compartments of the thorax (lungs, pleura, heart [see *Cardiac angiosarcoma*, p. 258], thymus, mediastinum) {3263,693}. They account for < 1% of mediastinal tumours {3348,2230}, usually occurring in the anterior (prevascular) mediastinum. In children, the mediastinum is the most common site {693}. Pulmonary angiosarcomas arise from pulmonary vessels.

Clinical features
Symptoms/signs include chest pain, dyspnoea, cough, haemoptysis, pleural thickening, effusion, haemothorax, and cardiac compression {1857,1944,3263}.

Epidemiology
Thoracic angiosarcomas are more common in males. There is a wide age range, with peak incidence in the seventh decade of life. Angiosarcomas are rare in children {693,2703}.

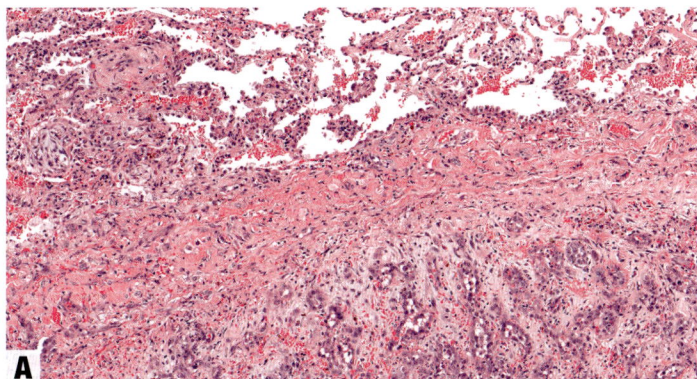
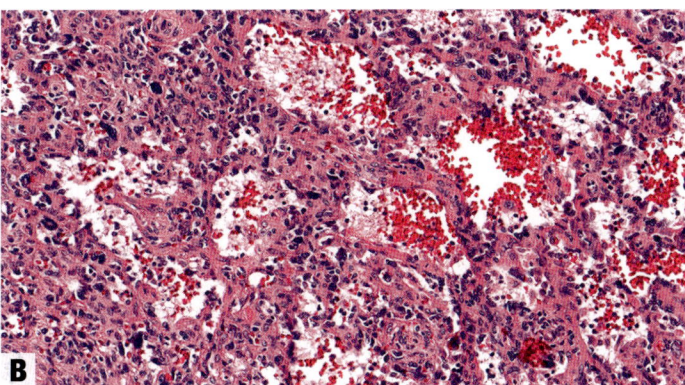

Fig. 4.21 Angiosarcoma. **A** This example of pulmonary angiosarcoma shows a proliferation of slightly angulated vessels lined by atypical endothelial cells in the lower half of the field; cellular atypia and areas of hobnailing can be seen at low magnification. **B** This tumour shows angulated, variably formed vascular channels, which are often ectatic and contain erythrocytes. Compressed, poorly formed vessels lined by markedly atypical endothelial cells give the neoplasm a more solid appearance in areas.

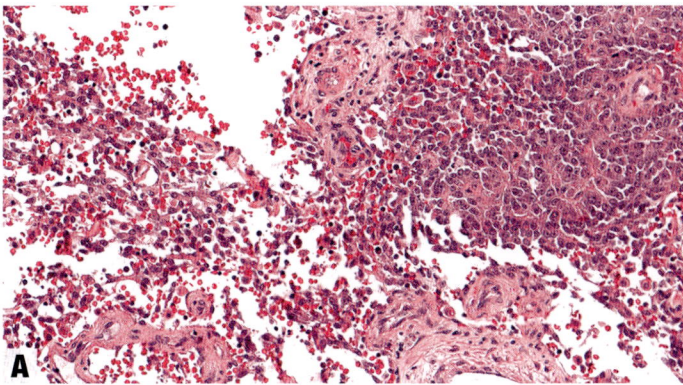
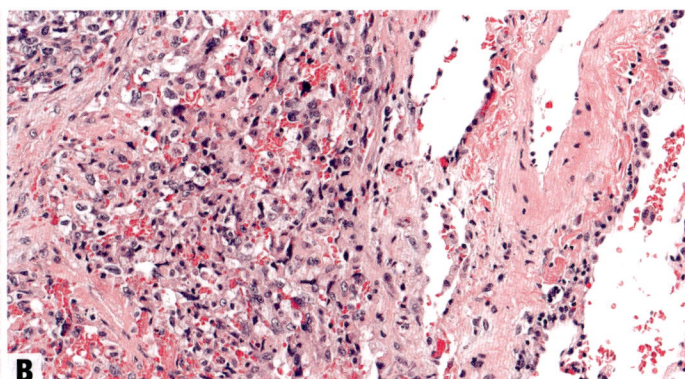

Fig. 4.22 Angiosarcoma. **A** This example shows vasoformative and solid areas. **B** Epithelioid angiosarcoma. There is a sheet-like proliferation of atypical epithelioid endothelial cells with intratumoural haemorrhage and focal vascular channel formation.

Etiology

For most cases, the etiology is unknown. A minority arise after radiation exposure {1435}. Angiosarcoma has been associated with implanted foreign material, pre-existing haemangioma / vascular malformation, prior trauma/surgery, chronic tuberculous pyothorax, syndromes (e.g. neurofibromatosis and Maffucci syndrome), and rarely asbestos {1457,1944,1303,3246, 1891,2547,605}.

Pathogenesis

Some harbour complex karyotypes {1022,3166}. Angiogenesis genes and vascular-specific receptor tyrosine kinases (*TIE1*, *TEK*, *KDR* [*VEGFR2*], *FLT4* [*VEGFR3*]) are frequently upregulated {90,1269}. A subset, typically younger patients, have *CIC* abnormalities {1202}. Approximately 40% harbour recurrent somatic mutations involving angiogenic signalling pathways (in *KDR*, *PTPRB*, *PLCG1*), and rare mutations occur in RAS genes, *PIK3CA*, *TP53*, *FLT4*, and *TIE1* {90,1270,194}. *MYC* amplifications occur in almost all postradiation/lymphoedema-associated angiosarcomas {1032,1786,1489,814}.

Macroscopic appearance

Angiosarcoma is frequently infiltrative, ranging from haemorrhagic and spongy to solid and fleshy {1878}.

Histopathology

Angiosarcomas range from anastomosing vessels to solid sheets of high-grade epithelioid or spindled cells with minimal vasoformation, often with mixtures of patterns. Vasoformative areas are lined by atypical endothelial cells, with frequent multilayering, hobnailing, or papillary-like projections. Epithelioid angiosarcomas typically have a sheet-like proliferation of cells with vesicular nuclei, prominent nucleoli, and abundant cytoplasm, and only focal vasoformation {841}. Pleural angiosarcomas can mimic mesothelioma or carcinoma {3493,793}. Mitotic activity, necrosis, and haemorrhage are common. Pleural angiosarcomas are positive for CD31 and ERG, and variably positive for CD34 {1912,1915,848}. Keratin expression is sometimes seen with the epithelioid pattern {42,841}. Radiation/lymphoedema-associated angiosarcomas are MYC-positive.

Cytology

Not clinically relevant

Diagnostic molecular pathology

MYC amplification is present in radiation/lymphoedema-associated angiosarcomas {814,1892,1032}.

Essential and desirable diagnostic criteria

Essential:
- Vasoformative to sheet-like
- Endothelial cell multilayering
- Nuclear atypia
- Mitotic activity
- CD31 and ERG positivity

Staging

Staging of angiosarcoma is not recommended, because the typically aggressive natural history of this tumour is not consistent with soft tissue staging systems.

Prognosis and prediction

These are aggressive neoplasms with a poor survival {618}. Anterior (prevascular) mediastinal angiosarcomas may have a more protracted course {3263}. For additional information, see the *Soft tissue and bone tumours* volume of this series {3298}.

Rhabdomyosarcoma of the thorax

Bridge JA
Hornick JL

Definition
Rhabdomyosarcoma is a family of sarcomas exhibiting morphological, immunophenotypic, and molecular features of skeletal myogenesis.

ICD-O coding
8900/3 Rhabdomyosarcoma, NOS
8910/3 Embryonal rhabdomyosarcoma
8912/3 Spindle cell rhabdomyosarcoma
8920/3 Alveolar rhabdomyosarcoma
8901/3 Pleomorphic rhabdomyosarcoma

ICD-11 coding
2B55.1 & XH0GA1 Rhabdomyosarcoma of respiratory or intrathoracic organs & Rhabdomyosarcoma, NOS
2B55.1 & XH83G1 Rhabdomyosarcoma of respiratory or intrathoracic organs & Embryonal rhabdomyosarcoma, NOS
2B55.1 & XH7099 Rhabdomyosarcoma of respiratory or intrathoracic organs & Alveolar rhabdomyosarcoma
2B55.1 & XH7NM2 Rhabdomyosarcoma of respiratory or intrathoracic organs & Spindle cell rhabdomyosarcoma
2B55.1 & XH5SX9 Rhabdomyosarcoma of respiratory or intrathoracic organs & Pleomorphic rhabdomyosarcoma, NOS

Related terminology
None

Subtype(s)
None

Localization
The chest wall and thoracic cavity are exceedingly rare primary sites for adult rhabdomyosarcoma {2118}. Similarly, no more than 7% of paediatric rhabdomyosarcomas arise in the chest wall or intrathoracically {878}.

Clinical features
Chest wall tumours are often asymptomatic or may be detected as masses. Dyspnoea, cough, pain, or other symptoms related to tumour location represent symptoms of intrathoracic tumours {1062,131}.

Epidemiology
Rhabdomyosarcomas commonly occur in children or young adults, but patients of any age can be affected. Pleomorphic rhabdomyosarcoma typically affects older adults.

Etiology
Embryonal rhabdomyosarcoma (ERMS) is associated with several syndromes, including Costello syndrome, neurofibromatosis type 1, and Noonan syndrome, among others {2787}.

Pathogenesis
ERMS features whole-chromosome gains (of 2, 8, 11, 12, 13, and/or 20) and losses (of 10 and 15) and loss of heterozygosity of 11p15.5 (inclusive of the imprinted genes *IGF2*, *H19*, and *CDKN1C*) {2729}. ERMS also frequently harbours mutations involving the RAS pathway, effectors of PI3K, or cell-cycle regulatory genes {2728,2787}.

Most alveolar rhabdomyosarcomas (ARMSs) exhibit a *PAX3-FOXO1* or *PAX7-FOXO1* fusion; rare cases show alternative fusions {2565,735,162,2896,1708,2728}.

Pleomorphic rhabdomyosarcomas demonstrate complex complements with recurrent numerical but not structural alterations (losses, gains, and amplifications) {1667}.

VGLL2, *SRF*, *TEAD1*, *NCOA2*, and *CITED2* are involved in fusions in congenital/infantile spindle cell rhabdomyosarcoma, whereas mutation of *MYOD1* is seen in tumours of adolescents / young adults and occasionally older adults {2010,44,2944,21}.

For additional details, see the *Soft tissue and bone tumours* volume of this series {3298}.

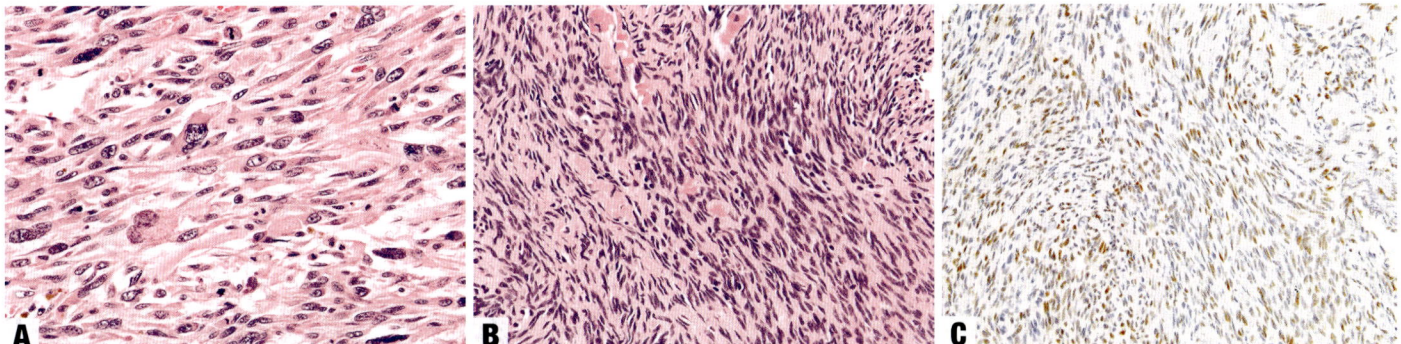

Fig. 4.23 Rhabdomyosarcoma. **A** Pleomorphic rhabdomyosarcoma. Fascicles and sheets of markedly atypical spindle cells and pleomorphic cells with eosinophilic cytoplasm and brisk mitotic activity. **B** Spindle cell rhabdomyosarcoma. This chest wall tumour is composed of highly cellular fascicles of uniform hyperchromatic spindle cells. Note the occasional brightly eosinophilic rhabdomyoblasts. **C** Spindle cell rhabdomyosarcoma. Diffuse nuclear staining for MYOD1 is a characteristic feature of spindle cell rhabdomyosarcoma.

Macroscopic appearance

Rhabdomyosarcomas form poorly circumscribed to well-marginated, tan-white soft tissue masses with variable amounts of fibrous tissue, necrosis, and haemorrhage.

Histopathology

ERMS and ARMS are composed of primitive round cells. Scattered differentiated rhabdomyoblasts are more common in ERMS. There is central loss of cellular cohesion within tumour nests in ARMS. Pleomorphic rhabdomyosarcomas demonstrate large round, polygonal, or spindled cells and scattered large rhabdomyoblasts with deeply eosinophilic cytoplasm. Spindle cell / sclerosing rhabdomyosarcomas (SCSRMSs) are composed of spindled and primitive round cells accompanied by occasional rhabdomyoblasts and a sclerotic matrix in varying proportions. Immunoreactivity (of variable extent) for desmin, myogenin, and MYOD1 can be detected in all types of rhabdomyosarcoma {2006,700,1184,2452}.

Differential diagnosis

The most important differential diagnosis is metastatic mesenchymal tumours. Distinguishing rhabdomyosarcoma from pleuropulmonary blastoma (see *Pleuropulmonary blastoma*, p. 160) is critical in this location {2240,2657}. The differential diagnosis also includes germ cell tumours and carcinosarcoma of lung and thymus, NUT carcinoma, thoracic SMARCA4-deficient undifferentiated tumour, triton tumour, and other sarcomas. The specific gene fusions can differentiate between various types of sarcomas.

Cytology

Cytology is not relevant for diagnosis.

Diagnostic molecular pathology

The specific genetic abnormalities are detectable by a variety of molecular approaches.

Essential and desirable diagnostic criteria

Essential:
- Primitive round, spindle, and/or pleomorphic cell morphology
- Variable immunolabelling for desmin, myogenin, and MYOD1

Desirable:
- Confirmation of defining genetic abnormalities (e.g. *PAX3/7-FOXO1* fusion in ARMS; various gene rearrangements [see above] or *MYOD1* mutations in SCSRMS)

Staging

For specific types of rhabdomyosarcoma, see the *Soft tissue and bone tumours* volume of this series {3298,1902}.

Prognosis and prediction

Prognosis and predictive factors relate to staging and fusion status for ERMS and ARMS {1139,1097,2787,2092}. Pleomorphic rhabdomyosarcoma is highly aggressive, and a metastatic lung presentation is much more common than a primary intrathoracic tumour {2144,892,899}. *MYOD1*-mutant SCSRMS has more-aggressive behaviour than fusion-positive SCSRMS {44,21,2453,23}.

Paraganglioma of the thorax

Jo VY
Hornick JL

Definition
Paragangliomas are neural crest neoplasms derived from para-ganglion cells of the autonomic nervous system.

ICD-O coding
8693/3 Extra-adrenal paraganglioma

ICD-11 coding
2F01 & XH1X68 Benign neoplasm of intrathoracic organs & Paraganglioma, benign
2F01 & XH2012 Benign neoplasm of intrathoracic organs & Gangliocytic paraganglioma
2C29.1 & XH1EN2 Other specified malignant neoplasms of other or ill-defined sites in the respiratory system or intrathoracic organs & Paraganglioma, malignant

Related terminology
None

Subtype(s)
None

Localization
In the thorax, paragangliomas are distributed along the prevertebral and paravertebral sympathetic chains and the sympathetic nerve fibres. Rarely, tumours may arise in the heart, where they are more common in the atria, the atrioventricular groove, and the atrial septum {1919,3209}.

Clinical features
Tumours occur as slow-growing, painless masses, although patients may have mass-related symptoms depending on the location and size of the tumour. Approximately 10% of patients have multifocal disease.

Paragangliomas of the sympathetic chain are capable of catecholamine synthesis, and patients may have symptoms secondary to elevated norepinephrine and dopamine. A subset of sympathetic paragangliomas (as many as 40%) are non-functioning and clinically silent {2689,3286}.

Epidemiology
Paragangliomas occur in patients of all ages, with peak incidence during the fourth through sixth decades of life. There is a slight female predominance {324}. Tumours arising in children are frequently bilateral and/or multifocal and associated with familial disease.

Etiology
Approximately 30% of cases arise in the setting of inherited disease, with mutations identified in numerous (at least 20) tumour susceptibility genes that appear to converge on the HIF signalling pathways {2229}.

Pathogenesis
As many as one third of paragangliomas arise in the setting of familial disease. Numerous hereditary tumour susceptibility genes have been identified, including *RET* (associated with multiple endocrine neoplasia type 2), *NF1*, and *VHL* (associated with von Hippel–Lindau syndrome); many sporadic

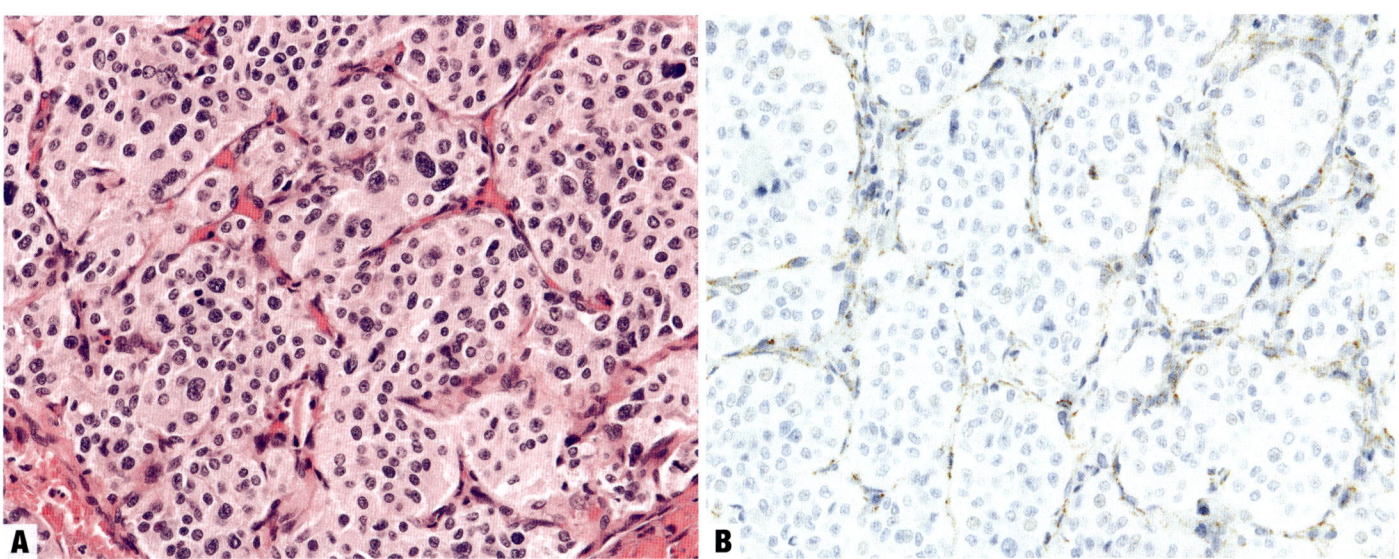

Fig. 4.24 Paraganglioma. **A** Tumour cell nests are surrounded by a delicate capillary vasculature. Note the rounded nuclei and syncytial, eosinophilic cytoplasm. **B** Immunohistochemistry for SDHB is a helpful screening method for detecting underlying SDH alterations; loss of cytoplasmic staining predicts a mutation (or hypermethylation).

paragangliomas have somatic mutations in these same genes {960,2087}. Notably, as many as 20% of all paragangliomas harbour SDH mutations and are referred to as succinate dehydrogenase (SDH)-deficient {206}. SDH deficiency occurs secondary to inactivating mutations in any of the four SDH subunit genes (*SDHA*, *SDHB*, *SDHC*, *SDHD*) or the related *SDHAF2* gene, or due to epigenetic events (i.e., *SDHC* promoter methylation).

Of these alterations, thoracoabdominal paragangliomas most commonly harbour *SDHB* mutations {205}. Hereditary paraganglioma-phaeochromocytoma syndromes occur secondary to germline SDH mutations {179}. Patients with the autosomal dominant Carney–Stratakis syndrome have germline SDH mutations and develop paragangliomas and gastrointestinal stromal tumour {2869}. Paragangliomas, gastrointestinal stromal tumour, and pulmonary chondroma are features of Carney triad; however, Carney triad is non-familial; tumours in affected patients have *SDHC* promoter hypermethylation {1054}.

Macroscopic appearance

Tumours are typically well circumscribed, with a smooth solid cut surface that varies in colour from tan to dark red-brown. Haemorrhage and cystic change may be seen. Most tumours are small, but they may occasionally be very large (≥ 100 mm in greatest dimension). Some tumours may be adherent to or invade into adjacent vessels, nerves, and soft tissue.

Histopathology

Paragangliomas show a characteristic nested (Zellballen) architecture of epithelioid tumour cells; the nests are round or oval in shape and invested by an extensive fibrovascular stroma. In many cases, the tumour cell nests are surrounded by supporting sustentacular cells that are not apparent on routine H&E staining but can be highlighted by S100 immunohistochemistry. Tumour cells may also be arranged in trabeculae and cords. Tumour cells have centrally or eccentrically located round nuclei and cytoplasm ranging from finely granular and eosinophilic to more basophilic. Notably, tumour nuclei may show variation in size and shape, are sometimes hyperchromatic, and may exhibit randomly bizarre pleomorphism; nucleoli may be inconspicuous or extremely large. Nuclear pseudoinclusions may be seen. Mitoses may be sparse, and frank necrosis is uncommon.

Rarely, other morphological appearances may be more prominent, including clear cell, spindled morphology, or angiomatoid patterns. The sclerosing pattern of paraganglioma is characterized by tumour cells arranged in irregular nests, cords, or strands within an extensively sclerotic stroma, which may mimic infiltrative growth worrisome for malignancy {2366}. Tumour cells of sclerosing paraganglioma may have more spindled morphology, a more prominent trabecular growth pattern, or distortion and crush artefact reminiscent of small cell carcinoma.

By immunohistochemistry, paragangliomas stain for the neuroendocrine markers chromogranin, synaptophysin, and INSM1 {2522,1533}. Keratin is consistently negative. The sustentacular cells at the periphery of tumour nests are positive for S100 and GFAP. SDH-deficient tumours (with mutations in any SDH subunit gene or *SDHC* promoter methylation) can be detected by immunohistochemical loss of SDHB expression {950}. Loss of SDHA expression correlates with *SDHA* mutations {1518}.

Cytology

On cytological preparations, paraganglioma shows tumour cells dispersed singly or in groups, often with acinar formation or syncytial arrangements {840}. Haemorrhage and naked nuclei in the background are common. Polygonal tumour cells are variably plasmacytoid or spindled, with pale, granular, or wispy cytoplasm; binucleated and multinucleated cells may be seen. Tumours often display endocrine atypia, with anisonucleosis and pleomorphism.

Diagnostic molecular pathology

Not clinically relevant

Essential and desirable diagnostic criteria

Essential:
- Nested (Zellballen) growth of epithelioid and polygonal cells

Desirable:
- Positivity for neuroendocrine markers (synaptophysin, chromogranin, INSM1, GATA3, tyrosine hydroxylase) and negative staining for keratin
- SDH-deficient tumours (with mutations in any SDH subunit gene or *SDHC* promoter methylation) can be detected by immunohistochemical loss of SDHB expression

Staging

Not clinically relevant

Prognosis and prediction

Most paragangliomas follow a benign course, particularly in the sporadic setting and with complete resection, with an overall recurrence rate of < 10%. Multifocal tumours and tumours arising in the familial setting may show increased recurrence {2140}. There are no histological criteria that accurately predict behaviour, and the sole determinant of malignancy is the presence of metastatic disease {1698}. Paragangliomas associated with inherited *SDHB* mutations are associated with the highest risk of metastasis {72,243} and shortest survival {71}. The most common sites of metastatic spread are regional lymph nodes, bone, liver, and lung {1458}. Even in the absence of family history, genetic counselling is recommended for affected patients given the high frequency of genetic susceptibilities.

Granular cell tumour of the thorax

Larsen BT
Glass C

Definition
Granular cell tumour is a Schwann cell neoplasm composed of large epithelioid cells with distinctive granular cytoplasm.

ICD-O coding
9580/0 Granular cell tumour
9580/3 Granular cell tumour, malignant

ICD-11 coding
2F01 & XH09A9 Benign neoplasm of intrathoracic organs & Granular cell tumour, NOS

Related terminology
Not recommended: granular cell schwannoma; granular cell nerve sheath tumour; granular cell myoblastoma; Abrikossoff tumour.

Subtype(s)
None

Localization
Most granular cell tumours arise in the dermis or subcutis, but granular cell tumours can also arise in deep soft tissues and visceral organs. Pulmonary granular cell tumours typically arise in large airways {643}. Cardiac granular cell tumours are usually epicardial near the sinoatrial node {3205}. Rarely, granular cell tumours can arise in the posterior (paravertebral) mediastinum {1756}.

Clinical features
Patients with pulmonary granular cell tumours may present with symptoms from airway obstruction (e.g. postobstructive pneumonia, atelectasis) in about half of cases or rarely with haemoptysis; other cases are asymptomatic {643}. Most cardiac granular cell tumours are discovered incidentally at autopsy or during surgery for other indications, and patients with mediastinal granular cell tumours may present with nonspecific cough or be asymptomatic {1756}. Most granular cell tumours are solitary, but multicentric granular cell tumours have also been reported {643,2399}.

Epidemiology
Most granular cell tumours occur in the fourth to sixth decades of life, but they can be encountered at any age. Granular cell tumours are more prevalent in men (M:F ratio: 2–3:1) {1576,232}. Malignant granular cell tumours are rare and more common in women {797}.

Etiology
The precise etiology of most granular cell tumours is unknown. Multiple granular cell tumours have been reported in the context of LEOPARD syndrome (multiple lentigines, electrocardiographic conduction abnormalities, ocular hypertelorism, pulmonic stenosis, abnormal genitalia, retardation of growth, and sensorineural deafness), due to a mutation in the *PTPN11* gene {2677}, as well as in neurofibromatosis type 1 and Noonan syndrome {1726,2420,2767}.

Pathogenesis
Loss-of-function mutations affecting the V-ATPase accessory genes *ATP6AP1* and *ATP6AP2*, or other V-ATPase–related genes, occur in most granular cell tumours and appear to be pathognomonic for this entity {2265,2700}. Mutations in *ASXL1*, *NOTCH2*, *PARP4*, and *ATM* have been reported in malignant granular cell tumours {3353,621}.

Macroscopic appearance
Grossly, granular cell tumours are firm, well-circumscribed, yellowish to pale-grey masses.

Histopathology
Granular cell tumours are composed of nests and sheets of large epithelioid cells with voluminous eosinophilic cytoplasm having a distinctive granular appearance. Current evidence indicates Schwannian differentiation. Despite their gross circumscription, granular cell tumours typically have ill-defined borders microscopically and appear to infiltrate adjacent tissue.

Malignant granular cell tumours may be overtly sarcomatous or deceptively bland. Malignant granular cell tumours typically show three or more of the following features: increased cellularity, prominent spindling, high N:C ratio, vesicular nuclei with prominent nucleoli, marked pleomorphism, increased mitotic activity (> 2 mitoses/2 mm²), and/or geographical necrosis {797}.

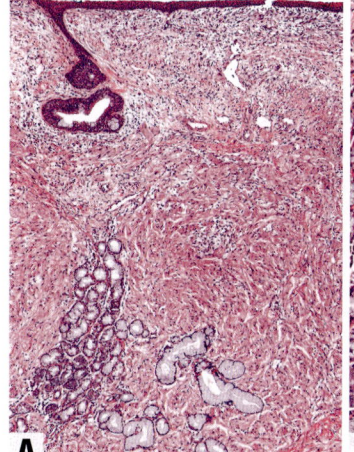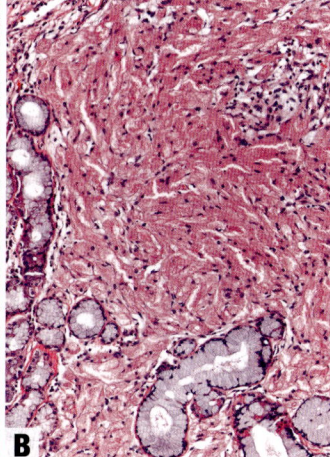

Fig. 4.25 Cardiac granular cell tumour. **A** This endobronchial granular cell tumour shows diffuse infiltration of the bronchial submucosa around the submucosal glands. **B** The tumour infiltrates around the submucosal glands, with epithelioid cells showing granular eosinophilic cytoplasm and small eccentrically situated nuclei.

Granular cell tumours show immunoreactivity for S100, SOX10, and NSE but not for NFP or GFAP. Granular cell tumours are also strongly immunoreactive for CD68 due to abundant intracytoplasmic lysosomes, but the more specific lineage-restricted histiocytic marker CD163 is negative. Nuclear immunoreactivity for TFE3 is often present in granular cell tumour, a potential diagnostic pitfall that can cause confusion with *TFE3*-rearranged tumours such as perivascular epithelioid cell tumours (PEComas) and alveolar soft part sarcoma.

The differential diagnosis of granular cell tumour includes tumefactive histiocytic proliferations such as juvenile xanthogranuloma and Rosai–Dorfman disease {1650,2128,1776}. The absence of giant cells and emperipolesis and the presence of SOX10 and NSE immunoreactivity can help distinguish granular cell tumour from these disorders.

Cytology
In cytological specimens, granular cytoplasm and bland nuclei are usual features {946}, but carcinomas and histiocytic processes must be considered.

Diagnostic molecular pathology
Not clinically relevant

Essential and desirable diagnostic criteria
Essential:
- Nests and sheets of epithelioid to polygonal cells
- Abundant, intensely eosinophilic, granular cytoplasm
- Positivity for S100 and SOX10 by immunohistochemistry

Staging
Not relevant

Prognosis and prediction
Granular cell tumours are usually benign, but they can recur locally if incompletely excised. Malignant granular cell tumour has a 50% rate of metastasis, with lungs and lymph nodes being the most common metastatic sites {797}. To date, no malignant primary cardiac granular cell tumours have been described; however, involvement of the heart and pericardium by metastases and disseminated congenital granular cell tumours has been reported {1016,621,2275}. Local recurrence, metastasis, larger tumour size, and older patient age are adverse prognostic factors for malignant granular cell tumour {797}.

Schwannoma of the thorax

Jo VY
Fishbein GA
Jain D
Perry A

Definition

Schwannoma is a benign nerve sheath tumour composed entirely or nearly entirely of neoplastic Schwann cells.

ICD-O coding

9560/0 Schwannoma

ICD-11 coding

2F3Y & XH98Z3 Benign non-mesenchymal neoplasms of other specified site & Schwannoma (neurilemmoma)

Related terminology

Not recommended: neurilemmoma.

Subtype(s)

Ancient schwannoma; cellular schwannoma; epithelioid schwannoma; microcystic/reticular schwannoma; plexiform schwannoma

Localization

In the thoracic cavity, most schwannomas arise in the posterior (paravertebral) mediastinum. Schwannomas can also occur in other mediastinal compartments and the pleura {259}. Rarely, tumours arise in visceral sites, including the heart {221}, with some predilection for the right atrium near the septum.

Clinical features

Schwannomas typically occur as slow-growing solitary tumours. Most are asymptomatic and are detected on imaging or at autopsy; however, some patients may present due to local mass effects.

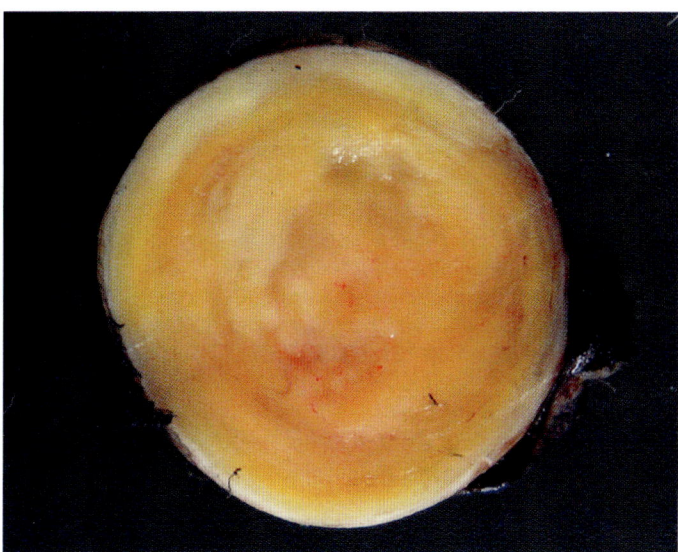

Fig. 4.26 Schwannoma. Well-circumscribed tumour arising in the pleura with a glistening, tan-white to yellow cut surface.

Schwannomas in the heart may cause shortness of breath, syncope, chest pain, murmurs, and atrial fibrillation {77,221}.

Epidemiology

The majority (90%) arise sporadically in patients of all ages, with peak incidence in adults in the fourth to sixth decades of life. Multiple schwannomas are a feature of neurofibromatosis type 2 and schwannomatosis.

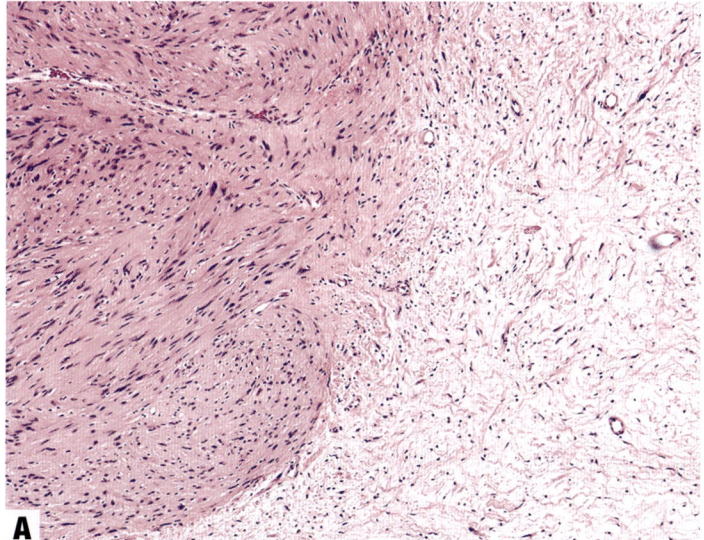
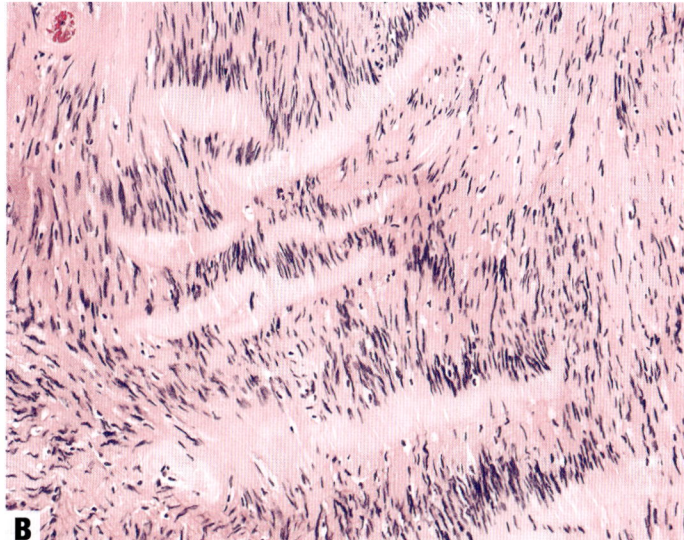

Fig. 4.27 Schwannoma. **A** Alternating compact (Antoni A; left) and loose (Antoni B; right) architectural patterns. **B** Verocay bodies (nuclear palisades) within Antoni A regions of the tumour.

Etiology

No etiological associations have been identified for sporadic schwannomas.

Pathogenesis

Inactivating mutations of *NF2* (located at 22q12.2) are detected in 50–75% of sporadic schwannomas {1283,1600,2155,1096}. Mutations in the genes *LATS1*, *LATS2*, *ARID1A*, *ARID1B*, and *DDR1* are also common, and 10% of tumours have recurrent *SH3PXD2A-HTRA1* fusions {2155,28}.

Neurofibromatosis type 2 is an autosomal dominant disease, with half of cases caused by sporadic (new) germline mutations. Vestibular schwannomas (often bilateral) are a key feature, and disease typically manifests before the age of 30 years.

Schwannomatosis typically occurs in adults, with germline *SMARCB1* or *LZTR1* mutations detectable in patients with familial (86%) and sporadic (40%) disease {1417}. *NF2* is also frequently inactivated somatically, supporting a three-hit or four-hit tumorigenesis model involving inactivation of two tumour suppressor genes on chromosome 22 {1417}.

Macroscopic appearance

Most tumours are 15–100 mm in greatest dimension. They are usually encapsulated, except in visceral sites, where they are still well circumscribed. Occasionally, an attached nerve is appreciated on the tumour capsule. The typical appearance is globoid with a glistening tan-white to yellow cut surface. Tumours often show cystic, haemorrhagic, calcific, and other degenerative changes.

Histopathology

Conventional schwannomas are spindle cell neoplasms showing alternating areas of compact (Antoni A) and hypocellular, loose (Antoni B) patterns. Areas of nuclear palisading (Verocay bodies) may be seen. Most tumours are surrounded by a perineurial capsule, with frequent subcapsular lymphoid aggregates; lymphoid aggregates may also be present at the periphery of unencapsulated tumours. The spindle cells have palely eosinophilic cytoplasm and ovoid or buckled nuclei with tapered ends. Lipid-laden and/or haemosiderin-laden histiocytes, vascular telangiectasias, and thick hyalinized blood vessels are common, especially in Antoni B regions. Some tumours may show nuclear inclusions, mild pleomorphism, and mitotic activity. Ancient schwannomas feature scattered atypical or bizarre nuclei with dark smudgy chromatin, considered a degenerative change. Cellular schwannomas show predominantly Antoni A architecture {3296,2299}, with absence of Verocay bodies, nuclear hyperchromasia, and increased mitotic activity, which may be concerning for malignancy. Other rare subtypes are epithelioid {1319}, microcystic/reticular {1677}, and plexiform {24} schwannomas.

All schwannomas show diffuse nuclear and cytoplasmic staining for S100, particularly in Antoni A areas. Tumours also show strong SOX10 nuclear staining {2131,1385}. GFAP and CD34 staining is variable, with the latter often accentuated in subcapsular areas. The perineurial capsule, if present, is positive for EMA. Intratumoural axons can be highlighted by NFP, typically at the periphery {2077}. Mediastinal tumours can show staining for keratin AE1/AE3 {796}.

Cytology

Schwannomas show cohesive fragments with fibrillary and fibrous stroma and a clean background {466}. Tumour nuclei have pointed ends and can show degenerative atypia or intranuclear inclusions. Because of the overlap with other low-grade spindle cell neoplasms, definitive diagnosis may require immunohistochemistry {34}.

Diagnostic molecular pathology

Not clinically relevant

Essential and desirable diagnostic criteria

Essential:

- Encapsulated or circumscribed tumour showing characteristic morphological features within a spectrum known to occur in tumours of well-differentiated Schwann cells

Desirable:

- Strong and diffuse S100 and SOX10 immunohistochemical staining supports the diagnosis

Staging

Not clinically relevant

Prognosis and prediction

Schwannomas follow a benign course after surgical resection and typically do not recur when removed with clear margins {259}. Malignant transformation is extremely rare, and reported transformed cases include epithelioid malignant peripheral nerve sheath tumour and epithelioid angiosarcoma {1865}.

Malignant peripheral nerve sheath tumour of the thorax

Boland JM
Folpe AL

Definition

Malignant peripheral nerve sheath tumour (MPNST) is a malignant neoplasm usually showing spindle cell morphology, which arises from a peripheral nerve, from a pre-existing benign nerve sheath tumour, or in a patient with neurofibromatosis type 1 (NF1). Outside of these settings, the diagnosis of sporadic or radiation-associated MPNST is challenging and requires histological and immunohistochemical evidence suggesting Schwannian differentiation.

ICD-O coding

9540/3 Malignant peripheral nerve sheath tumour

ICD-11 coding

2B5E & XH2XP8 Malignant nerve sheath tumour of peripheral nerves or autonomic nervous system, primary site & Malignant peripheral nerve sheath tumour

2B5E & XH4V81 Malignant nerve sheath tumour of peripheral nerves or autonomic nervous system, primary site & Malignant peripheral nerve sheath tumour, epithelioid

2B5E & XH2VV8 Malignant nerve sheath tumour of peripheral nerves or autonomic nervous system, primary site & Malignant peripheral nerve sheath tumour with rhabdomyoblastic differentiation

Related terminology

Not recommended: malignant schwannoma; neurofibrosarcoma; neurogenic sarcoma.

Subtype(s)

Malignant peripheral nerve sheath tumour, epithelioid

Localization

MPNSTs occur in the lung, chest wall, and all mediastinal compartments, most commonly in the paraspinal area; along the vagus nerve; or centred on the pleura, hilum, or bronchovascular bundle {259,1366,1248}.

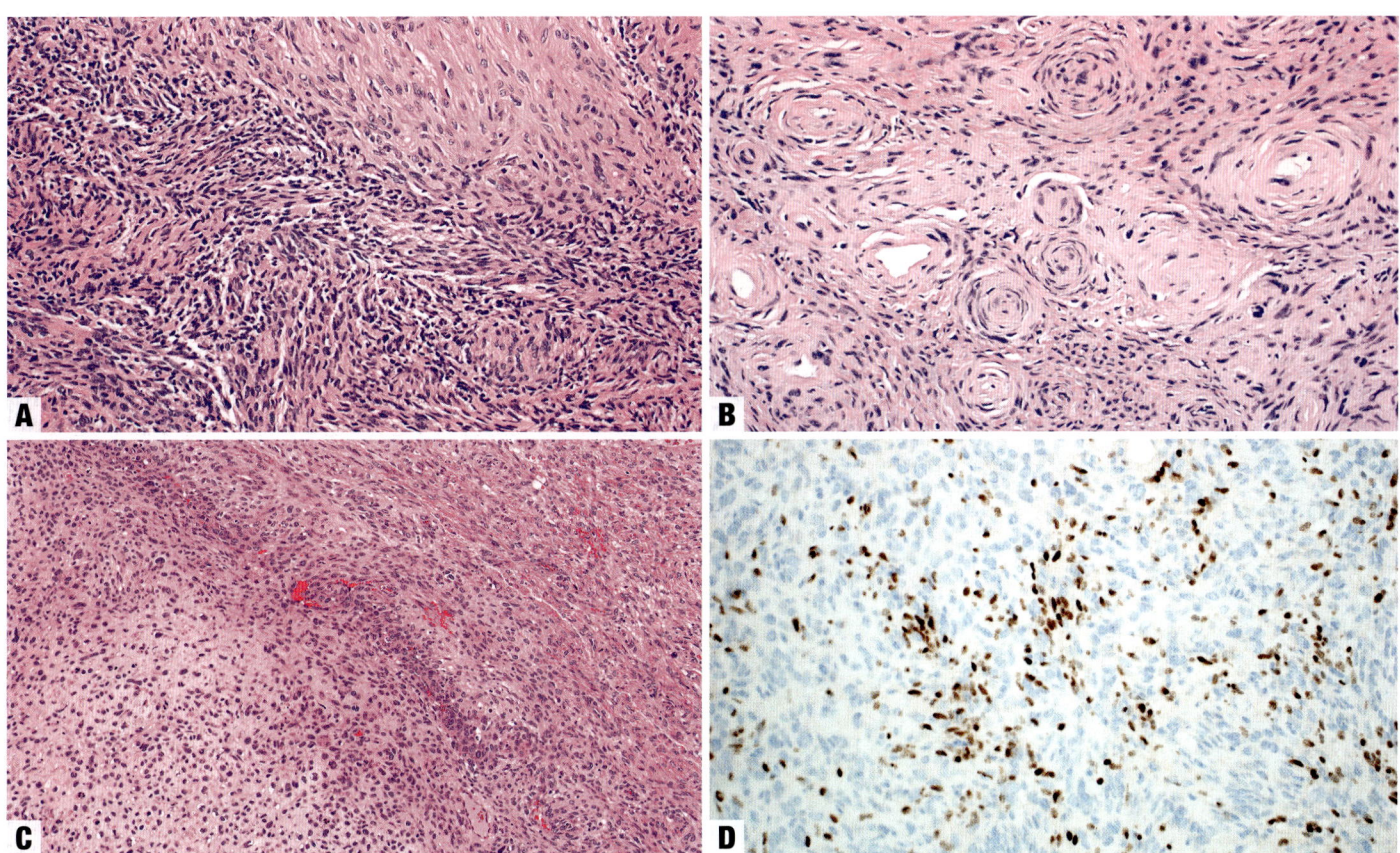

Fig. 4.28 Malignant peripheral nerve sheath tumour. **A** Spindle cell neoplasm showing alternating areas of hypercellularity and hypocellularity. **B** Whorls resembling Wagner–Meissner bodies. **C** Perivascular accentuation of cellularity and heterologous hyaline cartilage (lower left). **D** Immunohistochemistry for H3K27me3 shows abnormal loss of expression in the tumour cells, with retained normal staining in background inflammatory and endothelial cells.

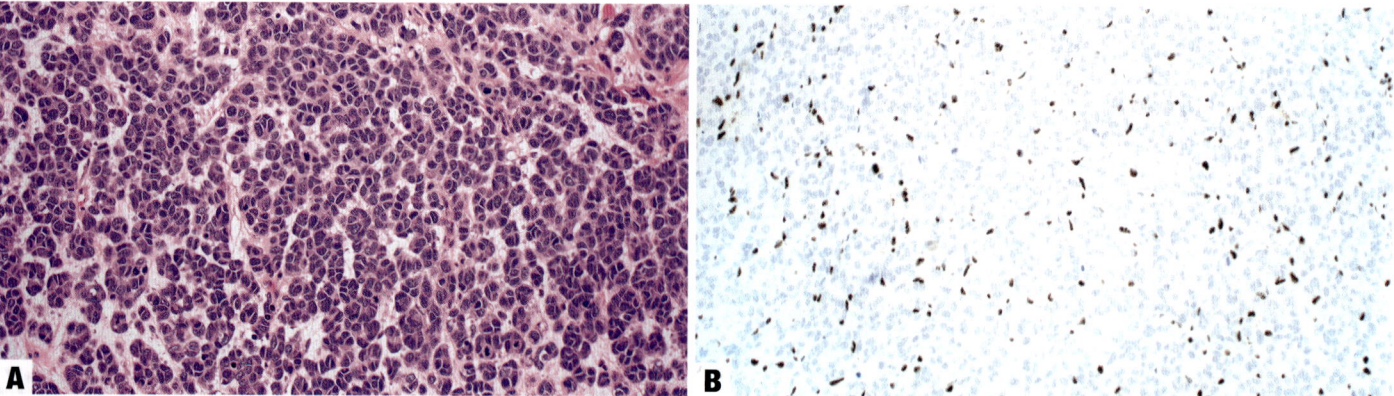

Fig. 4.29 Epithelioid malignant peripheral nerve sheath tumour. **A** Nested growth of malignant epithelioid cells with brisk mitotic activity. **B** Immunostain for SMARCB1 (INI1) shows abnormal loss of expression in the tumour cell nuclei, with retained normal staining in background inflammatory and endothelial cells.

Clinical features
Presenting symptoms include pain, dyspnoea, cough, and weight loss {259,2749}. Imaging shows a large, invasive, PET-avid mass {1366,2749}.

Epidemiology
The chest is an uncommon site for MPNSTs {2556}, which tend to occur in older adults (seventh decade of life) but have a wide age range {259}. About 50% of cases occur in patients with NF1, 10% are radiation-related, and the rest are sporadic {741}.

Etiology
MPNST may be associated with irradiation or NF1 {741}.

Pathogenesis
Complex structural and numerical chromosomal abnormalities and biallelic mutations in *NF1* are common in MPNST {1869, 292}. Frequent coexisting loss-of-function mutations occur in the genes of three pathways: *NF1*, *CDKN2A/CDKN2B*, and PRC2 core components (*EED* or *SUZ12*) {1645,638,3490,2319}. In NF1, histological progression from neurofibroma to MPNST is accompanied by progressive genomic alterations in these pathways, as well as increased copy-number variations {188, 1645,2319}. About 80% of conventional MPNSTs exhibit loss of PRC2 activity due to mutations in *EED* or *SUZ12*, as well as loss of H3K27me3 expression {2390,1645,2651}.

Epithelioid MPNSTs are genetically distinct. *SMARCB1* inactivation with SMARCB1 (INI1) loss by immunohistochemistry is observed in approximately 75% of cases {2649}, whereas these tumours rarely have alterations in the three pathways listed above {1645,1319}.

Macroscopic appearance
MPNSTs are large (up to 270 mm) circumscribed white-yellow masses {741,259,2749,1248}. They may be oblong, extending along a nerve {741,1366}.

Histopathology
Thoracic MPNSTs are usually composed of densely cellular monomorphic spindled cells growing in fascicles, with alternating cellularity, perivascular cellular condensation, and herniation into vascular lumina {741}. NF1-associated MPNSTs may arise from diffuse or plexiform neurofibromas {741} and may contain structures resembling Wagner–Meissner bodies {259}. Thoracic MPNSTs are usually high-grade, with numerous mitoses and necrosis. MPNSTs may show divergent differentiation, including rhabdomyoblasts, glands, bone, or cartilage {741}. Rare epithelioid MPNSTs consist of nests and sheets of relatively uniform epithelioid cells with prominent nucleoli.

Conventional spindled MPNSTs show patchy weak expression of S100 and SOX10, or they may be entirely negative. Loss of H3K27me3 expression is supportive in the appropriate morphological context, but it is not specific for MPNST {2651}. Epithelioid MPNSTs show diffuse S100 and SOX10 expression, retained H3K27me3, and loss of SMARCB1 (INI1) in a significant subset.

Cytology
Not clinically relevant

Diagnostic molecular pathology
Not clinically relevant

Essential and desirable diagnostic criteria
Conventional MPNST
Essential:
- Monomorphic fascicular spindle cell sarcoma with limited pleomorphism
- Sarcoma arising from nerve, pre-existing benign nerve sheath tumour, or in patient with NF1
- Sporadic soft tissue spindle cell sarcoma with evidence of Schwannian lineage (focal S100/SOX10)

Epithelioid MPNST
Essential:
- Sporadic malignant epithelioid neoplasm with diffuse S100/SOX10 expression and loss of SMARCB1

Staging
Not clinically relevant

Prognosis and prediction
Thoracic malignant peripheral nerve sheath tumours are aggressive sarcomas with a mortality rate of 60% {259,2749}. Truncal location, tumour size > 50 mm, local recurrence, high-grade morphology, association with NF1, and rhabdomyoblastic differentiation are adverse prognostic factors {1615}.

Peripheral neuroblastic tumours of the thorax

Shimada H

Definition

Peripheral neuroblastic tumours are a group of embryonal tumours arising from neural crest and include neuroblastoma; ganglioneuroblastoma, intermixed; ganglioneuroblastoma, nodular; and ganglioneuroma.

ICD-O coding

9490/0 Ganglioneuroma
9490/3 Ganglioneuroblastoma
9500/3 Neuroblastoma

ICD-11 coding

2F01 & XH03L9 Benign neoplasm of intrathoracic organs & Ganglioneuroma
2C29.1 & XH77W7 Other specified malignant neoplasms of other or ill-defined sites in the respiratory system or intrathoracic organs & Ganglioneuroblastoma
2C29.1 & XH85Z0 Other specified malignant neoplasms of other or ill-defined sites in the respiratory system or intrathoracic organs & Neuroblastoma, NOS

Related terminology

None

Subtype(s)

Neuroblastoma: undifferentiated; poorly differentiated; differentiating

Localization

Tumours are located in the posterior (paravertebral) mediastinum. Some cases show tumour extension into both mediastinal and abdominal cavities. Rarely, neuroblastoma and ganglioneuroma are diagnosed in the thymic gland of adults presenting with the syndrome of inappropriate antidiuretic hormone secretion (SIADH) {110,100,2151,2300} or with a thymic cyst {3117}.

Clinical features

Symptoms are often associated with mass effects caused by a large posterior (paravertebral) mediastinal tumour. Dumbbell-shaped tumour growth extending into the extradural space through intervertebral foramina may cause spinal cord compression leading to neurological emergency and laminectomy {655}. Unique paraneoplastic syndromes associated with this disease include Horner syndrome {1767}, opsoclonus-myoclonus-ataxia syndrome (likely immune-mediated mechanism) {1568}, Kerner–Morrison syndrome (due to the tumour secreting VIP) {1060}, and neurocristopathy syndromes (neuroblastoma associated with other neural crest disorders, e.g. congenital hypoventilation syndrome and Hirschsprung disease, due to *PHOX2B* gene mutations) {1111}. It is reported that only 3.6% of stage IV neuroblastoma cases had lung metastases at the time of initial diagnosis {739}.

Epidemiology

Peripheral neuroblastic tumours are the most common neoplasms in the first year of life and the most common extracranial solid tumours during the first 2 years of life. In the USA, 650–800 new cases are diagnosed each year (1 case per 7000 live births) {317,1044,1045}. Tumours in this group are diagnosed in the adrenal gland or sympathetic chain, and about 20% of them are found in the mediastinum.

Etiology

Unknown

Pathogenesis

The drivers for the development of these tumours are thought to be the molecular/genetic events taking place in the neural crest cells during pre-migratory, migratory, and/or postmigratory stages and leading to overexpression of MYC-family oncogenes (*MYCN*, *MYC*) {3212}, abnormal telomere maintenance/

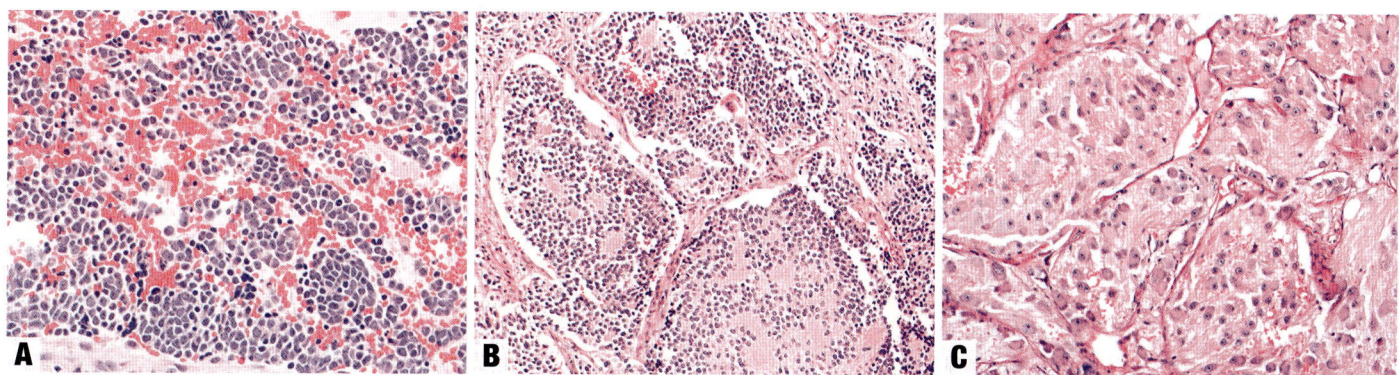

Fig. 4.30 Neuroblastoma. **A** The undifferentiated subtype has no clearly identifiable neurite formation. **B** The poorly differentiated subtype with rosette formation. **C** The differentiating subtype shows active neurite formation.

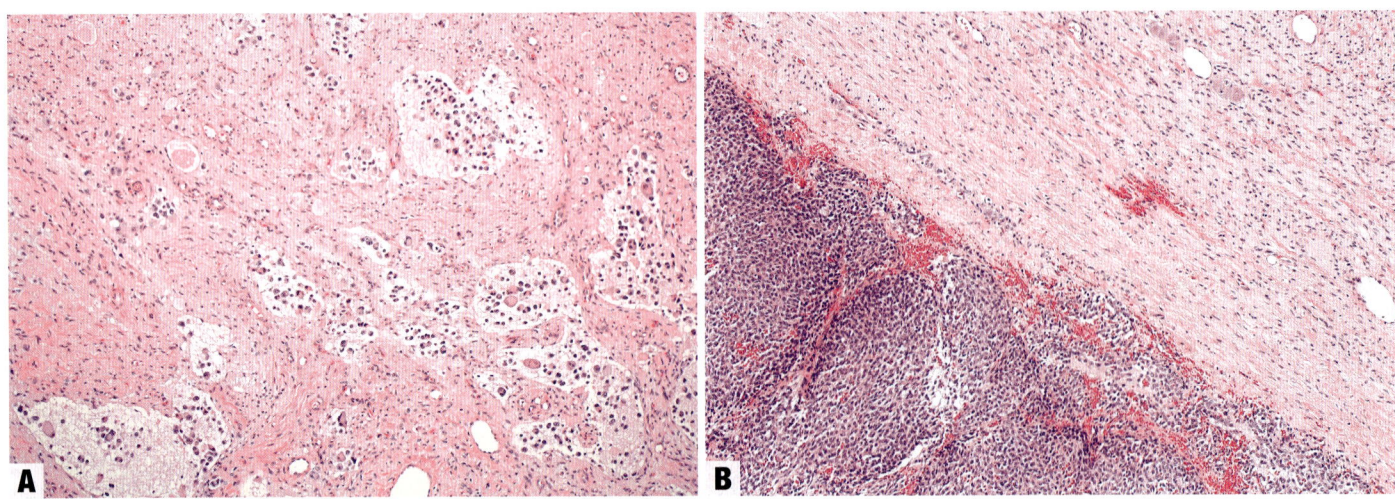

Fig. 4.31 Ganglioneuroblastoma. **A** Ganglioneuroblastoma, intermixed, shows microscopic foci of neuroblastic cells producing visible and naked neuritic processes in a ganglioneuromatous background supported by Schwannian stroma. **B** Ganglioneuroblastoma, nodular, is a composite tumour with a neuroblastoma component (lower left) and a ganglioneuroma component (upper right).

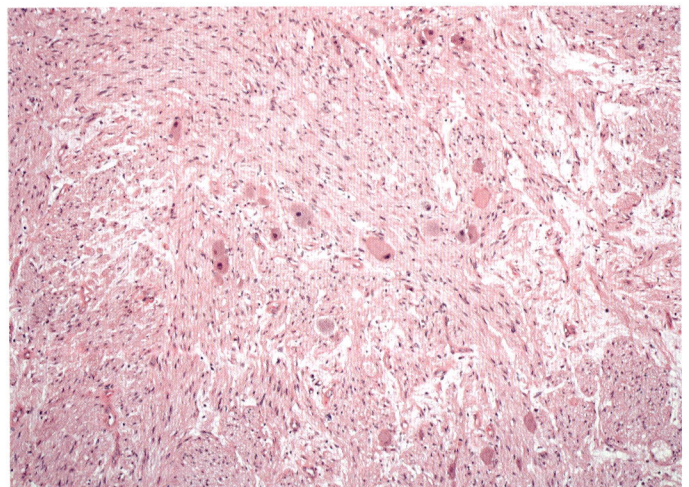

Fig. 4.32 Ganglioneuroma showing individual or small clusters of ganglion cells distributed in Schwannian stroma.

elongation (*TERT* rearrangement, *ATRX* mutation) {1134,736}, and overexpression of *ALK* gene due to mutation or amplification {2187,486}.

Important chromosomal changes include whole-chromosome gains without structural abnormalities, indicating a good prognosis {1730}, whereas diploid pattern and the presence of segmental chromosomal aberrations (1p deletion, 11q deletion, and/or 17q gain) indicate a poor prognosis {1730,2661}.

Macroscopic appearance

Neuroblastoma forms a soft, greyish-tan mass, which is often haemorrhagic, with or without foci of necrosis and calcification. Ganglioneuroblastoma and ganglioneuroma have firmer or elastic consistency and tannish-white cut surfaces. Complete resection of the primary tumour, even ganglioneuroma, is often difficult in this anatomical location, because the tumour firmly attaches to the vertebral column.

Histopathology

The histological appearances of the peripheral neuroblastic tumours are the same in various primary locations (e.g. adrenal gland and thoracic cavity) that are the destinations of neural crest cell migration. Neuroblastoma is composed of variably sized groups of primitive tumour cells irregularly demarcated by thin fibrovascular septal tissue. Neuroblastoma cells are characterized by their ability to produce neurites with or without Homer Wright rosette formation. During the maturation steps from neuroblastoma to ganglioneuroblastoma to ganglioneuroma, tumour cells show continuous differentiation from neuroblasts to ganglion cells, and the tumour tissues gradually become replaced by Schwannian stroma. It is believed that all ganglioneuromas were once neuroblastomas in their early stages of tumour development.

Immunohistochemically, neuronal markers (NSE, PGP9.5, synaptophysin, chromogranin, CD56, etc.) have been used to support the diagnosis of this disease. Because tumour cells in this group are of neural crest origin with neuronal differentiation, immunohistochemical detection of nuclear POX2B expression is one of the most reliable criteria for the diagnosis of this disease in routine practice. Tyrosine hydroxylase is another marker of neural crest cells with neuronal/neuroendocrine differentiation. However, tyrosine hydroxylase positivity is often lost after decalcification in metastatic neuroblastoma cells of bone marrow biopsy samples.

The International Neuroblastoma Pathology Committee defines four categories of peripheral neuroblastic tumours {2744}: neuroblastoma (Schwannian stroma–poor); ganglioneuroblastoma, intermixed (Schwannian stroma–rich); ganglioneuroma (Schwannian stroma–dominant); and ganglioneuroblastoma, nodular (composite, Schwannian stroma–rich/dominant and Schwannian stroma–poor). Within the neuroblastoma category, three subtypes are distinguished: undifferentiated, poorly differentiated, and differentiating. The committee also recommends determining the mitosis-karyorrhexis index (low: < 100/5000 cells; intermediate: 100–200/5000 cells; or high > 200/5000 cells) for each tumour in the neuroblastoma category and for neuroblastoma nodules in the ganglioneuroblastoma, nodular, category. The committee also established the International Neuroblastoma Pathology Classification for distinguishing favourable and unfavourable histology groups {2745,2341}.

Cytology
Not clinically relevant

Diagnostic molecular pathology
Recurrent genetic aberrations indicating aggressive tumour behaviour of this disease include *MYCN* amplification {319, 2694}, *ALK* mutation/amplification {2011}, *TERT* rearrangement {1200}, and *ATRX* mutation {497}. Important chromosomal changes include whole-chromosome gain without structural abnormalities, indicating a good prognosis {1730}, whereas diploid pattern and the presence of segmental chromosomal aberrations (1p deletion, 11q deletion, and/or 17q gain) indicate a poor prognosis {1730,2661}. Detecting these molecular/genetic abnormalities at the time of diagnosis is critical for patient stratification and protocol assignment in clinical trials.

Essential and desirable diagnostic criteria
Essential:
- Histological findings (grade of neuroblastic differentiation, mitosis-karyorrhexis index, Schwannian stromal development) for diagnosis and prognostic distinction (favourable vs unfavourable histology) according to the International Neuroblastoma Pathology Classification

Desirable:
- Molecular/genomic testing for *MYCN* oncogene status, *ALK* oncogene status, telomere maintenance gene (*TERT* and *ATRX*) status, DNA index, and segmental chromosomal aberrations for predicting clinical behaviours

Staging
There have been two major and widely used clinical staging systems: the International Neuroblastoma Staging System (INSS) {318} and the International Neuroblastoma Risk Group Staging System (INRGSS) {1963}. The former is a postsurgical staging system based on the surgical and pathological findings, and the latter is a presurgical staging system based on the presence or absence of image-defined risk factors.

Prognosis and prediction
Peripheral neuroblastic tumours are heterogeneous and classified into a biologically favourable group and a biologically unfavourable group. Practically, patients with this disease are stratified into different risk groups. There are two major risk-grouping systems: the Children's Oncology Group (COG) risk classification system {2272,2074} and the International Neuroblastoma Risk Group (INRG) classification system {557}. Both systems use a combination of various prognostic factors, such as clinical stage, age at diagnosis, histopathology, and molecular/genetic abnormalities {1236}.

Historically, the COG risk classification system (distinguishing low-risk, intermediate-risk, and high-risk groups) has contributed to actual patient stratification and protocol assignment. In contrast, the primary purpose of the INRG classification system (distinguishing very low, low-intermediate, and high risk) is to facilitate the comparison of risk-based clinical trials conducted in different regions and countries {2341,1963,557}.

Synovial sarcoma of the thorax

Yoshida A
Klebe S
Ladanyi M
Suurmeijer AJH

Definition

Synovial sarcoma (SS) is a monomorphic spindle cell sarcoma with variable epithelial differentiation and a specific *SS18*-SSX fusion gene.

ICD-O coding

9040/3 Synovial sarcoma, NOS

ICD-11 coding

2B5A.Y & XH9B22 Synovial sarcoma, other specified primary site & Synovial sarcoma, NOS

Related terminology

None

Subtype(s)

Synovial sarcoma, monophasic spindle cell; synovial sarcoma, biphasic; synovial sarcoma, poorly differentiated

Localization

Primary intrathoracic SS is uncommon. More than 80% of intrathoracic SSs affect pleura or pulmonary parenchyma. Mediastinum and heart are rarer primary sites {191,3210,1591, 3023}.

Clinical features

Patients usually present with chest pain, dyspnoea, cough, and haemoptysis. Some tumours are detected incidentally.

Epidemiology

Primary intrathoracic SS has a slight male predilection and affects all ages, with a peak in the fourth to fifth decades of life {191,1079,3210,3023}.

Etiology

Unknown

Pathogenesis

SS bears a unique chromosomal translocation that results in the formation of an oncogenic *SS18*-SSX fusion gene {371}. SS18-SSX protein exerts oncogenic activity by disrupting epigenetic control {154,1855}. For additional details, see the *Soft tissue and bone tumours* volume of this series {3298}.

Macroscopic appearance

Intrathoracic SS usually forms a large, well-circumscribed tumour. Cystic change, calcification, and necrosis may be present.

Histopathology

Monophasic SS consists of dense fascicles of monomorphic spindle cells with a high N:C ratio; entrapped pneumocytes

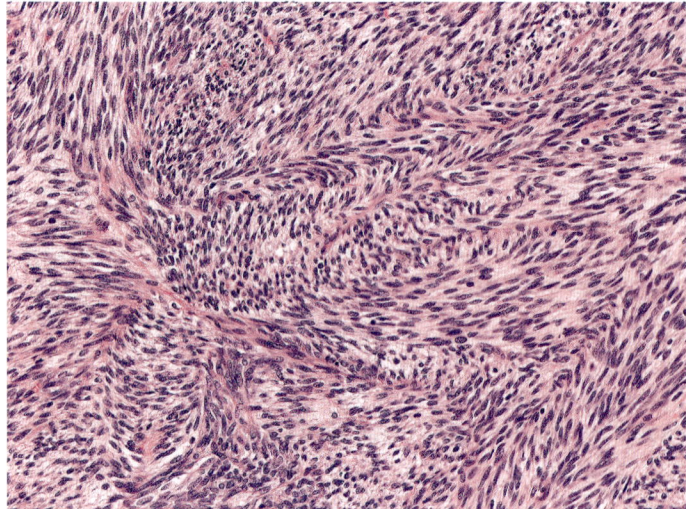

Fig. 4.33 Monophasic spindle cell synovial sarcoma. The tumour consists of fascicles of monomorphic spindle cells.

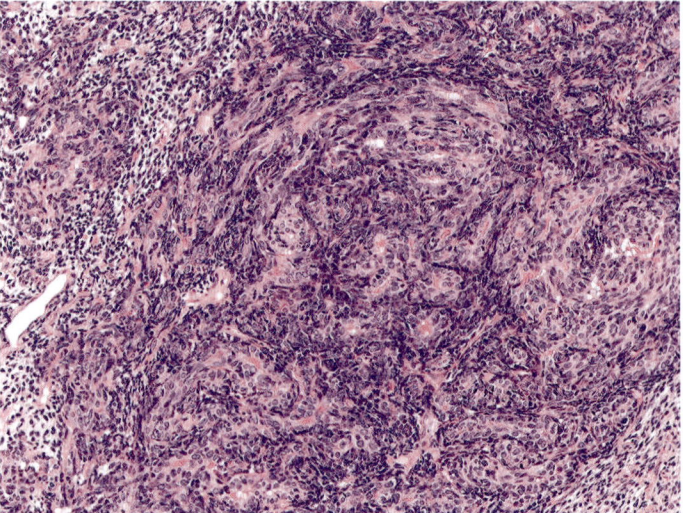

Fig. 4.34 Biphasic synovial sarcoma. The biphasic tumour consists of a glandular component showing intraluminal eosinophilic secretion and fascicles of spindle cell proliferation.

may mislead the diagnosis or determination of subtype. Biphasic SS has epithelial and spindle cell components, in varying proportions. Poorly differentiated SS with spindle or round cell morphology shows increased cellularity, greater nuclear atypia, and high mitotic activity {3136}.

Immunohistochemistry

Most SSs express EMA and/or cytokeratin {191}. TLE1 staining is characteristic {3024}, although it is not specific {1844,1519, 1477}. Expression of calretinin is common {1911,1079}. CD56 expression {1079}, rarely with focal synaptophysin {2639}, may lead to misdiagnosis as small cell carcinoma.

Cytology
For FNA, a cell block preparation is favoured.

Diagnostic molecular pathology
SS18-SSX fusion testing is recommended when histology and immunohistochemistry are insufficient to establish a diagnosis.

Essential and desirable diagnostic criteria
Essential:
- Monomorphic spindle cells showing variable epithelial differentiation

Desirable:
- Demonstration of *SS18*-SSX fusion

Staging
The American Joint Committee on Cancer (AJCC) or Union for International Cancer Control (UICC) TNM system may be used.

Prognosis and prediction
Intrathoracic SS is associated with poorer outcome than soft tissue SS {784,191,1079,1443,1591}. In general, prognostic factors include stage, size, grade, and poorly differentiated histology {3136,216,1023,3014,1532}.

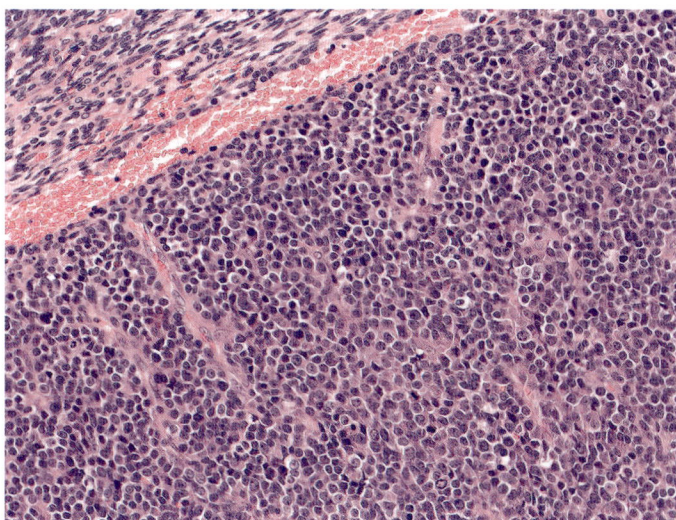

Fig. 4.35 Poorly differentiated synovial sarcoma. The poorly differentiated component consists of a uniform round cell proliferation. A spindle cell component is additionally present (upper left).

Undifferentiated small round cell sarcomas of the thorax

Yoshida A
Bridge JA

Definition
This generic category includes a select group of sarcoma entities composed of undifferentiated small round cells, including Ewing sarcoma, *CIC*-rearranged sarcoma, sarcoma with *BCOR* genetic alterations, and round cell sarcoma with *EWSR1*–non-ETS fusions.

ICD-O coding
9364/3 Ewing sarcoma
9367/3 *CIC*-rearranged sarcoma
9368/3 Sarcoma with *BCOR* genetic alterations
9366/3 Round cell sarcoma with *EWSR1*–non-ETS fusions

ICD-11 coding
2C29.1 & XH85G7 Other specified malignant neoplasms of other or ill-defined sites in the respiratory system or intrathoracic organs & Round cell sarcoma, undifferentiated

Related terminology
Not recommended: Askin tumour; Ewing-like sarcoma.

Subtype(s)
None

Localization
Ewing sarcoma and *EWSR1-PATZ1* sarcoma not infrequently involve the chest wall {314}, whereas the thoracic cavity is an uncommon primary site {3420,1845,3241,314,3419}.

Clinical features
Chest wall tumours may be detected as masses, whereas patients with intrathoracic tumours present with cough, dyspnoea, pain, or other symptoms related to tumour location {3271}. Some tumours are detected incidentally {1154}.

Epidemiology
These tumours typically occur in children or young adults, but patients of any age can be affected.

Etiology
Unknown

Pathogenesis
Ewing sarcoma characteristically exhibits a fusion of *EWSR1* or *FUS* to an ETS gene family member (e.g. *FLI1* or *ERG*). *CIC*-rearranged sarcomas harbour *CIC* rearrangement, most commonly *CIC-DUX4* {2826}. Sarcoma with *BCOR* genetic alterations features either *BCOR* fusions (to *CCNB3* or other partners) or internal tandem duplication (ITD) of *BCOR* exon 15 {2827, 1380,3419}. *EWSR1-NFATC2* (less commonly *FUS-NFATC2*) and *EWSR1-PATZ1* are the fusion genes seen in round cell sarcomas with *EWSR1*–non-ETS fusions.

Macroscopic appearance
Most undifferentiated round cell sarcomas are large, grey-tan soft masses with necrosis.

Histopathology
Ewing sarcoma consists of uniform small round cells, which are often positive for CD99 and NKX2-2 {3423}. *CIC*-rearranged sarcoma shows lobulated growth of minimally pleomorphic round to epithelioid cells, commonly immunopositive for ETV4 and WT1 {2826,3420,1211}. Sarcomas with *BCOR* genetic alterations are composed of uniform oval to spindle cells within

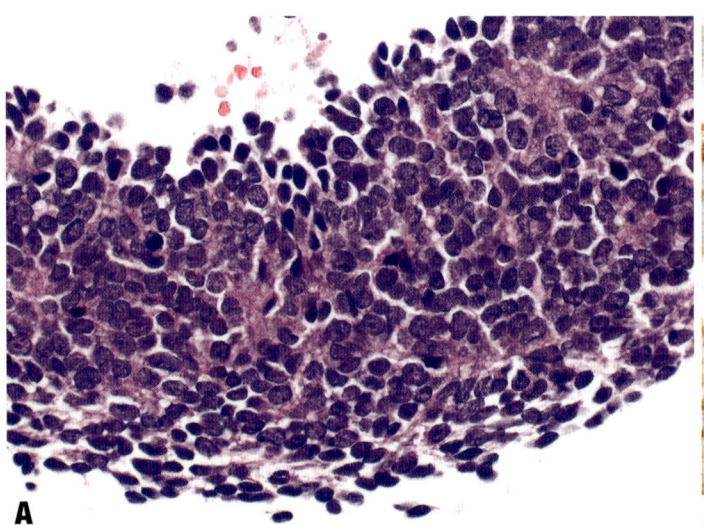 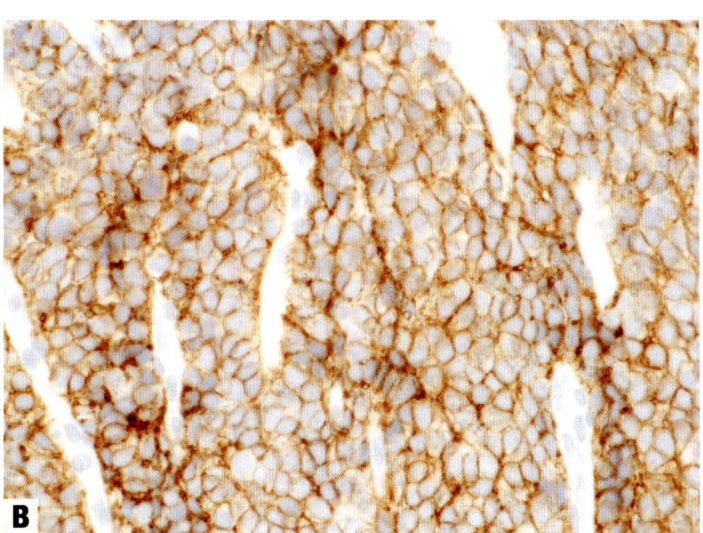

Fig. 4.36 Ewing sarcoma. **A** Diffuse proliferation of uniform round cells. **B** CD99 immunohistochemistry shows characteristic diffuse strong membranous staining.

variably vascular fibro-oedematous stroma, positive for BCOR {1378}. *EWSR1-PATZ1* sarcoma features round to spindle cells within a fibrous background and with variable expression of myogenic and neurogenic markers {314,517}. Cords/nests/trabeculae of round cells in a fibromyxoid stroma characterize *EWSR1-NFATC2* sarcomas {3202,701}.

For additional details, see the *Soft tissue and bone tumours* volume of this series {3298}.

Cytology
Not clinically relevant

Diagnostic molecular pathology
The specific genetic abnormalities are detectable by a variety of molecular methods.

Essential and desirable diagnostic criteria
Essential:
- Undifferentiated small round cell morphology
- Genetic confirmation for round cell sarcoma with *EWSR1–*non-ETS fusions

Desirable:
- Genetic confirmation for Ewing sarcoma, *CIC*-rearranged sarcoma, and sarcomas with *BCOR* genetic alterations

Staging
The Union for International Cancer Control (UICC) or American Joint Committee on Cancer (AJCC) TNM staging system may be used.

Prognosis and prediction
Undifferentiated small round cell sarcomas are generally associated with poor outcome. For Ewing sarcoma, stage, anatomical location, and pathological response to neoadjuvant chemotherapy are prognostic factors {49}. *CIC*-rearranged sarcomas have more aggressive behaviour than Ewing sarcoma {3420,88}.

EWSR1-FLI1 fusion protein

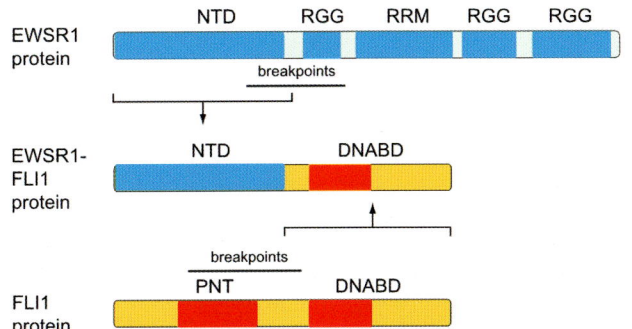

Fig. 4.37 EWSR1-FLI1 fusion proteins in Ewing sarcoma. The EWSR1 protein has an N-terminal domain (NTD) that is an intrinsically disordered domain and a C-terminal region that contains RGG domains and an RNA-recognition motif (RRM). The FLI1 protein has an N-terminal domain with a pointed protein–protein interaction domain (PNT) and an ETS-type DNA-binding domain (DNABD) within the C-terminus. The resulting EWSR1-FLI1 protein retains the EWSR1 NTD and the FLI1 DNABD.

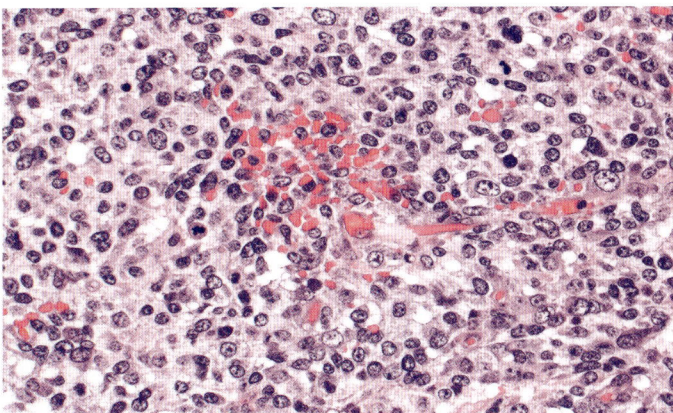

Fig. 4.38 *CIC*-rearranged sarcoma. Dense proliferation of minimally pleomorphic round to epithelioid cells.

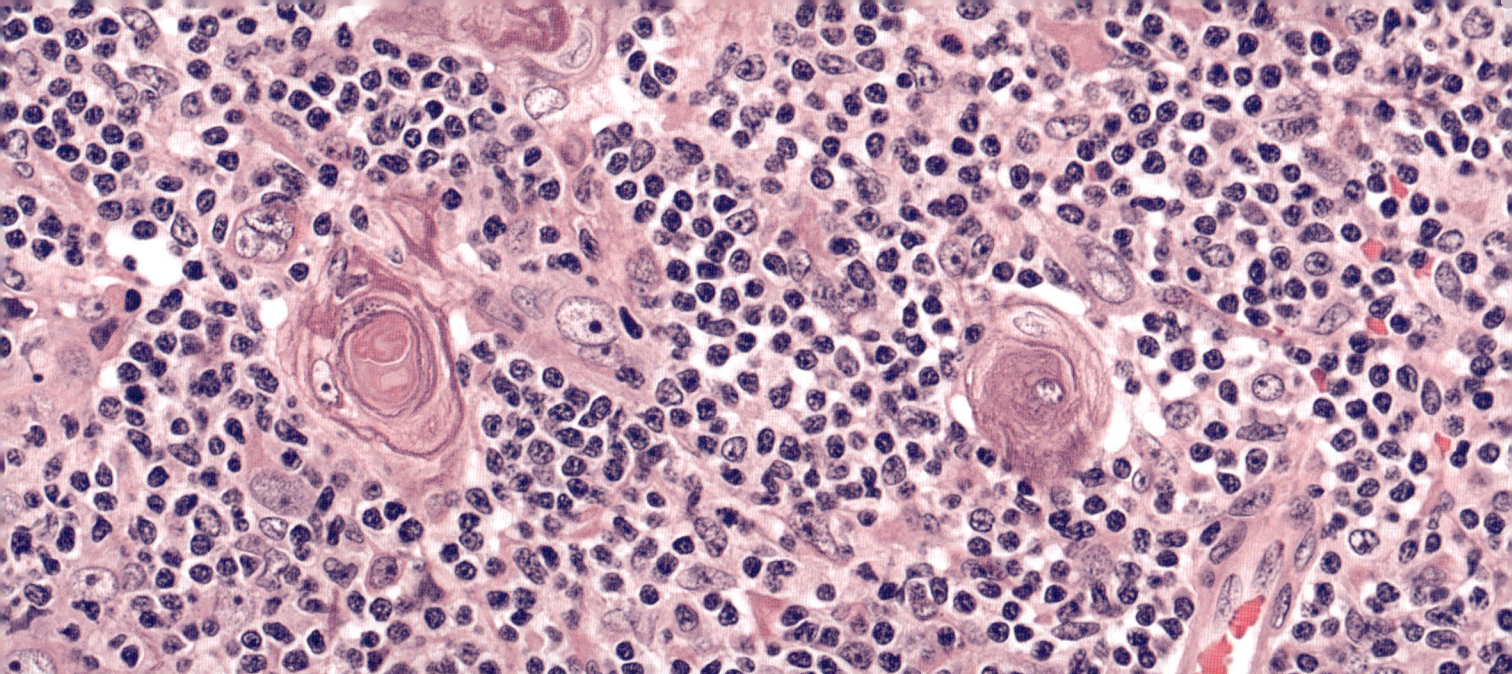

5

Tumours of the thymus

Edited by: Chan JKC, Lantuejoul S, Marx A

Thymoma
Lipofibroadenoma
Squamous cell carcinoma
Basaloid carcinoma
Lymphoepithelial carcinoma
NUT carcinoma of the thorax
Clear cell carcinoma
Low-grade papillary adenocarcinoma
Mucoepidermoid carcinoma
Thymic carcinoma with adenoid cystic carcinoma–like features
Enteric-type adenocarcinoma
Adenocarcinoma NOS
Adenosquamous carcinoma
Sarcomatoid carcinoma
Undifferentiated carcinoma
Thymic carcinoma NOS
Carcinoid/neuroendocrine tumour
Small cell carcinoma
Large cell neuroendocrine carcinoma

Thymoma: Introduction

Marx A
Detterbeck F
Marom EM
Rajan A
Ströbel P

Thymic epithelial tumours include thymomas, thymic carcinomas, and thymic neuroendocrine neoplasms. Thymomas are unique tumours of the mediastinal or ectopic thymus that are characterized by thymus-like organoid differentiation, including lobular growth, presence of perivascular spaces, and intratumoural infiltration of immature T cells. Only the epithelial component is neoplastic. The distinctive histology of thymomas is linked to highly prevalent autoimmune and immunodeficiency states and a distinct genomic landscape. The histological appearances of thymoma may be challenging in small biopsies, and typing may be impossible {1794}.

Epidemiology

Thymomas have an incidence of 0.13–0.26 cases per 100 000 population per year {1190,3252,628}, are commonest in the fifth and sixth decades of life (patient age range: 6–83 years; median: 58 years overall, but 48 years in the black population), and are exceedingly rare in children. They occur slightly more frequently in females than males (see Table 5.01). In the USA, thymomas are most prevalent in the Asian/Pacific Islander population, followed by the black population and the white population {1190,769}. In adults, thymic epithelial tumours account for 25–30% of mediastinal tumours, of which 75–85% are thymomas, 14–22% thymic carcinomas, and < 5% thymic neuroendocrine tumours (TNETs) {835,33,3508}. In children, thymic epithelial tumours constitute < 1% of thoracic tumours, and thymomas prevail over thymic carcinomas slightly {2552, 2503,2837}. Epidemiological and clinical findings of various thymoma types are shown in Table 5.01.

Etiology and pathogenesis

There are no known environmental factors triggering thymoma development {2409,769}. Like thymic carcinoma, thymoma may rarely arise in the wall of thymic cysts {2686,114}. Development of thymoma after irradiation, transplantation, or HIV infection is probably a coincidence {1621,1020,984,1860}. Familial

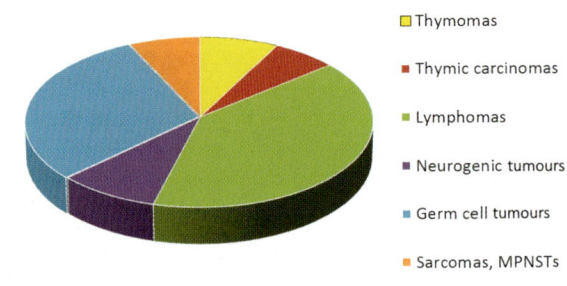

Primary mediastinal tumours in children (<18 y)

- Thymomas
- Thymic carcinomas
- Lymphomas
- Neurogenic tumours
- Germ cell tumours
- Sarcomas, MPNSTs

A

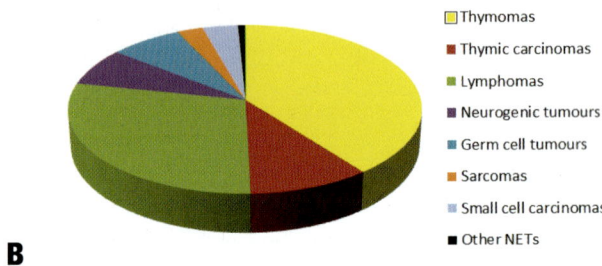

Primary mediastinal tumours (major groups) in adults

- Thymomas
- Thymic carcinomas
- Lymphomas
- Neurogenic tumours
- Germ cell tumours
- Sarcomas
- Small cell carcinomas
- Other NETs

B

Fig. 5.01 Frequency distribution of mediastinal tumours. **A** Primary mediastinal tumours in children (< 18 years old) reported to the German Childhood Cancer Registry from 2009 to 2018 (registered by 2020). In children, thymomas account for 7% of strictly mediastinal tumours (*n* = 77, shown here) and 1% of all thoracic neoplasms (*n* = 618, of which 54% are lymphomas). MPNST, malignant peripheral nerve sheath tumour. **B** Major groups of primary mediastinal tumours in adults, accounting for 56% of all mediastinal masses (*n* = 3308) {2505}. Of all mediastinal small cell carcinomas (2% of mediastinal masses), only 15% occur in the anterior mediastinum {2505}. NET, neuroendocrine tumour.

thymoma clustering {3496} or cancer susceptibility syndromes (e.g. Lynch syndrome, myotonic dystrophy type 1, and multiple endocrine neoplasia type 1) are rare {1920,2255,1916}. Patients

Table 5.01 Epidemiological and clinicopathological features of thymomas: proportion of thymoma types in relation to all thymomas

Thymoma type	Average relative frequency (range)[a]	Average age (range), in years[b]	M:F ratio[b]	Myasthenia gravis (+) mean (range)[b]	Average Masaoka stage[c]				
					I	II	III	IVa	IVb
Type A	11.5% (3.1–26.2%)	64 (8–88)	1:1.4	17% (0–33%)	60%	31%	8%	0.5%	0.5%
Type AB	25% (15–43.0%)	57 (11–89)	1:1.4	18% (6–42%)	67%	26%	6%	1%	0%
Type B1	17.5% (5.9–52.8%)	50 (4–83)	1:1.6	44% (7–70%)	50%	37%	9%	3%	1%
Type B2	26.0% (8.0–41.1%)	49 (4–83)	1:1	54% (24–71%)	32%	29%	28%	8%	3%[d]
Type B3	16.0% (3.4–35.1%)	55 (8–87)	1:0.8	50% (25–65%)	19%	36%	27%	15%	3%[e]
Micronodular	1.0%	65 (41–83)	1.2:1	Rare[f]	62%	36%	0%	2%	0%
Metaplastic[g]	< 1.0%	50 (28–71)	1:1.5	Very rare[h]	75%	17%	8%	0%	0%

[a]{679,1802,1040,1797,1798,628}. [b]{679,1287,427,1672}. [c]{472,2184,2273,2249,2873,1510,1440,628,1287}. [d]Range: 0–5%. [e]Range: 0–15%. [f]{2249}. [g]See *Metaplastic thymoma* (p. 347). [h]{1370}. Note: Union for International Cancer Control (UICC) staging not used in these publications.

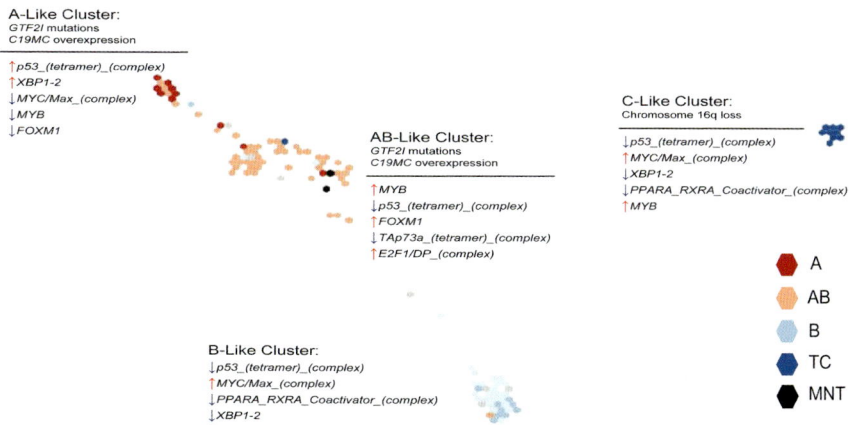

Fig. 5.02 Molecular subtypes of thymic epithelial tumours. Integrative unsupervised clustering of thymic epithelial tumour subtypes from 5 data platforms {2409}. Samples are placed according to similarities in their genomic profiles, integrating all platforms. For each cluster (A-like, AB-like, B-like, and "C-like" – representing thymic carcinomas [TCs]), single-platform hallmarks (e.g. the overexpressed microRNA cluster C19MC in the A-like and AB-like clusters) are listed above the thin line, whereas results of a multiplatform analysis that integrates copy-number alterations and RNA expression profiles are listed below the thin line. MNT, micronodular thymoma.

with thymomas have 3–4 times the risk of developing a synchronous or metachronous second solid or haematopoietic malignancy compared with controls {2415,769}. Whether this cancer susceptibility has a genetic or immunodeficiency-related basis is unknown {769}. Genetic overlap between type B3 thymomas and thymic squamous cell carcinoma suggests that the former can evolve into the latter {2877}.

Clinical features

Patients with thymoma are asymptomatic or present with symptoms attributable to the mass lesion, autoimmune diseases, or complications of thymoma-associated immunodeficiencies. Due to thymoma-derived autoreactive effector T cells {2876, 328} and defective regulatory T cells {2879}, autoimmune diseases develop preoperatively or postoperatively in 30–50% of thymoma patients, but rarely in thymic carcinomas {2409,1819}. Myasthenia gravis is the commonest autoimmune disease in patients with thymoma, and it occurs most often in the thymopoietically active type AB, B1, and B2 thymomas (25–40%) {1819}. Other organ-specific and systemic autoimmune diseases can occur with or without myasthenia gravis {3502} (see Table 5.02). Immunodeficiencies result from autoimmune B-cell and T-cell lymphopenia, hypogammaglobulinaemia (Good syndrome) {3467}, anti-cytokine autoantibodies {1469}, and thymoma-derived dysfunctional T cells {521}, and they often entail life-threatening infections {2026}. In children, autoimmune diseases are rarer than in adults, but the spectrum is similar {2293A,851}.

Imaging

Thymomas are usually well defined, round or lobulated, and homogeneous, although heterogeneity, calcifications, and cystic changes may be seen. CT can detect invasion into surrounding organs and distant metastases but cannot reliably distinguish between the WHO subtypes of thymoma. FDG PET-CT is not routinely used for thymic epithelial tumours, because some thymomas do not exhibit high FDG uptake. However, much higher FDG uptake is seen with type B3 thymomas and thymic carcinomas {396,1813}.

Table 5.02 Selected autoimmune and paraneoplastic disorders associated with thymoma; the 5 most commonly reported paraneoplastic syndromes are shown in bold {3502}

Category	Syndrome/disorder
Neuromuscular disorders	**Myasthenia gravis**
	Limbic encephalopathy
	Peripheral neuropathy
	Neuromyotonia (Isaacs syndrome)
	Stiff person syndrome
	Polymyositis
Haematological disorders	**Pure red cell aplasia**
	Pernicious anaemia
	Pancytopenia / aplastic anaemia
	Haemolytic anaemia
Collagen and autoimmune disorders	Systemic lupus erythematosus
	Rheumatoid arthritis
	Sjögren syndrome
	Scleroderma
	Graft-versus-host disease
	Interstitial pneumonitis
Immune deficiency disorders	**Good syndrome / hypogammaglobulinaemia**
	T-cell deficiency syndrome
Endocrine disorders	Autoimmune polyglandular syndrome
	Addison syndrome
	Thyroiditis
Dermatological disorders	**Lichen planus**
	Paraneoplastic pemphigus
	Chronic mucocutaneous candidiasis
	Alopecia areata
Miscellaneous disorders	Giant cell myocarditis
	Glomerulonephritis / nephrotic syndrome
	Ulcerative colitis
	Hypertrophic osteoarthropathy

Table 5.03 TNM classification and corresponding Masaoka–Koga stage

| TNM classification | | | Masaoka–Koga stage | Criteria {685,687} |
T	N	M		
1a	0	0	I	Grossly and microscopically completely encapsulated tumour
1a	0	0	IIa	Microscopic transcapsular invasion
1a	0	0	IIb	Macroscopic invasion into thymic or surrounding fatty tissue, or adherent to (but not breaking through) mediastinal pleura or pericardium
			III	Macroscopic invasion into neighbouring organs or mediastinal pleura
1b	0	0		- Mediastinal pleura
2	0	0		- Pericardium
3	0	0		- Lung, brachiocephalic vein, superior vena cava, phrenic nerve, chest wall, extra pericardial pulmonary artery or vein
4	0	0		- Aorta, arch vessels, intrapericardial pulmonary artery, myocardium, trachea, oesophagus
1–4	0	1a	IVa	Pleural or pericardial metastasis
			IVb	Lymphogenous or haematogenous metastasis
1–4	1	0–1b		- Perithymic lymph node involvement
1–4	2	0–1b		- Deep thoracic or cervical lymph node involvement
1–4	0–2	1b		- Pulmonary intraparenchymal or distant metastasis

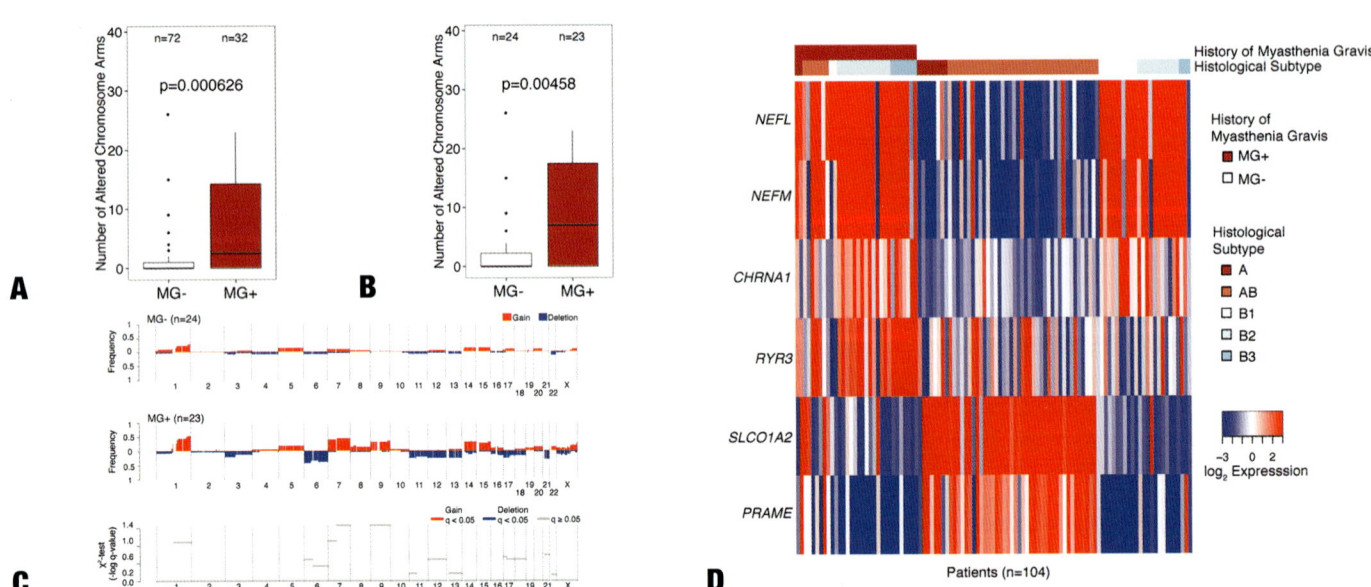

Fig. 5.03 Thymoma-associated autoimmunity. Patterns of somatic copy-number alterations and gene expression associated with myasthenia gravis (MG) {2409}.

Staging

All thymic epithelial tumours should be staged according to the TNM system {315,75,687} recently approved by the Union for International Cancer Control (UICC) / American Joint Committee on Cancer (AJCC) (see *TNM staging of epithelial tumours of the thymus*, p. 14) {315}). Optionally, the Masaoka–Koga system {685} may be used in parallel (see Table 5.03); its still-frequent use {2567} probably reflects the fact that current treatment guidelines (European Society for Medical Oncology [ESMO], Japan Lung Cancer Society [JLCS], National Comprehensive Cancer Network [NCCN]) {964,3405} take Masaoka–Koga stage information into account.

Histological classification: changes compared with the fourth edition

The histological classification, nomenclature, defining criteria, and reporting strategies for thymomas and thymic carcinomas are largely the same as in the fourth-edition WHO classification. This continuity is all the more justified given that molecular findings in the major thymoma types {2409,1632,2410} and rare entities {3176,2381,2380} strongly support the distinctiveness of the entities in the classification. However, two entities listed in the fourth edition are no longer included in this fifth edition: microscopic thymoma and sclerosing thymoma. The small thymic epithelial cell nests that characterize so-called

Table 5.04 Summary of genetic findings reported for the different WHO thymoma types and thymic squamous cell carcinoma (SCC); the recurrent loss of chromosome 6q25.2-q25.3 that is observed across the spectrum of thymomas and in thymic SCC and the hotspot mutation of the *GTF2I* gene are presented in bold; the microRNA data are given for comparison and are not recommended for diagnostic use at present

WHO type	Chromosomal gains	Chromosomal losses	Other mutations	MicroRNAs	Reference(s)
Type A thymoma		2, 4, 6p21, 6p25, 6q, **6q25.2-q25.3**, 13	***GTF2I* p.L424H (82–100%)** Activating *HRAS* mutation t(15;22)(p11;q11)	Expression of miR-34b, miR-34c, miR-130a, and miR-195 Overexpression of C19MC[a] Overexpression of C14MC[b]	{2334,2337,808,2409,965, 606,3479,1253,774}
Type AB thymoma		2, 4, 5q21-q22, 6p21, 6p25, **6q25.2-q25**, 7p15.3, 8p, 13q14.3, 16q, 18	***GTF2I* p.L424H (71–79%)** *HRAS* or *NRAS* mutation (rare) Ring chromosome 6 XX,+del(X)(q24),+i(5p),+?del(7)(q22),der(11)t(1;11)(q23;q25),t(11;?)(p15;?),-18,+r 46,XX,del(6)(p22p25) 46,XY,r(6),der(21)t(6;21)(p25;q22)	Overexpression of C19MC[a]	{2334,2337,808,2409,1253, 1540,1932,3137,1253}
Type B1 thymoma[c]	9q	1p, 2q, 3q, 4, 5, 6q, 8, 13, 18	***GTF2I* p.L424H (0–32%)**		{2334,808,2409,1629}
Type B2 thymoma	1q	1p, 3p, 6p25, **6q25.2-q25.3**	***GTF2I* p.L424H (0–22%)** Activating *KRAS* mutation (rare) *NRAS* mutation (rare) *TP53* mutation (rare) 44,XY,+X,inv(2)(p25q13),del(6)(q15),-8,-16,-17 57,X,2Y,+i(1)(q10),+add(4)(q12),+7,+8,+9,+14,+15, +16,der(17)t(9;17)(q13;p13),+20,+22 *KMT2A-MAML2* gene fusion		{2334,2337,808,2409,2321, 1540,2815,1253,965,1824A}
Type B3 thymoma	1q, 4[d], 5, 7, 8, 9q, 17q[d], X	3p, 6, 6p25, **6q25.2-q25.3**, 9p, 11q42.-qter, 13q, 16q, 17p	***GTF2I* p.L424H (10–21%)** *TP53* mutation (rare) *BCL2* copy-number gains (18q21.33) *CDKN2A/B* copy-number losses (9p21.3) Translocation t(11;X) *KMT2A-MAML2* gene fusion		{2334,2337,808,2409,2321, 2336,2335,3479,1253,965, 1824A}
Metaplastic thymoma			*YAP1-MAML2* gene fusion		{3176}
Thymic SCC	1q, 4, 5, 7, 8, 9q, 12, 15, 17q, 18, 20	3p, 6, 6p25, **6q25.2-q25.3**, 9p, 13q, 14, 16q, 17p	***GTF2I* p.L424H (0–8%)** Activating *KIT* mutation (2–11%) Activating *KRAS* mutation (rare) *NRAS* mutation (rare) *TP53* mutation Mutations in epigenetic regulatory genes (*BAP1, ASXL1, SETD2, SMARCA4, TET2, DNMT3A, WT1*) *BCL2* copy-number gains (18q21.33) *CDKN2A/B* copy-number losses (9p21.3) 52,XY,+4,+5,+8,+12,+16,der(16)t(1;16)(q12;q12.1) x2,+17	Expression of miR-21, miR-9-3, and miR-375	{2334,808,2409,2321,2875, 2335,3479,1253,2814,965, 774,3221}

[a]MicroRNA cluster on chromosome 19q13.42. [b]MicroRNA cluster on chromosome 14q32. [c]Only one available study. [d]Single cases {965,3479}.

microscopic thymoma are unlikely to be neoplastic {495}, and their role as precursors of thymomas could not be proved despite their description decades ago {2529}. Sclerosing thymoma does not appear to be a distinctive form of thymoma, but rather represents sclerotic change occurring in various types of conventional thymoma {1555,1556,1970}.

Chapter 5

Table 5.05 Routine immunohistochemical markers that are helpful for distinguishing (1) thymoma types from each other, (2) thymomas from thymic carcinomas, and (3) thymic carcinomas from non-thymic carcinomas, as well as special antibodies with differential labelling of cortical and medullary thymic epithelial cells (TECs) of the normal thymus and characteristic staining patterns in thymoma types {2874}

Marker	Antibody/clone	Reactivity
Conventional antibody targets		
Cytokeratins	AE1/AE3, MNF116, etc.	Pancytokeratin marker, positive in cortical and medullary TECs
CK19	RCK108	Cortical and medullary TECs
CK10	DE-K10	Terminally mature medullary TECs, Hassall corpuscles, squamous epithelial cells
		Focally positive in type B thymoma and thymic squamous cell carcinoma
		Negative in type A and AB thymomas
CK20	Ks20.8	Negative in normal and neoplastic TECs
		May be positive in thymic enteric-type adenocarcinoma (differential diagnosis: metastases to the mediastinum)
p40 or p63	11F12.1 (p40); SFI-6 (p63)	Cortical and medullary TECs
		Positive in thymomas, thymic carcinomas, and other carcinomas with squamous or myoepithelial differentiation
		Mediastinal large B-cell lymphoma is frequently p63-positive but p40-negative[a]
CD5	4C7	T cells
		Epithelial cells in ~70% of thymic squamous cell carcinomas and variably positive in thymic (and other) adenocarcinomas
CD20	L26	B cells
		Epithelial cells in ~50% of type A and AB thymomas
KIT (CD117)	Polyclonal (A4502)	Epithelial cells in ~80% of thymic squamous cell carcinomas
TdT	SEN28, polyclonal, etc.	Immature T cells in the normal thymic cortex
		Immature T cells in most thymomas
		T-lymphoblastic lymphoma
Desmin	D33	Myoid cells of thymic medulla, type B1 thymoma, rare type B2 and B3 thymomas and thymic carcinomas
Ki-67	MIB1, polyclonal, etc.	Any proliferating cells: immature T cells in normal thymic cortex, most thymomas, T-lymphoblastic lymphoma, etc.
Compartment-specific antibody targets		
Beta5t		Cortical TECs
PRSS16	Polyclonal (HPA017743)	Cortical TECs
Cathepsin V	BV55-1	Cortical TECs
Claudin-4	3E2C1	Subset of medullary TECs
CD40	11E9	Subset of medullary TECs
AIRE	ID326	Subset of medullary TECs
Involucrin	Polyclonal	Like CK10 but focally positive in type AB thymoma

[a]{501,1194}.

Nomenclature of heterogeneous and anaplastic tumours

For thymomas that exhibit more than one histological pattern, the diagnosis should list all observed histological types, starting with the predominant component, and minor components should be quantified in 10% increments {1818}. An example is "thymoma, with type B2 (80%) and type B3 (20%) components". This rule does not apply to type AB thymoma, because the diagnosis remains the same irrespective of the proportions of type A and type B–like components in the tumour.

If a heterogeneous tumour includes a thymic carcinoma component of any size along with one or more thymoma components, the diagnosis should be "thymic carcinoma" (with the percentage and histological type specified), followed by a list of the thymoma component(s) in the order of their relative proportions in the whole tumour. For further details, see *Thymic carcinoma: Introduction* (p. 351).

Anaplasia is a rare feature of unknown significance in otherwise conventional thymomas {14}; this feature alone should not lead to a diagnosis of thymic carcinoma.

Molecular classification

Multiomics analyses reveal three molecular thymoma subtypes that are very different from thymic carcinomas: an A-like subtype that overlaps with an AB-like subtype, and a distinct B-like subtype {2409}. These molecular subtypes are correlated with WHO tumour type, survival, and prevalence of myasthenia gravis {2409,1632,2334}. Thymomas show the lowest load of somatic mutations among adult cancers, although they show widespread copy-number variations that increase from type A and AB through B1 and B2 thymomas to B3 thymomas and thymic carcinomas {2409,2334,965,1253}. Rare cases of thymoma and thymic carcinoma exhibit microsatellite instability and a high mutation burden {2409,1253}.

The commonest recurrent genetic alteration in thymomas (in as many as 38% of cases) is missense mutation *GTF2I* p.L424H, which shows a significant association with enriched pathways affecting apoptosis, cell-cycle control, DNA damage response, and receptor tyrosine kinase signalling {2409}. This mutation has so far not been observed in other tumour types, is largely restricted to type A and AB thymomas, and is associated with a decreased prevalence of myasthenia gravis and a favourable prognosis {2409,1632,2334}. Mutation of the *HRAS* gene is also largely restricted to type A and AB thymomas, while *NRAS* and *TP53* mutations are much commoner in type B2 and B3 thymomas and thymic carcinomas. In contrast, genetic losses at 6q25.2-p25.3, which harbours the *FOXC1* tumour suppressor gene {2337}, occur across the whole spectrum of thymomas and thymic carcinomas {1253}. No targetable mutations (e.g. in the *EGFR* or *KIT* gene) have been detected in thymomas. Aneuploidy and intratumoural overexpression of genes sharing sequence similarity with autoimmune targets, including *CHRNA1*, *RYR3*, and *NEFM*, are more prevalent in thymomas from myasthenic patients {2409}. Overexpression of a large microRNA cluster on chromosome 19q13.42 is common and restricted to type A and AB thymomas {2410} (see Table 5.04, p. 323).

Diagnostic approaches: immunohistochemistry and molecular studies

Most thymic epithelial tumours do not require immunohistochemical or molecular studies for diagnosis. However, ancillary tests may be required for the distinction of type A thymomas from other spindle cell tumours; for the differential between type B1 thymoma and lymphoblastic lymphoma; or for the separation of atypical type A thymomas from type B3 thymomas with spindly cells, thymic squamous cell carcinomas, or TNETs {3273}. Immunostaining to determine the quantity of immature T cells in the tumour may also be required to distinguish some type AB thymomas from type A thymomas. Useful immunohistochemical and molecular markers are listed in Table 5.05.

Prognosis and predictive markers

Due to their potential for invasion and metastasis, all thymoma types are considered potentially malignant. Overall survival rates at 10 years range from 80–100% in type A, AB, and B1 thymomas, to 60–80% in type B2 and B3 thymomas {3252}, to 40% in thymic carcinomas and in TNETs {835}.

Most studies have shown the Masaoka–Koga stage {685,1498} to be the most relevant prognostic factor for overall survival in thymomas {1282,3252,2873} and thymic carcinomas {33} but not in TNETs {834}. TNM-based pathological staging also has significant prognostic value {687,2100,1509}, but tumour size does not {2100}. On multivariate analysis, WHO thymoma type is an independent prognostic marker of recurrence-free survival {2185,3252} but not overall survival {1282,3252}. Thymic carcinoma types are of no prognostic relevance {33}.

In regard to molecular markers, the *GTF2I* p.L424H mutation is associated with favourable disease-free and overall survival {1632,2334}, while high tumour mutation burden, chromosomal instability, and presence of *TP53* mutations are associated with unfavourable outcome {1632,3221,1670}. Whether high PDL1 expression is associated with poorer survival in thymoma patients is controversial {2812,1053,3257,3409}. Other prognostic biomarkers under evaluation for thymic epithelial tumours include expression of SOX2 and CAIX (CA9), as well as the methylation status of *KSR1*, *ELF3*, *IL1RN*, and *RAG1* {1627,2168, 1669}. Attempts have been made to develop gene signatures to predict survival and determine the risk of developing metastasis in patients with thymoma {1668,979}.

In terms of treatment-related factors, complete resection is of prognostic relevance in thymomas {1282,3252,2873}, thymic carcinomas {33}, and TNETs {834}. Adjuvant radiotherapy is a favourable prognostic factor in advanced-stage thymomas {1282,2488} and thymic carcinomas {33}. In contrast to other paraneoplastic autoimmune diseases, myasthenia gravis is of no adverse prognostic value or may even have a favourable prognostic value, probably due to earlier tumour detection {3502}.

Tissue-based predictive markers to guide targeted therapies have not been identified in thymic epithelial tumours, with the possible exception of the rare occurrence of *KIT* mutations predicting responses to KIT inhibitors in thymic carcinomas {2660}. PDL1 and PD1 are strongly expressed in most thymomas and somewhat less in thymic carcinomas {3257,2225,2554,2812, 1244}, but they poorly predict response to immune checkpoint inhibitors {2414,942}.

Type A thymoma
(including atypical subtype)

Ströbel P
Badve S
Chan JKC
Girard N
Matsuno Y
Nonaka D

Definition

Type A thymoma is a thymic epithelial neoplasm with variable growth patterns, composed of usually bland spindle/oval tumour cells with few or no admixed immature lymphocytes.

ICD-O coding

8580/3 Thymoma, NOS
8581/3 Thymoma, type A

ICD-11 coding

2C27.2 & XH6WN9 Malignant thymoma & Thymoma, type A

Related terminology

Not recommended: spindle cell thymoma.

Subtype(s)

Atypical type A thymoma

Localization

Type A thymoma is localized in the anterior (prevascular) mediastinum; ectopic occurrence is rare.

Clinical features

About 17–26% of patients with type A thymomas present with myasthenia gravis {679,1287,427,1672,3252}. Others present with symptoms related to the mass lesion or are incidentally discovered to have a mediastinal tumour on imaging examination. Association with pure red cell aplasia may occur, but is not restricted to type A thymoma {1556}.

Epidemiology

Type A thymoma is one of the rarer thymoma subtypes. In a review of > 2400 thymomas reported in multiple international studies, type A thymomas account for 11.5% (range: 3.1–26.2%) of all thymomas {679,1802,1040,1797,1798,628}. The patients' ages range from 8 to 88 years (average: 64 years) {679,1672}, being higher than those of patients with other thymomas (average: 50 years) {472,1561}. A slight female preponderance has been reported in most studies {679,1287}.

Etiology

The etiology of type A thymomas is unknown. A minor role of genetic risk factors appears possible given the rare occurrence of thymomas (including type A thymoma) with familial background {2553,297,3010}.

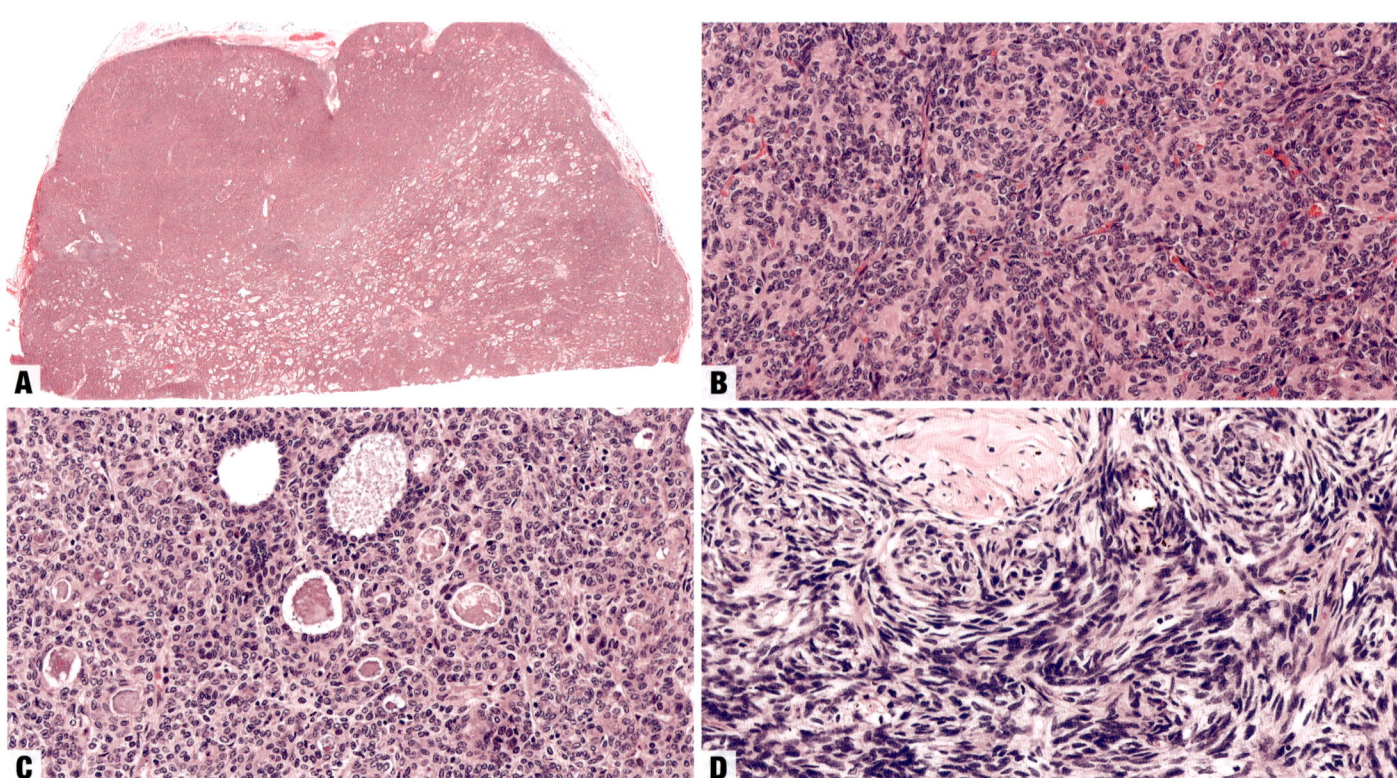

Fig. 5.04 Type A thymoma. **A** Type A thymomas are usually well circumscribed with pushing borders and vague lobular growth. **B** This example shows a rosetting pattern. **C** This example comprises sheets of uniform polygonal cells interspersed with glandular structures and microcysts. **D** This example shows spindle cells forming intersecting fascicles.

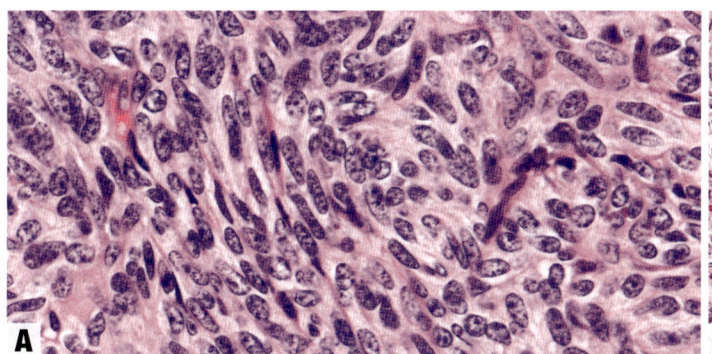
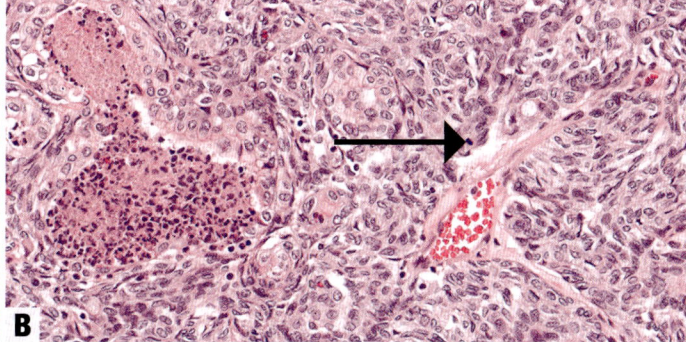

Fig. 5.05 Type A thymoma. **A** Type A thymoma ("typical"). Conventional type A thymoma shows slender, elongated nuclei with granular chromatin and small nucleoli. There are usually no or very few mitoses. **B** Type A thymoma (atypical). Atypical type A thymoma is characterized by increased cellularity, with nuclear crowding, more-prominent nucleoli, necrosis, and increased mitoses (arrow).

Pathogenesis

An origin of type A thymomas from a putative thymic epithelial cell precursor with minimal potential for corticomedullary differentiation has been proposed {2874}. In an unsupervised cluster analysis of five data platforms, type A thymomas constituted a distinct subtype related (but not identical) to type AB thymomas {2409}. Most type A thymomas harbour few genetic alterations {3479,1253,965,2409}, often involving chromosome 6q25.2 {1253}. Metastatic cases have a tendency to show slightly higher genetic instability than localized tumours {338}. Virtually 100% of type A thymomas, including metastatic cases, show mutations of *GTF2I* (p.L424H, which is considered a founder mutation) {2334,2409}. GTF2I is thought to be a positive regulator of cell morphogenesis, receptor tyrosine kinase signalling, retinoic acid receptors, neuronal processes, and WNT and sonic hedgehog signalling, and a negative regulator of apoptosis, cell cycle, DNA damage response, hormone receptor signalling, breast hormone signalling, RAS/MAPK, receptor tyrosine kinase, and TSC/mTOR signalling pathways {2409}. *HRAS* mutations are common (80%) in type A and rare in other types of thymoma {2409}. Overexpression of a large microRNA cluster on chromosome 19q13.42 {2410}, which is thought to enhance PI3K/AKT/mTOR signalling, is another characteristic feature of type A thymomas.

Macroscopic appearance

Type A thymoma is generally well circumscribed or encapsulated. The cut surface is homogeneous and light tan to white, with vague lobulation and occasionally focal cystic change. Average tumour size is 72 mm {1287,2249}.

Histopathology

The tumours are typically surrounded by a complete or incomplete fibrous capsule and may display coarse lobulation with thick fibrous bands. Microcystic change can occur but is often more pronounced in subcapsular areas. The tumours commonly show a fascicular, storiform, or haemangiopericytoma-like growth pattern {2249}. Other characteristic growth patterns include rosettes with or without a central lumen, glandular or glomeruloid structures, haemangioma-like papillary projections in cystic spaces, and meningioma-like whorls {1561,2024,2249, 1357}. Multiple patterns can occur in the same tumour. Perivascular spaces are less commonly seen than in other types of thymoma {436}. Hassall corpuscles are absent. The tumour cells are spindly and/or oval-shaped, with bland nuclei, finely dispersed "powdery" chromatin, and inconspicuous nucleoli. In some cases, subpopulations of tumour cells are polygonal, with uniform round nuclei exhibiting a similar chromatin pattern. Mitotic activity is low, with counts usually < 4 mitoses/2 mm². There should be no or only very few ("easily countable") immature lymphocytes throughout. Tumours with any lymphocyte-dense area ("not countable") or > 10% areas with moderate ("countable") infiltrate of TdT-positive T cells should be classified as type AB thymomas.

Immunohistochemistry

The tumour cells are strongly positive for AE1-defined acidic keratins and p63/p40 {501,724} and negative for AE3-defined basic keratins. They are always negative for CK20 {1558}. In general, keratin expression is stronger in the cystic and glandular structures. EMA is variably and only focally expressed. FOXN1 and CD205 are positive {3270,2132}, while CD5 and KIT (CD117) are negative {1163,2048}. A useful and frequent feature is aberrant expression of CD20 in the neoplastic epithelial cells, although the staining is often focal and may be missed in small biopsies. In very rare cases, single desmin-positive myoid cells may be seen. TdT-positive immature T cells may be completely absent or account for only a minority of CD3-positive T cells. CD20-positive B cells are usually absent.

Atypical type A thymoma

Rare type A thymomas can display some degree of atypia, such as hypercellularity, increased mitotic counts, and particularly focal necrosis. According to several published case series {2136,3177,1006,1968,338,1002}, these atypical features (perhaps with the exception of tumour necrosis) {3177,1006} are not associated with higher numbers of chromosomal alterations {338} or a more aggressive behaviour than conventional type A thymomas, and metastases can occur in the absence of such "atypical" histological features. Single atypical type A thymomas with *GTF2I* mutations are on record {1002}.

Differential diagnosis

The diagnosis of type A thymoma can be problematic in needle biopsies. As a spindle cell neoplasm in the mediastinum, its most important differential diagnoses are solitary fibrous tumour (cytokeratin–, STAT6+, CD34+) and synovial sarcoma (cytokeratin+/–, SS18-SSX+).

Cytology

Reliable classification of thymomas is generally not possible in cytological specimens {57,498,3186}. Smears of type A thymoma may contain only epithelial cells and thus can mimic other spindle cell lesions such as carcinoid, low-grade sarcoma, mesothelioma, and stromal cells in lymphoma {3186,3465}. The epithelial cells do not show vesicular nuclei and have inconspicuous nucleoli. Crush artefacts in clusters were reported to be less abundant than in type AB and type B thymomas {2581}.

Diagnostic molecular pathology

GTF2I mutations are highly characteristic, although not specific, for type A thymomas and may be helpful in problematic cases.

Essential and desirable diagnostic criteria

Essential:
- A thymic epithelial tumour with bland spindle and oval, and rarely polygonal, epithelial cells with a fascicular, storiform, or haemangiopericytomatous growth pattern
- Most cases lack areas of necrosis and have a low mitotic count and a low Ki-67 index
- Atypical type A thymomas may have higher mitotic count and focal necrosis

Desirable:
- Strong expression of epithelial markers (e.g. p63/p40)
- Paucity or absence of immature TdT-positive T cells throughout the tumour

Staging

Staging should follow the Union for International Cancer Control (UICC) TNM system {315,687}. However, because most published series and clinical stratification schemes have been based on the Masaoka–Koga system {685}, many experts still use and provide the Masaoka–Koga stage as additional information in their reports.

Most type A thymomas were diagnosed as limited disease, i.e. TNM stage I (corresponding to Masaoka stages I and II), in the International Thymic Malignancy Interest Group (ITMIG) cohort {3252} and an independent meta-analysis (see Table 5.01, p. 320).

Prognosis and prediction

The overall survival rate of patients with type A thymoma is close to 100% at 5 years and 10 years {2184,2873}, even though approximately 20% of these patients have Masaoka stage II or III tumours. Atypical cases tend to be at a higher stage at presentation {1006}.

In the ITMIG cohort, the overall survival rates of patients with R0-resected type A thymoma at 5 years and 10 years were 90% and 80%, respectively. The risk of recurrence is low if the tumour can be completely surgically removed {1561,2184, 2873}. Cases with local recurrences or distant metastases have been documented {1498,2249,1287}. The local recurrence rate after complete resection is in the range of 5–10% after 5 and 10 years {3252}. The association with myasthenia gravis has no significant effect on prognosis {436,2184,2406}.

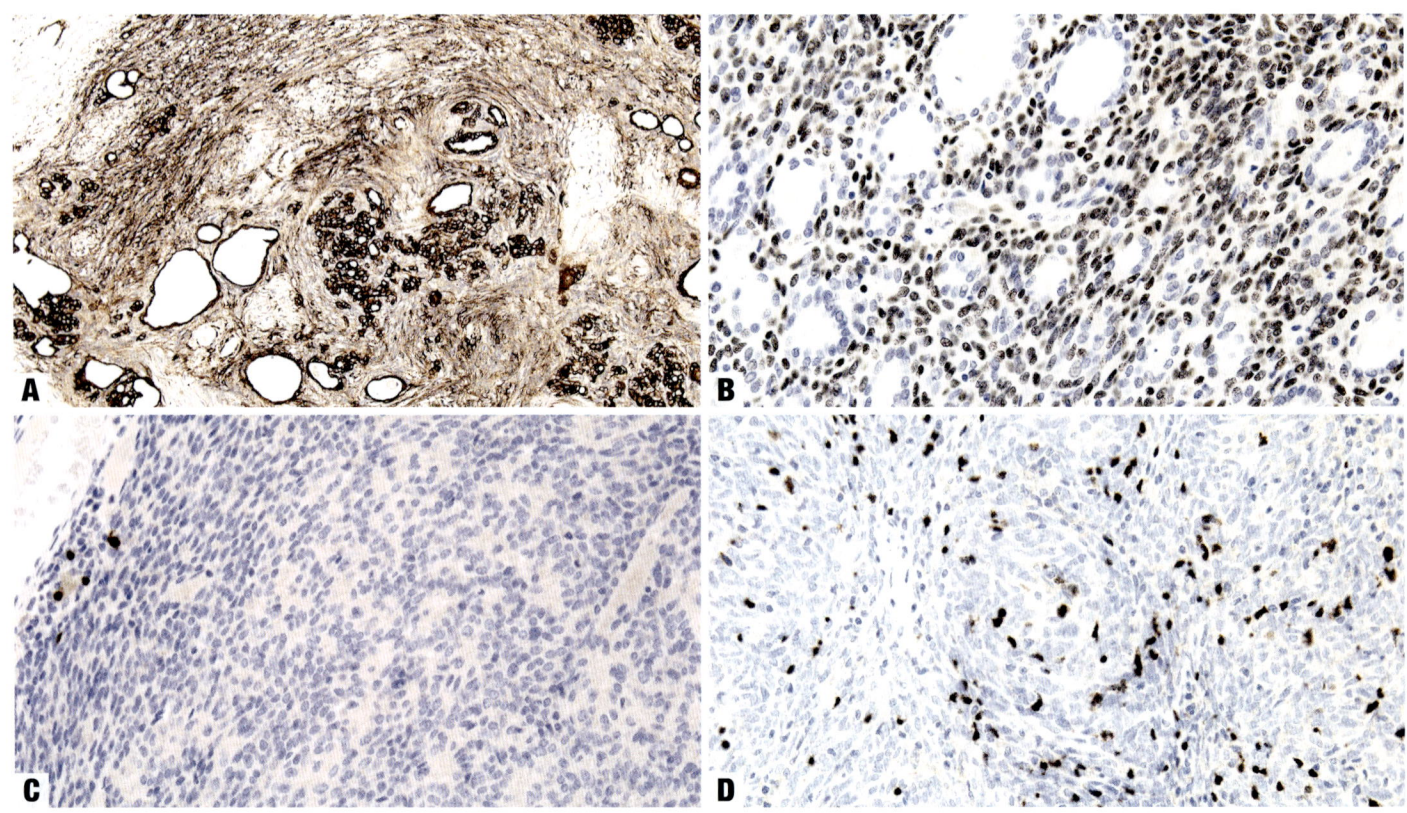

Fig. 5.06 Immunohistochemistry of type A thymoma. **A** Keratin stain highlights the glandular structures and cysts intensely, but it is also positive in most of the spindle cell areas. **B** Strong expression of p63 throughout is characteristic of type A thymoma. Note that the cells lining glandular structures are negative in this example. **C** There are usually no or only very few TdT-positive immature T cells in type A thymoma. **D** Moderate numbers of TdT-positive cells in as much as 10% of the tumour area are compatible with type A thymoma. Any lymphocyte-dense focus would result in a diagnosis of type AB thymoma.

Type AB thymoma

Ströbel P
Badve S
Chan JKC
Girard N
Matsuno Y
Nonaka D

Definition

Type AB thymoma is a thymic epithelial neoplasm composed of variable proportions a lymphocyte-poor spindle cell (type A) component and a lymphocyte-rich (type B–like) component with a significant population of immature T cells.

ICD-O coding

8582/3 Thymoma, type AB

ICD-11 coding

2C27.2 & XH0JH0 Malignant thymoma & Thymoma, type AB

Related terminology

Not recommended: mixed thymoma.

Subtype(s)

None

Localization

Type AB thymoma is localized in the anterior (prevascular) mediastinum.

Clinical features

Like other thymomas, type AB thymomas are frequently associated with a variety of paraneoplastic autoimmune disorders {1478,1819}, among which myasthenia gravis is by far the most frequent. Approximately 18–25% of type AB thymomas are associated with myasthenia gravis {3252}. Paraneoplastic pure red cell aplasia has also been reported {1556}. Other patients present with symptoms related to the mass lesion, or are incidentally discovered to have a mediastinal tumour on imaging examination. The imaging features of type AB thymoma have not been studied individually, but they seem to overlap with those of the other thymoma subtypes {2527}.

Epidemiology

Type AB thymoma is one of the most common thymoma subtypes and accounts for about 25% (range: 15–43%) of cases

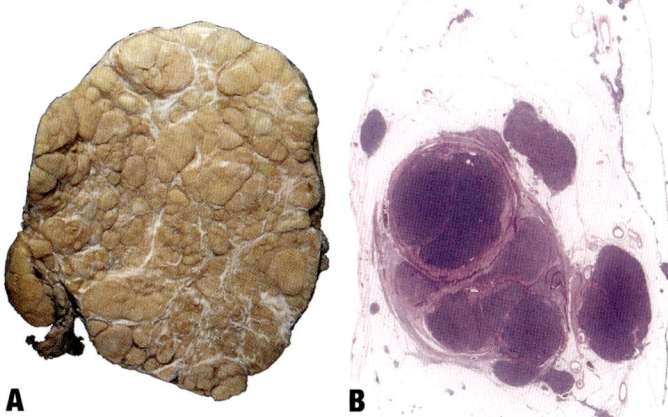

Fig. 5.07 Type AB thymoma. **A** Macroscopy shows a well-circumscribed tumour with prominent multiple nodules separated by white septa. **B** The low-power scan of a histological slide shows a small type AB thymoma with infiltration of the mediastinal fat and small thymic remnants at the margin on the right side. The dark blue nodules represent a lymphocyte-rich type B–like component, separated by pale spindle cell areas.

in most studies {679,1802,1040,1797,1798,628,3252}. The mean age at disease onset is 57 years (range: 11–89 years), with a slight female predominance {679,1287,427,1672}.

Etiology

Unknown

Pathogenesis

A putative thymic epithelial cell precursor with the potential for bilineage, corticomedullary differentiation and restricted terminal medullary maturation has been proposed as the cell of origin {2874}. An unsupervised cluster analysis of five data platforms suggested that type AB thymomas are related (but not identical) to type A thymomas {2409}. The most frequent genetic alterations in type AB thymoma overlap with those observed in type A thymoma but are more frequent and more complex. These shared alterations include losses of genetic

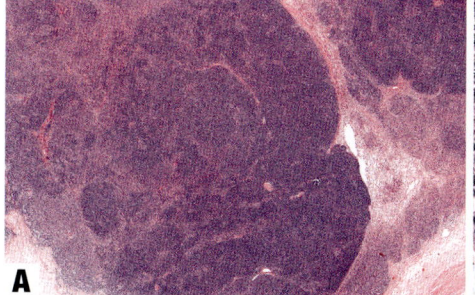 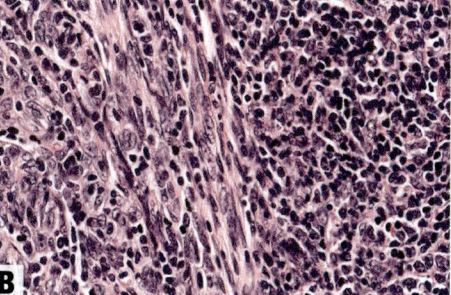 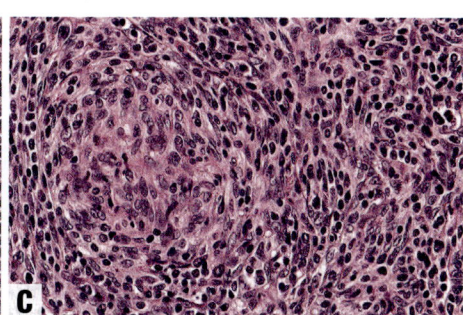

Fig. 5.08 Type AB thymoma. **A** Low magnification shows a nodular tumour with darker lymphocyte-rich and lighter lymphocyte-poor areas. **B** Higher magnification shows sharp transition between a lymphocyte-rich and a lymphocyte-poor area with spindle cell morphology of the epithelial cells. **C** This example shows more-diffuse distribution of lymphocytes over a background of spindle cells with focal nodules and rosetting.

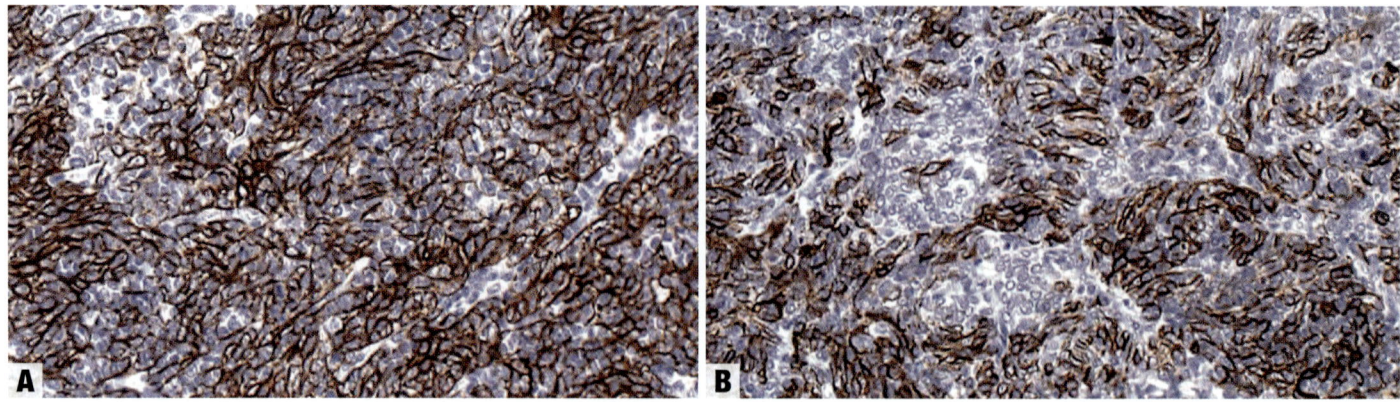

Fig. 5.09 Type AB thymoma. **A** CK19 immunostain highlights dense meshworks of epithelial cells. **B** Focal CD20 immunostaining in the neoplastic epithelium is a frequent observation in type A and AB thymomas.

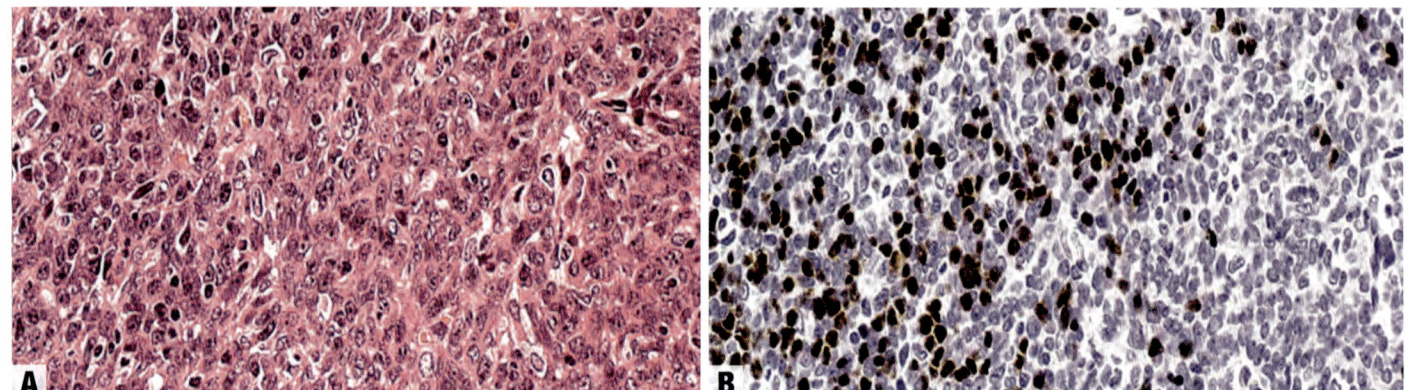

Fig. 5.10 Type AB thymoma. **A** H&E section shows spindle cell tumour with a moderate number of lymphocytes. **B** TdT immunostaining highlights a moderate number of scattered immature T cells. If such areas occupy > 10% of the investigated tumour material, this tumour would qualify as type AB thymoma.

material on chromosomes 2, 4, 6q25.2-q25.3, and 13 {1629, 981}. Moreover, type A and AB thymomas share frequent mutation of *GTF2I* (p.L424H) {2334,2409}, as well as overexpression of a microRNA cluster on chromosome 19q13.42 {2410}, which is thought to enhance PI3K/AKT/mTOR signalling.

Macroscopic appearance

Type AB thymomas are usually encapsulated. The cut surface is firm and shows multiple tan-coloured nodules of various sizes separated by white fibrous bands. The average tumour size is 70–80 mm.

Histopathology

Type AB thymomas are usually well demarcated and often encapsulated. They show a lobulated growth pattern and are composed of a highly variable mixture of a lymphocyte-poor type A component and a type B–like lymphocyte-rich component. These components can either form discrete, separate lobules or be intricately intermingled {2024}. All the diverse histological features of type A thymoma can be seen in the type A component. In addition, the type A component may comprise spindle cell fascicles that course around and among lymphocyte-rich nodules (type B–like component) like cellular fibrous septa. The type B–like areas are different from type B1, B2, or B3 thymoma. The tumour cells are small and oval, plump spindly, or polygonal in shape, with round to oval pale-staining

nuclei showing dispersed chromatin and inconspicuous nucleoli {1558,2024}. The large, vesicular nuclei with distinct nucleoli that are characteristic of the neoplastic cells in type B2 thymoma are only rarely seen {1558}. Medullary islands are rare and Hassall corpuscles are generally absent.

Immunohistochemistry

Immunostaining for pancytokeratin, CK19, and p63/p40 {724} highlights the dense and compact epithelial component, especially in the lymphocyte-rich areas. The elongated spindle cells are often strongly positive for vimentin and EMA, while weakly to moderately positive for cytokeratins (except the glandular structures, which are strongly positive). Tumour cells with aberrant expression of CD20 can be seen in both type A and type B–like areas. CD20-positive B cells and desmin-positive myoid cells are usually absent. The associated lymphocytes are mainly TdT-positive immature CD3-positive T cells. There is no epithelial expression of CD5. The Ki-67 proliferation index is usually low in the neoplastic epithelium, but interpretation can be difficult due to a high number of admixed proliferating immature T cells.

Differential diagnoses

Type A thymoma differs from AB thymoma in that it lacks the lymphocyte-rich component. Any thymoma that looks like a type A thymoma but with any lymphocyte-dense area (TdT-positive

T cells "impossible to count") or with > 10% area showing moderate infiltrate of TdT-positive T cells ("difficult to count") should be classified as type AB thymoma.

Micronodular thymoma with lymphoid hyperplasia shows segregation of the lymphocyte-poor epithelial nodules from a lymphocyte-rich stroma lacking epithelium. It also features large numbers of B cells.

Cytology

The few published descriptions state that the epithelial cells lack vesicular nuclei, show inconspicuous nucleoli and more prominent crush artefacts in cell clusters than type A thymoma and thymic carcinoma, and usually contain few lymphocytes {2581}.

Diagnostic molecular pathology

Molecular tests are not required for the diagnosis. In exceptional cases, when the clinical or anatomical situation is unusual (e.g. ectopic thymoma) {3515}, the demonstration of a *GTF2I* p.L424H mutation would strongly support the diagnosis.

Essential and desirable diagnostic criteria

Essential:

- A thymic tumour with a lobulated growth pattern
- Admixed spindle cell–predominant lymphocyte-poor component (type A) and lymphocyte-rich component (type B)
- Bland spindle, oval, and focally polygonal thymic epithelial cells and focal or diffuse abundance of immature T cells
- In type A tumours with focal lymphocytic stroma in which lymphocytes are difficult to count, ≥ 10% area showing infiltrate of TdT-positive T cells should be classified as type AB thymoma

Desirable:

- TdT immunostaining to assess TdT-positive cell density for differential diagnosis with type A thymoma

Staging

Staging should follow the Union for International Cancer Control (UICC) TNM system {315,687}. However, because most published series and clinical stratification schemes have been based on the Masaoka–Koga system {685}, many experts still use and provide the Masaoka–Koga stage as additional information in their reports.

In the International Thymic Malignancy Interest Group (ITMIG) cohort {3252} and an independent meta-analysis (see Table 5.01, p. 320), > 90% of type AB thymomas are in TNM stage I (corresponding to Masaoka–Koga stages I and II).

Prognosis and prediction

The overall survival rate is 80–100% at 5 years and 10 years {2184,472,2873}. Most type AB thymomas can be cured by radical surgery {1561,472,2873}. Recurrence and metastasis are rare {1498,2249} but do occur {1287}, justifying long-term clinical monitoring. The presence or absence of paraneoplastic myasthenia gravis has no major effect on prognosis {436, 2184,2406}. Limited data are available regarding platinum-based chemotherapy or radiosensitivity given the limited number of patients with advanced disease requiring adjuvant treatment.

Type B1 thymoma

Marx A
Jain D
Marchevsky AM
Marino M
Nicholson AG
Yang WI

Definition

Type B1 thymoma is a thymic epithelial tumour that recapitulates the cytoarchitectural features of the non-involuted normal thymic cortex, accompanied by regions of medullary differentiation.

ICD-O coding

8583/3 Thymoma, type B1

ICD-11 coding

2C27.2 & XH66U8 Malignant thymoma & Thymoma, type B1

Related terminology

Not recommended: organoid thymoma; predominantly cortical thymoma; lymphocytic thymoma.

Subtype(s)

None

Localization

Type B1 thymoma is typically localized in the anterior (prevascular) mediastinum; ectopic occurrence is commonest in the neck, followed by lung, pleura, thyroid, and pericardium {3274}.

Clinical features

Myasthenia gravis is the first presentation in 40% of patients. Pure red cell aplasia, hypogammaglobulinaemia (Good syndrome), or other autoimmune diseases occur alone or in combination with myasthenia gravis in 5% each {679,427,1672,3252}. Symptoms attributable to the mass lesion are uncommon. A third of patients are asymptomatic {686}. The imaging features of type B1 thymoma overlap with those of other thymoma types {2527}.

Epidemiology

In the International Thymic Malignancy Interest Group (ITMIG) cohort {3252} and an independent meta-analysis (see Table 5.01, p. 320), type B1 thymoma accounts for 17% of thymomas. It is the commonest type of thymoma in children {2837, 394}. The median age is 53 years (range: 4–83 years), and females predominate slightly {3252,679}.

Etiology

Unknown

Pathogenesis

A putative thymic epithelial cell precursor with the potential for bilineage, near-normal cortical and medullary maturation has been proposed as the cell of origin {2874}. An unsupervised cluster analysis of five genomic data platforms suggests that type B1 thymomas are related to B2 and B3 thymomas {2409}.

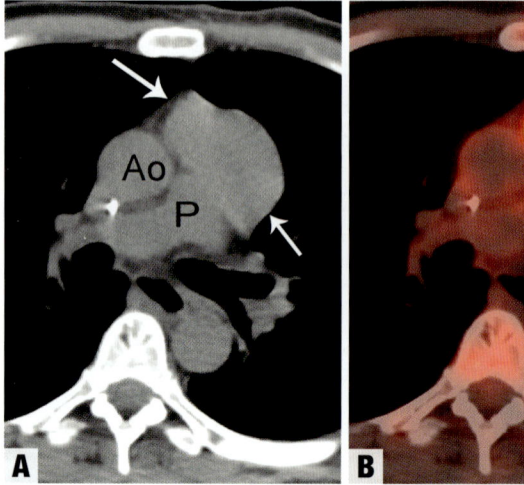

Fig. 5.11 Type B1 thymoma. **A** CT of type B1 thymoma. Unenhanced chest CT of a type B1 thymoma shows a homogeneous mass (arrows) separated by a fat plane from the aorta (Ao) but not from the main pulmonary artery (P). At surgery, a completely encapsulated stage I thymoma was seen with no adjacent fat involvement. Imaging is not accurate in determining adjacent fat involvement. **B** Fused PET-CT of type B1 thymoma. FDG PET-CT of this type B1 thymoma shows increased FDG uptake, above the mediastinal background activity, with a maximum standardized uptake value of 4.0.

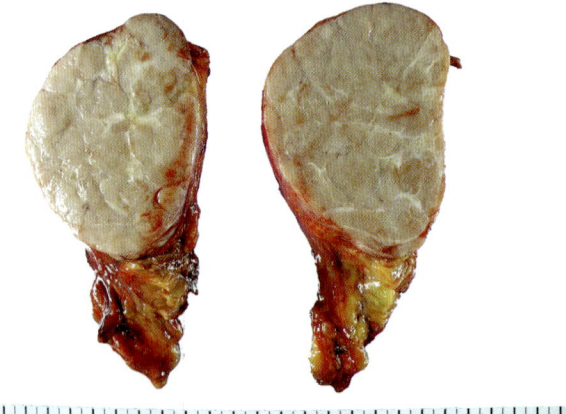

Fig. 5.12 Type B1 thymoma. Cut surface of type B1 thymoma specimen showing typical encapsulation and large lobules delineated by delicate fibrous septa.

Due to the low number of neoplastic epithelial cells among an overwhelming number of non-neoplastic thymocytes, molecular studies of type B1 thymomas have been difficult to perform. The reported genetic alterations are losses of genetic material on chromosomes 1p, 2q, 3q, 4, 5, 6q, 8, 13, and 18 and gain on 9q {1629}. No losses or gains of chromosomal arms were detected in The Cancer Genome Atlas (TCGA) series {2409}. Hotspot

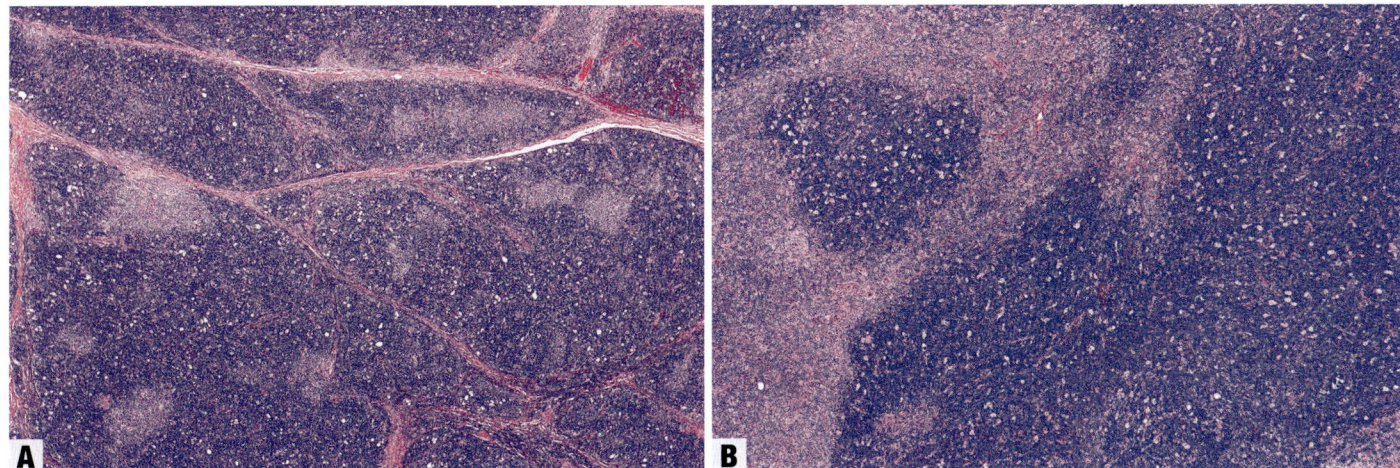

Fig. 5.13 Type B1 thymoma. **A** The tumour typically shows jigsaw puzzle–like lobulation. Pale-staining medullary islands are scattered in a dark-staining thymic cortex–like background. **B** More-extended, light-staining, irregular medullary areas surrounded by dark-staining cortical regions.

mutation of *GTF2I* (p.L424H) was observed (in 22–29% of cases) in some studies {808,2334} but not in others {2409,1632}.

Macroscopic appearance

Mean diameters range from 51 to 75 mm {436,3048}. Type B1 thymomas usually appear encapsulated or well circumscribed. The cut surface is soft, tan-pink, and lymph node–like or shows vague lobules that are delineated by septa. Necrosis or cystic changes may occur {2055,1988,1984,2926}.

Histopathology

Type B1 thymomas have a thymus-like architecture with lobules that are usually larger than normal thymic lobules, delineated by delicate, collagenous septa and dominated by thymic cortex–like areas. The neoplastic cells are individually interspersed among densely packed small lymphocytes and barely detectable at low power. An increase of epithelial cell density above that of the normal thymic cortex or the presence of epithelial cell clusters (defined as ≥ 3 contiguous epithelial cells) suggests a

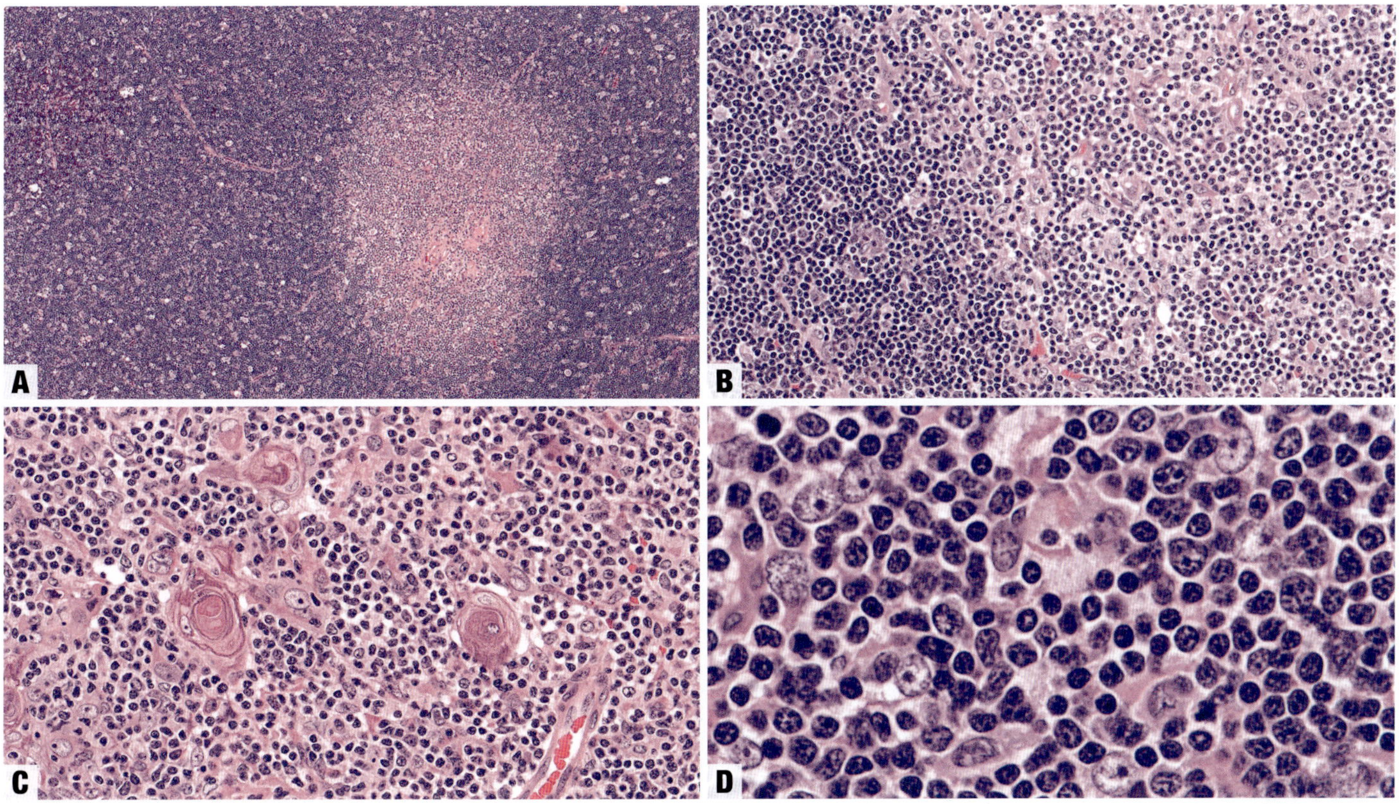

Fig. 5.14 Type B1 thymoma. **A** Classic light-staining nodular medullary island surrounded by a predominant cortical component. **B** Light-staining medullary island (upper-right corner) without Hassall corpuscles. **C** Medullary island with small Hassall corpuscles. **D** Neoplastic epithelial cells showing scant pale cytoplasm, round or oval vesicular nuclei, and distinct nucleoli among densely packed lymphocytes in the cortical component of a type B1 thymoma. They occur individually or in pairs (left-upper corner).

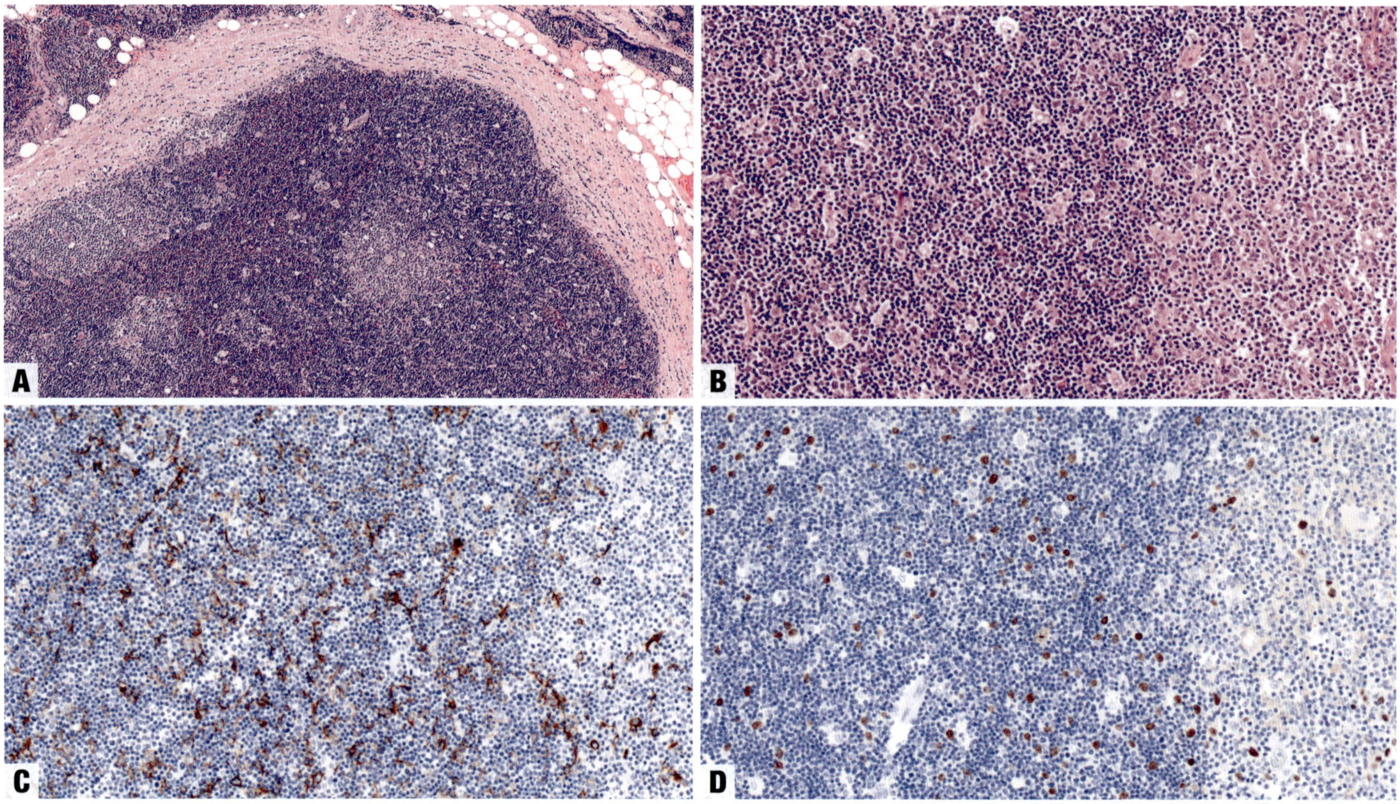

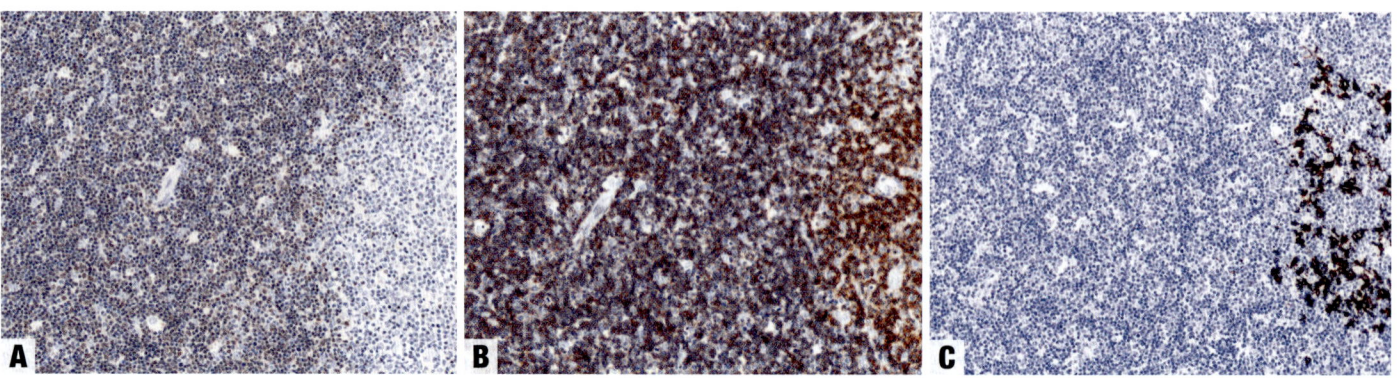

Fig. 5.15 Type B1 thymoma. **A** A lymphocyte-rich tumour surrounded by a thick capsule and showing light-staining medullary islands either surrounded by dark-staining cortical areas (centre) or abnormally arranged along the capsule (left). **B** Type B1 thymoma showing a light-staining medullary island (right) and dark-staining cortical region (left). **C** CK19 stain labelling a delicate epithelial cell meshwork in the light-staining medullary island (right) and darker-staining cortical region (left). **D** p40 stain labelling nuclei of widely dispersed thymic epithelial cells in the medullary island (right) and cortical region (left).

diagnosis of type B2 thymoma instead. The tumour cells have ill-defined, pale cytoplasm; round to oval nuclei with distinct membranes; clear chromatin; and small, variably conspicuous central nucleoli. Spindle cells should be absent, and their presence should raise the possibility of type AB thymoma. Pale nodular areas representing foci of medullary differentiation are obligatory for diagnosis, although they are not specific and may rarely be encountered in AB and B2 thymomas. These medullary islands consistently comprise a majority of lymphocytes that are less densely packed than in the cortical component. Hassall corpuscles and myoid cells are optional constituents. Poorly formed perivascular spaces are usually also present.

An admixture with type B2 thymoma occurs in 20%, and with type B3 thymoma more rarely {2873}.

Immunohistochemistry

Immunostaining is helpful in highlighting the delicate, keratin-positive epithelial meshwork and p40/p63-positive nuclei of the dispersed epithelial cells (in contrast to the higher density of positive cells in type B2 thymoma) {3190,14}. TdT staining highlights densely packed positive cells in the cortical areas and largely TdT-negative medullary islands. Some CD20-positive B cells are often present in the medullary islands, while the epithelial cells are typically CD20-negative (unlike in type AB thymomas).

Fig. 5.16 Type B1 thymoma. **A** TdT stain labelling densely packed immature T cells in the cortical region and rare cells in the medullary island. **B** CD5 stain labelling mature T cells in the medullary island (right) and immature T cells in the cortical region (left). **C** CD20 staining shows presence of B cells in the medullary island but not the cortical region.

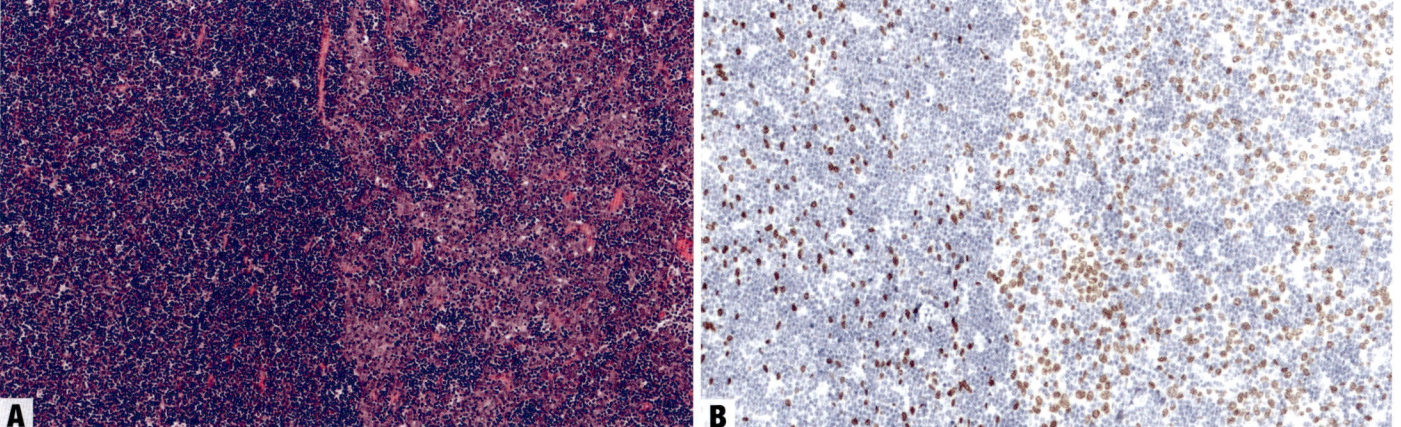

Fig. 5.17 Thymoma heterogeneity. **A** Type B1 thymoma component characterized by inconspicuous tumour cells among densely packed lymphocytes (left) sharply delineated from a lighter-staining type B2 thymoma component (right) with eosinophilic, clustered neoplastic cells. **B** p40 stain highlighting the small nuclei of dispersed tumour cells in the type B1 thymoma component (left) in contrast to the higher number of larger nuclei of the mostly clustered tumour cells in the type B2 thymoma component (right).

Differential diagnosis

The distinction from type B2 thymoma is addressed in *Type B2 thymoma* (p. 336). Lymphocyte-rich type AB thymomas are consistently more epithelial-rich and also contain a spindle cell component.

T-lymphoblastic lymphoma effaces the corticomedullary architecture and infiltrates septa and mediastinal fat {14}. Tumour cells are more monotonous, more atypical, and slightly larger than thymocytes, and they show many mitoses, apoptotic bodies, or necrosis. Monoclonal rearrangement of TR genes is almost consistently present, while abnormal immunophenotypes are less common {2942}.

Normal thymus shows distinct lobules delineated by adipose cells rather than fibrous septa. However, distinction may be impossible in small biopsies {14}.

Cytology

FNA yields cell-rich smears with abundant lymphocytes and rare epithelial cells with vesicular nuclei and variably conspicuous nucleoli. Published accuracies in diagnosis range from 77% to 100% {3465}. A distinction between type B1 and B2 thymoma is usually impossible {2581}.

Diagnostic molecular pathology

Not clinically relevant

Essential and desirable diagnostic criteria

Essential:
- A thymic epithelial tumour with organoid (corticomedullary) architecture with cortical predominance
- Dispersed, non-clustered thymic epithelial cells among densely packed lymphocytes
- Medullary islands are obligatory

Desirable:
- Cytokeratin and/or p40/p63 stains to highlight dispersed epithelial cells
- Sheets of TdT-positive immature T cells interspersed with TdT-negative nodular (medullary) areas

Staging

Type B1 thymomas should be staged according to the Union for International Cancer Control (UICC) TNM system {687} and, optionally, the Masaoka–Koga system {685}.

In the ITMIG cohort {3252} and an independent meta-analysis (see Table 5.01, p. 320), 80–90% of type B1 thymomas are in TNM stage I (corresponding to Masaoka–Koga stages I and II), while metastasis (mostly to the pleura) occurs in < 5%.

Prognosis and prediction

The overall survival rate is 80–100% at 5 years and 10 years {2184,472,2873}. Most type B1 thymomas can be cured by radical surgery {1561,472,2873}. Recurrence of TNM stage I tumours occurs in 10% of patients after 10 years of follow-up {3252}. The presence of myasthenia gravis has no major effect on prognosis {2237,829,436,2184}.

Type B2 thymoma

Marx A
Jain D
Marchevsky AM
Marino M
Nicholson AG
Yang WI

Definition
Type B2 thymoma is a lymphocyte-rich thymic epithelial tumour composed of polygonal tumour cells accompanied by numerous immature T cells. The tumour cells occur at a density higher than that of the normal thymus and type B1 thymoma.

ICD-O coding
8584/3 Thymoma, type B2

ICD-11 coding
2C27.2 & XH2G89 Malignant thymoma & Thymoma, type B2

Related terminology
Not recommended: cortical thymoma.

Subtype(s)
None

Localization
Type B2 thymoma is typically localized in the anterior (prevascular) mediastinum; ectopic occurrence is rare {3408}.

Clinical features
In the International Thymic Malignancy Interest Group (ITMIG) cohort {3252} and a meta-analysis (see Table 5.01, p. 320), myasthenia gravis is the first presentation in 50% of patients. Hypogammaglobulinaemia (Good syndrome), pure red cell aplasia, or other autoimmune diseases occur alone or in combination with myasthenia gravis in < 5% each {2406,679,1672, 3252}. A third of patients are asymptomatic {686,2406}. The imaging features overlap with those of other thymoma types {2527}.

Epidemiology
In the ITMIG cohort {3252} and a meta-analysis (see Table 5.01, p. 320), type B2 thymoma accounts for 26–28% of all thymomas. In these cohorts, the median age is 53 years {3252} and the mean age is 49 years (range: 4–83 years). Occurrence in children is rare {2837,394,1672}. There is no sex bias {3252, 679}.

Etiology
Unknown

Pathogenesis
A putative thymic epithelial cell precursor with the potential for bilineage, near-normal cortical and variably limited medullary maturation has been proposed as the cell of origin {2874}. An unsupervised cluster analysis of five genomic data platforms suggests that type B2 thymomas are related to B1 and B3 thymomas {2409}. Recurrent losses of chromosomes 1p, 3p, and

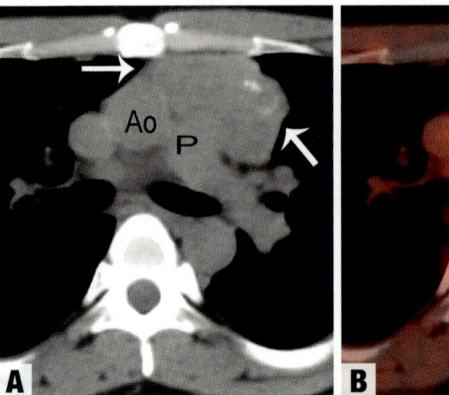

Fig. 5.18 WHO type B2 thymoma. **A** Unenhanced chest CT of a type B2 thymoma shows a heterogeneous primary tumour (arrows) with some calcifications within it and a lobular contour with the lung. The heterogeneous appearance and lobularity of the contour is worrisome for a more aggressive behaviour. There is no fat separating it from the pulmonary artery (P) and a small portion of the aorta (Ao). At surgery, the tumour encompassed the phrenic nerve and involved the adjacent lung (T3), but the pulmonary artery and aorta were not involved. **B** FDG PET-CT of this type B2 thymoma showed FDG uptake with a maximum standardized uptake value of 6.2.

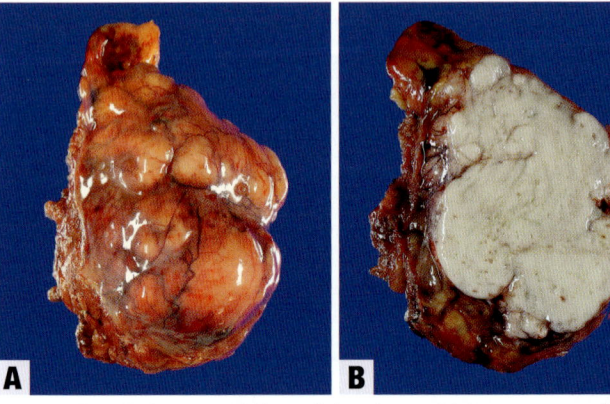

Fig. 5.19 Type B2 thymoma. **A** External view of a type B2 thymoma covered by mediastinal pleura showing a bosselated surface as is typical of an unencapsulated tumour with pushing-type, multifocal invasion. **B** Cut surface of the same type B2 thymoma showing a light-grey to white tumour with variably sized lobules incompletely delineated by delicate septa and smooth contours towards the mediastinal fat.

6q25.2-q25.3 and gain of 1q are found in both type B2 and B3 thymomas {2321,1253,3479,965,1629,2336}. As many as 6% of cases exhibit *KMT2A-MAML2* gene fusion {1824A}. A high frequency of altered chromosome arms is associated with myasthenia gravis {2409}. Activating *KRAS* {965} and *NRAS* mutations, inactivating *TP53* mutations {2409}, and microsatellite instability {1253} are rare. No gain of *BCL2*, loss of *CDKN2A/B* {2335}, or mutations of *KIT* or *EGFR* have been observed {2877}. Hotspot

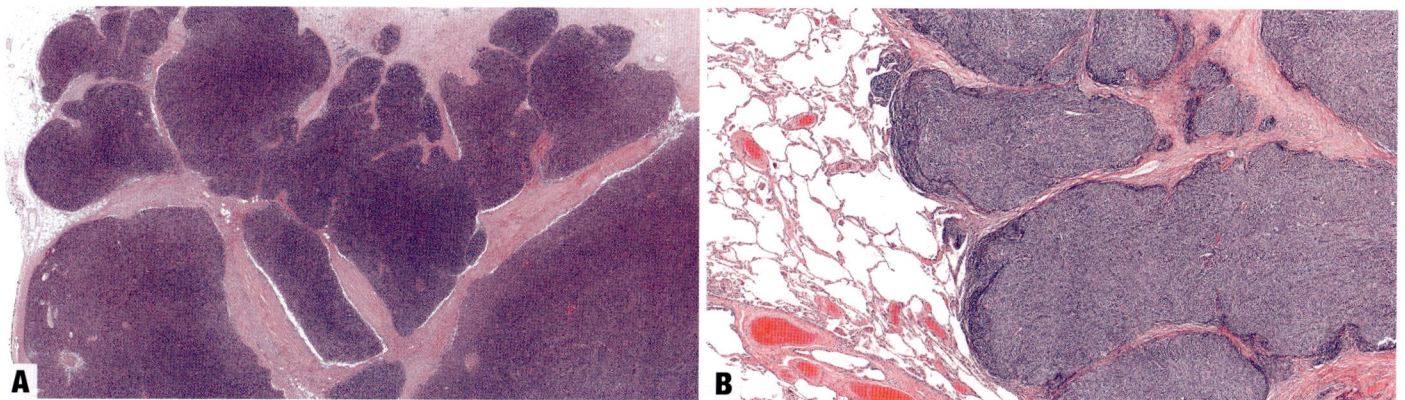

Fig. 5.20 Type B2 thymoma. **A** Type B2 thymoma showing a lobular and multinodular growth pattern and a smooth-contoured, pushing-type invasion front reaching into mediastinal fat. **B** Tumour showing a smooth-contoured, pushing-type invasion front reaching into lung.

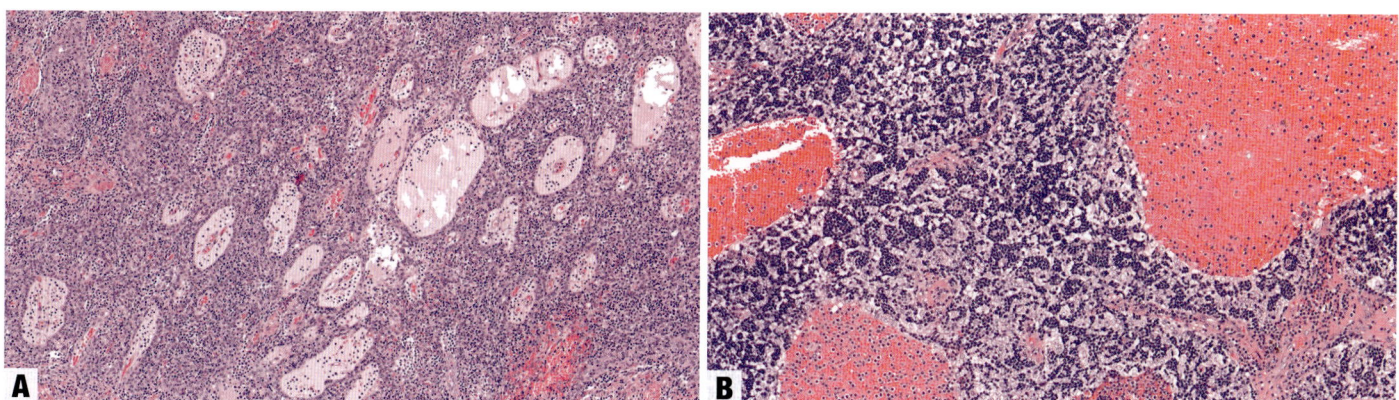

Fig. 5.21 Type B2 thymoma. **A** Perivascular spaces composed of a central venule surrounded by a clear space containing proteinaceous fluid and variable numbers of lymphoid cells. **B** Perivascular spaces are often prominent, and in this example they are filled with blood.

mutation of *GTF2I* (p.L424H) is observed (in 10–22% of cases) in some studies {808,2334} but not in others {2409,1632}.

Macroscopic appearance

The tumours are encapsulated or partially circumscribed or show invasion of mediastinal fat or adjacent organs. The mean diameters range from 40 to 62 mm {3252,3048,436}. The cut surface is tan and soft to firm, with multiple lobules delineated by white fibrous septa. Necrosis, cystic changes, and haemorrhage may be present {2055,1984,2926}.

Histopathology

At low power, type B2 thymomas appear blue in H&E-stained slides due to the abundance of lymphocytes. Lobules of irregular size and shape are delineated by fibrous septa. Polygonal/oval epithelial cells occur among the lymphocytes as interspersed

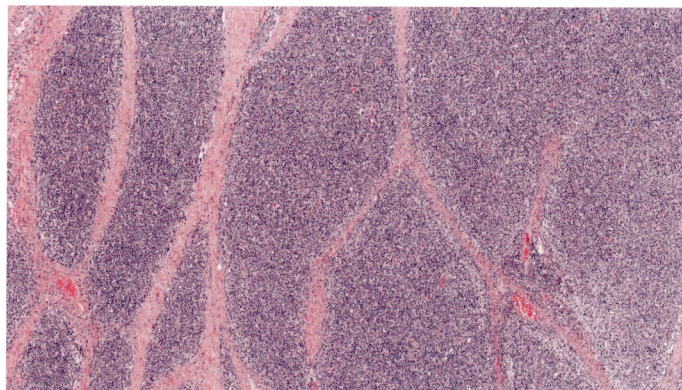

Fig. 5.22 Type B2 thymoma. Distinct lobular growth pattern with delicate fibrous septa delineating tumour lobules with angulated shapes and sharp angles.

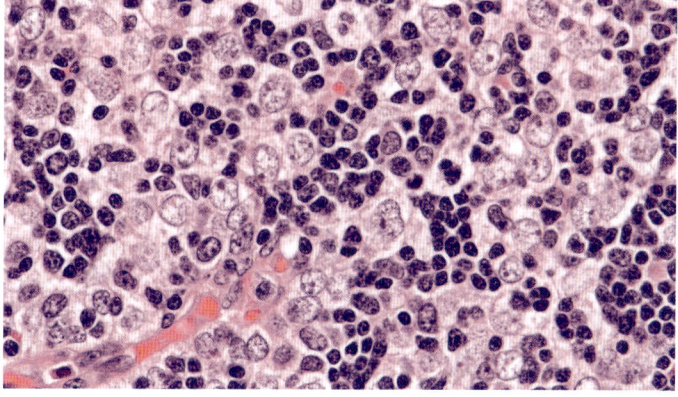

Fig. 5.23 Type B2 thymoma. Single and clustered epithelial cells are found among numerous lymphocytes. The epithelial cells have round to oval nuclei, vesicular chromatin, and distinct nucleoli.

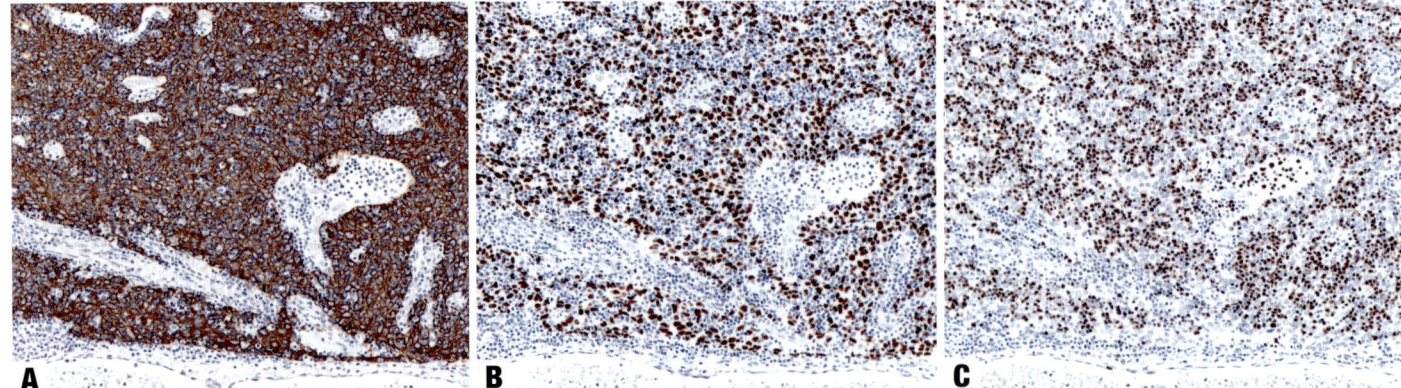

Fig. 5.24 Type B2 thymoma. **A** CK19 stain highlights perivascular spaces and an epithelial cell meshwork that is much denser than in a type B1 thymoma. **B** p40 stain highlights numerous nuclei of dispersed and clustered neoplastic epithelial cells. **C** TdT stain labelling abundant immature T cells in between neoplastic epithelial cells in the surrounding of perivascular spaces; note a few TdT-positive cells also inside perivascular spaces.

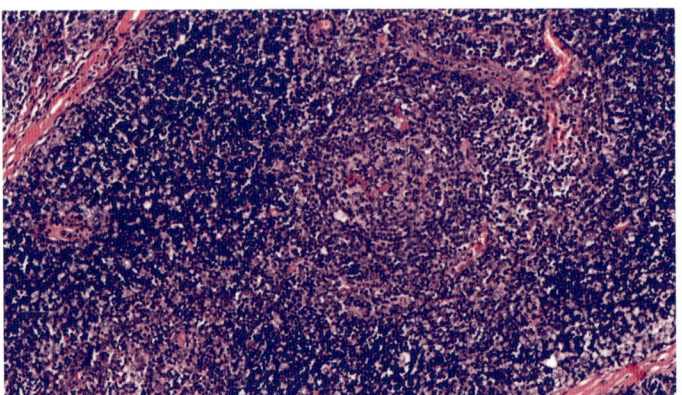

Fig. 5.25 Type B2 thymoma. Lymphoid follicle in the perivascular space of a myasthenia gravis–associated tumour.

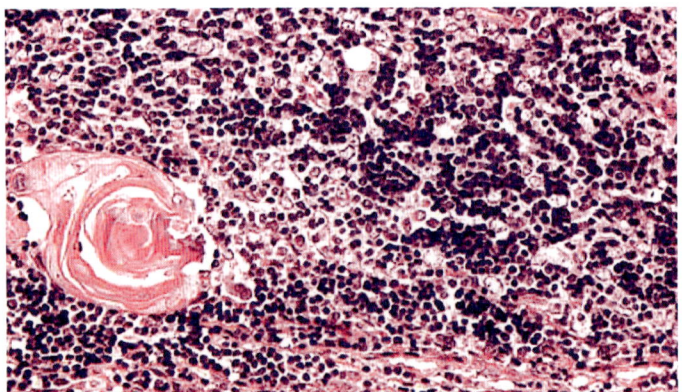

Fig. 5.26 Type B2 thymoma. A Hassall corpuscle; abundance and clustering of epithelial cells in the nearby cortical area argue against type B1 thymoma.

single cells or clusters (i.e. ≥ 3 contiguous cells). They have round nuclei with vesicular chromatin and small, conspicuous central nucleoli and lightly eosinophilic cytoplasm. Focal anaplasia is rare. Perivascular spaces are common. Inconspicuous medullary islands with or without Hassall corpuscles are sometimes present. Germinal centres mainly occur in fibrous septa and/or perivascular spaces in patients with myasthenia gravis. Corticosteroid or neoadjuvant treatment may elicit histiocytic infiltration, lymphocyte depletion, and necrosis. An admixture with type B3 or B1 thymoma occurs in 43% and 4%, respectively {2873}; an admixture with thymic carcinoma occurs exceptionally {2919,1559}.

Immunohistochemistry

Immunostaining is helpful in highlighting the increased density of the keratin-positive epithelial meshwork and increased number of p40/p63-positive nuclei of tumour cells, compared with the normal thymic cortex or type B1 thymoma. TdT staining labels numerous immature T cells. Some CD20-positive B cells are often present in the rare medullary islands, while the epithelial cells are CD20-negative.

Differential diagnosis

Type B1 thymoma shows few epithelial cells, lacks epithelial cell clusters, and consistently shows conspicuous medullary islands. Perivascular spaces are usually less prominent.

Type B3 thymoma is a lymphocyte-poor tumour characterized by sheets of tumour cells sprinkled with immature T cells. Therefore, H&E-stained sections of type B3 thymoma show a pink colour instead of the blue colour that is characteristic of type B2 thymoma.

T-lymphoblastic lymphoma can mimic lymphocyte-rich thymomas (see *Type B1 thymoma*, p. 332). T-lymphoblastic lymphoma may rarely arise in type B2 thymoma {782}.

Type B2 thymoma with anaplasia is distinguishable from thymic carcinoma by the maintenance of typical thymoma features: lobular growth pattern, perivascular spaces, TdT-positive immature T cells, and absence of CD5/KIT (CD117) expression {14}.

Cytology

FNA yields cell-rich smears with isolated or clustered epithelial cells intermingled with abundant lymphocytes. A distinction between type B1 and B2 thymoma is often impossible {2581,3465}.

Diagnostic molecular pathology

Not clinically relevant

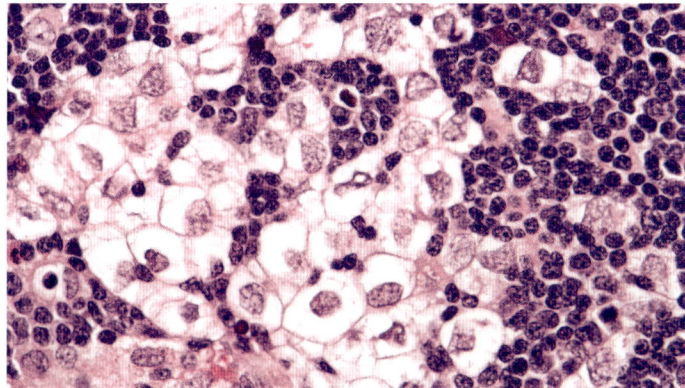

Fig. 5.27 Type B2 thymoma. Some neoplastic epithelial cells in this example have water-clear cytoplasm.

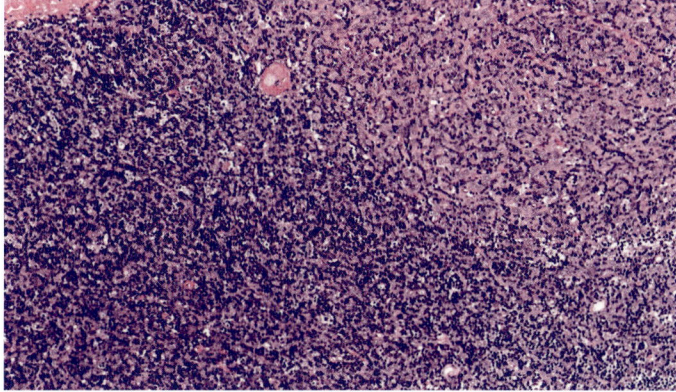

Fig. 5.28 Thymoma heterogeneity. Sharp transition between the blue-staining type B2 thymoma component (left and lower part) and the pink-staining, epithelial cell–predominant type B3 component (upper-right part).

Chapter 5

Essential and desirable diagnostic criteria

Essential:
- Lobulated architecture
- Abundance of lymphocytes
- Polygonal/oval neoplastic epithelial cells that are more numerous than in the normal thymic cortex and often present in clusters

Desirable:
- Keratin and/or p40/p63 stains to highlight the increased density of dispersed and/or clustered epithelial cells compared with the normal thymic cortex

Staging

Type B2 thymomas should be staged according to the Union for International Cancer Control (UICC) TNM system {315,687} and, optionally, the Masaoka–Koga system {685}.

In the ITMIG cohort {3252} and an independent meta-analysis (see Table 5.01, p. 320), 60–65% of type B2 thymomas are in TNM stage I (corresponding to Masaoka–Koga stages I and II), while pleural and distant metastasis occurs in 8–10% and 3–5%, respectively.

Prognosis and prediction

The overall survival rate is 70–100% at 5 years and 45–82% at 10 years {472,2873,1074}. Complete resection is achieved in 70–90% of cases {2184,436,2873,2273}, and most patients can be cured by radical surgery {1561,472,2873}. In the ITMIG cohort, recurrence rates of TNM stage I tumours after R0 resection are 14% and 32% after 5 years and 10 years, respectively {3252}. Advanced stage (Masaoka–Koga stages III and IV) is a poor prognostic factor for tumour-related death {2873}. The presence of myasthenia gravis has no effect on prognosis {2237,436,2184,2406,829}.

Type B3 thymoma

Marx A
Jain D
Marchevsky AM
Marino M
Nicholson AG
Yang WI

Definition

Type B3 thymoma is a thymic epithelial tumour predominantly composed of mildly or moderately atypical polygonal tumour cells, accompanied by small numbers of non-neoplastic immature T cells.

ICD-O coding

8585/3 Thymoma, type B3

ICD-11 coding

2C27.2 & XH4EW9 Malignant thymoma & Thymoma, type B3

Related terminology

Not recommended: atypical thymoma; well-differentiated thymic carcinoma.

Subtype(s)

None

Localization

Type B3 thymoma is typically localized in the anterior (prevascular) mediastinum; ectopic occurrence is rare {3408}.

Clinical features

One third of patients are asymptomatic. Others have chest pain, cough, dyspnoea, or superior vena cava syndrome. In the International Thymic Malignancy Interest Group (ITMIG) cohort {3252} and an independent meta-analysis (see Table 5.01, p. 320), myasthenia gravis and other autoimmune disorders occur in 40–50% and about 5% of patients, respectively {436, 679,3252,3502}.

Imaging

The imaging features overlap with those of other thymoma types {2527}, but type B3 thymomas are more likely to be of higher stage and show higher FDG uptake {1814,210}.

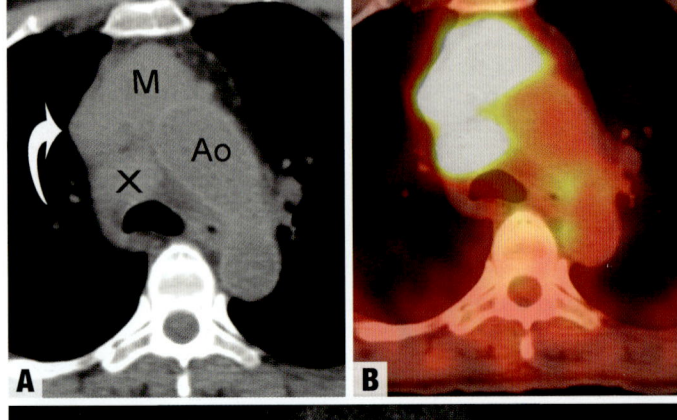

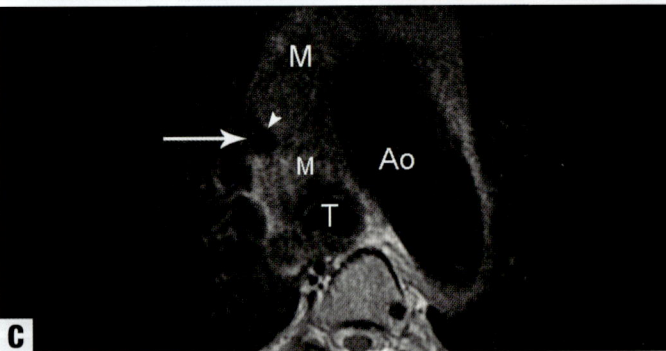

Fig. 2.29 Type B3 thymoma. **A** Unenhanced chest CT of a type B3 thymoma shows an aggressive-looking prevascular mass (M) abutting and inseparable from the aorta (Ao) and superior vena cava (curved arrow). Soft tissue is also seen in the lower right paratracheal region (X), which by imaging is worrisome for an N2 lymph node. The lack of intravenous contrast does not enable one to identify vascular involvement. **B** FDG PET-CT of a type B3 thymoma showing marked FDG uptake with a maximum standardized uptake value of 14.3. **C** Selected image from a thoracic spine MRI obtained at the same time. The image was obtained in a black-blood sequence; thus, vessels with blood flow (e.g. the aorta [Ao]) as well as air (e.g. the trachea [T]) are depicted as black. The prevascular mass replaces the left brachiocephalic vein and directly invades (arrowhead) the superior vena cava (arrow). The mass continues to the right paratracheal region. Exploratory thoracotomy showed that the right paratracheal soft tissue was due to tumour insinuating itself along the pericardial recess. Mediastinal lymph nodes were not involved.

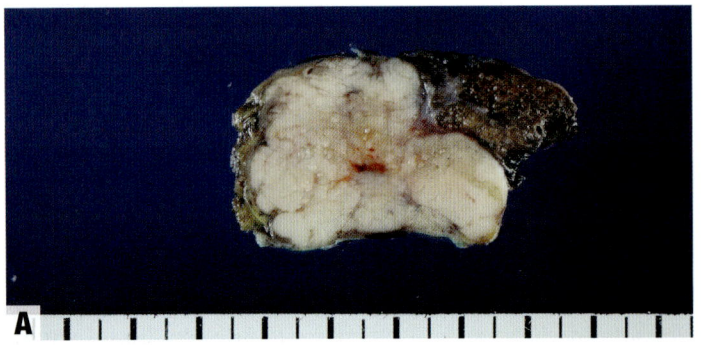

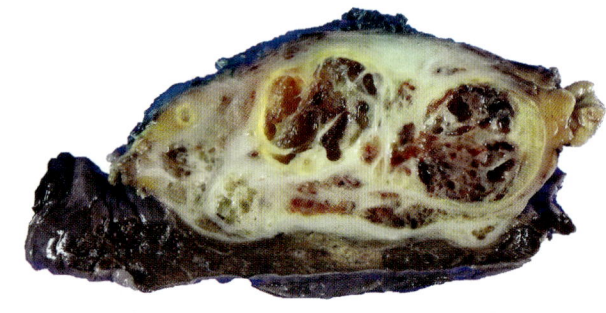

Fig. 5.30 Type B3 thymoma. **A** Cut surface of a grey-white tumour composed of poorly delineated tumour nodules with bosselated, smooth borders. The tumour abuts the adherent lung. **B** Cut surface of a delineated, grey-white tumour invading the lung. After neoadjuvant therapy, there are many cysts, as well as necrotic and sclerotic regions.

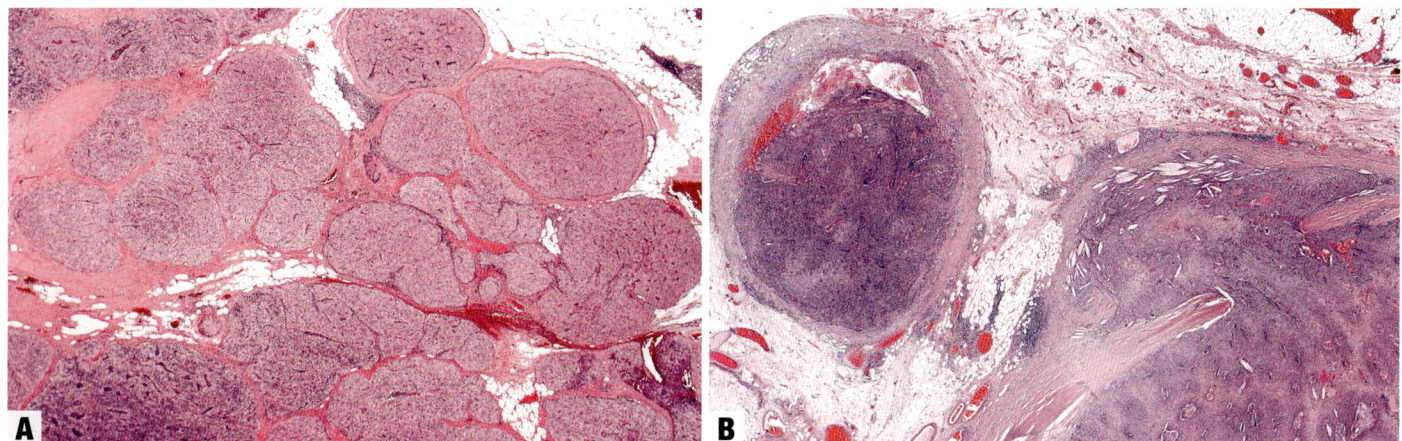

Fig. 5.31 Type B3 thymoma. **A** The lobulated tumour shows pushing-type invasion into mediastinal fat. Note the pink appearance due to sheets of eosinophilic tumour cells. **B** Transcapsular invasion into mediastinal fat, in the form of an encapsulated satellite nodule.

Epidemiology

In the ITMIG cohort {3252} and an independent meta-analysis (see Table 5.01, p. 320), type B3 thymoma accounts for 16–21% of thymomas. In these cohorts, the median and mean ages are 52 years and 55 years (range: 8–87 years), respectively. There is a slight male predominance {679,1287}. Occurrence in children is exceptionally rare {2837,394,1672}.

Etiology

Unknown

Pathogenesis

An origin from a putative thymic epithelial cell precursor with minimal corticomedullary differentiation has been proposed {2874}. An unsupervised cluster analysis of five genomic data

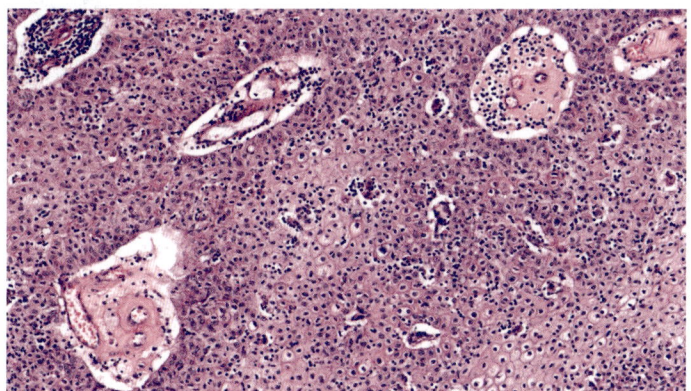

Fig. 5.32 Type B3 thymoma. Sheets of tumour cells surrounding perivascular spaces. Note the paucity of lymphocytes in between tumour cells but variably numerous lymphocytes in perivascular spaces.

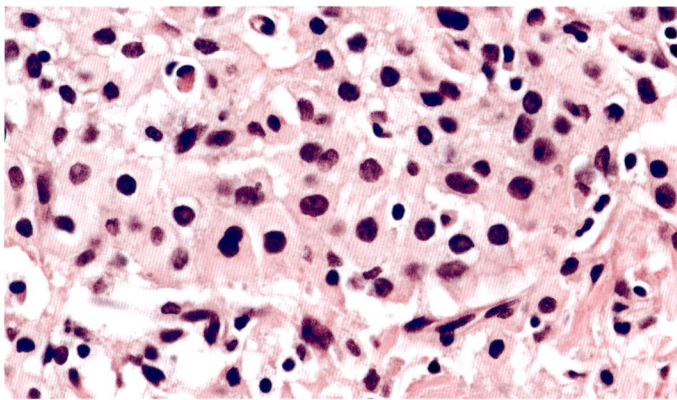

Fig. 5.33 Type B3 thymoma. This example is composed of cells with indistinct cell borders, showing moderate pleomorphism; the nucleoli are indistinct.

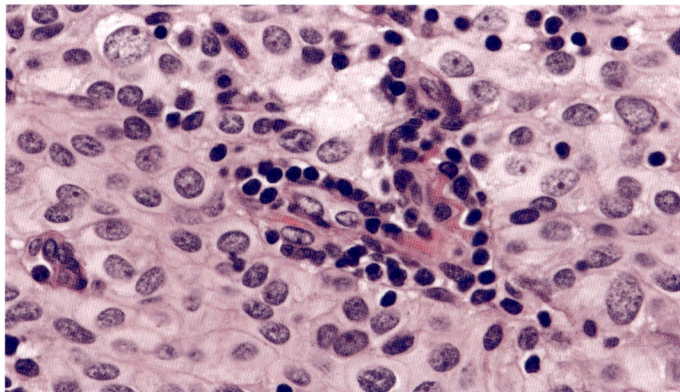

Fig. 5.34 Type B3 thymoma. Polygonal tumour cells with distinct cell borders and abundant eosinophilic cytoplasm. The nuclei are oval and have small indistinct nucleoli. A perivascular space is seen in the centre.

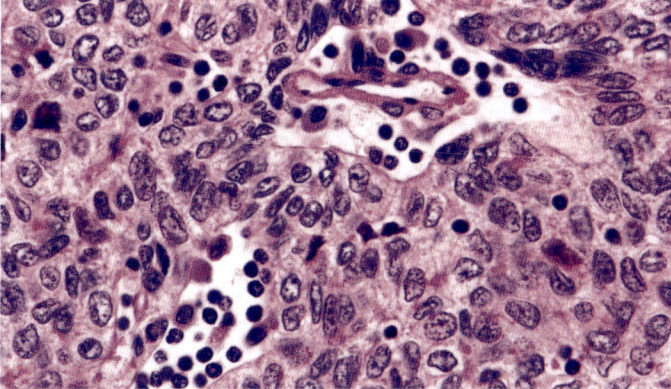

Fig. 5.35 Type B3 thymoma. This example is composed of cells that are polygonal or show indistinct cell borders. Nuclear atypia is mild, and nucleoli are inconspicuous. Perivascular spaces are seen.

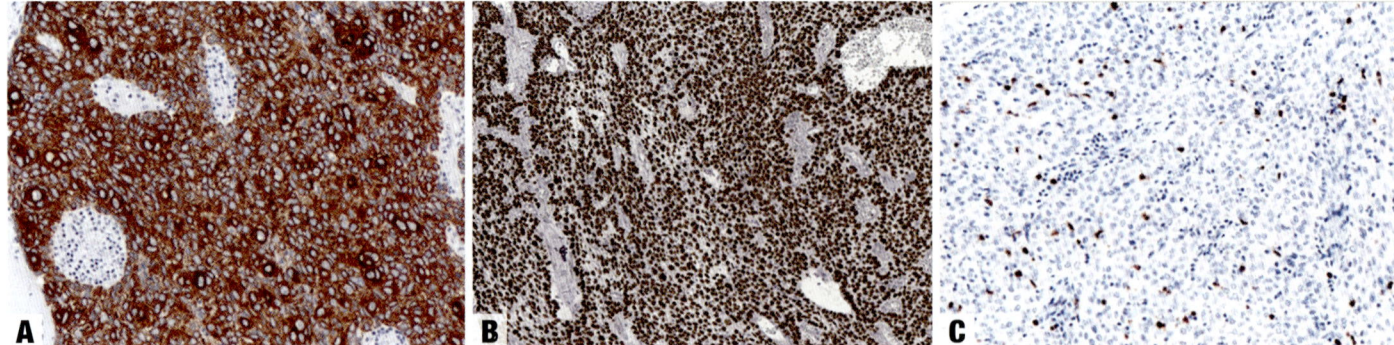

Fig. 5.36 Type B3 thymoma. **A** Type B3 thymoma showing diffuse expression of CK19 throughout the tumour around a perivascular space. **B** Type B3 thymoma showing strong nuclear expression of p40 throughout the tumour. **C** Type B3 thymoma showing expression of TdT in the nuclei of the scattered non-neoplastic immature T cells.

platforms suggests that type B3 thymomas are closely related to type B2 thymomas {2409}. Recurrent gene copy-number alterations are commoner in type B3 thymomas than other thymoma types {2321,3479,965,1629}. Recurrent losses of chromosomes 6q25.2–q25.3 and 3p and gains of chromosome 1q are found in both type B2 and B3 thymomas, while losses of 13q, 16q, and 17p and gains of 4p and 17q are found only in type B3 thymomas and thymic carcinomas {2321,3479,965, 2336,2335}. *KMT2A-MAML2* gene fusion has been detected in 6% of cases {1824A}. Copy-number gain of *BCL2* and copy-number loss of *CDKN2A/B* are associated with a poor outcome {2335}. Inactivating *TP53* mutations {2409} and microsatellite instability {1253} are rare. While there are no activating mutations in the *EGFR* gene {2409,1879,965} or *KIT* gene {2409,965, 961}, genes in the EGFR (HER1) pathway (*PIK3CA*, *AKT1*) are rarely mutated {2604}. Hotspot mutation of *GTF2I* (p.L424H) is reported in 10–21% of cases {2409,808,2334}.

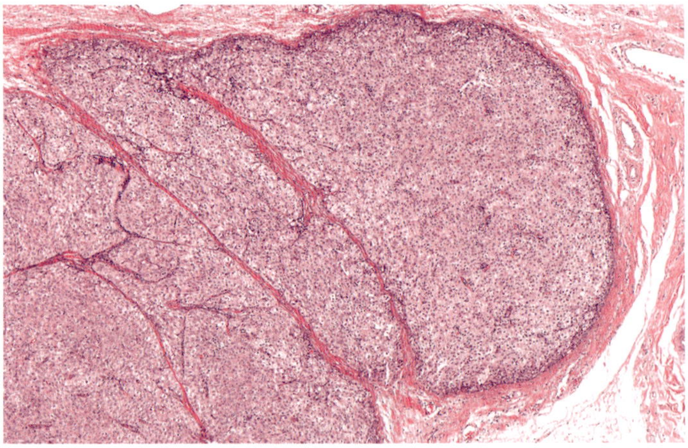

Macroscopic appearance

The tumours usually appear poorly circumscribed, with smooth extensions into mediastinal fat or adjacent organs. Mean diameters range from 51 to 68 mm {436,3048}. The cut surface is firm and grey or yellow, with tumour nodules separated by fibrous bands. Necrosis and haemorrhage may be present {1988,2926}.

Histopathology

Type B3 thymoma comprises variably sized and shaped lobules delineated by fibrous septa, and it often shows smooth invasive fronts. At low power, the tumour appears pink in H&E-stained

Fig. 5.37 Type B3 thymoma. Lobular growth pattern of a smoothly contoured tumour. Note sheets of tumour cells with clear cytoplasm.

slides due to the abundance of polygonal tumour cells that show eosinophilic or clear cytoplasm and form sheets. Intercellular bridges between tumour cells are absent except in rare Hassall corpuscles or squamous eddies. The mildly to moderately atypical, round to elongated, sometimes grooved or raisinoid nuclei can be smaller or larger than those of type B2 thymoma. Nucleoli may be inconspicuous or prominent. Perivascular spaces with epithelial palisading are prominent. Sparse immature T cells are almost always interspersed among the tumour cells, although they may be missing in < 5% of cases. Lymphoid

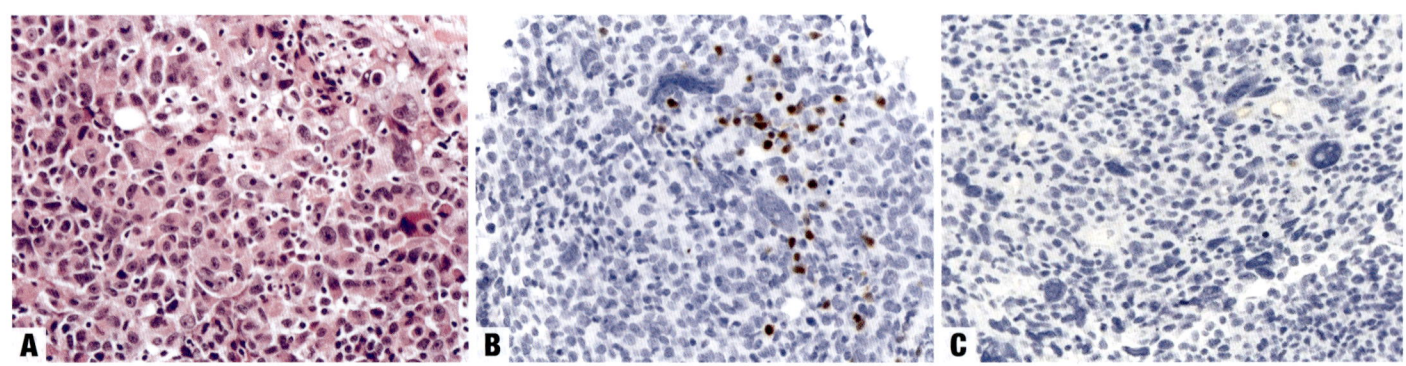

Fig. 5.38 Type B3 thymoma with anaplasia. **A** Occurrence of some bizarre tumour cells in a core needle biopsy. **B** TdT stain highlights small numbers of immature T cells adjacent to bizarre tumour cells, which suggests a diagnosis of type B3 thymoma with anaplasia rather than thymic carcinoma. **C** Absence of KIT (CD117) expression again suggests a diagnosis of type B3 thymoma with anaplasia rather than thymic carcinoma.

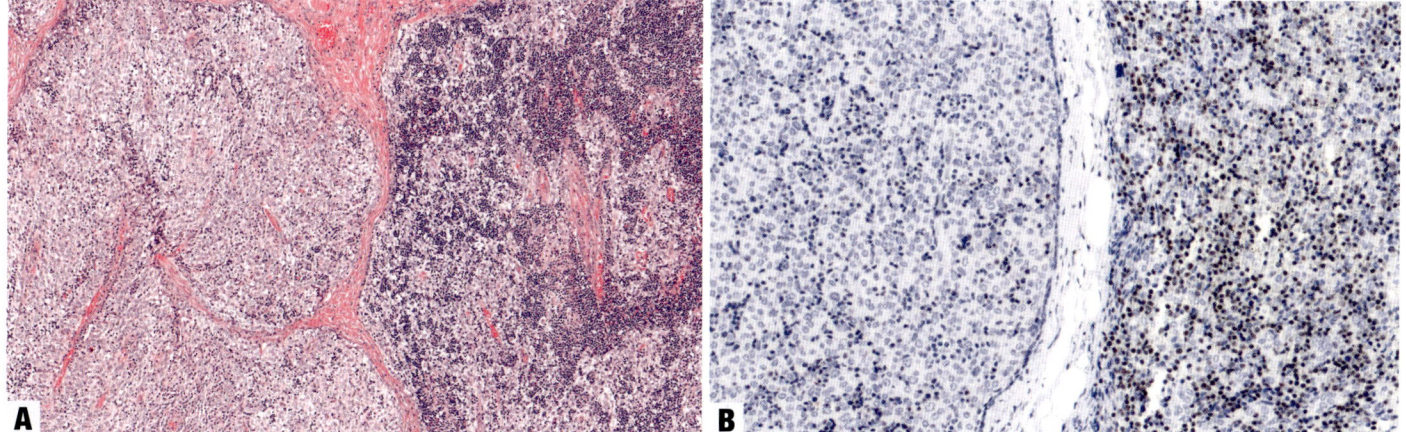

Fig. 5.39 Heterogeneity in type B3 thymoma. **A** Epithelial cell–predominant type B3 thymoma areas (left) sharply delineated from a lymphocyte-rich type B2 thymoma component (right). **B** Rare TdT-positive immature T cells in the type B3 thymoma area (left) as compared with the many TdT-positive immature T cells in the type B2 thymoma component (right).

follicles in association with perivascular spaces are common in cases associated with myasthenia gravis.

Thymomas comprising type B3 and B2 components are common (2–16% of all thymomas) and may exceed the frequency of pure type B3 thymomas {472,2873,628}. Combined thymic carcinomas with a type B3 thymoma component are rare (0.2–1% of thymic epithelial tumours) {2873,628}.

Immunohistochemistry

The tumour cells usually stain with pancytokeratin antibodies, as well as antibodies to CK19, CK5/6, CK7, CK8, and CK10 but not to CK20. p40 and p63 are almost always positive {501,3342, 724,3190}. Focal expression of EMA {885} is typical. PAX8 is often positive using polyclonal antibody {3270}, but negative using monoclonal antibody {3055}. TTF1, CD20, and thymic carcinoma markers (CD5, KIT [CD117], EZH2) are almost always negative {1119,1504,1436} or only focally expressed (GLUT1 and EMA [MUC1]) {1504,1347}. TdT labels low numbers of immature T cells in > 95% of cases.

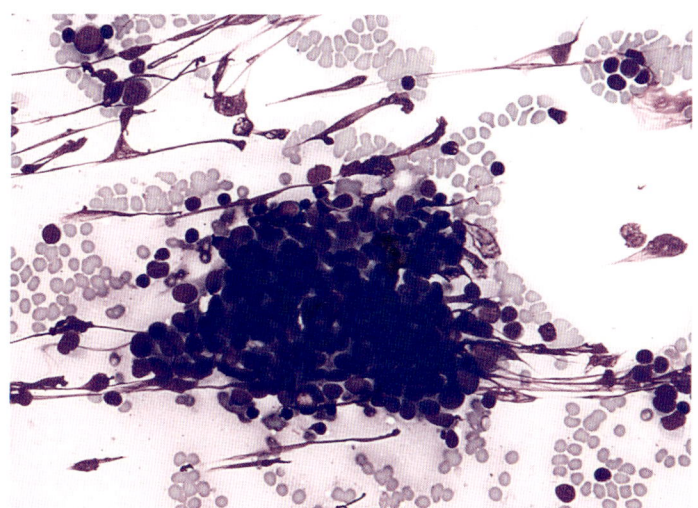

Fig. 5.40 Type B3 thymoma. FNA smear showing sheets of relatively monotonous, medium-sized cells with round nuclei and inconspicuous small nuclei; lymphocytes are virtually missing (Giemsa stain).

Rare features in type B3 thymoma

Spindle cells can occur focally in an otherwise typical B3 thymoma. Whether a pure spindle cell subtype of type B3 thymoma exists is unclear, and distinction from atypical type A thymoma is difficult.

Rare type B3 thymomas exhibit anaplasia characterized by the presence of bizarre or giant tumour cells. In contrast to thymic carcinomas, such tumours maintain typical thymoma features such as lobular growth pattern, perivascular spaces, and presence of TdT-positive T cells, and they lack CD5 and KIT (CD117) expression in tumour cells.

Rare tumours showing typical histological features of type B3 thymomas but either exhibiting (usually focal) expression of CD5 or KIT (CD117) {1098,2048} or lacking TdT-positive T cells should still be classified as type B3 thymomas.

Differential diagnosis

Type B2 thymomas are lymphocyte-rich tumours, appearing blue rather than pink in H&E-stained sections. However, because there is a morphological continuum between type B2 and B3 thymomas, rare cases at the B2/B3 boundary may defy clear-cut classification {2920,2598}.

Thymic squamous cell carcinoma (SCC) is distinguished from type B3 thymoma by the absence of a lobular growth, infiltrative rather than pushing-type invasion, lack of perivascular spaces, more-prominent nuclear atypia, and frequent presence of intercellular bridges. Thymic SCCs commonly express CD5 (in ~75% of cases), as well as KIT (CD117) and EZH2 (each in > 80%), whereas B3 thymomas do not {1119,1504,1436}, with rare exceptions {2170,1098}. CD205 is more frequently positive in thymic SCC than in type B3 thymomas {1436,2132}. GLUT1 expression is more common in thymic SCC (in > 90% of cases) than in type B3 thymomas (~50%) {1119,1504,1347,1098}; staining is typically diffuse in thymic SCC but patchy in B3 thymoma {3029}. The cortical epithelial cell marker beta5t may be positive in B3 thymomas but is typically negative in thymic SCC {3358}. With rare exceptions, TdT-positive immature T cells are absent in thymic SCC {1430}.

Cytology

Smears show sheets of tumour cells with some size variation, round nuclei and inconspicuous nucleoli, and rare admixed lymphocytes {3465}.

Diagnostic molecular pathology

Not clinically relevant

Essential and desirable diagnostic criteria

Essential:

- Lobulated tumour
- Sheets of mildly/moderately atypical, polygonal tumour cells
- Interspersed perivascular spaces
- Paucity of lymphocytes

Desirable:

- TdT immunostain to highlight the small population of immature T cells

Staging

Type B3 thymomas should be staged according to the Union for International Cancer Control (UICC) TNM system {315,687} and, optionally, the Masaoka–Koga system {685}.

In the ITMIG cohort {3252} and an independent meta-analysis (see Table 5.01, p. 320), 43–55% of type B3 thymomas are in TNM stage I (i.e. Masaoka–Koga stages I and II), while pleural and distant metastasis occurs in 14–15% and 3–5%, respectively.

Prognosis and prediction

The reported 5-year, 10-year, and 20-year overall survival rates are 60–86%, 50–70%, and 25–36%, respectively {472,2184, 2873,1074}. In the ITMIG cohort, the overall survival rates with R0-resected type B3 thymoma at 5 years and 10 years were 89% and 81%, respectively. Complete resection rates range from 53% to 92% {2873,436,2184}. Recurrence occurs in as many as 44% of cases overall {2873}. After an R0 resection, recurrences occur in 23% and 29% of cases across all tumour stages within 5 years and 10 years, respectively (11% for Masaoka–Koga stage I/II and 28% for stage III within 10 years) {3252}. Advanced Masaoka–Koga stage (III/IV) is a poor prognostic factor for tumour-related death {2873}. The prognostic significance of resection status, tumour size, and recurrence has not been reported for single WHO thymoma types, including type B3 thymomas {686,678,436,2184,628}. Age, sex, and myasthenia gravis have no effect on prognosis {2237,829,2873, 2184,2406}. High PDL1 expression in type B3 thymoma cells is correlated with better overall survival in some studies {2554,95} but not others {1053,3257,3409,1395,2236}. PDL1 expression levels are a poor predictor of the response to immune checkpoint inhibitor therapies {3500}.

Micronodular thymoma with lymphoid stroma

Tateyama H
Girard N
Roden AC
Ströbel P

Definition
Micronodular thymoma with lymphoid stroma is characterized by multiple small discrete nodules of bland spindle or oval cells disposed in an epithelial cell–free lymphoid stroma.

ICD-O coding
8580/1 Micronodular thymoma with lymphoid stroma

ICD-11 coding
4B40.Y & XH56K5 Other specified diseases of thymus & Micro-nodular thymoma with lymphoid stroma

Related terminology
Not recommended: micronodular thymoma with lymphoid B-cell hyperplasia.

Subtype(s)
None

Localization
Most cases occur in the anterior (prevascular) mediastinum, rare cases in the cervical region {1883,3521,3454}.

Clinical features
Most tumours are incidental findings. Myasthenia gravis is usually absent {2249,2999}. CT and MRI findings overlap with those of other types of thymoma {1449,425,1364}.

Epidemiology
Micronodular thymoma with lymphoid stroma accounts for 1–5% of thymomas. The patient ages range from 41 to 83 years (mean: 63.8 years), with a slight male predominance (M:F ratio: 1.2:1) {2917,2999,2878,1266,1947}.

Etiology
Unknown

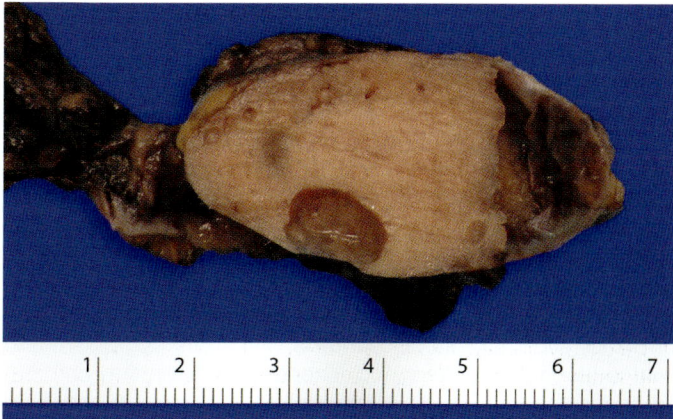

Fig. 5.41 Micronodular thymoma with lymphoid stroma. Macroscopy shows a light-tan, well-circumscribed tumour with several cysts.

Pathogenesis
Of two published cases {2409}, only one case showed genetic alterations: a *GTF2I* p.L424H mutation (which is otherwise characteristic of type A and type AB thymomas) and losses of 6q and chromosome 10.

Langerhans cells within the tumour nodules {1266} and chemokines expressed by the tumour cells {2878} may play a role in the formation of lymphoid stroma.

Macroscopic appearance
Tumours are usually well circumscribed and often encapsulated, soft, and friable. Diameters range from 12 to 150 mm. The cut surface is homogeneous and light tan, with occasional cystic spaces.

Histopathology
Micronodular thymoma with lymphoid stroma is characterized by multiple, discrete and/or coalescing small nodules of tumour

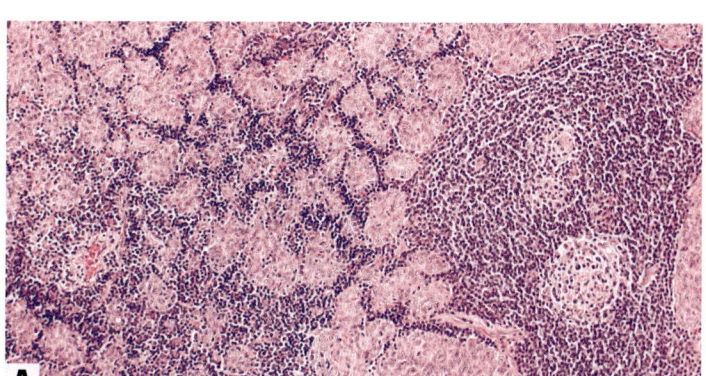
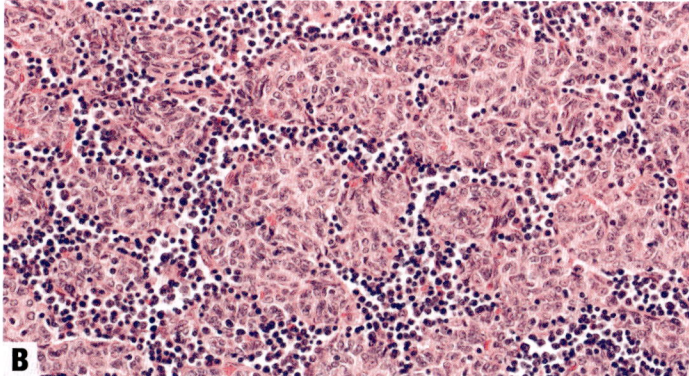

Fig. 5.42 Micronodular thymoma with lymphoid stroma. **A** Multiple small tumour nodules separated by abundant lymphoid stroma with lymphoid follicles showing germinal centres. **B** Higher magnification shows epithelial micronodules composed of bland-looking spindle and oval cells.

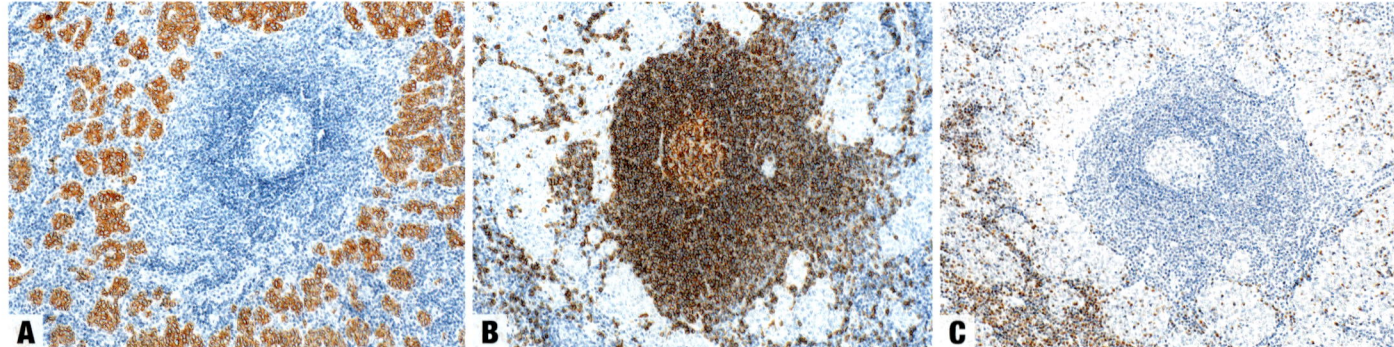

Fig. 5.43 Micronodular thymoma with lymphoid stroma. **A** Immunostaining for pancytokeratin shows discrete epithelial micronodules but absence of a meshwork of epithelial cells in the lymphoid stroma. **B** Stromal lymphoid cells with a lymphoid follicle between small epithelial nodules show positive immunostaining for CD20. **C** Immunostaining for TdT shows a narrow band of immature lymphocytes surrounding the tumour nodules and scattered lymphocytes within the nodules.

cells separated by abundant lymphoid stroma, which usually contains lymphoid follicles with or without germinal centres and variable numbers of plasma cells. The nodules are composed of bland, short spindle or oval cells with scant cytoplasm and oval to elongated uniform nuclei containing dispersed chromatin and indistinct nucleoli. Mitotic activity is minimal. Some lymphocytes may be interspersed within the nodules. Microcystic and macrocystic changes are common. Rosette-like structures and glandular formation may be seen. Hassall corpuscles and perivascular spaces are absent. Associated multilocular thymic cysts have been reported {2404,1364}.

Areas corresponding to type A thymoma occur in as many as 30% of cases {2999,2878,1947}. Associations with type AB thymoma {2249,2878,1947}, type B2 thymoma {3033,1947}, and thymic carcinoma {2917} are rare.

Immunohistochemistry

The epithelial component shows a pancytokeratin+/CK5/6+/CK19+/CD20– immunophenotype. The lymphoid stroma is devoid of keratin-positive epithelial cells and contains mostly mature CD20+/CD79a+ B cells mixed with some CD3+/TdT– T cells, but it typically also harbours a population of CD3+/CD1a+/CD99+/TdT+ immature T cells around the tumour nodules. Within the epithelial nodules, TdT+ T cells are scarce. Germinal centres in reactive follicles show CD20+/CD10+/BCL2– B cells and CD23+ follicular dendritic cell networks. Many CD1a+/langerin+ Langerhans cells are diffusely distributed within the tumour nodules, while fascin-positive mature dendritic cells are present mainly in the stroma. Plasma cells are usually polyclonal, but rare cases harbour monoclonal B and/or plasma cells and even various low-grade intratumorous lymphomas {2878}.

Differential diagnosis

Thymic follicular hyperplasia is typically associated with myasthenia gravis and shows lymphoid follicles in the medulla and perivascular spaces. Rarely, epithelial cells adjacent to lymphoid follicles become hyperplastic {253} to the extent that there is a resemblance to micronodular thymoma with lymphoid stroma. However, the lobular thymic architecture and Hassall corpuscles are maintained in thymic follicular hyperplasia.

Type AB thymoma is composed of spindle cells in variable lymphocyte-rich and lymphocyte-poor areas. However, the lymphocyte-rich areas of type AB thymoma invariably contain a meshwork of keratin-positive epithelial cells; the lymphocytes are predominantly immature, TdT-positive T cells; and B cells are sparse or absent.

Micronodular thymic carcinoma with lymphoid hyperplasia mimics micronodular thymoma with lymphoid stroma, but tumour cells demonstrate high-grade nuclear atypia and increased mitotic activity, and the lymphoid stroma lacks immature T cells {3268}.

Rare tumours show a micronodular thymoma-like growth pattern and stroma, but the nodules are composed of polygonal epithelial cells resembling the tumour cells of type B2 thymoma {2999,1947}. It is unclear whether these tumours represent an atypical subtype of micronodular thymoma with lymphoid stroma or a micronodular subtype of type B thymoma.

Cytology

Not available

Diagnostic molecular pathology

Not clinically relevant

Essential and desirable diagnostic criteria

Essential:
- Multiple small discrete nodules composed of bland spindle or oval epithelial cells
- Abundant epithelial cell–free lymphoid stroma

Desirable:
- Predominant CD20-positive B cells in stroma

Staging

Micronodular thymoma with lymphoid stroma should be staged according to the Union for International Cancer Control (UICC) TNM system {315,687} and, optionally, the Masaoka–Koga system {685}.

Prognosis and prediction

Almost all patients present with localized, Masaoka stage I/II disease (55% encapsulated, 42% minimally invasive), representing pT1a in TNM classification {2917,2249,2999,3033,2878}. Only 1 case showed wide invasion and pleural implants {2917}. There have been no reports of recurrences, distant metastases, or tumour-related deaths after surgical resection {1947}.

Metaplastic thymoma

Sholl LM
Chan JKC
Liu B
Marx A

Definition
Metaplastic thymoma is a biphasic tumour of the thymus comprising islands of epithelial cells in a background of bland-looking spindle cells, with sharp or gradual transitions between the two components.

ICD-O coding
8580/3 Metaplastic thymoma

ICD-11 coding
2C27.2 & XH3DX0 Malignant thymoma & Metaplastic thymoma

Related terminology
Not recommended: thymoma with pseudosarcomatous stroma; low-grade metaplastic carcinoma; biphasic thymoma, mixed polygonal and spindle cell type.

Subtype(s)
None

Localization
Metaplastic thymoma is localized in the anterior (prevascular) mediastinum.

Clinical features
Signs and symptoms
Most patients are asymptomatic, being incidentally found to have an anterior (prevascular) mediastinal mass, but some patients present with cough, dyspnoea, or chest pain {1704}. Patients rarely present with myasthenia gravis {1370,2950,3176}.

Imaging
CT features are similar to those of type A thymoma: a well-defined, smooth, homogeneous anterior (prevascular) mediastinal mass {1370,1704}. In one case report, the tumour was highly FDG-avid, with uptake similar to that found in more aggressive tumours such as thymic cancer {1265}.

Epidemiology
Metaplastic thymoma is an extremely rare type of thymoma, with < 40 cases reported in the English-language literature. It occurs in adult patients with a median age of 50 years (range: 28–71 years) and a slight female sex predilection (M:F ratio: 1:1.5) {2923,3411, 3412,2127,472,2002,1744,1704,1370,1265,2950,3176}.

Etiology
The etiology is unknown. Occasional examples appear to arise in the wall of thymic cysts {2373,2002}.

Pathogenesis
Metaplastic thymoma harbours a distinctive *YAP1-MAML2* rearrangement, fusing exon 2 or 5 of *YAP1* with exon 2 of

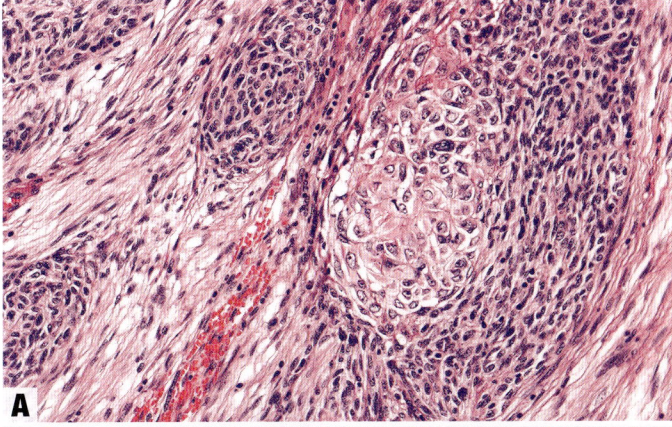

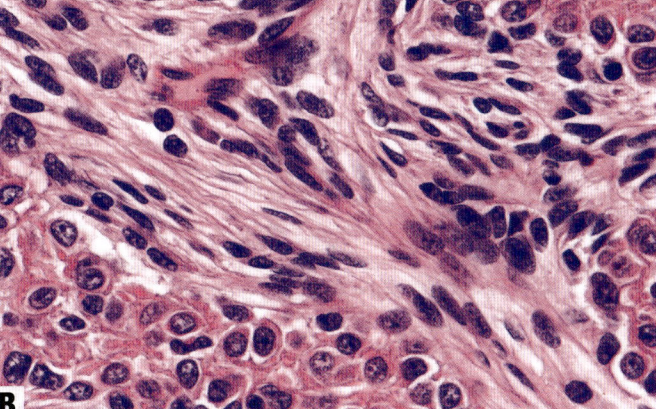

Fig. 5.44 Metaplastic thymoma. **A** The typical biphasic pattern of metaplastic thymoma. Nuclear pleomorphism is visible in the epithelial cells. **B** Cytological details of epithelial and spindle cells.

MAML2 {3176}. Comparative genomic hybridization, microsatellite studies, and targeted next-generation sequencing studies have shown no or few other genetic alterations {1704,3176}. Metaplastic thymoma does not show the *GTF2I* c.74146970T>A mutation frequently present in type A or type AB thymoma {3176}. EBV is negative {1704}.

Macroscopic appearance
The tumours are well circumscribed or encapsulated, but some may show invasive buds focally. The cut surfaces show homogeneous, solid, rubbery, grey-white to yellow tumour with fascicular appearance. Reported maximum size ranges from 30 to 180 mm {1370,1704,3411,3176}.

Histopathology
The tumours appear biphasic, with a solid epithelial component merging gradually or abruptly with a spindle cell component. The two components are present in highly variable proportions. A lobular growth pattern and perivascular spaces are absent.

Chapter 5

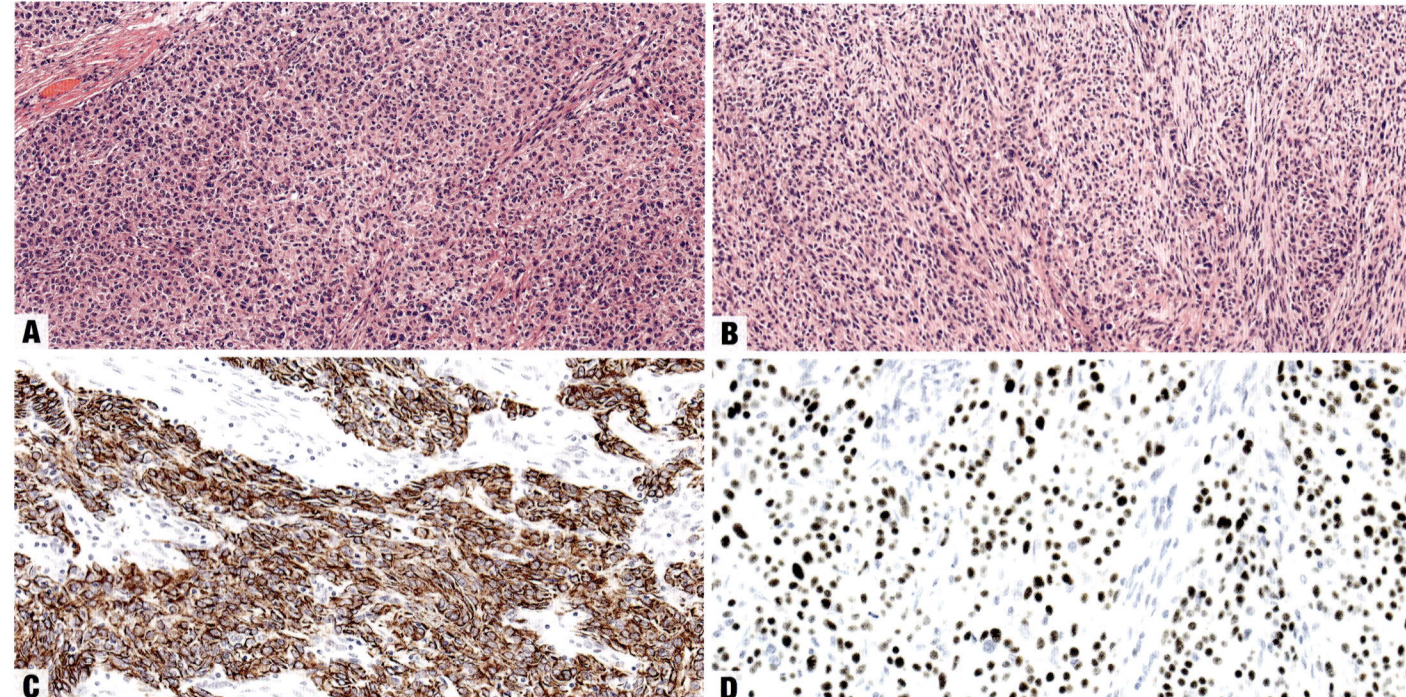

Fig. 5.45 Metaplastic thymoma. **A** An epithelium-rich area. **B** A spindle cell–rich area. **C** Cytokeratin stain highlights the epithelial elements. **D** p40 stain highlights epithelial cells and is negative in the spindle cells.

The epithelial cells form anastomosing islands or broad trabeculae, and they may exhibit a squamoid or whorled quality. They are oval, polygonal, or plump spindly, with oval or grooved nuclei, granular chromatin, small nucleoli, and a moderate amount of eosinophilic cytoplasm. Some cells can exhibit enlarged pleomorphic nuclei with pseudoinclusions, but mitotic figures are usually absent. Epithelial islands are commonly traversed by twigs of eosinophilic hyaline material.

Between the epithelial islands, slender, bland fibroblast-like spindle cells form short fascicles or storiform arrays. Their elongated nuclei have fine chromatin. Lymphocytes are usually sparse; an exceptional reported case with associated myasthenia gravis harboured abundant TdT-positive lymphocytes {2950}. Plasma cells can be present in occasional cases. Focal tumour necrosis has rarely been reported {1704}.

Rarely, areas of sarcomatoid carcinoma have been described in association with metaplastic thymoma, suggesting high-grade transformation {2002,1744}.

The epithelial islands are positive for cytokeratins and p63/p40, variably positive for EMA, and negative for vimentin {1370}. The spindle cells are negative or focally positive for cytokeratins, negative for p63/p40, focally positive for EMA and actin, and positive for vimentin. Both components are negative for CD5, CD20, CD34, and KIT (CD117). The Ki-67 index is low (< 5%) in both components. TdT-positive T cells are typically absent but may be encountered in adjacent thymic remnants {2127}.

The differential diagnosis includes sarcomatoid carcinoma (carcinosarcoma), which invariably shows a high-grade spindle cell component with significant nuclear atypia, frequent mitotic figures, prominent coagulative necrosis (commonly), and occasional heterologous differentiation {757}.

Type A thymoma can show variable epithelial cell growth patterns, mimicking a biphasic growth pattern. It is also often devoid of immature T cells. However, it is basically a monophasic tumour, lacks the anastomosing solid squamoid epithelial islands, and strongly expresses keratin and often CD20 but not vimentin in spindle cells.

Cytology
Not available

Diagnostic molecular pathology
Not clinically relevant

Essential and desirable diagnostic criteria
Essential:
- Biphasic thymic tumour
- Anastomosing islands of polygonal epithelial cells, which may show variable nuclear atypia
- Background of bland-looking spindly cells

Staging
Most tumours are localized and non-invasive, although occasional examples can show infiltration of adjacent tissues. Metastasis has not been reported {2127,2923,3411,3412,1704}.

Prognosis and prediction
Among reported patients with follow-up information, the majority have remained well at 1.5–20 years (median: 10 years) after surgical excision {2127,2923,3411,3412,1704,2950,3176}. One patient developed local recurrence at 14 months and died at 6 years {3412}. In two patients there was progression to sarcomatoid carcinoma at presentation, but the clinical course was uneventful after complete resection in one patient and unknown in the other {2002,1744}.

Lipofibroadenoma of the thymus

Chalabreysse L

Definition
Lipofibroadenoma is a benign thymic tumour that resembles fibroadenoma of the breast.

ICD-O coding
9010/0 Lipofibroadenoma

ICD-11 coding
4B40.Y & XH5854 Other specified diseases of thymus & Lipofibroadenoma

Related terminology
None

Subtype(s)
None

Localization
Lipofibroadenoma of the thymus is localized in the anterior (prevascular) mediastinum.

Clinical features
Of the 6 patients reported so far, 3 were asymptomatic and 2 presented with cough (one with fever and the other with expectoration). The remaining patient, in whom lipofibroadenoma was associated with type B1 thymoma, had dyspnoea and pure red cell aplasia {1556}. All cases reported were TNM stage I tumours.

Epidemiology
Only 6 tumours have ever been reported, all in men aged 20–62 years {1556,2195,2403,3223,1770,1207}.

Etiology
Unknown

Pathogenesis
It is uncertain whether the epithelial or the lipofibromatous component (or both) is neoplastic, or whether the lesion is a hamartoma. Because the tumours in 3 reported cases were associated with an adjacent type B1 thymoma {1556,3223,1207}, a putative thymic epithelial cell precursor is hypothesized to contribute to tumour development.

Macroscopic appearance
The tumours are oval and well circumscribed, with maximal diameters ranging from 30 to 230 mm. The cut surface is solid, grey, and firm.

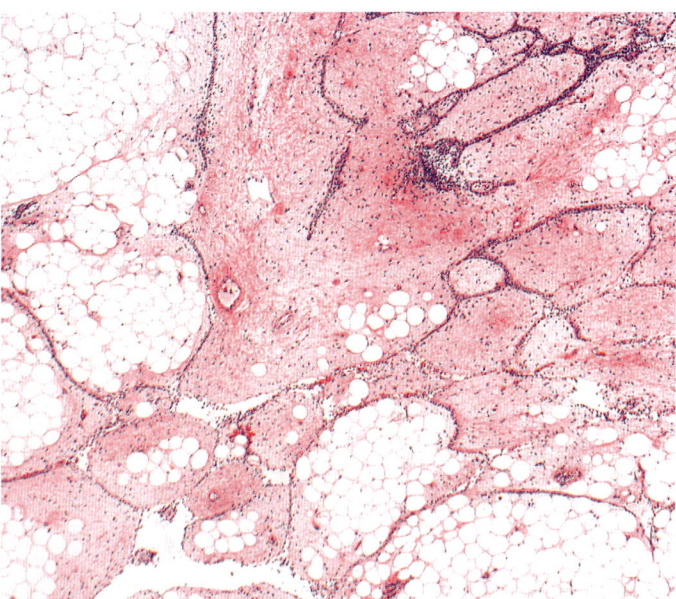

Fig. 5.46 Lipofibroadenoma of the thymus. Strands of epithelial cells separated by a fibrous tissue–predominant fibrolipomatous stroma.

Histopathology
The tumour resembles fibroadenoma of the breast. Fibrotic and hyaline stroma predominates over narrow strands of bland-looking epithelial cells, single or multiple fat cells, and few lymphocytes. Hassall corpuscles (reminiscent of thymic parenchyma) and calcifications can occur. Three cases arose adjacent to a type B1 thymoma {1556,3223,1207}.

Immunohistochemistry
The epithelial cells are positive for AE1/AE3 and CK19. Lymphocytes express either CD3 or CD20, but not TdT.

Differential diagnosis
Thymolipoma is characterized by a predominance of fatty tissue over epithelial cell strands with or without (usually minimal) thymic parenchyma and absence of a fibrous tissue component {2482}. Thymofibrolipoma has been described as a subtype of thymolipoma with a substantial fibrous component {1989}. It is currently unclear whether thymolipoma, thymofibrolipoma, and lipofibroadenoma constitute a spectrum of neoplastic or hamartomatous entities.

Sclerosing thymomas are distinguished by the presence of large islands of polygonal cells in a dense collagenous stroma without intermixed adipose tissue. Tumour cell palisades around perivascular spaces and lymphocytes may occur.

Cytology

Not available

Diagnostic molecular pathology

Not clinically relevant

Essential and desirable diagnostic criteria

Essential:

- A benign thymic tumour resembling fibroadenoma of the breast with a predominance of fibrous tissue over adipocytes and delicate strands of epithelial cells

Staging

Not applicable

Prognosis and prediction

All patients were disease-free after complete resection, by video-assisted thoracoscopy in one case {1770}.

Thymic carcinoma: Introduction

Chan JKC
Detterbeck F
Marino M
Marom EM

Marx A
Rajan A
Ströbel P

Overview

Thymic carcinomas are much less common than thymomas, accounting for 14–22% of all thymic epithelial tumours. Patients with thymic carcinoma are often symptomatic, presenting with symptoms referable to the mass lesion in the mediastinum. Paraneoplastic syndromes that are commonly present in patients with thymoma are very rare. The clinicopathological features that distinguish thymic carcinomas from thymomas are listed in Table 5.06.

On imaging studies, thymic carcinoma often appears as an anterior (prevascular) mediastinal mass that is more likely than thymoma to exhibit poorly defined, irregular lobular margins and necrotic or cystic changes that on CT manifest as low-attenuation regions and on MRI as greater tumour heterogeneity. Accompanying lymphadenopathy and pleural effusion may also be evident. The imaging features are similar across the various thymic carcinoma types, including the rare thymic adenocarcinomas {514,2951}.

Table 5.06 Comparison of the clinicopathological features of thymoma and thymic carcinoma

Feature	Thymoma	Thymic carcinoma
Nature	An epithelial tumour unique to the thymus, showing variable resemblance to the cytoarchitecture of the normal thymus	Thymic epithelial tumour with histological features of invasive carcinoma as observed in other anatomical sites
Frequency	75–85% of all thymic epithelial tumours	14–22% of all thymic epithelial tumours
Association with myasthenia gravis	Common	Very rare
Salient histological features	Exhibiting variable organotypic features: jigsaw puzzle–like lobulation, perivascular spaces, medullary differentiation, presence of intermingled immature T cells; nuclear atypia usually mild to at most moderate	Morphology of conventional carcinomas, usually with overt nuclear atypia and pleomorphism
Distinctive immunophenotypic features	Most thymomas have a component of non-neoplastic immature T cells, which can be highlighted by TdT immunostain; immature T cells are also present in the tumour in metastatic sites	Often exhibits immunostaining for CD5 and KIT (CD117), markers uncommonly expressed in conventional carcinomas
Behaviour	Indolent malignant neoplasm that can be non-invasive or invasive, with some cases exhibiting invasion of surrounding anatomical structures; a small proportion of cases can show pleural implant; lymph node metastasis and distant metastasis are very rare	Frankly malignant neoplasm that invades surrounding anatomical structures; a significant proportion of cases develop metastasis to lymph nodes and distant sites

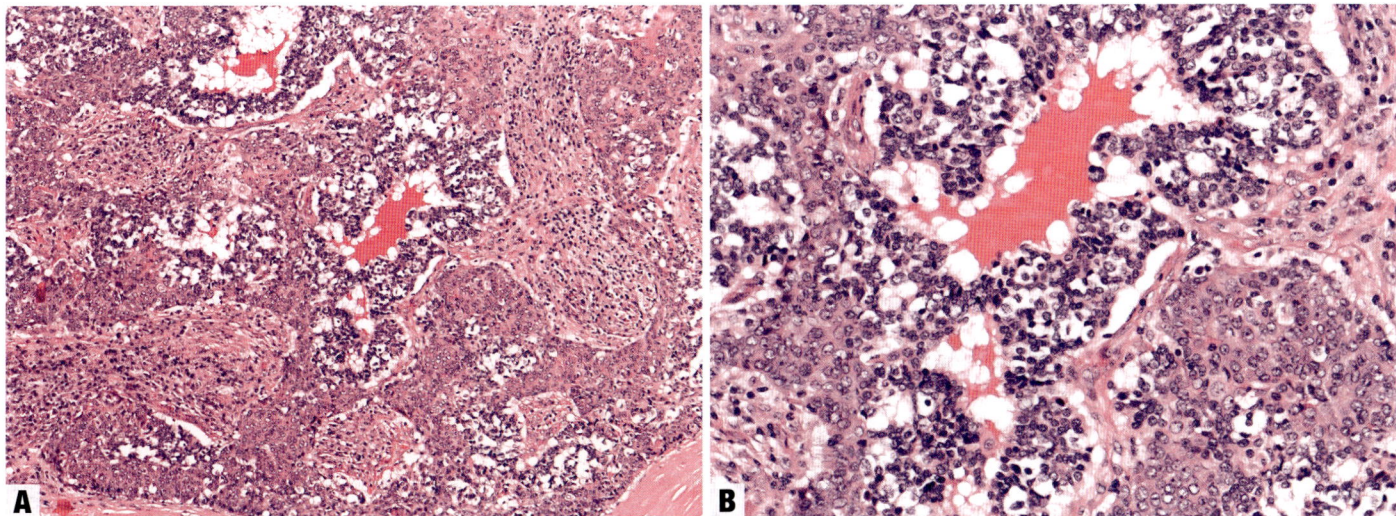

Fig. 5.47 Combined thymic squamous cell carcinoma and carcinoid. **A** Note intricately intermingled eosinophilic-staining squamous cell carcinoma and basophilic-staining carcinoid. **B** The squamous cell carcinoma component is sharply delineated from the dark-staining carcinoid component.

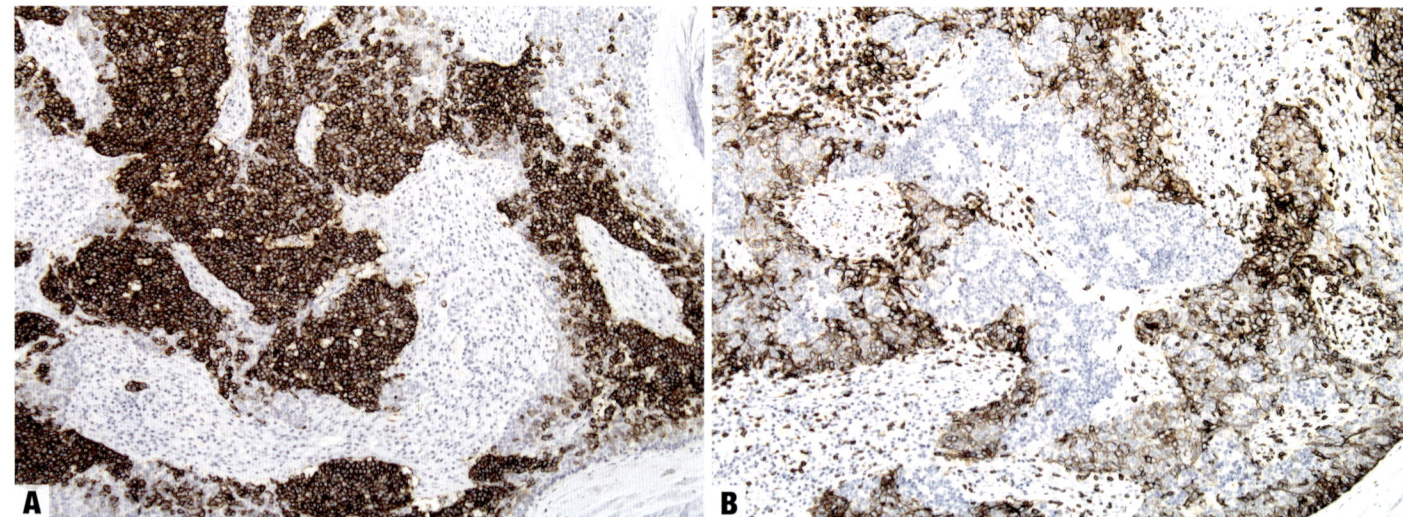

Fig. 5.48 Combined thymic squamous cell carcinoma and carcinoid. **A** Synaptophysin stain highlights the carcinoid component. **B** Reciprocal staining of the thymic squamous cell carcinoma component for CD5.

Etiology and pathogenesis

The etiology of thymic carcinomas is largely unknown. Rarely, a thymic carcinoma may show a concomitant component of thymoma, suggesting transformation from the latter.

The pathogenesis of thymic carcinomas is varied. The commonest type, thymic squamous cell carcinoma, shows a highly prevalent recurrent loss of chromosome 16p, various other copy-number alterations, or (rarely) microsatellite instability {2409}. Thymic mucoepidermoid carcinoma (with *MAML2* gene fusion) {2504}, NUT carcinoma (with *NUTM1* gene fusion), and a subtype of clear cell carcinoma (hyalinizing clear cell carcinoma, with *EWSR1* gene fusion) {865} are "translocation carcinomas" showing distinctive and therefore diagnostic gene fusions. Information on other types of thymic carcinomas is limited.

Classification of thymic carcinomas: changes in the fifth edition

The classification of thymic carcinomas in this fifth edition of the WHO classification is basically similar to that in the fourth edition. The three minor changes are as follows: (1) Micronodular thymic carcinoma with lymphoid hyperplasia is provisionally added as a subtype of squamous cell carcinoma. (2) For clear cell carcinoma, a hyalinizing subtype characterized by *EWSR1* gene translocation is recognized, analogous to hyalinizing clear cell carcinoma of salivary gland; further studies are required to re-evaluate the nosological nature of clear cell carcinoma of the thymus. (3) For primary thymic adenocarcinoma, the various subtypes are maintained, but with minor changes in terminology, from "papillary adenocarcinoma" to "low-grade papillary

Table 5.07 Reporting of heterogeneous tumours showing more than one histological type of thymic epithelial tumour

Component 1	Component 2	Terminology / reported diagnosis
Thymoma	Thymoma of a different type	Thymoma (state the components in 10% increments; start reporting with the most prevalent component)
Thymic carcinoma	Thymoma	Combined thymic carcinoma and thymoma
Thymic carcinoma	Thymic carcinoma of a different type	Combined thymic carcinoma (state the components in 10% increments; start reporting with the most prevalent component)
Thymic carcinoma	Carcinoid	Combined thymic carcinoma and carcinoid
Carcinoid	Thymoma	Combined carcinoid and thymoma
Small cell carcinoma	Thymic carcinoma	Combined small cell carcinoma and thymic carcinoma
Small cell carcinoma	Thymoma	Combined small cell carcinoma and thymoma
Small cell carcinoma	Carcinoid	Combined small cell carcinoma and carcinoid
Small cell carcinoma	LCNEC (< 10%)	Small cell carcinoma
Small cell carcinoma	LCNEC (≥ 10%)	Combined small cell carcinoma and LCNEC
LCNEC	Thymic carcinoma	Combined LCNEC and thymic carcinoma
LCNEC	Thymoma	Combined LCNEC and thymoma
LCNEC	Carcinoid	Combined LCNEC and carcinoid

LCNEC, large cell neuroendocrine carcinoma.

adenocarcinoma", and from "mucinous adenocarcinoma" to "enteric-type adenocarcinoma".

Reporting of heterogeneous tumours

Thymomas composed of more than one histological type of thymoma are common {2873,1977}, but combined thymic carcinomas are rare. By definition, these tumours are composed of at least one type of thymic carcinoma or thymic neuroendocrine neoplasm (NEN) and another thymic epithelial tumour. Examples comprise thymic squamous cell carcinoma associated with type B2/B3 thymoma {2919,3276} or micronodular thymoma with lymphoid stroma {2917}, low-grade papillary adenocarcinoma associated with type A or AB thymoma {1840, 3276}, sarcomatoid carcinoma associated with type A or metaplastic thymoma {2921,3276,3275,2002,1744}, and lymphoepithelial carcinoma associated with type B thymoma {2914, 3276}. Small cell carcinoma combined with thymoma {3068}, thymic carcinoma {1560,2796}, or carcinoid {3068} may rarely be encountered in the thymus.

Whereas the reporting of heterogeneous thymomas is exclusively based on the prevalence of the different thymoma components, the reporting of combined thymic carcinomas takes the aggressiveness of the various components into account, when applicable (see Table 5.07).

Squamous cell carcinoma of the thymus

Chan JKC
Chen G
Molina TJ
Ströbel P

Definition

Thymic squamous cell carcinoma (SCC) is a primary malignant neoplasm of the thymus with morphological features of SCC as seen in other organs.

ICD-O coding

8070/3 Squamous cell carcinoma, NOS

ICD-11 coding

2C27.0 & XH0945 Carcinoma of thymus & Squamous cell carcinoma, NOS

Related terminology

Not recommended: epidermoid keratinizing carcinoma; epidermoid non-keratinizing carcinoma; type C thymoma.

Subtype(s)

Micronodular thymic carcinoma with lymphoid hyperplasia

Localization

Thymic SCC originates in the thymus. The most frequently invaded mediastinal structures are the pericardium (40%), lung (40%), pleura (30%), and innominate veins and superior vena cava (20%) {3276,3508}. Mediastinal, cervical, and axillary lymph node metastases are common. Systemic metastases occur most frequently in the bone, liver, lung, adrenal glands, and brain {3276}.

Clinical features

Signs and symptoms

The most frequent symptoms are related to mediastinal compression: chest pain, cough, and shortness of breath {3276, 2152,1707,3508}. Less common symptoms include fever, superior vena cava syndrome, hoarseness, and haemoptysis {3276, 2152,436,3384,2927}. One third of patients are incidentally found to have the thymic tumour {3276,3508,2152}. Less than 5% of patients have associated myasthenia gravis {3508}, which is related to the presence of a coexisting thymoma component in at least some cases {2927,1563,1452}. Paraneoplastic polymyositis has been rarely reported {1429}. Approximately 12% of patients have a history of an extrathymic malignancy {33}.

Imaging

Thymic SCCs appear as an anterior (prevascular) mediastinal mass and are more likely than thymomas to show poorly defined, irregular lobular margins or necrotic or cystic changes that on CT manifest as low-attenuation regions and on MRI as greater tumour heterogeneity. Accompanying lymphadenopathy, pleural effusion, and distant metastases are more common than with thymoma {2527,1250}.

Epidemiology

Thymic carcinomas account for approximately 20% of thymic epithelial neoplasms {3508}, with SCC accounting for 70–80% of all cases {3283,3508,2581,519,3277,2181,33,1162}. Thymic SCC occurs in patients of various ages, but it is most common in the sixth decade of life. It is slightly more frequent in men {519,3277,3276}.

Etiology

There is no known association with cigarette smoking or other environmental factors. A small proportion of cases appear to arise from unilocular or multilocular thymic cysts or pre-existing thymomas {3275}.

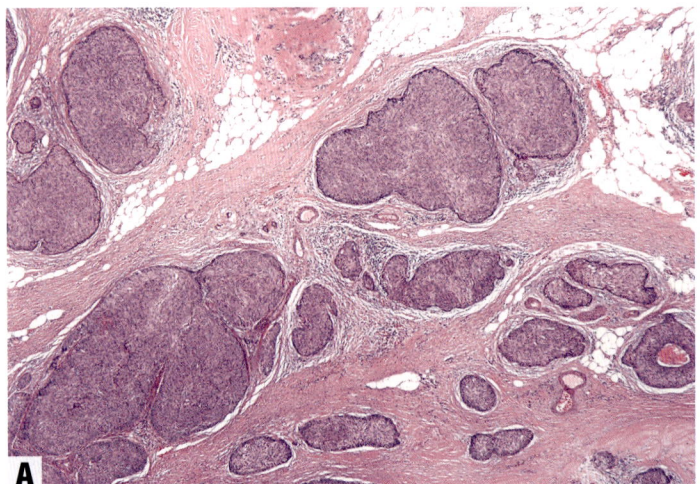
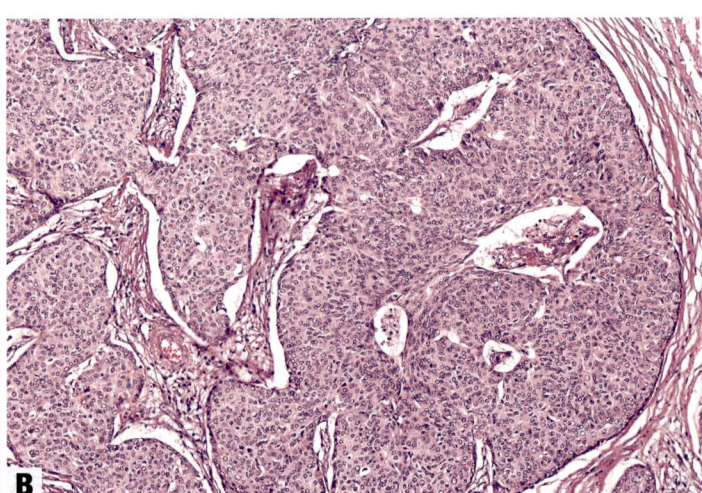

Fig. 5.49 Thymic squamous cell carcinoma. **A** The carcinoma may invade in the form of smooth-contoured islands, resembling the growth pattern of invasive thymoma. **B** Growth in the form of anastomosing smooth-contoured islands, traversed by thin fibrovascular septa.

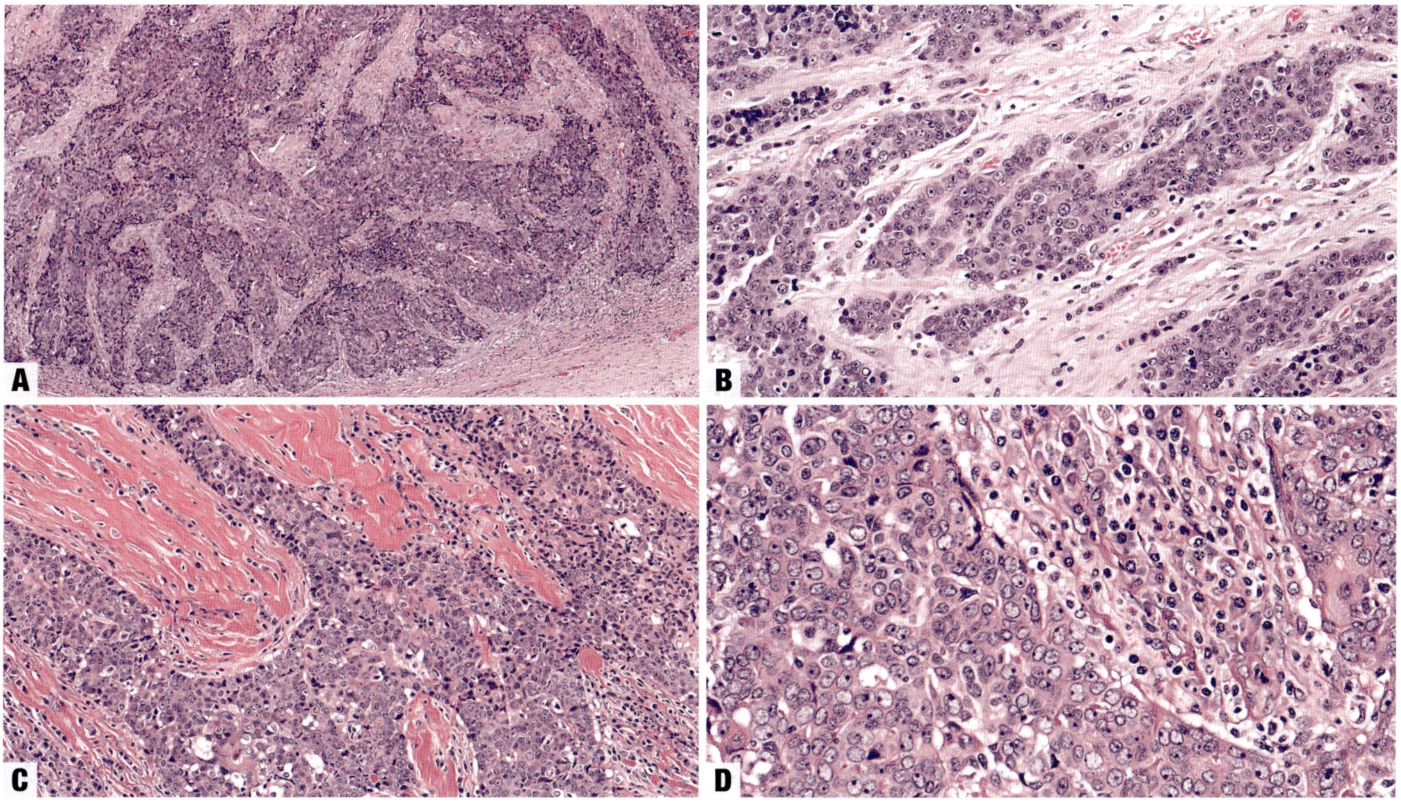

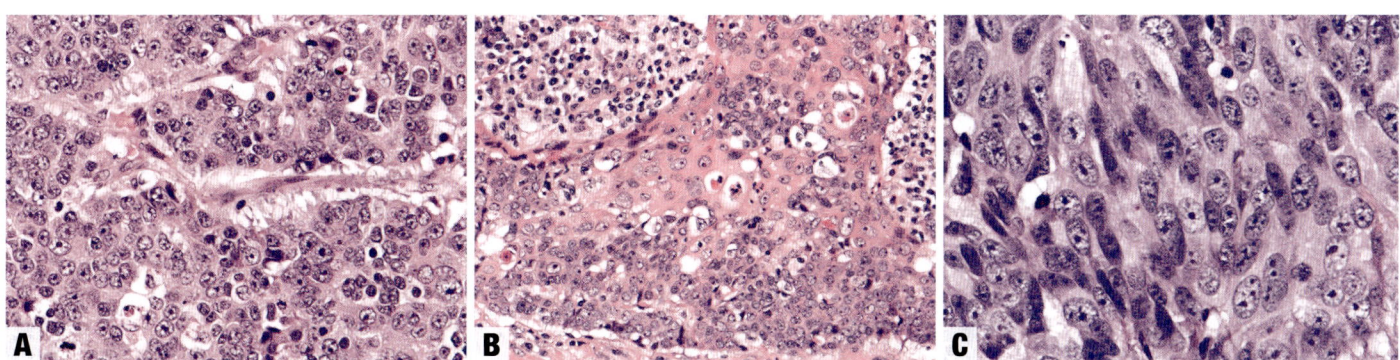

Fig. 5.50 Thymic squamous cell carcinoma. **A** Anastomosing irregularly shaped islands and sheets of tumour cells, in a sclerotic to desmoplastic stroma. **B** Irregular jagged islands and trabeculae of tumour cells in a sclerotic to desmoplastic stroma. **C** Presence of prominent sclerohyaline stroma. **D** The fibrovascular septa may resemble perivascular spaces as typical of thymoma, but there are plasma cells in addition to lymphocytes, and there is no epithelial cell palisading around the focus.

Pathogenesis

Loss of chromosomes 3p, 6, 6q25.2-q25.3, 16q, and 17p and gain of 1q, 17q, and 18 are frequently observed in thymic SCC {965,2877,3479,2409}. Among these aberrations, deletion of chromosome 6 and gain of 1q are shared with type B3 thymoma {1251}. The pattern of chromosome gains and losses in thymic SCC has been found to be different from that in pulmonary SCC {965}. The tumour mutation burden is significantly higher than that of thymomas {2409}.

KIT mutation has been reported in as many as 11% of thymic SCCs {3404, 3095, 965, 2872, 2338, 2246, 2659, 3028}. *TP53* mutation is found in about 20% of cases {1151, 2998, 3251,

965, 3292, 3221}. Copy-number gain of *BCL2* and deletion of *CDKN2A* (p16) are common; loss of immunostaining for p16 has been reported to be associated with a worse outcome {1151, 1544, 3281, 2335, 18}. *KRAS/HRAS/NRAS* mutations have been reported in 13.6% of cases {2604}.

GTF2I, *EGFR*, *BRAF*, *PIK3CA*, *APC*, *RET*, or *PTEN* gene mutations are rare or absent {2334, 3404, 965, 2872, 2930, 3359, 1879, 3293, 3281, 3292, 2409}. Mutations in epigenetic regulatory genes (*BAP1*, *ASXL1*, *SETD2*, *SMARCA4*, *TET2*, *DNMT3A*, *WT1*) {3221} are common, and DNA methylation of *GHSR*, *GNG4*, *HOXD9*, and *SALL3* is a common epigenetic alteration {1470}.

Fig. 5.51 Thymic squamous cell carcinoma. **A** Poorly differentiated carcinoma comprising polygonal cells with significant nuclear pleomorphism. There is no overt evidence of squamous differentiation. **B** In some areas, squamous differentiation is evident, with a greater amount of eosinophilic cytoplasm and intercellular bridges. **C** Neoplastic spindle cells can be present in some areas.

Macroscopic appearance

Thymic SCCs are frankly invasive tumours, lacking the encapsulation or internal fibrous septation characteristic of thymomas. The cut surfaces show firm to hard tan-coloured tumour with frequent foci of necrosis and haemorrhage. The mean maximum dimension is 72 mm (range: 20–170 mm) {3508}.

Histopathology

Thymic SCCs consist of infiltrative sheets, islands, and cords of large polygonal cells, accompanied by broad zones of desmoplastic to sclerohyaline stroma that is variably infiltrated by chronic inflammatory cells. Unlike in SCC of non-thymic origin, the tumour islands tend to be smooth-contoured, although invasion in jagged islands can occur. The tumour islands are frequently traversed by delicate blood vessels.

The polygonal tumour cells have large vesicular or hyperchromatic nuclei and distinct nucleoli. The cytoplasm is eosinophilic, and vague to obvious intercellular bridges can be identified in areas. Keratinization is present in some cases, and the keratinizing whorls may resemble Hassall corpuscles. The mitotic count is variable from case to case. Foci of coagulative necrosis are common.

Thymic SCCs can range from well to moderately to poorly differentiated, on the basis of nuclear pleomorphism, extent of squamous cell differentiation, and keratinization. The relevance of grading is controversial {2927,2152,3384,3508,3028}.

The cystic well-differentiated pattern is characterized by prominent cysts lined by squamous epithelium with different degrees of atypia. The intervening fibrous stroma is infiltrated

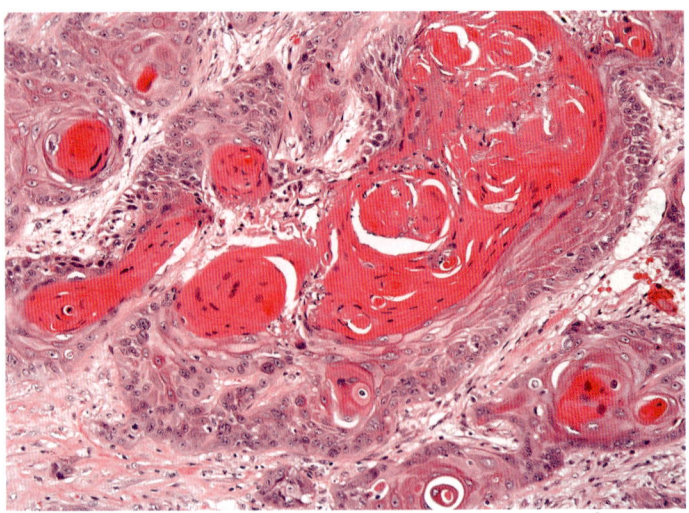

Fig. 5.52 Thymic squamous cell carcinoma. Overt keratinization is uncommon.

by islands and trabeculae of carcinoma. Focal keratinization is present. This variant is possibly associated with a better prognosis than conventional thymic SCC {3261}.

Subtypes

Micronodular thymic carcinoma with lymphoid hyperplasia, a carcinoma with marked morphological resemblance to micronodular thymoma with lymphoid hyperplasia, is provisionally considered a subtype of thymic SCC {2999,3268,1947}. Discrete small tumour nodules are separated by abundant lymphoid stroma

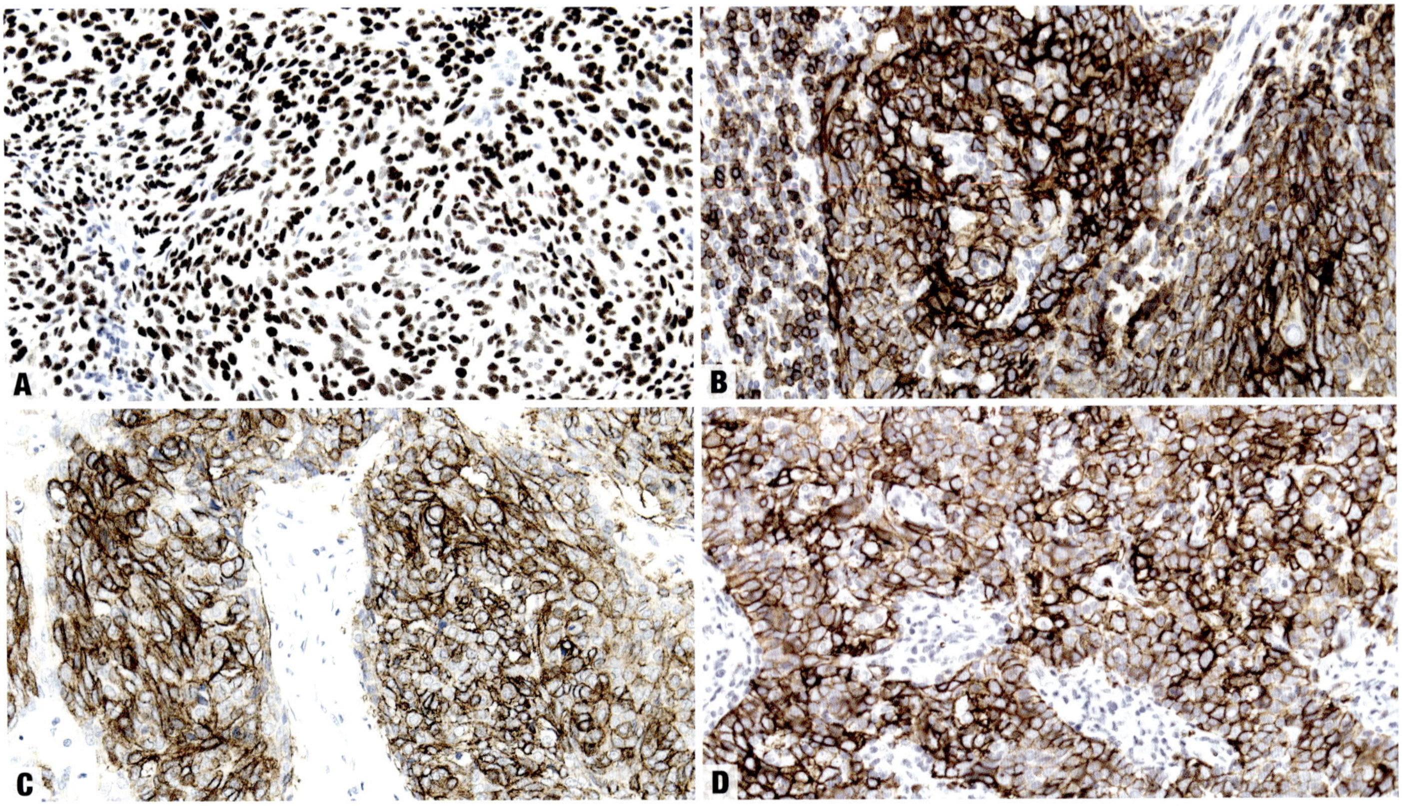

Fig. 5.53 Thymic squamous cell carcinoma. **A** Positive staining for p63 supports the squamous nature of the neoplasm. **B** The carcinoma cells show membranous staining for CD5. Many of the lymphocytes (T cells) in the stroma are also positive. **C** Carcinoma cells show membranous staining for KIT (CD117). **D** Diffuse positive staining for GLUT1.

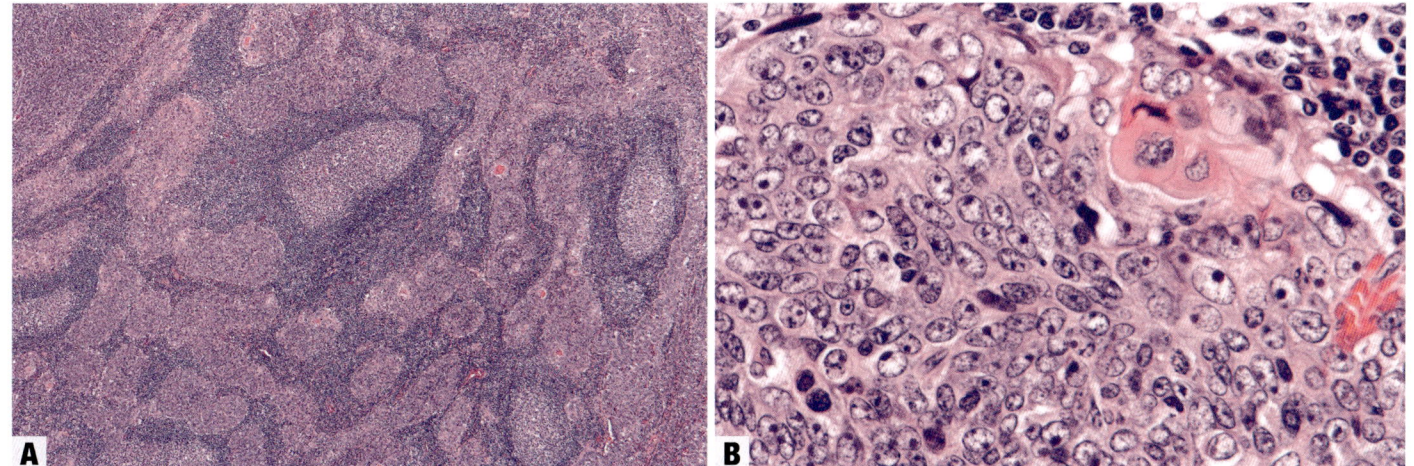

Fig. 5.54 Micronodular thymic carcinoma with lymphoid hyperplasia. **A** Round, oval to elongated nodules of carcinoma are disposed in a lymphoid cell–rich stroma containing reactive lymphoid follicles. **B** The poorly differentiated carcinoma cells focally show morphological evidence of squamous differentiation. The nuclei are pleomorphic and nucleoli are prominent.

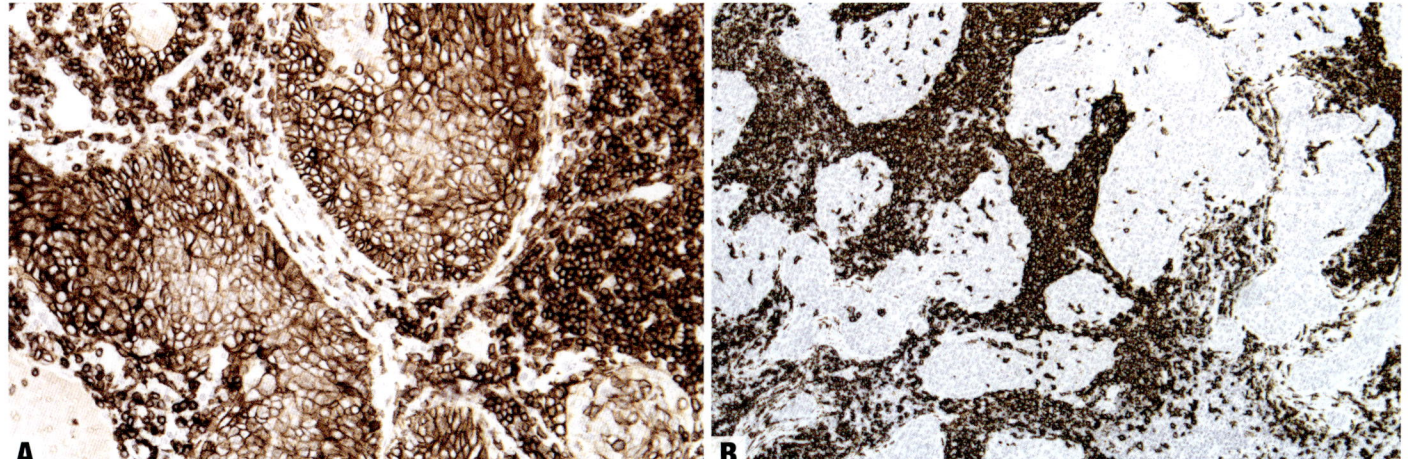

Fig. 5.55 Micronodular thymic carcinoma with lymphoid hyperplasia. **A** The nodules of carcinoma cells are immunoreactive for CD5. Some lymphoid cells (T cells) in the background are also positive. **B** CD20 immunostaining highlights numerous B cells in the lymphoid stroma.

with reactive lymphoid follicles; coalescence of tumour nodules to form large islands and sheets can be present in areas. The cytologically atypical oval to spindly tumour cells show vesicular nuclei, conspicuous nucleoli, and mitotic activity. Focal keratinization is often present. Unlike in micronodular thymoma, the tumour cells often coexpress CD5 and KIT (CD117), and there are no immature TdT-positive T cells surrounding the tumour islands.

Immunohistochemistry

Thymic SCCs are immunoreactive for pancytokeratins, and most are positive for p63/p40 {2248,724,3190}. PAX8 is positive in about 75% of cases when immunostaining is performed using polyclonal antibodies {117,3270,3276}, but it is negative when PAX8-specific monoclonal antibody is used {2929,3055}.

CD5, KIT (CD117), EMA (MUC1), and EZH2 are frequently expressed in thymic SCCs (75–85%) but rarely expressed in thymomas (usually < 5%), and thus may be of value in the differential diagnosis of these tumours in difficult cases {2132,1348, 1504, 1098, 3028, 2247, 2048, 117, 434, 719, 3358, 2997, 212,

1517, 3276, 3404, 3095, 1436}. GLUT1 is frequently expressed by the majority of tumour cells in thymic SCCs, unlike in type B3 and type A thymomas {1504,3029,734,2887}.

Proteasome subunit beta5t is not expressed in thymic carcinoma, in contrast to its almost universal expression in type B thymomas {3358,1098}. FOXN1 and CD205 (thymic epithelial markers important for thymic organogenesis) are expressed in almost all thymomas and in 68–76% and 10–59% of thymic carcinomas, respectively {2132,3276}. Because these markers are uncommonly expressed in carcinomas of non-thymic origin, they are of value for confirming the thymic origin of a carcinoma {2132}.

Focal expression of neuroendocrine markers is common in thymic carcinomas (seen in 64% of cases), but it is rare in thymomas {1606,1164}. PDL1 is commonly expressed, and tumour response to immune checkpoint inhibitor therapy has been reported {1804,2603,3115}. Unlike in thymomas, the infiltrating lymphocytes include mature T cells and B cells but not TdT-positive immature T cells (with very rare exceptions).

Differential diagnosis

Pulmonary SCC invading or metastasizing to the mediastinum can be difficult to distinguish from thymic SCC. Clinical and radiological assessment is crucial for the distinction. Positive immunostaining for CD5, KIT (CD117), FOXN1, and/or CD205 can be of help, because these markers are uncommonly expressed in non-thymic SCC {117,1535}. In contrast, EMA (MUC1) is not helpful for this purpose.

Distinction from type B3 thymoma, which can be difficult, is addressed in the section *Type B3 thymoma* (p. 340).

Other types of thymic carcinomas can show focal squamous differentiation or keratinization, such as lymphoepithelial carcinoma, basaloid carcinoma, NUT carcinoma, and sarcomatoid carcinoma. However, they exhibit features characteristic of these tumour types in areas not showing squamous differentiation.

Atypical carcinoid or large cell neuroendocrine carcinoma (LCNEC) can be in the differential diagnosis because thymic SCC frequently shows endocrine tumour–like vasculature and focal expression of neuroendocrine markers. However, atypical carcinoid shows a more prominent delicate vasculature and extensive immunoreactivity for neuroendocrine markers in > 50% of tumour cells.

Cytology

Cytological smears show overt malignant features. Clustered or single large cells show enlarged nuclei, coarse chromatin, discrete macronucleoli, and a moderate amount of cytoplasm. Immunohistochemistry may help in confirming the diagnosis.

Diagnostic molecular pathology

Assay of *KIT* mutation may be helpful to identify a potential therapeutic target.

Essential and desirable diagnostic criteria

Essential:
- Invasive SCC of the thymus, often accompanied by desmoplastic to sclerohyaline stroma
- Exclusion of invasion from adjacent pulmonary carcinoma or metastasis

Desirable:
- Positive immunostaining for p63/p40, CD5, KIT (CD117), FOXN1, and/or CD205
- Assay of *KIT* mutation may be helpful to identify a potential therapeutic target

Staging

Thymic SCC should be staged according to the TNM system {315,687} and, optionally, the Masaoka–Koga system {685}. The Masaoka–Koga stage distribution at diagnosis is as follows: stage I/II: ~20%; stage III: ~50%; stage IVA: ~15%; and stage IVB: ~20% {3276,1508,3384,628,1707,3508,33}.

Prognosis and prediction

The 5-year overall survival rate is 57.6–67.1% {59,291,436, 472,628,875,2566,1162}. Most large series (including analysis of the SEER and International Thymic Malignancy Interest Group [ITMIG] databases) have found a significant association between tumour stage and survival {33,3283}. Multivariate analysis of thymic carcinomas revealed that stage, R0 resection, and postoperative chemotherapy/radiotherapy were independent prognostic factors, whereas sex was not {33,875}. *KIT* mutation has been reported in as many as 11% of thymic SCCs {3404,3095,965,2872,2338,2246,2659,3028}, and some dramatic responses to tyrosine kinase inhibitors have been recorded for *KIT* mutation–positive cases {2875,2549}.

Basaloid carcinoma of the thymus

Papotti M
Marx A
Mukai K
Soares FA

Definition

Basaloid carcinoma of the thymus is a squamous cell carcinoma characterized by solid and cystic papillary nests of medium-sized to small cells with a high N:C ratio and peripheral palisading.

ICD-O coding

8123/3 Basaloid carcinoma

ICD-11 coding

2C27.0 & XH3GS1 Carcinoma of thymus & Basaloid squamous cell carcinoma

Related terminology

Acceptable: basaloid squamous cell carcinoma.

Subtype(s)

None

Localization

Basaloid carcinoma of the thymus is localized in the anterior (prevascular) mediastinum.

Clinical features

About 60% of cases are discovered incidentally {321}. The remaining patients present with mediastinal compression symptoms {321,2599,2891}. CT or MRI typically shows a multicystic mass with solid components {2992,2599,2891}.

Epidemiology

Basaloid carcinoma accounts for < 5% of all thymic carcinomas {2927}. Forty cases are reported in the English literature

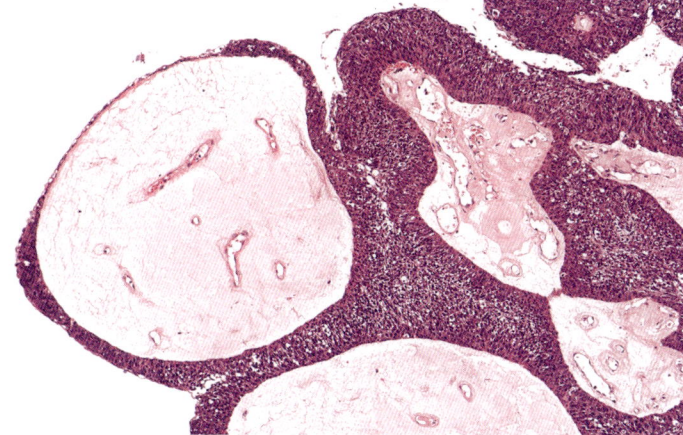

Fig. 5.56 Basaloid carcinoma. Cystic-papillary pattern with endoluminal frond-like growth.

{321, 2599, 2891, 3099, 3275, 3357, 331, 1789, 1841, 1938, 2766}. The tumour occurs in adults (mean age: 58 years; range: 34–77 years), with an M:F ratio of about 2:1. The International Thymic Malignancy Interest Group (ITMIG) database documents 19 basaloid carcinomas among 6097 thymic epithelial neoplasms {33}.

Etiology

Multilocular thymic cysts were observed in 45% of cases {321, 2599,2891,3099,3275,3357,331,1789,1841,1938,2766} and may represent precursor lesions {1230,2599}.

Pathogenesis

Unknown

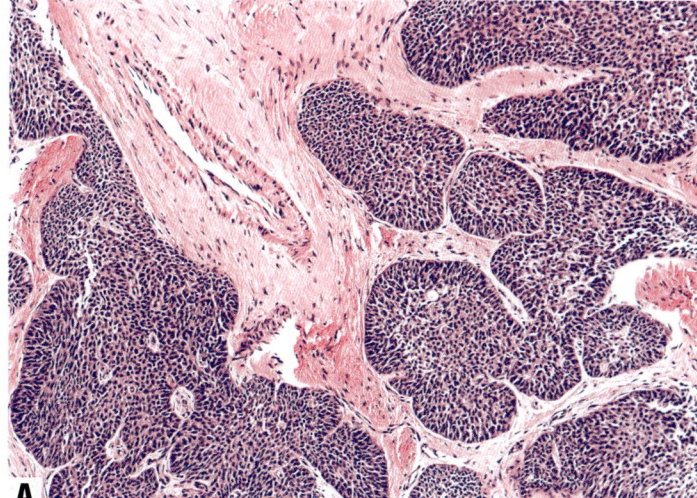
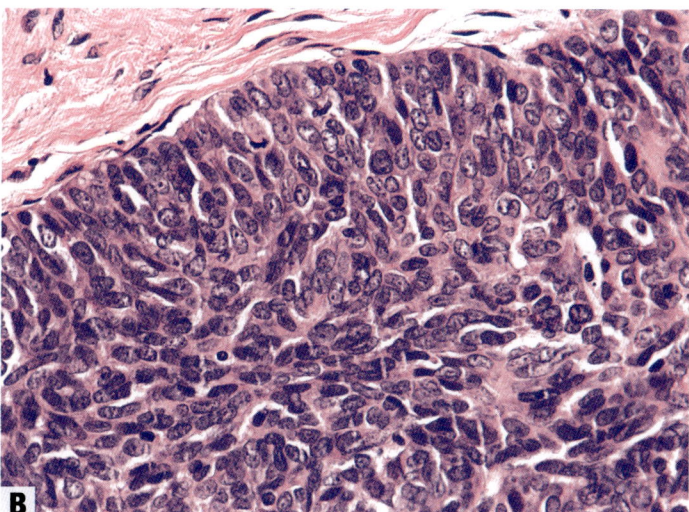

Fig. 5.57 Basaloid carcinoma. **A** Nesting growth pattern with peripheral palisading. **B** Tumour nest containing atypical basaloid cells with a high N:C ratio.

Chapter 5

Macroscopic appearance

Basaloid carcinoma is a well-circumscribed greyish tumour with solid and cystic areas and a mean size of 80 mm (range: 28–200 mm) {321,2599,2891}.

Histopathology

Basaloid carcinoma usually shows an admixture of two growth patterns {321}. The cystic-papillary pattern is characterized by cystic spaces lined by multilayered tumour cells, which occasionally generate papillary protrusions. The nesting pattern is characterized by variably sized, compact nests of monotonous small or medium-sized tumour cells with peripheral palisading, in a desmoplastic stroma {3275}. The tumour cells are rounded or spindly, with indistinct cell borders, a high N:C ratio, hyperchromatic nuclei, and distinct nucleoli. The mitotic count varies from 0 to > 30 mitoses/2 mm² {321,2382}. Comedonecrosis is common. Focal abrupt squamous differentiation occurs in 40% of cases {321}. Small glandular spaces and deposits of amorphous basement membrane–like material may be present within the tumour nests. Cystic changes can result from pre-existing multilocular thymic cysts or cystic tumour degeneration. Rarely, there is transformation to sarcomatoid carcinoma {321}.

Immunohistochemistry

Basaloid carcinomas are immunoreactive for pancytokeratin and CK5/6. About 75% of cases are positive for p40/p63 and KIT (CD117), while < 50% of cases express CD5 {321,331}.

Differential diagnosis

Thymic carcinoma with adenoid cystic carcinoma–like features is characterized by nests of basaloid cells arranged in a cribriform and microcystic pattern, lacking KIT (CD117)-positive luminal cells and lacking myoepithelial marker expression in the basaloid cells. Palisading is a feature of neuroendocrine carcinomas (NECs) as well, but the lack of neuroendocrine markers in a p40-positive tumour favours basaloid carcinoma. NUT carcinomas can resemble basaloid carcinomas due to the small tumour cell size and transitions to squamous differentiation, but they show nuclear NUT expression. Poorly differentiated squamous cell carcinoma lacks the conspicuous peripheral palisading of basaloid carcinoma {321}.

Cytology

Smears show a necrotic background with single and cohesive sheets of small monomorphic cells with a high N:C ratio. The cells have round nuclei, granular chromatin, and prominent nucleoli {2382}.

Diagnostic molecular pathology

Not clinically relevant

Essential and desirable diagnostic criteria

Essential:
- A basaloid carcinoma of the thymus with nests or cystic spaces lined by basaloid neoplastic cells with peripheral palisading

Desirable:
- Immunostaining positive for p63/p40 and/or KIT (CD117) and negative for TTF1, neuroendocrine markers, and NUT

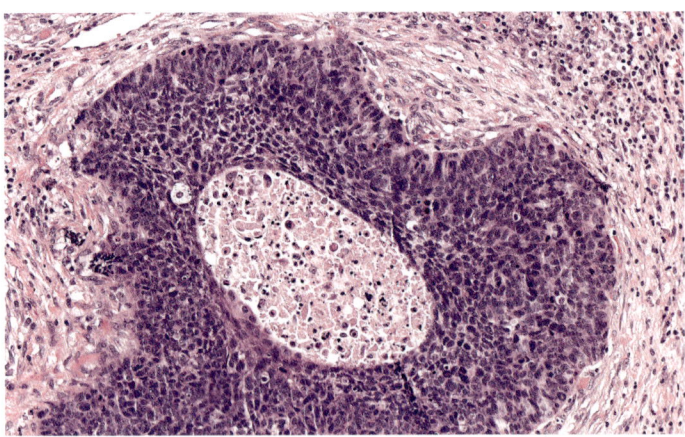

Fig. 5.58 Basaloid carcinoma. Tumour nest composed of basaloid cells with scant cytoplasm, peripheral palisading, and central necrosis.

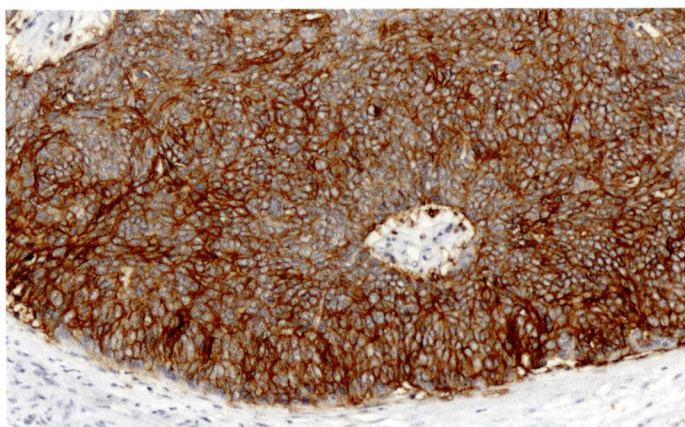

Fig. 5.59 Basaloid carcinoma of the thymus. Strong expression of CD5 by the tumour cells of a basaloid carcinoma.

Staging

Basaloid carcinomas should be staged according to the TNM system {315,687} and, optionally, the Masaoka–Koga system {685}. In the ITMIG cohort, 35%, 35%, and 30% of basaloid carcinomas are in stages I/II, III, and IV, respectively {33}.

Prognosis and prediction

Fatal outcome due to pleural, liver, and lung metastases occurs in approximately 50% of cases {321,2927}. Successful combined surgical treatment, chemotherapy, and radiotherapy was reported in one case {2946}. A durable response to platinum-based chemotherapy (up to 24 months) was reported in 3 advanced cases {331,1789,1938}. In the ITMIG cohort, survival and recurrence rates overlap with those of other thymic carcinoma types {33}.

Lymphoepithelial carcinoma of the thymus

Chan JKC
Chalabreysse L
Mukai K
Tateyama H

Definition

Lymphoepithelial carcinoma is a primary thymic undifferentiated or poorly differentiated squamous cell carcinoma (SCC) accompanied by a prominent lymphoplasmacytic infiltrate, morphologically similar to nasopharyngeal non-keratinizing SCC.

ICD-O coding

8082/3 Lymphoepithelial carcinoma

ICD-11 coding

2C27.0 & XH1E40 Carcinoma of thymus & Lymphoepithelial carcinoma

Related terminology

Acceptable: lymphoepithelioma-like carcinoma.

Subtype(s)

None

Localization

Lymphoepithelial carcinoma of the thymus is localized in the anterior (prevascular) mediastinum (thymus).

Clinical features

Signs and symptoms

Although some patients are asymptomatic, most present with symptoms related to the mediastinal mass, such as dull chest pain, cough, and dyspnoea {1080,3306}. Superior vena cava syndrome can occur in patients with more-advanced disease {1080,1191, 1238,3306}. There is no association with myasthenia gravis, pure red cell aplasia, or hypogammaglobulinaemia, but rare cases can

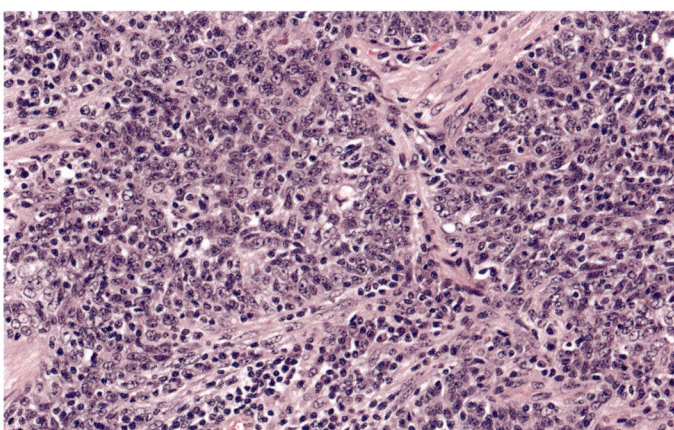

Fig. 5.60 Thymic lymphoepithelial carcinoma. Discrete islands of carcinoma with admixed lymphocytes and plasma cells.

be complicated by hypertrophic osteoarthropathy, polymyositis, or nephrotic syndrome {1191,1238,2113,1516,1434}.

Imaging

Lymphoepithelial carcinoma tends to be large at presentation and locally aggressive. On CT, low-attenuation regions within the tumour correspond to necrosis {1516}.

Tumour spread

The tumour shows local spread into surrounding tissues and organs, with frequent invasion of pleura, lung, diaphragm, and pericardium {3389}. Lymph node, lung, liver, and bone are frequent sites for metastasis.

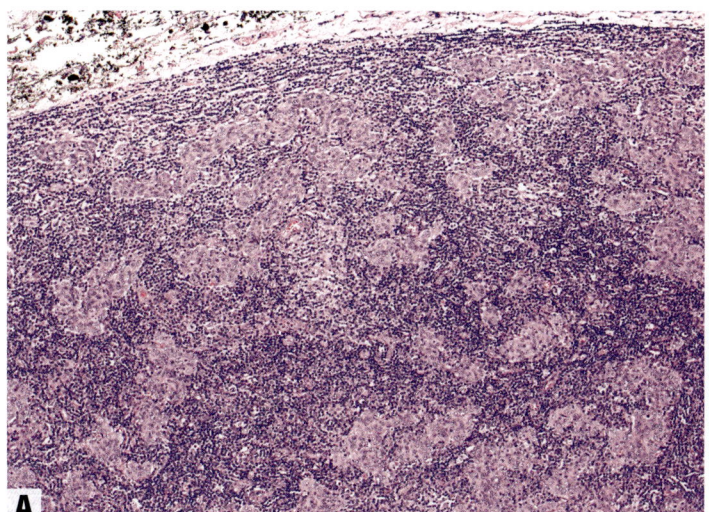
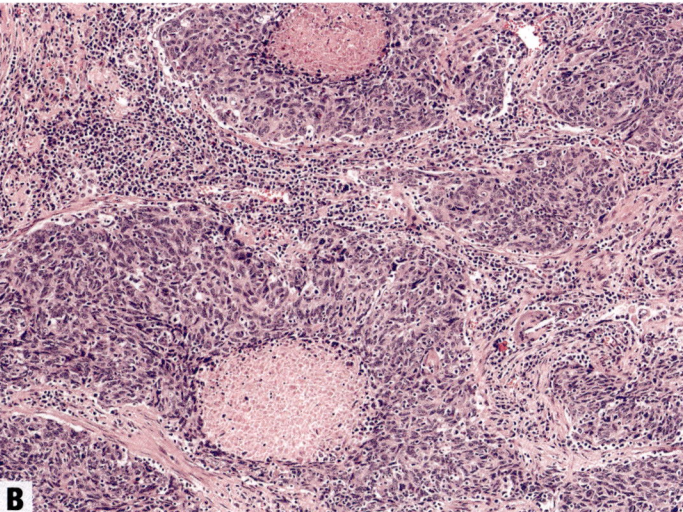

Fig. 5.61 Thymic lymphoepithelial carcinoma. **A** Irregular islands of carcinoma accompanied by a dense lymphoid infiltrate. **B** Irregular islands of carcinoma with coagulative necrosis, accompanied by a stroma heavily infiltrated by lymphocytes and plasma cells.

Chapter 5

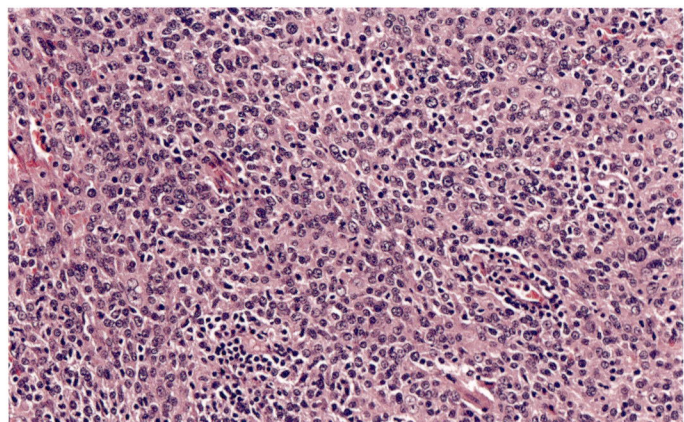

Fig. 5.62 Thymic lymphoepithelial carcinoma. The intimate intermingling of carcinoma cells with lymphocytes and plasma cells may render the epithelial nature of the tumour difficult to recognize.

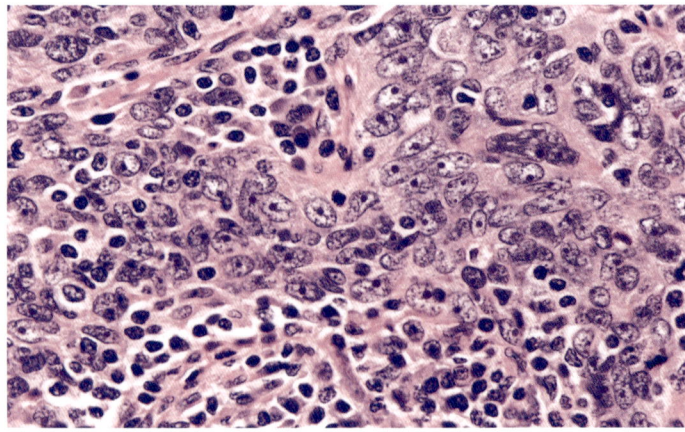

Fig. 5.63 Thymic lymphoepithelial carcinoma. The carcinoma cells typically show indistinct cell borders (a syncytial appearance), overlapping vesicular nuclei, and conspicuous nucleoli. Lymphocytes and plasma cells are present within the tumour islands and in the stroma.

Epidemiology

Thymic lymphoepithelial carcinomas are rare, accounting for 1.3–6% of all thymic carcinomas {1162,2566,1199}. The patients range in age from 4 to 76 years, with a median age of 41 years and bimodal age peaks at 14 years and 48 years. The M:F ratio is approximately 2:1 {1080,1560,1229,2855,1191,1238,3306,3345, 2113,2927}.

Etiology

Approximately half of all cases show association with EBV {3485}; EBV is almost always positive in children and young adults, but it is uncommonly positive in adults aged > 30 years. The association with EBV is apparently not related to geographical or ethnic factors {1191,2113,2855,1229,478,1402,2914}.

Exceptionally, there is a concomitant component of thymoma, raising the possibility of transformation of lymphoepithelial carcinoma from thymoma {3276}.

Pathogenesis

Unknown

Macroscopic appearance

The tumours typically show invasive borders. The cut surfaces are solid and yellow-white, with areas of necrosis.

Histopathology

The tumour comprises anastomosing sheets, nests, and cords of carcinoma cells accompanied by abundant lymphocytes and plasma cells, both in the fibrous stroma and intimately admixed with the carcinoma cells. The carcinoma cells have indistinct cell borders, large vesicular nuclei, and one or more distinct nucleoli. The nuclei are unevenly crowded and may appear overlapping. In general, there is no striking nuclear size variation or anaplasia {434,1191,3276,1560}.

In some cases, focal squamous differentiation can be present. The carcinoma cells are polygonal, with a greater amount of eosinophilic cytoplasm and vague intercellular bridges. The carcinoma cells can also appear spindly. Mitotic activity is variable but often pronounced. Coagulative necrosis is common. Germinal centres, eosinophils, and granuloma may be present.

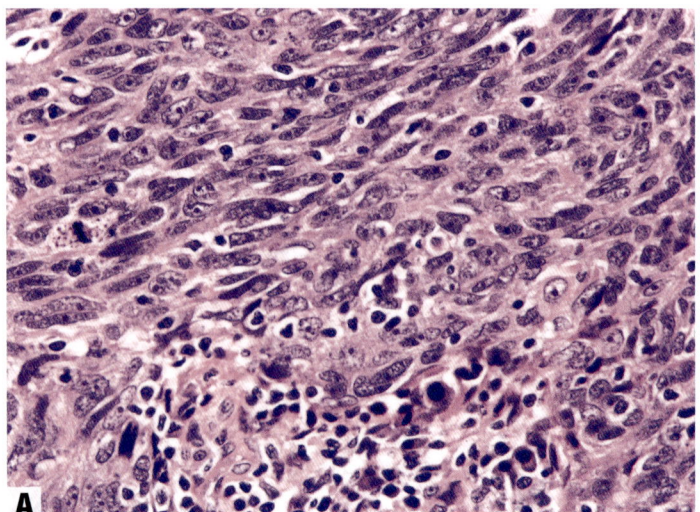

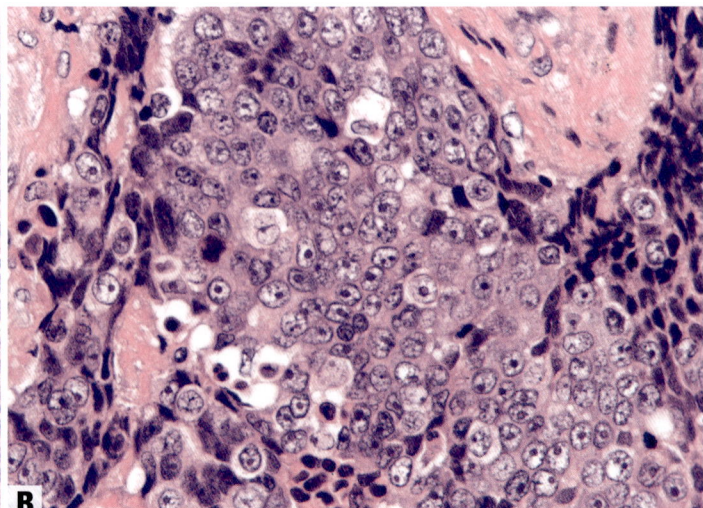

Fig. 5.64 Thymic lymphoepithelial carcinoma. **A** The carcinoma cells can be spindly. **B** Lymphocyte-poor and EBV-positive lymphoepithelial carcinoma lacking prominent lymphoid stroma but showing a syncytial appearance of the large tumour cells, with overlapping vesicular nuclei and prominent nucleoli.

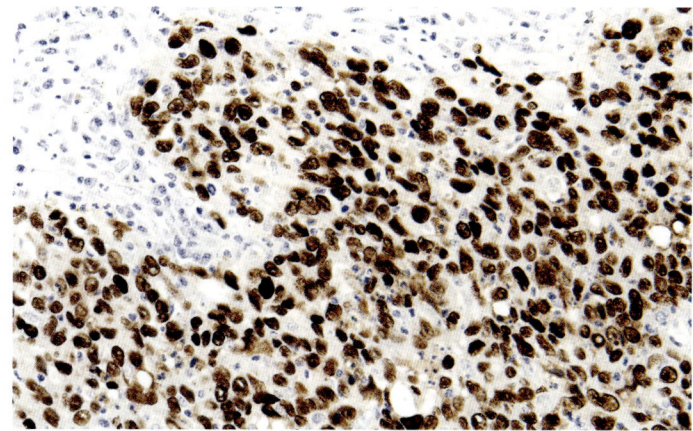

Fig. 5.65 Thymic lymphoepithelial carcinoma. The tumour cells show positive nuclear labelling for EBV-encoded small RNA (EBER) on in situ hybridization.

Poorly differentiated carcinomas with the above-described histological features but not accompanied by a significant lymphoplasmacytic infiltrate and shown to harbour EBV are provisionally classified as lymphoepithelial carcinoma, although it is currently unclear whether these tumours are more related to lymphoepithelial carcinomas or SCCs.

Immunohistochemistry

Tumour cells are positive for pancytokeratins, CK5/6, p63, and p40. There is variable immunoreactivity for CD5 and frequent immunoreactivity for KIT (CD117) {719,2247,2914}. PDL1 is commonly expressed {2913}. In tumours associated with EBV, in situ hybridization shows EBV-encoded small RNA (EBER) labelling of the tumour cells. The admixed lymphocytes include mature T cells and B cells, and the plasma cells are polyclonal.

Differential diagnosis

The differential diagnosis includes thymic undifferentiated carcinoma (with significant nuclear pleomorphism; EBV-negative), SCC (overt squamous differentiation; lacking syncytial quality

of tumour cells; EBV-negative), micronodular thymic carcinoma with lymphoid hyperplasia (nodular rather than diffuse growth; lacking syncytial quality; few lymphocytes in tumour islands), and metastatic lymphoepithelial carcinoma (clinical correlation required).

Cytology
Not available

Diagnostic molecular pathology
Not clinically relevant

Essential and desirable diagnostic criteria
Essential:
- Primary thymic carcinoma
- Sheets, nests, and cords of carcinoma cells with syncytial appearance, vesicular chromatin, and prominent nucleoli
- Many admixed lymphocytes and plasma cells

Desirable:
- Immunohistochemistry for pancytokeratins, p63/p40
- In situ hybridization for EBER – the result does not affect diagnosis of cases with typical lymphoepithelial carcinoma morphology, but EBER positivity supports the diagnosis in lymphocyte-poor cases

Staging

Lymphoepithelial carcinoma should be staged by the TNM system {315,687} and, optionally, the Masaoka–Koga system {685}. In the International Thymic Malignancy Interest Group (ITMIG) cohort, the Masaoka stage distribution is as follows: stage I/II: 25%; stage III: 43%; and stage IV: 32%.

Prognosis and prediction

Thymic lymphoepithelial carcinoma is a highly malignant neoplasm with a poor prognosis {3276,434}. The median survival time is 36 months {1402}, but patients with low-stage, completely resected tumour appear to have a favourable outcome {2914}. The EBV status has no effect on prognosis.

NUT carcinoma of the thorax

French CA
Badve S
den Bakker MA
Jain D

Definition
NUT carcinoma is a poorly differentiated carcinoma genetically defined by the presence of nuclear protein in testis (*NUTM1*) gene rearrangement.

ICD-O coding
8023/3 NUT carcinoma

ICD-11 coding
2C27.0 & XH2855 Carcinoma of thymus & NUT carcinoma

Related terminology
Not recommended: NUT midline carcinoma; NUT-rearranged carcinoma; t(15;19) carcinoma; thymic carcinoma with t(15;19); carcinoma with t(15;19) translocation; aggressive t(15;19)-positive carcinoma; midline lethal carcinoma; midline carcinoma of children and young adults with NUT rearrangement.

Subtype(s)
None

Localization
Thoracic/mediastinal NUT carcinoma accounts for 51% of all cases {464}, but due to the involvement of both lung and mediastinum in most cases at presentation, it is not possible to determine the fraction of these cases that originated within the mediastinum/thymus {175}. Head and neck primary sites account for 41% of NUT carcinomas, and bone and soft tissue primary sites account for 6% {464}. Rare cases arise within kidney {237,703}, pancreas {2724}, thyroid {1592}, and bladder {867}.

Clinical features
Signs and symptoms
NUT carcinoma is usually at an advanced stage at presentation, with pleuritic chest pain, non-productive cough, weight loss, and shortness of breath {1624,2083,3015}.

Imaging
Chest X-rays usually demonstrate a widened mediastinum with partial or complete opacification of the hemithorax due to pulmonary extension of tumour. Extremely rapid disease progression is reported, with complete opacification of the thorax occurring within 2–8 weeks from initial presentation {2371}. By CT, NUT carcinoma appears as a hypoattenuating, heterogeneously enhancing, often extensively necrotic mass with poorly defined, infiltrative borders {2083,2371,2854}. Invasion of adjacent structures, necrosis, and calcifications are frequent {2371,2083,3015}. MRI reveals a hypointense T1-weighted and hyperintense T2-weighted lesion {2371}. High FDG uptake by NUT carcinoma is characteristic, thus PET-CT is the modality of choice to determine the systemic disease burden in patients in whom the diagnosis of NUT carcinoma has been established

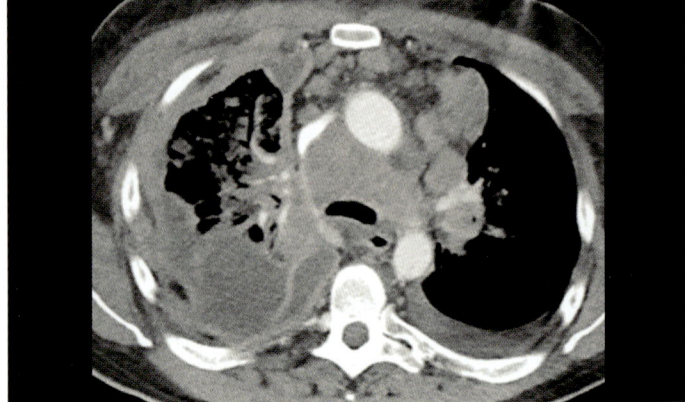

Fig. 5.66 NUT carcinoma. CT demonstrates a large, heterogeneous, widely infiltrative tumour with associated mediastinal adenopathy.

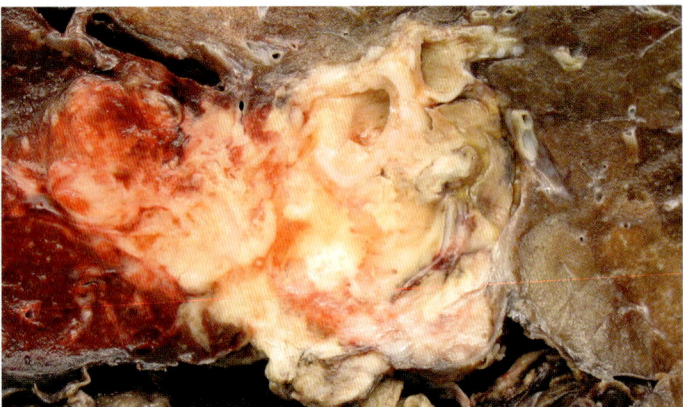

Fig. 5.67 NUT carcinoma. Pneumonectomy specimen reveals an extensively infiltrative tumour with abundant necrosis.

{2112,2683,2533}, and it is helpful in monitoring response to treatment.

Tumour spread
NUT carcinoma commonly spreads by local invasion and lymphatic and haematogenous metastasis {175,464}. There is often invasion of the pleura. Distant metastases are common; bone metastases are observed early, and multiorgan dissemination (e.g. to ovaries, liver, and brain) is seen later in the course of disease {3152,2724,773,151,2983,2396,2371}.

Epidemiology
More than 200 cases have been reported. NUT carcinoma affects males and females equally. Originally thought to be a disease of children and younger adults (median age: 23.6 years) {867}, NUT carcinoma can affect people of any age (range: 0–80 years) {866,2724,2853,464}. Whether the

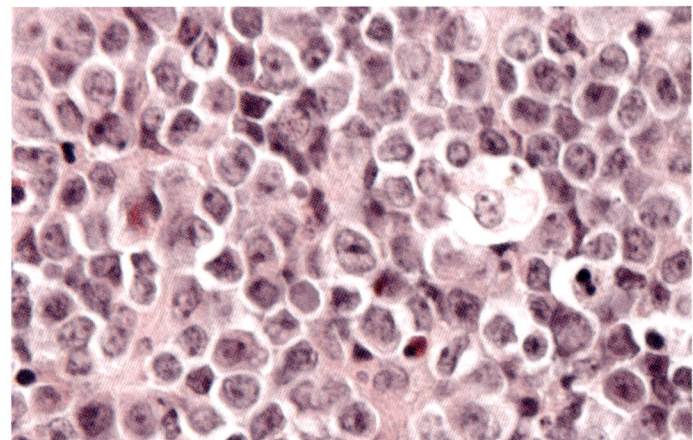

Fig. 5.68 NUT carcinoma. A sheet-like proliferation of monomorphic, small to medium-sized cells demonstrating separation artefacts and a conspicuous lack of nuclear moulding.

observed increasing frequency of NUT carcinomas in patients aged > 18 years is due to the higher awareness of the disease is unknown {175,463}. Based on a series of 14 107 consecutive tumours analysed by next-generation sequencing, the estimated frequency of *NUTM1* rearrangement was 0.06% of solid malignancies; the majority of these were NUT carcinomas {2861}. NUT carcinoma has been reported to account for 4–18% of poorly differentiated carcinomas {786,867,2853}, 0.6% of lung carcinomas lacking glandular differentiation {2761}, and 2.7–4% of mediastinal/thymic carcinomas in limited series {786, 2339,980,978}.

Etiology
The etiology is unknown. No associations with environmental factors have been demonstrated.

Pathogenesis
NUT carcinoma is characterized by chromosomal translocation t(15;19)(q14;p13.1) and resulting fusion of *NUTM1* to *BRD4* (> 75% of cases) or by fusion of *NUTM1* to genes coding for BRD4-interacting proteins, such as *BRD3* (9q34.2; ~15% of cases), *NSD3* (8p11.23; ~5%), and others (*ZNF532*, *ZNF592*, and other unidentified gene[s]; ~5%) {868,870,2756,54,869}.

The *BRD4-NUTM1* and *BRD3-NUTM1* fusions occur by chromosomal translocation resulting from highly complex genomic rearrangements, often resulting in multiple rearrangements that occur during a single catastrophic event, termed chromoplexy {1638}. The host cell is believed to be an otherwise normal, dividing somatic cell. NUT-fusion oncoproteins, most commonly BRD4-NUT {868}, act as single drivers of NUT carcinoma that function by blocking differentiation and maintaining proliferation {870}. Few, if any, additional oncogenic mutations have been demonstrated {1638,464,2841}. BRD4-NUT binds to acetylated histones of chromatin through the dual bromodomains of BRD4, and NUT recruits histone acetyltransferase p300 to form massive, BRD4-NUT/acetyl-histone/p300-enriched regions, termed megadomains {2472,53,1005,54}. Megadomains drive transcription of adjacent coding and non-coding DNA. Key transcriptional targets of BRD4-NUT required to maintain viability, growth, and the blockade of differentiation include the epithelial stem cell–associated transcription factor *TP63* and the oncogene *MYC* {53,1005}. Other members of the BRD4-NUT chromatin complex that interact with BRD4 and are required for growth and the blockade of differentiation include NSD3, ZNF532, and ZNF592 {54,869}. All of these BRD4-NUT complex proteins are encoded by genes that are fused to *NUTM1* in variant cases of NUT carcinoma, including *NSD3-NUTM1*, *ZNF532-NUTM1*, and *ZNF592-NUTM1* {54,2756,869}. The interchangeability of these proteins with BRD4-NUT suggests that a subset of core BRD4-interacting proteins, when fused to NUT, can link NUT to BRD4 in a manner that recapitulates BRD4-NUT function. In support of this idea, ectopic expression of NSD3-NUT can fully rescue NUT carcinoma cells depleted of BRD4-NUT {869}.

Macroscopic appearance
Thoracic NUT carcinoma is typically widely invasive at the time of diagnosis, precluding surgical resection. Patients usually present with one or more large pulmonary or mediastinal masses that extend into the hilum, pleura, and/or chest wall. The cut surface of NUT carcinoma is tan to white, often with extensive geographical necrosis {2983}.

Histopathology
NUT carcinoma typically shows sheets and nests of small to intermediate-sized undifferentiated cells with a monomorphic

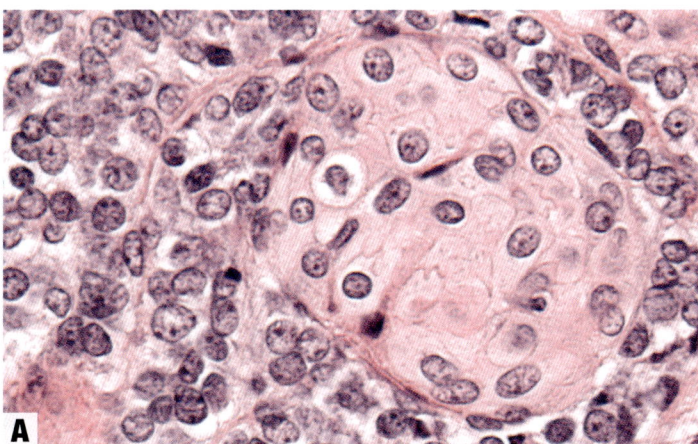

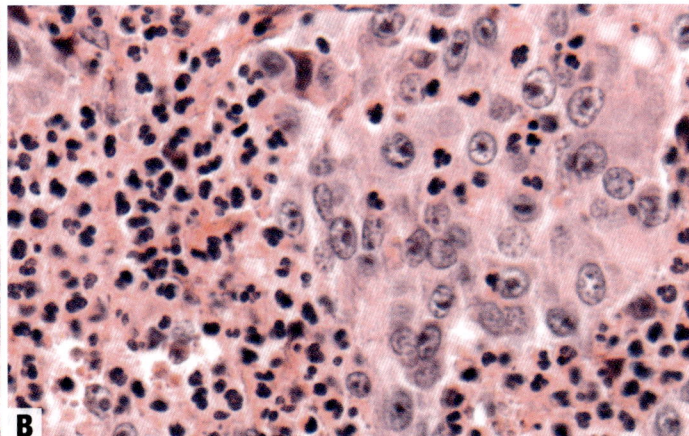

Fig. 5.69 NUT carcinoma. **A** Abrupt keratinization is evident within a sea of otherwise undifferentiated cells. **B** Extensive neutrophilic infiltrates are common in this cancer.

appearance. The cells have evenly sized nuclei with irregular outlines, vesicular chromatin, and prominent nucleoli. The cytoplasm varies from pale eosinophilic to basophilic and may have a granular appearance. A characteristic feature of the sheet-like growth pattern is even spacing of cells, often with separation between cells evident, and a lack of nuclear moulding. There is brisk mitotic activity and necrosis is often present. NUT carcinomas demonstrate characteristic abrupt foci of keratinization; however, this is evident in only 33% of cases {464}. A prominent neutrophilic infiltrate, with or without associated necrosis, is commonly admixed with the tumour cells, although in some cases only minor chronic inflammation is seen. Definitive glandular differentiation is not seen in NUT carcinoma, and it can be used as an exclusionary criterion. Mesenchymal differentiation, which can occur in salivary gland {657} and soft tissue and bone primary sites {703}, has not been described in thoracic NUT carcinoma. The histological features alone are those of an undifferentiated carcinoma, poorly differentiated squamous carcinoma, or undifferentiated small round blue cell malignancy, and are not specific for NUT carcinoma.

Immunohistochemistry

NUT carcinoma is positive for NUT protein in 87% of cases by immunohistochemistry using a highly specific rabbit anti-human monoclonal NUT antibody (clone C52B1) {1048}. The staining is typically punctated. With the exception of weak, focal staining in seminomas, dysgerminomas, and embryonal carcinomas, staining with this antibody is limited to NUT carcinoma, and is thus diagnostic {1048}. Pancytokeratin is positive in the majority of cases, although rare cases are negative {786,3519}. Variable results are obtained with other epithelial markers such as EMA, BerEP4, and CEA. Most cases show nuclear staining for p63/p40, indicating squamous differentiation. Occasional NUT carcinomas can stain for chromogranin, synaptophysin, or even TTF1 {2983}. NUT carcinomas often stain for the haematopoietic stem cell marker CD34, which may lead to a misdiagnosis of acute leukaemia {867}. Germ cell, lymphoid, and myeloid markers are negative. Ki-67 expression is often very high.

Differential diagnosis

NUT carcinoma needs consideration in the differential diagnosis of poorly differentiated squamous cell carcinoma, small cell carcinoma, and combined small cell and squamous cell carcinoma, particularly when there is abrupt transition from small cell tumour areas to foci of squamous differentiation. Expression of TTF1 and neuroendocrine markers in a subset of NUT carcinomas is a potential pitfall {2983}. Undifferentiated carcinomas and the spectrum of small round blue cell tumours (including leukaemias) can enter the differential diagnosis in a subset of NUT carcinomas expressing CD34 and CD99 and/or lacking expression of p40 and keratin {2053,867}. An emerging heterogeneous group of NUTM1-rearranged malignancies with histological features of sarcoma and novel NUTM1 fusion partners remain unclassified {2861,703,711}. Differentiation from SMARCA4-deficient tumours requires SMARCA4 immunohistochemistry.

Cytology

Aspirates yield cellular smears mainly composed of discohesive clusters and solitary cells that are distinctly monomorphic

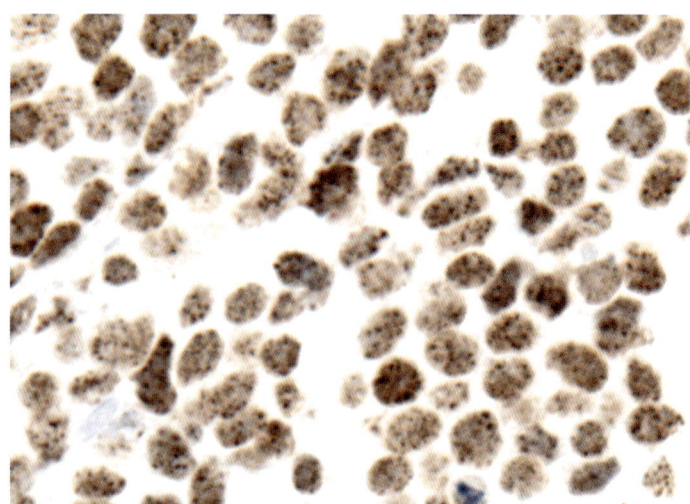

Fig. 5.70 NUT carcinoma. Staining with the C52B1 rabbit monoclonal antibody demonstrating > 50% nuclear staining is diagnostic of NUT carcinoma. The nuclear speckled pattern of staining is characteristic but not required for the diagnosis.

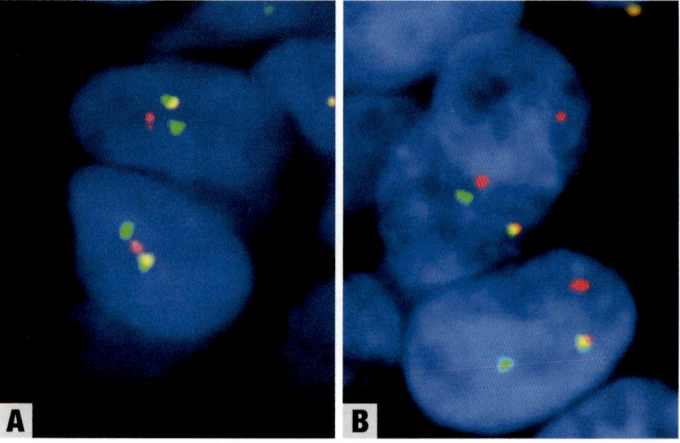

Fig. 5.71 NUT carcinoma. FISH using red and green probes flanking the BRD4 (**A**) and NUTM1 (**B**) loci reveals signal splitting of the probes. Together, these findings are diagnostic of NUT carcinoma with BRD4-NUTM1 fusion.

and of intermediate size, with irregular nuclear contours, variable granular to vesicular chromatin, and discrete nucleoli. Cells may be rounded or spindled depending on the degree of squamous differentiation. The cytoplasm varies from pale to dense eosinophilic and may be vacuolated but does not contain mucin. Larger sheets may be present. Mitotic figures, necrotic debris, and crush artefacts are common {202,3519,237}. The cytological characteristics are similar to those of other undifferentiated carcinomas or poorly differentiated squamous carcinomas and are not specific for NUT carcinoma.

Diagnostic molecular pathology

Demonstration of NUTM1 rearrangement is required, such as by positive immunostaining (e.g. with clone C52B1) for nuclear NUT expression in > 50% of nuclei, which achieves 100% specificity and 87% sensitivity {1048}. In the remaining cases, cytogenetic analysis, in situ hybridization (FISH), RT-PCR, or next-generation sequencing may be necessary {2756,2861,703}.

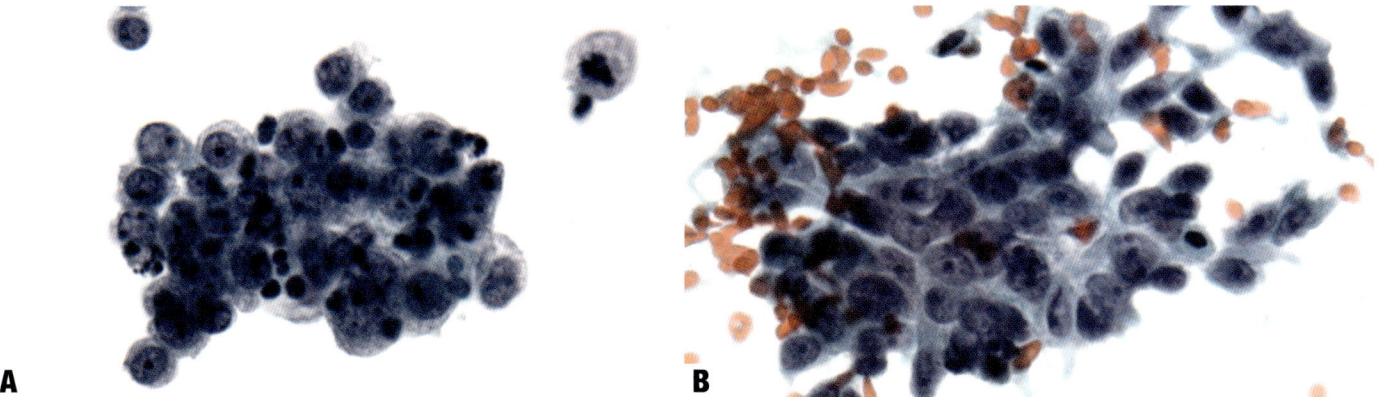

Fig. 5.72 NUT carcinoma. **A** Cytology of a malignant pleural effusion reveals discohesive clusters of primitive round cells (Pap stain). **B** This FNA specimen reveals some spindling indicative of squamous differentiation (Pap stain).

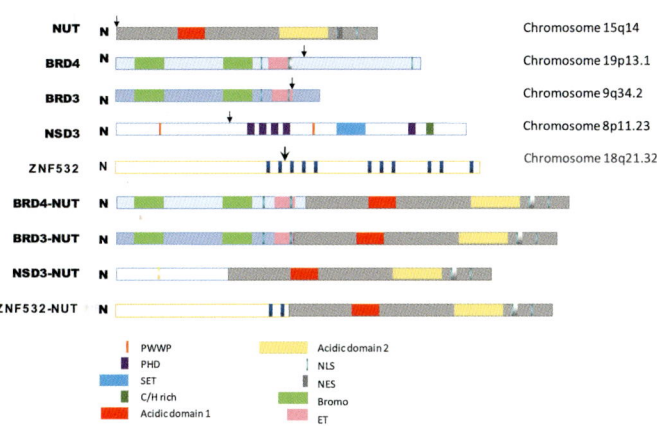

Fig. 5.73 NUT carcinoma. Schematic of various *NUTM1* fusions associated with NUT carcinoma.

Essential and desirable diagnostic criteria

Essential:

- Demonstration of *NUTM1* rearrangement by molecular methods or NUT-positive immunohistochemistry in a poorly differentiated squamous cell carcinoma or other poorly differentiated carcinoma

Staging

Not yet available

Prognosis and prediction

NUT carcinoma is an extremely aggressive cancer, with patients having a median survival time of 6.5 months across all molecular subsets and anatomical sites {464}. Median overall survival is particularly poor in the thoracic *BRD4-NUTM1* NUT carcinoma subset (4.4 months) compared with non-thoracic *BRD4-NUTM1* NUT carcinomas (10 months) and non-thoracic, non–*BRD4-NUTM1* NUT carcinomas (36.5 months) ($P < 0.0001$). Complete resection and initial treatment with radiotherapy are independently significantly associated with prolonged survival (both progression-free and overall survival) {175}. Overall survival is significantly worse in the presence of metastasis but not significantly correlated with age or sex {464}. Most chemotherapeutic regimens have failed to provide durable responses in NUT carcinoma patients; however, small series have suggested that ifosfamide-based regimens, in particular the Ewing sarcoma Scandinavian Sarcoma Group (SSG) IX protocol, can lead to long-term complete responses or even cure in a small subset of paediatric cases {1897,2866}. Trials investigating the treatment of NUT carcinoma with BET small molecule inhibitors that target BRD4 (belonging to the BET family of proteins) are in progress {546}.

Clear cell carcinoma of the thymus

Porubsky S
Marino M

Definition
Clear cell carcinoma is a thymic carcinoma composed predominantly or totally of clear cells.

ICD-O coding
8310/3 Clear cell carcinoma

ICD-11 coding
2C27.0 & XH6L02 Carcinoma of thymus & Clear cell adenocarcinoma, NOS
2C27.0 & XH9DC1 Carcinoma of thymus & Squamous cell carcinoma, clear cell type

Related terminology
None

Subtype(s)
Carcinoma of the thymus with clear cell features; hyalinizing clear cell carcinoma

Localization
Clear cell carcinoma of the thymus occurs in thymus or ectopic thymus {2183}.

Clinical features
Symptoms comprise dyspnoea, chest pain, and superior vena cava syndrome. No association with autoimmunity or myasthenia gravis has been observed. Locally invasive growth and metastases to mediastinal lymph nodes, lung, and bone are common {2381,1092,2796}.

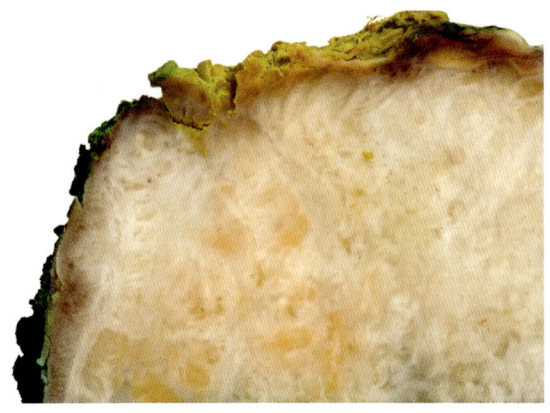

Fig. 5.74 Hyalinizing clear cell carcinoma. Solid, infiltrative tumour with a grey to yellowish cut surface.

Epidemiology
The tumour is rare, with about 25 cases reported so far. The average age is 55 years (range: 33–84 years), with an M:F ratio of approximately 2:1 {2381,3334,2796,1092}.

Etiology
Unknown

Pathogenesis
EWSR1-ATF1 gene fusion, the characteristic molecular change of salivary gland–type hyalinizing clear cell carcinoma, has been found selectively in cases exhibiting prominent stromal hyalinization {86,2381}. It is currently unclear whether clear cell carcinomas lacking hyalinization and *EWSR1* translocation

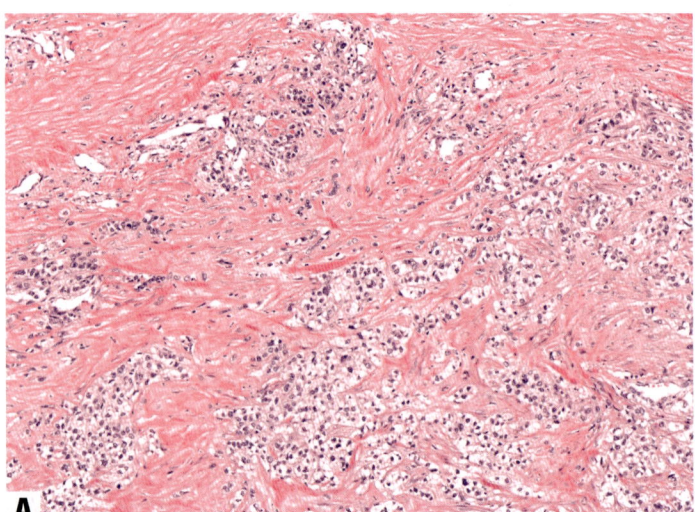
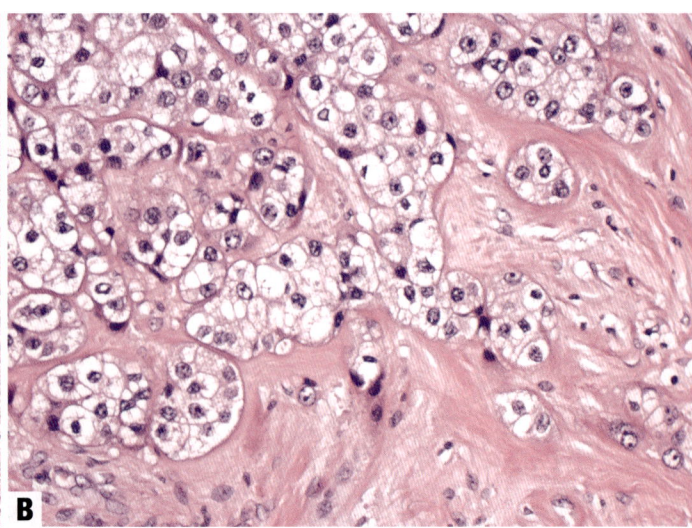

Fig. 5.75 Hyalinizing clear cell carcinoma. **A** Sheets and islands of clear cells are embedded in variable amounts of stroma with hyaline character. **B** Higher-power view showing sheets and islands of clear cells embedded in variable amounts of stroma with hyaline character.

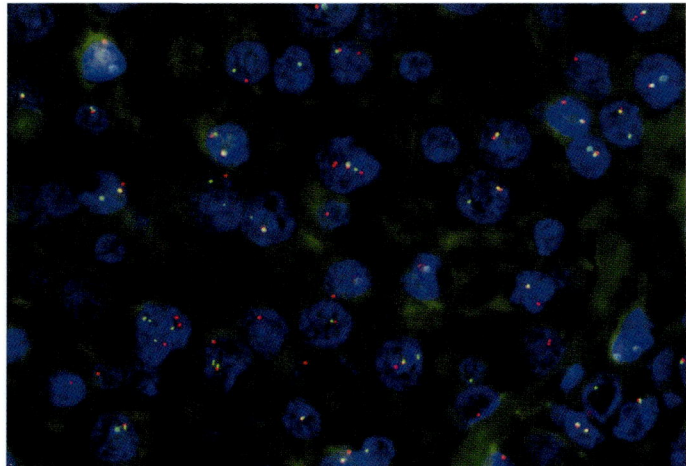

Fig. 5.76 Hyalinizing clear cell carcinoma. Cases exhibiting hyalinized stroma show rearrangement of the *EWSR1* locus as visualized by splitting of green and red signals as contrasted with the normal locus appearing in yellow.

represent a distinct entity or merely other specific types of thymic carcinoma with clear cell change.

Macroscopic appearance
The tumour is firm and often infiltrative, measuring 40–120 mm, with a greyish, mostly solid but occasionally cystic and haemorrhagic cut surface {2381,2796,1092}.

Histopathology
The infiltrative tumour is composed of sheets, islands, and trabeculae of polygonal clear cells with well-defined cell membranes {1658,2381}. The nuclei are small to medium-sized and moderately pleomorphic, with fine chromatin and small nucleoli. Focal squamous differentiation can occur but is rare. Variable amounts of fibrous stroma are present, but some cases have voluminous hyalinized stroma around the tumour islands, reminiscent of hyalinizing clear cell carcinoma of major/minor salivary glands {2381}. The mitotic count is usually low {1092}.

Immunohistochemistry
The tumour is typically positive for low- and high-molecular-weight cytokeratins (e.g. CK5, CK6, CK8, CK18, and CK19), p40, and p63. CD5, KIT (CD117), and GLUT1 are expressed in a minority of cases {719,1559,2381,1092}. Immature, TdT-positive T lymphocytes are absent.

Differential diagnosis
Distinction from hyalinizing clear cell carcinoma of salivary gland or lung requires clinical correlation {2381}. Clear cell renal cell carcinoma often shows focal glandular/tubular formations and is typically PAX8-positive and p40/CK5/6-negative. Thymomas with focal clear cell change exhibit typical morphology of thymoma, do not show nuclear pleomorphism as is seen in clear cell carcinoma, and show at least sparse TdT-expressing immature T cells. Mediastinal large B-cell lymphoma and mediastinal seminoma can be rich in clear cells but can be readily distinguished from clear cell carcinoma by the morphology and immunophenotype. Clear cell sarcoma, although also positive for the *EWSR1-ATF1* fusion, typically expresses S100, HMB45, and melan-A (MART1) but not cytokeratins, and it usually does not primarily arise in the mediastinum.

Cytology
The experience is limited to one report of clusters of vacuolated, signet-ring–like cells {1586}.

Diagnostic molecular pathology
Demonstration of *EWSR1* gene translocation may help to identify the hyalinizing clear cell carcinoma.

Essential and desirable diagnostic criteria
Essential:
- Islands and trabeculae of carcinoma cells with clear cytoplasm
- Abundant hyalinized stroma in hyalinizing clear cell carcinoma

Desirable:
- Cytokeratin and p40/p63 immunostaining
- *EWSR1* translocation for hyalinizing clear cell carcinoma

Staging
Thymic clear cell carcinoma should be staged according to the Union for International Cancer Control (UICC) TNM staging system {315,687} and, optionally, the Masaoka–Koga system {685}. Most cases are at an advanced stage at presentation.

Prognosis and prediction
This is an aggressive neoplasm. Local recurrence and intrathoracic and extrathoracic metastases are common. Surgery and radiochemotherapy are the standard approaches.

Low-grade papillary adenocarcinoma of the thymus

Marino M
Marx A
Matsuno Y
Mukai K

Definition

Low-grade papillary adenocarcinoma is a primary thymic carcinoma composed of well-formed tubulopapillary structures, often associated with type A thymoma.

ICD-O coding

8260/3 Low-grade papillary adenocarcinoma

ICD-11 coding

2C27.0 & XH6LV9 Carcinoma of thymus & Papillary adenocarcinoma, NOS

Related terminology

Not recommended: papillary adenocarcinoma.

Subtype(s)

None

Localization

Low-grade papillary adenocarcinoma of the thymus is localized in the anterior (prevascular) mediastinum.

Clinical features

Patients may be asymptomatic {2174,1181,893,1840} or have cough, chest pain, and dyspnoea {1352,1840}. High serum levels of CEA may occur {2174}.

Imaging

Imaging reveals well-circumscribed, partially cystic or solid lesions in the anterior (prevascular) mediastinum, as well as tumours with invasion into the lung and intrathoracic dissemination {1840,1181,2174}.

Epidemiology

Papillary adenocarcinoma represents 3% in a series of 65 thymic carcinomas {3276}. The mean age of presentation was 52 years, with no sex predilection {893}.

Etiology

A subset of papillary adenocarcinomas appear to arise from type A or AB thymoma or from multilocular thymic cysts {1840, 3275,3276,1998}.

Pathogenesis

Unknown

Macroscopic appearance

Tumours may be completely or partially encapsulated and show cystic and solid areas. In multilocular cysts they may form nodular protrusions {3276}. The mean size is 65 mm {893}.

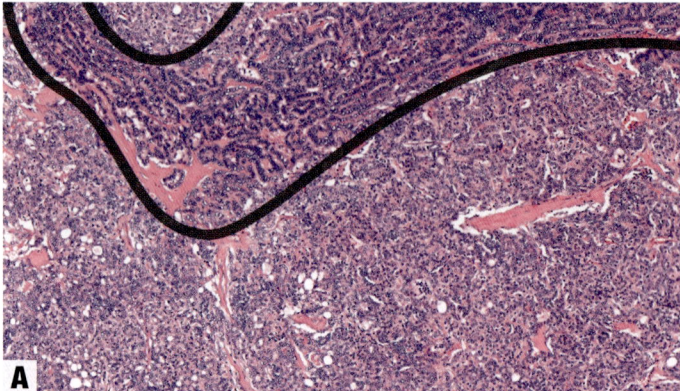
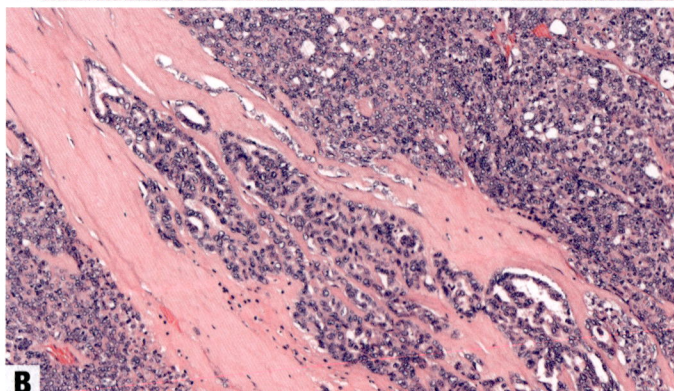
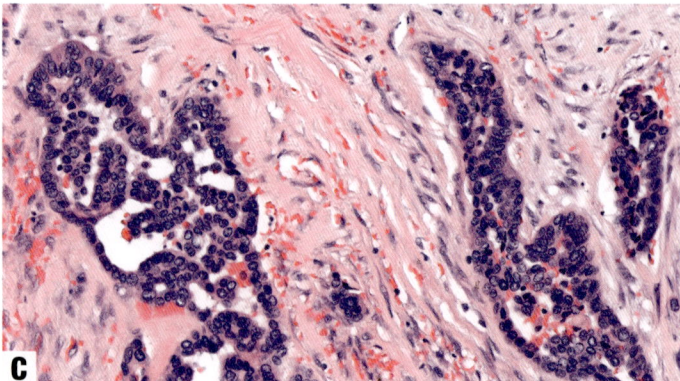

Fig. 5.77 Low-grade papillary adenocarcinoma and type A thymoma. **A** Association of low-grade papillary adenocarcinoma (outlined) with type A thymoma. **B** Papillary adenocarcinoma (centre) and type A thymoma (upper-right and lower-left corners). **C** Area of low-grade papillary adenocarcinoma at higher magnification.

Histopathology

Tubulopapillary structures are lined by cuboidal or polygonal cells with mildly atypical round to oval nuclei, small distinct nucleoli, and eosinophilic or clear cytoplasm. Nuclei may show grooves and irregularities; mitotic figures can be present {3276}.

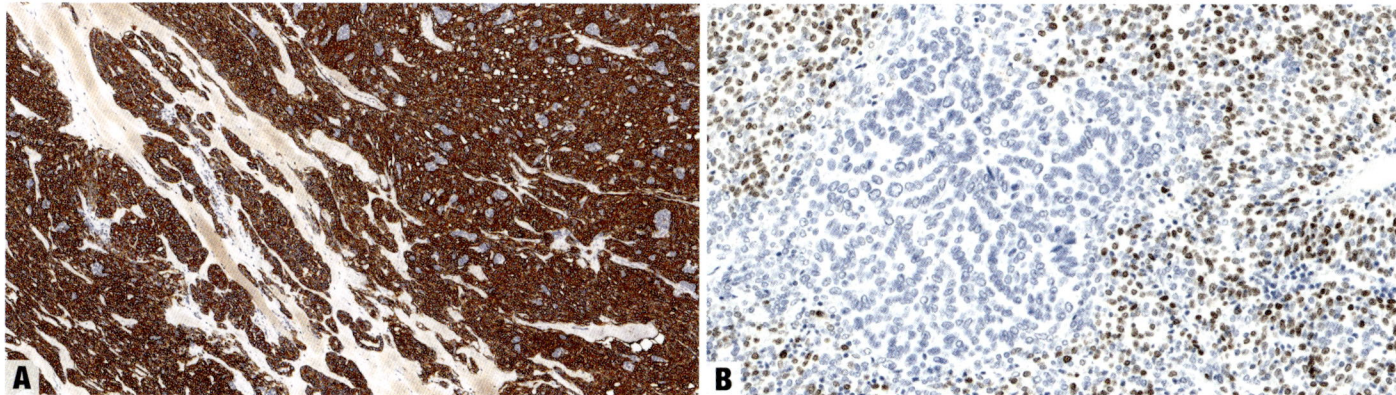

Fig. 5.78 Low-grade papillary adenocarcinoma and type A thymoma. **A** CK19 stains both low-grade papillary adenocarcinoma (centre) and type A thymoma (upper-right and lower-left corners). **B** p40 is expressed in type A thymoma but not in the low-grade papillary adenocarcinoma.

Fibrovascular cores are present in some papillae. Psammoma bodies and coagulative necrosis can be present. Discernible type A or AB thymoma elements may be found within a main tumour.

Immunohistochemistry
The tumour shows positivity for cytokeratins (including CK8 and CK7), EMA, BerEP4, and vimentin; variable and focal positivity for CD5, CEA, calretinin, CD15, and KIT (CD117) {1840,3432, 1352}; and negativity for CK20, CDX2, thyroglobulin, TTF1, calcitonin, FOXN1, p63, p40, CD20, and PAX8 {1352,1181,893}.

Differential diagnosis
Thymic carcinomas with papillary features and high-grade atypia are classified as thymic adenocarcinomas NOS instead. Ectopic or metastatic thyroid carcinoma, mesothelioma, mediastinal extension of papillary adenocarcinoma of the lung, and metastasis from other organs must be excluded. Of note, unlike in squamous or squamous-related carcinomas, CD5 expression in adenocarcinomas is not indicative of a thymic origin {2974}.

Cytology
Not available

Diagnostic molecular pathology
Not clinically relevant

Essential and desirable diagnostic criteria
Essential:
- A primary thymic low-grade adenocarcinoma with areas of tubulopapillary growth
- Tubulopapillary structures lined by cuboidal or polygonal cells

Desirable:
- Immunostains to exclude papillary neoplasms of the thyroid, pleura, lung, and extrathoracic sites

Staging
Low-grade papillary adenocarcinomas should be staged according to the TNM system {315,687} and, optionally, the Masaoka–Koga system {685}.

Prognosis and prediction
About 50% of cases recur, but tumour-related death is uncommon {1840,893,1352}.

Mucoepidermoid carcinoma of the thymus

Inagaki H
Roden AC

Definition
Mucoepidermoid carcinoma (MEC) is a primary thymic carcinoma characterized by a combination of mucus-producing cells, intermediate cells, and squamoid cells, analogous to the salivary gland counterpart.

ICD-O coding
8430/3 Mucoepidermoid carcinoma

ICD-11 coding
2C27.0 & XH1J36 Carcinoma of thymus & Mucoepidermoid carcinoma

Related terminology
Not recommended: mucoepidermoid tumour.

Subtype(s)
None

Localization
MEC of the thymus is localized in the anterior (prevascular) mediastinum.

Clinical features
Patients may present with dyspnoea or chest discomfort, although half of the patients are asymptomatic. A rare case associated with myasthenia gravis has been documented {3336}.

Imaging
Most cases show a well-demarcated mass with varying combinations of solid and cystic areas {2122}.

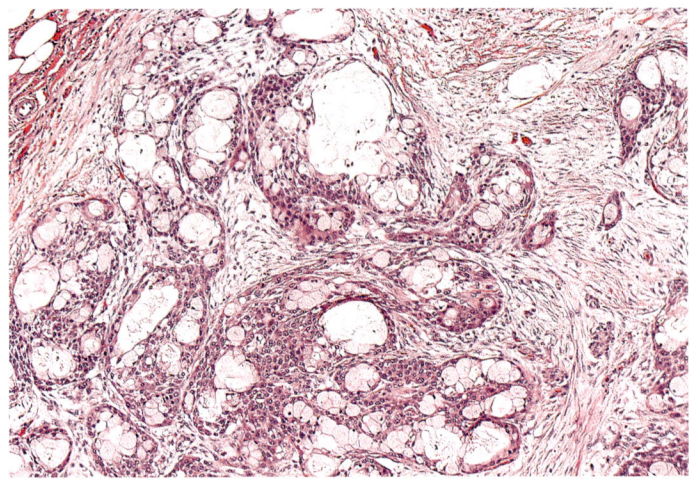

Fig. 5.79 Low-grade mucoepidermoid carcinoma of the thymus. Tumour nests are composed of an admixture of mucus-producing, intermediate, and squamoid cells.

Epidemiology
Primary thymic MECs are rare. According to the International Thymic Malignancy Interest Group (ITMIG) database, they account for 2.5% of thymic carcinomas {33}. The median age of the patients is in the sixth decade of life, with a wide age range (8–87 years) {1058}. There is a slight male predominance {1058}.

Etiology
Some cases may arise from multilocular thymic cysts {1975}. Rarely, this tumour has been associated with a thymoma {3344}, suggesting possible derivation from a putative thymic epithelial precursor.

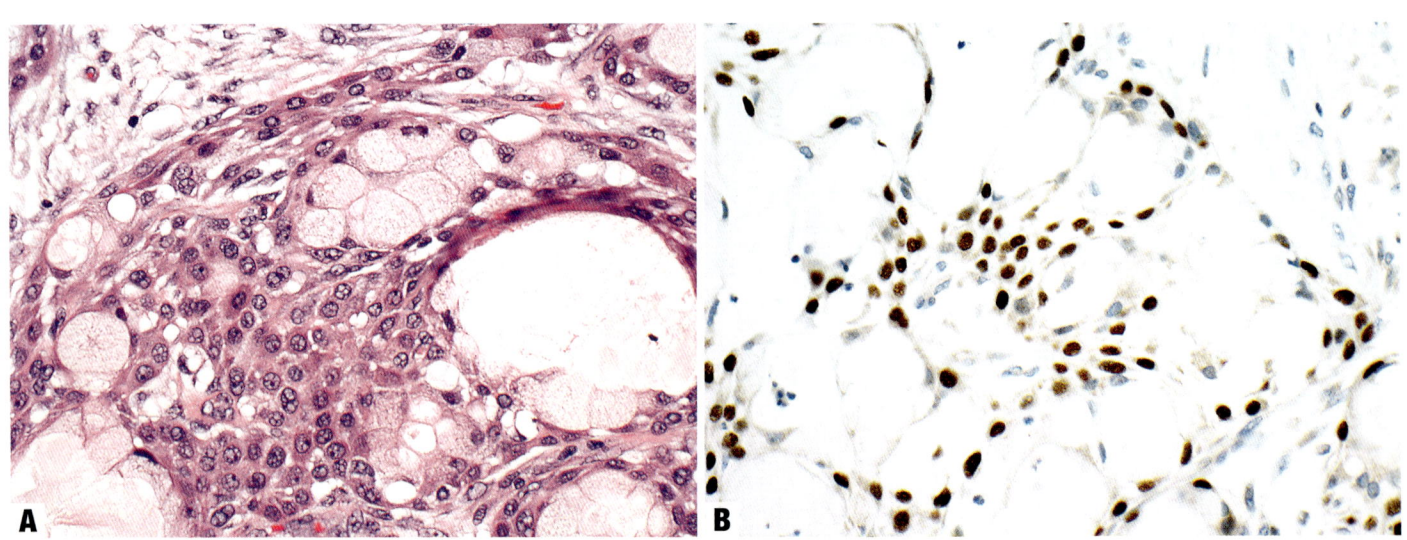

Fig. 5.80 Low-grade mucoepidermoid carcinoma of the thymus. **A** Higher magnification shows cystic areas lined by mucus-producing cells and surrounded by intermediate and squamoid cells. **B** Intermediate and squamoid cells, but not mucus-producing cells, are positive for p40.

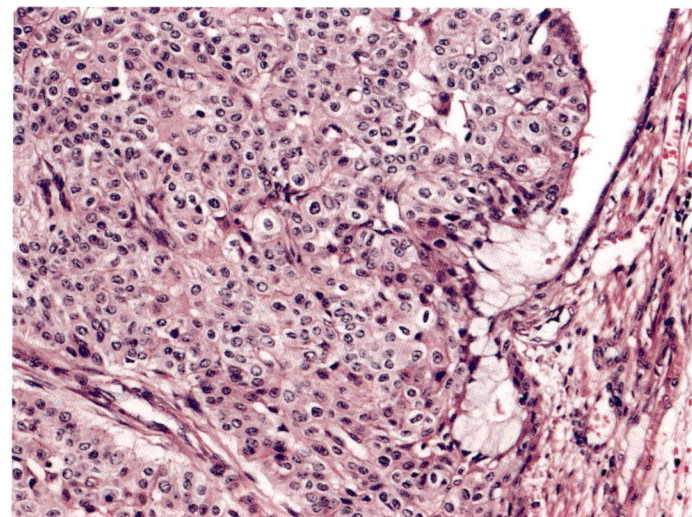

Fig. 5.81 High-grade mucoepidermoid carcinoma of the thymus. Solid growth of tumour cells with focal mucus-producing cells.

Pathogenesis

CRTC1-MAML2 gene fusion, which causes disruption of cell-cycle regulation and differentiation, is a hallmark of salivary gland MECs and is found in some but not all thymic MECs {2504,2389}.

Macroscopic appearance

Tumour size ranges from 40 to 110 mm. The tumours are well circumscribed but may be adherent to the pleura and show invasion into perithymic adipose tissue. The cut surface is solid, with or without cystic areas, and shows a granular and mucoid appearance {2133,1975}.

Histopathology

The tumour shows features similar to those of salivary gland MEC. Variable combinations of mucus-producing (goblet) cells,

intermediate cells, and squamoid cells are observed. Intermediate cells are the predominant cell type in most cases, and they form sheets or solid islands. Mucus-producing cells contain intracytoplasmic mucin, which can be highlighted by mucicarmine or PAS / Alcian blue stain. These cells line cystic spaces or occur as single cells. Keratinization is, in general, absent. Approximately 70% of cases are histologically low-grade {1058}. Some histological patterns described in salivary gland MEC, including clear cell and oncocytic patterns, have not been well documented in thymic MEC.

Immunohistochemistry

The tumour cells are consistently positive for pancytokeratins, CK5/6, p63, and p40 and negative for CD5, KIT (CD117), TTF1, and neuroendocrine markers.

Differential diagnosis

Thymic squamous cell carcinoma lacks mucin (in contrast to most high-grade MECs), while keratin pearls and prominent nuclear pleomorphism in a tumour with a glandular component in ≥ 10% of the tumour area suggest adenosquamous carcinoma. Detection of a *MAML2* fusion gene is helpful for diagnosis of MEC, but its absence does not exclude MEC. In some *MAML2* fusion–negative high-grade tumours, a distinction between high-grade MEC, adenosquamous carcinomas, and squamous cell carcinoma may be arbitrary.

Cytology

In low-grade MEC, aspiration cytology smears show cohesive clusters of small-sized cells in a mucoid background. Nuclei have smooth nuclear membranes, coarse chromatin, and inconspicuous nucleoli. In high-grade MEC, nuclear membranes are irregular and necrosis may be present {1382}.

Diagnostic molecular pathology

Detection of *MAML2* rearrangement may be helpful for definitive diagnosis in problematic cases {2504,2389}.

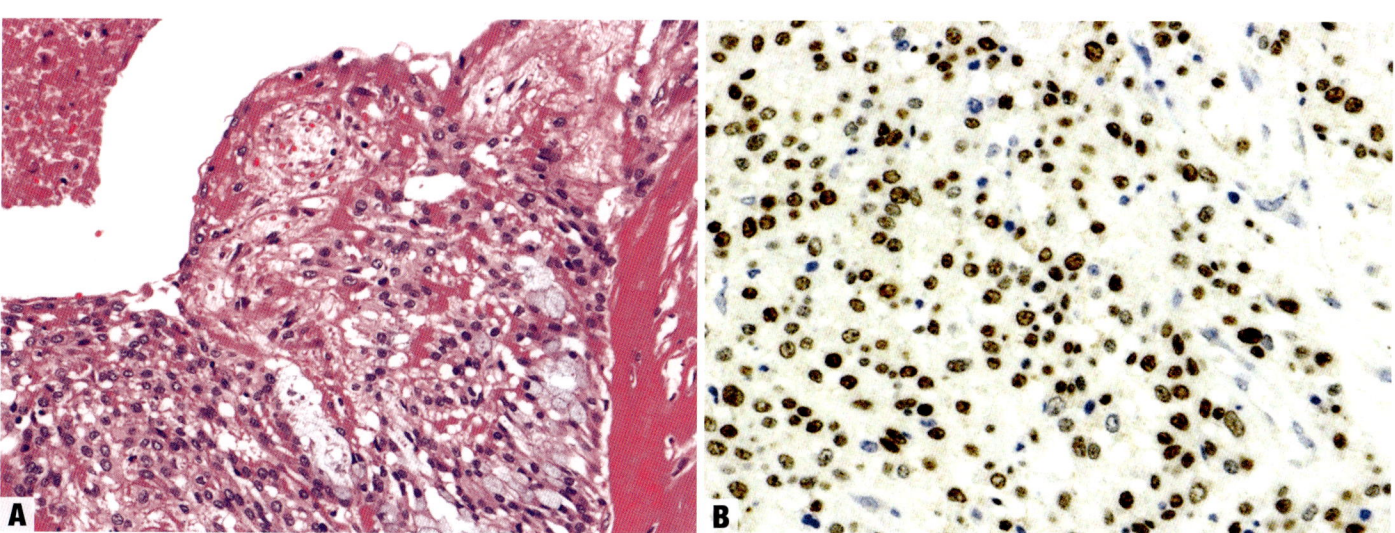

Fig. 5.82 High-grade mucoepidermoid carcinoma of the thymus. **A** Sheets of tumour cells are admixed with mucus-producing cells. Hyalinized stroma (right) and necrosis (upper-left corner) are present. **B** Tumour cells are positive for p63.

Essential and desirable diagnostic criteria

Essential:

- A primary thymic carcinoma characterized by a combination of mucus-producing, intermediate, and squamoid cells growing in nests and cystic structures
- In high-grade MEC, the diagnosis requires the presence of at least focal intracellular mucin

Desirable:

- Immunohistochemistry positive for pancytokeratins, CK5/6, p63/p40
- *MAML2* rearrangement studies might be helpful in difficult cases, in particular high-grade cases, although negative results do not rule out the diagnosis.

Staging

Thymic MECs should be staged according to the TNM system {315,687} and, optionally, the Masaoka–Koga system {685}. Most MEC cases (68%) are in Masaoka–Koga stages I and II, and the remaining 32% are stage III or IV disease {1058}.

Prognosis and prediction

The mainstay of treatment is surgical resection with or without chemotherapy or radiation. The prognosis is dependent on histological grade and possibly tumour stage. Survival is favourable in patients with low-grade tumours after complete resection, whereas patients with high-grade tumours have a poor prognosis {2133}.

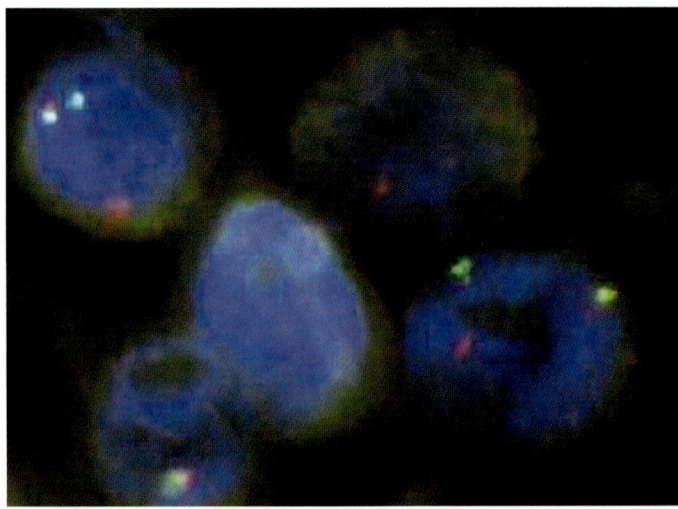

Fig. 5.83 Low-grade mucoepidermoid carcinoma of the thymus. FISH image shows rearrangement of the *MAML2* locus (separation of the red and green signals) in tumour nuclei found in the upper-left and lower-right corners.

Thymic carcinoma with adenoid cystic carcinoma–like features

Marino M
Di Tommaso L
Matsuno Y
Mukai K

Definition
Thymic carcinoma with adenoid cystic carcinoma–like features is a primary thymic carcinoma resembling salivary gland adenoid cystic carcinoma.

ICD-O coding
8200/3 Thymic carcinoma with adenoid cystic carcinoma–like features

ICD-11 coding
2C27.0 & XH92Y9 Carcinoma of thymus & Thymic carcinoma with adenoid cystic carcinoma–like features

Related terminology
Not recommended: adenoid cystic carcinoma–like tumour; adenoid cystic carcinoma of the thymus.

Subtype(s)
None

Localization
Thymic carcinoma with adenoid cystic carcinoma–like features is localized in the anterior (prevascular) mediastinum.

Clinical features
Patients are usually asymptomatic. In one case, multiple bone and pulmonary metastases were found {1375}.

Epidemiology
This is a very rare tumour, with < 10 cases reported in the literature {1358}. The patients' ages ranged from 47 to 77 years. Male patients predominate.

Etiology
Unknown

Pathogenesis
Comparative genomic hybridization revealed an isolated gain of chromosome 8 in one single case {695}.

Macroscopic appearance
The tumours are solid to solid-microcystic, mostly with pushing margins, rarely infiltrative, and 40–130 mm in diameter, with haemorrhagic areas {695}.

Histopathology
The tumour shows marked histological similarities to adenoid cystic carcinoma {1358,695,1375}. It consists of nests of basaloid cells arranged in a cribriform pattern, with the microcysts containing mucoid matrix (basement membrane–like, mucicarmine-positive, and collagen IV–positive) and formed by two cell rows. Intracellular mucin is not found. Nuclear atypia is slight

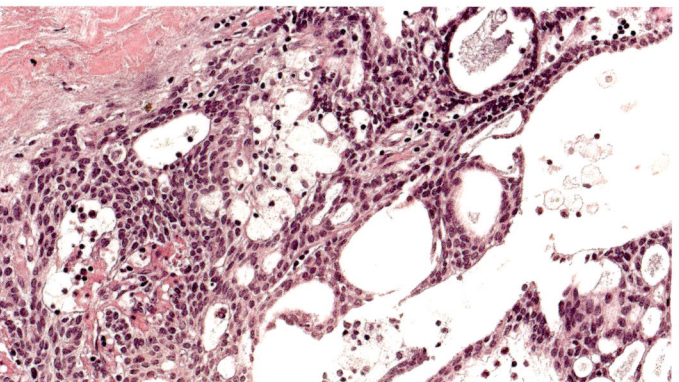

Fig. 5.84 Thymic carcinoma with adenoid cystic carcinoma–like features. Bland-looking cuboidal tumour cells showing a cribriform growth pattern.

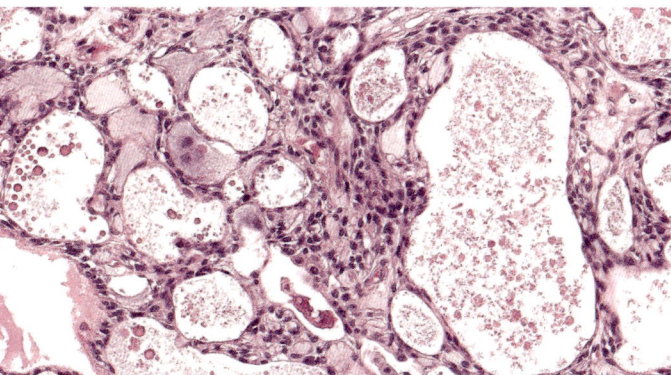

Fig. 5.85 Thymic carcinoma with adenoid cystic carcinoma–like features. Cystic spaces filled with debris or basal membrane–like material.

to moderate, and mitotic activity is minimal. Unlike in adenoid cystic carcinoma, true glands, containing PAS-positive, diastase-resistant material, are rarely seen within the basaloid islands. Tumour necrosis and vascular invasion are occasionally present.

Immunohistochemistry
The tumour shows positivity for p63, high-molecular-weight cytokeratin, pancytokeratin, CK19, and CK5/6; there are scattered CD5-positive cells and scattered S100-positive cells {695,2427}. Unlike in adenoid cystic carcinoma, KIT (CD117) is negative, and myoepithelial markers (e.g. SMA) are negative. Neuroendocrine markers are negative {1375}.

Cytology
Not available

Diagnostic molecular pathology
Not clinically relevant

Essential and desirable diagnostic criteria
Essential:
- Thymic carcinoma morphologically similar to adenoid cystic carcinoma, but generally lacking true glands within the cribriform-basaloid islands
- Exclusion of metastasis from salivary gland, lung, or breast

Desirable:
- Immunohistochemistry positive for pancytokeratins, CK5/6, p63/p40
- Negative staining for SMA, KIT (CD117)

Staging
Tumours should be staged according to the TNM system {315,687} and, optionally, the Masaoka–Koga system {685}.

Prognosis and prediction
In the few reported cases, the disease followed an indolent course (follow-up of < 3 years) {1358}. However, one patient had

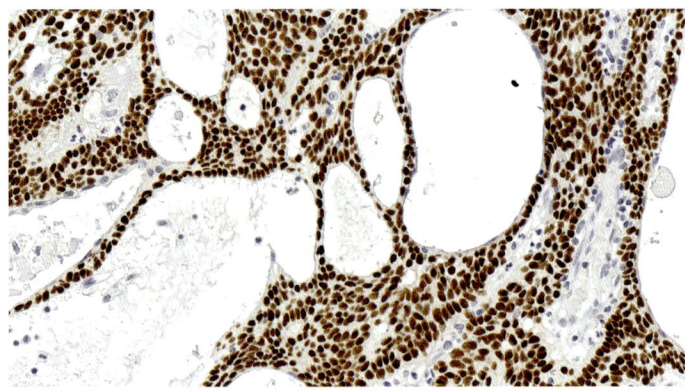

Fig. 5.86 Thymic carcinoma with adenoid cystic carcinoma–like features. p63 stain highlights not only basal cells but all tumour cell nuclei throughout the tumour.

Masaoka–Koga stage III disease {155} and one patient showed distant metastases {1375}.

Enteric-type adenocarcinoma of the thymus

Marino M
Di Tommaso L
Marx A
Matsuno Y
Mukai K

Definition
Enteric-type adenocarcinoma is a primary thymic neoplasm having the same histological and immunohistochemical features as colorectal adenocarcinoma.

ICD-O coding
8144/3 Adenocarcinoma, enteric-type

ICD-11 coding
2C27.0 & XH0349 Carcinoma of thymus & Adenocarcinoma, intestinal type

Related terminology
Not recommended: intestinal-type adenocarcinoma; mucinous (colloid) adenocarcinoma.

Subtype(s)
None

Localization
Enteric-type adenocarcinoma of the thymus is localized in the anterior (prevascular) mediastinum.

Clinical features
Some patients have chest pain, cough, and dyspnoea {1571, 1759}; others are asymptomatic {2008}. CEA serum levels may be elevated {1759}.

Epidemiology
Enteric-type adenocarcinomas account for < 5% of all thymic carcinomas {1352}. The average age is 45 years, with male predominance {1352}.

Etiology
Unknown

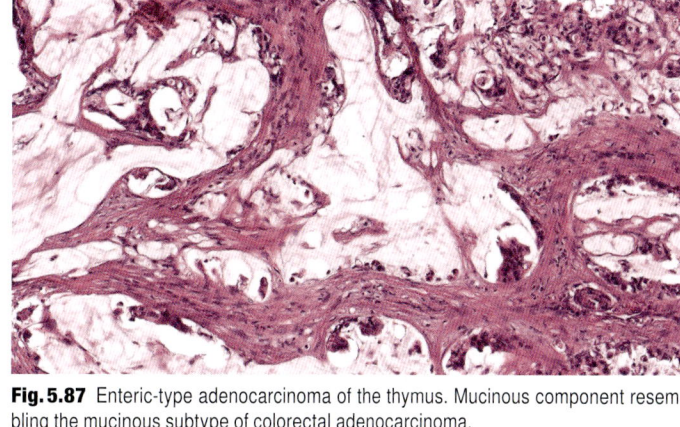

Fig. 5.87 Enteric-type adenocarcinoma of the thymus. Mucinous component resembling the mucinous subtype of colorectal adenocarcinoma.

Pathogenesis
An origin from the glandular structures of involuted thymus {514} or derivation from thymic cysts has been suggested in selected cases {1759}. Single cases show mutations of *KRAS*, *TP53*, *TGFB2*, *TNFSF15*, and *MYC* and losses of HLA loci at 6p21.32 {2606,1647,1763}.

Macroscopic appearance
Tumours are large, solid or solid-cystic, and at times ill defined, with white to yellowish-white cut surfaces and variable mucin (colloid) content. Most cases are associated with thymic cysts.

Histopathology
The tumour exhibits a mucinous and/or papillotubular morphology or small tumour cell clusters floating in pools of extracellular mucin. Intracellular mucin can occur. Expression of at least one marker of enteric differentiation (CK20, CDX2, MUC2) {1571} is mandatory. Expression of CK7 and CD5 is variable {2008}; TTF1 and KIT (CD117) are negative {1759,2008}.

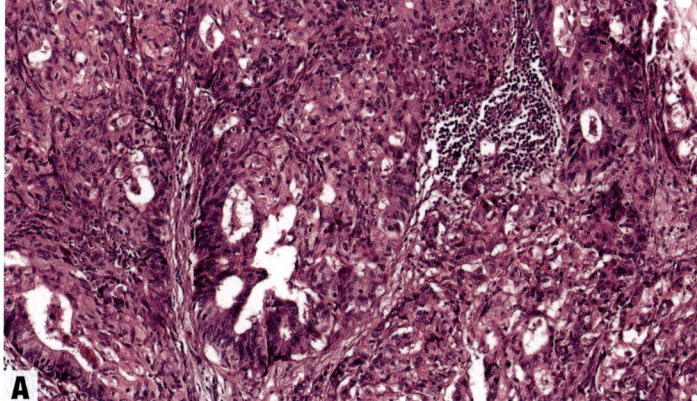
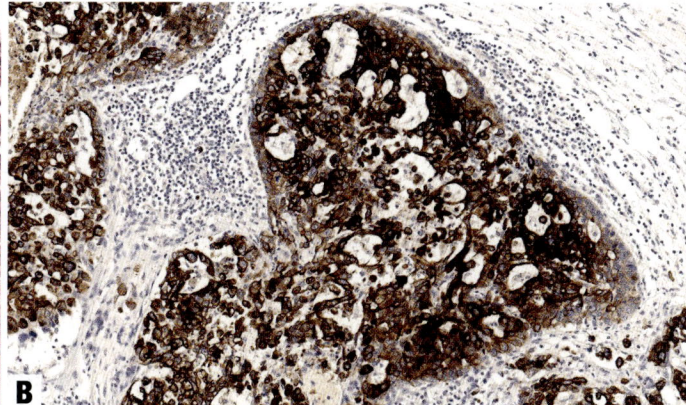

Fig. 5.88 Enteric-type adenocarcinoma of the thymus. **A** Tumour resembling colorectal adenocarcinoma NOS. **B** Tumour cells are positive for CK20.

Cytology

In smears, tumour cells show nuclear crowding and form clusters within extracellular mucin {1570}. Immunostaining for enteric markers may help to confirm the diagnosis {1571,2977}.

Diagnostic molecular pathology

Not clinically relevant

Essential and desirable diagnostic criteria

Essential:

- A primary thymic tumour mimicking colorectal adenocarcinoma
- Exclusion of metastasis from an enteric primary

Desirable:

- Expression of at least one marker of enteric differentiation (CK20, CDX2, MUC2)

Staging

Enteric-type adenocarcinomas should be staged according to the TNM system {315,687} and, optionally, the Masaoka–Koga system {685}. Most tumours are in Masaoka–Koga stages III and IV {1571}.

Prognosis and prediction

In a recent series, 2 of 9 patients died of the tumour; all others were alive with disease {1571}.

Adenocarcinoma NOS of the thymus

Marino M
Marx A
Matsuno Y
Mukai K

Definition
Adenocarcinoma NOS of the thymus is a heterogeneous group of primary thymic carcinomas showing glandular differentiation and/or mucin production, and not conforming to low-grade papillary adenocarcinoma or enteric-type adenocarcinoma.

ICD-O coding
8140/3 Adenocarcinoma, NOS

ICD-11 coding
2C27.0 & XH74S1 Carcinoma of thymus & Adenocarcinoma, NOS

Related terminology
Not recommended: non-mucinous adenocarcinoma; tubular adenocarcinoma; tubulopapillary carcinoma; high-grade papillary carcinoma.

Subtype(s)
None

Localization
Adenocarcinoma NOS of the thymus is localized in the anterior (prevascular) mediastinum.

Clinical features
Patients either present with symptoms related to the thymic mass lesion or are asymptomatic {1763}. Lymph node and distant metastases are common. Paraneoplastic syndromes have not been described.

Imaging
The imaging features of adenocarcinoma NOS of the thymus are similar to those of other thymic carcinomas {514,2951}. Whole-body FDG PET-CT is helpful to exclude metastasis from a primary elsewhere.

Epidemiology
Thymic adenocarcinomas are rare, with approximately 70 cases having been reported in the literature {1352}. In the International Thymic Malignancy Interest Group (ITMIG) cohort, only 11 of 706 patients (1.6%) with thymic epithelial malignancy (carcinoma) have thymic adenocarcinoma {1571}. The mean age is 45 years {1352}. Males predominate.

Etiology
Unknown

Pathogenesis
Unknown

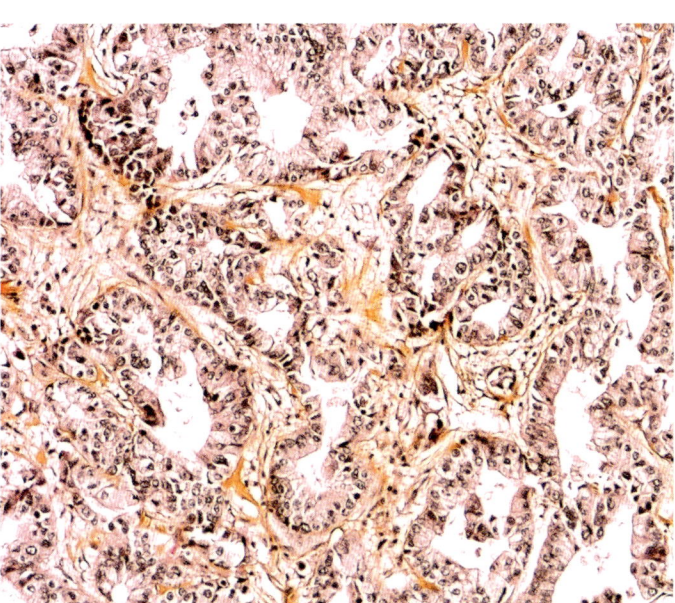

Fig. 5.89 Adenocarcinoma NOS. Crowded individual and fused glands with moderate cytological atypia (Van Gieson stain). Enteric differentiation was excluded by immunostaining.

Macroscopic appearance
The tumours are usually large, soft, and invasive, measuring 50–140 mm in greatest dimension. Necrosis, cystic changes, and mucinous areas can be present {1352}.

Histopathology
Provisionally, adenocarcinoma NOS includes tubular adenocarcinoma, non-mucinous adenocarcinoma, high-grade papillary adenocarcinoma, and signet-ring cell carcinoma with a gastric immunophenotype. Histologically, the tumours show variable combinations of tubules and tubulopapillary structures lined by columnar cells {2646,3019}. Mucinous areas may be present. Rarely, a solid component is present, with sheets of neoplastic cells and only a limited glandular component. Nuclear pleomorphism and coagulative necrosis are common {1352}.

Immunohistochemistry
Adenocarcinomas NOS are positive for pancytokeratins and sometimes also CD5. By definition, they lack expression of enteric markers (CK20, CDX2, and MUC2) {2646,514,1763}. Other markers, such as CEA or CA19-9, may be positive {1763, 3}. Some cases express CK7 {2951,2407,2558}.

Cytology
Not available

Diagnostic molecular pathology
Not clinically relevant

Essential and desirable diagnostic criteria
Essential:
- Adenocarcinoma of thymus after exclusion of mediastinal metastasis from other sites and defined types of thymic adenocarcinoma (low-grade papillary, enteric-type)

Desirable:
- Immunophenotyping to rule out mediastinal metastasis or defined types of thymic adenocarcinoma

Staging
Adenocarcinomas NOS should be staged according to the TNM system {315,687} and, optionally, the Masaoka–Koga system {685}.

Prognosis and prediction
Adenocarcinomas NOS tend to be advanced-stage and aggressive tumours, with poor prognosis {1763}.

Adenosquamous carcinoma of the thymus

Nonaka D
Tateyama H
Weissferdt A

Definition

Adenosquamous carcinoma is a primary thymic carcinoma showing both squamous and glandular differentiation, analogous to its pulmonary counterpart – i.e. each component constitutes ≥ 10% of the tumour.

ICD-O coding

8560/3 Adenosquamous carcinoma

ICD-11 coding

2C27.0 XH7873 Carcinoma of thymus & Adenosquamous carcinoma

Related terminology

None

Subtype(s)

None

Localization

Adenosquamous carcinoma of the thymus is localized in the anterior (prevascular) mediastinum.

Clinical features

Symptoms are related to an anterior (prevascular) mediastinal mass, such as chest pain {3088}.

Epidemiology

There are no data available.

Etiology

Unknown

Pathogenesis

The pathogenesis is unknown. Unlike in mucoepidermoid carcinoma, *MAML2* rearrangement has not been detected {2504}. *KIT* mutation is only occasionally seen {3095}.

Macroscopic appearance

Not reported

Histopathology

Adenosquamous carcinoma is a high-grade carcinoma with areas closely resembling non-keratinizing squamous cell carcinoma (SCC) and areas of adenocarcinoma with definite glandular formations and often containing mucins {2493,3088}. The presence of mucin can be highlighted by mucicarmine staining {2504}. A minor glandular component (< 10%) may be observed in otherwise typical SCC, and such cases should be diagnosed as SCC. Definitive diagnosis requires a resection specimen, but the diagnosis may be suggested based on findings in small biopsies, cytology, or excisional biopsies.

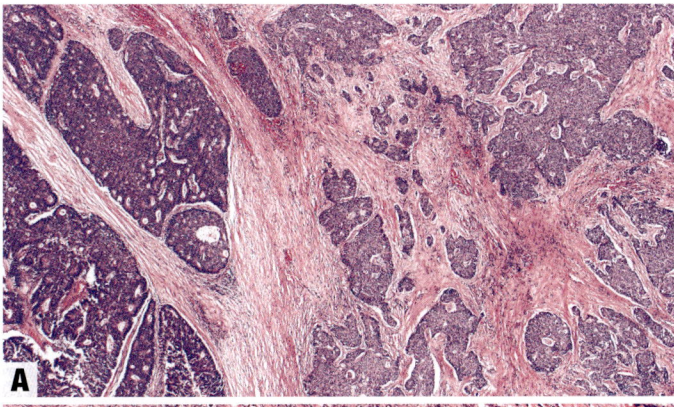
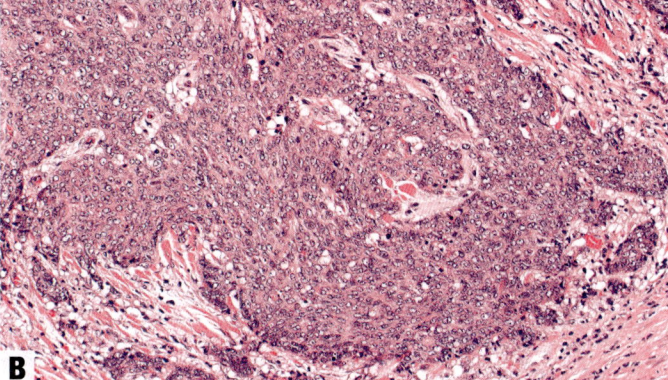
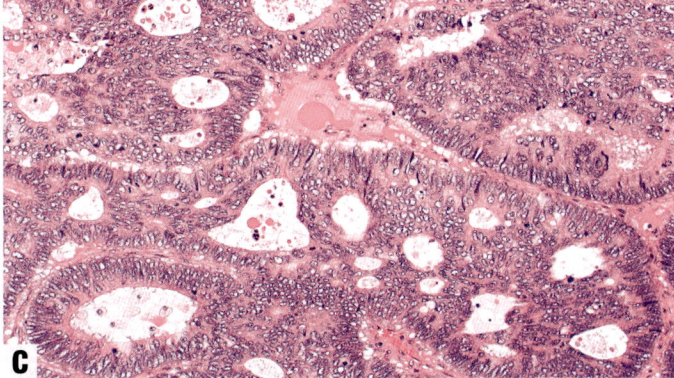

Fig. 5.90 Adenosquamous carcinoma of thymus. **A** Adenocarcinoma component (left) and squamous cell carcinoma component (right). **B** Squamous cell carcinoma component. **C** Adenocarcinoma component.

One case of adenosquamous cell carcinoma with a rhabdomyomatous component {637} and one case with a sarcomatous component {1716} have also been reported.

Immunohistochemistry

The tumour is positive for epithelial markers such as cytokeratins and EMA {637,3088}, and it can be variably positive for

CD5 and KIT (CD117) {2504,3095}. The squamous component should be positive for p63/40 and/or CK5/6.

Differential diagnosis

Thymic SCC by definition lacks a glandular component in ≥ 10% of the tumour area. Poorly differential mucoepidermoid carcinoma lacks frank squamous differentiation (keratinization, intercellular bridges) and may show *MAML2* translocations {2504}.

Cytology

Not available

Diagnostic molecular pathology

Not clinically relevant

Essential and desirable diagnostic criteria

Essential:
- A primary thymic carcinoma with both squamous and glandular differentiation in which each component constitutes ≥ 10% of the tumour within a resection specimen
- Exclusion of mucoepidermoid carcinoma

Desirable:
- The squamous component should be positive for p63/40 and/or CK5/6

Staging

Adenosquamous carcinoma of the thymus should be staged according to the TNM system {315,687} and, optionally, the Masaoka–Koga system {685}.

Prognosis and prediction

Not reported

Sarcomatoid carcinoma of the thymus

Marino M
Di Tommaso L
Mukai K

Definition

Sarcomatoid carcinoma is a primary thymic carcinoma partly or completely composed of spindle-shaped epithelial cells. Tumours with heterologous sarcomatous elements are called carcinosarcomas.

ICD-O coding

8033/3 Sarcomatoid carcinoma
8980/3 Carcinosarcoma

ICD-11 coding

2C27.0 & XH35M3 Carcinoma of thymus & Pseudosarcomatous carcinoma

Related terminology

Acceptable: spindle cell or metaplastic carcinoma; carcinosarcoma.

Subtype(s)

Sarcomatoid carcinoma; carcinosarcoma

Localization

Sarcomatoid carcinoma of the thymus is localized in the anterior (prevascular) mediastinum.

Clinical features

The commonest symptoms include chest pain, cough, shortness of breath, and superior vena cava syndrome {3068}. No autoimmune diseases are reported in the International Thymic Malignancy Interest Group (ITMIG) cohort {33}.

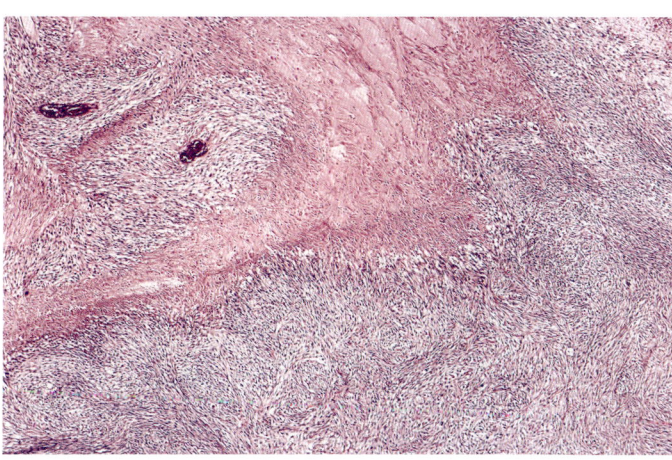

Fig. 5.91 Sarcomatoid carcinoma. Spindle cells predominate, and there are areas of geographical necrosis.

Imaging

The tumours, large and lobular, usually show poorly defined borders. Areas of low attenuation on CT correlate with necrotic areas {2117,1744}. Extensive local invasion occurs {2175}. Metastases to regional lymph nodes and lung are common.

Epidemiology

Sarcomatoid carcinoma accounts for 2.5–10% of all thymic carcinomas, occurring mostly in the fourth to eighth decades of life. In the ITMIG cohort, 18 of 6097 patients with thymic epithelial neoplasm (including 706 patients with thymic carcinomas) have sarcomatoid carcinoma. The average age is 47 years {33}.

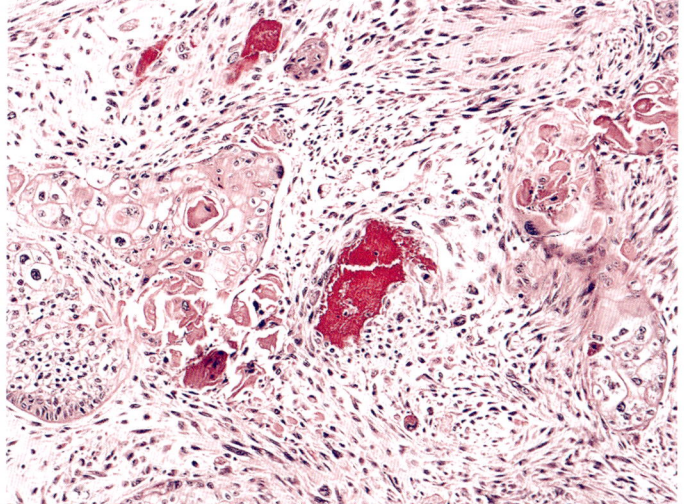

Fig. 5.92 Sarcomatoid carcinoma. A biphasic area composed of a squamous cell component that gradually merges into a spindle cell (sarcomatoid) component.

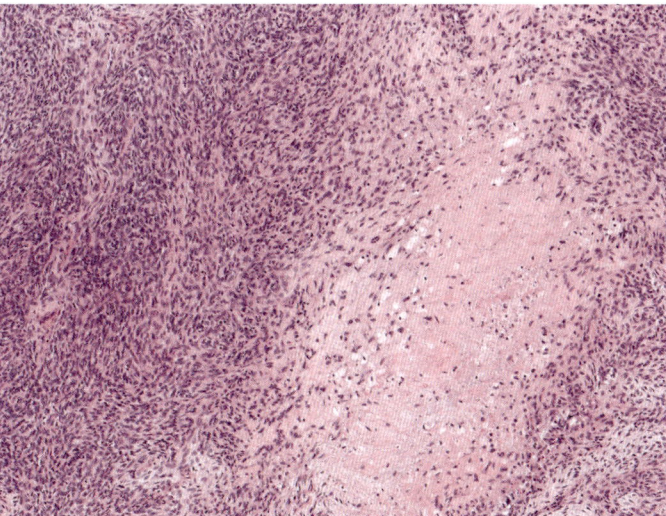

Fig. 5.93 Sarcomatoid carcinoma. Spindle cell carcinoma with area of necrosis.

Chapter 5

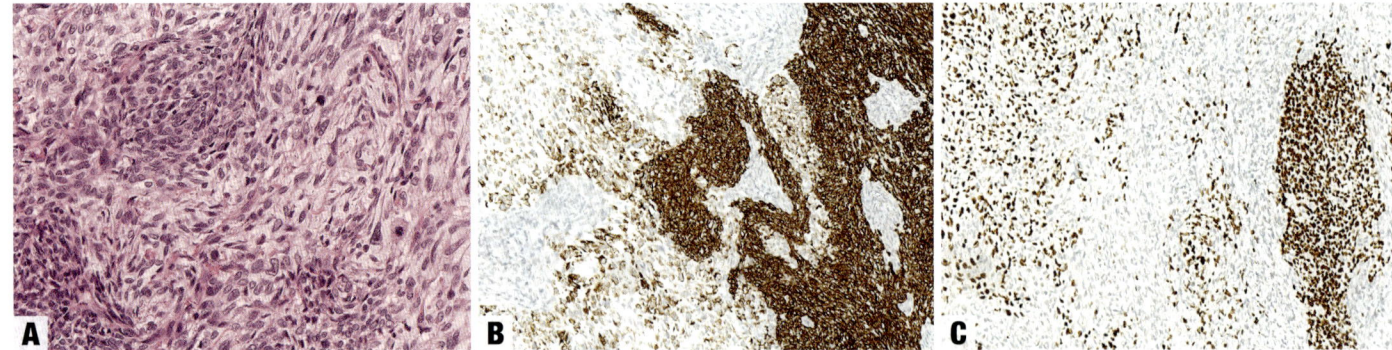

Fig.5.94 Sarcomatoid carcinoma. **A** Biphasic tumour, region resembling metaplastic thymoma with epithelioid and spindle cell areas and mitotic activity. **B** Immunostaining for keratin (AE1/AE3) reveals strong expression in epithelioid area and faint or no expression in the spindle cell (sarcomatoid) component. **C** Immunostaining for p63 reveals strong expression in epithelioid area and variable or no expression in the spindle cell (sarcomatoid) component.

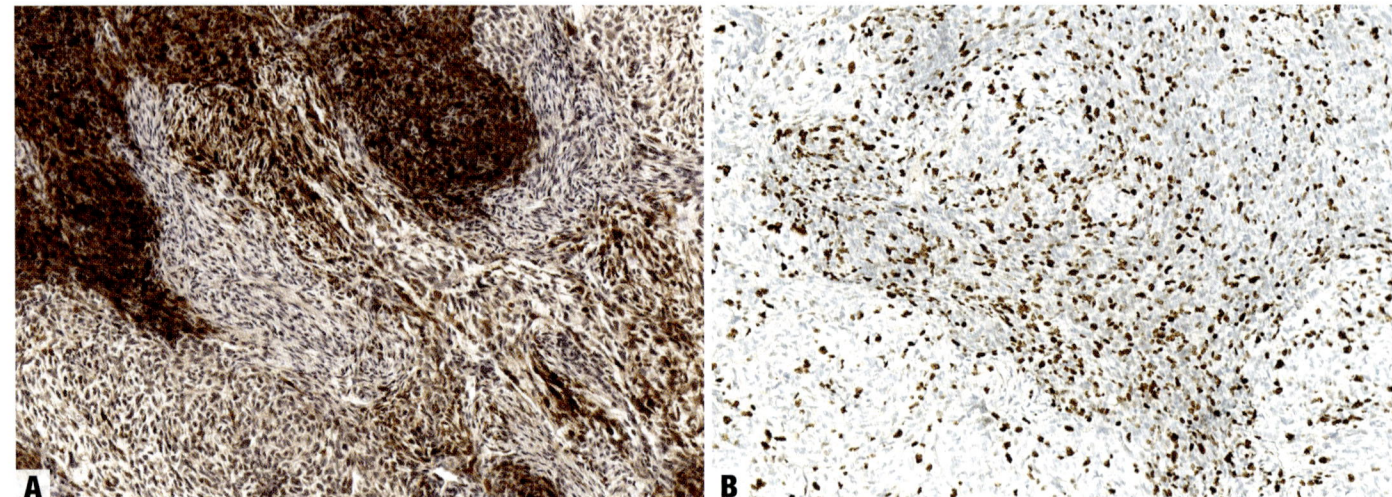

Fig.5.95 Sarcomatoid carcinoma. **A** Immunostaining for KIT (CD117) reveals strong expression mainly in the epithelioid area; this is not a feature of metaplastic thymoma. **B** High Ki-67 index, much in excess of what is encountered in metaplastic thymoma.

Etiology

A subset of sarcomatoid carcinomas co-occur with type A thymoma, metaplastic thymoma, other thymic carcinomas, or multilocular thymic cysts, from which they may arise {2921,2915, 3276,3275}. In other cases the etiology is unknown.

Pathogenesis

One case of sarcomatoid carcinoma has been reported that showed a complex chromosomal abnormality including der(16) t(1:16)(q12;q12.1), similar to a case of thymic squamous cell carcinoma {757}.

Macroscopic appearance

The tumours are often large, with infiltrative borders. The fleshy white or grey cut surfaces often show areas of haemorrhage, necrosis, and cystic degeneration {3068}.

Histopathology

Tumours may consist entirely of malignant spindle cells with moderately to highly atypical features, arranged in fascicles or storiform arrays {2921}. They are mitotically active {3276}. Some cases are admixed with type A thymoma {2921} or metaplastic thymoma {1744} or have a rhabdomyomatous component {1353}.

In sarcomatoid transformation of thymic carcinoma, both malignant epithelial (carcinomatous) and spindle cell (sarcomatous/sarcomatoid) components may occur {2927}. Tumours with heterologous mesenchymal elements such as rhabdomyosarcoma, osteosarcoma, or chondrosarcoma (carcinosarcoma) may occur {3068}. In some cases, the epithelial nature of the tumour can be demonstrated only by immunohistochemistry or electron microscopy {757}.

Differential diagnosis

Atypical type A thymoma usually shows low-grade nuclear atypia, is CD5-negative, and may harbour rare TdT-positive immature T cells {338}. Metaplastic thymoma is a biphasic tumour with consistently bland, mitotically inactive spindle cells; variably atypical epithelial islands; and common *YAP1-MAML2* gene fusion {3176}.

Thymic neuroendocrine tumours (NETs) with spindle cell features are distinguished by a prominent vasculature and synaptophysin and/or chromogranin expression {1982,710}.

Other biphasic tumours, such as mesothelioma, synovial sarcoma, or metastases may require appropriate ancillary studies for recognition.

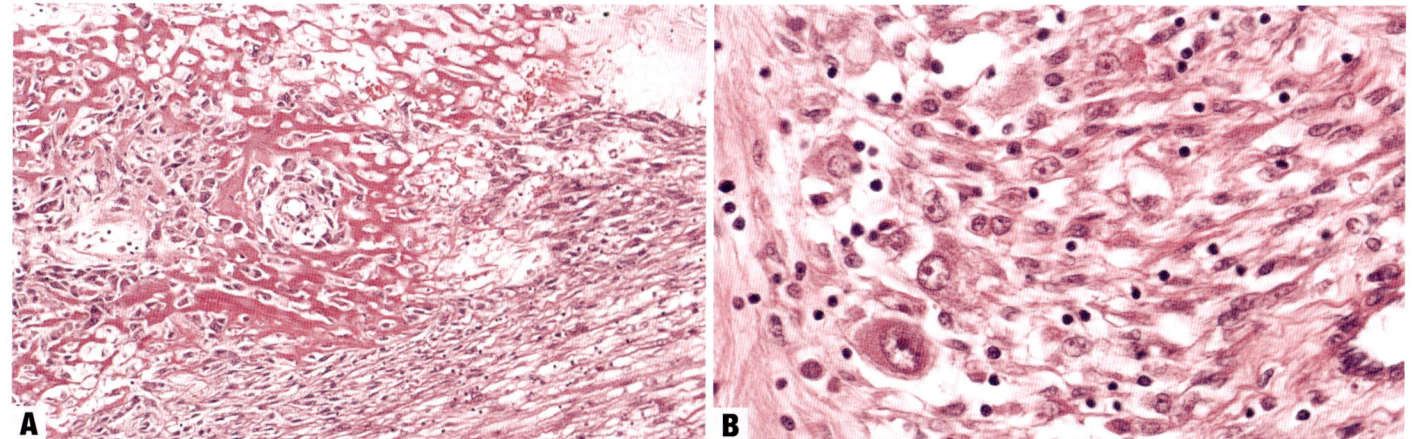

Fig. 5.96 Carcinosarcoma. **A** Malignant osteoid formation. **B** Skeletal muscle differentiation characterized by round rhabdomyoblasts with eosinophilic cytoplasm.

Cytology

Atypical spindle cells in smears can hint to thymic sarcomatoid carcinoma {3186}.

Diagnostic molecular pathology

Not clinically relevant

Essential and desirable diagnostic criteria

Essential:

- A thymic epithelial carcinoma either partly or completely composed of atypical spindle cells with at least focal epithelial features; carcinosarcoma includes heterologous sarcomatous elements

Desirable:

- Epithelial components may stain with characteristic markers

Staging

Sarcomatoid carcinomas should be staged according to the TNM system {315,687} and, optionally, the Masaoka–Koga system {685}. In the ITMIG cohort, 17% of sarcomatoid carcinomas are in stage I/II, 33% in stage III, and 50% in stage IV {33}.

Prognosis and prediction

This tumour type is highly aggressive. In the ITMIG cohort, the survival and outcome indicators are similar to those for other thymic carcinoma types {33}.

Undifferentiated carcinoma of the thymus

Thomas de Montpréville V
Marx A
Porubsky S

Definition

Thymic undifferentiated carcinoma is a primary carcinoma of the thymus lacking morphological or immunohistochemical differentiation other than epithelial differentiation. This is a diagnosis of exclusion.

ICD-O coding

8020/3 Carcinoma, undifferentiated, NOS

ICD-11 coding

2C27.0 & XH1YY4 Carcinoma of thymus & Carcinoma, undifferentiated, NOS

Related terminology

Not recommended: anaplastic carcinoma.

Subtype(s)

None

Localization

Undifferentiated carcinoma of the thymus is localized in the anterior (prevascular) mediastinum.

Clinical features

Symptoms are related to local tumour growth or metastases {3264}. Some cases are asymptomatic.

Epidemiology

Only 2.5% of non-neuroendocrine thymic carcinomas (18 of 706) are of undifferentiated type {33}. The largest reported series included 7 cases {2927}. The patients are adults, with no sex predominance and a median age of 54 years {434,2135, 3028,3264}. One case has been reported in a 2-year-old girl {1548}.

Etiology

The rare coexistence of undifferentiated carcinoma and thymoma {3028} suggests a possible derivation from pre-existing more differentiated tumours.

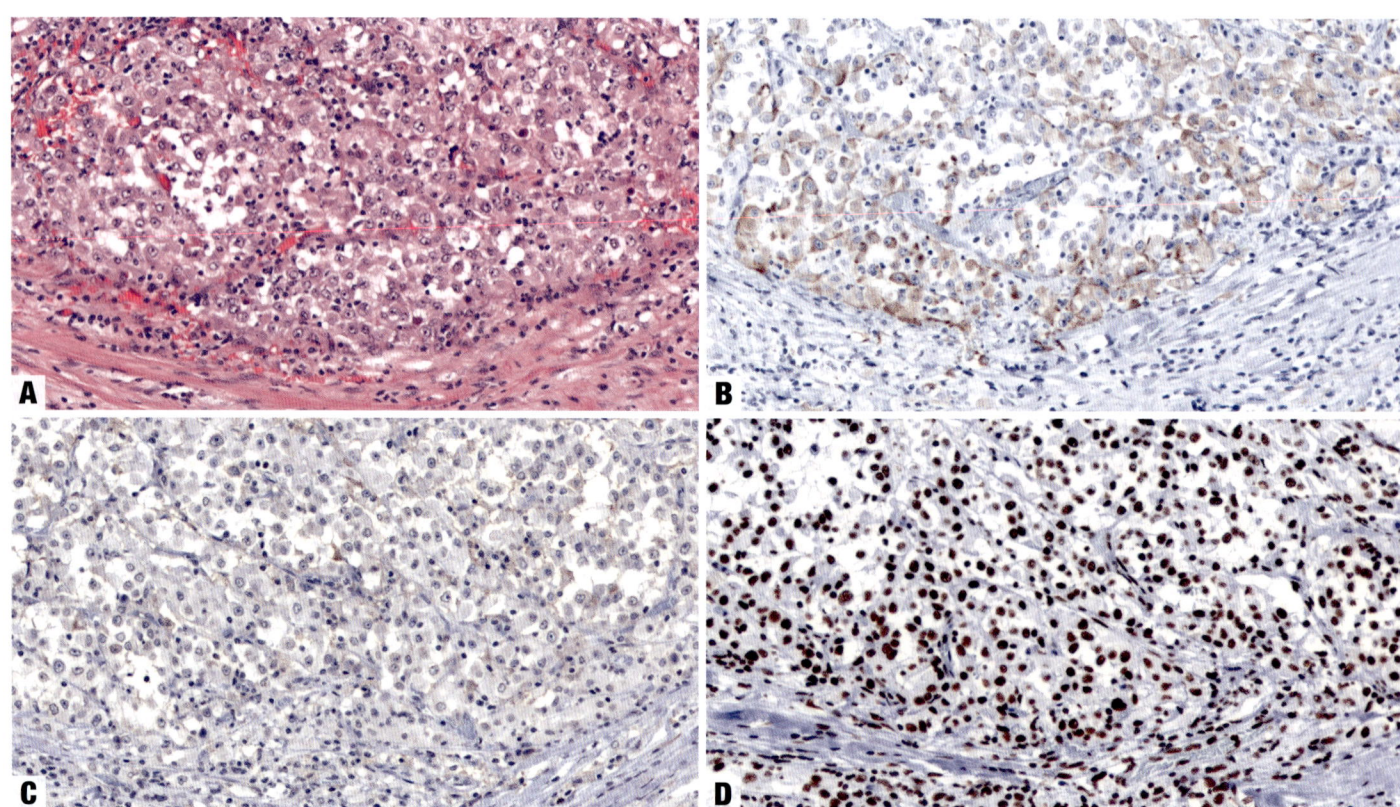

Fig. 5.97 Undifferentiated carcinoma of the thymus. **A** The tumour comprises sheets of poorly cohesive, large tumour cells with conspicuous nucleoli. Some cells with eccentric nuclei show rhabdoid features. **B** Pancytokeratin stain (AE1/AE3) labels the majority of the tumour cells. **C** Tumour cells do not show nuclear p63 expression (and were also negative for TTF1, CD5, and KIT [CD117], not shown). **D** Strong nuclear expression of SMARCA4 (and SMARCA2, not shown) excludes the diagnosis of a SMARCA4-deficient neoplasm.

Pathogenesis
Unknown

Macroscopic appearance
The tumours are often infiltrative and large {3264}.

Histopathology
Tumour cells are large and polygonal, with nuclear atypia, mitotic activity, and necrosis {2927,3028,3264}. Squamous, glandular, or sarcomatoid features should be absent. Rarely, there can be admixed bland-looking myoid cells. Tumour cells are positive for pancytokeratins {434,3028,3264}. Unlike in poorly differentiated thymic squamous cell carcinoma, there is no expression of CK5/6, p40/p63, or CD5 {3028}. Expression of KIT (CD117) and PAX8 is reported in 60% and 40% of cases, respectively {2048, 3028,3264}. Malignant germ cell tumour markers (e.g. OCT3/4 and SALL4) and neuroendocrine markers are negative.

Differential diagnosis
The main differential diagnoses are poorly differentiated squamous cell carcinoma, poorly differentiated neuroendocrine carcinomas (NECs), sarcomatoid carcinoma, NUT carcinoma, malignant germ cell tumours, other malignancies (e.g. melanoma, large cell lymphoma, or SMARCA4-deficient neoplasms {2324}), invasion from a large cell or pleomorphic carcinoma of the lung, and metastatic undifferentiated carcinoma. Cases associated with prominent inflammatory reaction mimicking Castleman disease {2135} are probably related to micronodular carcinoma with lymphoid hyperplasia {3268}.

When immunohistochemistry or molecular studies are not available or appropriate, the diagnosis may be rendered provisionally.

Cytology
Not available

Diagnostic molecular pathology
Immunohistochemical and/or molecular studies for NUT and *SMARCA4* genes are helpful for the exclusion of other poorly differentiated tumours {786,865,2324}.

Essential and desirable diagnostic criteria
Essential:
- Primary malignant thymic tumour showing only epithelial differentiation and not conforming to any other defined entity
- Immunohistochemistry and molecular studies required to exclude other diagnoses

Staging
Thymic undifferentiated carcinoma should be staged according to the TNM system {315,687} and, optionally, the Masaoka–Koga system {685}.

Prognosis and prediction
Undifferentiated carcinoma has a poor prognosis {434,2135, 3028,3264}. In the International Thymic Malignancy Interest Group (ITMIG) database, the survival and recurrence rates are similar to those for other types of thymic carcinoma {33}.

Thymic carcinoma NOS

Nonaka D
Tateyama H
Weissferdt A

Definition

Thymic carcinoma NOS is a heterogeneous group of carcinomas of thymic origin that cannot be categorized under other thymic carcinoma entities.

ICD-O coding

8586/3 Thymic carcinoma, NOS

ICD-11 coding

2C27.0 Carcinoma of thymus

Reports of hepatoid carcinoma {859} and rhabdoid carcinoma {3053} occurring as a primary tumour in the thymus are rare. These tumours show features analogous to those in other organs.

Undifferentiated large cell carcinoma associated with Castleman disease–like reaction is a rare tumour characterized by solid nests or cords of undifferentiated large tumour cells separated by abundant lymphoid stroma with prominent germinal centres. These germinal centres exhibit features closely resembling the late stage of hyaline-vascular Castleman disease {2135,2999}. This entity shows morphological overlap with micronodular thymic carcinoma with lymphoid hyperplasia (provisionally considered a subtype of thymic squamous cell carcinoma), and their clinical courses appear less aggressive than expected from their high-grade histology.

Two thymic carcinomas with sebaceous differentiation have been described, morphologically characterized by medium-sized to large tumour cells arranged in nests, which are intermingled with areas of vacuolated, clear, and focally keratinized cells {1354,2380}. The tumour is diffusely positive for CK5/6 and p63, and the cells with sebaceous differentiation express adipophilin. *FGFR2* amplification was found in one of the cases {2380}.

Thymic carcinoma NOS should be staged according to the TNM system {687} and, optionally, the Masaoka–Koga system {685}.

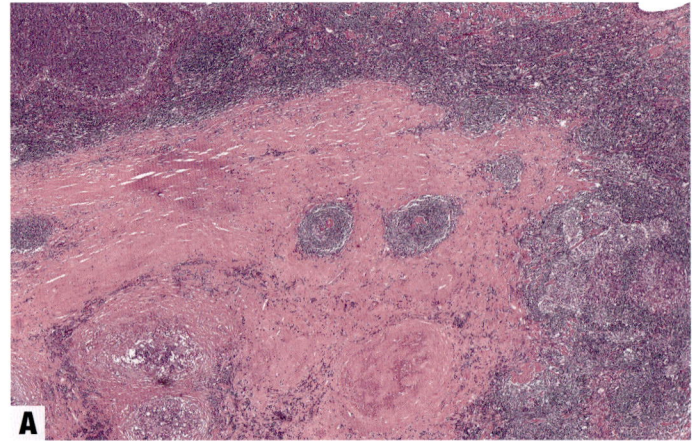
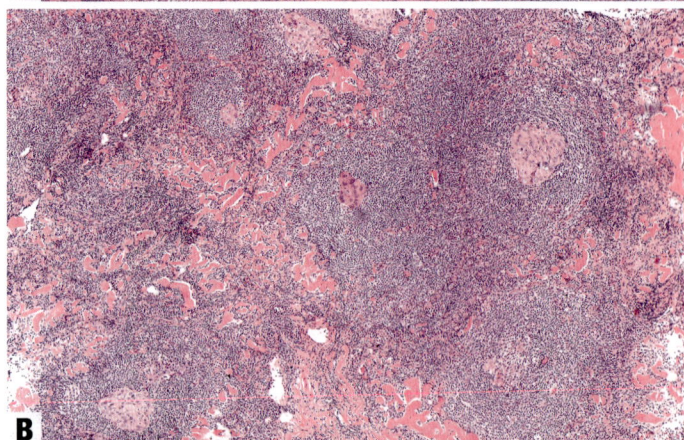
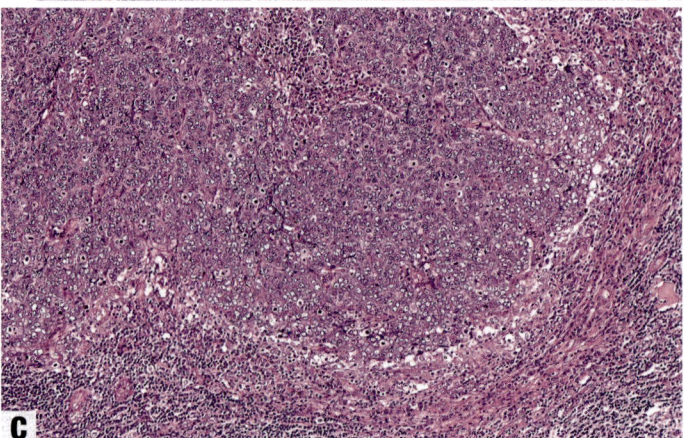

Fig. 5.98 Undifferentiated large cell carcinoma associated with Castleman disease–like reaction. **A** Abnormal follicles within diffusely hyalinized and fibrotic stroma. **B** Clusters of highly malignant epithelial cells in lymphoid follicles. **C** Cohesive sheets of undifferentiated epithelioid tumour cells surrounded by dense inflammation.

Thymic neuroendocrine neoplasms: Introduction

Ströbel P
Marchevsky AM
Marom EM
Pelosi G

Classification of neuroendocrine neoplasms of the thymus

Thymic neuroendocrine neoplasms (TNENs) account for 2–5% of all thymic neoplasms and only 0.4% of all neuroendocrine neoplasms (NENs) {993,1976,923,2801}. Most occur in adult patients. All TNENs share a propensity for recurrence, lymph node or distant metastasis, and tumour-associated death, with increasing risk from low-grade to high-grade tumours {884, 2801,2880}. Their radiological appearance is indistinguishable from that of thymic carcinomas. The approach taken in previous editions of the WHO classification (i.e. the use of the same nomenclature and criteria as for lung tumours) is maintained in this edition (see Table 5.08), although recent data have shown that this morphological approach reflects the underlying molecular biology of these tumours only imperfectly {710}.

Epidemiology of thymic neuroendocrine tumours in comparison to lung

Pulmonary NENs and TNENs share many similarities. First, all of the four histological subtypes found in the lung (typical carcinoid [TC], atypical carcinoid [AC], large cell neuroendocrine carcinoma [LCNEC], and small cell carcinoma [SmCC]) are also observed in the thymus, with virtually identical morphology. Second, patients with multiple endocrine neoplasia type 1 are at risk of developing TC and AC in both their lungs and thymus {3008}, although the genotype–phenotype correlation is weaker in the thymus. Third, smoking is not a risk factor for the development of pulmonary and thymic TCs and ACs. Fourth, the propensity for lymph node and distant metastases increases incrementally from TC to AC to LCNEC to SmCC. However, despite these similarities, there are also notable differences: thymic TC and AC show a strong male predominance, whereas pulmonary

Table 5.08 Neuroendocrine neoplasms (NENs) of the thymus

	Low-grade	Intermediate-grade	High-grade	
Classification of tumours with neuroendocrine morphology	Typical carcinoid	Atypical carcinoid	Large cell neuroendocrine carcinoma	Small cell carcinoma
	No necrosis < 2 mitoses/2 mm² (mean: 1 mitosis/2 mm²)	Necrosis present (any) and/or 2–10 mitoses/2 mm² (mean: 6.5 mitoses/2 mm²)	Non-small cell cytology Neuroendocrine markers > 10 mitoses/2 mm² (mean: 45 mitoses/2 mm²) Frequent necrosis	Small cell cytology > 10 mitoses/2 mm² (mean: 110 mitoses/2 mm²)

Current classification

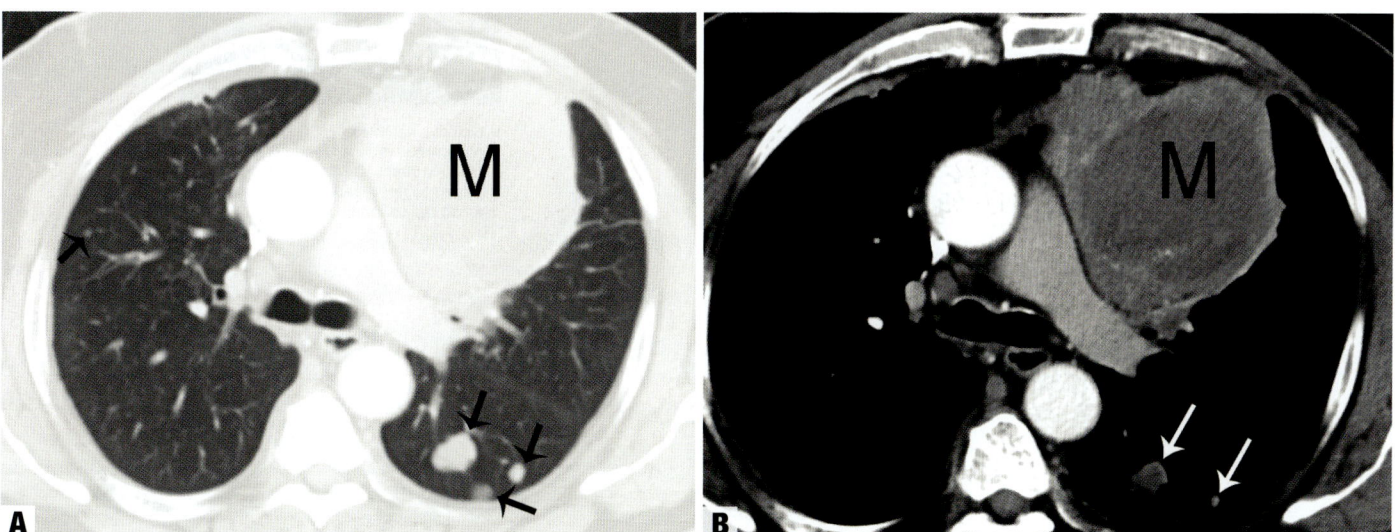

Fig. 5.99 Thymic neuroendocrine neoplasm (NEN). Similar to thymic carcinoma, thymic NENs may demonstrate aggressive behaviour such as invasion of adjacent structures, mediastinal lymph node involvement, and other visceral metastases at presentation. On contrast-enhanced chest CT, lung windows (**A**) and soft tissue windows (**B**) demonstrate a heterogeneous prevascular mass (M) with multiple pulmonary nodules (arrows) consistent with metastatic disease at presentation. Note that the larger pulmonary nodule in panel B has a heterogeneous low attenuation in appearance similar to the primary mass.

carinoids occur more often in females. AC and LCNEC are by far the most frequent subtypes in the thymus, whereas TC and SmCC prevail in the lung. Most patients with pulmonary LCNEC and SmCC are heavy smokers, whereas there is no established role of smoking in the development of any neuroendocrine tumour (NET) type in the thymus. The reasons for these differences are currently unknown, but molecular findings indicate that thymic and pulmonary carcinoids are different at the molecular level {1679,2880}, while thymic and pulmonary LCNECs and SmCCs appear to be more similar.

Molecular classification

Studies looking at chromosomal alterations in TNENs have found increasing numbers of gains and losses from TC to AC to LCNEC and SmCC that reflect the increasing clinical aggressiveness of these tumours. However, defining the optimal cut-off points for the histological distinction of the four subtypes, especially between AC and LCNEC, has been a constant challenge. The addition of Ki-67 is not helpful in this context {710}.

Atypical carcinoid tumours with elevated mitotic counts

Similar to grade 3 (G3) NETs in the pancreas, cases with carcinoid-like morphology but mitotic counts above the threshold currently allowed for AC (> 10 mitoses/2 mm²) also occur in the lung and thymus, and they are probably more frequent in the thymus than in the lung {710,1806,2405,1391,2463}.

On the basis of the frequency of chromosomal alterations, TNENs seem to fall into three molecular clusters: with low, intermediate, and high numbers of chromosomal changes. Cases with carcinoid morphology but increased mitotic counts were found in the clusters with low and intermediate numbers of chromosomal changes. A few patients whose primary tumours had been classified as TC or AC had metastases or recurrences of tumours that showed higher mitotic counts and evidence of slight morphological and molecular progression {710}, suggesting that TC, AC, and AC-like tumours with increased mitotic activity fall into the same spectrum of low- to intermediate-grade NETs. These intermediate-grade tumours were clearly different from poorly differentiated, high-grade LCNEC at the morphological, immunohistochemical, and molecular levels: intermediate-grade tumours showed carcinoid morphology and intermediate mitotic counts, were positive for chromogranin and negative for EZH2, and showed mutations of ATRX, whereas high-grade LCNEC showed the inverse immunohistochemical profile and had markedly higher mitotic counts {710}. Remarkably, tumours of both groups harboured NF1 gene mutations {710,789}. In the current edition of the WHO classification, such tumours are still classified as LCNEC, but the report should state that the histological appearance is that of a carcinoid tumour with increased mitotic counts, that such tumours appear to be distinct from

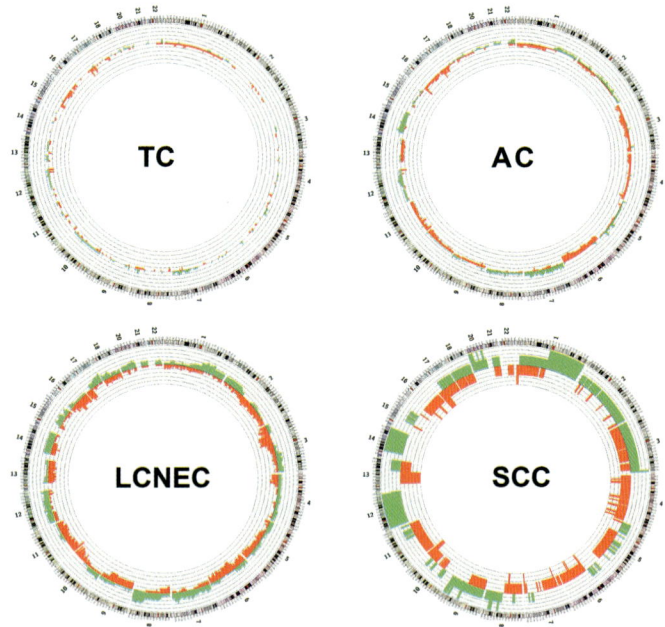

Fig. 5.100 Chromosomal changes in thymic neuroendocrine neoplasms (NENs). Synopsis of chromosomal gains and losses in thymic NENs (Circos plot, low-coverage whole-genome sequencing results). AC, atypical carcinoid; LCNEC, large cell neuroendocrine carcinoma; SCC, small cell carcinoma; TC, typical carcinoid.

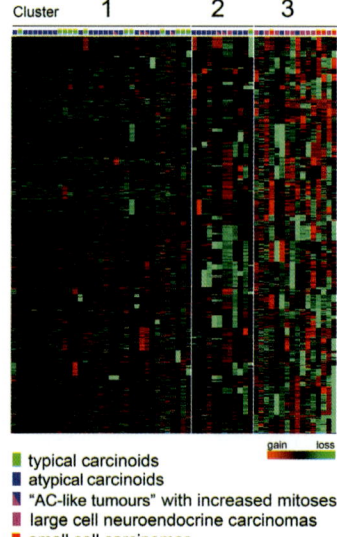

Fig. 5.101 Molecular clusters in thymic neuroendocrine neoplasm (NEN). Clustering of data from low-coverage whole-genome sequencing of thymic NENs reveals three major molecular clusters {710}. AC, atypical carcinoid.

conventional types of LCNEC, and that systemic management (e.g. the effectiveness of immunotherapies) may also differ.

Carcinoid/neuroendocrine tumour of the thymus

Ströbel P
Marchevsky AM
Nicholson AG
Osamura RY

Definition

Carcinoid/neuroendocrine tumour (NET) of the thymus is a neuroendocrine epithelial neoplasm of thymic origin with low-grade nuclear features; typical carcinoid (TC) has < 2 mitoses/2 mm^2 and lacks necrosis, whereas atypical carcinoid (AC) has 2–10 mitoses/2 mm^2 and/or foci of necrosis.

ICD-O coding

8240/3 Carcinoid tumour, NOS / neuroendocrine tumour, NOS
8240/3 Typical carcinoid / neuroendocrine tumour, grade 1
8249/3 Atypical carcinoid / neuroendocrine tumour, grade 2

ICD-11 coding

2C27.1 & XH9LV8 Carcinoid tumour or other neuroendocrine neoplasms of thymus & Neuroendocrine tumour, grade 1
2C27.1 & XH51K1 Carcinoid tumour or other neuroendocrine neoplasms of thymus & Neuroendocrine tumour, grade 2

Related terminology

Acceptable: carcinoid tumour; atypical carcinoid.

Subtype(s)

Typical carcinoid (grade 1 NET); atypical carcinoid (grade 2 NET)

Localization

Carcinoid/NET of the thymus is localized in the anterior (prevascular) mediastinum.

Clinical features

About 50% of patients present with chest pain, cough, dyspnoea, or superior vena cava syndrome {993,1976,2801}.

Paraneoplastic manifestations due to hormone production include Cushing syndrome (17–30% of adult and > 50% of childhood carcinoids) {636,2801,2918}, with or without cutaneous hyperpigmentation {919}; hypercalcaemia/hypophosphataemia due to production of PTHrP {3429} or from primary hyperparathyroidism in the context of multiple endocrine neoplasia type 1 (MEN1) {3009}; acromegaly {1292}; and inappropriate production of antidiuretic hormone or atrial natriuretic peptide {2178}. Carcinoid syndrome is exceedingly rare (< 1%) {2801}.

The clinical presentation of ACs is indistinguishable from that of TCs and includes the same paraneoplastic manifestations. About 40–50% of patients already have mediastinal, cervical, or supraclavicular lymph node metastasis at presentation {993, 3131,1976}. Invasion into adjacent organs (40–50%) or pleural or pericardial cavity (10%) is common {993,3131}. Sites of distant metastasis include lung, brain, lumbar spine, bone, liver, kidney, adrenals, skin, and soft tissues {993,1976,2801,35}. Late recurrences occurring as late as 9 years after resection have been reported {3096}.

Epidemiology

The average age at presentation for patients with typical carcinoids is 49 years {2801}, with a marked male predominance. MEN1-associated thymic neuroendocrine neoplasms (NENs) have all been carcinoids and occurred almost exclusively in adult men (age range: 31–66 years; mean: 44 years) {3008,518, 2778}.

In the thymus, ACs are far more common than TCs, and they occur in a slightly older age group {993,1976,35,2880,710}. They usually occur in adults, with an average patient age of 48–55 years (range: 18–82 years) {993,1976,2801,3131}, but

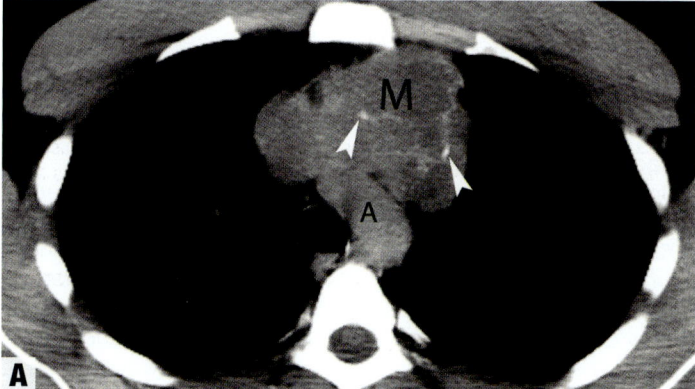
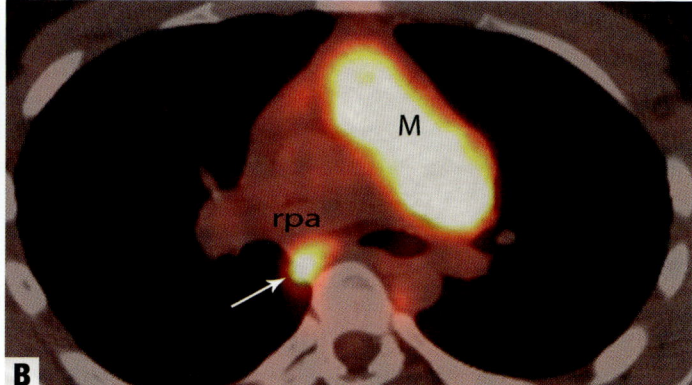

Fig. 5.102 CT of thymic carcinoid. **A** Unenhanced chest CT at the level of the transverse aorta (A) shows a lobular heterogeneous anterior (prevascular) mediastinal mass with areas of low attenuation corresponding to necrosis (M) and fine calcifications (arrowheads). **B** An axial fused image from FDG PET-CT at the level of the right pulmonary artery (rpa) shows that the primary mass (M) is markedly FDG-avid (with a maximum standardized uptake value of 25.7) and is associated with a mildly enlarged subcarinal FDG-avid lymph node consistent with a metastasis (arrow). This tumour shows aggressive imaging features commonly found in patients with neuroendocrine tumours (NETs), such as low-attenuation regions corresponding to areas of necrosis, calcifications, and avid FDG uptake. Imaging with FDG PET-CT is useful in patients with NETs and other forms of thymic cancer because it highlights lymph nodes and distant metastases, which can be overlooked with morphological imaging early in the disease, when small.

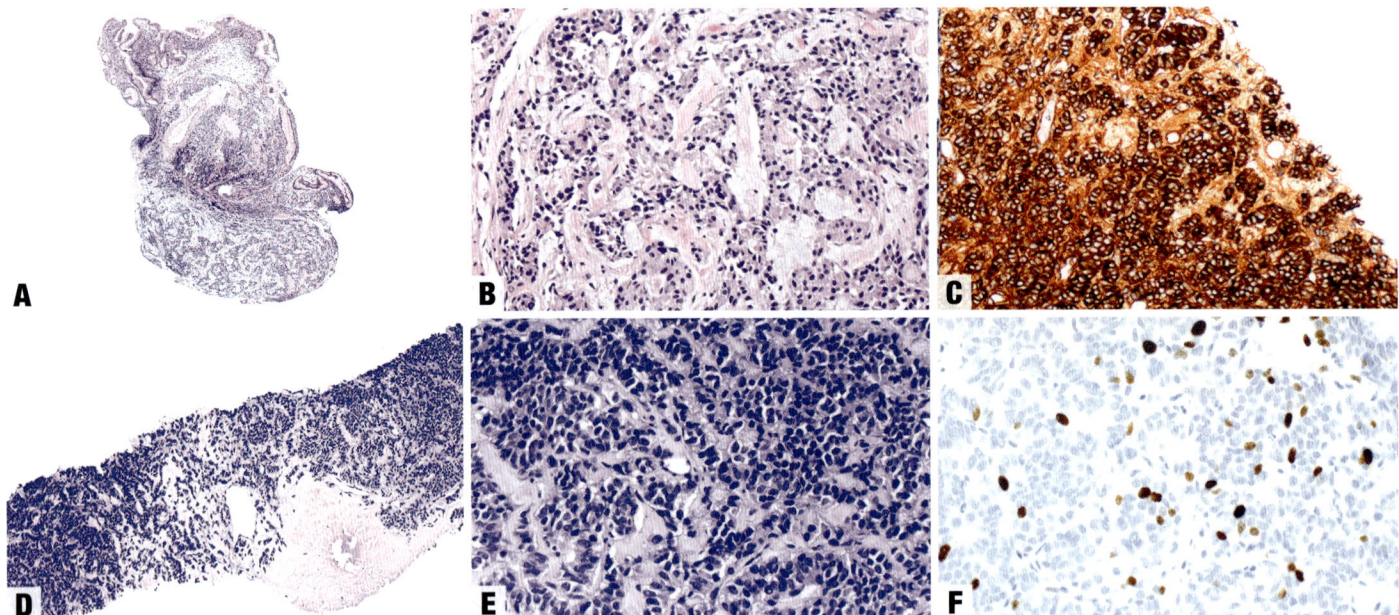

Fig. 5.103 Typical carcinoid. A 45-year-old man with multiple endocrine neoplasia type 1 had separate primary typical carcinoids in his stomach (**A,B**) and thymus (**D,E**). Both tumours showed strong chromogranin staining (**C**) and low/moderate Ki-67 labelling (**F**).

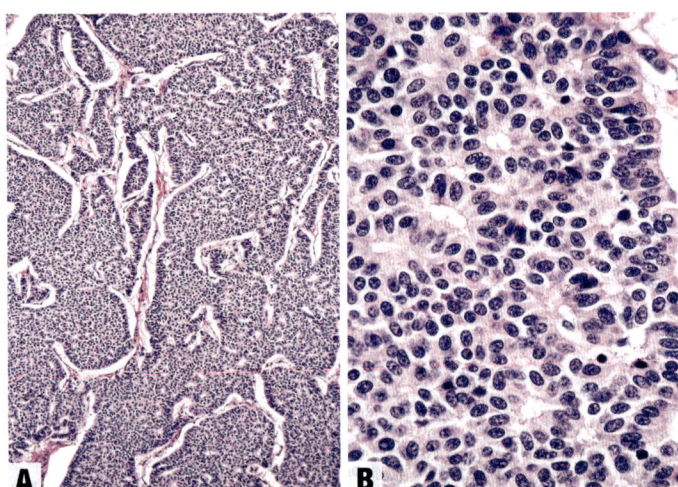

Fig. 5.104 Histology of typical carcinoid of the thymus. **A** A solid and trabecular growth pattern; note the delicate vasculature between tumour masses; necrosis is absent. **B** High-power magnification showing rosettes, bland cytology, and no mitoses.

they have also been rarely observed in children {919,1684}. There is a strong male predominance, with the M:F ratio ranging from 2:1 to 7:1 {752,993,1976,2801,710}.

Etiology

About 25% of patients with thymic carcinoids have a family history of MEN1 {3006}. Conversely, among MEN1 patients, thymic carcinoids occur in 8% of cases {947}. In MEN1, smoking has been reported to be a risk factor in males {947,820,994} but not females {2609}.

Pathogenesis

TCs / grade 1 (G1) NETs show the lowest number of genetic alterations among thymic NETs. Recurrent aberrations include gains on chromosomes 1q, 5, 6q, 7q, 8q, 10, 11q, 12q, 13q,

18q, 20, 21q, and 22q and losses on chromosomes 1, 2p, 4p, 8, 10p, 11p, 15q, 17p, 18p, and 22q {2250,2480,2880}. The gene locus of *MEN1* on chromosome 11q13 is consistently unaltered {947,2250,3007,3009}. These alterations are different from those described in pulmonary TC. Moreover, copy-number alterations in gene loci of tumour suppressor and driver genes with reported frequent alterations in pulmonary NETs are very rare in thymic TC {3187,816,710}. There are no published reports on specific gene mutations in TC.

ACs / grade 2 (G2) NETs show higher numbers of chromosomal alterations than TCs {2880}, and the percentage of alterations shared between AC and TC is lower than the percentage shared between AC and large cell and small cell neuroendocrine carcinomas (NECs) {710}. A small study comparing histological and molecular features in primary and metastatic ACs {710} suggests that TC and AC belong to a spectrum of neoplasms that can further progress at least to intermediate-grade tumours with mitotic counts exceeding those allowed for AC (see also *Thymic neuroendocrine neoplasms: Introduction*, p. 389, and *Large cell neuroendocrine carcinoma of the thymus*, p. 397). Single cases with *CTNNB1* gene mutations are on record {789}.

Macroscopic appearance

Most tumours are unencapsulated and either circumscribed or grossly invasive. The size ranges from 20 to 200 mm (mean: 80–100 mm) {656,1976,2801}. Cases associated with Cushing syndrome tend to be smaller (30–50 mm) due to earlier detection. They are grey-white and firm on cut section, can have a gritty consistency, and usually lack the characteristic lobulated growth pattern of thymomas. Oncocytic tumours may show a tan or brown cut surface. Calcifications are more frequent in thymic than extrathymic NETs {1976}.

Histopathology

Tumour cells are uniform and polygonal, with relatively small, round nuclei; finely granular chromatin; and pale eosinophilic

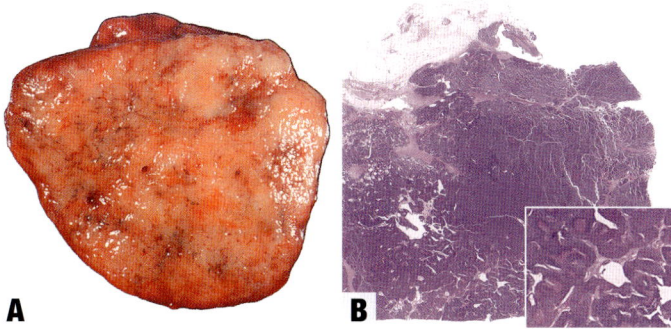

Fig. 5.105 Atypical carcinoid of the thymus. A macroscopic image (**A**) and a low-power H&E section (**B**) of a thymic atypical carcinoid. The H&E section shows vague circumscription and infiltrative growth of the tumour. The inset figure highlights multiple microscopic foci of necrosis.

cytoplasm. Most tumours show trabecular and rosetting growth patterns, but several other patterns, such as festoons, solid nests, glandular structures, and nuclear palisades, are also common. A delicate endocrine tumour–type vasculature between the nests and trabeculae is characteristic. Lympho-vascular invasion is frequent. There are several recognized patterns, including spindle cell {1657,3304,1982}, pigmented {1167, 1479,1585}, with amyloid {1657}, oncocytic {1980,3360}, muci-nous {2159,2922}, angiomatoid {1971}, and sarcomatous (with fibrosarcomatous, myoid, osseous, or chondroid differentiation) {1557,2289}. Calcifications are also frequent {1976}.

In ACs, all architectural features of TCs can occur. Even small punctate area of necrosis (comedonecrosis) in an otherwise-typical carcinoid justify a diagnosis of AC. Compared with TCs, ACs more frequently show some degree of nuclear pleomor-phism, including rare anaplastic cells {993}, a focal diffuse growth pattern (so-called lymphoma-like) {993,1976,3131}, or extensive desmoplastic stroma with single-cell filing of tumour cells {3302}.

Immunohistochemistry
Both TC and AC show strong expression of keratins and neuroen-docrine markers (e.g. synaptophysin and chromogranin) but are usually negative for TTF1.

Atypical carcinoid tumours with elevated mitotic counts
Similar to grade 3 (G3) NETs in the pancreas, cases with car-cinoid-like morphology but mitotic counts above the threshold currently allowed for AC (> 10 mitoses/2 mm²) also appear in the lung and thymus and are probably more frequent in the thymus than in the lung {710,1806,2405,1391,2463}. Please see *Thymic neuroendocrine neoplasms: Introduction* (p. 389) for more detailed information. In the current edition of the WHO classifica-tion, such tumours are still classified as large cell neuroendocrine carcinoma (LCNEC), but the report should state that the histo-logical appearance is that of a carcinoid tumour with increased mitotic counts, that such tumours appear to be distinct from con-ventional types of LCNEC, and that systemic management (e.g. the effectiveness of adjuvant therapies) may also differ.

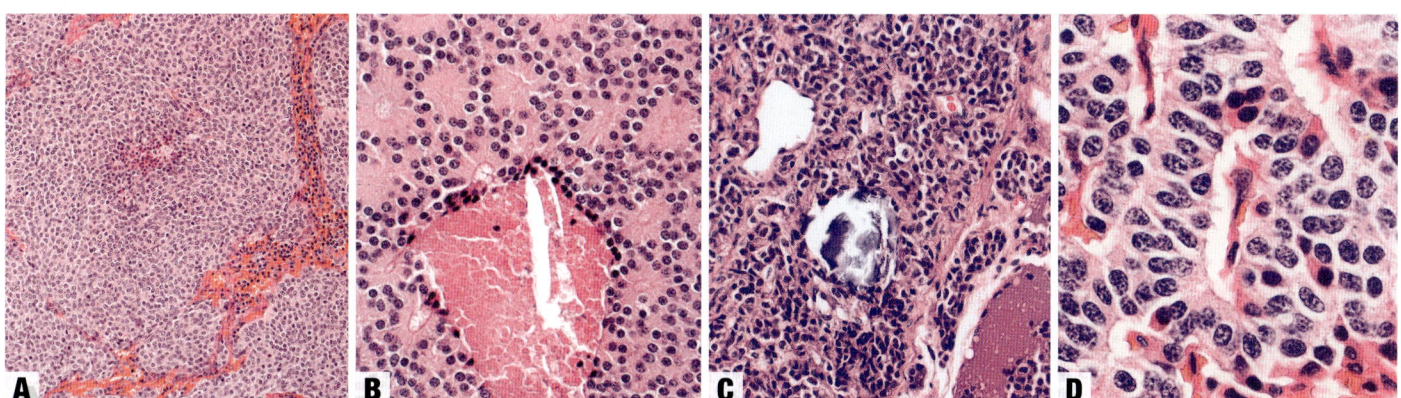

Fig. 5.106 H&E morphology of atypical carcinoid of the thymus. **A** Solid growth pattern with a small central focus of comedonecrosis. **B** Striking rosette formation with central comedonecrosis. **C** Calcification is a common finding. **D** High magnification shows trabecular growth and the delicate vasculature, as well as salt-and-pepper chromatin of the tumour cells.

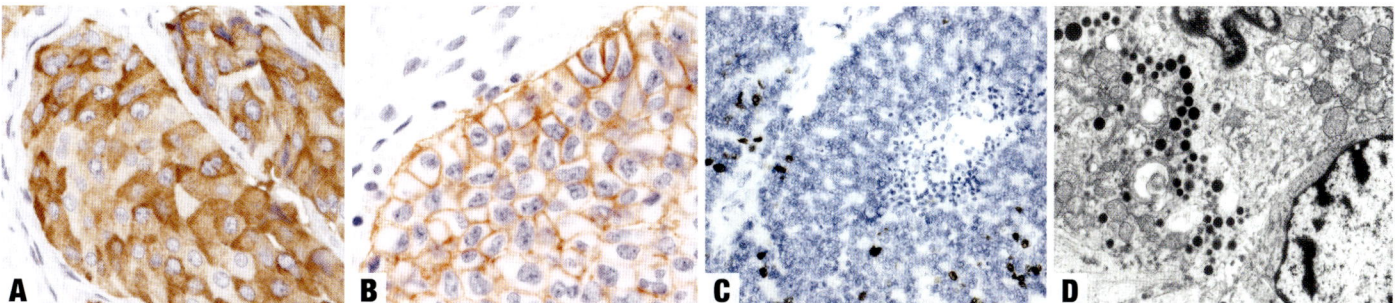

Fig. 5.107 Immunohistochemistry of atypical carcinoid of the thymus. **A** Chromogranin staining. **B** Strong membranous staining of CD56. **C** Low Ki-67 index. **D** Transmission electron microscopy shows distinct electron-dense neurosecretory granules of variable sizes in the cytoplasm of a tumour cell.

Cytology

Characteristic cells lie in loose clusters or small strands showing indistinct cell borders. They are uniformly small and round to oval with scant cytoplasm, sometimes interspersed with larger cells with abundant granular cytoplasm {3197}. ACs cannot be distinguished from TCs on the basis of cytological features.

Diagnostic molecular pathology

Not clinically relevant

Essential and desirable diagnostic criteria

Essential:

- TC: primary thymic NET with low-grade nuclear features, neuroendocrine morphology (e.g. trabecular or rosetting), absence of any necrosis, and mitotic count of < 2 mitoses/2 mm^2
- AC: same as TC, but with comedonecrosis and/or mitotic count of 2–10 mitoses/2 mm^2

Desirable:

- Both TC and AC: strong expression of keratins and neuroendocrine markers (e.g. synaptophysin and chromogranin), usually negative for TTF1
- Ki-67 can be useful in distinguishing carcinoids from high-grade LCNEC and small cell carcinoma, particularly in small crushed biopsies

Staging

TC and AC should be staged according to the Union for International Cancer Control (UICC) TNM system {315,687}.

Prognosis and prediction

There are few published data on the prognosis of thymic carcinoids. The available data suggest that the clinical course of TCs is similar to that of ACs {2880,710}. Reported 5-year overall survival rates of ACs vary in published series, from 20–70% {1976,2801,2880} up to 80% {590,993}, with a median survival time of 59 months {2880,710,834}.

Surgery and postoperative radiotherapy improve the outcome {2218,3285}. Published 5-year survival rates are in the range of 50–70% {1976,2801,2880,710,834}, with a median survival time of 126 months {2880}.

Small cell carcinoma of the thymus

Travis WD
Marchevsky AM
Nicholson AG
Ströbel P

Definition

Small cell carcinoma (SmCC) is a high-grade thymic carcinoma of neuroendocrine origin. Combined SmCC has an additional component of other thymic epithelial tumours (including thymoma and/or thymic carcinoma).

ICD-O coding

8041/3 Small cell carcinoma
8045/3 Combined small cell carcinoma

ICD-11 coding

2C27.Y & XH0YB0 Other specified malignant neoplasms of thymus & Small cell carcinoma, NOS

Related terminology

Not recommended: oat cell carcinoma; poorly differentiated (high-grade) neuroendocrine carcinoma (obsolete).

Subtype(s)

Small cell carcinoma; combined small cell carcinoma

Localization

SmCCs occur in the anterior (prevascular) mediastinum.

Clinical features

Symptoms include weight loss, sweating, chest pain, cough, and superior vena cava syndrome {3043,1560,3305,3306}. Exceptional patients may present with Cushing syndrome due to ectopic ACTH production {1113}. Most tumours show invasion of neighbouring structures such as the lung, pericardium, pulmonary artery, phrenic nerve, or aortic arch {1560,1113,3305, 3306}, or distant metastases to the lung, bone, brain, liver, and abdominal lymph nodes {2880,3043,1560,3088,3305,3306}.

Epidemiology

SmCCs account for approximately 10% of all thymic neuroendocrine neoplasms (NENs) {435,901,1976,2880,3043}, with an

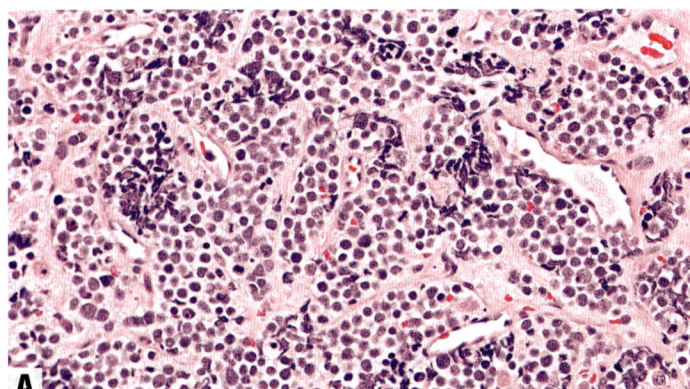
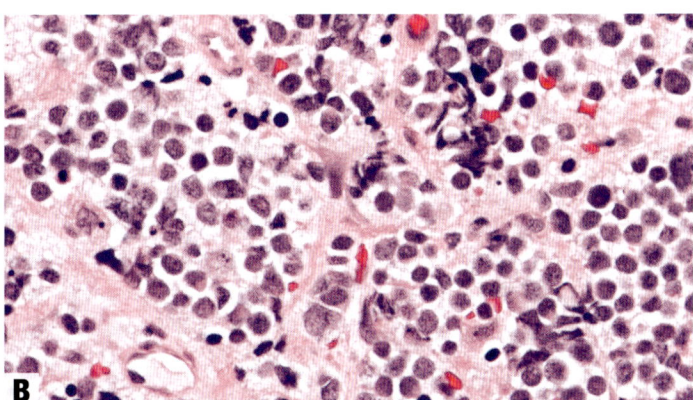

Fig. 5.108 Thymic small cell carcinoma. **A** This tumour consists of diffuse sheets and organoid nests of small tumour cells with scant cytoplasm and finely granular nuclear chromatin. Nucleoli are inconspicuous or absent. Mitotic count is high. **B** This tumour consists of nests and sheets of small cells with scant cytoplasm, finely granular nuclear chromatin, and frequent mitoses.

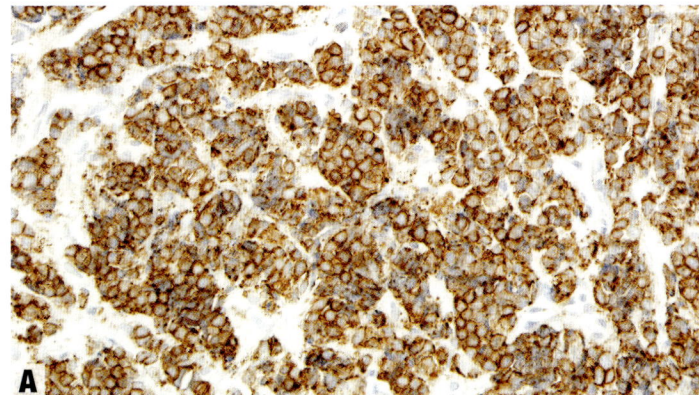
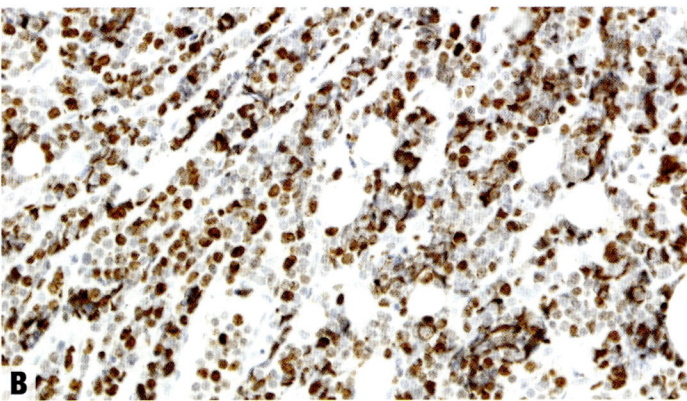

Fig. 5.109 Thymic small cell carcinoma. **A** This tumour is strongly positive for CD56. **B** The Ki-67 proliferation index is 80–90%.

estimated incidence of 1 case per 50 million individuals per year {923}. Men and women are equally affected, and the median patient age is 58 years (range: 37–63 years) {2880,1560,1113, 3088,3305,3306}.

Etiology

The etiology of SmCC is unknown. SmCCs do not occur in multiple endocrine neoplasia type 1 {3043,820,947,994,2609}. There are no data on the etiological role of smoking.

Pathogenesis

The pathogenesis of thymic SmCC is unknown. The tumour does not appear to evolve from thymic carcinoid tumours, in line with other NENs {2490}. There are limited genetic data available. Two studied tumours were highly aberrant, showing multiple chromosomal gains and losses that were mostly overlapping with the more stable thymic carcinoid tumours and large cell neuroendocrine carcinomas (LCNECs) {2880}. In addition, SmCCs show a high copy-number instability score by whole-genome sequencing {710}.

Macroscopic appearance

The macroscopy of SmCC is similar to that of other thymic NENs, but necrosis and haemorrhage can be extensive. The tumours may be large, measuring 100–150 mm in diameter {1560,3305,3306}.

Histopathology

The histology of thymic SmCC is identical to that of SmCCs in other organs (see *Small cell lung carcinoma*, p. 139). Tumour cells are small (usually < 3 times the size of a small resting lymphocyte), with scant cytoplasm. Nuclei can be round, oval, or spindle-shaped; the chromatin is finely granular, and nucleoli are inconspicuous or absent. Apoptotic bodies are often numerous. Mitotic count is high, > 10 mitoses/2 mm^2 but averaging > 50 mitoses/2 mm^2. Neuroendocrine differentiation can be demonstrated in some cases by electron microscopy {3043, 3088}.

Combined SmCC with thymoma, squamous cell carcinoma, or adenosquamous cell carcinoma has been reported.

Immunohistochemistry

Most cases stain for keratins, with rare exceptions {1560,1113, 3088}, and most tumours stain with neuroendocrine markers such as chromogranin, synaptophysin, or CD56 {3043,1560, 1113,3088}, although expression of neuroendocrine markers is not required for the diagnosis. ACTH may be expressed. The Ki-67 index is high, usually > 50% and often 80–100%.

Differential diagnosis

The main differential diagnosis is metastasis from pulmonary SmCC, which requires careful correlation with clinical findings and imaging. TTF1 staining can be positive in thymic SmCC as in other extrapulmonary SmCCs {225}. The diagnosis of SmCC with negative keratin should be made with great caution after

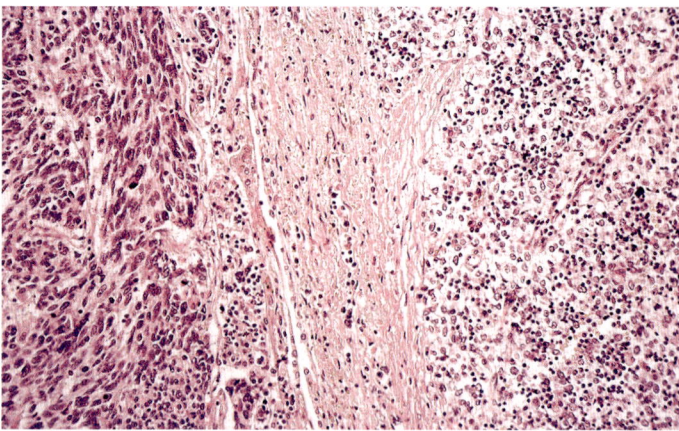

Fig. 5.110 Combined small cell carcinoma and thymoma. Small cell carcinoma of the thymus (left) adjacent to a type B3 thymoma (right). Such tumours should be classified as combined small cell carcinoma.

exclusion of lymphoma (CD45, TdT, and CD3) and Ewing sarcoma (e.g. CD99 or *EWSR1* translocation).

Cytology

The tumour cells show a high N:C ratio, scant cytoplasm, nuclear moulding, and finely granular nuclear chromatin. The nucleoli are inconspicuous or absent. Crush artefacts, nuclear breakdown, and apoptotic bodies are common.

Diagnostic molecular pathology

Not clinically relevant

Essential and desirable diagnostic criteria

Essential:
- Radiological evidence of thymic origin
- Exclusion of a tumour spreading from the lung or metastatic from another extrapulmonary site to the thymus
- A tumour consisting purely of small cells with characteristic morphology similar to lung SmCCs
- Combined SmCC: a small carcinoma combined with another histology such as thymoma or other type of thymic carcinoma

Desirable:
- Positive immunohistochemistry for cytokeratins and neuroendocrine markers, as well as elevated Ki-67 (usually > 50%)

Staging

Tumours are staged according to the eighth-edition TNM classification {315,687}.

Prognosis and prediction

Prognosis is poor, with a 5-year survival rate of 0% {2880,1983}. Median survival time is 14 months (range: 13–26 months) {2880, 3043,1560,3305,3306}.

Large cell neuroendocrine carcinoma of the thymus

Nicholson AG
Marchevsky AM
Osamura RY
Ströbel P

Definition

Large cell neuroendocrine carcinoma (LCNEC) is a high-grade thymic tumour comprising large cells with neuroendocrine morphology and positive neuroendocrine immunohistochemistry.

ICD-O coding

8013/3 Large cell neuroendocrine carcinoma

ICD-11 coding

2C27.Y & XH0NL5 Other specified malignant neoplasms of thymus & Large cell neuroendocrine carcinoma

Related terminology

Not recommended: high-grade (grade 3) neuroendocrine tumour of the thymus.

Subtype(s)

None

Localization

LCNECs arise in the anterior (prevascular) mediastinum.

Clinical features

About 50% of patients are asymptomatic at presentation; the remainder present with chest pain, dyspnoea, or superior vena cava obstruction {35,3043}. Cushing syndrome is very rare {2594}. About 50% of patients present with local spread or distant metastasis {923}.

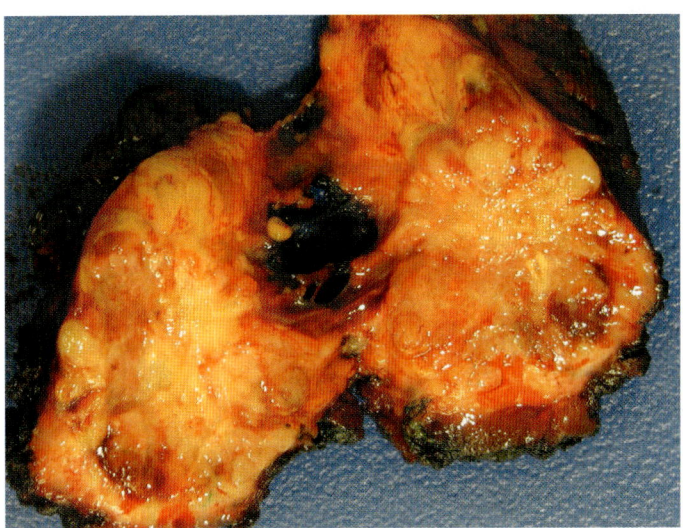

Fig. 5.111 Large cell neuroendocrine carcinoma (LCNEC) of the thymus. There is an infiltrative thymic mass within the mediastinum.

Epidemiology

LCNECs are more common in males, with a median age of 57 years (range: 16–79 years). They account for 14–26% of thymic neuroendocrine neoplasms (NENs) {710,35,3043,2880}, with an estimated incidence of 1 case per 20 million individuals per year {923}.

Etiology

The etiology is unknown. There is no association with multiple endocrine neoplasia type 1.

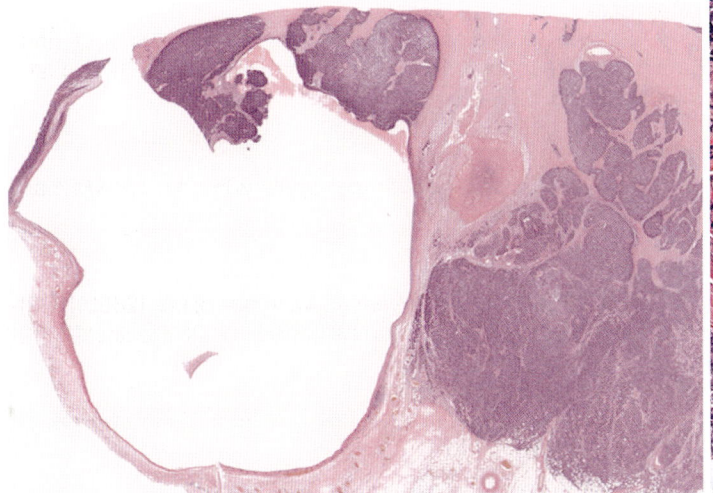

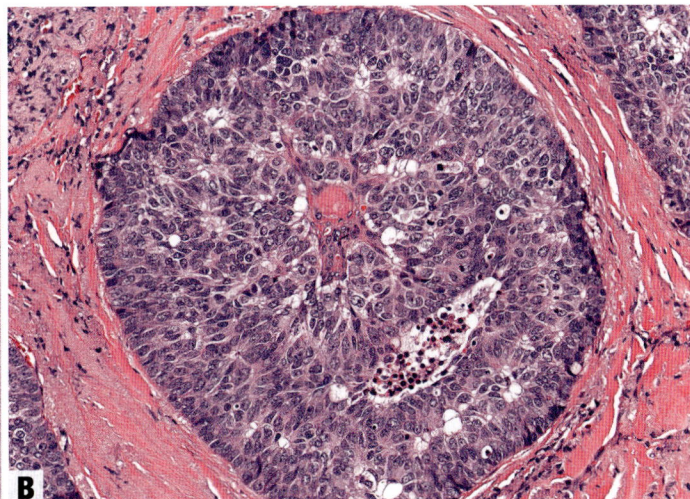

Fig. 5.112 Large cell neuroendocrine carcinoma (LCNEC) of the thymus. **A** Multinodular tumour adjacent to a thymic cyst. **B** The tumour shows neuroendocrine morphology, which stained for both INSM1 and synaptophysin.

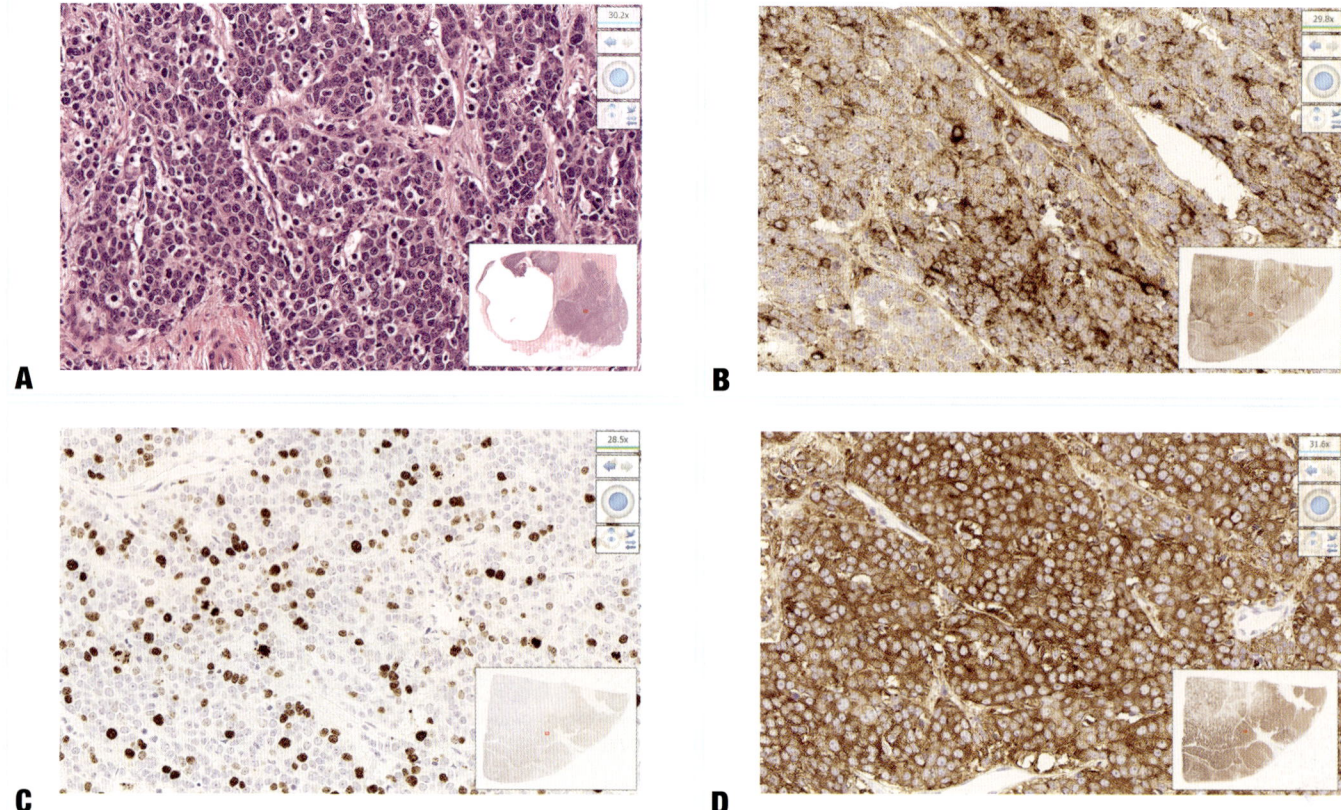

Fig. 5.113 Large cell neuroendocrine carcinoma (LCNEC) of the thymus. **A** H&E. **B** Chromogranin A. **C** Ki-67 index of up to 40%. **D** Synaptophysin.

Pathogenesis

Chromosomal aberrations are similar to those seen in pulmonary counterparts, such as gains in 2p, 9p, and 17q and losses at 4p, 8p, 9p, and 18p {2880}. Copy-number instability is high in LCNECs {710}.

Macroscopic appearance

LCNECs are unencapsulated, infiltrative, and generally solid tumours, sometimes with focal calcification. Necrosis may be present. Tumour lobulation, as seen in thymomas, is absent.

Histopathology

LCNECs comprise sheets of non-small cell epithelial cells with neuroendocrine morphology and a high mitotic count of > 10 mitoses/2 mm^2 {1976,710}, usually much higher. Necrosis is nearly always seen and often extensive. Architecture varies between solid sheets and neuroendocrine morphology (nesting, trabeculae, and rosettes), the latter often poorly developed.

There is staining for at least one neuroendocrine marker (chromogranin, synaptophysin, CD56). However, if morphological features are convincing for LCNEC, any extent of expression of even a single neuroendocrine marker is accepted to support the diagnosis (see *Large cell neuroendocrine carcinoma of the lung*, p. 144) {3390,710,3269}. Staining for CD5 is negative, although occasional cases stain with KIT (CD117). Staining for TTF1 is usually negative {1976,3043}. If there is a small cell component of ≥ 10%, the tumour should be classified as a combined small cell carcinoma and LCNEC.

Cytology

Cytological features are the same as those in primary pulmonary LCNEC (see *Large cell neuroendocrine carcinoma of the lung*, p. 144).

Diagnostic molecular pathology

Not clinically relevant

Essential and desirable diagnostic criteria

Essential:
- Neuroendocrine morphology
- Mitotic count of > 10 mitoses/2 mm^2
- Necrosis, often geographical
- Positive neuroendocrine immunohistochemistry

Desirable:
- High Ki-67 index: > 30%, generally 40–80%; negative p40 immunohistochemistry

Staging

Staging is according to the Union for International Cancer Control (UICC) TNM classification {315,687}.

Prognosis and prediction

The 5-year overall survival rate ranges from 0% to 66% {3043, 387,2880,710}.

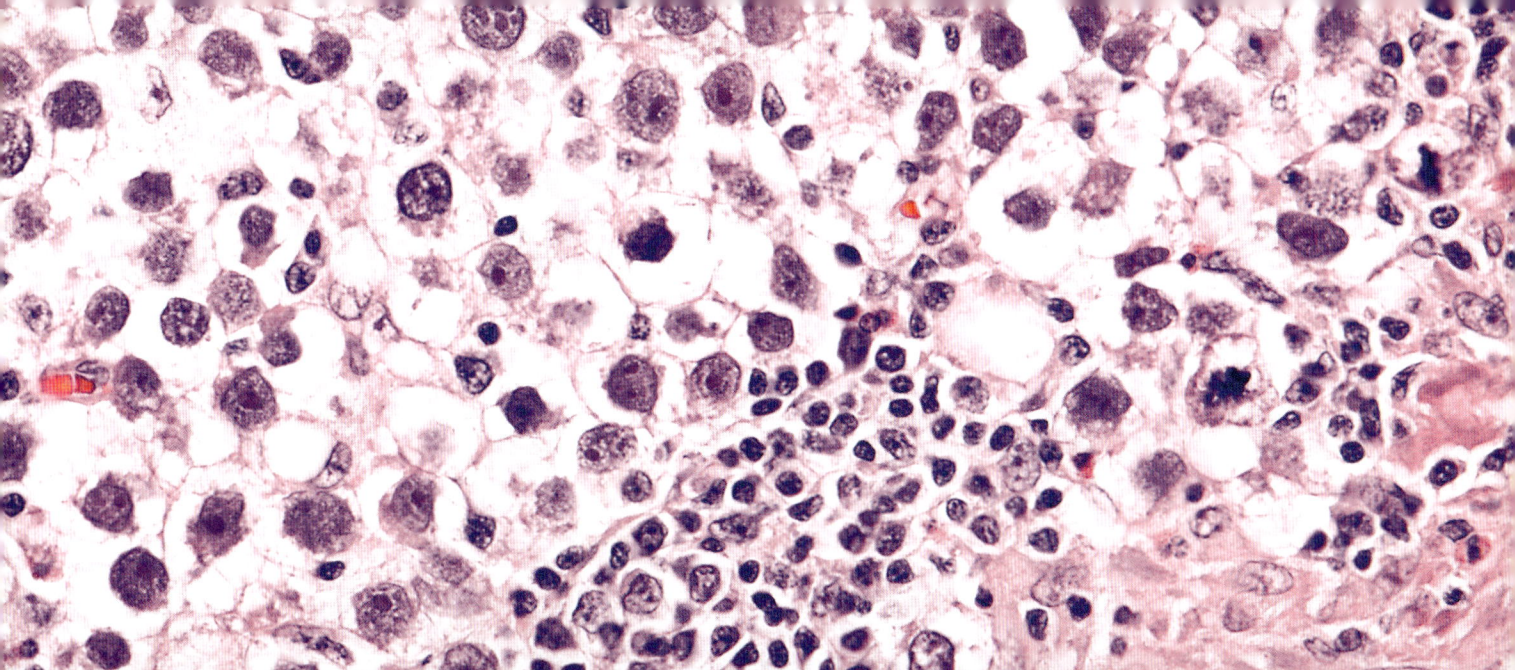

6

Germ cell tumours of the mediastinum

Edited by: Borczuk AC, Lax SF

Seminoma
Embryonal carcinoma
Yolk sac tumour
Choriocarcinoma
Teratoma
Mixed germ cell tumours
Germ cell tumours with somatic-type solid malignancy
Germ cell tumours with associated haematological malignancy

Germi cell tumours of the mediastinum: Introduction

Roden AC
Marom EM
Moreira AL
Ulbright TM

Primary mediastinal germ cell tumours account for 1–15% of all mediastinal neoplasms in adults and 11–20% in children {1010,2505}. The age range spans from birth to at least 79 years (mean age: 40 years). The incidence increases after puberty. Mediastinal germ cell tumours account for 16.3% of all solitary mediastinal lesions among people aged 18–29 years; in the fourth, fifth, and sixth decades of life and beyond they account for 9.9%, 2.8%, and 0.2–1.1% of all mediastinal lesions, respectively {2505}. There is a strong correlation between some tumour types and patient age {2147,258,1978}. For instance, whereas mature teratomas and yolk sac tumours are the almost exclusive tumour types in very young patients, seminomas are almost always diagnosed in patients aged ≥ 10 years {2668}. Mixed mediastinal germ cell tumours are more common in adults, with a marked male predominance. The vast majority of these tumours (81–100%) occur in the anterior (prevascular) mediastinum {2505,1951,2719,2147,616}.

Germ cell tumours are histologically classified as seminomas, non-seminomatous germ cell tumours (choriocarcinoma, yolk sac tumour, embryonal carcinoma, or mixed germ cell tumour), and teratomas {1978,2965}. A seminoma with any component of a non-seminomatous tumour is considered a non-seminomatous germ cell tumour. The majority of the morphological and genetic features are similar to those of these tumours' gonadal counterparts; however, a few histological and molecular characteristics are unique to the mediastinum, including common cystic changes and lack of *PDGFRA* gene mutations in mediastinal seminomas, among others {1987}. Furthermore, the prognosis of malignant mediastinal germ cell tumours is worse than that of their gonadal counterparts {1863}. In fact, the mediastinal location of a non-seminomatous germ cell tumour is a major adverse prognostic factor {1257}. The only known risk factor appears to be Klinefelter syndrome, which has been identified in 8–33% of male patients with primary mediastinal germ cell tumour {2093, 691,1088,258,2965,2889,3314,1089,211}. Furthermore, Klinefelter syndrome is associated with a 67-fold increased risk for primary mediastinal germ cell tumour, which occurs mostly in patients who are younger (age range: 4.5–31 years) than those without the syndrome.

Mediastinal germ cell tumours usually occur as a large anterior mediastinal (prevascular) mass, often discovered secondary to reports of chest pain, chronic cough, or dyspnoea. On CT, the presence of fat in a prevascular mass is suggestive of teratoma, but the identification of a fat–fluid level or bone is pathognomonic of teratoma. Seminomas tend to be homogeneous, whereas non-seminomatous germ cell tumours are more heterogeneous {2528}.

The immunophenotype of primary mediastinal germ cell tumours is similar to that of their gonadal counterparts {1987}. Although many markers are sensitive for these tumours, no marker is specific for a single type of germ cell tumour, with immunophenotypic overlap among germ cell tumours for many

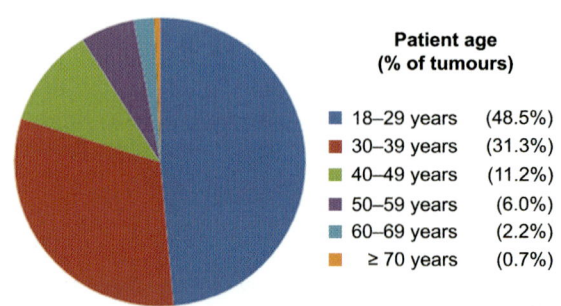

Patient age (% of tumours)

- 18–29 years (48.5%)
- 30–39 years (31.3%)
- 40–49 years (11.2%)
- 50–59 years (6.0%)
- 60–69 years (2.2%)
- ≥ 70 years (0.7%)

Fig. 6.01 Germ cell tumours of the mediastinum. Distribution of mediastinal germ cell tumours in adults, by age (N = 134) {2505}.

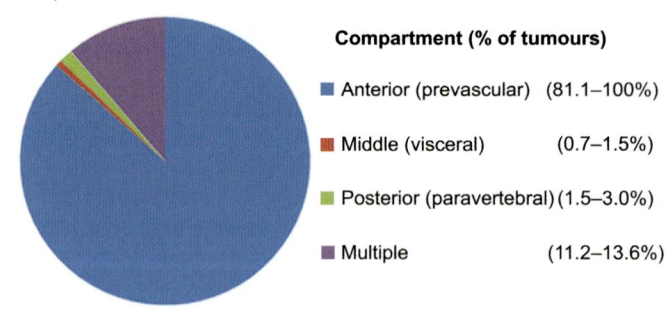

Compartment (% of tumours)

- Anterior (prevascular) (81.1–100%)
- Middle (visceral) (0.7–1.5%)
- Posterior (paravertebral) (1.5–3.0%)
- Multiple (11.2–13.6%)

Fig. 6.02 Germ cell tumours of the mediastinum. Distribution of mediastinal germ cell tumours in adults, by mediastinal compartment (N = 134) {2505}.

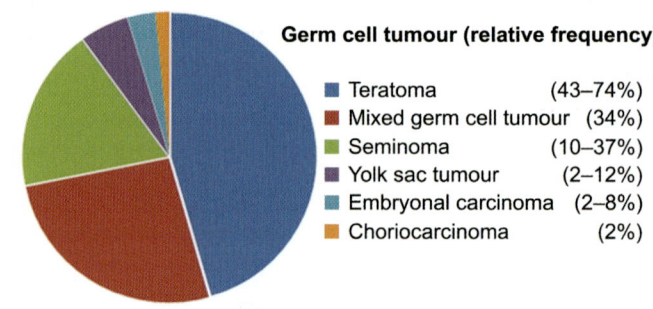

Germ cell tumour (relative frequency)

- Teratoma (43–74%)
- Mixed germ cell tumour (34%)
- Seminoma (10–37%)
- Yolk sac tumour (2–12%)
- Embryonal carcinoma (2–8%)
- Choriocarcinoma (2%)

Fig. 6.03 Germ cell tumours of the mediastinum. Relative frequency of germ cell tumours in the mediastinum {2965,1978,742}.

markers. Therefore, a panel of immunostains is recommended to secure a diagnosis, with the composition of the panel dependent on the morphological features of the tumour. There is a strong histological correlation with clinical, radiographic, and serological findings, including levels of AFP, β-hCG, and LDH, which are important clinical data. The immunohistochemical profiles of primary mediastinal germ cell tumours are summarized in Table 6.01.

Primary mediastinal germ cell tumours are thought to arise either from germ cells that aberrantly migrated during embryonic development or from stem cells in the thymus {2123,2199, 862,1261,160}. Some evidence suggests that the epithelial cells of the thymus might provide an appropriate microenvironment for germ cells {659}. Type I tumours encompass infantile teratomas and yolk sac tumours that develop as immature teratomas during embryonic life. Somatic mutations are usually not identified in type I teratomas. Type II germ cell tumours are malignant, include seminomas and non-seminomatous germ cell tumours, and occur in adolescents and adult men. Type II tumours are characterized by gain of chromosome 12p, commonly as an isochromosome of 12p {431,2907,2392,2393,1376}. In addition, in seminomas, activating *KIT* mutations and a rare case with *KRAS* mutation are described {2392}.

There is no official staging system for primary mediastinal germ cell tumours.

The outcome of primary mediastinal germ cell tumours depends on the subtype of the tumour, with overall survival rates ranging from 85–88% for seminomas to 40–45% for non-seminomatous tumours. The latter rate is lower than that for testicular non-seminomatous germ cell tumours {258,1257}. The survival of patients with mediastinal non-seminomatous germ cell tumours is also worse than that of patients with other extragonadal non-seminomatous germ cell tumours. Reasons for

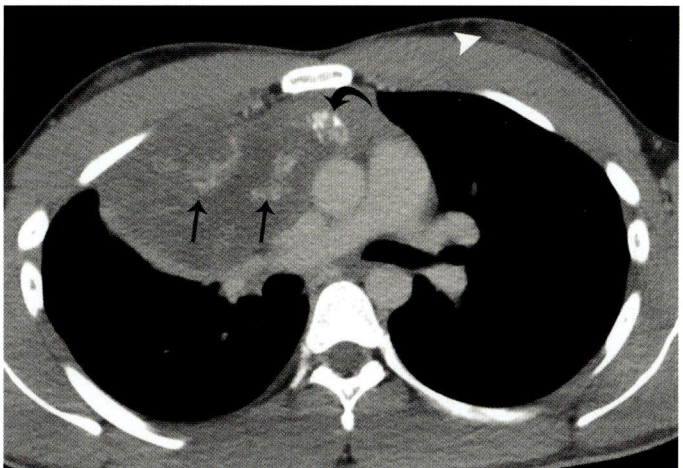

Fig. 6.04 Contrast-enhanced chest CT of a non-seminomatous germ cell tumour. There is a heterogeneous prevascular mass that shows areas of enhancement (straight arrows) and calcifications (curved arrow). Distinction from seminoma is not specific by imaging. Both tumour types may occur as a large enhancing prevascular mass with or without pulmonary metastases. However, seminomas tend to be more homogeneous, whereas non-seminomatous germ cell tumours tend to be more heterogeneous {2528}. The areas of low attenuation represent necrosis or haemorrhage. A clue favouring non-seminomatous germ cell tumour on CT is the incidental finding of gynaecomastia (white arrowhead). Gynaecomastia in these patients correlates with higher β-hCG levels, distant haematogenous metastases, and worse prognosis {1474}.

this worse survival may include, at least in part, larger tumour size at presentation because of delayed clinical manifestation. An overall higher rate of somatic-type malignancies probably also contributes to the worse outcome {1772}.

Table 6.01 Immunohistochemical profiles of primary mediastinal germ cell tumours {1333,3278,2907,764,1094,1324,3262,1702,908,2924,1655,1410,377,1863,1987,2520,3121,1226,1986}

Marker	Frequency of expression (%)				
	Teratoma	Seminoma	Embryonal carcinoma	Yolk sac tumour	Choriocarcinoma
OCT3/4, OCT4	0	91–100	100	0	0
CD30	NR	0–2	33–100	7–11	0
KIT (CD117)	NR	75–100	< 1	21–43	NR
SALL4	28–79	91–100	100	100	0–80
Glypican-3 (GPC3)	NR	0	NR	71–100	NR
PLAP	NR	43–100	0 to expressed	0–40, focal in 100	0
NANOG	0	100	66	0	0
Keratin (AE1/AE3 and CAM5.2)	NR	43–88[a]	100	100	100
CK7	NR	35	NR	NR	NR
High-molecular-weight cytokeratin	NR	39	NR	NR	NR
GATA3	NR	0	NR	36	NR
PAX8	NR	6	NR	NR	NR
AFP	NR	0	0	55–100	0
β-hCG	NR	2	33[b]	0	100
CDX2	Expressed	NR	NR	29	NR
SOX2	57	0	100	0	0

NR, not reported in the mediastinum.

[a]In most cases, keratin highlights only a small proportion of tumour cells, with variable intensities; there is usually a dot-like paranuclear staining pattern in seminoma {3278}. [b]Scattered syncytiotrophoblasts are positive for β-hCG in embryonal carcinomas.

Seminoma of the mediastinum

Roden AC
Chan JKC
Ulbright TM

Definition
Seminoma is a primary malignant germ cell tumour of the mediastinum, composed of seminomatous germ cells.

ICD-O coding
9061/3 Seminoma

ICD-11 coding
2C28.0 & XH9FM4 Malignant germ cell neoplasms of heart or mediastinum, or non-mesothelioma of pleura & Seminoma, NOS

Related terminology
Acceptable: germinoma.

Subtype(s)
None

Localization
Seminoma occurs in the anterior (prevascular) mediastinum or rarely in the middle (visceral) mediastinum {3352}.

Clinical features
Most patients (61–75%) are symptomatic (see Table 6.02).

Radiology
CT usually reveals a bulky, lobular, homogeneous soft tissue opacity with only slight contrast enhancement in the anterior (prevascular) mediastinum {2881,1015}.

Epidemiology
Mediastinal seminomas account for 10–37% of malignant primary mediastinal germ cell tumours and occur almost exclusively in postpubertal males (≥ 10 years of age; reported median:

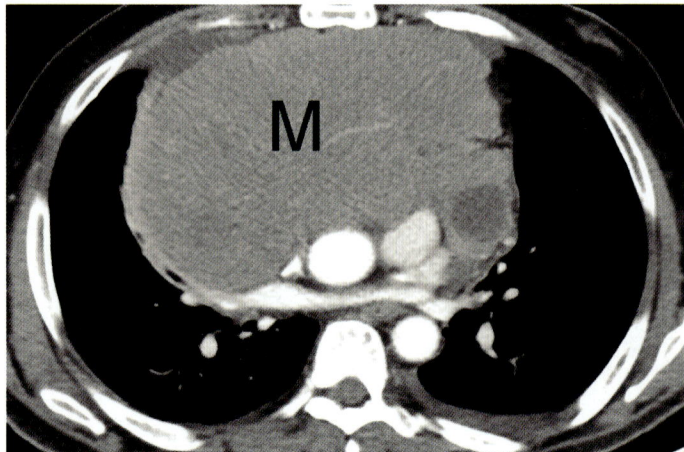

Fig. 6.05 Seminoma of the mediastinum. Contrast-enhanced chest CT. There is a large homogeneous anterior (prevascular) mass (M) displacing the mediastinum posteriorly.

27.6–46.5 years; range: 9–79 years) {760,1432,2368,322,2965, 132,1987,3279,908,1978,2147,258,307,2668,2392,2072}.

Etiology
Seminomas are type II germ cell tumours {2198}, usually arising from the thymic gland {2392,1321}. Metastatic disease should be ruled out, because testicular seminomas may metastasize to mediastinal lymph nodes {3295,254}. Confinement of the tumour to the anterior (prevascular) mediastinal compartment is good evidence of its primary nature {1321}.

Pathogenesis
Common genetic abnormalities and their frequencies in primary mediastinal seminomas are summarized in Table 6.03 {431,2907,2392,3017}. A single case with *KRAS* mutation in codon 13 has been reported {2393}.

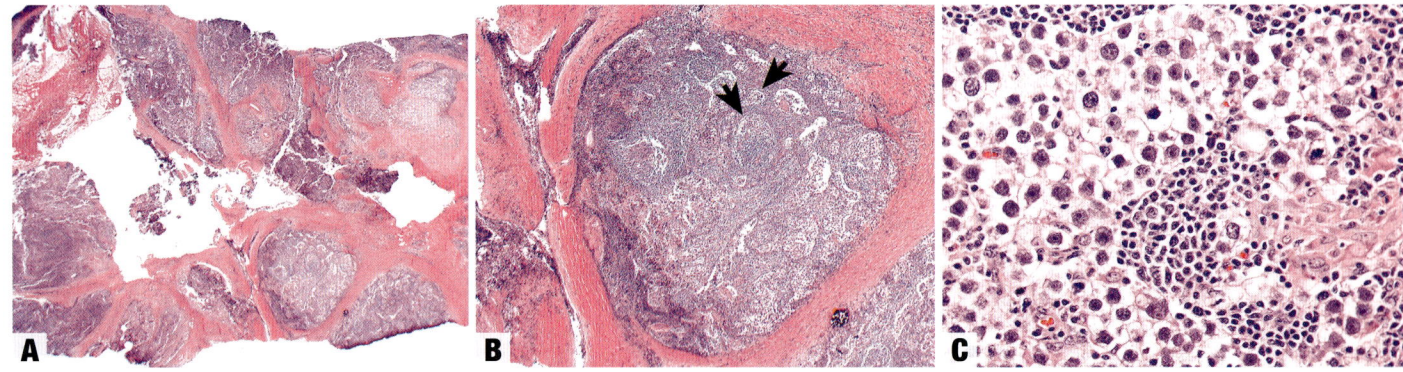

Fig. 6.06 Seminoma of the mediastinum. **A** Seminoma of the mediastinum showing cellular nodules intersected by fibrous stroma. **B** The cellular areas consist of nests of neoplastic cells (arrows) in a lymphoid background with follicles and germinal centres, which may mask the tumour cells. **C** The polygonal tumour cells have clear or focally eosinophilic cytoplasm, distinct cell membranes, and round to polygonal nuclei with prominent nucleoli.

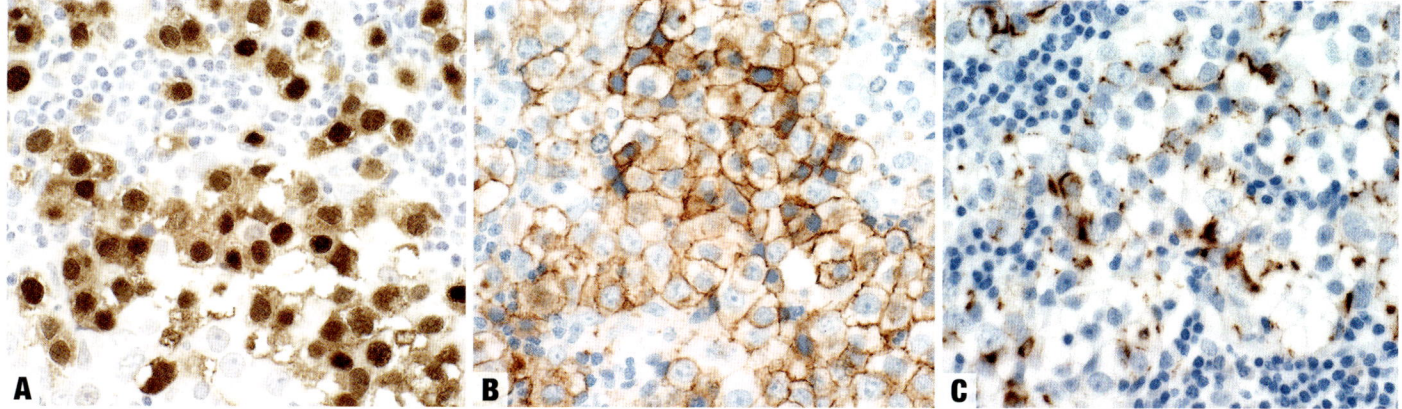

Fig. 6.07 Seminoma of the mediastinum. **A** The tumour cells express nuclear OCT4. **B** The tumour cells express KIT (CD117) in a membranous pattern. **C** The tumour cells express keratin in a dot-like pattern.

Macroscopic appearance

The median tumour size is 50 mm (up to 200 mm) {908,258}. The outer surface is smooth, glistening, or lobulated. The cut surface is white to light tan and coarsely lobular or nodular. Cystic spaces and necrosis may be seen.

Histopathology

Seminomas are composed of round to polygonal, fairly uniform tumour cells with round to oval nuclei showing vesicular chromatin and large nucleoli. The tumour cells commonly have abundant glycogen-rich, clear to lightly eosinophilic cytoplasm and distinct cell membranes, although they may have dense eosinophilic cytoplasm. They grow in confluent sheets, multinodular clusters, cords, or irregular lobules. Morphological characteristics are summarized in Table 6.04 (p. 404) {1974, 2907}. Seminomas are in general not associated with somatic-type malignancies {1082}. Synchronous or combined thymomas and seminomas have been described {1631,3260}.

Seminomas are typically positive for OCT4, SALL4, and KIT (CD117), and they frequently express D2-40, PLAP, and CD99. As many as 70% of seminomas may stain for keratins, but the staining is often focal and weak, usually with a paranuclear distribution. KIT (CD117) expression may be absent in cases with *KIT* mutations {2392}. Immunostains are shown in Table 6.01 (p. 401) in *Germ cell tumours of the mediastinum: Introduction*.

The differential diagnosis includes other germ cell tumours (e.g. embryonal carcinoma, solid pattern yolk sac tumour), thymic carcinomas (e.g. squamous cell carcinoma, clear cell carcinoma), lymphomas, metastases, thymomas, and cystic tumours of the mediastinum. Characteristic morphological and immunohistochemical features permit distinction in almost all cases, although a potential pitfall is spurious immunohistochemical staining for TdT, which may lead to a misdiagnosis of lymphoblastic lymphoma {316,1284}.

Cytology

Seminoma cells are discohesive, with round to polygonal nuclei having one or more prominent nucleoli and pale cytoplasm. Lymphocytes, plasma cells, and the characteristic tigroid

Table 6.02 Symptoms and serology of primary mediastinal seminomas {258,3279, 2044A}

Symptoms/serology	Frequency
Symptoms due to compression of adjacent structures (trachea, mainstem bronchi, phrenic nerve, superior vena cava)	
Dyspnoea	29–46%
Chest pain	39%
Superior vena cava syndrome	10–31%
Cough/haemoptysis	15–22%
Hoarseness	8%
Systemic symptoms	
Weight loss	19%
Fever	6%
Nausea	6%
Gynaecomastia	Case report
Serology	
β-hCG, mildly elevated (median: 8.5 IU/L; ≤ 100 IU/L in adults, ≤ 25 IU/L in children)[a]	~1 in 3 patients

[a] β-hCG > 1000 IU/L is usually indicative of non-seminomatous tumour elements; AFP is usually not elevated.

Table 6.03 Common genetic abnormalities and their frequencies in primary mediastinal seminomas

Genetic abnormality	Frequency
Isochromosome 12p and/or 12p amplification {431,2907}	96%
12p amplification	87%
Isochromosome 12p	65%
KIT mutations {2392}, almost all in exon 17, rarely in exon 9 {3017}	38–50%

stripes are seen in the background. Necrosis and giant cells may be present {1574,2521}.

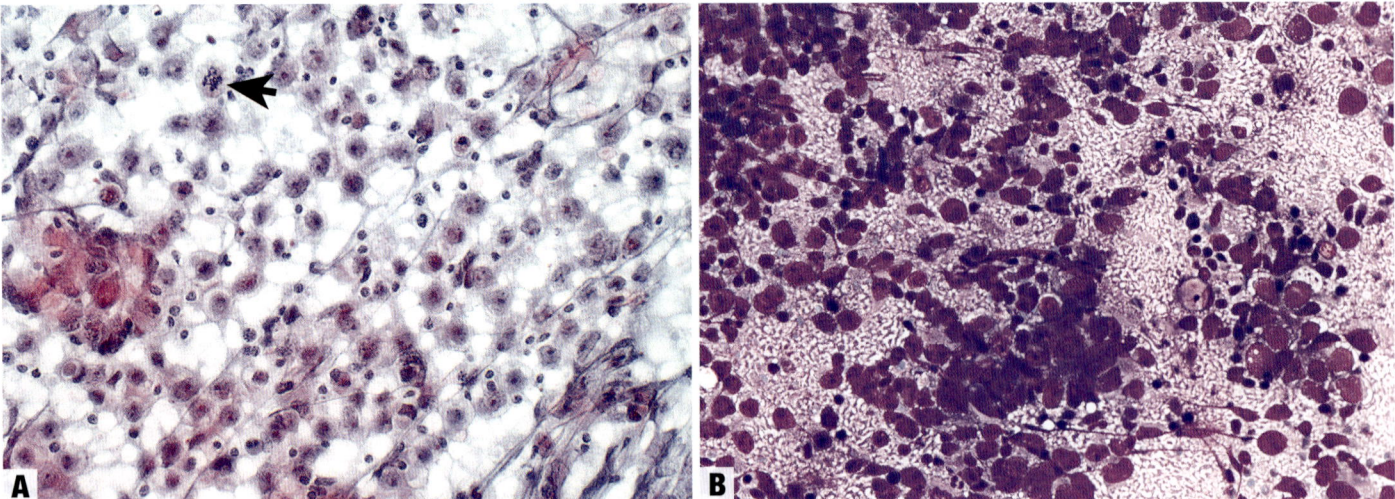

Fig. 6.08 Seminoma of the mediastinum, cytology preparation. **A** Pap stain. Large, polygonal tumour cells with round to ovoid, single nuclei (with vesicular chromatin and prominent nucleoli) and clear, occasionally vacuolated, abundant cytoplasm are predominantly in a single-cell pattern. Mitotic activity is present (arrow). The background shows lymphocytes and plasma cells. **B** Diff-Quik stain. The tigroid background pattern can be seen.

Diagnostic molecular pathology
Not clinically relevant

Essential and desirable diagnostic criteria
Essential:
- Clusters and small sheets of large polygonal epithelioid cells with clear to eosinophilic cytoplasm
- Lymphocytic and/or granulomatous background
- Male sex
- No testicular lesion by imaging

Desirable:
- Postpubertal male patient
- Tumour cells express OCT4 and KIT (CD117)
- FISH studies for 12p abnormalities may be performed but are rarely needed for diagnosis

Staging
No official staging system is currently in place.

Prognosis and prediction
Of the patients with mediastinal seminomas, 94% were classified as having a good prognosis and 6% an intermediate prognosis (defined by absence or presence of non-pulmonary visceral metastases, respectively, and normal AFP with any β-hCG and LDH {258,1257}). Many patients (37.5–41%) have metastases at presentation, most often to cervical lymph nodes, or less commonly to other lymph node sites, lungs, bone, liver, spleen, brain, tonsils, and subcutaneous tissue {258,132,2072}.

Table 6.04 Morphological features of primary mediastinal seminomas

Morphological characteristic {1974,2907,2392,3267,3279,1987}	Frequency
Lymphocytic infiltration	100%
Fibrous septa/stroma	91%
Prominent tumour cell nucleoli	91%
Clear tumour cell cytoplasm	87%
Distinct tumour cell borders	87%
Non-necrotizing granulomas	46–74%
Cellular pleomorphism	43%
Necrosis	35%
Thymic remnant	27%
Florid lymphoid hyperplasia (may mask tumour cells)	13%
Prominent cystic changes	8%
Intercellular oedema	4%
Syncytiotrophoblast	4%
Mitotic activity: mean of 4.4 mitoses/2 mm² (range: 0–16 mitoses/2 mm²)	

The 5-year progression-free and overall survival rates are 75–88% and 88–100%, respectively {258,2072,2965}. The prognosis is better than for non-seminomatous malignant germ cell tumours {1257}.

Embryonal carcinoma of the mediastinum

Roden AC
Marx A
Ulbright TM

Definition

Embryonal carcinoma of the mediastinum is a malignant, non-seminomatous germ cell tumour arising in the mediastinum, characterized by embryonal type cells.

ICD-O coding

9070/3 Embryonal carcinoma

ICD-11 coding

2C28.0 & XH8MB9 Malignant germ cell neoplasms of heart, mediastinum, or non-mesothelioma of pleura & Embryonal carcinoma, NOS

Related terminology

None

Subtype(s)

None

Localization

Embryonal carcinoma of the mediastinum occurs in the anterior (prevascular) mediastinum.

Clinical features

Patient symptoms include chest pain, dyspnoea, cough, and superior vena cava syndrome. Although there are reports of highly elevated serum AFP and LDH levels with mediastinal embryonal carcinomas {2029,1013}, the former almost certainly reflects associated yolk sac tumour elements in the same neoplasm and does not reflect production by embryonal carcinoma elements.

Epidemiology

Embryonal carcinomas account for 2–8% of primary mediastinal germ cell tumours {1986,2965}. They are predominantly tumours of young men, with a median age of 28 years (range: 4–39 years) {2029,1013,3356}.

Etiology

The etiology is the same as in other non-seminomatous germ cell tumours (see *Germ cell tumours of the mediastinum: Introduction*, p. 400).

Pathogenesis

An aberrant midline migration of primordial germ cells has been hypothesized {3316,2199}, but origin from local embryonic stem cells is an alternative theory.

Macroscopic appearance

Tumours are often infiltrating and large, with reported sizes of up to 220 mm {1013,1482}. The cut surface may be haemorrhagic and necrotic {2521}.

Histopathology

Tumour cells are large and polygonal (or sometimes columnar) and have moderate amounts of eosinophilic, amphophilic, basophilic, or clear cytoplasm and mostly indistinct cell borders. Mitoses are numerous and often atypical {1986}. Tumour cell nuclei harbour large single or multiple eosinophilic nucleoli. Solid, tubular/glandular, and/or papillary growth patterns can occur {1986}. Tumour necrosis is common. Scattered single or small groups of syncytiotrophoblasts can be seen in about one third of cases {1986}. Somatic-type malignancies including sarcoma, adenocarcinoma, and acute myeloid leukaemia have been reported {2029}. The differential diagnosis is summarized in Table 6.05 (p. 406).

OCT4, SALL4, CD30, SOX2, and CAM5.2 are very sensitive immunohistochemical markers for embryonal carcinoma (see Table 6.01, p. 401, in *Germ cell tumours of the mediastinum: Introduction*). However, they are not specific and can also be expressed by other germ cell tumours or other tumours that enter the differential diagnosis, such as seminoma (OCT4, SALL4, keratin), thymic carcinoma (keratin), and lymphoma (CD30). Therefore, a panel of immunostains is recommended for the diagnosis

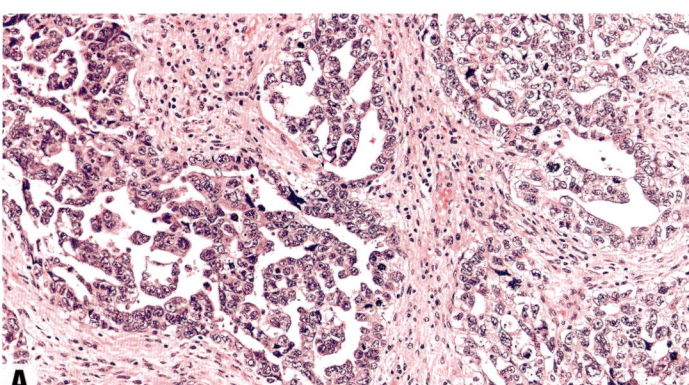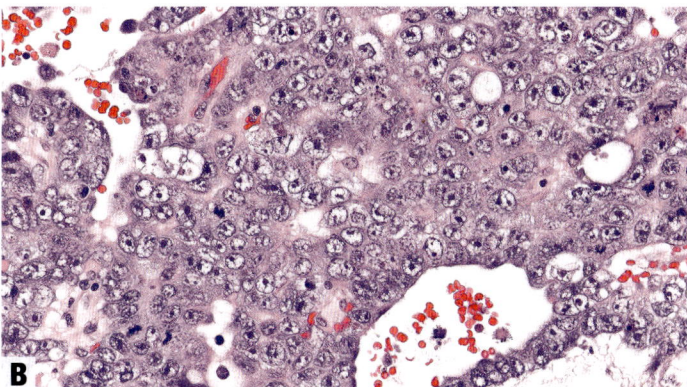

Fig. 6.09 Embryonal carcinoma of the mediastinum. **A** Tumour cells, arranged in solid nests and glandular structures, are in a desmoplastic stroma. **B** The tumour cells are large and polygonal, with amphophilic cytoplasm, indistinct cell borders, and large round nuclei with prominent nucleoli. Mitotic activity is easily identifiable.

Table 6.05 Differential diagnosis of primary embryonal carcinomas of the mediastinum {2521}

Differential diagnosis	Distinguishing features of the differential diagnosis[a]
Seminoma (germinoma)	Lymphocytic infiltration, fibrous septa/stroma, clear tumour cell cytoplasm, distinct tumour cell borders, non-necrotizing granulomas
	Lack of tubular/glandular or papillary growth and less pleomorphic nuclei than in embryonal carcinoma
Yolk sac tumour	Usually multiple morphological patterns (microcystic, macrocystic, glandular-alveolar, papillary, endodermal sinus–like, myxomatous, hepatoid, enteric, polyvesicular-vitelline, solid, and/or spindle cell)
Thymic carcinoma	Squamous differentiation and distinct cell borders for squamous subtype
	Glandular architecture and mucin-containing cells for adenocarcinoma or mucoepidermoid carcinoma subtypes
NUT carcinoma	Sometimes abrupt squamous differentiation
	Tumour cells usually monotonous
	Tumour cells express NUT
	t(15;19) in majority of tumours
SMARCA4-deficient undifferentiated tumour	Focal rhabdoid morphology in at least a subset of cases
	Loss of immunoreactivity for SMARCA4 (BRG1)
Large B-cell lymphoma, primary mediastinal large B-cell lymphoma	Tumour cells usually more discohesive
	Distinct immunophenotype

[a]For distinguishing immunophenotypic features, see Table 6.01 (p. 401) in *Germ cell tumours of the mediastinum: Introduction.*

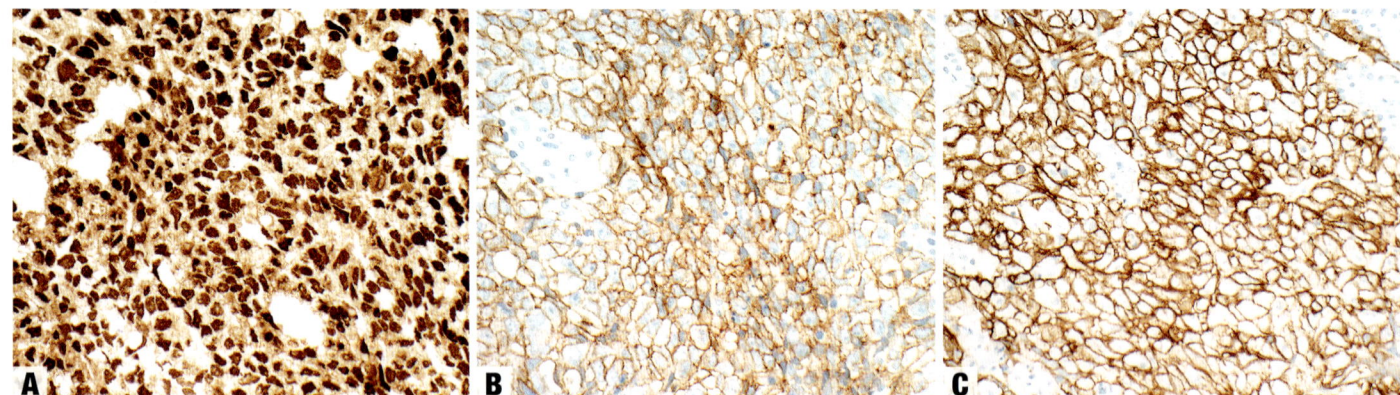

Fig. 6.10 Embryonal carcinoma of the mediastinum. **A** These tumour cells express OCT4. **B** The tumour cells express CD30. **C** The tumour cells express wide-spectrum-molecular-weight keratins (OSCAR).

of embryonal carcinoma. Scattered syncytiotrophoblasts express β-hCG and should not lead to confusion with choriocarcinoma.

Cytology
Syncytial cohesive clusters of pleomorphic epithelial cells show frequent mitotic figures; necrosis and haemorrhage are seen in many cases {2521}.

Diagnostic molecular pathology
Diagnostic molecular pathology is not reported in primary mediastinal embryonal carcinomas.

Essential and desirable diagnostic criteria
Essential:
- Large polygonal tumour cells with eosinophilic or amphophilic cytoplasm, indistinct cell borders, and single or multiple prominent nucleoli
- Solid, papillary, tubular/glandular growth pattern

Desirable:
- Young male patient
- Panel of immunohistochemical stains including SALL4 (expressed), OCT4 (expressed), CD30 (expressed), SOX2 (expressed), keratin (expressed), KIT (CD117; negative), and CD45 (negative)

Staging
No official staging system is currently in place.

Prognosis and prediction
Both haematogenous and lymphatic-based metastases may be seen. In a series of 11 mediastinal embryonal carcinomas, 4 cases (including 2 pure embryonal carcinomas, 1 with seminoma, and 1 with choriocarcinoma) had pulmonary metastases {2965}. Among 5 patients with primary mediastinal embryonal carcinoma, 3 patients died (2 of disease) within 11–22 months.

Yolk sac tumour of the mediastinum

Marx A
Marom EM
Moreira AL
Roden AC
Ulbright TM

Definition

Yolk sac tumour (YST) of the mediastinum is a malignant non-seminomatous germ cell tumour arising in the mediastinum, characterized by numerous patterns that recapitulate the yolk sac, allantois, and extraembryonic mesenchyme.

ICD-O coding

9071/3 Yolk sac tumour

ICD-11 coding

2C28.0 & XH09W7 Malignant germ cell neoplasms of heart, mediastinum, or non-mesothelioma of pleura & Yolk sac tumour

Related terminology

Not recommended: endodermal sinus tumour.

Subtype(s)

None

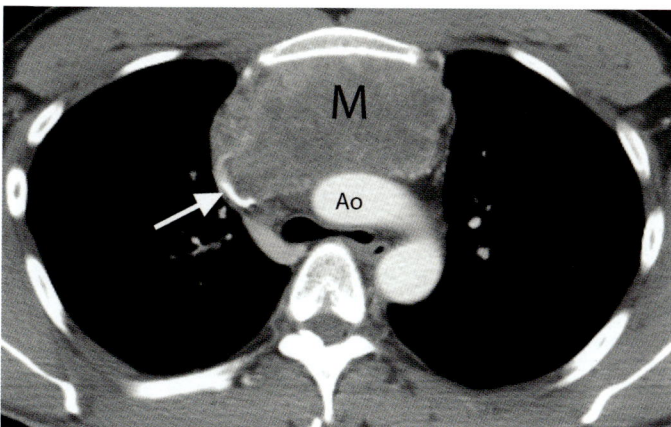

Fig. 6.11 Yolk sac tumour of the mediastinum. Contrast-enhanced chest CT of a 40-year-old man, at the level of the main bronchi, shows a lobulated, poorly marginated, heterogeneous anterior (prevascular) mediastinal mass (M) invading the superior vena cava (arrow). The mass displaces the aorta (Ao) and airways posteriorly. Involvement of the superior vena cava by the tumour was confirmed at surgery.

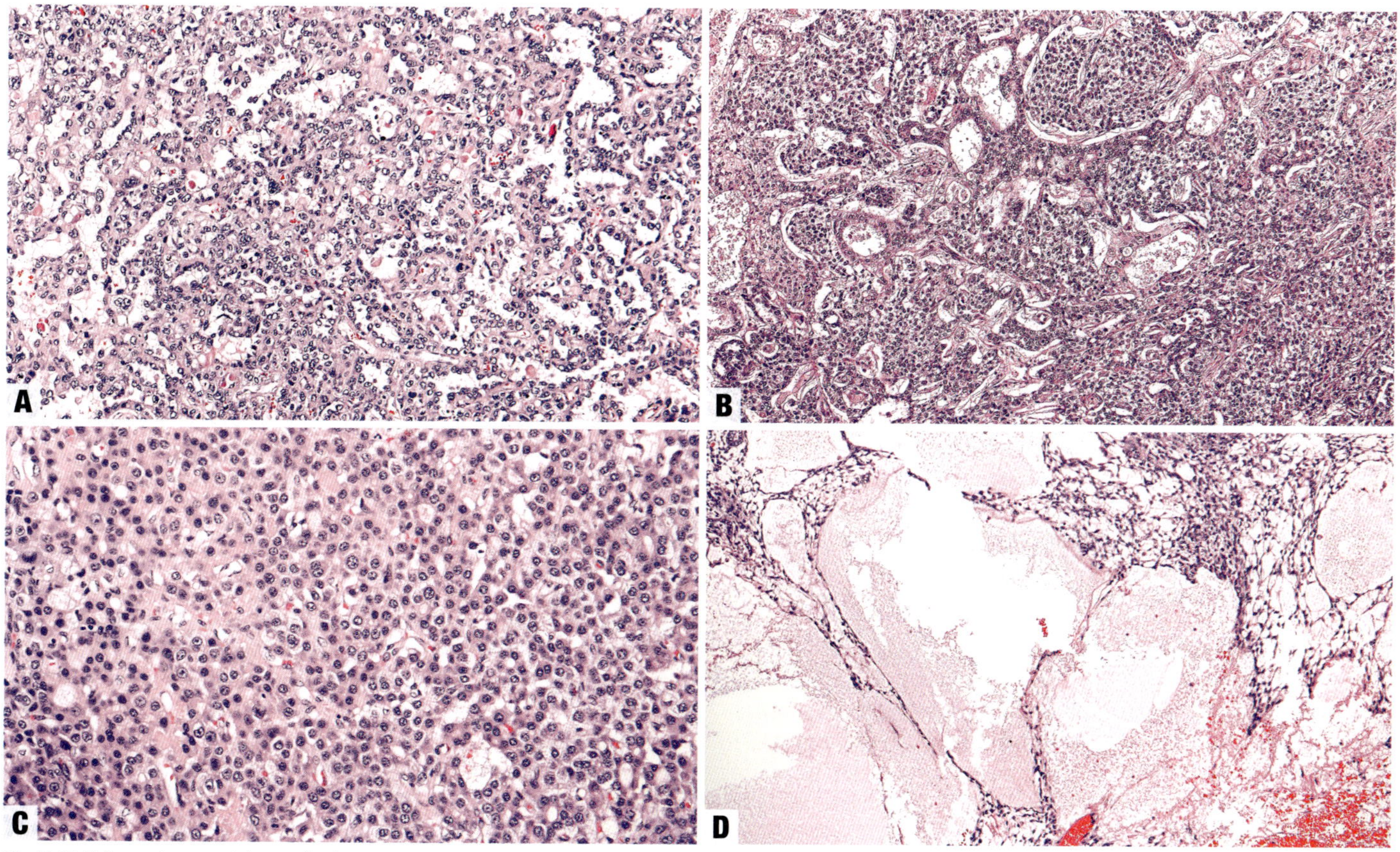

Fig. 6.12 Yolk sac tumour of the mediastinum, spectrum of growth patterns. **A** Alveolar pattern. **B** Admixture of glandular and solid patterns. **C** Hepatoid pattern. **D** Macrocystic and microcystic patterns.

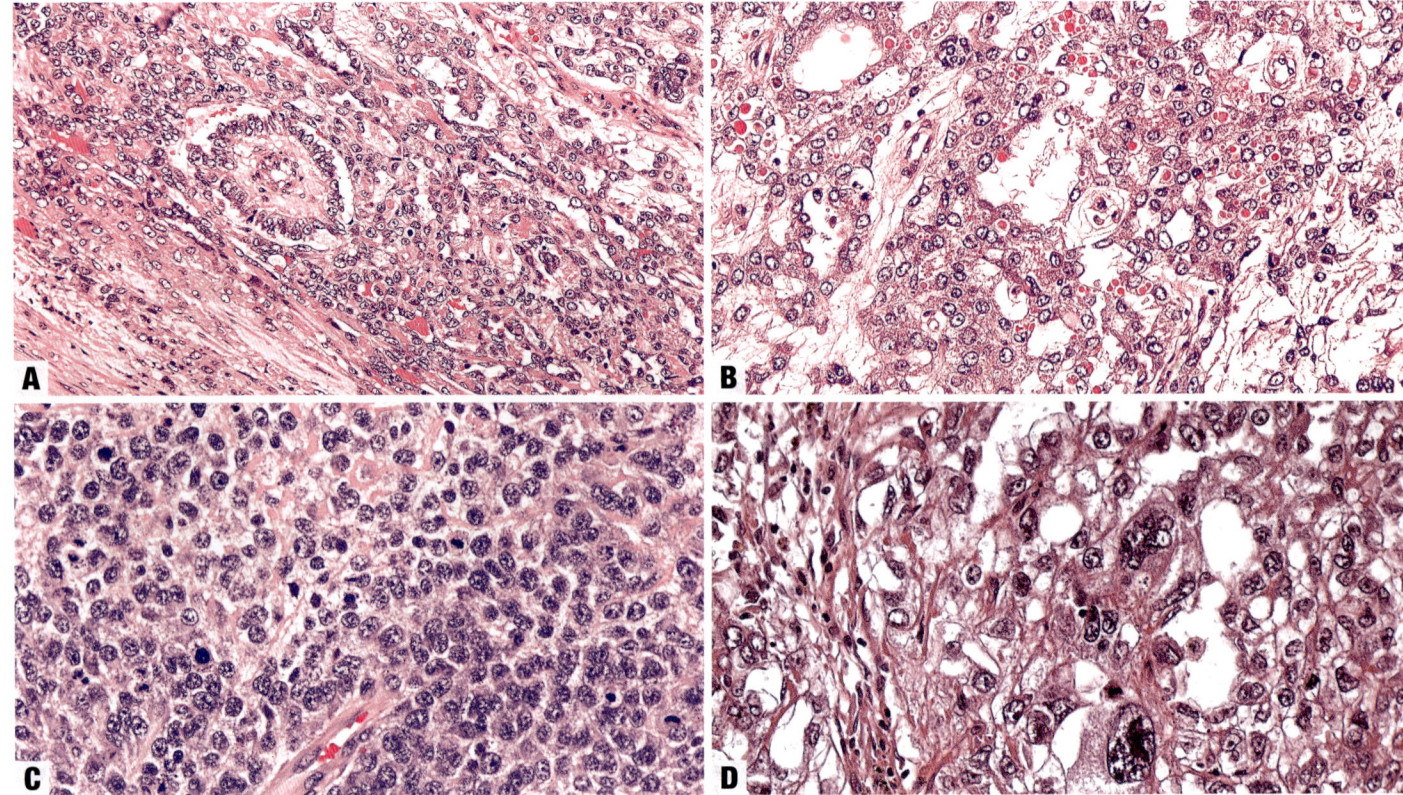

Fig. 6.13 Yolk sac tumour of the mediastinum, special histological features. **A** Schiller–Duval body. **B** Alveolar growth pattern with hyaline globules. **C** Solid growth pattern with intercellular basement membrane material. **D** Cellular anaplasia.

Localization

YST of the mediastinum occurs in the anterior (prevascular) mediastinum or rarely in the posterior (paravertebral) mediastinum {967}.

Clinical features

Patients may present with chest pain, dyspnoea, chills, fever, and superior vena cava syndrome {2964,2965,1986}. Serum level of AFP is almost always elevated.

There are no specific imaging features. FDG PET may detect tiny occult primary tumours or recurrences {1711,2952}.

Epidemiology

After puberty, YST is restricted to men, with rare exceptions {3379,1400}. Its incidence peaks in the third decade of life and declines thereafter {2575}. Between 15 and 59 years, its incidence is 0.3 cases per 1 million per year {2575}. Pure YST accounts for 2–12% of mediastinal germ cell tumours in adults, being the fourth commonest germ cell tumour, after seminomas, mixed germ cell tumours, and teratomas {1978,2630,1426, 2965}.

In young children, the epidemiology is different. YST has an incidence of 0.25 cases per 100 000 children (aged < 15 years) per year, being the most common malignant germ cell tumour before puberty, with a peak incidence at 1 year {2668}. Up to the age of 5 years, YST is virtually the only malignant germ cell tumour of the mediastinum {2671}. There is a strong female preponderance (70–80%) {2668}. After the age of 6 years, pure YST is rare {2668}.

Etiology

Klinefelter syndrome is a risk factor after puberty, for unknown reasons {3179}.

Pathogenesis

An aberrant midline migration of primordial germ cells has been hypothesized {3316,2199}, but origin from local embryonic stem cells is an alternative theory. Mediastinal YSTs in children aged < 8 years exhibit genetic losses at 1p, 4q, and 6q and gains at 1q, 3, 20q, and 20, but neither isochromosome 12p nor sex-chromosomal alterations {1192,2671,2670}. In contrast, YSTs occurring after the age of 8 years show isochromosome 12p (in 60%), gain of chromosomes 21 and X (in 50% each), and loss of chromosome 13 (in 30%) {2671}. Age-related genetic alterations are accompanied by distinct imprinting patterns {2672,2198, 2771} and gene expression profiles {2245}.

Macroscopic appearance

Pure YSTs are solid and soft, and the cut surface is typically pale grey or grey-white, with a gelatinous or mucoid quality. After neoadjuvant treatment, haemorrhage and necrosis are common. Cyst formation may be treatment-related or may indicate a mixed germ cell tumour (YST and teratoma).

Histopathology

YST usually shows different histological patterns: microcystic (reticular), macrocystic, glandular-alveolar, endodermal sinus (pseudopapillary), myxomatous, hepatoid, enteric, polyvesicular-vitelline, solid, and spindle {3011,1986,1863,1377}. The

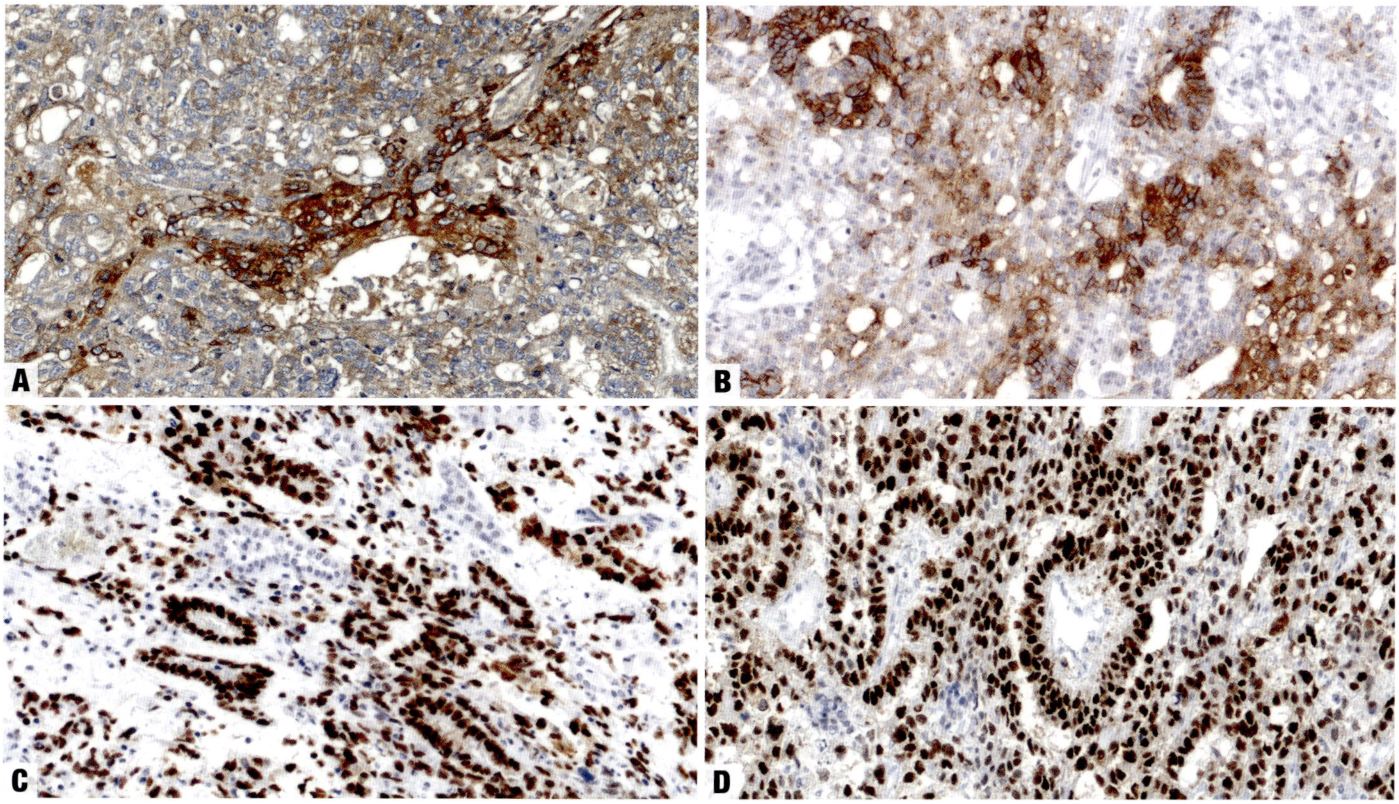

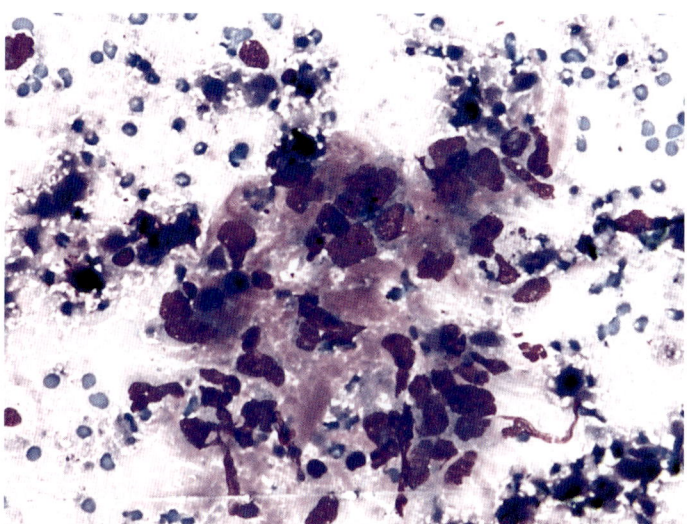

Fig. 6.14 Yolk sac tumour of the mediastinum. **A** Expression of AFP. **B** Expression of glypican-3 (GPC3). **C** Expression of SALL4. **D** Expression of GATA3.

microcystic/reticular pattern is characterized by a loose network of cystic spaces and channels lined by flat or cuboidal cells with scant cytoplasm. In myxomatous areas, epithelial cells are in a mucinous stroma. The endodermal sinus pattern shows pseudopapillary structures and Schiller–Duval bodies. The polyvesicular-vitelline pattern is defined by cysts that are lined by cuboidal to flat tumour cells surrounded by a dense fibrous stroma. The solid pattern resembles embryonal carcinoma or seminoma, but cells are smaller and less

pleomorphic than those of embryonal carcinoma and more pleomorphic than seminoma cells, and they typically retain the usual immunohistochemical profile of YST, although commonly with negative or weak and focal staining for AFP {1377}. YST with a hepatoid pattern {3120,1972} has cells with abundant eosinophilic cytoplasm resembling fetal or adult liver {2383}. The enteric and endometrioid patterns show glandular features resembling the fetal human gut and secretory endometrial glands, respectively {542,553}. Syncytiotrophoblasts can occur in rare YSTs and do not change the diagnosis to mixed germ cell tumour {1863}.

Sarcoma development in YST represents somatic-type malignancy; it is rare in pure mediastinal YST {1772} but more common in mixed germ cell tumour {3119,2470}. Associated, clonally related haematological malignancies (mainly acute leukaemias and myelodysplastic syndromes) {2096,1580,725,1082} occur only in adults and are commonest in mixed germ cell tumour with a YST component (58%) or pure YST (25%) {1863,1082}.

Immunohistochemistry

YSTs are consistently immunoreactive for keratins (AE1/AE3), glypican-3 (GPC3) {3529}, SALL4 {1702,3201,376}, and LIN28 {3289,378}, whereas they are consistently negative for OCT4, NANOG {1729,141}, SOX2 {1702,2624,1728,2130}, and D2-40 {1226,1604,141}. Single syncytiotrophoblastic cells in rare YSTs are positive for β-hCG {1986}.

YSTs may variably express AFP and PLAP in as many as 70% of cases, KIT (CD117) in as many as 43% {1226}, and CD30 in as many as 11% {1377,378,1702,377,3201,2924}, whereas < 25% of cases are EMA-positive in a minority of tumour cells {3201,1226}.

Fig. 6.15 Yolk sac tumour of the mediastinum, cytology. A high-grade neoplasm with large irregular nuclei. Note the presence of metachromatic material around tumour cells (hyaline balls) and necrotic background.

Table 6.06 Differential diagnosis of yolk sac tumours of the mediastinum: distinguishing histological, immunohistochemical, and molecular criteria

Differential diagnosis	Morphological features	Immunohistochemistry[a]
Seminoma (germinoma)	Homogeneous morphology with relatively uniform polygonal tumour cells, usually with clear to eosinophilic cytoplasm and distinct cell membranes Lacks variety of morphological patterns	Positive: OCT4, NANOG, keratin (dot-like) Negative: glypican-3 (GPC3), AFP
Embryonal carcinoma	Tumour cells in general larger and more atypical	Positive: CD30, OCT4, NANOG (+/−) Negative: AFP
Choriocarcinoma	Biphasic pattern, haemorrhagic background	Positive: β-hCG
Immature teratoma	Usually has a component of embryonic-appearing neuroepithelium	
Thymic carcinoma	Can mimic solid growth pattern of yolk sac tumour Lacks variety of morphological patterns	Positive: PAX8 (polyclonal; +/−), CD5 (+/−) Negative: OCT4, AFP, glypican-3 (GPC3), SALL4 Pitfall: KIT (CD117) is expressed in many thymic carcinomas
Metastatic carcinoma	Morphological features and immunophenotype suggestive of the origin History required Metastasis from a gonadal or retroperitoneal pure yolk sac tumour or mixed germ cell tumour requires clinicoradiological correlation	Immunophenotype depends on the site of origin Usually lacks 12p amplification Negative for isochromosome 12p
Lymphoma	Discohesive tumour cells Tumour cells in general are more homogeneous	Characteristic immunophenotype; keratin negative Pitfall: CD30 expression in some mediastinal lymphomas common
All differential diagnoses	Lack of Schiller–Duval bodies	

[a]See also Table 6.01 (p. 401) in *Germ cell tumours of the mediastinum: Introduction*.

Differential diagnosis

The typical morphological and molecular features of potential mimics of mediastinal YSTs are given in Table 6.06.

Seminomas can resemble solid areas of YST. A pitfall is their common (80%) dot-like keratin expression {1987}. Unlike YST, seminoma is typically positive for OCT4 and D2-40 and negative for GPC3.

Embryonal carcinoma shows larger and more atypical tumour cells, is less varied, and lacks microcystic areas and Schiller–Duval bodies. Unlike YSTs, embryonal carcinomas are positive for OCT4 and SOX2.

Choriocarcinoma is a biphasic tumour with haemorrhagic background. Pitfalls are the consistent shared immunoreactivity for SALL4 {377} and LIN28 {958} and rare occurrence of β-hCG–positive syncytiotrophoblasts in YST {1986}.

Immature teratoma may mimic the varied growth patterns of YST and may focally express GPC3, AFP, SALL4, LIN28, Hep-Par-1, and CDX2 in endodermal components {2124,375,1863}. However, immature teratoma typically harbours CD56-positive and/or OCT4-positive neuroectodermal cells {8} or EMA-positive components.

Thymic carcinoma and YST may share a solid growth pattern and expression of KIT (CD117), and both may lack AFP expression {1377,2247,1119,1226}. However, thymic carcinoma is often positive for CD5 {1163} and negative for GPC3 {1702}, SALL4 {1276}, and LIN28 {378}.

Metastases of hepatocellular and hepatoid carcinomas and gonadal germ cell tumour to the mediastinum must be excluded {890}, because they may share expression of GPC3, AFP, CDX2, and HepPar-1 {1424,141}. Hepatocellular carcinoma is SALL4-negative {3124}, and most metastatic carcinomas are negative for SALL4 and LIN28 {141,2124}, with rare exceptions {1914,378,377}.

Cytology

Smears of YST show aggregates of medium-sized to large cells with variable nuclei, prominent nucleoli, and moderate to occasionally abundant cytoplasm, with a variable background of debris, mucoid material, or metachromatic material. Lymphoid cells and granulomas are typically absent. The presence of hyaline globules is typical of YST, but distinction between non-seminomatous germ cell tumours is often not reliable {3379,3185}.

Diagnostic molecular pathology

Diagnostic molecular pathology is usually not relevant. Rarely, identification of chromosome 12p alterations may help to exclude SALL4-positive OCT4-negative carcinomas {1914} or identify somatic-type malignancy.

Essential and desirable diagnostic criteria

Essential:
- A malignant germ cell tumour characterized by numerous patterns that recapitulates the yolk sac, allantois, and extra-embryonic mesenchyme
- Growth pattern: usually multiple within a single tumour, including microcystic, macrocystic, glandular-alveolar, endodermal sinus, myxomatous, hepatoid, enteric, polyvesicular-vitelline, solid, and spindle cell

Desirable:
- Schiller–Duval bodies are a hallmark of the disease but might be absent
- Serology: AFP markedly increased
- Coexpression of keratins, SALL4, glypican-3 (GPC3), and variably AFP
- Negative staining for GATA3 and OCT4

Staging

There is no validated staging system for mediastinal germ cell tumours. Mediastinal YSTs almost always extend into adjacent structures, including the lung, while pleural dissemination is rare {3379,1986}. Before puberty, pure and mixed mediastinal YSTs have a 30% risk for distant metastasis {2671}, mainly to lung, lymph nodes, liver, bone, and brain {976,977,2669,2150}. After puberty, 50% of mediastinal YSTs metastasize to lung or intrathoracic lymph nodes, while extrathoracic metastasis occurs in < 10% of cases {1978,1986}.

Prognosis and prediction

The 5-year event-free and overall survival rates of all children aged < 15 years with malignant non-seminomatous mediastinal germ cell tumours are 83% and 87%, respectively, with no difference between YST and mixed germ cell tumours {2669}. The most important favourable prognostic factor is complete resection of the primary lesion; following incomplete resection, the 5-year survival rate drops to 42% {2669}. Primary brain metastasis is a poor prognostic sign {976,977}.

After the age of 15 years, the 5-year overall survival rate in mediastinal non-seminomatous tumours is 45–54% {1083, 2509,2630,806}. Lack of metastasis {2630,2509,1978,1986}, completeness of resection and postoperative normalization of tumour markers {2630,1369}, low preoperative β-hCG levels {2509}, pure YST histology {2509}, and complete tumour necrosis after chemotherapy {1426} are favourable prognostic factors. Somatic-type malignancy and clonally related haematological malignancies are refractory to therapy and portend a poor prognosis {2096,1580,725,1082}.

Choriocarcinoma of the mediastinum

Ströbel P
Moreira AL

Definition

Choriocarcinoma of the mediastinum is a highly malignant trophoblastic neoplasm arising in the mediastinum, composed of syncytiotrophoblast, cytotrophoblast, and variably intermediate trophoblast.

ICD-O coding

9100/3 Choriocarcinoma

ICD-11 coding

2C28.0 & XH8PK7 Malignant germ cell neoplasms of heart, mediastinum or non-mesothelioma of pleura & Choriocarcinoma, NOS

Related terminology

None

Subtype(s)

None

Localization

Choriocarcinoma of the mediastinum occurs in the anterior (prevascular; majority) and posterior (paravertebral) mediastinum {1979,3506}.

Clinical features

Choriocarcinomas grow rapidly {3460}, and early lung invasion is typical. Reported symptoms at presentation include shortness of breath, chest pain, cough, superior vena cava syndrome, syncopal episodes, persistent headache, and cardiac tamponade {1979,1394,1642,615}. Some patients present with gynaecomastia (see Fig. 6.04, p. 401) {372} due to hCG production {1978,742,2765,372,922}. Some patients develop thyrotoxicosis due to TSH-like effects of hCG {2003,1642,2658}.

Epidemiology

Almost all reported cases of choriocarcinoma have occurred in adult male patients (age range: 17–63 years) {742,2765, 372,2965,1979,1394,922}. Only 3% of mediastinal germ cell tumours are pure choriocarcinomas {1425,1482,1978,1986}; however, estimates are probably biased by the referral patterns of the reporting institutions. The crude estimated incidence of choriocarcinomas is 1 case per 12 million individuals per year {2965}.

Etiology

For unknown reasons, choriocarcinoma, either pure or as part of a mixed germ cell tumour, tends to be particularly frequent in patients with Klinefelter syndrome {3108,2867,598,2802,1642, 2658}.

Pathogenesis

An aberrant midline migration of primordial germ cells has been hypothesized {3316,2199}. Mediastinal choriocarcinomas have been described to harbour an isochromosome 12p characteristic of postpubertal malignant germ cell tumours at all sites {431}.

Macroscopic appearance

Most tumours are large (average size: 100 mm), soft, friable, extensively haemorrhagic, and with foci of necrosis {1979,1394}.

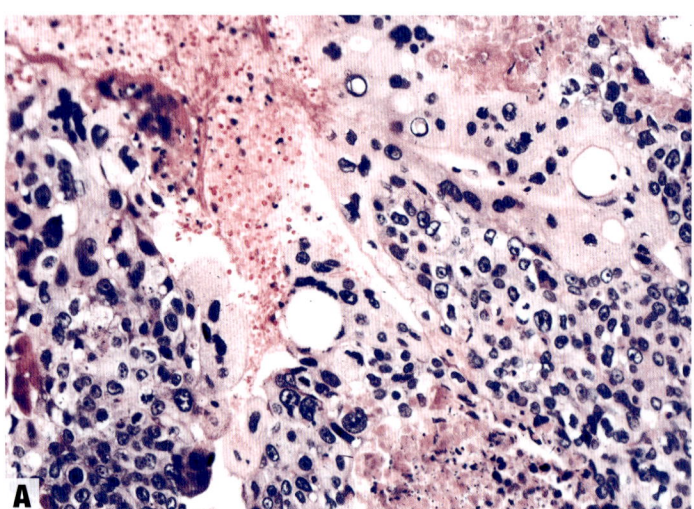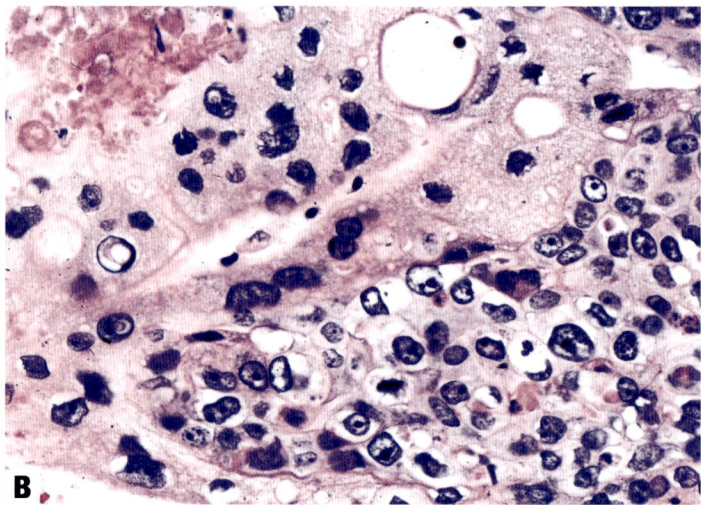

Fig. 6.16 Choriocarcinoma of the mediastinum. **A** Choriocarcinoma is characterized by the presence of two cell types: syncytiotrophoblasts and cytotrophoblasts. Syncytiotrophoblasts are large pleomorphic cells with irregular hyperchromatic nuclei; the cells are often multinucleated. Cytoplasm is abundant and eosinophilic. Mononucleated cytotrophoblasts are medium-sized cells with vacuolated, basophilic cytoplasm and eccentric nuclei. The tumour also shows necrosis and haemorrhage. **B** Higher power highlights the cytological features of both the syncytiotrophoblasts and cytotrophoblasts.

Histopathology

Mediastinal choriocarcinoma can occur in a pure form or as part of a mixed germ cell tumour. Most choriocarcinomas occur as a component of mixed germ cell tumours. The histology is the same as that of its gonadal counterpart. Syncytiotrophoblasts and cytotrophoblasts are typically intermingled in a bilaminar plexiform pattern or in disordered sheets. Occasionally, scattered clusters of syncytiotrophoblasts cap cytotrophoblast nodules. Syncytiotrophoblasts are large multinucleated cells with numerous, pleomorphic, dark-staining nuclei; variably distinct nucleoli; and abundant densely eosinophilic or amphophilic cytoplasm (which may contain cytoplasmic lacunae). Cytotrophoblasts are uniform, polygonal cells with round nuclei, prominent nucleoli, and clear or eosinophilic cytoplasm. Atypical mitosis and cellular atypia are common. There can be sheets of nondescript mononuclear cells that resemble intermediate trophoblast. Choriocarcinomas are typically intimately associated with dilated vascular sinusoids. Partial or complete replacement of the walls of blood vessels is common. There are often vast areas of haemorrhage and necrosis {1979,1394,922}.

Choriocarcinomas are positive for keratins, SALL4, and GATA3, and they are negative for OCT3/4, PLAP, AFP, CEA, CD30, and vimentin. The syncytiotrophoblastic cells express hCG {1394,922,2924}, glypican-3 (GPC3) {3530}, and α-inhibin {2299A}.

Differential diagnosis

Sarcomatous carcinomas with giant cell features may mimic choriocarcinoma. However, in contrast to choriocarcinomas that consist of two cell populations of cytotrophoblasts and syncytiotrophoblasts, giant cell carcinomas show a continuum between smaller or medium-sized tumour cells and the larger giant cells.

Cytology

The cytology is characterized by abundant necrosis and haemorrhage. Clusters or isolated pleomorphic cells with large and often multiple nuclei and abundant eosinophilic cytoplasm are seen (syncytiotrophoblasts). Mononucleated cytotrophoblasts are rarely recognized and are composed of medium-sized cells with vacuolated, basophilic cytoplasm and eccentric nuclei {1836,857}.

Diagnostic molecular pathology

Not clinically relevant

Essential and desirable diagnostic criteria

Essential:
- Atypical and proliferating syncytiotrophoblasts and cytotrophoblasts with dilated vascular sinusoids, often with areas of haemorrhage and necrosis

Desirable:
- The immunohistochemical profile should show positivity for keratins, SALL4, and GATA3, as well as hCG in syncytiotrophoblasts

Staging

There is currently no established staging system for mediastinal germ cell tumours. Most patients with choriocarcinoma present with infiltration of neighbouring organs (e.g. the great vessels, lung, and chest wall) and/or with intrathoracic and extrathoracic metastases {922,1979} into the lungs, liver, kidney, and spleen {1979}, but also the brain, choroids, heart, adrenals, and bone {1482,1530,1979,2765}.

Prognosis and prediction

In most reported cases, patients died of disseminated disease shortly after diagnosis (average survival time: 1–2 months) {1979,2765,1986,372,922}. However, treatment with cisplatin-based chemotherapy may improve the outcome {2965,258,742, 1642,615}.

Teratoma of the mediastinum

Moreira AL
Roden AC
Ströbel P
Ulbright TM

Definition
Teratoma of the mediastinum is a neoplasm of pluripotent cell origin that forms differentiated somatic-type tissues, which may be exclusively mature (adult-type), exclusively immature (embryonal and/or fetal), or a combination of both.

ICD-O coding
9080/0 Mature teratoma
9080/1 Immature teratoma of the thymus

ICD-11 coding
2C28.0 & XH3GV5 Malignant germ cell neoplasms of heart, mediastinum or non-mesothelioma of pleura & Teratoma, benign
2C28.0 & XH7YZ9 Malignant germ cell neoplasms of heart, mediastinum or non-mesothelioma of pleura & Teratoma, malignant, NOS

Related terminology
None

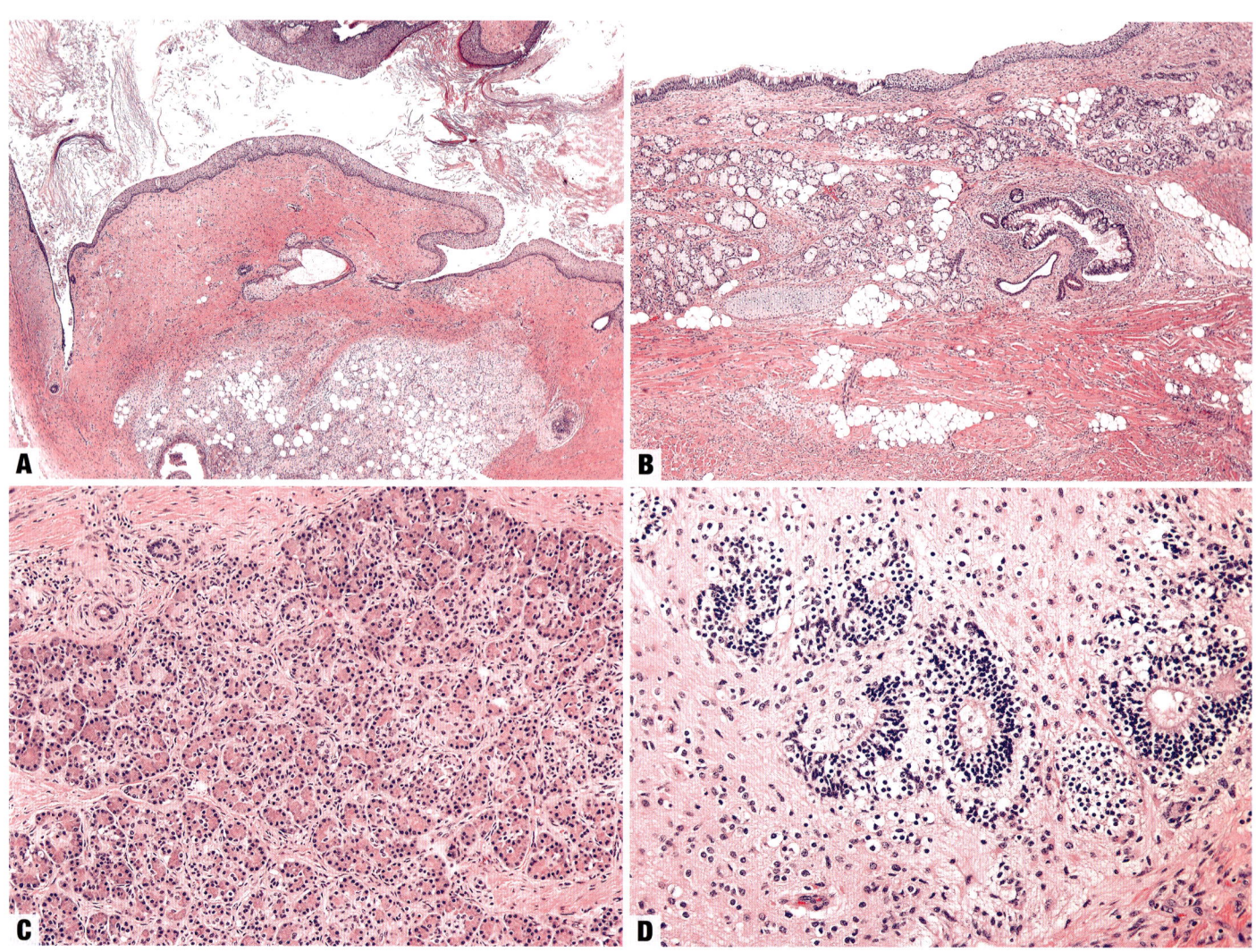

Fig. 6.17 Teratoma from the anterior (prevascular) mediastinum of a 27-year-old man, with mature tissues. **A** Cysts are lined by stratified squamous epithelium with associated pilosebaceous units, surrounded by adipose tissue with apocrine glands. **B** Other areas show transition from squamous to respiratory epithelium (top), with numerous seromucinous glands and a small focus of cartilage in the underlying stroma. **C** Pancreatic acinar tissue and occasional ducts are seen. **D** An immature area with a small focus of neuroepithelial rosettes embedded in neuropil, with numerous astrocytic cells.

Subtype(s)

None

Localization

Teratoma of the mediastinum occurs in the anterior (prevascular) mediastinum, often arising in the thymus, and rarely in the posterior (paravertebral) mediastinum {2330,1978,196,1222}.

Clinical features

Postpubertal mature teratomas are often asymptomatic; they are found incidentally on imaging studies or thoracotomy in 36–59% of patients {1659,2965,196}. Symptoms, when present, are due to compression or obstruction of adjacent structures and include chest pain, shortness of breath, wheezing, and cough. Superior vena cava syndrome, haemoptysis, dysphagia, nausea, and hoarseness are less common {1659,2669,258,1019}. Systemic symptoms are rare {2965}. Teratomas rarely erode into pericardium, pleura, adjacent vascular structures, or bronchus (leading to trichoptysis [coughing of hair]), or through the skin to form fistula {1019,2433,65,1705}. An endocrine pancreatic component can cause hyperinsulinism and hypoglycaemia {783,30,37}. Serum tumour markers (AFP and β-hCG) are not elevated {2669}. In children, teratomas are more symptomatic than in postpubertal patients {2965}. Hydrops fetalis is a complication of congenital mediastinal teratoma, often associated with immature teratomas {2079,1057,2580,1894}. Rare cases of mature or immature teratoma may be associated with paraneoplastic limbic encephalitis caused by auto-antibodies against NMDAR {2809,1405,1403}.

Radiology

Mature teratomas are well-demarcated tumours. Multilocular cysts are present in 90% of cases {1659,2965,2283,2881, 1951}. Attenuation is heterogeneous, with varying combinations of soft tissue, fluid, fat, and calcification {1951,2965,2283, 2881}. Eggshell calcifications occur in 26–53% {1659,1951}. Bone and teeth occur in as many as 8% of cases and are pathognomonic findings {1659,1951}. On MRI, fat-saturation techniques may reveal small foci of macroscopic fat. Rupture into the pericardium or pleura leads to pleuropericardial effusions {2433,2197,1705}. Immature teratomas are more often solid masses {2881}.

Epidemiology

Teratomas account for < 10% of all mediastinal masses. They occur in both prepubertal and postpubertal patients, with no sex predominance {1659,1978,2669}. Pure teratomas account for 58% of all mediastinal germ cell tumours in prepubertal patients and for 60–93% in postpubertal patients {2965,3249, 2881,742}. Teratoma can occur in fetuses {2298,1894}. Mature and immature teratomas can be associated with other germ cell tumours (mixed germ cell tumours) and can occur in patients with Klinefelter syndrome {2886,663,3179}. Immature teratomas are much rarer than mature teratomas and occur more frequently in men than in women {1978,3021}.

Etiology

Unknown

Pathogenesis

The pathogenesis is similar to that of other germ cell tumours. The tumours most likely arise from migrating embryonic cells arrested in the midline during embryogenesis. Somatic mutations are usually not identified {2521}.

There are few data about the molecular biology and genetic features of primary mediastinal teratomas; two studies failed to show any overrepresentation of chromosome 12p in 38 pure mature or immature teratomas {1376,1644}. In contrast, pure teratomas after chemotherapy for mixed germ cell tumours have frequent 12p overrepresentation {1376}. Fourteen pure mediastinal paediatric teratomas analysed by comparative genomic hybridization showed no abnormalities {2671}. The DNA methylation status is non-contributory {894}. One report of immature teratoma of the posterior mediastinum showed rearrangement of chromosomes 6 and 11 and a lack of 12p anomalies {3140}.

Macroscopic appearance

Mature teratomas are usually encapsulated masses ranging from 30 to 250 mm {2470,3249}; adhesions to the surrounding organs may occur {2470,196,2433}. Cut surface is variegated, showing unilocular or multilocular cysts varying from millimetres to several centimetres. The cysts can contain clear fluid, mucoid material, sebaceous and keratinaceous debris, hair, fat, cartilage, and (rarely) teeth or bone {2881,2521}. Immature teratomas have a similar size distribution {1515} and have a soft to fleshy consistency or are extensively fibrous or cartilaginous. Haemorrhage and necrosis are common {2470}.

Histopathology

The hallmark of mature teratoma is haphazard distribution of mature somatic tissues. Skin and cutaneous appendages are common, often lining cysts. Monodermal teratomas (dermoid cysts) are rare in the mediastinum, and struma has not been reported {1863}. Bronchial mucosa and glands, gastrointestinal mucosa, nerves and mature brain tissue, smooth muscle, adipose tissue, and pancreatic tissues (including both exocrine and endocrine glands) are found in 60–80%. Skeletal muscle, bone, cartilage, salivary glands, prostate, liver, and melanocytes are less common.

Extensive granulomatous inflammation may be seen in association with ruptured cysts. Remnant thymic tissue is found outside of the capsule in 75% of cases.

Immature teratomas are composed of immature tissues corresponding to embryonal and/or fetal tissues either exclusively or in addition to mature tissues varying from 20–50% {1719,1515, 1978,3249}. The most common component is neuroectodermal tissue, with neuroepithelial cells forming tubules and rosettes {3249,1863}. Immature glands lined by tall columnar cells, fetal lung, mesenchymal and primitive cartilage, bone, rhabdomyoblasts, or blastemal-like stromal cells can be present. There are insufficient data to support a grading system for immature teratomas of the mediastinum, and some studies show no prognostic significance of grading in children {2669,1810}.

Cytology

The diagnosis of teratoma in cytological specimens or small biopsies should be made only after careful correlation with imaging and serological studies to exclude mixed germ cell tumour. Anucleated squamous cells and macrophages in a cystic background {547} are commonly found. The presence of ciliated bronchial epithelium, smooth muscle, and cartilage can be mistaken for contamination by bronchopulmonary tissue or bronchogenic cyst. Presence of pancreatic acini and intestinal-type mucosa is suggestive of a teratomatous lesion {2888,6}.

Immature teratomas may show a pattern of small blue cell tumour with small, round, hyperchromatic nuclei with inconspicuous nucleoli and a high N:C ratio. Rosettes with neuropils are rarely seen, as are rhabdomyoblasts, immature cartilage, and blastema-like stromal cells {6,2417,1234,1962}.

Diagnostic molecular pathology

Not clinically relevant

Essential and desirable diagnostic criteria

Essential:

- A tumour composed entirely of differentiated somatic-type tissue, which may be mature (adult-type), immature, or a combination

Staging

There is no agreed-upon staging system for teratoma.

Prognosis and prediction

Mature teratomas are benign {1376,1644,635,3021,742}, although they may rarely be fatal secondary to local compressive effects on vital structures. Immature teratomas have malignant potential, with some evidence suggesting that greater amounts of immature tissue correlate with malignant behaviour {742,625}. A variety of somatic-type malignancies may occur in mature teratomas and determine the prognosis {2582,1376,1447}, with complete surgical resection generally being the best therapeutic option {1447}.

Mixed germ cell tumours of the mediastinum

Moreira AL
Roden AC
Ströbel P
Ulbright TM

Definition
Mixed germ cell tumours of the mediastinum are neoplasms composed of two or more types of germ cell tumours.

ICD-O coding
9085/3 Mixed germ cell tumour

ICD-11 coding
2C28.0 & XH2PS1 Malignant germ cell neoplasms of heart, mediastinum or non-mesothelioma of pleura & Mixed germ cell tumour

Related terminology
Not recommended: malignant teratoma.

Subtype(s)
None

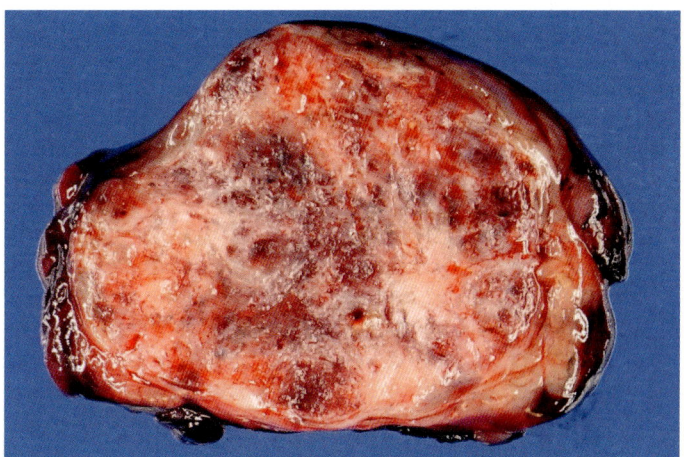

Fig. 6.18 Mixed germ cell tumour of the mediastinum. Cut surface of a mediastinal mixed germ cell tumour, after chemotherapy. Note the areas of fibrosis and haemorrhage.

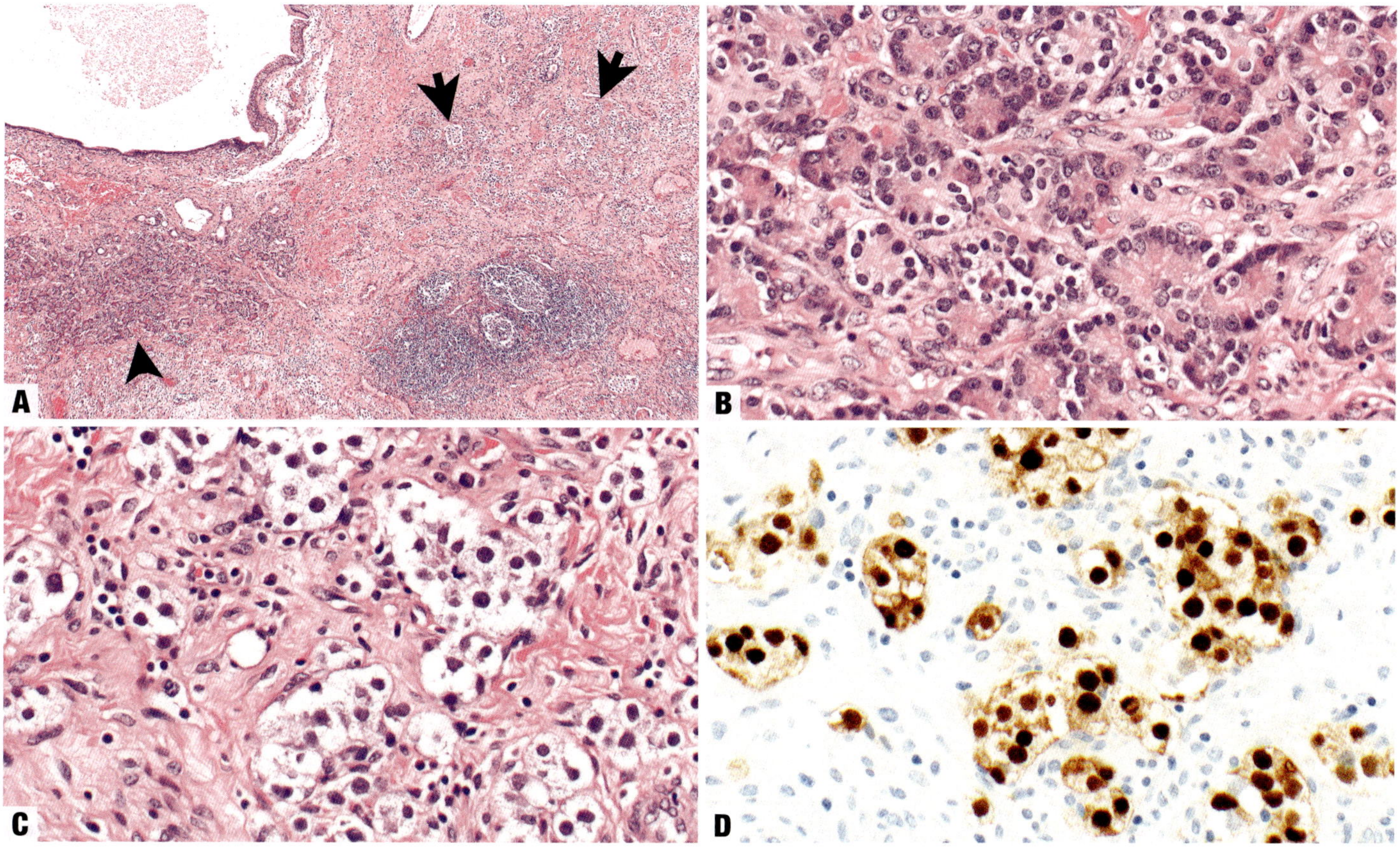

Fig. 6.19 Mixed germ cell tumour of the mediastinum. **A** Tumour consisting of glandular teratomatous structures (arrowhead) and a focal seminomatous component (arrows). **B** Teratomatous component of a mixed germ cell tumour resembling gastrointestinal glandular tissue. **C** Seminomatous component of a mixed germ cell tumour consists of nests of large polygonal cells with clear cytoplasm. **D** The seminomatous component expresses OCT3/4.

Chapter 6

Localization

Mixed germ cell tumours of the mediastinum occur in the anterior (prevascular) mediastinum.

Clinical features

Most patients present with symptoms similar to those of other mediastinal germ cell tumours, as well as elevated serum tumour markers {3338}. Imaging studies typically show a large, heterogeneous mass with necrosis, haemorrhage, and often infiltration of adjacent structures. The presence of cystic spaces or adipose tissue suggests the presence of a teratomatous component {2881}. Common sites of metastasis include the lung, pleura, lymph node, liver, bone, and brain {1433,2671,403,2965}.

Epidemiology

In adult patients, virtually all of whom are men {1433,1978}, the two most common tumour components are teratoma and embryonal carcinoma. In children, yolk sac tumour and teratoma (mature or immature) are more common {742,1433,2965,2198}.

Etiology

The etiology is similar to that of other germ cell tumours.

Pathogenesis

Mixed germ cell tumours of the mediastinum in children (teratoma and yolk sac tumour) {2198} lack the 12p overrepresentation characteristic of the malignant tumours in older males, but they often show chromosomal gains involving 1q, 3, and 20q and chromosomal losses involving 1p, 4q, and 6q {2671}. Because the teratoma elements in these tumours have a normal karyotype, the anomalies are thought to be due to the yolk sac tumour component {2198,2671}. In adults, frequent 12p gain is found {2671, 2618}. Patients with Klinefelter syndrome, who are at greatly increased risk, show extra copies of the X chromosome {3314}.

Macroscopic appearance

Mixed germ cell tumours are resected after chemotherapy. The tumours show a heterogeneous cut surface, with solid fleshy tumour interspersed with areas of haemorrhage and necrosis. The presence of cystic spaces usually indicates the presence of a teratomatous component.

Histopathology

Various types of germ cell tumours can occur in any combination, and their morphologies are identical to those of pure germ cell tumours. Most histological diagnoses are made on small biopsy specimens.

Cytology

The cytomorphological features of the germ cell tumour components are similar to those described for pure germ cell tumours.

Diagnostic molecular pathology

Not clinically relevant

Essential and desirable diagnostic criteria

Essential:
- Presence of more than one type of germ cell tumour

Staging

There is no agreed-upon staging system.

Prognosis and prediction

Mixed germ cell tumours have an unfavourable prognosis {1257}. The overall 5-year survival rate is 45% {258}. The most favourable outcomes are in patients aged < 30 years with localized disease to the mediastinum and normal hCG levels {258,1083,2550,2509}. Children have a better prognosis {2889,635}.

Mediastinal germ cell tumours with somatic-type solid malignancy

Roden AC
Ströbel P
Ulbright TM

Definition

Germ cell tumour with somatic-type solid malignancy of the mediastinum is a mediastinal germ cell tumour with a component of a malignant neoplasm resembling those seen at somatic sites.

ICD-O coding

9084/3 Teratoma with somatic-type malignancies

ICD-11 coding

2C28.0 Malignant germ cell neoplasms of heart, mediastinum or non-mesothelioma of pleura

Related terminology

Not recommended: teratoma with malignant transformation; teratoma with non-germ cell malignancy.

Subtype(s)

None

Localization

Mediastinal germ cell tumours with somatic-type solid malignancy occur in the anterior (prevascular) mediastinum.

Clinical features

These tumours occur in male patients, predominantly white men, at reported median ages of 21 and 31 years (range: 8–76 years) {111,1772,987,2653,1491,803,1049}. As many as 30% of non-seminomatous germ cell tumours develop a solid somatic-type malignancy {111}, most of which are metastatic at the time of diagnosis {1491}. Somatic-type malignancies may occur synchronously as a component of the primary germ cell tumour, months or more after the primary germ cell tumour, or in metastases. Various serum tumour markers other than those typical of germ cell tumours may be elevated.

Epidemiology

The epidemiological features are similar to those of non-seminomatous germ cell tumours {111,1772}.

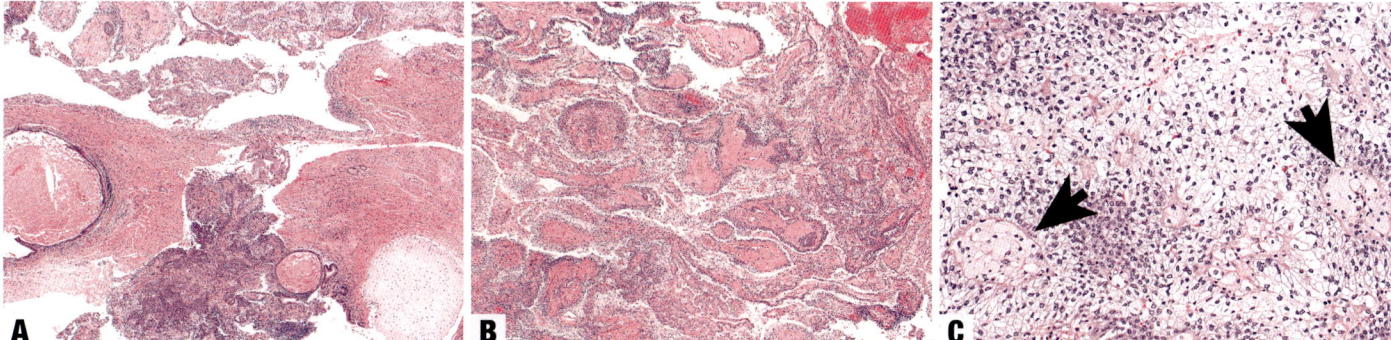

Fig. 6.20 Clear cell renal cell carcinoma with papillary pattern arising in mature teratoma. **A** Elements of mature teratoma (cartilage, columnar epithelium lining cysts) are adjacent to the papillary neoplasm. **B** The carcinoma expands over at least an entire low-power field and is characterized by a papillary and solid growth pattern. **C** The tumour cells have clear cytoplasm. Clusters of foamy macrophages are present (arrows).

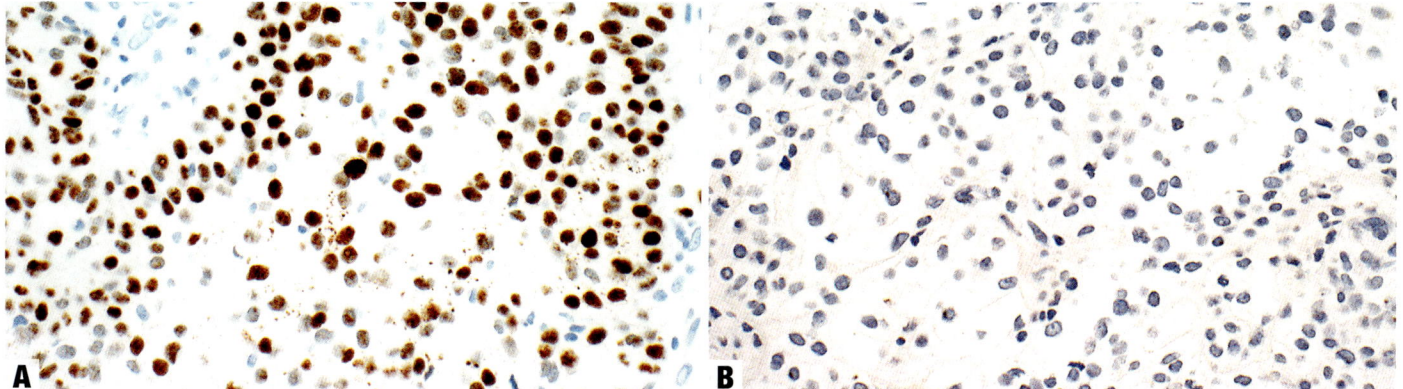

Fig. 6.21 Clear cell renal cell carcinoma arising in mature teratoma. **A** The tumour cells are positive for PAX8. **B** The tumour cells lack staining with OCT4.

Chapter 6

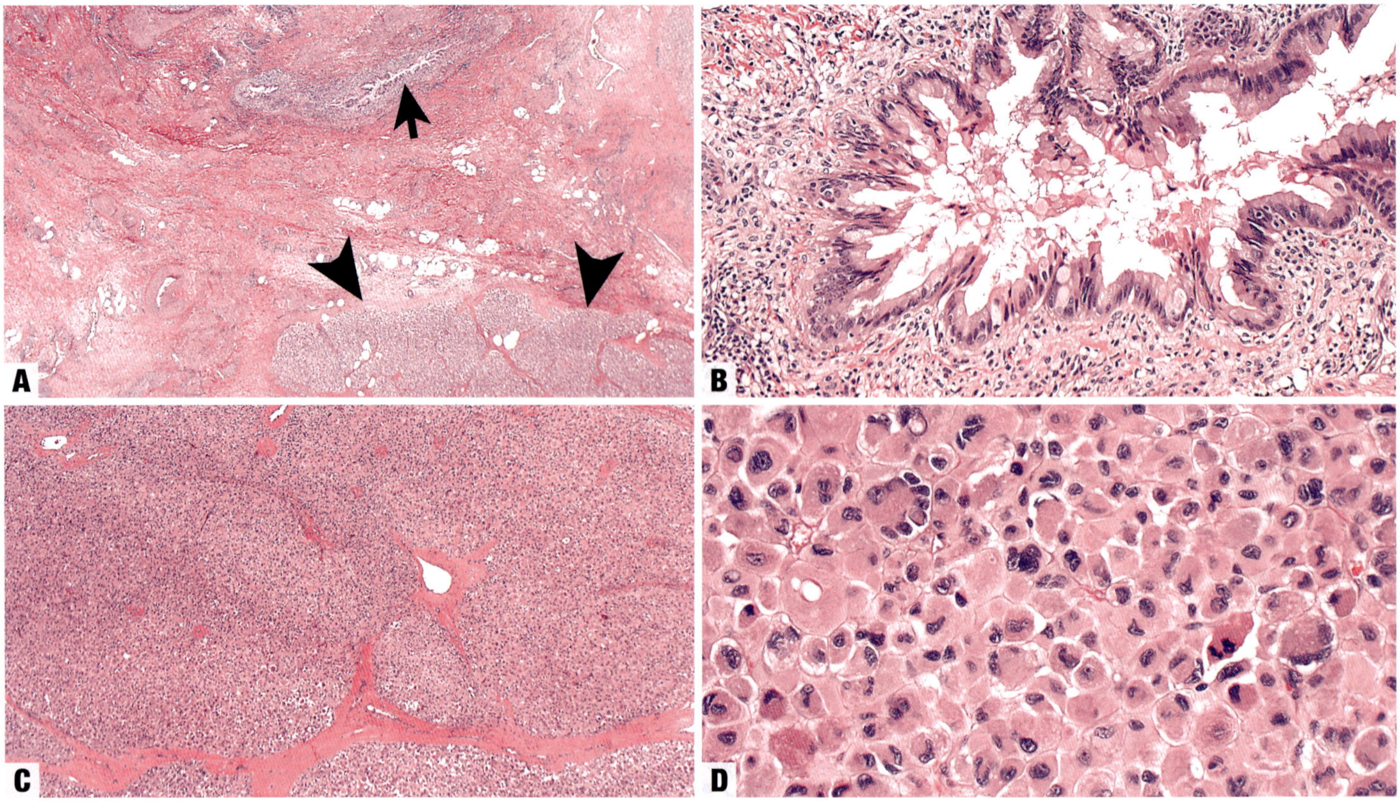

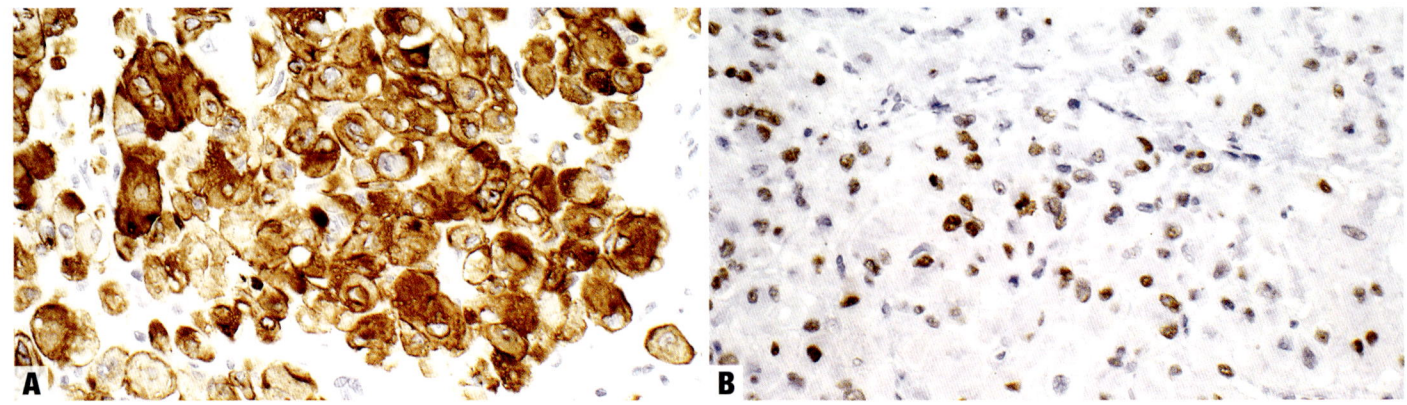

Fig. 6.22 Teratoma with rhabdomyosarcoma. **A** The tumour is composed of glandular structures (arrow) indicative of a teratomatous component and a sarcomatous component (arrowheads). **B** The glands are surrounded by a cellular spindle cell component. **C** The sarcomatous component expands over more than a low-power field, without an intervening teratoma component. **D** The sarcomatous component is composed of large round to oval cells with ample eosinophilic cytoplasm.

Etiology
Unknown

Pathogenesis
The pathogenesis is not well established. Many cases are likely to arise from corresponding somatic elements in teratomas, representing progression and overgrowth of teratomatous elements {2123}. This may be the result of activation of the same oncogenes as in the somatic counterparts {2017,2510}. Derivation from the germ cell tumour is indicated by the presence of identical 12p abnormalities, including isochromosome 12p, in both the somatic and the germ cell components of at least some tumours {1546,2017,2510,2897,1376}. The role of chemotherapy

is unclear, because these tumours are also found in patients without previous chemotherapy. Chemotherapy probably destroys chemosensitive elements of the germ cell tumour, thus allowing pre-existing somatic malignancies, which are not responsive to chemotherapy, to progress {140,3119}.

Macroscopic appearance
Tumour size ranges from 60 to 150 mm.

Histopathology
Somatic-type malignancies most commonly occur in association with mature teratomas and less commonly with immature teratomas, choriocarcinomas, yolk sac tumours, and embryonal

Fig. 6.23 Teratoma with rhabdomyosarcoma. The sarcoma cells express desmin (**A**) and myogenin (**B**).

carcinomas but not seminomas {111,1772,2653,1082,1783}. The somatic-type tumours include sarcomas and carcinomas. Rhabdomyosarcoma is the most frequent sarcoma (60%); angiosarcoma, leiomyosarcoma, primitive neuroectodermal tumour {1376}, glioblastoma multiforme {1709}, and malignant peripheral nerve sheath tumour have also been reported {1772}. Epithelial malignancies associated with germ cell tumours are mostly colonic-type adenocarcinomas {2612,1999,447,1906, 1447,2244} but also include adenosquamous and squamous cell carcinomas {3119,2470} and rarely neuroendocrine tumours {2653,1643,1039}. The percentage of all somatic-type malignancies of the entire tumour should be reported {1772}.

The differential diagnosis includes sarcoma and carcinoma independent of germ cell tumour and pure teratoma with cytological atypia but without a somatic-type malignancy (almost exclusively a finding in postchemotherapy resections). Distinction relies on the presence of a typical germ cell tumour component and sufficient overgrowth of the somatic-type malignancy (at least a 4× microscopic field or overtly invasive growth for carcinoma), respectively. The somatic-type malignancy shows the same immunophenotype as analogous tumours without associated germ cell tumour and usually lacks germ cell tumour markers.

Cytology
Not clinically relevant

Diagnostic molecular pathology
Not clinically relevant

Essential and desirable diagnostic criteria
Essential:
- Presence of a germ cell tumour such as teratoma, immature teratoma, choriocarcinoma, embryonal carcinoma, yolk sac tumour
- Presence of at least a component of a sarcoma or carcinoma

Desirable:
- Immunophenotype of the corresponding germ cell tumour
- Immunophenotype of the corresponding sarcoma or carcinoma

Staging
There is no agreed-upon staging system.

Prognosis and prediction
The prognosis for these patients is worse than for patients without somatic-type malignancies; some die within 6 months of diagnosis {1772}. The reported mean and median survival times are 14 and 9 months, respectively; only rare patients survive > 3 years {1772,987}. These tumours have a worse outcome than their gonadal counterparts, even though metastases are less common in the mediastinal cases {1772}. The somatic-type malignancy is generally resistant to chemotherapy that is targeted at the germ cell tumour. Local tumour progression is common, and some patients develop metastases, commonly to the lung and lymph nodes, among others {1049}.

Mediastinal germ cell tumours with associated haematological malignancy

Orazi A
Moreira AL
Roden AC

Definition

Germ cell tumour with associated haematological malignancy of the mediastinum is a germ cell tumour in the mediastinum associated with a clonally related haematological malignancy.

ICD-O coding

9086/3 Germ cell tumour with associated haematological malignancy

ICD-11 coding

2C28.0 & XH9QP9 Malignant germ cell neoplasms of heart, mediastinum or non-mesothelioma of pleura & Germ cell tumour with associated haematological malignancy

Related terminology

None

Subtype(s)

None

Localization

Mediastinal germ cell tumours with associated haematological malignancy occur in the anterior (prevascular) mediastinum.

Clinical features

The most common clinical features at diagnosis include pancytopenia, hepatosplenomegaly, and thrombocytopenia, each occurring in 20–35% of cases. Bleeding and infections arise due to cytopenias in myelodysplastic syndromes. Acute leukaemias are also common events. Thromboembolic complications due to thrombocytosis {2096} and mediastinal mass formation (due to myeloid sarcoma) are rare {2593}. Other clinical signs are leukaemic skin lesions, flushing {1082}, and the development of haemophagocytic syndromes {3123}. Haematological complications can accompany, follow {258,3123,3178}, or precede local symptoms. Leukaemias most commonly become apparent within the first year after diagnosis of germ cell tumours (at a median of 6 months; range: 0–122 months) {650, 1082,2017,2096,2202}.

Epidemiology

Haematological malignancies develop in 2–6% of malignant non-seminomatous mediastinal germ cell tumours {1081,2082}, but they virtually never occur in germ cell tumours of other sites {1809}. Patients are typically adolescents or young adults (patient age range: 9–48 years), and virtually all patients are male {430,650,2096,2823}. About 10–20% of cases have been associated with Klinefelter syndrome {183,691,2096}.

Etiology

It is hypothesized that a totipotent or pluripotent primordial germ cell gives rise to a leukaemic clone, independent of prior chemoradiation {2094,2095}. Alternatively, the presence of foci of extramedullary haematopoiesis within the yolk sac tumour component suggests that these haematological malignancies may develop from more-committed, somatic-type haematopoietic cells {2202}.

Pathogenesis

Genetic studies have demonstrated chromosomal aberrations (particularly isochromosome 12p) shared between germ cell tumours and associated haematological malignancies {430, 1580}, providing evidence of a clonal relationship. The predilection for mediastinal germ cell tumours remains unexplained.

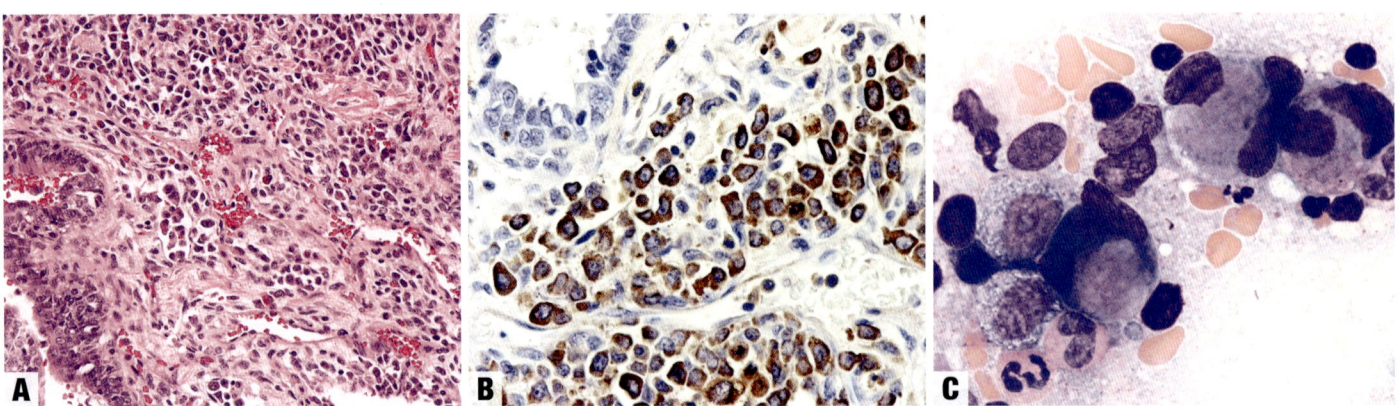

Fig. 6.24 Mediastinal germ cell tumours with associated haematological malignancy. **A** A germ cell tumour showing high-grade myelodysplastic syndrome (myelodysplastic syndrome with excess blasts); note the increased number of blasts and the presence of severe dysmegakaryopoiesis. **B** Mediastinal germ cell tumour with haematopoietic differentiation. Intravascular proliferation of immature myeloid precursors showing myeloperoxidase immunoreactivity. **C** Myelodysplastic syndrome with excess blasts. Bone marrow touch preparation of the same biopsy, showing high-grade myelodysplastic syndrome (myelodysplastic syndrome with excess blasts); note the presence of severe dysmegakaryopoiesis.

It has been speculated that the expression of haematopoietic growth and differentiation factors in some mediastinal germ cell tumours could drive the differentiation of primordial germ cells into haematopoietic progeny. The profile of differentiation factors expressed may also underlie the preferred commitment to the megakaryocytic and monocytic lineages {2082,2202}. Concomitant mediastinal and extramediastinal leukaemias show a comparable immunophenotype and genotype, suggesting the spread of haematopoietic tumour cells from germ cell tumours to blood, bone marrow, and extramedullary sites {430,1580,2017}.

Macroscopic appearance
The gross findings are identical to those of non-seminomatous malignant germ cell tumours.

Histopathology
The germ cell tumours underlying the haematological malignancies are typically non-seminomatous malignant germ cell tumours, most often yolk sac tumours or mixed germ cell tumours with a yolk sac component, although immature teratomas and mixed germ cell tumours with somatic-type sarcomas have also been observed {430,1082,1579,2017,2096}. Reported haematological malignancies include acute leukaemias {258, 1598} and histiocytic sarcoma (malignant histiocytosis) {116,183, 650,1579,2096}, as well as (rarely) localized histiocytic proliferations {3525}, myelodysplastic syndromes {520,2082,2806,3178}, myeloproliferative neoplasms {430,1580,2096}, and mastocytosis {457}. Among the acute leukaemias, acute megakaryoblastic leukaemia and acute myeloid leukaemia with monocytic differentiation {995,1580,2020,3154,3455} are most common, accounting for about half of all cases {258,2096,2202}. Acute myeloid leukaemia, differentiated {3178}; erythroleukaemia {2082,2615}; acute undifferentiated leukaemia {2096}; and acute lymphoblastic leukaemia {1598,2096} have also been described. Myelodysplastic syndromes include myelodysplastic syndrome with excess blasts, as well as other subtypes {520,2094,2806}. Myelodysplasia can precede acute myeloid leukaemias {520,3178}. Essential thrombocythaemia and primary myelofibrosis are the types of myeloproliferative neoplasms encountered in association with mediastinal germ cell tumours {918,2096}. Leukaemias may diffusely or focally infiltrate the underlying germ cell tumour {2202}, or they can form tumorous lesions (myeloid sarcoma) in the mediastinum {2021,2593}. Extramediastinal manifestations (e.g. organomegaly and leukaemia) can occur in the presence or absence of detectable haematopoietic malignancy in the mediastinal germ cell tumour {2202}.

Immunohistochemistry
CD34 and TdT can be used to identify the presence of blasts. Useful immunohistochemical stains for myeloid-associated antigens include myeloperoxidase, CD33, KIT (CD117), CD68, CD14, CD163, lysozyme, CD61 (or CD42b), and CD71 (or glycophorin). Additionally, CD10, CD19, CD79a, CD7, and CD3 may be useful for excluding the possibility of acute lymphoblastic leukaemia. If blastic plasmacytoid dendritic cell tumour is under consideration, then CD123 (and/or CD303), CD4, and CD56 must be added.

Cytogenetics
Isochromosome 12p is the most specific and most common chromosomal marker shared by germ cell tumours and the associated haematological malignancies {430,520,2017, 2096,3455}. The haematological malignancies can also harbour other genetic alterations more typically seen in various haematological malignancies, such as del(5q) and trisomy 8, suggesting that aberrations not specific to germ cell tumour determine the phenotype of the associated haematological malignancy {2017}.

Differential diagnosis
Clonally related haematological malignancies must be distinguished from secondary myelodysplastic syndromes and acute myeloid leukaemias that are related to chemotherapy regimens – especially salvage therapy (including etoposide treatment) {1505,2593}. In one large series, secondary myelodysplastic syndromes and acute myeloid leukaemias occurred in 0.7% and 1.3% of cases, respectively {1505}. Chemotherapy-related acute myeloid leukaemias do not show isochromosome 12p, and they usually manifest later (25–60 months after chemotherapy) than germ cell tumour–related acute myeloid leukaemias (which have a median time to onset after chemotherapy of 6 months; range: 0–122 months) {1082,2096}.

Cytology
Not clinically relevant

Diagnostic molecular pathology
Cytogenetic investigation may be helpful in selected cases.

Essential and desirable diagnostic criteria
Essential:
- Malignant germ cell tumour of the mediastinum
- Haematological malignancy in the same tumour or external to the mediastinum

Desirable:
- Complete characterization of the mediastinal germ cell tumour–associated leukaemia process
- Cytogenetics may be helpful in both tumours in selected cases

Staging
There is no agreed-upon staging system.

Prognosis and prediction
The occurrence of a clonally related acute leukaemia in a patient with mediastinal germ cell tumour is among the most adverse prognostic factors. In a published series, none of the reported patients survived for > 2 years after the onset of leukaemia; the median survival time was 6 months {1082}. These leukaemias appear to be refractory to current treatment protocols, including aggressive induction chemotherapy and allogeneic bone marrow transplantation {1233,3501}. However, the clinical course in patients with myeloproliferative neoplasms may be more protracted {918}.

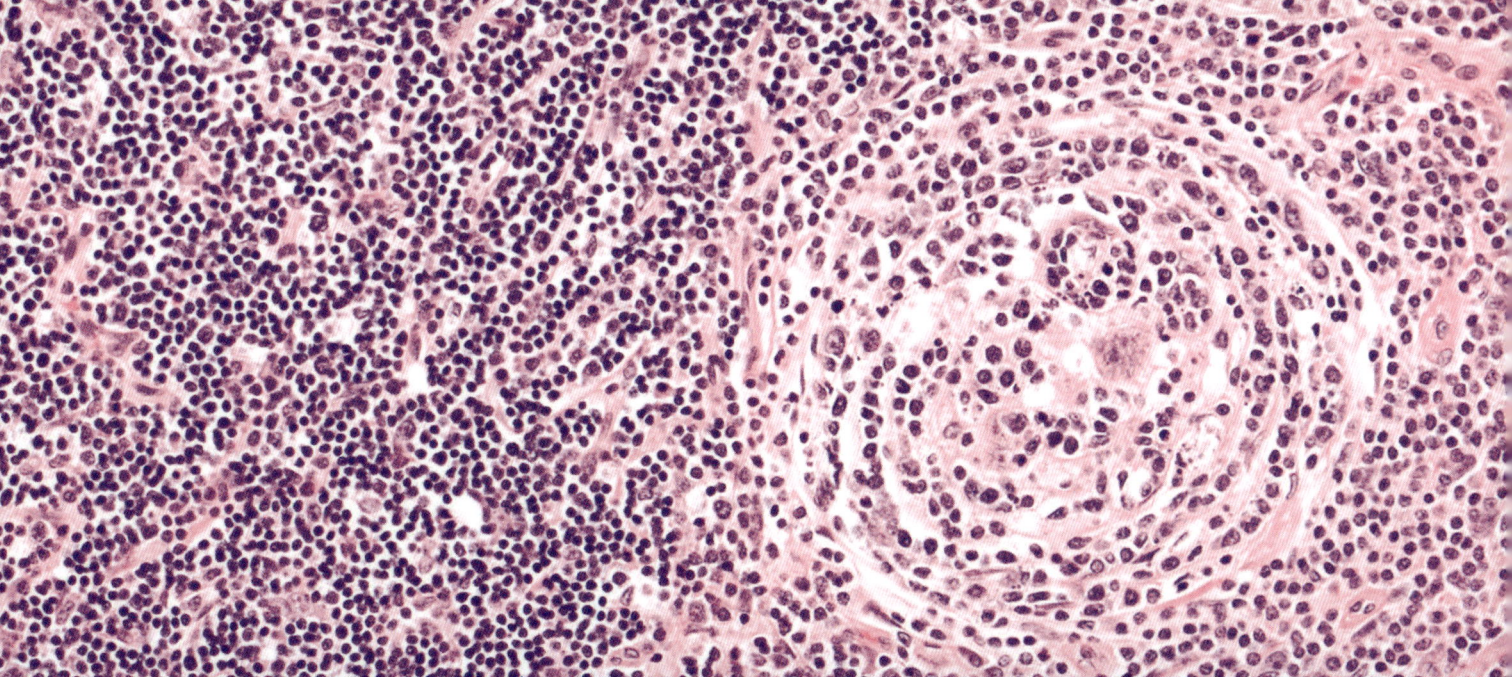

7

Haematolymphoid tumours of the mediastinum

Edited by: Chan JKC, Marx A

Primary mediastinal large B-cell lymphoma
MALT lymphoma
T-lymphoblastic leukaemia/lymphoma
Classic Hodgkin lymphoma
Mediastinal grey zone lymphoma
Follicular dendritic cell sarcoma
Myeloid sarcoma

Haematolymphoid tumours of the mediastinum: Introduction

Chan JKC
Cooper WA

Overview

Primary haematolymphoid neoplasms of the mediastinum may arise in the thymus, mediastinal lymph nodes, or mediastinal soft tissues. In an individual case, it is often difficult, if not impossible, to determine from which mediastinal component the neoplasm originated. A proportion of haematolymphoid neoplasms of the mediastinum likely arise in mediastinal lymph nodes, and are thus expected to share the same broad repertoire of lymphoma types as seen in conventional nodal lymphomas.

Lymphomas of the mediastinum

Lymphomas account for 12–25% of all primary mediastinal lesions (including tumours, cysts, and thymic hyperplasia) {1170,551,398,2505}. Mediastinal lymphomas account for 2.4% of all extranodal lymphomas {864}.

Several distinctive types of lymphomas arise primarily in the thymus / anterior (prevascular) mediastinum, including nodular sclerosis classic Hodgkin lymphoma, primary mediastinal (thymic) large B-cell lymphoma, mediastinal grey zone lymphoma, and T-lymphoblastic leukaemia/lymphoma. Extranodal marginal zone lymphoma of mucosa-associated lymphoid tissue (MALT lymphoma) of the thymus, although rare, exhibits some clinicopathological features distinct from those of extranodal marginal zone lymphomas of other anatomical sites. Other types of B-cell and T-cell lymphomas can also occur as primary thymic tumours {426,2351,1252,1268,2972,1350,647}, but they are so rare that they are not covered in this volume on thoracic tumours; detailed information about these other lymphoma types is available in the 2017 volume on tumours of haematopoietic and lymphoid tissues {2941}.

Histiocytic, dendritic cell, and myeloid neoplasms of the mediastinum

Histiocytic, dendritic cell, and myeloid neoplasms of the mediastinum are very rare. Among them, only follicular dendritic cell sarcoma occurs with some frequency, and this entity is therefore discussed within this fifth-edition volume on thoracic tumours. Myeloid sarcoma is also covered. Other histiocytic and dendritic cell neoplasms that were covered in the fourth edition of the thoracic tumours volume (Langerhans cell lesions {740,2768}, histiocytic sarcoma {1363}, interdigitating dendritic cell sarcoma {2647}, fibroblastic reticular cell tumour {440,2647}, and hybrid dendritic cell tumour {706}) are extremely rare in the mediastinum, and are therefore not covered in the fifth-edition of this volume; detailed information is available in the 2017 volume on tumours of haematopoietic and lymphoid tissues {2941}. See *Pulmonary Langerhans cell histiocytosis* (p. 186) and *Pulmonary Erdheim–Chester disease* (p. 189) for those histiocytic lesions that primarily involve the lung parenchyma.

Primary mediastinal large B-cell lymphoma

Klapper W
Gaulard P
Rosenwald A

Definition
Primary mediastinal (thymic) large B-cell lymphoma (PMBCL) is a mature aggressive large B-cell lymphoma of putative thymic B-cell origin, arising in the mediastinum, with distinctive clinical, immunophenotypic, genotypic, and molecular features.

ICD-O coding
9679/3 Mediastinal large B-cell lymphoma

ICD-11 coding
2A81.0 Primary mediastinal large B-cell lymphoma

Related terminology
Not recommended: primary mediastinal clear cell lymphoma of B-cell type {1958} (obsolete); mediastinal diffuse large cell lymphoma with sclerosis {1885} (obsolete).

Subtype(s)
None

Localization
PMBCL involves the anterior-superior mediastinum (thymus) {15}. Infiltration of the lung, chest wall, pleura, and pericardium is frequent. Regional involvement of supraclavicular and cervical lymph nodes may occur {3523}. At progression, dissemination to extranodal sites including kidney, adrenal, liver, or CNS is common, contrasting with the low frequency of bone marrow involvement {1612,411}.

Clinical features
The commonest symptom is superior vena cava syndrome, followed by airway obstruction and pleural and pericardial effusions. B symptoms may be present.

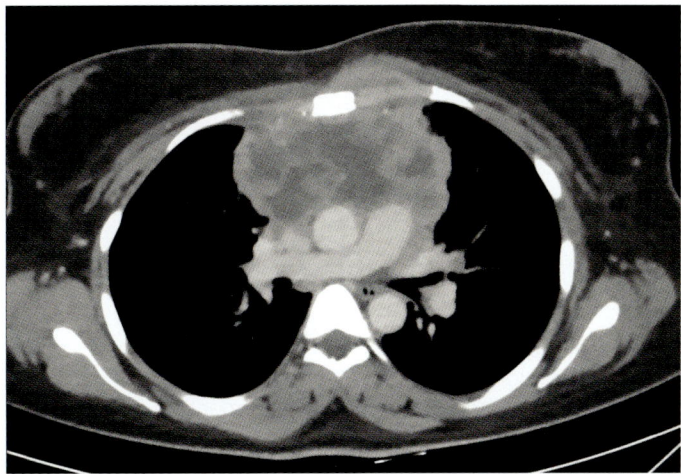

Fig. 7.01 Primary mediastinal large B-cell lymphoma. CT of a patient with a primary mediastinal large B-cell lymphoma forming a large anterior (prevascular) mediastinal mass.

Imaging
A characteristic feature of PMBCL at first diagnosis is the regular contour of the primary tumour and the (near) absence of lymphadenopathy {2996}.

Epidemiology
PMBCL accounts for 2–3% of non-Hodgkin lymphomas and occurs predominantly in young adults (third and fourth decades of life), with a female predominance {3027,411,1611,3523,1078}.

Etiology
The etiology is unknown. Rare familial clustering suggests *KMT2A* (previously called *MLL*) as a candidate predisposition gene {2585}.

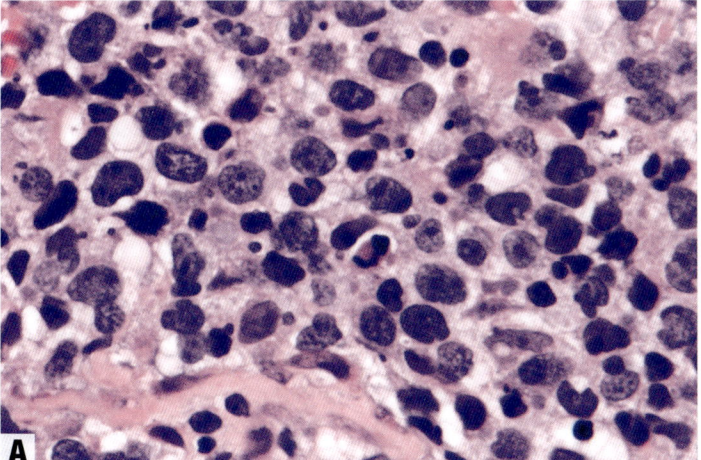
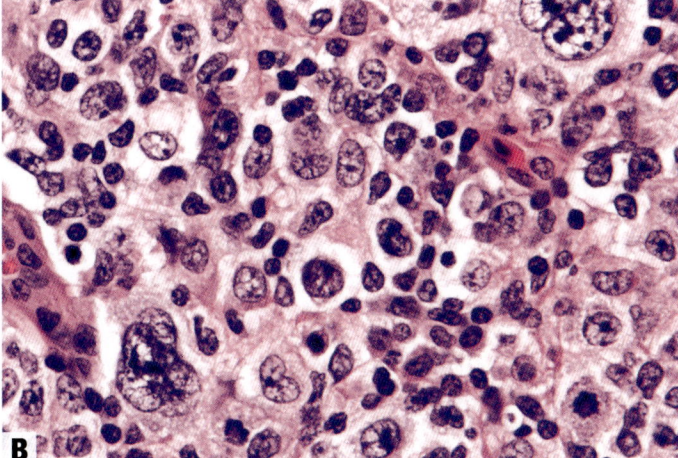

Fig. 7.02 Primary mediastinal large B-cell lymphoma. **A** An example with a monotonous population of large lymphoma cells. **B** An example showing marked variation in the size of lymphoma cells. The larger cells show some resemblance to Reed–Sternberg cells.

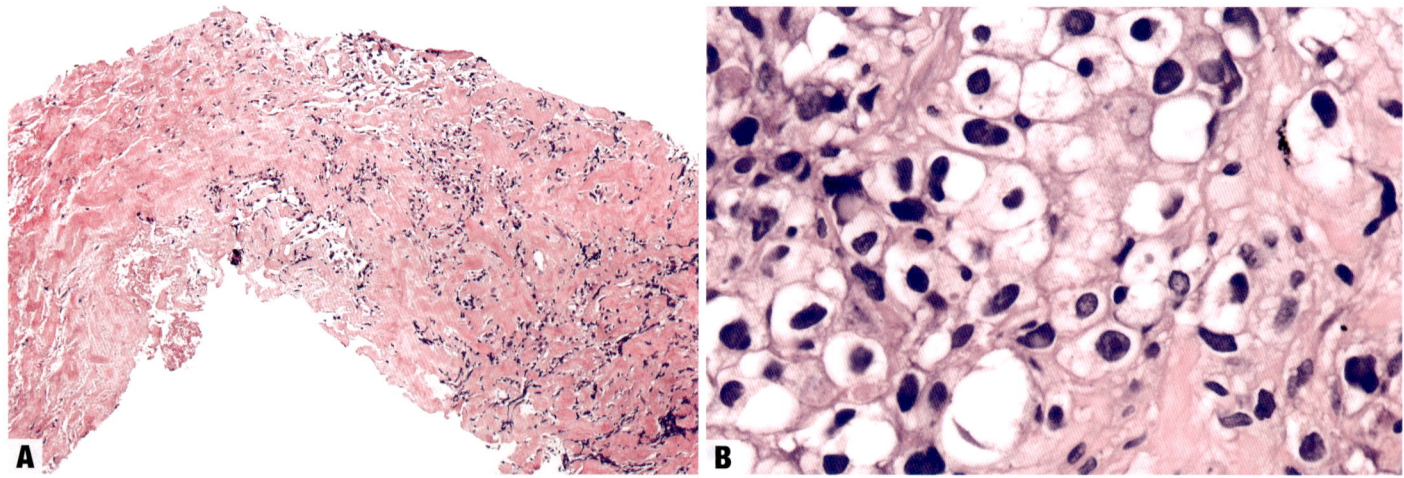

Fig. 7.03 Primary mediastinal large B-cell lymphoma. **A** In this mediastinal biopsy, the lymphoma cells are found in a densely sclerotic stroma. **B** These malignant large B cells have clear cytoplasm.

Pathogenesis

PMBCL is thought to be derived from thymic B cells. IG genes are clonally rearranged {1651}. Rearrangements of *BCL2*, *BCL6*, and *MYC* are absent or rare {3091}. Breaks in the MHC class II transactivator *CIITA* at 16p13.13 result in downregulated expression of MHC class II molecules and overexpression of PDL1 (CD274) and PDL2 (PDCD1LG2) {2850}. The genomic profile typically contains gains including amplified regions in chromosome 9p24.1, including the *JAK2/PDCD1LG2* (*PD-L2*) locus, and 2p16.1, including the *REL/BCL11A* locus, but also in chromosomes Xp11.4-p21 and Xq24-q26 {1325,209,3288}. Among lymphomas, copy-number gains and high-level amplification, as well as rearrangements of *CD274* (*PD-L1*) or *PDCD1LG2* (*PD-L2*), occur almost exclusively in PMBCL {2015,1007,3112}. PMBCL has a unique transcriptional signature that is distinct from that of other forms of diffuse large B-cell lymphoma, but it shares similarities with classic Hodgkin lymphoma (CHL) {2644, 2535}. PMBCL has constitutively activated NF-κB {827} due to deleterious mutations in the *TNFAIP3* gene {2665}. Recurrent mutations of *STAT6* (or *PTPN1*) and *SOCS1* are found {1029}. Comprehensive molecular profiling emphasizes immune evasion and interferon response factor, as well as mutations in XPO1 pathways, as relevant pathogenic mechanisms {2014, 455,738,1293}.

Macroscopic appearance

PMBCL occurs as a solid mass lesion, tan to light brown, sometimes with central necrosis.

Histopathology

The growth pattern is diffuse and the large tumour cells usually form clusters or sheets. The centre of the lesion contains predominantly neoplastic cells, while a variable number of admixed reactive lymphocytes, macrophages, and granulocytes may be present at the periphery. A frequent feature is distinctive stromal fibrosis made up of irregular collagen bands, compartmentalizing the lymphomatous infiltrate into variably sized aggregates {1958,2291,3445}. This stromal component is frequently absent in involved lymph nodes. The pattern of involvement in lymph nodes is carcinoma-like, starting from marginal sinuses, followed by infiltration and replacement of the nodal parenchyma.

PMBCL has a broad range of cytomorphology. The cells range from medium-sized to large (2–5 times the size of a small lymphocyte) and have abundant, frequently clear cytoplasm and irregularly round or ovoid (occasionally multilobated) nuclei, usually with small nucleoli {2291}. Some cases contain cells with pleomorphic nuclei and abundant amphophilic cytoplasm, resembling Hodgkin lymphoma or non-lymphoid tumours {2291,3063}.

Rarely, there are grey zone (borderline) lesions combining features of PMBCL and CHL {2350}. Examples of composite PMBCL and nodular sclerosis CHL have been described, and PMBCL may occur before, concurrent with, or at relapse of nodular sclerosis CHL {3063}.

Immunohistochemistry

PMBCL expresses B-cell lineage antigens such as CD19 and CD20. It lacks immunoglobulin expression despite a functional IG gene rearrangement and expression of relevant transcription factors {1367,2348,1725}. CD30 is present in > 80% of cases, but unlike in CHL, it is usually weak and heterogeneous and often without membranous staining {1144,2348}. Tumour cells frequently express IRF4 (MUM1; 75%) and CD23 (70%), and variably BCL2 and BCL6. CD10 expression is uncommon {362, 632,2348}. PMBCL often lacks HLA class I and/or class II molecules {1959,1958}.

Differential diagnosis

Diffuse large B-cell lymphoma involving the mediastinum often shows involvement of mediastinal lymph nodes rather than the thymic area, as well as widespread extramediastinal involvement including extrathoracic lymph nodes and bone marrow. Expression of CD30, CD23, MAL, and PDL1; rearrangements/ mutations of *CIITA*; and copy-number gains of the *CD274* (*PD-L1*) or *PDCD1LG2* (*PD-L2*) locus in PMBCL are helpful to exclude diffuse large B-cell lymphoma but not CHL, which shares these features with PMBCL {2015,1007,3112,571}.

CHL can be ruled out by detection of surface B-cell antigens such as CD79a and CD19, as well as CD45. However, grey zone lymphomas sharing features of CHL and PMBCL have been described {3063} (see *Classic Hodgkin lymphoma of the mediastinum*, p. 435).

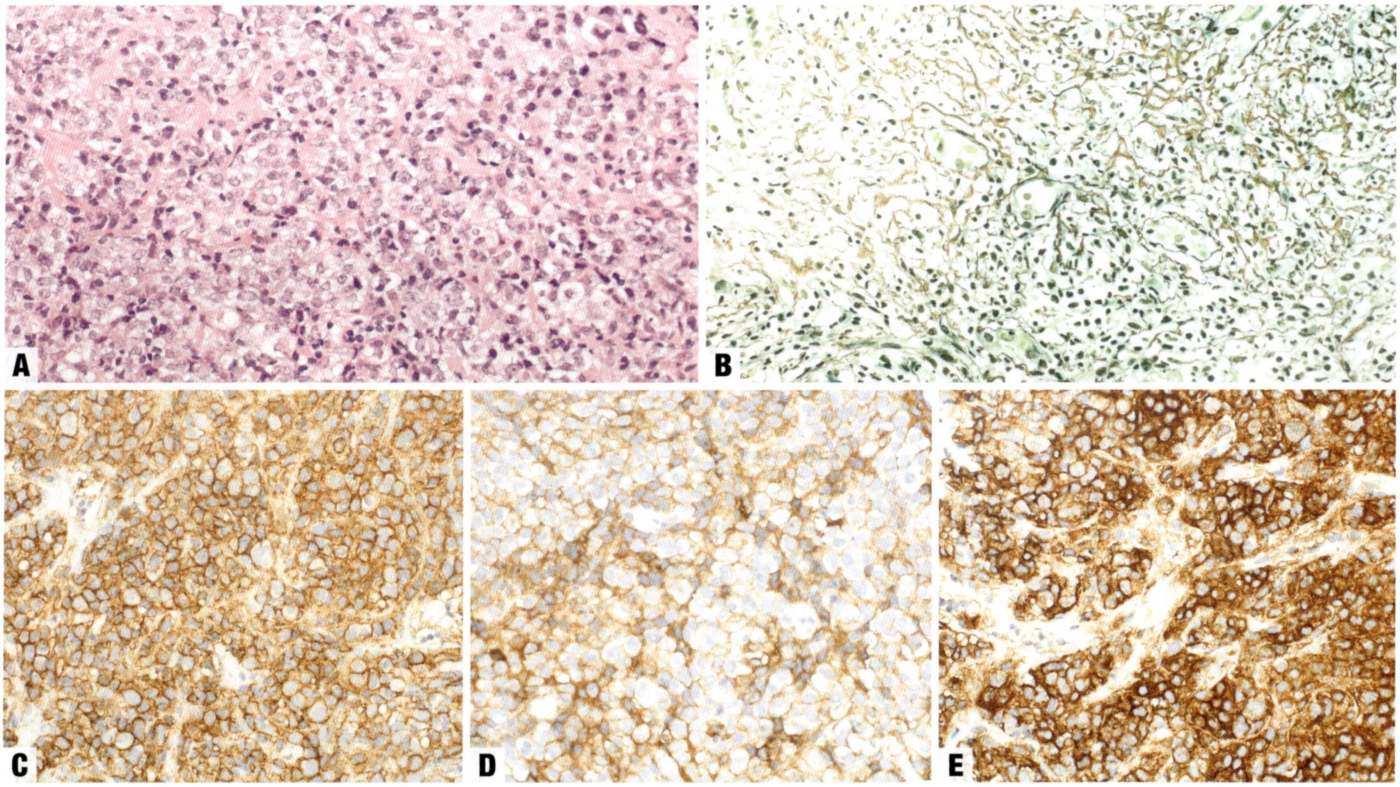

Fig. 7.04 Primary mediastinal large B-cell lymphoma (PMBCL). **A,B** Histopathology of a typical PMBCL showing diffuse sheets of blasts with clear or pale eosinophilic cytoplasm and accompanying sclerosis: H&E stain (**A**) and Gomori silver stain (**B**). **C–E** PMBCL immunophenotype with expression of CD20 (**C**), CD30 (**D**), and CD23 (**E**).

PMBCLs arising outside the mediastinum lacking the typical clinical presentation are uncommon. Extramediastinal PMBCLs may be identified by genomic or transcriptional analysis, but not by current clinical practice {2016,3222}.

Cytology
FNA can be used successfully in most cases to differentiate between lymphoma and other malignant tumours, but further subclassification of lymphoma is not advised on FNA alone.

Diagnostic molecular pathology
Usually not required

Essential and desirable diagnostic criteria
Essential:
- Large B-cell lymphoma in the anterior (prevascular) mediastinum with no or only minor extramediastinal spread
- Mature B-cell phenotype, accompanied by at least partial expression of CD23 and/or CD30

Desirable:
- Distinctive sclerosis
- Absence of *MYC*, *BCL2*, and *BCL6* rearrangements and copy gain of *CD274* (*PD-L1*) or *PDCD1LG2* (*PD-L2*) locus

Staging
Staging is performed according to the Lugano modification of the Ann Arbor scheme for lymphomas (Union for International Cancer Control [UICC]). Staging is established using both standard radiological procedures and PET, which is helpful in assessing response to treatment {1880}.

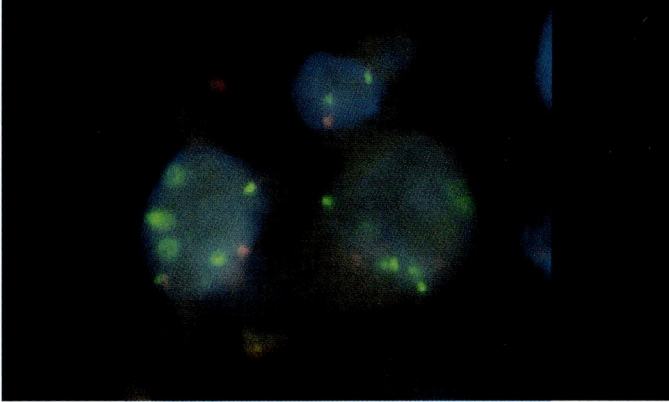

Fig. 7.05 Primary mediastinal large B-cell lymphoma. FISH for the *CD274* (*PDCD1LG1*) locus (PDL1 [CD274], green signal) and centromere of chromosome 9 (red signal), indicating a copy-number gain.

Prognosis and prediction
Histopathological patterns of PMBCL are not associated with outcome {2291}. Extension into adjacent thoracic viscera, pleural or pericardial effusion, and poor performance status are associated with inferior outcome {411,1611,1612,2644}. Positive interim or end-of-treatment PET is associated with inferior outcome {1880,1215}. Patients with PMBCL treated with immuno-chemotherapy show a 5-year progression-free survival rate of approximately 80% {971,2479,1215}.

MALT lymphoma of the mediastinum

Inagaki H
Cook JR
Cooper WA

Definition

Extranodal marginal zone lymphoma of mucosa-associated lymphoid tissue (MALT lymphoma) is a low-grade primary extranodal B-cell lymphoma recapitulating the features of mucosa-associated lymphoid tissue.

ICD-O coding

9699/3 MALT lymphoma

ICD-11 coding

2A85.3 & XH3FE9 Extranodal marginal zone B-cell lymphoma, primary site excluding stomach or skin & Mature B-cell lymphomas

Related terminology

Acceptable: primary thymic extranodal marginal zone lymphoma; thymic extranodal marginal zone B-cell lymphoma of mucosa-associated lymphoid tissue.

Subtype(s)

None

Localization

Thymic MALT lymphomas occur in the anterior (prevascular) mediastinum.

Clinical features

Thymic MALT lymphomas are usually found incidentally, although some patients present with chest-related symptoms {1241}. A multiloculated or cystic mass in the anterior (prevascular) mediastinum is discovered on chest X-ray, CT, or MRI. Most tumours are of low stage (I or II) at presentation. Concurrent sites of MALT lymphoma, including the lung or salivary glands, are found in about 20% of cases. Monoclonal gammopathy (usually of the IgA type) is common.

Epidemiology

Thymic MALT lymphoma is rare, with a higher incidence in Asian populations. Most patients are in their sixth or seventh decade of life, with ages ranging from 14 to 75 years. There is a female predominance (M:F ratio: 1:3). Male patients are about 10 years older than female patients on average {974}.

Etiology

Thymic MALT lymphoma is strongly associated with autoimmune diseases, especially Sjögren syndrome {1241}, but may also complicate lymphoepithelial sialadenitis–like thymic hyperplasia in the absence of autoimmunity {2380A}. There is no direct association with EBV or any other microorganisms. Currently, there is no evidence suggesting a histogenetic link with primary mediastinal large B-cell lymphoma.

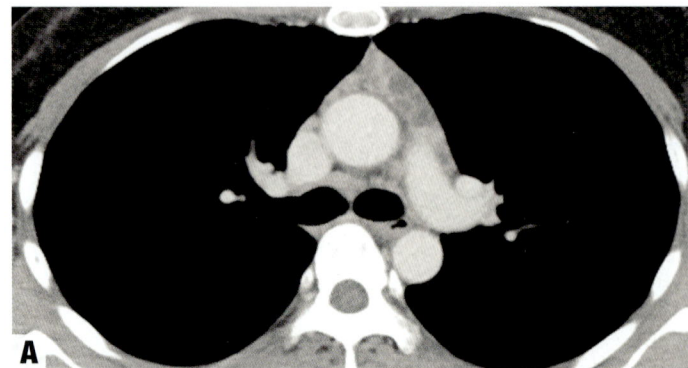

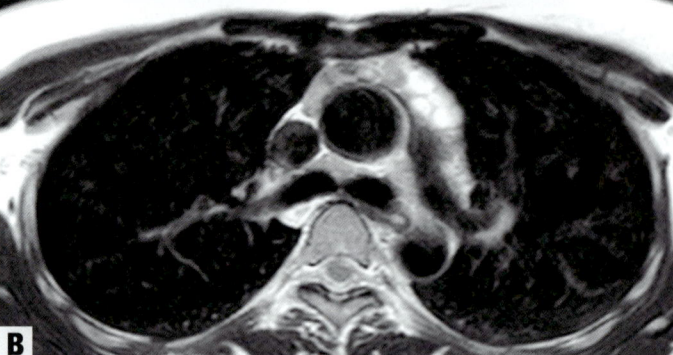

Fig. 7.06 Thymic extranodal marginal zone lymphoma of mucosa-associated lymphoid tissue (MALT lymphoma). **A** Contrast-enhanced CT of the chest shows an anterior (prevascular) mediastinal mass with solid and cystic components. **B** T2-weighted MRI of the chest shows a multiloculated mass in the anterior (prevascular) mediastinum.

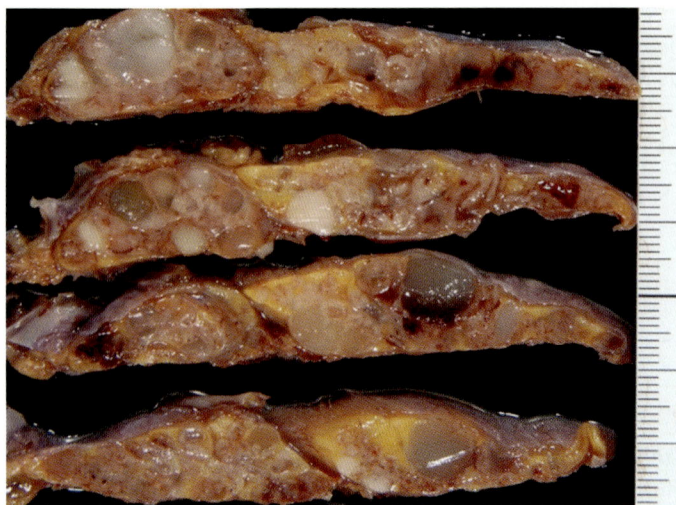

Fig. 7.07 Thymic extranodal marginal zone lymphoma of mucosa-associated lymphoid tissue (MALT lymphoma). The cut surface of the tumour shows fleshy, tan-coloured tumour tissue interspersed with multiple cystic spaces containing white or greyish material.

Pathogenesis

A biased use of IGHV (VH) genes suggests that this tumour may originate from specific subsets of B cells {3426}. Cytogenetically, one case each with 46,X,dup(X)(p11p22) and with add(8)(q24.1) has been reported {1073,1960}. Some tumour suppressor genes are frequently methylated {2975}. Translocations involving the *MALT1* or IGH genes, which are frequently found in MALT lymphomas at other sites, are absent {1506}.

Macroscopic appearance

Grossly, thymic MALT lymphoma is often well circumscribed and consists of fleshy, tan-coloured tissue, commonly interspersed with multiple variably sized cysts filled with proteinaceous material.

Histopathology

The normal thymic architecture is effaced. There are commonly many interspersed epithelium-lined cystic spaces. Reactive lymphoid follicles are surrounded by small lymphocytes with cleaved nuclei (centrocyte-like cells), monocytoid cells, plasmacytoid lymphocytes, plasma cells, and few scattered centroblast-like cells. The residual thymic epithelium, including Hassall corpuscles and the epithelium lining the cysts, is variably preserved and is often expanded by infiltrates of lymphoma cells, forming lymphoepithelial lesions. These areas impart a pale nodular appearance at low power. Rare cases may be accompanied by crystal-storing histiocytosis. Large cell transformation is very rare.

Tumour cells are typically positive for CD20, CD19, and CD79a and negative for CD5, CD10, CD23, BCL6, and cyclin D1. Monotypic cytoplasmic immunoglobulin is demonstrable in tumour cells with plasmacytic differentiation. Expression of IgA is common {1241}.

Flow cytometry for biopsied or resected tumour specimens is useful for detecting a CD5-negative, CD10-negative, and light chain–restricted monoclonal B-cell population. The main differential diagnoses include multilocular thymic cyst and thymic follicular hyperplasia.

Cytology

Features overlap with reactive lymphoid processes.

Diagnostic molecular pathology

Demonstration of clonal IG gene rearrangement may be helpful in supporting a diagnosis of lymphoma in problematic cases.

Essential and desirable diagnostic criteria

Essential:
- Interfollicular to diffuse infiltrate of centrocyte-like cells and small lymphoid cells, with or without monocytoid cells, effacing normal thymic architecture
- Positivity for B-lineage markers
- Exclusion of other small B-cell lymphomas

Desirable:
- Demonstration of clonal IG gene rearrangement
- Lymphoepithelial lesions
- Plasmacytic differentiation with monotypic immunoglobulins

Staging

Thymic MALT lymphoma is staged according to the Lugano classification, which has been adopted by the eighth-edition Union for International Cancer Control (UICC) TNM classification {492}.

Prognosis and prediction

Patients are typically free of disease after complete tumour resection and have an excellent prognosis.

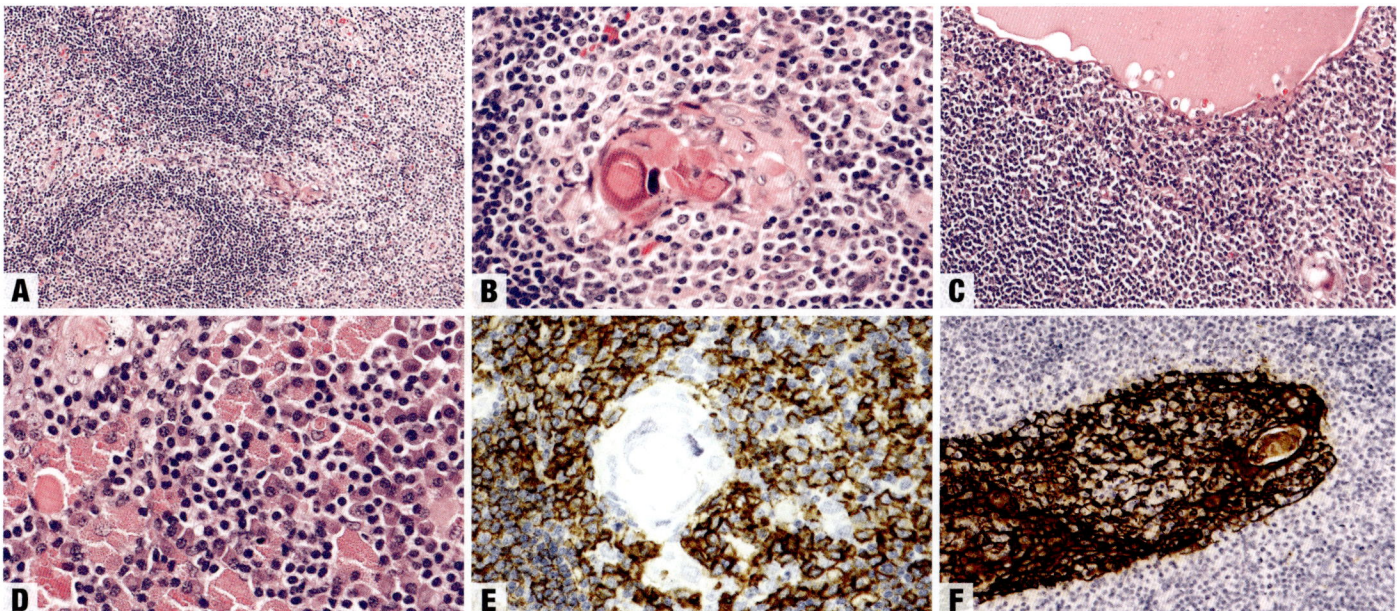

Fig. 7.08 Thymic extranodal marginal zone lymphoma of mucosa-associated lymphoid tissue (MALT lymphoma). **A** The pale areas between reactive lymphoid follicles with intact mantle zone consist of thymic epithelium heavily infiltrated by lymphoma cells with pale cytoplasm. **B** A Hassall corpuscle surrounded by neoplastic B cells and plasma cells. **C** A large cystic space containing eosinophilic proteinaceous fluid is lined by thymic epithelium, which is invaded by neoplastic B cells, forming a lymphoepithelial lesion. **D** This case is accompanied by crystal-storing histiocytosis. **E** Dense infiltrate of CD20-positive neoplastic B cells around a Hassall corpuscle. **F** Immunostaining for cytokeratin highlights lymphoepithelial lesions.

Mediastinal T-lymphoblastic leukaemia/lymphoma

Ferry JA
Molina TJ

Definition

T-lymphoblastic leukaemia/lymphoma (T-ALL/LBL) is a neoplasm of precursor lymphoid cells committed to T lineage, occurring either as a mass lesion with no or minimal blood or marrow involvement (T-lymphoblastic lymphoma [T-LBL]) or with extensive blood and/or marrow involvement (T-lymphoblastic leukaemia [T-ALL]).

ICD-O coding

9837/3 T-lymphoblastic leukaemia/lymphoma

ICD-11 coding

2A90 & XH50W7 Mature T-cell lymphoma, specified types, nodal or systemic & T lymphoblastic leukaemia/lymphoma

Related terminology

Not recommended: precursor T-lymphoblastic leukaemia/lymphoma.

Subtype(s)

None

Localization

Patients with T-LBL present with involvement of the thymus, less often of peripheral lymph nodes, and rarely of other extranodal sites. T-ALL involves peripheral blood and bone marrow, with or without extramedullary involvement.

Clinical features

T-LBL patients present with rapidly enlarging, anterior (prevascular) mediastinal (thymic) masses and/or peripheral lymphadenopathy. Mediastinal masses are associated with respiratory distress and/or chest pain, as well as (often) pleural and/or pericardial effusions {2355}. T-ALL patients typically have marked leukocytosis with a predominance of lymphoblasts. About 5–15% of cases are of early T-cell precursor (ETP) type {581, 3435}, usually occurring as T-ALL, but occasionally as T-LBL {1286}.

Epidemiology

Most patients with mediastinal T-ALL/LBL are children and young adults, although older adults may be affected. The M:F ratio is 2.5–3:1 {349,350,2355,2904}. T-LBL accounts for 15–20% of

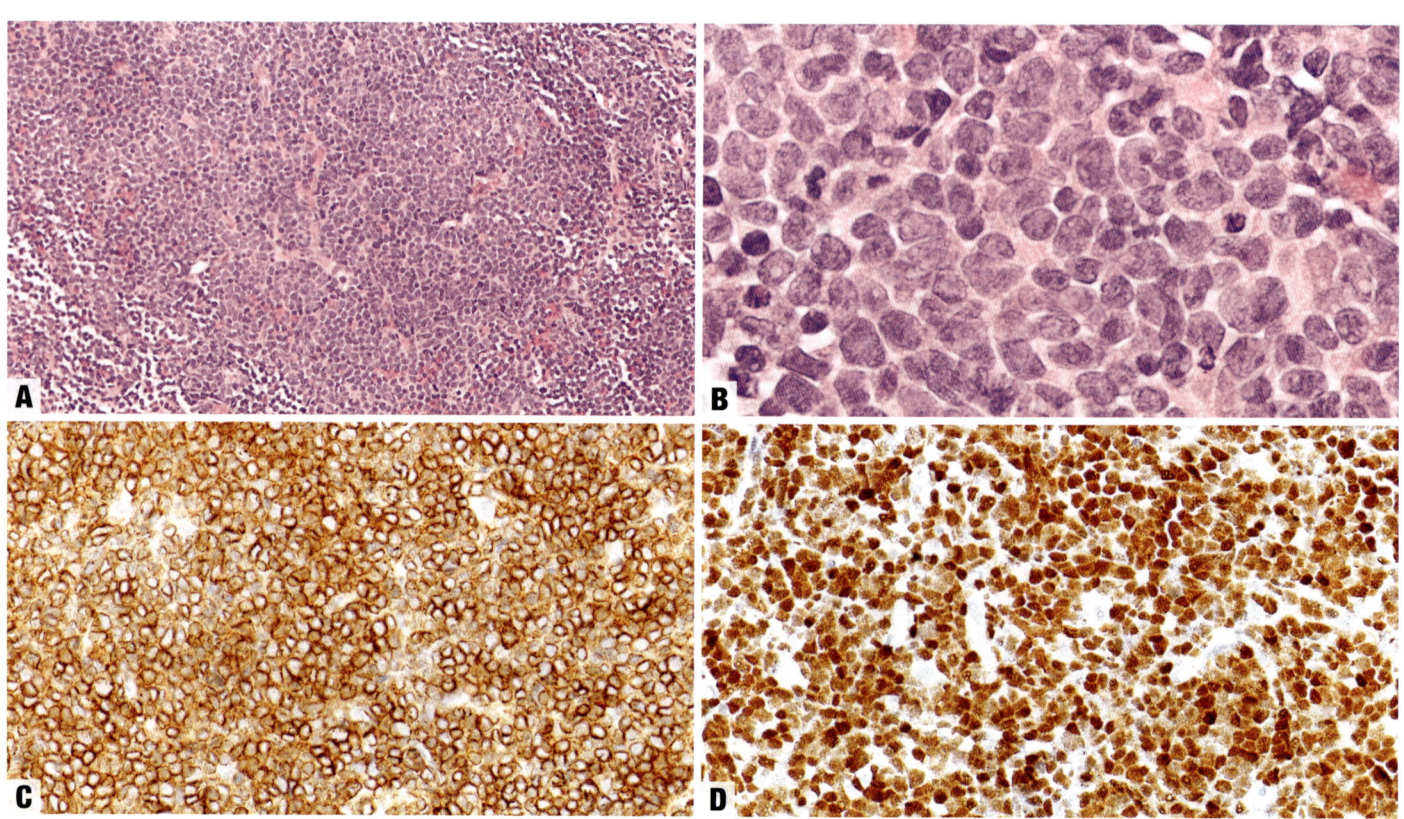

Fig. 7.09 T-lymphoblastic lymphoma. **A** The mediastinal core biopsy shows a diffuse, monotonous infiltrate of atypical lymphoid cells. **B** The core biopsy, on high magnification, shows medium-sized atypical lymphoid cells with irregular nuclei, fine chromatin, small nucleoli, and scant cytoplasm. **C** The atypical cells are CD3-positive. **D** The atypical cells are TdT-positive. By flow cytometry, the atypical cells were sCD3–, cCD3+, TdT+, CD1a+, CD5+, CD2+, CD4/CD8+, CD7+, CD10+/–.

non-Hodgkin lymphomas in children and adolescents {349, 350}, and for 85–90% of lymphoblastic lymphomas. T-LBL is the second most common paediatric non-Hodgkin lymphoma, after Burkitt lymphoma {350}. T-ALL represents approximately 15% of paediatric lymphoblastic leukaemia and 25% of adult lymphoblastic leukaemia {2941}. Most patients in the USA are white, but Asians and black people are also affected {349}.

Etiology
Unknown

Pathogenesis
T-LBL is thought to derive from a thymic T-cell lymphoid precursor. Diverse genetic changes lead to T-ALL/LBL {3151,2941}. TRB or TRG genes are almost always clonally rearranged; concurrent clonal IGH is found in as many as about 20% of cases {581,2353,2943}. Karyotype is abnormal in about 60% of cases, with structural and numerical changes including translocations, pseudodiploidy, hyperdiploidy, hypodiploidy, and partial losses of chromosomes {2699,2355}. Translocations often involve TR genes (TRA/TRD at 14q11, TRB at 7q34, TRG at 7p14) {1875, 3147,3435}.

Group A genetic changes associated with arrest of T-cell maturation at various stages of differentiation can be divided into five main subgroups {1875,3147}: (1) the TAL/LMO subgroup, with abnormalities of TAL1, TAL2, LMO1, and LMO2; (2) the TLX1 activation subgroup; (3) the TLX3 subgroup, with ectopic expression of TLX3; (4) the HOXA subgroup, with elevated expression of members of the HOXA gene cluster, including cases with PICALM-MLLT10 translocations and KMT2A (MLL) rearrangements; and (5) the MYB subgroup, with activation of the MYB oncogene {3147}. Group B abnormalities are shared among different T-ALL/LBL subgroups and include cell-cycle defects such as del(9p21)/CDKN2A/B (in 60–70% of cases), Notch activation due to mutated NOTCH1 (in ~60% of cases) or mutated FBXW7 (negative regulator of NOTCH1), T-cell receptor signalling abnormalities (affecting LCK, RAS genes, NF1, PTEN), JAK/STAT activation, tyrosine kinase activation, and others {1875,3147,149,270}. ETP T-ALL/LBL is characterized by high LYL1 expression {1875}; changes overlap with those of acute myeloid leukaemia, with less frequent changes typical of T-ALL/LBL {3435,349}.

Macroscopic appearance
Not relevant

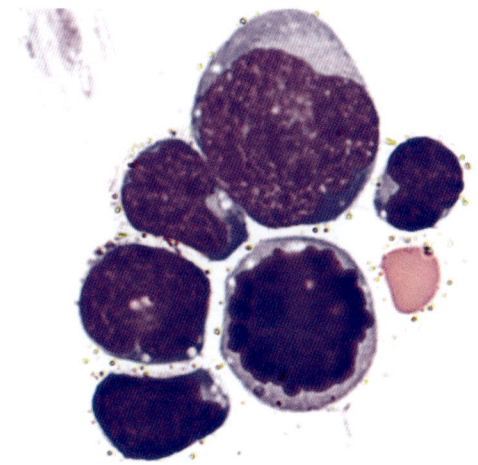

Fig. 7.10 Mediastinal T-lymphoblastic lymphoma involving pleural fluid. The patient had a pleural effusion containing T lymphoblasts with the same cytomorphology and immunophenotype by flow cytometry as seen in the mediastinal biopsy. A mitotic figure is present.

Histopathology
Thymus, lymph nodes, and/or bone marrow are partially or entirely replaced by a diffuse proliferation of lymphoblasts. Partially involved lymph nodes often show preferential paracortical involvement {2355}. Lymphoblasts are mostly small to medium-sized, with round, irregular, clefted, or convoluted nuclei; moderately condensed or fine chromatin; small or absent nucleoli; and scant cytoplasm {2355}. On touch or smear preparations, the scant cytoplasm is agranular and occasionally vacuolated. Mitotic figures are frequent. Tingible-body macrophages may be present {349,2941}. The presence of eosinophils should prompt investigation for myeloid/lymphoid neoplasms with eosinophilia. Among these, presentation as T-LBL is most common with FGFR1 gene rearrangement (8p11), less common with PDGFRA rearrangement, and rare with PDGFRB rearrangement {2941}.

Immunohistochemistry
Neoplastic cells variably express T-cell–associated markers (CD1a, CD2, CD3, CD5, CD7), CD10, CD34, and CD45, and they usually express TdT. By flow cytometry, cCD3 is typically positive; sCD3 is often negative. CD4 and CD8 are often coexpressed (double-positive), but both may be negative (double-negative) or one may be positive. In some cases, there is expression of CD13, CD33, KIT (CD117), or B-cell markers (weak). If T-cell receptor is expressed, it is usually TCRαβ;

Table 7.01 Immunophenotype of T-lymphoblastic leukaemia/lymphoma (T-ALL/LBL) and stages of intrathymic differentiation {2355,886,349,581}

Intrathymic stage	Immunophenotype[a]	Comments
Pro-T	cCD3+, CD7+, CD2–, CD5–, CD1a–, CD4–, CD8–, CD34+/–	
Pre-T	cCD3+, CD7+, CD2+, CD5+/–, CD1a–, CD4–, CD8–, CD34+/–	
Cortical T	cCD3+, CD7+, CD2+, CD1a+, CD4+, CD8+, CD34–	Most common immunophenotype for T-ALL/LBL
Medullary T	cCD3+, sCD3+, CD7+, CD2+, CD1a–, CD4 or CD8+, CD34–	
Early T-precursor	CD1a–, CD8– CD5– or expressed by < 75% of blasts ≥ 1 myeloid or stem cell antigen expressed by ≥ 25% of blasts (CD11b, CD13, CD33, CD34, CD65, KIT [CD117], HLA-DR)	Corresponds to some cases with pro-T or pre-T immunophenotype

[a]The immunophenotype of neoplastic cells may deviate from the normal T-cell maturation pattern.

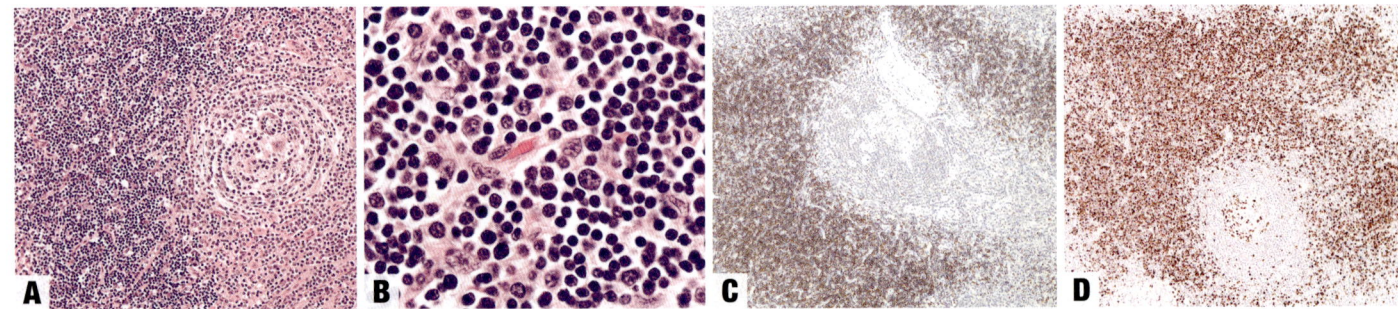

Fig. 7.11 Castleman disease and indolent T-lymphoblastic proliferation. **A** A lymphoid follicle with an involuted germinal centre with a centrally located large dysplastic follicular dendritic cell is adjacent to an aggregate of dark, closely packed lymphoid cells. **B** Higher power of the dark cells shows a predominance of small cells with some variation in cell size. **C** TdT-positive indolent T-lymphoblastic proliferation surrounds a hyaline-vascular follicle. **D** The Ki-67 proliferation index of the indolent T-lymphoblastic proliferation is very high.

TCRγδ expression is rare {2355}. Proliferation index is high (often > 90%). T-LBL has a more mature immunophenotype than T-ALL, with some overlap {3253}. The immunophenotype of T-ALL/LBL roughly corresponds to stages of intrathymic T-cell differentiation (see Table 7.01, p. 433) {2355,886,1875, 204}. ETP T-ALL/LBL has a distinct immunophenotype (see Table 7.01, p. 433) {349,581}.

Differential diagnosis
Type B thymomas, particularly type B1 thymomas, have many non-neoplastic, polyclonal, immunophenotypically immature T cells, masking the sparse neoplastic epithelial cells and potentially mimicking T-LBL, especially on a needle biopsy. Unlike T-LBL, type B1 thymomas contain regularly dispersed cytokeratin-positive neoplastic epithelial cells forming a delicate network. Clinical presentation is crucial, because type B1 thymomas are almost always localized at presentation, and they do not involve the bone marrow. T-LBL is typically positive with antibody to NOTCH1, whereas T cells in thymomas are negative {1300}.

Indolent T-lymphoblastic proliferation is a rare disorder characterized by a proliferation of sheets or clusters of polyclonal TdT-positive immature T cells (usually small in size) and distorting but not obliterating architecture. TR genes are not clonally rearranged {3165,2871,2162,2161}. Indolent T-lymphoblastic proliferation usually involves head and neck sites and rarely occurs in association with hyaline-vascular Castleman disease, follicular dendritic cell sarcoma, and other neoplasms {2161, 2163,3189}.

Cytology
Pleural and pericardial effusions often contain numerous lymphoblasts with admixed mesothelial cells and histiocytes {2355}. The lymphoblasts are medium-sized cells with round or convoluted nuclei, fine to homogeneous chromatin, inconspicuous nucleoli, and scant cytoplasm.

Diagnostic molecular pathology
Demonstration of clonal TR rearrangement, as well as cytogenetic and mutation analysis showing features of T-ALL/LBL, may be helpful.

Essential and desirable diagnostic criteria
Essential:
- Diffuse proliferation of lymphoblasts expressing T-lineage markers but not myeloperoxidase, and with no strongly expressed B-lineage markers

Desirable:
- Demonstration of clonal TR rearrangement
- Cytogenetic and mutation analysis showing features of T-ALL/LBL

Staging
Almost all patients have stage III or IV disease {2451,2904} according to Union for International Cancer Control (UICC) or Murphy staging {2034}. Staging requires history; physical examination; complete blood count with differential; bone marrow biopsy with flow cytometric, karyotypic, and molecular genetic analysis; lumbar puncture with cerebrospinal fluid cytology and flow cytometry; LDH; imaging studies; and in males, testicular ultrasound {349}. At presentation, < 10% have CNS involvement and < 5% have testicular involvement {2451,576, 350}. Among patients presenting with an extramedullary mass, marrow involvement is common {576,350}. Although arbitrary, marrow involvement of ≥ 25% is usually used as the threshold to diagnose T-ALL {2034}.

Prognosis and prediction
Optimal treatment is intensive: lymphoblastic leukaemia–type chemotherapy with CNS prophylaxis {576}. Paediatric T-ALL/LBL patients have a 75–90% 5-year event-free survival rate with current treatment; relapse predicts a poor outcome {349,886, 2451,2904}. ETP T-ALL/LBL was previously associated with an inferior prognosis {581}, but with current therapy, prognosis is similar to that of other T-ALL/LBL {349,267}. Detectable minimal residual disease after induction/consolidation is a significant risk factor for relapse {576,166}. An oncogenetic classifier comprising mutations of *NOTCH1/FBXW7* combined with wildtype *RAS/PTEN* helps to identify a favourable prognostic group in both paediatric and adult T-ALLs {2331,3086}. Most deaths are due to tumour progression; a minority are due to complications of therapy or second malignancies {2451,2904}.

Classic Hodgkin lymphoma of the mediastinum

Fend F
Nakamura S

Definition

Classic Hodgkin lymphoma (CHL) is a clonal, malignant B-cell lymphoid proliferation in which a minority of malignant cells with a characteristic immunophenotype, termed Hodgkin/Reed–Sternberg (H/RS) cells, reside in a mixed inflammatory background {2843,1829}.

ICD-O coding

9650/3 Classic Hodgkin lymphoma, NOS
9663/3 Classic Hodgkin lymphoma, nodular sclerosis
9652/3 Classic Hodgkin lymphoma, mixed cellularity
9651/3 Classic Hodgkin lymphoma, lymphocyte-rich
9653/3 Classic Hodgkin lymphoma, lymphocyte depletion

ICD-11 coding

2B30.1 Classical Hodgkin lymphoma

Related terminology

Acceptable: Hodgkin disease.

Subtype(s)

Nodular sclerosis; mixed cellularity; lymphocyte-rich; lymphocyte-depleted

Localization

CHL most commonly involves the anterior (prevascular) mediastinum, including the thymus, as well as cervical, supraclavicular, mediastinal, and hilar lymph nodes {747}. Lung involvement may occur independently {3444}.

Clinical features

Most patients present with painless, frequently indurated lymphadenopathy. Mediastinal involvement may be asymptomatic and detected on a routine chest X-ray or may occur as bulky disease with symptoms related to the local mass, such as dyspnoea or superior vena cava syndrome {747,2354}. Laboratory findings are nonspecific and can include leukocytosis, eosinophilia, and elevated LDH. About 30–40% of patients have B symptoms.

Epidemiology

CHL accounts for about 15–25% of all malignant lymphomas. In the mediastinum, nodular sclerosis classic Hodgkin lymphoma (NSCHL) constitutes 50–70% of all lymphomas, which represent 20% of all mediastinal tumours {2354}. NSCHL shows a slight female preponderance, and it is most prevalent between the ages of 15 and 34 years {969,3031,1294}.

Etiology

The etiology of CHL is unknown, but 20% to almost 100% of cases of CHL are associated with EBV, depending on age, ethnicity, socioeconomic status, subtype, and presence of immunosuppression {3254,2037}. In EBV-positive cases, the virus is present in episomal form in H/RS cells and shows viral type II latency with expression of LMP1, indicating an etiological role of the virus {1126}.

Pathogenesis

H/RS cells are germinal-centre B cells with somatically hypermutated IG genes, absence of immunoglobulin expression, and lack of a B-cell gene expression programme {2843,1829, 2688}. Thymic CHL is thought to originate from specialized thymic B cells {2535,3063,2632}. H/RS cells show constitutive activation of NF-κB and other growth- and survival-promoting signalling pathways and produce a plethora of cytokines and chemokines responsible for the inflammatory infiltrate, systemic symptoms, and generation of a protective microenvironment {2850,2848,1829}.

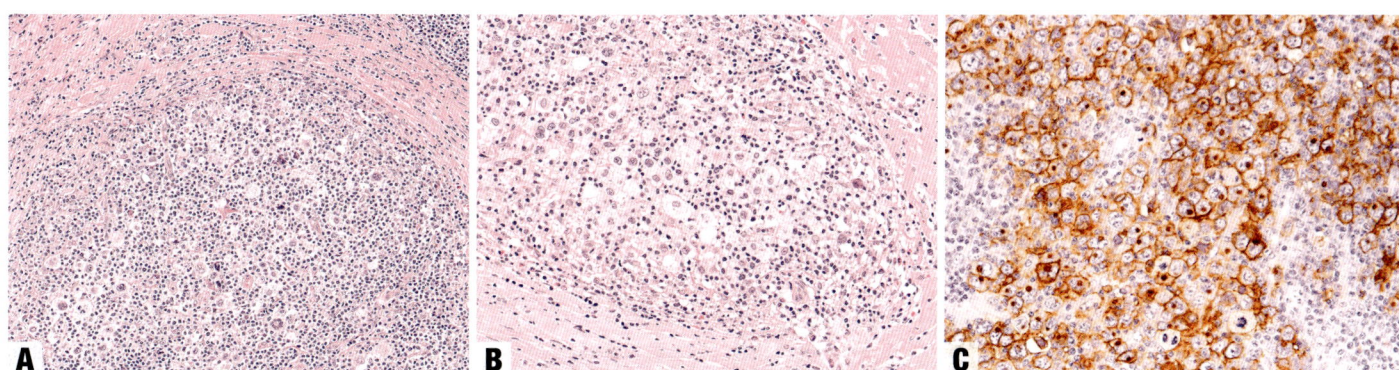

Fig. 7.12 Nodular sclerosis classic Hodgkin lymphoma. **A** A cellular nodule with many typical Hodgkin and Reed–Sternberg cells and inflammatory background. **B** Fibrous bands surround the cellular nodule, with many neoplastic cells, predominantly lacunar cells with ample, clear cytoplasm and sometimes folded nuclei with medium-sized nucleoli. **C** Strong expression of CD30 in Hodgkin/Reed–Sternberg cells.

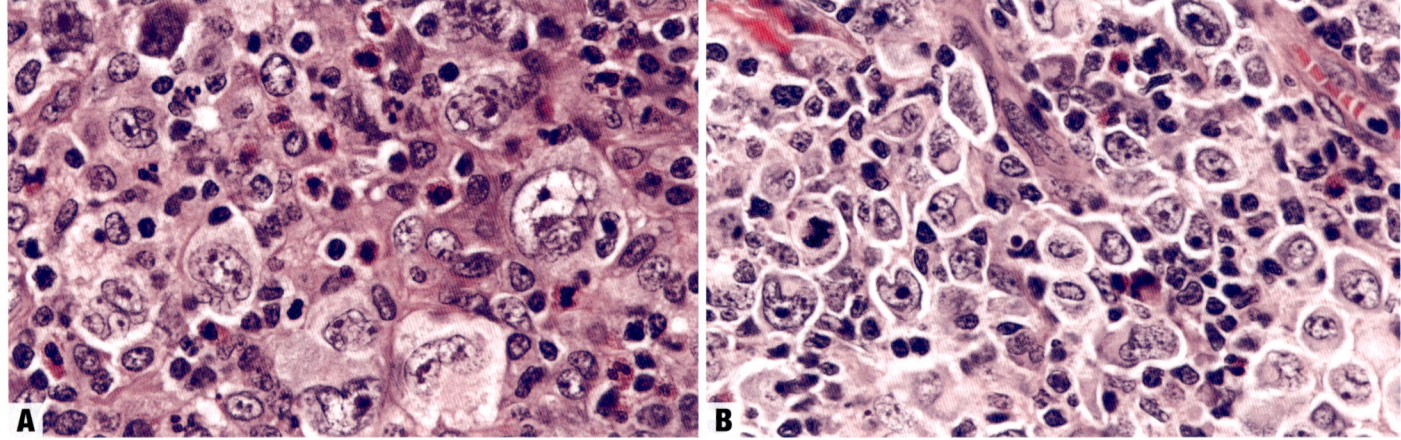

Fig. 7.13 Mediastinal nodular sclerosis classic Hodgkin lymphoma. **A** Lacunar cells and Hodgkin/Reed–Sternberg cells are scattered in a background rich in small lymphocytes, histiocytes, and eosinophils. **B** An example rich in neoplastic cells.

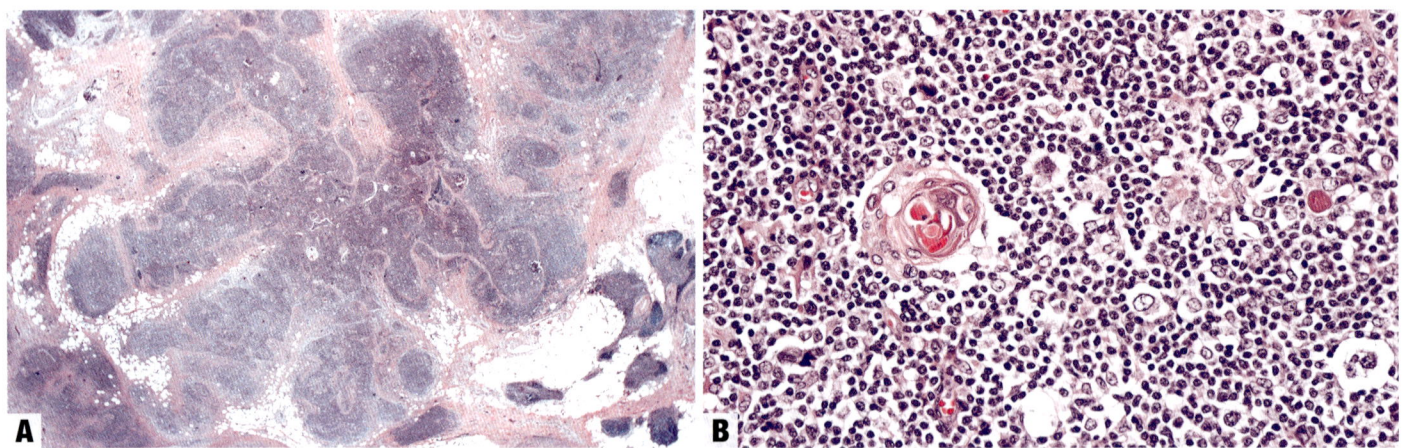

Fig. 7.14 Mediastinal nodular sclerosis classic Hodgkin lymphoma. **A** Low power. This case shows lobulation, with fibrous bands surrounding some of the tumour nodules. **B** High power shows thymic involvement, with tumour surrounding a Hassall corpuscle and showing scattered lacunar Reed–Sternberg cells with multinucleated morphology and prominent nucleoli.

Macroscopic appearance

Lymph nodes involved by CHL may have a nodular appearance, with fibrotic bands and induration in NSCHL. Thymic involvement may manifest as a multilocular cystic mass {1694,1542,2354}.

Histopathology

The main feature of CHL is the presence of pathognomonic H/RS cells and variants in a mixed inflammatory background. Classic Reed–Sternberg cells are binucleated or multinucleated large cells showing nuclei with open chromatin and large, eosinophilic nucleoli and eosinophilic or amphophilic cytoplasm. The mononuclear variant is called a Hodgkin cell. In NSCHL, the dominant neoplastic cell is the lacunar cell, characterized by spiderweb-like retracted cytoplasm surrounded by a clear space, as well as frequently lobulated nuclei with less prominent nucleoli. The frequency of neoplastic cells and the composition of the background may vary significantly, depending on the CHL subtype. The most common subtype is NSCHL, especially in mediastinum, with cellular nodules containing H/RS cells, lymphocytes, eosinophils, neutrophils, and histiocytes, surrounded by dense collagen fibres {749,2941}. Necrosis and microabscesses are frequent. Cases with dominant fibrosis and rare neoplastic elements may present a diagnostic challenge, especially in core needle biopsies {2788,27}.

Immunohistochemistry

The most useful immunophenotypic markers for H/RS cells are CD30 and CD15, which are positive in almost 100% and 75–85% of cases, respectively. H/RS cells typically show weak to moderate positivity for PAX5, whereas other B-cell markers, including CD20 and the transcription factors OCT2 and BOB1, are either negative or weakly positive in a minority of tumour cells. They express IRF4 (MUM1) and fascin. LMP1 is expressed in EBV-positive cases, with NSCHL showing a positivity rate of 10–25%. CD45, ALK, and EMA are negative {749}. PDL1 expression is activated by genetic alterations and represents a potential therapeutic target {2513,2597,3204}. The background lymphoid population in NSCHL shows a dominance of CD4+ T cells {76}.

Differential diagnosis

H/RS-like cells can occur in a variety of non-Hodgkin lymphomas and reactive conditions, including EBV-associated lymphoid proliferations {717,716}. In the mediastinum, the presence

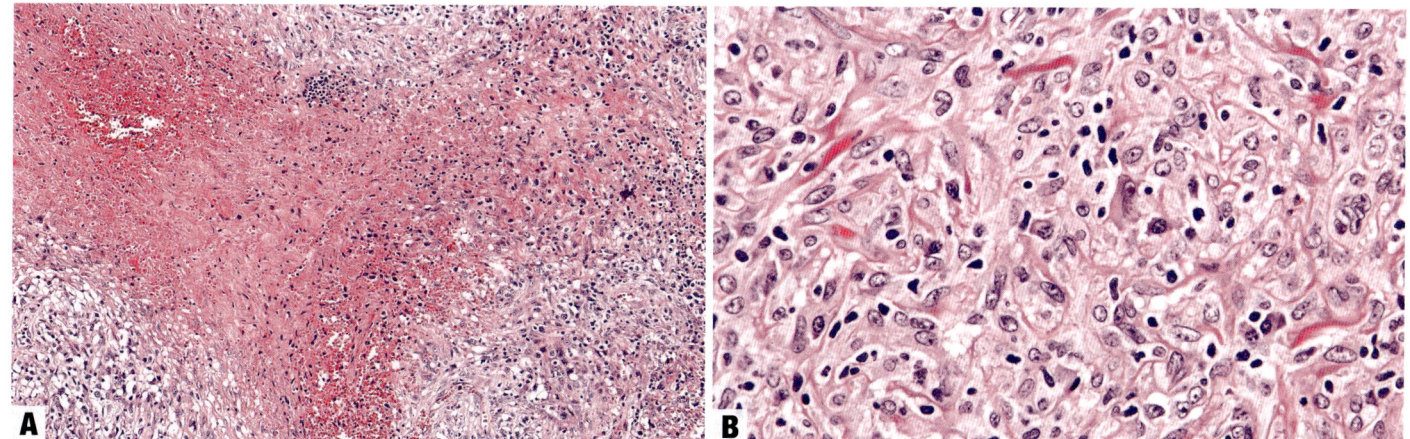

Fig. 7.15 Mediastinal nodular sclerosis classic Hodgkin lymphoma. **A** Geographical coagulative necrosis may be present. **B** So-called fibrohistiocytic pattern, characterized by large neoplastic cells accompanied by numerous spindly fibrohistiocytic cells.

of sheets of tumour cells with a preserved B-cell programme raises the differential diagnosis of primary mediastinal large B-cell lymphoma or mediastinal grey zone lymphoma {1077, 2632,2633,3063}. Cases with distinct, separate areas of both CHL and primary mediastinal large B-cell lymphoma should be diagnosed as composite lymphoma.

Cytology
FNA specimens show H/RS cells in a mixed inflammatory background, but cytology and flow cytometry are of limited use for diagnosis of CHL {3185}.

Diagnostic molecular pathology
Molecular studies are not required and are currently of limited diagnostic use. Although the presence of a major clonal B-cell or T-cell population argues against a CHL diagnosis, clonal B-cell populations can be detected in a substantial percentage of CHL cases by sensitive PCR techniques {337,536}.

Essential and desirable diagnostic criteria
Essential:
- Scattered H/RS cells with typical immunophenotype (CD30+, CD15+/–, PAX5+ [weak], CD20–/+, ALK–)
- An appropriate inflammatory background

Staging
Staging is performed according to the Lugano classification and relevant for the selection of therapy {492}. About 75–80% of patients present with stage I or II; the spleen is involved in 10% of all cases, and bone marrow involvement is rare (< 5%) {2028,2477}.

Prognosis and prediction
With modern chemotherapy regimens, 80–90% of patients with CHL can be cured {2715}. Stage is the most important predictor of outcome, but complete remission is also achieved in the majority of stage IV patients, and avoidance of complications (including second neoplasms) is of major importance. Neither the histological subtype nor the many investigated biological and histological parameters are relevant for prognostication in clinical practice {3145,1462}.

Mediastinal grey zone lymphoma

Rosenwald A
Campo E
Nakamura S

Definition

Mediastinal grey zone lymphoma (MGZL) is an otherwise unclassifiable B-cell lymphoma with features intermediate between diffuse large B-cell lymphoma (DLBCL) and classic Hodgkin lymphoma (CHL).

ICD-O coding

9596/3 Grey zone lymphoma

ICD-11 coding

2A86.Y Other specified B-cell lymphoma, mixed features

Related terminology

Acceptable: B-cell lymphoma, unclassifiable, with features intermediate between DLBCL and CHL.

Not recommended: Hodgkin-like anaplastic large cell lymphoma (obsolete).

Subtype(s)

None

Localization

The most common presentation is a large anterior (prevascular) mediastinal mass, with or without involvement of the supraclavicular lymph nodes. Other peripheral lymph node groups are less commonly involved. There may be spread to the lung by direct extension, as well as spread to the liver, spleen, and (less commonly) bone marrow. Non-lymphoid organs are rarely involved, unlike in primary mediastinal large B-cell lymphoma (PMBCL) {743}.

Clinical features

Most patients present with a large mediastinal mass, which may be associated with superior vena cava syndrome. The mass may cause tracheal compression and respiratory distress {910,3063}.

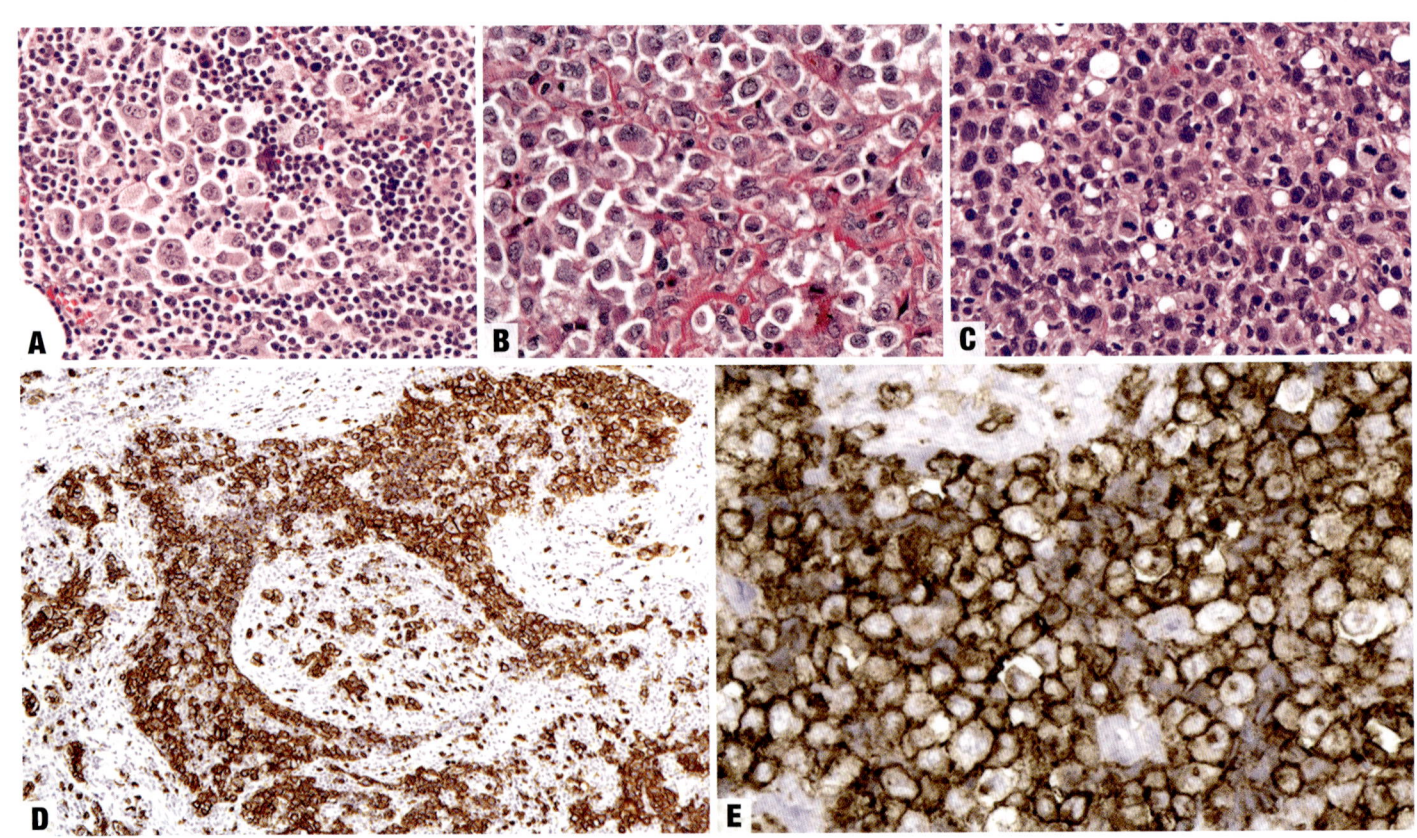

Fig. 7.16 Mediastinal grey zone lymphoma, thymus gland. **A** Large aggregates of atypical cells, some of which resemble lacunar cells. However, CD20 was strongly and uniformly positive. **B** The lymphoma is composed of sheets of cells with clear cytoplasm and fine sclerosis. The appearance resembles that of primary mediastinal large B-cell lymphoma. **C** There is a sheet-like growth of pleomorphic lymphoid cells. Some binucleated cells are present, but there is marked variation in cell size and shape. The biopsy was taken from a 28-year-old man with a mediastinal mass and supraclavicular lymph node involvement. **D** The neoplastic cells are strongly and uniformly positive for CD20. **E** The tumour cells are strongly CD15-positive and also CD30-positive (not shown).

Epidemiology

The epidemiology of MGZL is similar to that of nodular sclerosis classic Hodgkin lymphoma (NSCHL), except that MGZL is more common in males than females {910,3063}. MGZL usually occurs in patients aged 20–40 years. Cases occurring outside the mediastinum are seen in older patients {751}. Most cases have been reported from North America. Like NSCHL, the disease appears to be less common in black people and Asians.

Etiology

The etiology is unknown. Like NSCHL, MGZL is infrequently positive for EBV {910,3063}, and EBV positivity should prompt suspicion for EBV-positive DLBCL {2350}.

Pathogenesis

Clonal IG gene rearrangement is often positive. The tumour cells show many of the genetic aberrations reported in PMBCL and NSCHL. {2849}. In particular, gains at 2p16.1 (*REL* locus) and alterations at 9p24.1 involving the *JAK2/PDCD1LG2* (*PD-L2*) locus are common {751}. Increased expression of PDL1 (CD274) may occur as a result. Genetic and epigenetic profiling shows differences from both CHL and PMBCL {750,3149}.

Macroscopic appearance

The tumour has a tan, fish-flesh appearance, often with extensive areas of necrosis. Areas of fibrosis may also be present.

Histopathology

The tumour is composed of a confluent, sheet-like growth of pleomorphic tumour cells in a diffusely fibrotic stroma. Focal fibrous bands may be seen in some cases. The cells are larger and more pleomorphic than in the typical case of PMBCL, although some centroblast-like cells may be present. Pleomorphic cells resembling lacunar cells and Hodgkin cells are readily seen. A characteristic feature is the broad spectrum of cytological appearances, with different areas of the tumour showing variations in cytological appearance. The background inflammatory infiltrate is less evident than in NSCHL, although scattered eosinophils, lymphocytes, and histiocytes may be present. Necrosis is usually evident {910,3063}.

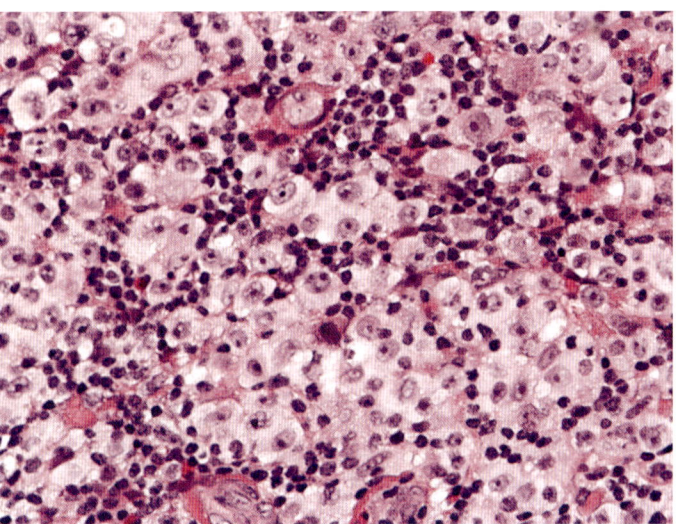

Fig. 7.17 Mediastinal grey zone lymphoma, thymus gland. Sheets of tumour cells resembling lacunar cells are present, with a minimal inflammatory background.

Immunohistochemistry

On immunohistochemical stains, the B-cell programme is often preserved, with expression of both CD20 and CD79a. Both CD30 and IRF4 (MUM1) are usually positive, but CD15 is less commonly expressed. Surface and cytoplasmic immunoglobulins are absent. The transcription factors PAX5, OCT2, and BOB1 are usually positive. BCL6 is variable, and CD10 and ALK are negative. The background lymphocytes are predominantly CD3/CD4-positive, as seen in CHL.

The spectrum of MGZL ranges from cases with a morphology more closely related to CHL but showing a strong B-cell phenotype to cases in which morphology is more closely related to DLBCL but with a CHL-like immunophenotype {2632}. The diagnosis of MGZL should be considered only if the criteria for the diagnosis of other entities (especially CHL and EBV-positive DLBCL) are not met {2350}.

Cytology

Cytological features are not reliable for distinguishing this tumour from other mediastinal lymphomas.

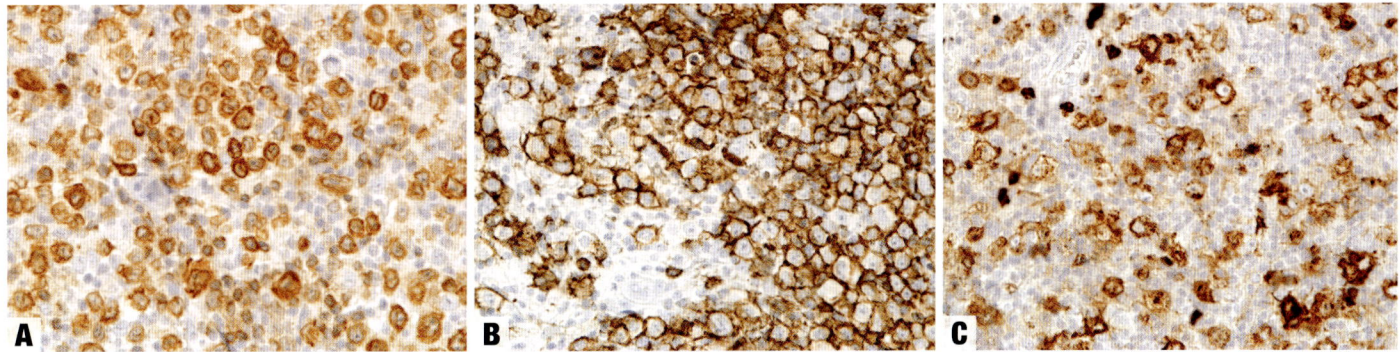

Fig. 7.18 Mediastinal grey zone lymphoma, thymus gland. **A** CD79a is uniformly positive. **B** The tumour cells are strongly positive for CD20. **C** CD15 is positive, but the sheet-like growth and strong staining for CD20 and CD79a favour mediastinal grey zone lymphoma.

Diagnostic molecular pathology

IG gene rearrangement is usually present.

Essential and desirable diagnostic criteria

Essential:
- Pleomorphic cells resembling lacunar and Hodgkin cells
- Expression of B-cell antigens

Desirable:
- CD30 positivity

Staging

Staging is done according to the Lugano classification {492}.

Prognosis and prediction

These lymphomas generally have a more aggressive clinical course and worse outcome than either CHL or PMBCL. There is no consensus on the optimal treatment, although there is evidence that combined-modality treatment is required, with both chemotherapy and radiation therapy used for patients with a residual PET-positive mass at the completion of the chemotherapy regimen {743,3322}.

Follicular dendritic cell sarcoma of the mediastinum

Pileri SA
Chan JKC

Definition

Follicular dendritic cell (FDC) sarcoma is a neoplasm showing the morphological and phenotypic characteristics of FDCs, which are stromal-derived cells normally found in the germinal centres.

ICD-O coding

9758/3 Follicular dendritic cell sarcoma

ICD-11 coding

2B31.5 Follicular dendritic cell sarcoma

Related terminology

Acceptable: follicular dendritic cell tumour.

Subtype(s)

None

Localization

In a comprehensive review of the literature, 75 of 343 FDC sarcomas affected thoracic structures (mediastinal nodes: 21; lung: 31; mediastinum: 20; chest wall: 2; pleura: 1) {2647}.

Clinical features

Most patients present with a localized slow-growing mass, which over time can produce chest discomfort, mediastinal syndrome, or shortness of breath {2647}. Occasionally, patients have paraneoplastic pemphigus {790}.

Epidemiology

FDC sarcoma is a rare disease that more often affects adults (median age: 50 years), with no sex predilection {2323A,2647, 609}.

Etiology

A proportion of cases develop in the setting of hyaline-vascular Castleman disease, which can co-occur with or precede FDC sarcoma {2349,790,3174}. In concurrent cases, possible transition from hyaline-vascular Castleman disease to FDC sarcoma can be seen with proliferation of dysplastic FDCs outside the hyaline-vascular follicles {790,3174}.

Pathogenesis

IGHV and TR are occasionally clonally rearranged {481}. *BRAF* p.V600E mutation is found in a small proportion of cases {975}. Limited cytogenetic studies showed a complex karyotype {2325}. Next-generation sequencing has revealed recurrent alterations in NF-κB regulatory genes {1009}. Studies on transcriptional profile have shown (1) highly specific expression of the genes encoding FDCSP and SRGN and (2) a microenvironment enriched in T follicular helper (TFH) cell and T regulatory (Treg) cell populations, with special reference to the inhibitory receptor PD1 and its ligands PDL1 and PDL2 {1584,1735}.

Macroscopic appearance

FDC sarcoma has a fleshy appearance with no distinctive features.

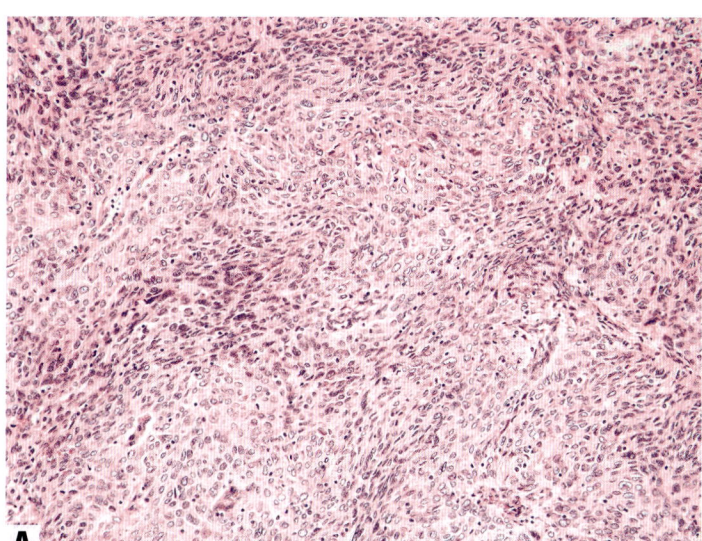
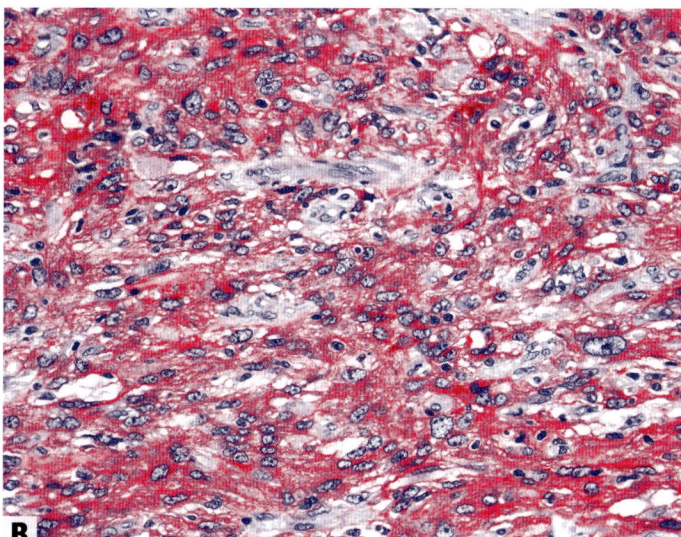

Fig. 7.19 Follicular dendritic cell sarcoma. **A** Spindle-ovoid neoplastic cells show indistinct cytoplasmic borders and oval nuclei with finely dispersed chromatin arranged in fascicles, storiform arrays, and whorls. **B** The spindle-ovoid neoplastic cells express CD21 antigen immunohistochemically.

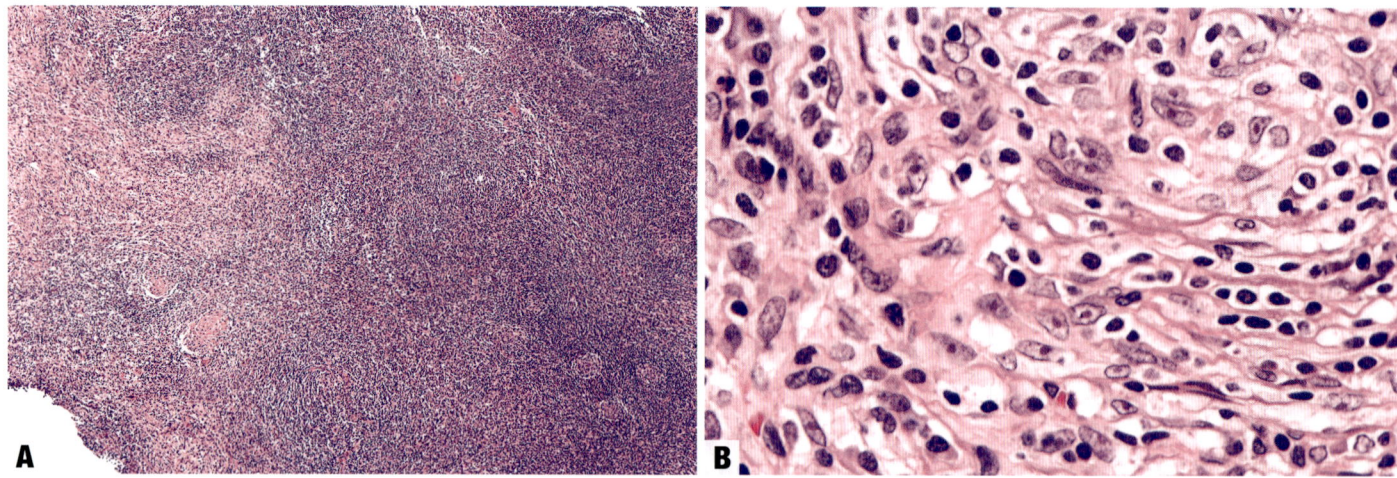

Fig. 7.20 Mediastinal follicular dendritic cell sarcoma, arising in hyaline-vascular Castleman disease. **A** Hyaline-vascular Castleman disease is evident in the right side of the field, and the follicular dendritic cell sarcoma is evident on the left. **B** The follicular dendritic cell sarcoma comprises spindly cells with indistinct cell borders, elongated nuclei with vesicular chromatin, and distinct nucleoli. There are typically intermingled small lymphocytes.

Histopathology

FDC sarcoma consists of spindled-ovoid cells forming fascicles, storiform arrays, whorls, diffuse sheets, or vague nodules. The neoplastic cells usually have indistinct borders, a moderate amount of eosinophilic cytoplasm, and oval or elongated nuclei, with finely dispersed chromatin, small but distinct nucleoli, and a delicate nuclear membrane. Nuclear pseudoinclusions and multinucleated tumour cells are common. Ultrastructurally, tumour cells display long processes connected by scattered desmosomes {2349}. Some cases can show significant cytological atypia, high mitotic counts, atypical mitoses, and coagulative necrosis. The tumour is typically infiltrated by small lymphocytes. Occasionally, neoplastic cells are scattered singly in a background of small lymphocytes, mimicking Hodgkin lymphoma. Rare cases may show jigsaw puzzle–like lobulation and perivascular spaces, mimicking thymoma or carcinoma showing thymus-like elements {2349,2167,609,790}. Other differential diagnoses include interdigitating dendritic cell sarcoma, Langerhans cell sarcoma, classic Hodgkin lymphoma, thymoma, carcinoma showing thymus-like elements, peripheral nerve sheath tumour, and melanoma {2349,609,790}.

Immunohistochemistry

The neoplastic cells are positive for one or more of the FDC markers CD21, CD23, CD35, CXCL13, and podoplanin, and new FDC markers such as FDCSP and SRGN. Expression of clusterin, desmoplakin, vimentin, fascin, EGFR, and HLA-DR is usually observed. Variable positivity for EMA, S100, and CD68 can be present, and exceptionally for CD20, CD45, CD30, or cytokeratins. PDL1 is commonly expressed. CD1a, lysozyme, myeloperoxidase, CD34, CD3, CD79a, and HMB45 are negative {2349,3168,2167,609,790}. The Ki-67 index ranges from 1% to 25%. The admixed small lymphocytes include mixed B cells and T cells.

Cytology

Not clinically relevant

Diagnostic molecular pathology

Not clinically relevant

Essential and desirable diagnostic criteria

Essential:

- Spindly-ovoid cell tumour with variable growth pattern and intermingled small lymphocytes
- Extensive immunophenotyping to demonstrate one or more FDC markers (CD21, CD23, CD35, CXCL13, podoplanin, FDCSP, and SRGN)

Staging

FDC sarcoma is usually localized at presentation {2647}. No staging system has been adopted.

Prognosis and prediction

FDC sarcoma usually follows an indolent course. Most patients are treated by surgical excision with or without radiotherapy and/or chemotherapy. Local recurrences and metastases are recorded in 50% and 25% of patients, respectively, with 10–20% of them ultimately dying of FDC sarcoma {2349,2647, 609,608,790}. Cases showing significant cytological atypia, extensive coagulative necrosis, high proliferation, and tumour size > 60 mm can run a rapidly fatal course {2349}.

Myeloid sarcoma of the mediastinum

Orazi A
Pileri SA

Definition

Myeloid sarcoma is a mass-forming neoplastic proliferation of myeloblasts with or without maturation, occurring in an extramedullary site. Interstitial infiltration of myeloid blasts without a nodular mass is termed extramedullary acute myeloid leukaemia.

ICD-O coding

9930/3 Myeloid sarcoma

ICD-11 coding

2A60.39 Myeloid sarcoma

Related terminology

Acceptable: granulocytic sarcoma.
Not recommended: extramedullary myeloid cell tumour; chloroma.

Subtype(s)

None

Localization

Most documented cases arose in the anterior (prevascular) mediastinum.

Clinical features

Mediastinal myeloid sarcoma has been reported in association with superior vena cava syndrome {2418,2441}. Most mediastinal cases occur simultaneously with acute myeloid leukaemia or are followed shortly by acute myeloid leukaemia. All patients who presented with primary mediastinal myeloid sarcoma without concurrent acute myeloid leukaemia eventually relapsed with frank leukaemia if not given systemic therapy {525}.

Epidemiology

In a large series of myeloid sarcomas, a mediastinal location was seen in approximately 21% of the cases {1409}.

Etiology

The etiology is the same as that of acute myeloid leukaemia and myeloid sarcoma occurring in other locations. Most cases arise de novo, but some may be therapy-related {539}. Rare cases have been reported in association with mediastinal germ cell tumours and those may share a common germ cell precursor {2202}. Some cases transform from myeloproliferative neoplasm, myelodysplastic/myeloproliferative neoplasm, or myelodysplastic syndrome {1409}.

Pathogenesis

The pathogenesis of mediastinal myeloid sarcoma is the same as that of acute myeloid leukaemia and myeloid sarcoma occurring in other locations.

Macroscopic appearance

Macroscopically, there is a tumour mass in the anterior (prevascular) mediastinum.

Histopathology

The most common type of mediastinal myeloid sarcoma is granulocytic sarcoma {3369}, a tumour composed of myeloblasts and promyelocytes. The degree of maturation varies in different cases. The blastic tumours are entirely composed of

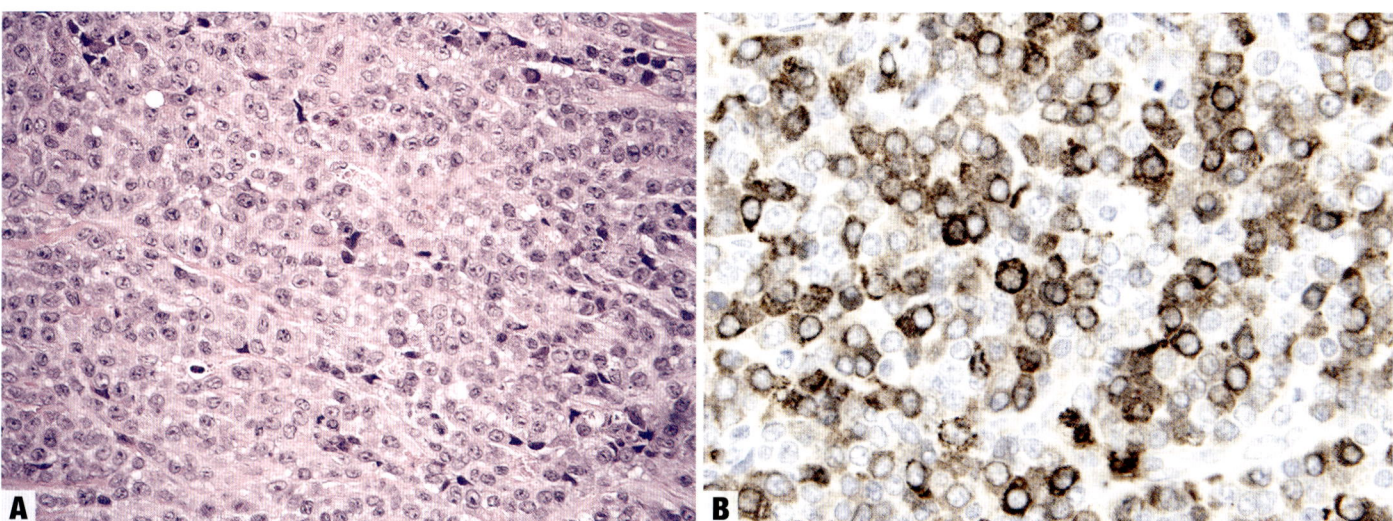

Fig. 7.21 Mediastinal myeloid sarcoma. **A** Note a diffuse proliferation of poorly differentiated myeloblasts. In the absence of immunohistochemistry confirming myeloid lineage, the histological appearance could easily be mistaken for that of a large cell lymphoma. **B** The neoplastic cells show granular cytoplasmic staining for myeloperoxidase.

Chapter 7

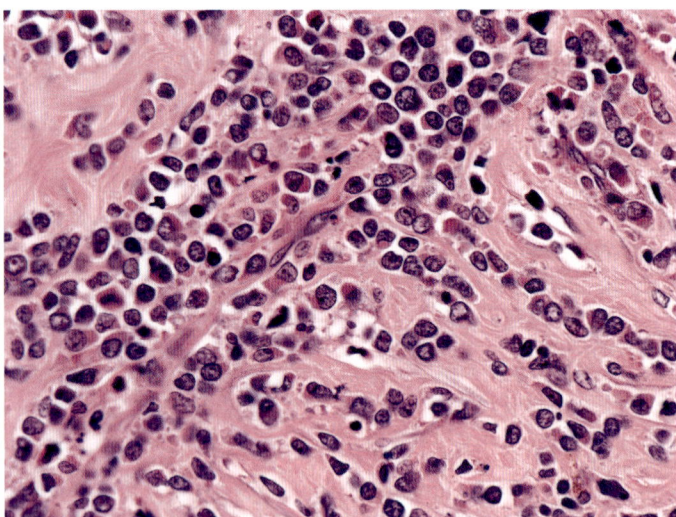

Fig. 7.22 Mediastinal myeloid sarcoma. This example shows prominent sclerosis, mimicking mediastinal large cell lymphoma. Some of the neoplastic cells show fine eosinophilic cytoplasmic granules.

myeloblasts; in the more differentiated tumours, promyelocytes are also present {2941}. Cases composed of monoblasts and/or promonocytes (monoblastic sarcoma), can also occur in this location. Cases associated with acute transformation of an underlying myeloproliferative neoplasm may show areas containing a preponderance of mature myeloid cells (e.g. granulocytes) or foci of trilineage extramedullary haematopoiesis in association with the blastic proliferation. Some cases can show prominent sclerosis.

Cytochemistry and immunophenotype
The histochemical stain for CAE is helpful in identifying promyelocytes present in better-differentiated cases of myeloid sarcoma. Flow cytometry is also useful in demonstrating myeloid antigen expression. Paraffin-reactive markers helpful in confirming the diagnosis include CD34, KIT (CD117), lysozyme, myeloperoxidase, CD33, CD43, and CD68, as well as CD61/CD42b for megakaryoblastic differentiation and CD71/E-cadherin for erythroid differentiation. The lack of expression of lymphoid-associated antigens helps in the differential diagnosis with lymphoma. If blastic plasmacytoid dendritic cell tumour is

under consideration, then CD123, TCL1 (and/or CD303), CD4, and CD56 must be added.

Differential diagnosis
The major differential diagnoses are with non-Hodgkin lymphomas, especially lymphoblastic lymphoma, and diffuse large cell lymphoma; in children, the differential diagnosis also includes various metastatic small round cell tumours. Cases with prominent sclerosis may mimic primary mediastinal (thymic) large B-cell lymphoma.

Cytology
Blasts can be identified in touch preparation or in FNA material.

Diagnostic molecular pathology
A significant proportion of mediastinal myeloid sarcomas have complex cytogenetic abnormalities {2418}. Most of the complex cytogenetic abnormalities occurring in acute myeloid leukaemia can also be seen {2346}.

Essential and desirable diagnostic criteria
Essential:
- Mass-forming infiltrate of myeloblasts or monoblasts with or without maturation

Desirable:
- Cytogenetics and molecular genetic tests, following the usual guidelines for diagnosis of patients with acute myeloid leukaemia as outlined in the 2017 volume on tumours of haematopoietic and lymphoid tissues {2941}

Staging
Not clinically relevant

Prognosis and prediction
Mediastinal myeloid sarcoma is an aggressive disease. Patients treated with local irradiation only (before developing acute myeloid leukaemia) eventually all relapsed with frank leukaemia and died soon after {525}. In contrast, patients who were considered to have acute myeloid leukaemia and given upfront systemic chemotherapy had better outcomes, their prognosis being that associated with the underlying leukaemia {525}. Allogeneic bone marrow transplantation is the only available potentially curative treatment {1639,1409,1613}.

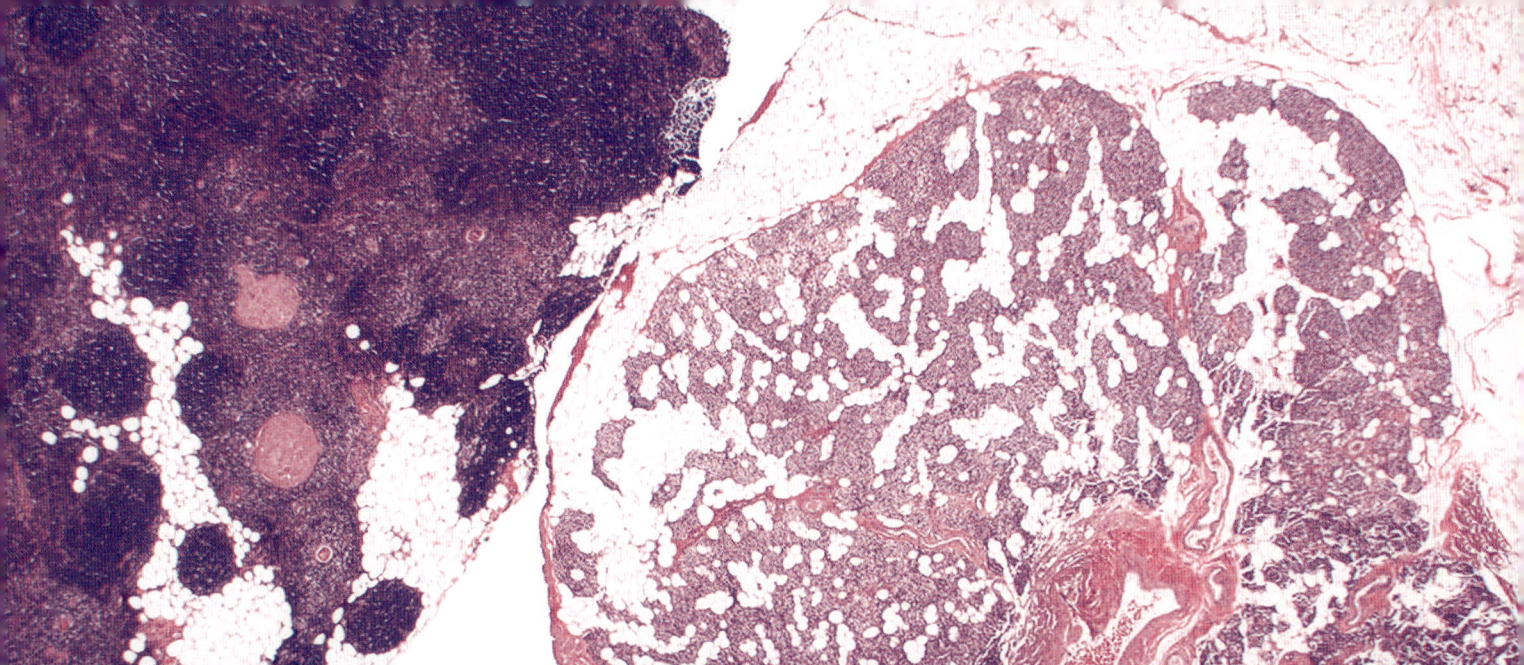

8

Ectopic tumours of thyroid and parathyroid origin

Edited by: Chan JKC, Marx A

Ectopic thyroid tumours
Ectopic parathyroid tumours

Ectopic thyroid tumours

Weissferdt A
Chalabreysse L
Weis CA

Definition
Ectopic thyroid tumours are those neoplasms of thyroid origin that occur in sites other than their typical location in the anterior neck.

ICD-O coding
8260/3 Papillary carcinoma of thyroid
8330/0 Follicular adenoma
8330/3 Follicular carcinoma
8345/3 Medullary thyroid carcinoma

ICD-11 coding
2F9A Neoplasms of unknown behaviour of endocrine glands

Related terminology
None

Subtype(s)
None

Localization
Ectopic thyroid tumours are most commonly found in the anterior (prevascular) and superior mediastinum.

Clinical features
Ectopic thyroid tumours may be incidental lesions, or patients can present with signs and symptoms related to compression of adjacent anatomical structures, such as chest pain, shortness of breath, or cough.

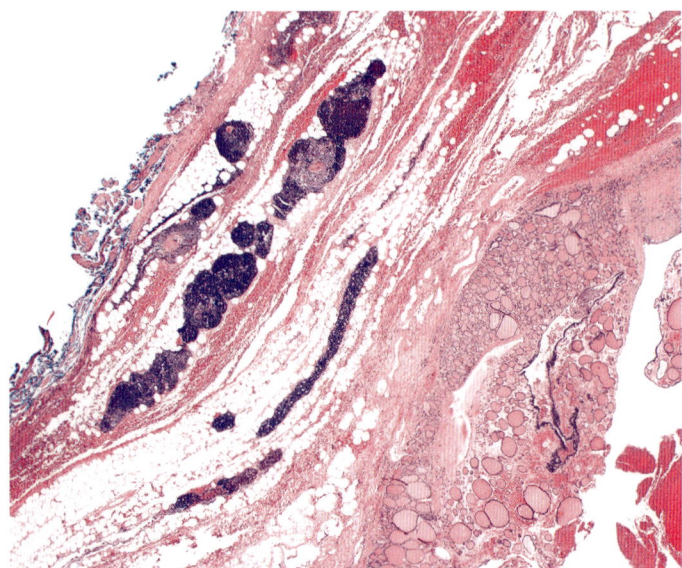

Fig. 8.01 Ectopic goitre. Low-power view of a retrosternal goitre (right) in the anterior (prevascular) mediastinum. Note the rim of thymic tissue (left).

Epidemiology
Ectopic thyroid tissue in the mediastinum is very rare. The most common lesion of thyroid origin is retrosternal goitre, followed by follicular adenoma. Malignant transformation to papillary, follicular, or medullary thyroid carcinoma is uncommon and typically occurs in ectopic goitres {2740,2090}. In most cases of ectopic thyroid tissue, a thin connection to the orthotopic thyroid gland in the neck can be identified. Mediastinal thyroid lesions without connection to the thyroid proper are exceedingly rare.

Etiology
The etiology is unknown, but it is likely to be similar to that of orthotopic thyroid neoplasms.

Pathogenesis
Ectopic mediastinal thyroid tissue and resultant tumours develop from aberrant migration of the thyroid anlage to the mediastinum during embryological descent. The exact reason that thyroid lesions develop in these embryological rests is uncertain.

Macroscopic appearance
Ectopic thyroid lesions are typically well-demarcated and circumscribed lesions, especially those that are benign. Substernal goitres often have a nodular, semitranslucent and tan-brown cut surface, which can demonstrate areas of fibrosis, haemorrhage, and cystic degeneration. Malignant ectopic thyroid tumours, on the other hand, show more infiltrative growth, with or without extension into adjacent anatomical structures, as well as areas of haemorrhage and necrosis.

Histopathology
The cytological, histopathological, and molecular features of ectopic thyroid lesions in the mediastinum closely resemble those of the thyroid gland proper, and nomenclature and diagnostic criteria should follow the *WHO classification of tumours of endocrine organs* {1718}. As mentioned above, substernal goitre is the most common ectopic thyroid lesion, followed by follicular adenoma {2740,2090}. Papillary, follicular, and medullary thyroid carcinomas are the most common malignant tumours in this context {1933,2224,2344,2882,3219}. Immunohistochemically, thyroid tumours of follicular origin are positive for pancytokeratin, thyroglobulin, TTF1, and PAX8, while medullary thyroid carcinomas are positive for chromogranin A and calcitonin and variably positive for TTF1 and PAX8. Malignant ectopic thyroid tumours may be difficult to differentiate from primary thymic carcinomas, especially neuroendocrine carcinomas, due to similar histopathological and immunohistochemical features. In addition, a metastatic process to the thymus must always be excluded by close clinical and radiological correlation.

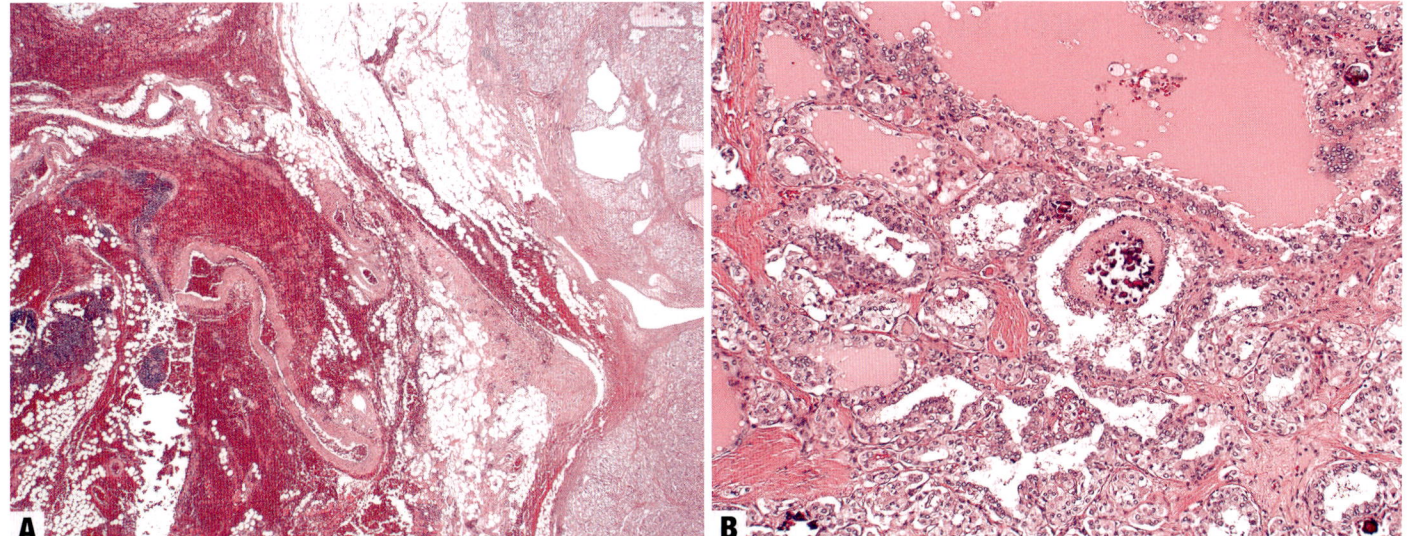

Fig. 8.02 Ectopic papillary thyroid carcinoma. **A** Ectopic papillary thyroid carcinoma arising in the anterior (prevascular) mediastinum. **B** The tumour shows the typical papillary architecture and contains numerous psammoma bodies.

Cytology
There are insufficient cytology data.

Diagnostic molecular pathology
Diagnostic molecular pathology is not clinically relevant in most cases (see the *WHO classification of tumours of endocrine organs* volume {1718}).

Essential and desirable diagnostic criteria
Essential:
- Thyroid tumour ectopic to the normal location of the thyroid gland
- Diagnosis according to standard criteria for goitre or WHO criteria for papillary, follicular, or medullary carcinoma or follicular adenoma (see the *WHO classification of tumours of endocrine organs* volume {1718})

Desirable:
- Immunohistochemical staining for TTF1, PAX8, and thyroglobulin is typically positive for follicular neoplasms; for medullary carcinoma, calcitonin and CEA are typically positive, with variable TTF1 positivity, and PAX8 is typically negative; Congo red staining is positive in medullary carcinoma when amyloid stroma is present

Staging
Like other thyroid tumours, ectopic thyroid tumours should be staged according to the eighth-edition Union for International Cancer Control (UICC) TNM classification, when applicable.

Prognosis and prediction
Although information on the prognosis and outcome of ectopic thyroid tumours in the mediastinum is limited, their biological behaviour probably resembles that of their orthotopic counterparts {3300}.

Ectopic parathyroid tumours

Weissferdt A
Chalabreysse L
Weis CA

Definition

Ectopic parathyroid tumours are those neoplasms of parathyroid origin that occur in sites other than their typical location in the neck.

ICD-O coding

8140/0 Parathyroid adenoma
8140/3 Parathyroid carcinoma

ICD-11 coding

2F9A Neoplasms of unknown behaviour of endocrine glands

Related terminology

None

Subtype(s)

None

Localization

Most ectopic parathyroid lesions occur in the anterior (prevascular) and/or superior mediastinum close to the thymic gland or the great vessels. Posterior (paravertebral) mediastinal locations have also been described.

Clinical features

The majority of mediastinal parathyroid neoplasms are functional tumours, and patients present with signs and symptoms of hyperparathyroidism (hypercalcaemia, weakness, nephrolithiasis, myalgia, polyuria, polydipsia, and osteoporosis). Patients with non-functional tumours are usually asymptomatic and the lesions are found incidentally {3194,1981,2576,2536}.

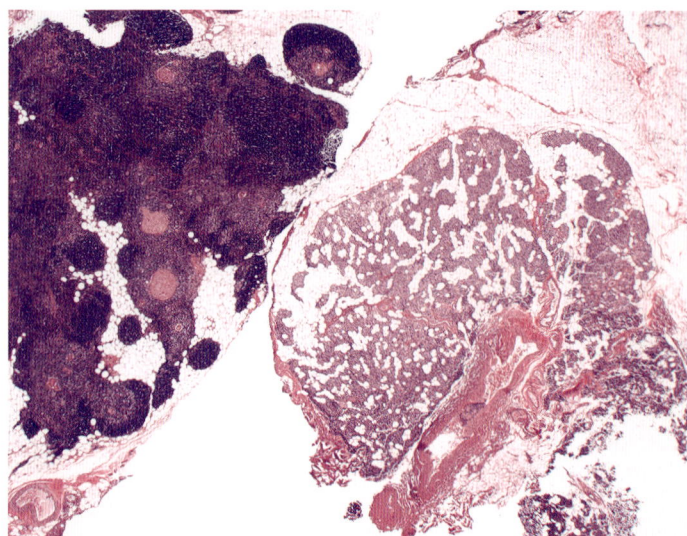

Fig. 8.03 Ectopic parathyroid tissue. Ectopic parathyroid gland (right) in close association with the thymus (left).

Epidemiology

Ectopic parathyroid glands in the mediastinum are estimated to occur in 3–4% of the population, and parathyroid neoplasms have been reported in 1.2–14% of affected individuals {3194, 2231,1071}.

Etiology

The etiology is unknown, but it is likely to be similar to that of orthotopic parathyroid neoplasms.

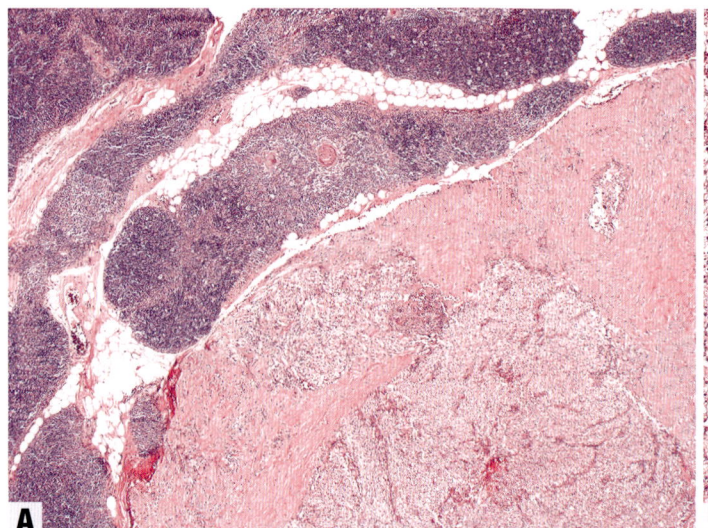

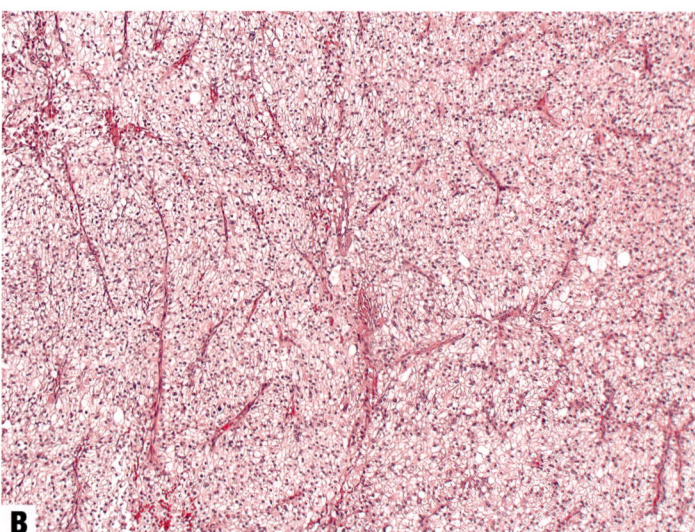

Fig. 8.04 Ectopic parathyroid carcinoma. **A** The tumour (right) is seen in close association with the thymic gland (left). **B** The tumour is composed of sheets of polygonal cells with clear cell features. It is accompanied by a rich vasculature.

Pathogenesis

Ectopic parathyroid gland tissue is thought to be the result of misplacement of the inferior parathyroid glands during embryological development. The common origin of ectopic parathyroid tumours from the third branchial pouch is attributed to its close association with the thymic gland {570,2739,2080}. Ectopic parathyroid glands may also represent supernumerary glands that may remain clinically unsuspected.

Macroscopic appearance

Mediastinal parathyroid adenomas are usually well-circumscribed tumours that range in size from 20 to 60 mm and have a tan-brown homogeneous cut surface without a demonstrable fatty component. Parathyroid carcinomas are typically larger tumours (up to 150 mm); show more invasive growth; and often contain areas of haemorrhage, calcification, and necrosis {1981}.

Histopathology

Mediastinal parathyroid adenomas generally consist of monotonous tumour cells arranged in solid sheets, cords, acini, follicles, or microcysts traversed by a delicate vascular network. Individual tumour cells are round and have uniform nuclei and eosinophilic (chief cells) to clear (water clear cells) or granular eosinophilic (oxyphilic cells) cytoplasm. In some cases, nuclear pleomorphism can be seen, but mitoses should be absent {1981}. Mediastinal parathyroid carcinomas are usually infiltrative tumours characterized by fibrous bands, areas of necrosis, and mitotic activity. Nuclear atypia can be highly variable, ranging from minimal to significant {1981}. Immunohistochemically, ectopic parathyroid neoplasms express pancytokeratin, synaptophysin, and chromogranin A {778}. In addition, staining for PTH is a valuable and important tool to confirm the diagnosis.

Loss of staining for parafibromin favours a diagnosis of parathyroid carcinoma over parathyroid adenoma {778,2981}. The differential diagnosis primarily includes thymic neuroendocrine carcinomas and ectopic medullary thyroid carcinoma. Demonstration of PTH in the tumour by immunohistochemistry usually aids in confirming the diagnosis.

Cytology

Not clinically relevant

Diagnostic molecular pathology

Not clinically relevant

Essential and desirable diagnostic criteria

Essential:

- Parathyroid tumour ectopic to the normal location of the parathyroid glands
- Diagnosis according to WHO criteria for parathyroid adenoma and carcinoma (see the *WHO classification of tumours of endocrine organs* volume {1718})

Desirable:

- PTH is a valuable and important tool to confirm the diagnosis

Staging

Like other parathyroid tumours, ectopic parathyroid neoplasms should be staged according to the eighth-edition Union for International Cancer Control (UICC) TNM classification, when applicable (i.e. carcinoma).

Prognosis and prediction

While ectopic parathyroid adenomas are benign tumours that are treated by complete surgical resection, ectopic parathyroid carcinomas have the potential to recur and metastasize {1981,1219}.

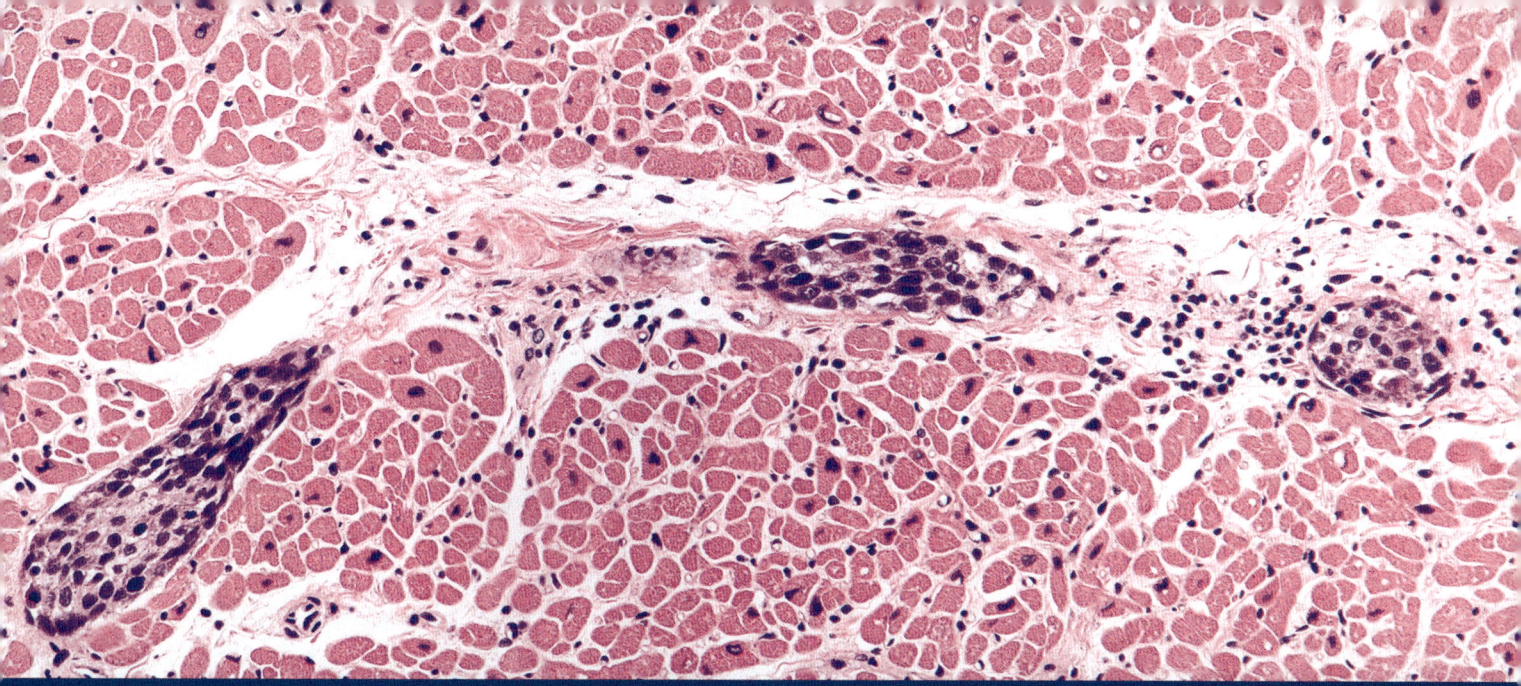

9

Metastases

Edited by: Kerr KM, Maleszewski JJ, Marx A, Nicholson AG, Travis WD

Metastasis to the lung
Metastasis to the pleura
Metastasis to the thymus and mediastinal lymph nodes
Metastasis to the heart and pericardium

Metastasis to the lung

Joubert P
Chang JC
Glass C
Hiroshima K
Lin DM

Padera RF
Poleri C
Sholl LM
Soares FA

Definition
Metastasis to the lung represents a malignancy that has spread to the lung from an extrapulmonary site of origin.

ICD-O coding
8000/6 Neoplasm, metastatic

ICD-11 coding
2D70 Malignant neoplasm metastasis in lung

Related terminology
None

Subtype(s)
None

Localization
Pulmonary metastases typically affect the lower lobes and periphery, with equal distribution in the right and left lungs {1674,2675}. They are often multiple and bilateral, but they can be solitary. Because pulmonary lymphatics are concentrated in the bronchovascular bundles and the interlobular septal/pleural areas, metastatic disease is often observed in these locations {2675}. Metastatic cells within the lymphatics or vasculature can exit these structures and infiltrate into the lung parenchyma. They can then grow as pulmonary nodules anywhere in the lung parenchyma or even as endobronchial masses, often with rounded, pushing borders rather than the infiltrative pattern of primary lung malignancies {2675,1796}.

Clinical features
Signs and symptoms
Most patients with metastatic lung disease are asymptomatic, even in the presence of fulminant metastases that occupy almost an entire lung {1289}. When present, common symptoms include cough, haemoptysis, wheezing, dyspnoea, and fever. Vascular/thromboembolic or lymphatic spread may mimic symptoms of an interstitial pneumonia, tuberculosis, and/or cor pulmonale, leading to delayed diagnoses.

Imaging
CT, often with simultaneous PET (PET-CT), is the most sensitive imaging modality for detecting pulmonary metastases {2705}. Typical radiological findings include solitary or multiple peripherally located, round, variably sized nodules (haematogenous metastasis) or diffuse thickening of the interstitium (lymphangitic carcinomatosis) {622,1153,2705}. Metastases are usually well circumscribed, with expanding growth and smooth margins, but irregular contours can also be present {1153,896}. Squamous cell carcinomas (SCCs) are regarded as the most common type of cavitating metastases {1153,2705}. In general, calcification in a nodule suggests that it is a benign lesion

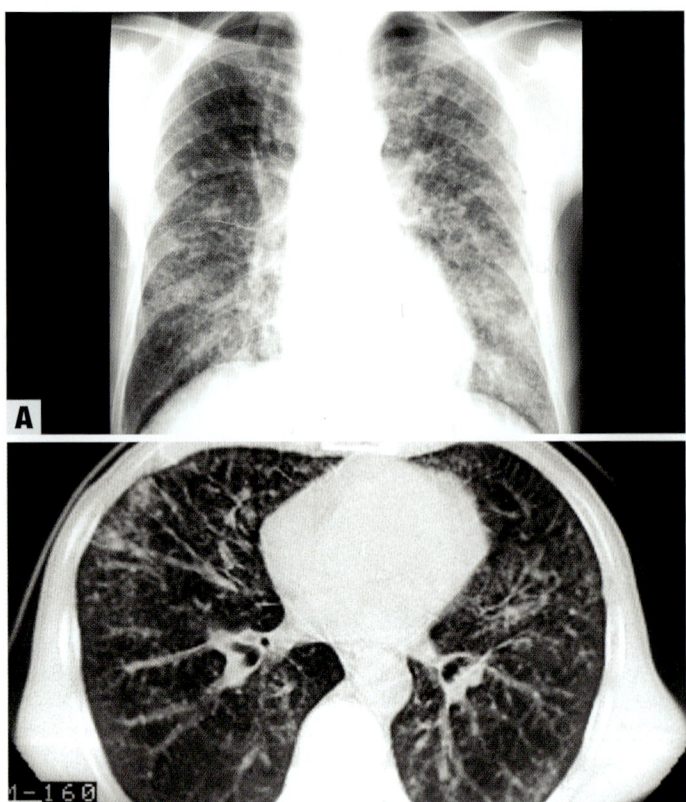

Fig. 9.01 Metastasis to the lung. **A** Pulmonary metastases from a gastric adenocarcinoma. The chest X-ray shows multiple small nodules representing foci of haematogenous metastasis. Thickening of interlobular septa and interlobar fissure represent lymphatic involvement. **B** Lymphangitic carcinomatosis from metastatic gastric adenocarcinoma. CT shows diffuse thickening of bronchovascular bundles and interlobular septa, suggesting lymphatic involvement (lymphangitic carcinomatosis) by metastatic tumour. Discrete nodules may represent foci of haematogenous metastasis.

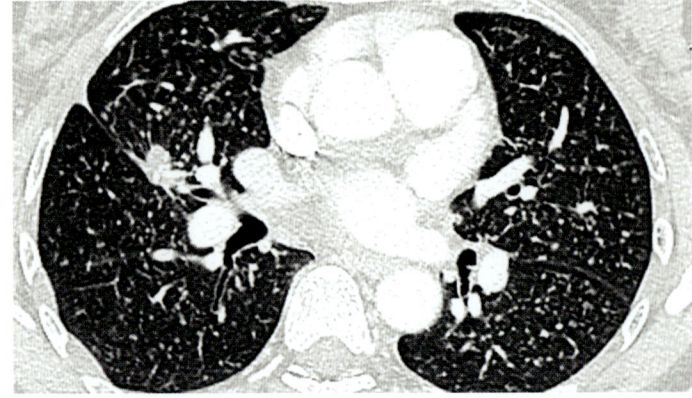

Fig. 9.02 Diffuse pulmonary metastases. High-resolution chest CT shows a primary lung adenocarcinoma with *EGFR* p.L858R mutation manifesting as extensive bilateral intrapulmonary metastases.

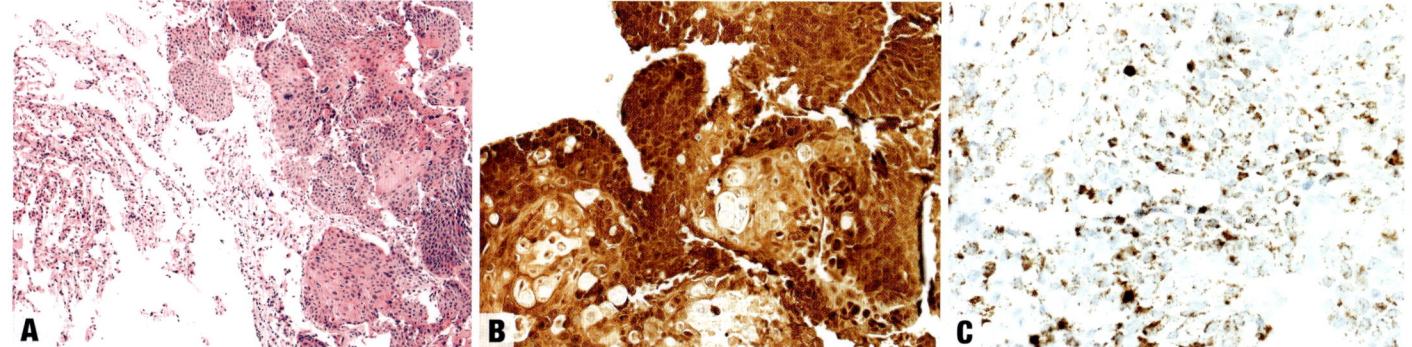

Fig. 9.03 Pulmonary metastasis from a squamous cell carcinoma. **A** A 49-year-old man with a history of squamous cell carcinoma of the base of the tongue presented with a left upper lobe lung nodule, confirmed as a squamous cell carcinoma on biopsy. **B** p16 immunostain is positive. **C** In situ hybridization for high-risk HPV with probes for HPV16 and HPV18 was positive.

such as a granuloma or hamartoma. However, this can also be seen in a metastatic sarcoma or adenocarcinoma {2705,1153}. Pneumothorax commonly occurs in metastases from an osteosarcoma {2705}. Chest X-rays are normal in 50% of cases with lymphangitic carcinomatosis, but CT shows beaded or nodular interstitial thickening {1153}. Endobronchial metastasis may lead to partial or complete bronchial obstruction, with atelectasis or obstructive pneumonia {2705}.

Epidemiology

The lung is a common site for metastases from a wide spectrum of primary malignant tumours from different lineages, including sarcomas, carcinomas, and melanomas. A series of autopsies on patients with extrapulmonary malignancies showed the presence of pulmonary metastases in 20–54% of patients {2705}. Carcinomas (76%) represent the majority, while sarcoma (16.3%), melanoma (5.5%), and germ cell tumours (2.2%) are less frequently encountered {402}. Among epithelial tumours, gastrointestinal, urothelial, and breast carcinomas are the most frequent sites of origin {402}. Germ cell tumours, sarcomas, and melanoma have a high rate of lung metastases, although the prevalence of these malignancies remains relatively low {573}. The majority of patients diagnosed with metastases in the lung initially present with multiple lesions rather than a solitary nodule {402}. Patient age and sex vary depending on the histological type and the origin of the metastasis. Metastases from germ cell tumours and some sarcomas are diagnosed mostly in young adults and children, while metastatic carcinomas are generally seen in older adults. Intrapulmonary metastases of lung cancer have a prevalence of 0.2–20% in patients undergoing lung resection {2186,2188,810,3343,3242}.

Etiology

Etiology depends on the primary origin of the tumour.

Pathogenesis

Tumour dissemination

There are six major modalities for the spread of lung metastases: intrapulmonary aerogenous, haematogenous, lymphangitic, endobronchial, and pleural spread, and direct invasion from adjacent organs and local sites such as the chest wall and mediastinum. Haematogenous spread is the most common form of dissemination and results in micronodular (miliary), macronodular, solitary, cavitary, and thromboembolic lesions

{573}. The lungs are frequent targets of metastases because of their central role in circulation. In addition, pulmonary capillaries are fenestrated, which facilitates the extravasation of the tumour cells into the lung {1036}.

The tumour/lung microenvironment is an important determinant of lung metastases {3439}. The capacities of the tumour cells to undergo epithelial–mesenchymal transition and to

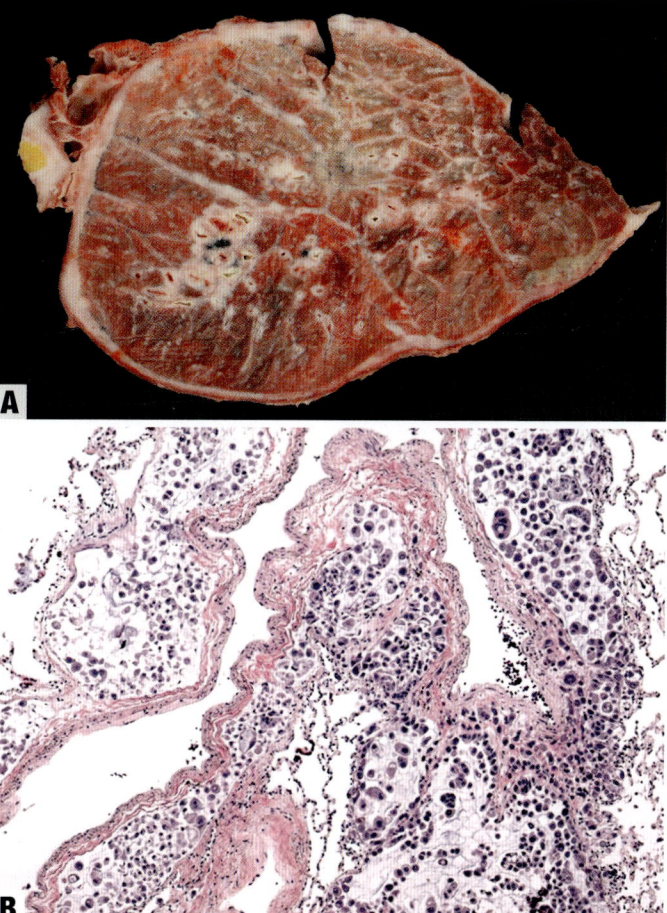

Fig. 9.04 Lymphangitic carcinomatosis. Diffuse pulmonary metastases from a gastric adenocarcinoma. The lung parenchyma shows lymphangitic carcinomatosis with thickening of the alveolar septa and the subpleural space (**A**). These findings correspond to the presence of tumour cells in the lymphatics (**B**).

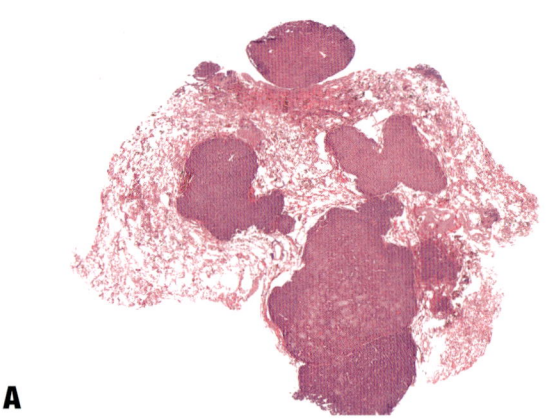

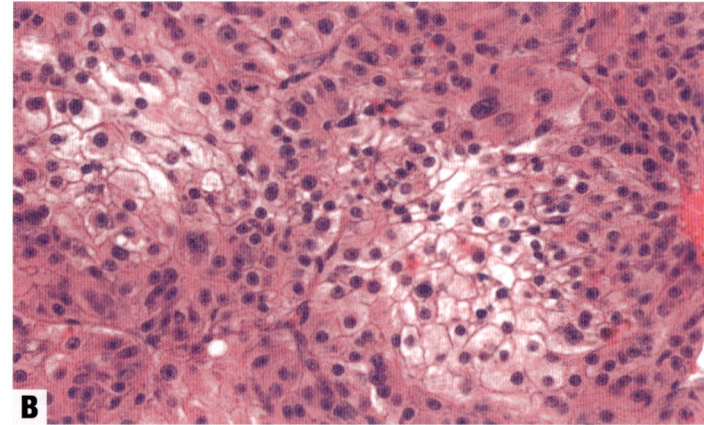

Fig. 9.05 Pulmonary metastasis from a hepatocellular carcinoma. **A** Metastatic hepatocellular carcinoma showing several pulmonary subcentimetre nodules at low power. **B** At high power, the tumour cells display mild to moderate atypia with abundant eosinophilic and focal clear cytoplasm.

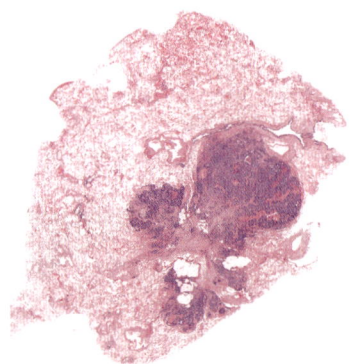

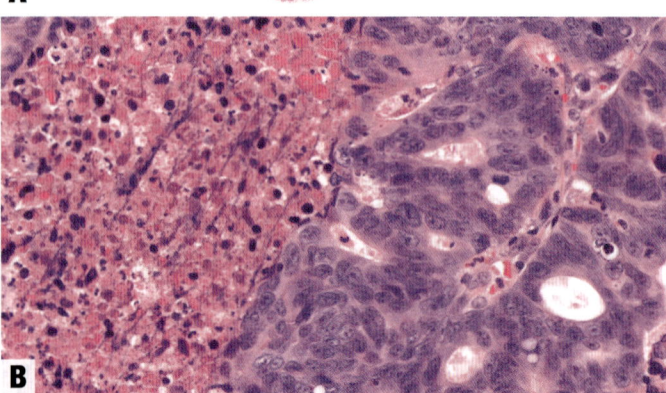

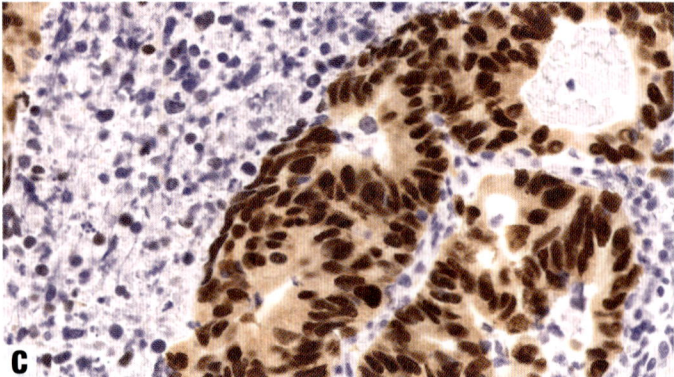

Fig. 9.06 Pulmonary metastasis from a colon adenocarcinoma. **A** Lung parenchyma with a well-circumscribed lesion with areas of dirty necrosis, consistent with a metastasis from a colon adenocarcinoma. **B** At higher power, a cribriform pattern with an area of dirty necrosis is seen. **C** The tumour cells are strongly and diffusely positive for CDX2.

acquire stem cell–like characteristics are key determinants of lung invasion, as is the reprogramming of lung macrophages by chemokines, which facilitates tumour growth {3013,1936,3486}. More recently, tumour cell exosomes have also been shown to play a pivotal role in lung metastases through the creation of metastatic niches {1182,3248,3247}. These factors explain the propensity of tumours arising from certain sites to generate lung metastases.

Macroscopic appearance

Metastatic tumour nodules are generally firm due to increased interstitial tumour pressure, and they stand up above the surrounding normal lung parenchyma on cut section. Metastases are typically round, tan-white in colour, variably sized, and well demarcated from the surrounding parenchyma {1674}. There may be haemorrhage and necrosis, which may represent outgrowth of the tumour from the vascular supply or may reflect systemic treatment effect. Cystic changes may rarely be prominent, especially in indolent disease {2217}. Tumours with typical macroscopic appearances at their primary sites commonly show these features at metastatic sites as well. Metastatic melanoma may appear brown or black, and metastatic renal cell carcinoma often appears golden yellow.

Histopathology

In general, lung metastases share overlapping histological characteristics with the primary tumour, which underscores the importance of obtaining slides from the previous primary to compare the morphology. For example, in metastatic colon carcinoma, it is common to observe cribriform glands with areas of dirty necrosis and columnar cells with basally located nuclei. Likewise, tumour cells from a metastatic renal clear cell carcinoma typically exhibit abundant and clear cytoplasm. However, it is not uncommon for a high-grade component of a primary malignant tumour (e.g. a sarcomatoid component in a clear cell carcinoma of the kidney) to be overrepresented in the corresponding metastasis. In these cases, ancillary immunohistochemistry or molecular profiling is useful to confirm the origin. It is also important to point out that there are distinct histopathological features that should raise suspicion for pulmonary metastases, such as multiple well-defined and round nodules and distribution in the subpleural space and/or surrounding a

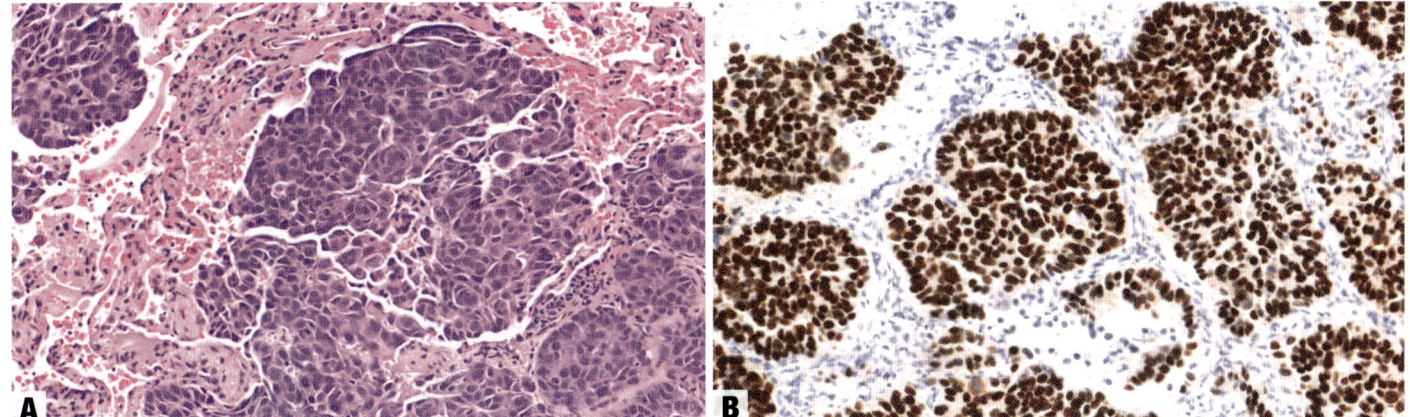

Fig. 9.07 Pulmonary metastasis from a breast carcinoma. **A** Poorly differentiated tumour cells organized in solid nests. The cells are strongly positive for SOX10 (**B**) and negative for ER, PR, and ERBB2, consistent with a triple-negative breast carcinoma.

bronchovascular bundle. Tumour cells can also be seen mainly in the lymphatic compartment, which can sometimes mimic an interstitial disease {595,2851}. It is also worth mentioning that the presence of a lepidic pattern of growth in a lung tumour does not rule out metastasis, because the presence of such a pattern has been described in various types of metastatic malignancies {2608,2044,1946}.

Synchronous primary lung cancer vs intrapulmonary metastases

Patients with multifocal lung tumours are increasingly seen in clinical practice, possibly as a result of changes in imaging practices {683}. Pathological features that have been proposed to suggest the same origin of two or more lung tumours (intrapulmonary metastases) include the presence of lymphovascular invasion, solid growth pattern, and matching histological appearance {3071,2104,680,962}. In contrast, features proposed to suggest clonal independence (synchronous tumours) include distinct histological type, lepidic growth, and different biomarker patterns {683}. This is addressed further in *Diagnostic molecular pathology*, below.

Immunohistochemistry

Immunohistochemistry is valuable in addressing whether a tumour is a lung primary or a metastasis. A variety of antibodies can be used to favour either lung origin or a metastasis from an extrapulmonary site (see Table 9.01). Most primary lung adenocarcinomas are positive for TTF1 and/or napsin A, except mucinous adenocarcinomas. Because of overlapping expression profiles, immunohistochemistry (TTF1, napsin, CDX2, SMAD4, HNF4α, CK7, CK20) is of limited utility in distinguishing metastatic mucinous tumours of gastrointestinal or pancreatobiliary origin from mucinous lung adenocarcinoma {3391,523,2864, 1552,2459}. It is important to keep in mind that 20–25% of primary pulmonary adenocarcinomas do not stain for TTF1 {3390}. In addition, TTF1 expression has also been reported at a low frequency in carcinomas originating from several other sites, such as the stomach, bile duct, pancreas, colorectum, prostate, ovary, liver, breast, and urothelial cells {513A,3180A,3169A}.

Cytology

Cytology has become an important diagnostic modality in the evaluation of lung lesions. The cytological features of metastatic carcinomas vary according to the type of lesion. Metastatic colonic carcinomas occur as gland-forming cohesive clusters, with columnar cells, palisading nuclei, and abundant necrosis {1503}. Breast cancer cells of ductal type often form rounded cell clusters (so-called cannonballs), whereas linear arrays of uniform small tumour cells may suggest metastasizing breast lobular carcinoma. The distinction between metastatic and primary SCC is unreliable by cytology. Pancreas or biliary adenocarcinoma is often especially challenging, because it closely resembles pulmonary mucinous adenocarcinoma. Melanoma shows discohesive tumour cells with cytoplasmic melanin, with primary lung melanoma being extremely rare {3320} (see

Table 9.01 Non-exhaustive list of immunohistochemical markers for identification of the most common origins of pulmonary metastases

Common origins of lung metastases	Useful immunohistochemical stains
Epithelial	
Bladder	GATA3, CK7, CK20, uroplakin
Breast	GATA3, ER, PR, SOX10, GCDFP-15, mammaglobin
Gastrointestinal tract and pancreatobiliary system	CDX2, CK7, CK20, SMAD4
Kidney	PAX8, RCCm, CK7, CK20, KIT (CD117), CD10
Liver	Arginase-1 (ARG1), glypican-3 (GPC3), HepPar-1
Lung	TTF1, napsin A, CK7, CK20
Ovary	PAX8, ER, WT1, CK7, CK20
Prostate	NKX3-1, PSA, AMACR
Thyroid	PAX8, thyroglobulin, TTF1, CEA
Uterus	PAX8, ER, CK7, CK20
Others	
Melanoma	SOX10, S100, melan-A, HMB45, MITF

Table 9.02 Cytological features of the most common primary tumours to result in lung metastases

Primary tumour	Cytological features
Breast carcinoma	Cohesive and discohesive aggregates of tumour cells, with the presence of 3D cell balls; nuclei are round and enlarged, and the cytoplasm is moderately abundant {1791}
Colon carcinoma	Presence of variable amount of necrosis in the background, with glandular formation and at least some foci of columnar cells and elongated, pseudostratified nuclei {1791}
Melanoma	In the epithelioid type, cells are polygonal or plasmacytoid in shape, with or without intracellular melanin pigment; nuclei are large and sometimes binucleated, nucleoli are prominent, and there are occasional intranuclear inclusions Spindle cell morphology can also be seen {1381} – when this is present, the differential diagnosis includes metastatic sarcomas or sarcomatoid carcinoma
Renal carcinoma	Aggregates of tumour cells with abundant vacuolated cytoplasm, indistinct cytoplasmic outlines, bland round nuclei with single micronucleoli, or enlarged nuclei with prominent nucleoli {1791}; a sarcomatoid component composed of atypical spindle cells can also be seen The differential diagnoses include other clear cell tumours such as lung adenocarcinoma with clear cell changes, benign or malignant perivascular epithelioid cell tumour (PEComa), melanoma, etc. {3301}
Urothelial carcinoma	Small syncytial clusters or papillary fragments of squamoid cells with enlarged round nuclei, increased N:C ratio, and dense cytoplasm; presence of spindle, pyramidal, and/or racquet-shaped cells; intracytoplasmic vacuoles can be seen {374}

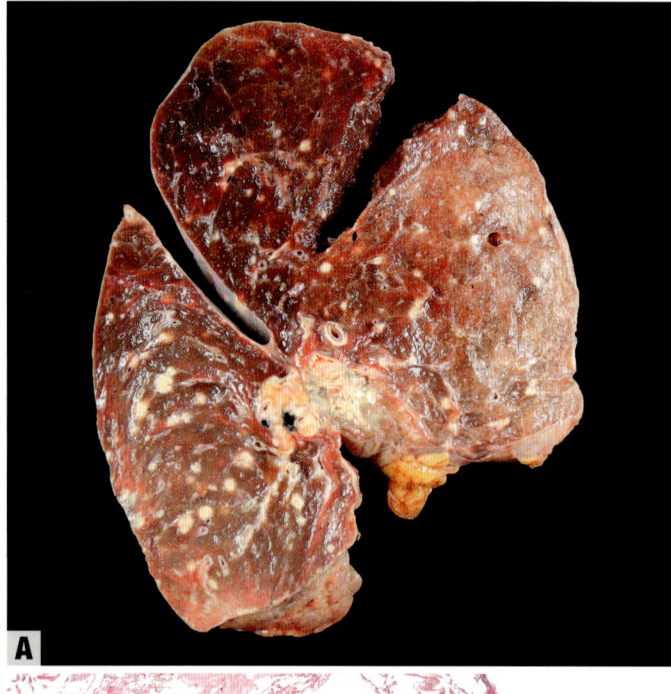

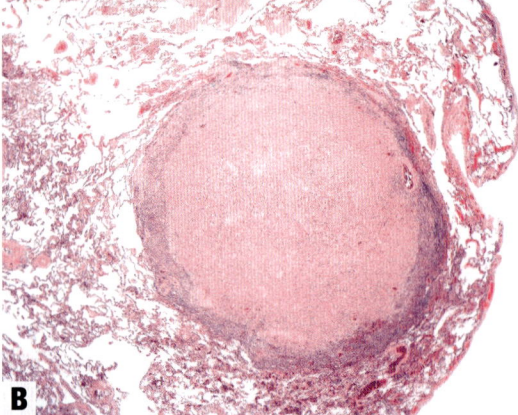

Fig. 9.08 Diffuse pulmonary metastasis from a melanoma. **A** Diffuse lung metastases from a melanoma showing multiples small round nodules. **B** Each lesion corresponds microscopically to a well-delineated intraparenchymal tumour.

Melanoma of the lung, p. 150). Both liquid-based cytology and cell block preparations can be used for immunohistochemical, cytogenetic, and molecular tests {1524}. Because cytology is commonly the only specimen available for diagnosing a lung lesion, immunohistochemistry and molecular profiling are frequently required to confirm the origin of the lesion and to guide the treatment of the patient, necessitating cell block preparation {2642} (see *Small diagnostic samples*, p. 29).

Cytological features of the most common sites of lung metastases are summarized in Table 9.02.

Diagnostic molecular pathology

There are no routine molecular tests that exist to differentiate primary from metastatic tumours of the lung; rather, a more comprehensive approach, as described here, is required to inform this decision.

Molecular pathology may be useful when metastatic tumours share the same lineage as a lung primary. Common primary sites of SCC metastatic to lung include head and neck, oesophagus, gynaecological/genitourinary tract, and skin. In general, lung SCC shares more genomic similarities with squamous carcinomas of other sites than with lung adenocarcinomas {367,2681,2868,29}. In the appropriate context, HPV testing may be useful to distinguish between primary lung SCC and metastasis from head and neck, cervical, or anal primary sites {603}. Given the relative paucity of specific molecular biomarkers for lung SCC, evolving transcriptomic, epigenomic, and proteomic signatures may be informative {368,2706,2863}.

Mutation profiles of mucinous lung tumours can also overlap substantially with those of mucinous tumours arising at other sites. Pancreatic adenocarcinoma, in particular, shares not only morphological features but also molecular features with lung invasive mucinous adenocarcinomas, with common mutations in *TP53*, *SMAD4*, *CDKN2A*, *KRAS*, and *GNAS* {3182,142,2494}. SMAD4 loss is identified in > 50% of pancreatic carcinomas but is also seen in 10% of lung adenocarcinomas {2495}. Certain *KRAS* mutations (p.G12C) are significantly more common in but not exclusive to primary lung tumours {1528}. Molecular alterations that are enriched in certain tumour types may help to distinguish primary from metastatic poorly differentiated or dedifferentiated

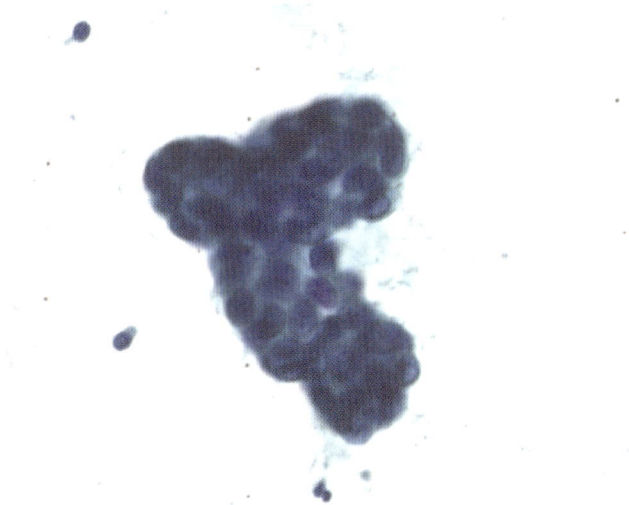

Fig. 9.09 Pulmonary metastasis from a urothelial carcinoma. Bronchial wash smear shows tight clusters of tumour cells with an increased N:C ratio.

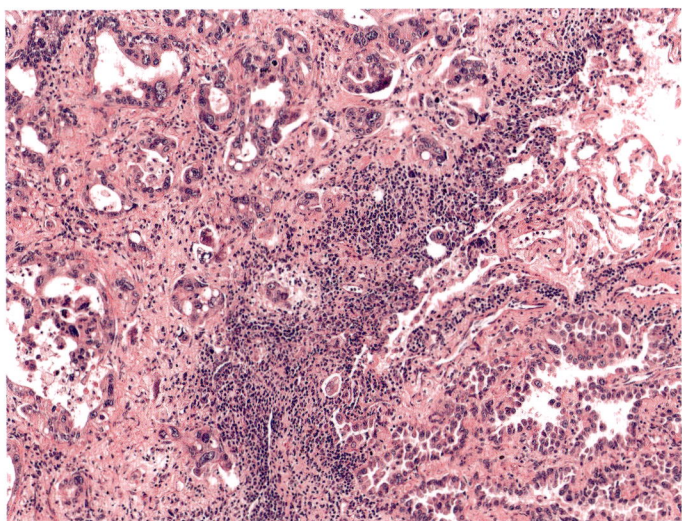

Fig. 9.10 Pulmonary metastasis from a prostate carcinoma. Metastatic high-grade prostate carcinoma (left) with reactive pneumocyte hyperplasia (right).

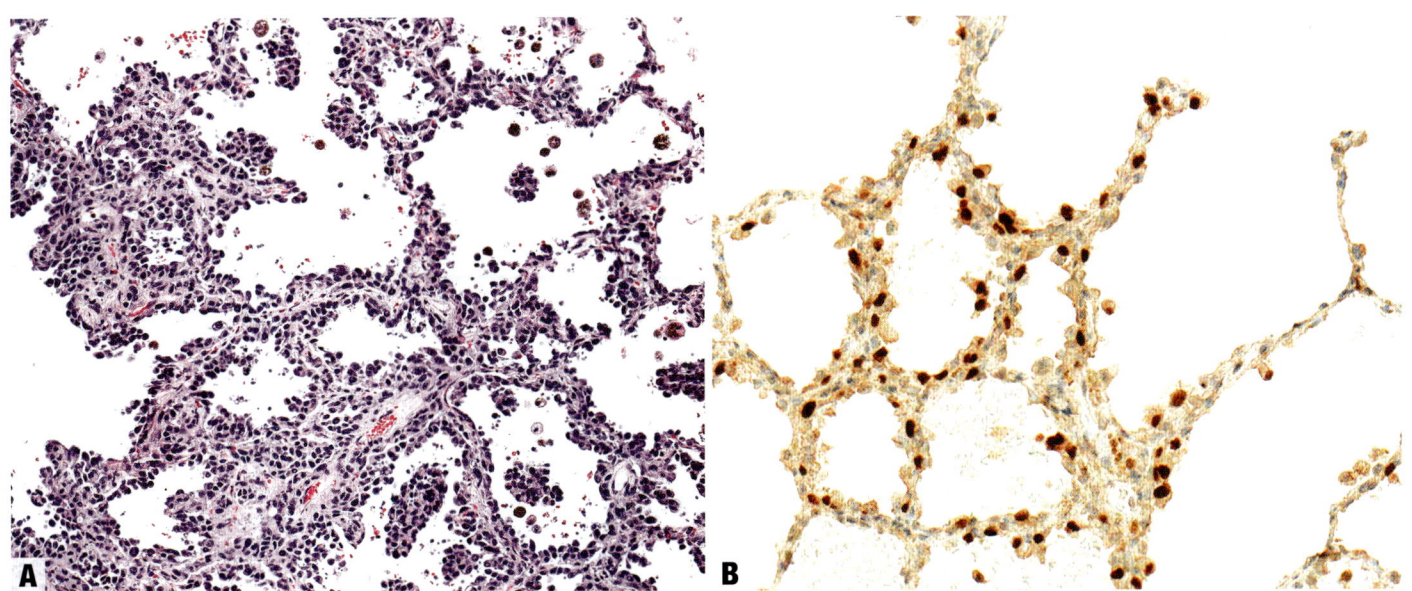

Fig. 9.11 Metastatic melanoma. **A** This patient had bilateral lung metastasis from melanoma, including multiple areas of ground-glass infiltrates, which on biopsy showed lepidic growth. Metastatic melanoma tumour cells are seen growing in a lepidic pattern along the surface of alveolar walls. **B** The metastatic melanoma tumour cells growing along the alveolar wall surface are highlighted by nuclear positivity for MITF.

tumours (carcinomas of unknown primary) but should be interpreted in the clinical context. A combination of *BAP1*, *NF2*, and/or *CDKN2A* mutations may help to distinguish mesothelioma, sarcomatoid pattern, which frequently loses mesothelial markers, from pleomorphic/sarcomatoid lung carcinoma {330,2256}.

Synchronous primary lung cancer vs intrapulmonary metastases

Molecular analysis of paired specimens for determination of clonal relatedness is most informative when carried out using a broader sequencing panel or comparative genomic hybridization {2035,2036,443,3173,963}. However, to date few studies have demonstrated a significant difference in stage-adjusted survival outcomes when stage is predicated on molecular as compared with histological comparisons {2287}. In a substantial number of cases, however, molecular analysis contradicts histologically driven conclusions regarding clonal relatedness, for both lung adenocarcinomas and SCCs {2673,3173,443}. This may have implications for accurate interpretation of tumour stage and choice of therapy {2613,682,680,684}.

Essential and desirable diagnostic criteria

Essential:

- Pathological diagnosis of a tumour compatible with origin in an extrapulmonary site according to diagnostic histological, immunohistochemical, and/or molecular criteria for that tumour
- Exclusion of primary lung tumour on the basis of clinical history, imaging, and histopathological findings

Desirable:

- Histological, immunohistochemical, and molecular profiling of metastatic tumour and comparison with any previous tumours (if available)
- Multidisciplinary discussion of the case, such as at a tumour board

Staging

According to the current pathological TNM system and the Union for International Cancer Control (UICC), metastatic tumours are generally considered stage III or IV disease {315,75}.

Prognosis and prediction

Lung metastases from extrapulmonary malignancies usually have a dismal prognosis. Patient outcomes typically depend on the type of primary tumour and its sensitivity to chemotherapy. Germ cell tumours and differentiated thyroid cancer are associated with better prognoses after metastasectomy {402,2811}, whereas the prognoses of carcinomas (colonic, renal, breast, and others), sarcomas, and melanoma are less favourable. Rare cases of metastatic lung disease may show an indolent course, especially when the primary tumour is a low-grade neoplasm, for example benign metastasizing leiomyoma {161} and metastatic cellular fibrous histiocytoma {2217}.

Multiple studies indicate that complete metastasectomy improves the outcomes for a variety of tumours, especially for patients with a single pulmonary metastasis {1232,496,1695, 2833,2342,2755,510}, with a shorter disease-free interval, thoracic lymph node metastasis, incomplete metastasectomy, and multiple metastases being unfavourable prognostic factors {1232,1695,2342,2755,510,642}.

For patients with recurrent lung metastases from sarcoma or colorectal cancer, repeat metastasectomy in selected patients can prolong survival {496,2833,2342}. Other factors reported as affecting prognosis are elevated pre-thoracotomy CEA serum levels in patients with pulmonary metastases from colorectal cancer, with > 5 ng/mL suggesting poor prognoses. Overexpression of PDL1 in patients with metastasis from head and neck SCC may be an independent predictor for poor outcomes {1232,2685,2177}. In metastatic colorectal adenocarcinoma, aerogenous spread with floating cancer cell clusters, similar to spread through airspaces described in lung cancers, is associated with poor prognosis {2754}.

Metastasis to the pleura

Sholl LM
Kadota K
Sauter JL

Definition
Pleural metastases represent spread to the pleura from a tumour that originated at an extrapleural site.

ICD-O coding
8000/6 Neoplasm, metastatic

ICD-11 coding
2D72 Malignant neoplasm metastasis in pleura

Related terminology
Acceptable: malignant pleural effusion.

Subtype(s)
None

Localization
Both visceral and parietal pleurae are commonly involved {1900}.

Clinical features
Patients present with cough, chest pain, and dyspnoea on exertion but may be asymptomatic {490,1214}. Imaging shows focal to diffuse nodularity, masses, or circumferential pleural or fissural thickening {1214}. Malignant effusions are moderate to large (500–2000 mL); in primary lung cancer, effusions localize to the ipsilateral pleural space. As many as 15% of lung cancer patients with malignant pleural effusions also have pleural nodules visible on CT; most show FDG uptake on PET {326}, but this is not specific for malignancy {2379}.

Epidemiology
Pleural involvement is seen in 4% of male and 8% of female cancer patients with metastatic disease {2486}. Malignant pleural effusions reportedly affect > 150 000 individuals per year in the

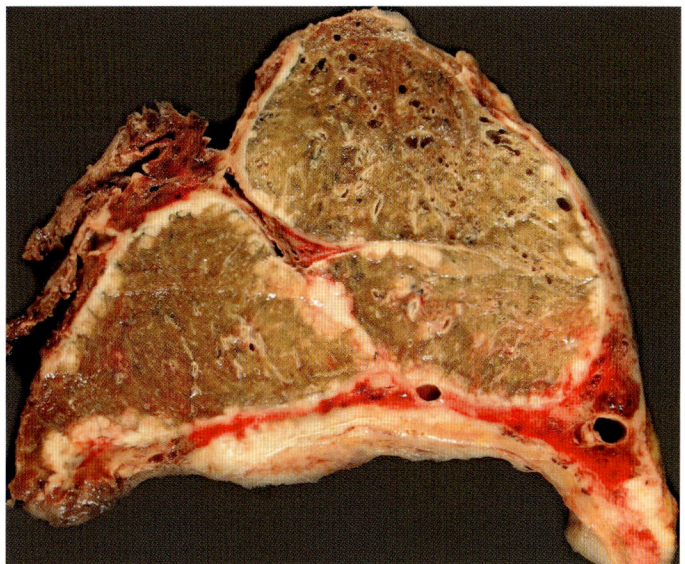

Fig. 9.12 Pseudomesotheliomatous spread of small cell lung carcinoma. Cross-section of an autopsied lung with near-complete involvement of the pleura by confluent tumour nodules.

USA and 40 000 per year in the United Kingdom {3030,754}. Common sources of pleural metastases are lung adenocarcinoma and haematolymphoid neoplasms in men and invasive breast carcinoma, Müllerian carcinomas, and lung adenocarcinoma in women {1323,2691,1189,672}. However, the majority do not have a known primary tumour site at the time of presentation {672}. Malignant pleural effusion is the presenting manifestation in 15% of cancer patients {3469}. Between 7% and 26% of patients with primary lung cancers present with malignant pleural effusions, and another 14% develop malignant pleural effusions during follow-up {490,2378}.

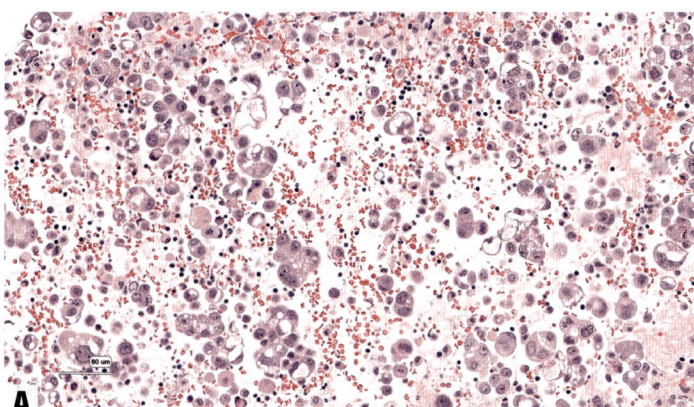
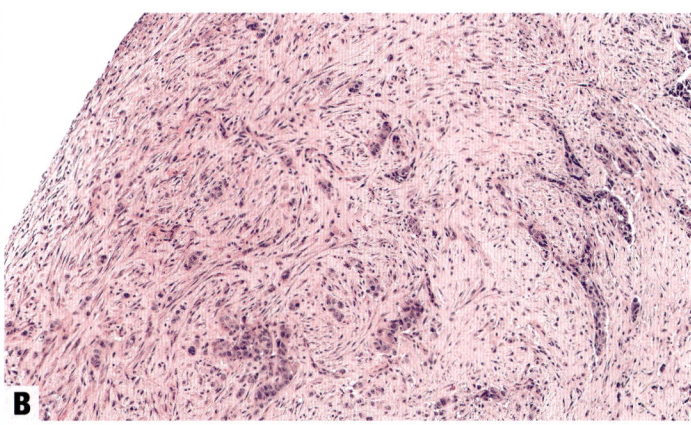

Fig. 9.13 Metastasis to the pleura. **A** Malignant pleural effusion. Metastatic lung adenocarcinoma diagnosed in an effusion specimen. Malignant cells are present as large single cells and micropapillary clusters in a background of smaller reactive mesothelial cells, lymphocytes, and red blood cells. **B** Pleural metastasis of lung adenocarcinoma. Parietal pleura contains infiltrating nests of lung adenocarcinoma. The pleura demonstrates a pronounced fibroproliferative stromal response.

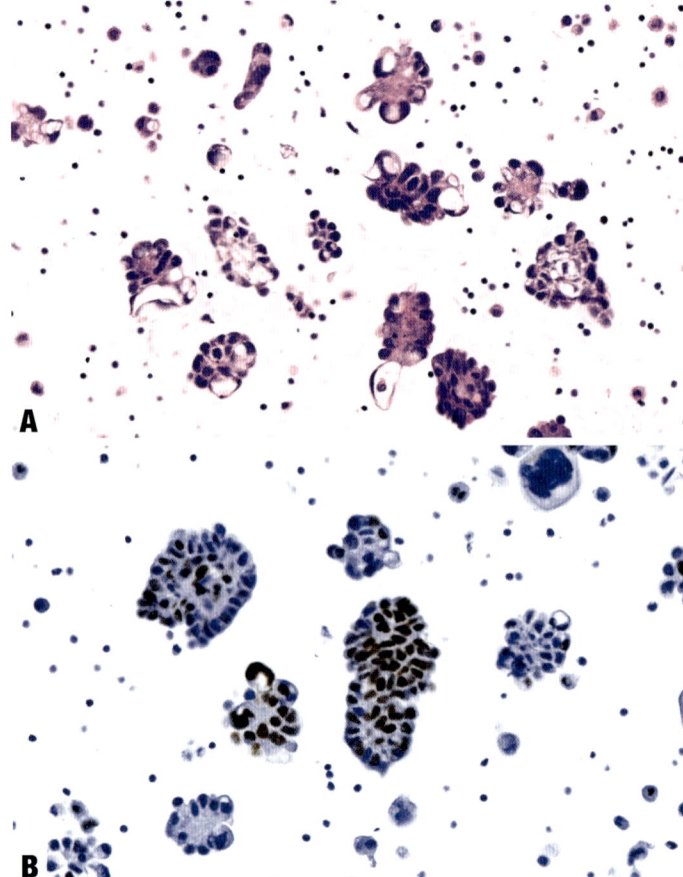

Fig. 9.14 Pleural metastasis of ovarian carcinoma. **A** Cell block from recurrent bilateral pleural effusions showing small clusters of malignant cells. **B** The ovarian carcinoma cells are strongly and multifocally positive for PAX8.

Table 9.03 Selected immunohistochemistry markers that may aid in the distinction of metastatic carcinoma from mesothelioma

Mesothelial markers		
Marker	**Sensitivity**	**Specificity vs lung adenocarcinoma**
Calretinin	95%	90–95%
CK5/6	85%	80–90%
WT1	86%	95–100%
D2-40	90–100%	85%
Adenocarcinoma (positive epithelial markers)		
Marker	**Sensitivity**	**Specificity vs mesothelioma**
Claudin-4	90–96%	80–100%
MOC31	95–100%	80–91%
BerEP4	95–100%	83–93%
BG8 (LewisY)	90–100%	92–98%
B72.3	25–85%	86–100%
Monoclonal CEA	80–100%	> 95%
Squamous cell carcinoma markers[a]		
Marker	**Sensitivity**	**Specificity vs mesothelioma**
CK5/6	75–95%	10–50%
p63	> 95%	~85%
p40	> 95%	~95%
Organ specific – lung		
Marker	**Sensitivity**	**Specificity vs mesothelioma**
TTF1 (8G7G3/1)	~80%	> 95%
Napsin A	~80%	High
Organ specific – breast		
Marker	**Sensitivity**	**Specificity vs mesothelioma**
ERα	~80%	> 95%
PR	n/a	n/a
GCDFP-15	30–40%	High
Mammaglobin	50–85%	High
Organ specific – renal		
Marker	**Sensitivity**	**Specificity vs mesothelioma**
PAX8	70–100%	High
PAX2	80%	Unknown
RCCm	Up to 85%	75–90%
CD15 (LeuM1)	60%	High

n/a, not applicable.
[a]{2022A,2760A,3353A,239,452A,1567A}.

Etiology

Etiology depends on the primary origin of tumour.

Pathogenesis

Tumour spreads to pleura via lymphatic and haematogenous routes or direct invasion. About 55–60% of patients with pleural metastases develop a malignant effusion {1900,2591}. Multiple factors probably contribute to development of an effusion, including lymphatic blockage, inflammatory response, extent of angiogenesis, and vascular leakage; the burden of pleural metastasis does not appear to correlate {3475,3385,2842,1683, 2591}. Molecular alterations are specific to tumour type.

Macroscopic appearance

Resected pleural metastases may appear smooth and lobulated or plaque-like and infiltrative. Carcinomas, thymic tumours, and angiosarcomas can manifest rarely with diffuse disease mimicking mesothelioma, so-called pseudomesotheliomatous growth {3493,121,122,788}.

Histopathology

Tumour infiltrates pleural fibrous tissue and may invade chest wall soft tissue or lung tissue in parietal or visceral pleural biopsies, respectively {1213,1388}. For primary lung carcinomas, elastic stains may be helpful to distinguish between a discrete intrapleural metastasis and visceral pleural invasion from an intrapulmonary tumour.

General carcinoma markers such as claudin-4, BerEP4, and CEA are useful in the distinction from mesothelioma (see Table 9.03; see also *Diffuse pleural mesothelioma*, p. 204).

Table 9.04 Differential diagnosis of pleural metastases

Entity	Differential diagnostic features
Neoplastic	
Mesothelioma	Positive mesothelial markers; malignant features (see the sections on mesothelial tumours, beginning on p. 196)
Primary pleural lymphoma	Positive lymphoid markers (see the sections on haematolymphoid tumours, beginning on p. 220)
Primary pleural mesenchymal tumours	Positive mesenchymal markers (see Chapter 4: *Mesenchymal tumours of the thorax*)
Reactive/benign entities	
Pleural fibrosis +/− talc pleurodesis	Fibrosis +/− polarizable talc crystals; no cytological malignant features
Reactive mesothelial hyperplasia	Positive mesothelial markers; no cytological malignant features (although sometimes cells are entrapped in superficial fibrosis)
Rounded atelectasis	Localized pleural scar with adjacent collapsed lung
Endometriosis	Presence of endometrial stroma +/− glands; no cytological malignant features; history of endometriosis
IgG4-related disease	Increased IgG4-positive cells and IgG4:IgG ratio; no clonality
Amyloidosis	Congo red–positive material
Granulomatous/tuberculous pleuritis	Granulomas (+/− necrosis); fibrosis; no cytological malignant features (organisms detected on culture or acid-fast bacilli stains for tuberculosis)
Apical cap	Hypocellular, intrapulmonary fibroelastotic scar with entrapped benign reactive pneumocytes; often bilateral

Site-specific markers can help to determine tumour origin, including for adenocarcinomas of lung (TTF1, napsin A), breast (ER, PR, GCDFP-15, mammaglobin, SOX10), kidney and Müllerian origin (PAX8), gastrointestinal tract (CDX2), prostate (PSA, NKX3-1), melanoma (S100, HMB45, melan-A), and haematopoietic processes (CD20, CD45) {1213,2211,2212,758,1043,1605}. SOX10 is expressed in melanomas and triple-negative breast cancers {2751,2084,3059,1605}. GATA3 is commonly expressed in tumours of breast and urothelial origin; however, it is also expressed in more than half of mesotheliomas {1913}. p40/p63 aids in distinction between squamous cell carcinoma and mesothelioma with pseudosquamous morphology; however, very rare mesotheliomas with true squamous differentiation have been reported {2982,2620}.

The differential diagnosis includes primary pleural neoplasms (see Chapter 2: *Tumours of the pleura and pericardium* and Chapter 4: *Mesenchymal tumours of the thorax*), which can be excluded using appropriate immunohistochemistry for mesothelial, lymphoid, and mesenchymal markers (see Table 2.05, p. 215) and reactive pleural diseases, the latter all lacking malignant cytology (see Table 9.04).

Cytology

Pleural fluid cytology is diagnostic in 60% of cases in the context of malignant pleural effusions {673}. In metastatic carcinoma, tumour cells are admixed with benign mesothelial cells and inflammatory cells, resulting in a second, separate population of cells distinct from benign mesothelial cells. Carcinomas may appear as single cells or clusters and can be distinguished from benign mesothelial cells by nuclear atypia; however, reactive mesothelial cells can sometimes show marked atypia {2906}. Lobular breast carcinoma can mimic histiocytes or mesothelial cells. Individual tumour types may display distinct cytomorphological features in effusion fluids that suggest primary origin. However, immunohistochemistry is often essential to distinguish metastases from mesothelial origin and suggest site of origin {1654,2906,1318}.

Diagnostic molecular pathology

The need for molecular analysis is informed by the suspected site of origin.

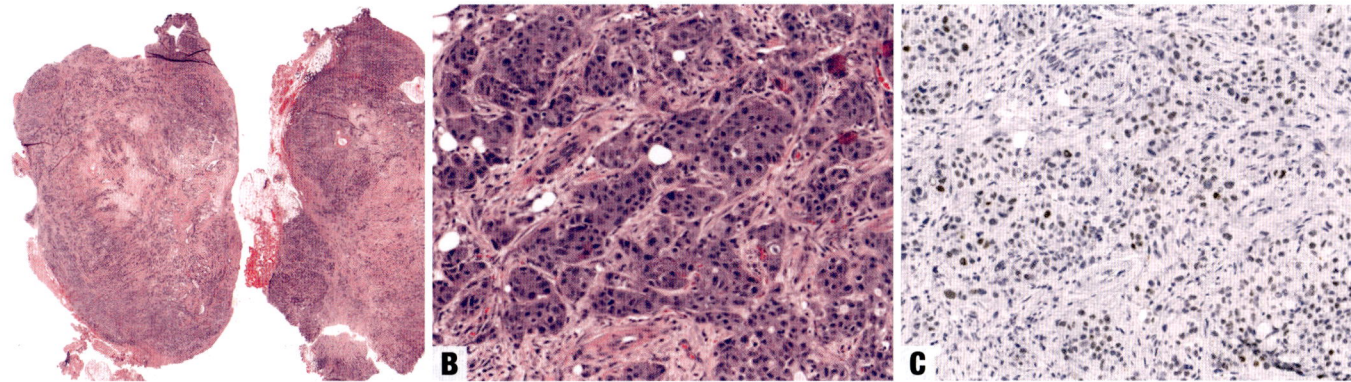

Fig. 9.15 Pleural metastasis of gastric adenocarcinoma. **A** Solid nodules from the pleura in a patient with diffuse and bilateral pleural carcinomatosis. The malignant cell nodules show solid and acinar patterns (**B**) and weak and focal positivity for CDX2 (**C**).

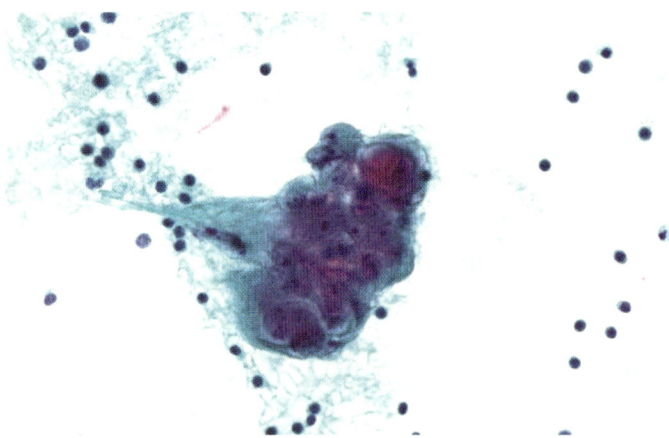

Fig. 9.16 Malignant pleural effusion. Metastatic breast carcinoma diagnosed in an effusion specimen. Malignant cells are present as a large cell cluster in a background of smaller mesothelial cells and lymphocytes.

Essential and desirable diagnostic criteria

Essential:

- Pathological diagnosis of a tumour compatible with origin in an extrapleural site according to diagnostic histological, immunohistochemical, and/or molecular criteria for that tumour
- Exclusion of benign entities and mesothelioma on the basis of clinical and radiographic presentation, histopathological findings, and immunohistochemistry

Desirable:

- Histological and immunohistochemical comparison with prior specimens (if available)
- If histological results are unclear, comparative molecular testing may be helpful
- Multidisciplinary discussion of the case, such as at a tumour board

Staging

Staging is based on the Union for International Cancer Control (UICC) TNM classification, according to the site of origin of the metastasis. Pleural metastases from lung cancer or thymic epithelial tumours are staged as M1a disease. Pleural spread from other sites is distant metastasis and should be staged according to criteria for tumour type.

Prognosis and prediction

Across all tumour types, survival time from diagnosis of malignant pleural effusion is a median of 5 months, although it can be variable. As an example, for ovarian metastases it is 21 months {3469}. The clinical status at time of diagnosis is significantly associated with outcomes {3469}. Pseudomesotheliomatous spread of carcinoma is associated with a median survival time of 8 months {122}.

Metastasis to the thymus and mediastinal lymph nodes

Roden AC

Definition
Metastasis to the thymus and mediastinal lymph nodes is spread of malignant tumours originating outside the mediastinum to the thymus or the mediastinum.

ICD-O coding
8000/6 Neoplasm, metastatic

ICD-11 coding
2D71 Malignant neoplasm metastasis in mediastinum
2D7Y Malignant neoplasm metastasis in other specified thoracic organs

Related terminology
None

Subtype(s)
None

Localization
Metastasis to mediastinal lymph nodes can occur in any mediastinal compartment; metastasis to the thymus is generally found in the anterior (prevascular) mediastinum.

Clinical features
Metastases might be incidentally identified during surveillance imaging or unrelated surgery {1030}. Symptoms can occur due to compression or obstruction of surrounding structures and organs. Serum tumour markers (dependent on primary tumour) may be increased. Although multiple lesions in the thymus/mediastinum favour metastasis, multiple thymic tumours do not exclude primary disease {1995,2137}. No specific imaging findings distinguish primary from metastatic disease or suggest the primary site of the tumour.

Epidemiology
Metastatic disease to the mediastinum is not uncommon. In an imaging-based study, 5.1% of all solitary mediastinal lesions were metastases; most occurred in the central (visceral) mediastinum, accounting for 14.8% of all solitary lesions {2505}.

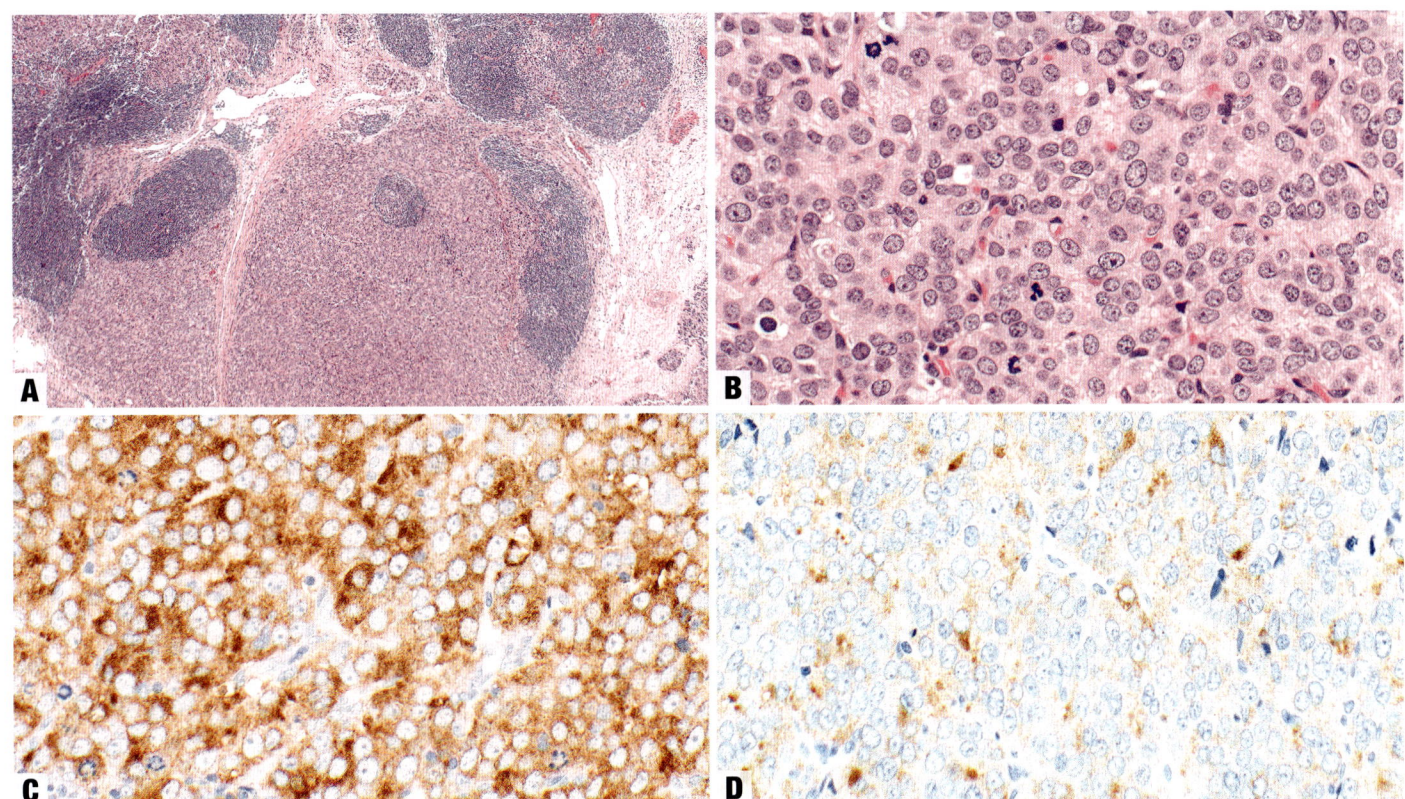

Fig. 9.17 Mediastinal lymph nodes involved by metastatic prostate carcinoma. **A** Sheets of tumour cells partially replace a lymph node. **B** The tumour cells are growing in a vague cribriform pattern, harbour prominent nucleoli, and exhibit high mitotic activity. **C** They are positive for PSA. **D** Scattered tumour cells express PAP.

Table 9.05 Immunohistochemical stains that aid in the distinction between thymic carcinoma and metastasis

Immunohistochemical marker	% of cases expressing marker		
	Thymic carcinoma	Non-thymic SCC	Non-lymphoid metastasis other than SCC
CD5[a]	20–100	Lung: 0–15 Skin: 0	Lung adenocarcinoma: 9–26 Prostatic adenocarcinoma: 22 Ductal breast carcinoma: 27 Pancreatic adenocarcinoma: 46 Colon adenocarcinoma: 50 Cholangiocarcinoma: 86
KIT (CD117)	60–90	Lung: 0[b]–20 Oesophagus: 15 Head and neck: 71	Lung adenocarcinoma: 6–16 Serous carcinoma: ~80 Adenoid cystic carcinoma: up to 100 Seminoma: up to 100
CD5 and KIT (CD117)	65	Lung: 0	Lung adenocarcinoma: 4
PAX8	Poly: 4–69 Mono: 0	Lung (poly): 0–2 Lung (mono): 0 Skin (poly): 0	Lung adenocarcinoma (poly): 0–2 NSCLC (poly): 6 Thyroid carcinoma (poly, mono): 80–100 Clear cell RCC (poly): 95 Breast carcinoma (poly): 0 Gastrointestinal and pancreatic adenocarcinoma (poly): 0 Endometrioid carcinoma (poly): 93 Serous carcinoma (poly): 99
PAX8 (poly) and KIT (CD117)	69	Not reported	CK7+ chromophobe RCC with papillary architecture (mono): 87 NEC of the endometrium (poly): 4 Thyroid CASTLE[c] (poly): 100 (1 report) NSCLC: 0
PAX8 (poly) and CD5	49	Not reported	NSCLC: 0

CASTLE, carcinoma showing thymus-like elements; mono, monoclonal PAX8; NEC, neuroendocrine carcinoma; NSCLC, non-small cell lung carcinoma; poly, polyclonal PAX8; RCC, renal cell carcinoma; SCC, squamous cell carcinoma.
[a]Clones 4C7, SP19, NCL-CD5–4C5. [b]Rarely cytoplasmic. [c]Primary or metastatic CASTLE might involve the upper mediastinum {3338A,1276A,442A}.
Table references: {1905A,2366A,2887,1535,3055,117,2929,2914,1308A,1098,2048,1991A,522A,2854A,2192A,356A,2227A,2140A,230A,3222A}

Metastatic disease to the thymus or ectopic thymic gland, including from the breast, colorectum, and thyroid gland, among others, is very rare {1030,888,882,2274,2328,2038}. Metastases can occur simultaneously with the primary tumour {2274,2328,2038} or up to 22 years later {1030,888,882}, and as either single {888} or multiple lesions, or together with metastases in other organs {882}.

Etiology
Etiology depends on the primary origin of tumour.

Pathogenesis
Tumours usually spread to mediastinal lymph nodes by haematogenous or lymphangitic routes. Metastatic tumour to the thymus may occur through blood vessels, lymphatics, and nerves within the capsule and interlobular septa {2038}.

Macroscopic appearance
Metastases can manifest as single or multiple nodules/masses, sometimes forming conglomerates of lymph nodes.

Histopathology
Metastases usually resemble, morphologically and immunophenotypically, their primary tumour. They can mimic primary thymic malignancies, because many subtypes of thymic carcinomas are similar in morphology and immunophenotype to carcinomas elsewhere. A panel of immunohistochemical markers may be helpful. Expression of PAX8 (polyclonal), CD5, and KIT (CD117) might aid in the distinction of primary thymic squamous cell carcinoma from its pulmonary counterpart (see Table 9.05). Expression of TTF1 (lung or thyroid), GATA3 (breast or urothelial), hormone receptors (breast or serous), and WT1 (serous) favours metastatic adenocarcinoma; CDX2 and CK20 may be expressed in metastatic colorectal adenocarcinoma, but they can also be positive in rare cases of primary thymic adenocarcinoma with enteric differentiation {1352}. Although not entirely specific, PAX8 (polyclonal) is more commonly expressed in thymic carcinoid tumours, while TTF1 is more often present in lung carcinoid tumours {3280}. TTF1 can also be expressed in some type A and AB thymomas {3258}. Ultimately, clinicoradiological correlation is often necessary.

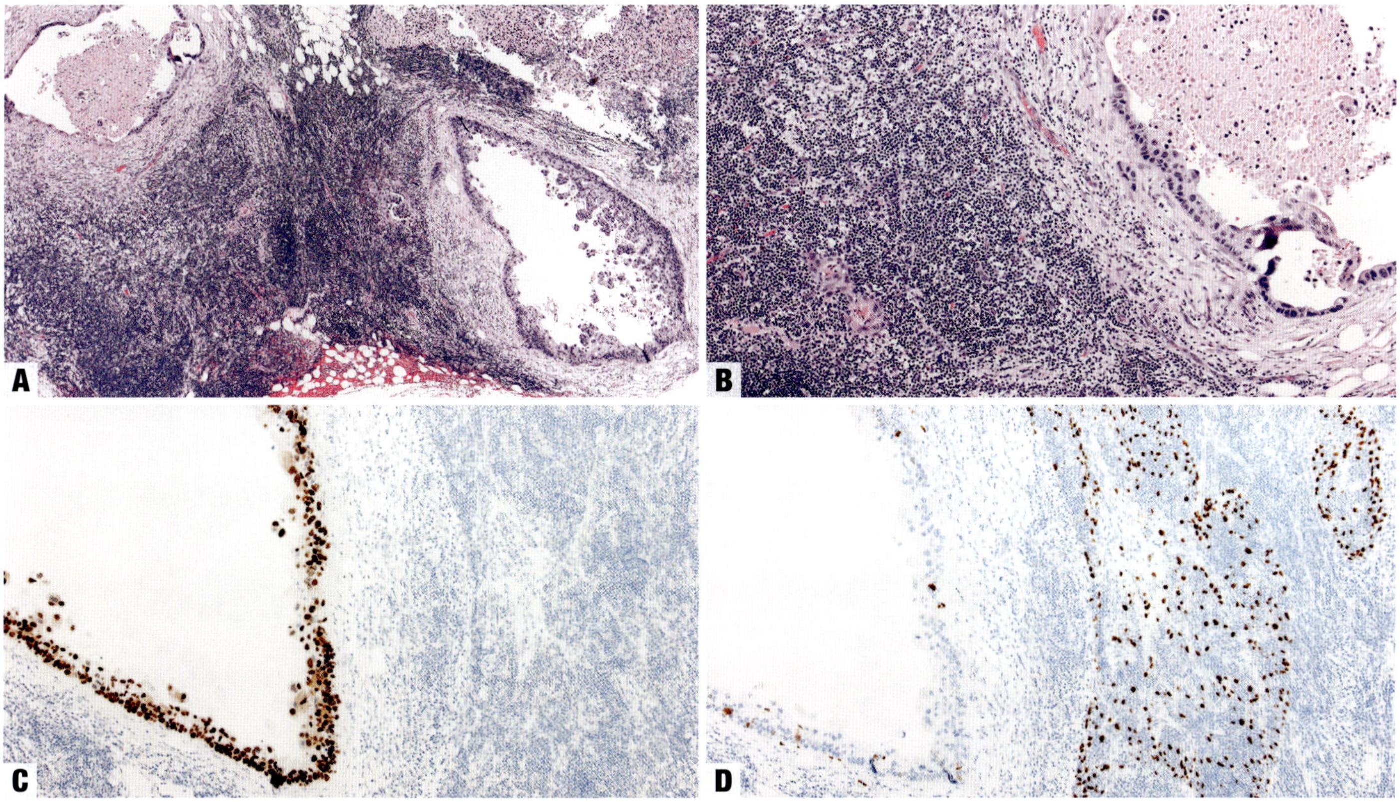

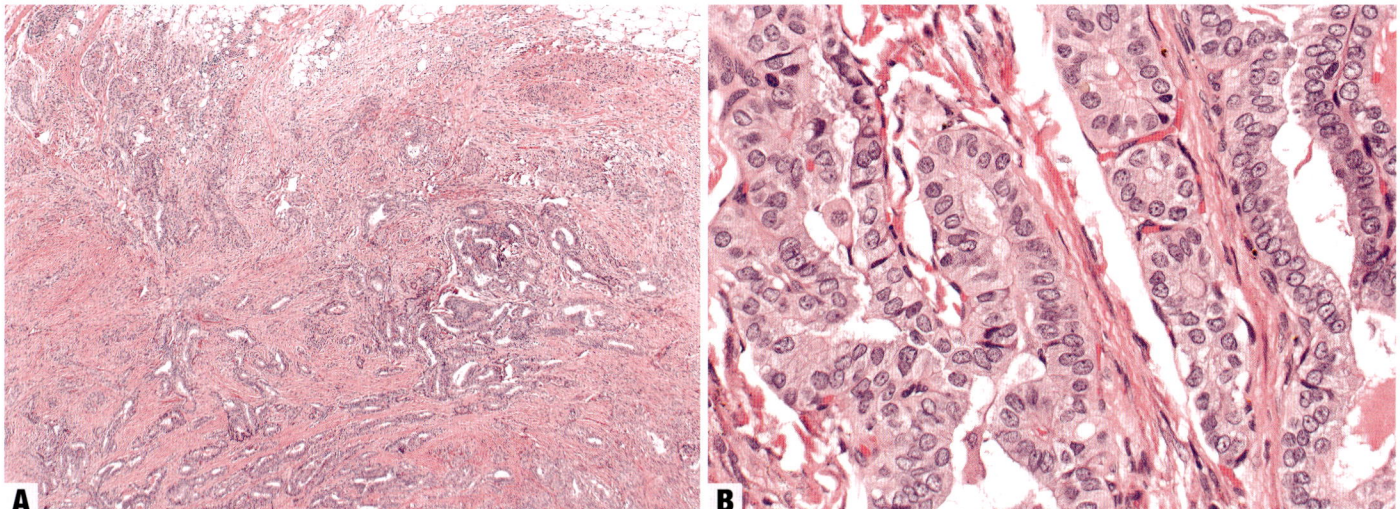

Fig. 9.18 Metastasis to the thymus. **A** The thymus is infiltrated by metastatic lung adenocarcinoma forming cystic structures lined by cuboidal to micropapillary malignant glandular epithelium. **B** A cystic and necrotic focus of metastatic adenocarcinoma infiltrates the thymus. A Hassall corpuscle is seen in the thymic tissue (lower left). The adenocarcinoma consists of cytologically atypical glandular cells growing along the wall of the cystic and necrotic tumour. Some micropapillary tumour clusters are seen in the cyst lumen. **C** TTF1 immunohistochemistry: the lung adenocarcinoma tumour cells show positive nuclear staining for TTF1. **D** p40 immunohistochemistry: p40 stains the thymic epithelial cells but is negative in the tumour cells.

Fig. 9.19 Papillary thyroid carcinoma forming a tumour deposit in the mediastinum. **A** Tumour is growing in a fibrotic background and extending into adjacent adipose tissue. Lymph node tissue is not apparent. **B** The tumour cells have oval nuclei, some with nuclear grooves. Nuclear overlap is focally noted.

Cytology
Cytological features are similar to those of the primary tumour.

Diagnostic molecular pathology
Distinct genetic aberrations that might aid in the distinction between primary thymic and metastatic squamous cell carcinomas include gains of 1q and loss of 6 and 16q, which favour primary thymic carcinoma {3479}.

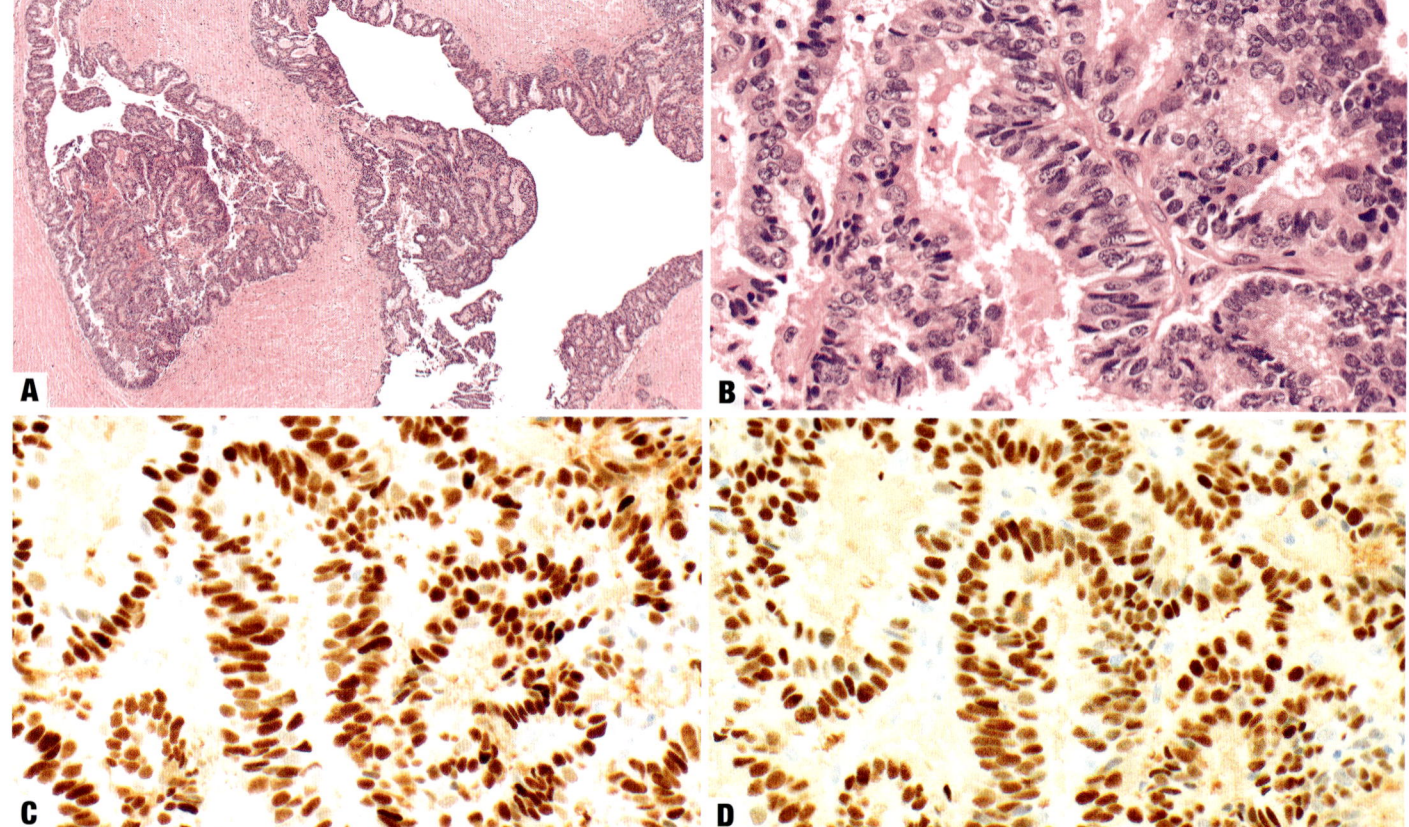

Fig. 9.20 Metastatic endometrioid adenocarcinoma manifesting as a solitary, > 60 mm mediastinal mass > 8 years after primary tumour. **A** Complex malignant glands are in a fibrotic background consistent with adenocarcinoma. **B** While some tumour cells have a polygonal shape, others are columnar and show pseudostratification. **C** The neoplastic cells are strongly and diffusely positive for ER. **D** The neoplastic cells are strongly and diffusely positive for PR.

Essential and desirable diagnostic criteria

Essential:

- Pathological diagnosis of a tumour compatible with origin outside the mediastinum according to diagnostic histological, immunohistochemical, and/or molecular criteria for that tumour
- Exclusion of primary thymic tumour on the basis of clinical history, imaging, and histopathological findings

Desirable:

- Histological, immunohistochemical, and molecular profiling of the metastatic tumour and comparison with any previous tumours (if available)
- Multidisciplinary discussion of the case, such as at a tumour board

Staging

Staging is based on the Union for International Cancer Control (UICC) TNM staging of the primary tumour.

Prognosis and prediction

Prognosis depends on primary disease and whether a single metastasis or oligometastases can be surgically removed.

Metastasis to the heart and pericardium
Padera RF

Definition
Metastasis to the heart and pericardium represents a malignancy that has spread to these sites from an extracardiac/extrapericardial site of origin.

ICD-O coding
8000/6 Neoplasm, metastatic

ICD-11 coding
2D7Y Malignant neoplasm metastasis in other specified thoracic organs

Related terminology
Not recommended: secondary malignant neoplasm of heart and pericardium.

Subtype(s)
None

Localization
The pericardium is the most frequently involved site of cardiac metastasis, accounting for 64–69% of all cardiac metastases in two recent large case series {352,354,9}. Epicardial (25–34%) and myocardial (29–32%) involvement represents the second and third most common sites of cardiac metastasis. Endocardial and intracavitary metastases are rare, accounting for 3–5% of cardiac metastases on autopsy. Pericardial and epicardial metastatic deposits tend to favour the base of the heart and atria rather than the apical ventricular areas.

Clinical features
The nature of the clinical presentation is dictated by the location and extent of the metastatic tumour, with some cardiac metastases being clinically silent and detected only at postmortem examination. Tumour metastasis to the pericardium may initially result in pericarditis, with subsequent development of serosanguinous or haemorrhagic malignant pericardial effusions {1661}. Depending on their size and rate of accumulation, malignant pericardial effusions may be symptomatic or silent. Although less common than pericardial effusions, deposits of pericardial metastases may also compromise cardiac output via constrictive pericarditis. However, this condition may also result from pericardial adhesions caused by radiation therapy or any prior surgery requiring sternotomy. Patients with pericarditis and/or pericardial effusions often report chest discomfort and dyspnoea on exertion. Epicardial or myocardial metastases may result in a variety of life-threatening complications, including arrhythmias (atrial fibrillation with rapid ventricular response, complete atrioventricular block, or ventricular fibrillation), chest pain mimicking acute coronary syndromes, myocardial ischaemia from direct involvement or spasm of coronary arteries, congestive heart failure, cardiac rupture, and sudden death. Endocardial and intracavitary

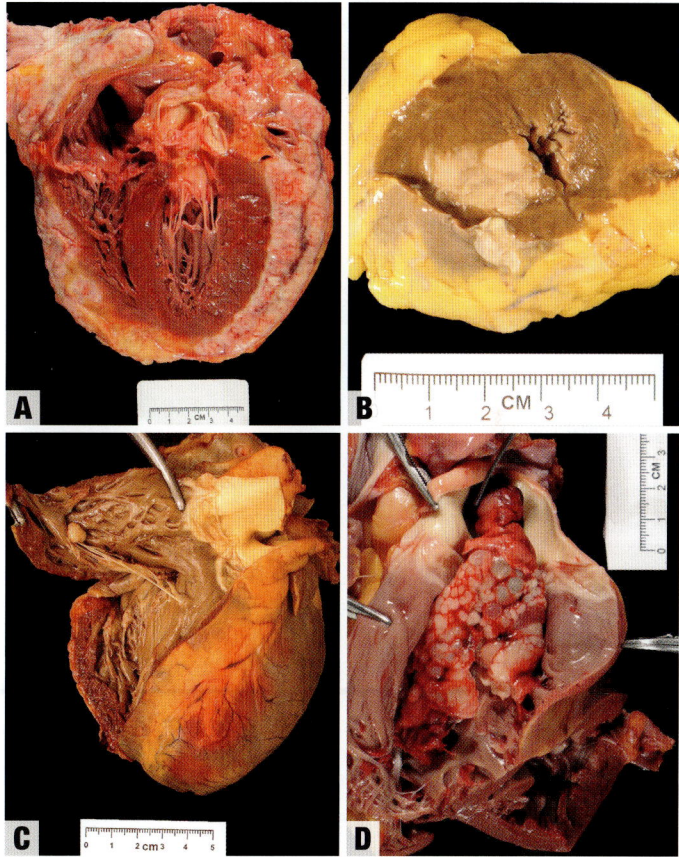

Fig. 9.21 Metastasis to the heart and pericardium. **A** Metastasis to the pericardium. Metastatic lung adenocarcinoma diffusely filling the pericardial space and causing restrictive physiology. **B** Metastasis to the myocardium. Metastatic breast cancer forming a nodule within the left ventricular free wall near the apex. **C** Metastasis to the endocardium. Metastatic pancreatic adenocarcinoma occurring as a nodule in the anterior right ventricular endocardium. **D** Metastasis to the endocardium. Metastatic malignant peripheral nerve sheath tumour occurring as an intracavitary mass in the right ventricular outflow tract, causing obstruction.

metastases can have dramatic clinical consequences such as heart failure and/or cardiogenic shock from bulky inflow tract (e.g. right or left atrial) or outflow tract (e.g. right or left ventricular) obstruction, as well as cardioembolic phenomenon including pulmonary emboli and stroke {400,2322,915}. Involvement of the superior or inferior vena cava can be a prelude to cardiac metastasis. In particular, renal cell and hepatocellular carcinomas may spread via an endovascular route from the inferior vena cava to the right atrium, with potential haemodynamic and embolic consequences as described above. Superior vena cava involvement can result in superior vena cava syndrome, an oncological emergency that may manifest with presyncope or syncope, dilated chest wall veins, upper extremity oedema, periorbital oedema, and headache if superior vena cava obstruction is subacute. Superior vena cava syndrome is classically associated with thoracic tumours such as lung cancer, breast cancer, lymphoma, thymoma, and germ cell tumours. Echocardiography is the initial imaging modality for the detection of pericardial effusions, as well as to assess for the presence and clinical consequences of any cardiac metastasis {329}. Cardiac MRI, CT, and PET can provide additional non-invasive characterization of cardiac masses {982, 2018}.

Clinical diagnosis of cardiac metastasis can sometimes be made on imaging, but tissue histology remains the most definitive method for differentiating neoplastic from non-neoplastic masses and for planning definitive or palliative therapy {1652}. Although exploratory thoracotomy and open biopsy are sometimes necessary to identify cardiac metastases, various techniques for obtaining tumour cells do not require thoracic surgery. Malignant cells can be identified in the majority of malignant pericardial effusions drained by pericardiocentesis, and the cytology of malignant cells has an extraordinarily high correlation with the histological diagnosis. Another approach to more definitively obtain tissue is endomyocardial biopsy, which is especially useful for right-sided cardiac masses showing infiltration or obstruction {1652}.

Epidemiology

The frequency of metastatic tumours to the pericardium, myocardium, great vessels, or coronary arteries has been reported as 0.7–3.5% at autopsy in the general population, 9.1% in patients with known malignancies, and up to 14.2% in patients with multiple distant metastases {1774,982,1775}. This rate has been increasing in recent decades, probably secondary to increased life expectancy in oncological patients as a result of modern advances in cancer diagnosis and treatment.

Although any type of tumour can affect the heart, the probability of cardiac involvement is a function of anatomical considerations, stage of disease, and individual tumour and host biology {352,325,3461,64}. Primary lung cancer represents 36–39% of cardiac metastases, followed by breast cancer (10–12%) and haematological malignancies (10–21%) {354, 60,355,9}. These numbers reflect the high prevalence of these tumours in the general population and their aggressive nature; in contrast, prostate cancer, although more prevalent in men than any of the above tumours, rarely metastasizes to the heart. Pleural mesothelioma and melanoma have an unusual proclivity to involve the heart, with an estimated 28–56% of patients with metastatic melanoma having some cardiac involvement. Other tumours with high rates of cardiac metastasis include ovarian, gastric, renal, and pancreatic carcinomas; lymphomas; and angiosarcomas {1774,982,1775}.

Etiology

The etiology of the malignancy varies depending on the specific nature of primary tumour.

Pathogenesis

Tumours can reach the heart and pericardium via four main pathways: haematogenous spread, lymphatic spread, transvenous extension, and direct extension {982}. Spread by the haematogenous route generally gives rise to myocardial or endocardial metastasis, as is common with melanoma, lymphoma, and sarcoma, whereas spread by the lymphatic route often results in pericardial and epicardial tumour involvement,

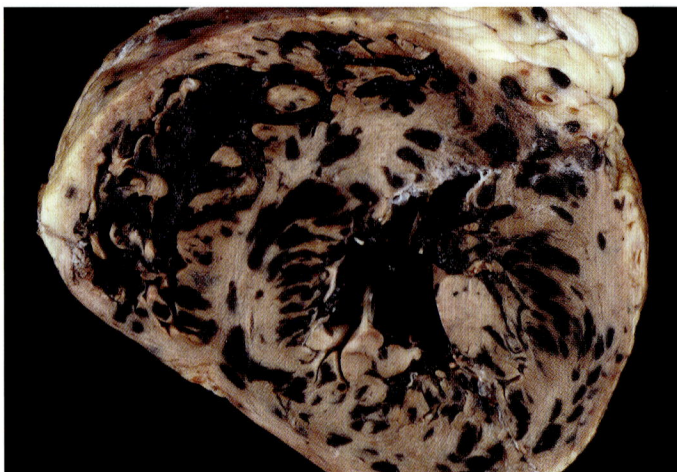

Fig. 9.22 Metastatic melanoma. Numerous metastatic deposits can be seen involving the epicardium, myocardium, and endocardium. Tumour thrombus is also present within the right ventricle.

as with many epithelial tumours such as of the lung and breast. Certain tumours such as renal cell carcinoma and hepatocellular carcinoma can extend into the inferior vena cava and grow into the right atrium via transvenous extension. Locally aggressive mediastinal and pleural tumours such as mesothelioma can directly invade the pericardial sac {982}.

Macroscopic appearance

Metastatic tumours to the pericardium can be grossly subtle, involving the pericardial lymphatics without forming a discrete mass. In these situations, they often cause a fibrinous pericarditis that can be haemorrhagic or a pericardial effusion that can range from serous to serosanguinous. Metastatic tumours can form firm, white nodules on the pericardium or epicardium, and they can grow to completely fill the pericardial space, encasing the heart with areas of haemorrhage and necrosis. Metastatic tumours to the myocardium can range from millimetre-sized miliary-like nodules to larger (centimetre-sized) firm white nodules that may have associated haemorrhage and necrosis. Myocardial involvement by leukaemia or lymphoma can occur as a diffuse infiltrate with or without associated haemorrhage. Metastatic tumours to the endocardium and intracavitary masses may manifest as firm white nodules that are affixed to the endocardial surface, most commonly in the right atrium or right ventricle, or they may be more loosely adherent tumour emboli that can obstruct blood flow through the heart {352}.

Histopathology

The histological morphology of the metastatic site usually mimics that of the primary site, so review of any histological slides from a potential primary site can be helpful in establishing the correct diagnosis. Pericardial metastases may not form a discrete grossly identifiable mass but may line the pericardial surface, form small nests within the pericardial interstitium, or be present only in lymphovascular spaces within the pericardium. This is also true of tumours metastatic to the epicardial surface or epicardial adipose tissue. There may be an associated fibrinous pericarditis, acute and/or chronic inflammation, reactive mesothelial cell hyperplasia, and possibly haemorrhage. Distinguishing this reactive hyperplasia from metastatic tumour may be difficult on purely

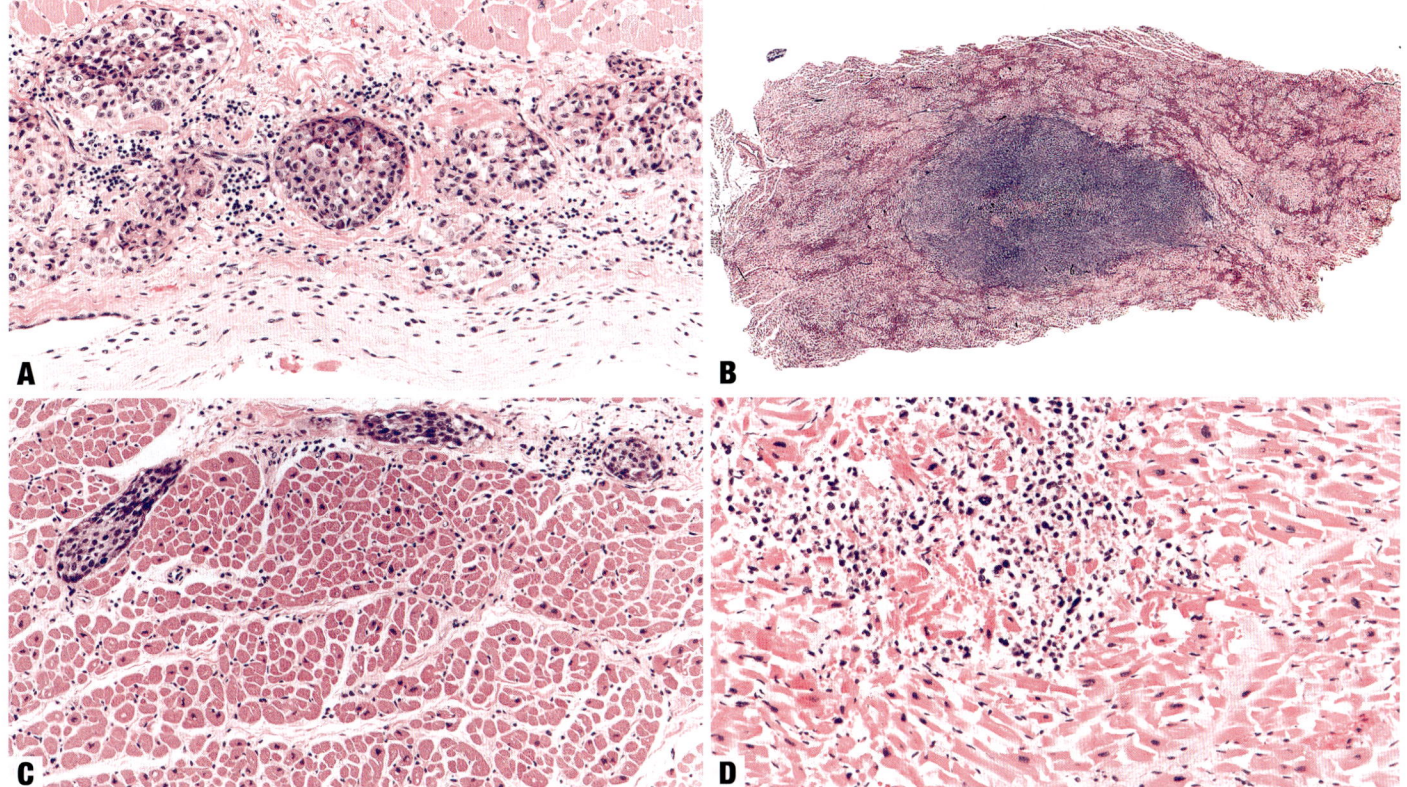

Fig. 9.23 Metastasis to the heart and pericardium. **A** Metastasis to the pericardium. Metastatic renal cell carcinoma involving angiolymphatic spaces in the pericardium without forming a discrete mass. **B** Metastasis to the myocardium. Small nodule of metastatic melanoma within the myocardium, which is also diffusely involved by amyloidosis. **C** Metastasis to the myocardium. Metastatic lung squamous cell carcinoma within angiolymphatic spaces in the myocardium, not causing myocardial damage. **D** Metastasis to the myocardium. Metastatic ovarian serous carcinoma involving the myocardium, with destruction of myocytes.

morphological grounds, so immunohistochemistry can be helpful. Metastatic tumours within the myocardium proper may form nodules with infiltrative or expansile borders that cause necrosis of the cardiac myocytes. Often, individual tumour cells or small tumour cell clusters may be present only in small blood vessels or lymphatics within the myocardium without exiting into the myocardial interstitium. Tumours involving the endocardial surface may have associated mural thrombus secondary to the loss of overlying intact, functional endothelium {352}.

Cytology
Although most pericardial effusions in the general population are benign, malignancy may be responsible for as many as 30% of effusions in large cancer centres {730}. Benign effusions can occur in cancer patients as well, the most common etiologies of which are secondary to treatment such as radiation or secondary to infection. Cytological evaluation of pericardial effusions can be instrumental in the diagnosis of pericardial or epicardial metastatic disease, with high specificity and sensitivity (varying from 40% to 95%) {2292}. Additional studies such as immunohistochemistry and molecular diagnostics on cytology material can be useful to establish a diagnosis and confirm the likely primary site.

Diagnostic molecular pathology
The genetic profile of the malignant cells from the metastatic site depends on the biology of the primary tumour. In cases of a poorly differentiated malignancy where morphology and immunohistochemistry are not definitive, characteristic mutations or genetic signatures (e.g. associated with smoking or ultraviolet [UV] light) may allow identification of the likely primary site.

Essential and desirable diagnostic criteria
Essential:
- Histopathological or cytological diagnosis of malignancy, with exclusion of primary cardiac, vascular, or pericardial malignancy on the basis of clinical history, histopathological or cytological findings, immunohistochemistry, and molecular profile

Desirable:
- Histological and immunohistochemical comparison with biopsy of any previous primary malignancies (if available) and discussion of the clinical case with caregivers

Staging
According to the current pathological TNM system and the Union for International Cancer Control (UICC) staging guidelines, metastatic tumours are generally characterized as stage IV disease.

Prognosis and prediction
Cardiac metastases are most often found in patients with multiple metastases and a profound burden of disseminated disease. Therefore, the prognosis is generally poor and long-term survival is rare, with a median survival time of about 3.5 months without treatment {2471,2966,856}.

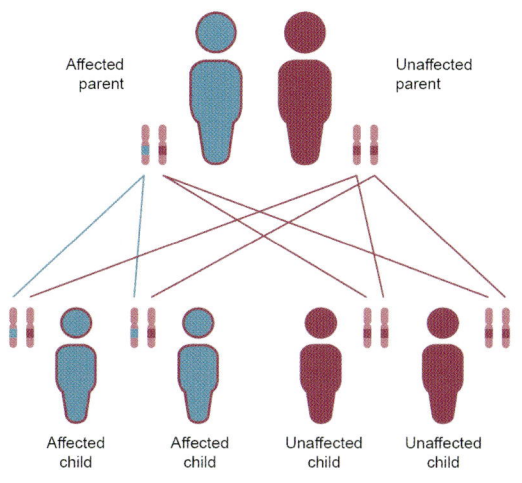

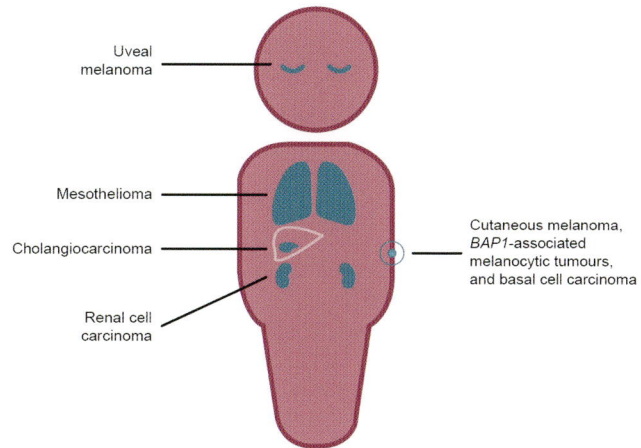

10

Genetic tumour syndromes involving the thorax

Edited by: Cooper WA, Dacic S, Jain D, Lazar AJ

Li–Fraumeni syndrome
BAP1 tumour predisposition syndrome
Carney complex

Genetic tumour syndromes involving the thorax: Introduction

Lazar AJ
Cooper WA

Hereditary factors can contribute to the development of thoracic tumours. These genetic variants may have other phenotypic consequences as well, resulting in clinically recognizable tumour-predisposing syndromes. However, with the rapidly increasing use of massively parallel (next-generation) sequencing of DNA in both diagnostic pathology and clinical genetics, constitutional pathogenetic variants can now be routinely screened for and identified with great precision. This in turn makes it possible to identify at-risk individuals in affected families, who can then be offered genetic counselling. Information on underlying genetic variants can also have an important effect on the choice of therapy and surveillance guidelines. The unbiased nature of sequencing studies will undoubtedly continue to widen the spectrum of known predisposing genetic variants among patients with thoracic tumours, also encompassing monogenic and polygenic variants with only a moderate effect on tumour risk.

This chapter provides detailed descriptions of three selected disease syndromes, which are summarized in Table 10.01. These syndromes have been covered in detail because their clinical, histopathological, and genetic characteristics are well characterized in the thorax, or because their associated neoplasms have features that are different from those of their sporadic counterparts.

There is a broader range of hereditary genetic disorders that are associated with familial predisposition to a variety of thoracic neoplasms (see Table 10.02). These hereditary syndromes are associated with a range of benign and malignant neoplasms involving multiple organ systems and are not limited to the thorax. While Li–Fraumeni syndrome, *BAP1* tumour predisposition syndrome, and Carney complex are briefly discussed in this chapter, with focus on thoracic manifestations, other hereditary tumour syndromes are covered in separate WHO classifications, because they are predominantly associated with non-thoracic tumours. Germline *EGFR* p.T790M and *ERBB2* mutations are addressed below due to the distinct connection of the germline *EGFR* status with lung cancer.

Non-small cell lung carcinomas, by far the commonest type of thoracic malignancy, are only rarely associated with a hereditary tumour syndrome, such as Li–Fraumeni syndrome,

Peutz–Jeghers syndrome, and germline *EGFR* p.T790M and *ERBB2* mutations {390,3341A,1745A}. Several germline mutations within or adjacent to the kinase domain of *EGFR* have been reported to potentially predispose to lung carcinoma {1745A}, with p.T790M being the best characterized. Germline *EGFR* p.T790M mutations account for a rare lung cancer hereditary syndrome with dominant inheritance that predisposes to the development of lung adenocarcinoma, regardless of smoking status and sometimes associated with an additional *EGFR* activating mutation {925}. The germline mutation is estimated to occur in < 1 person per 7500 {925}, and the estimated risk for lung cancer development is 31% in never-smokers, although the familial penetrance, lifetime risk, and resultant clinical syndrome are not well characterized {925}. The *EGFR* p.T790M mutation commonly occurs as an acquired resistance mutation after treatment with EGFR tyrosine kinase inhibitors but is rarely found in pretreatment tumour samples. Approximately 50% of de novo *EGFR* p.T790M mutations are thought to be germline {2226}, and this could be considered an indication for definitive germline testing. Germline *EGFR* p.T790M is an emerging entity that will probably be granted a dedicated section in the next edition, as additional data emerge and mature.

Peutz–Jeghers syndrome is an autosomal dominant syndrome caused by germline mutations in the tumour suppressor gene *STK11* (*LKB1*), which is involved in cell-cycle regulation. The syndrome is associated with gastrointestinal polyps, mucocutaneous pigmentation, and increased risk of gastrointestinal tract carcinomas, as well as a variety of non-gastrointestinal malignancies including lung carcinoma {3341A}.

Several other hereditary tumour syndromes are associated with a variety of thoracic neoplasms, and these are discussed in other chapters. They include germline pathogenic *DICER1* loss-of-function variations that are found in the majority of patients with pleuropulmonary blastoma (see *Pleuropulmonary blastoma*, p. 160) {1445,2862}. Because *DICER1* is a tumour suppressor gene, an acquired variant is required in the second *DICER1* allele – usually a missense variant in the RNase IIIb domain of the protein. These patients also commonly develop cystic nephroma, Sertoli–Leydig cell tumours, thyroid neoplasms, and lung cysts {1427,2862}.

Table 10.01 Hereditary tumour syndromes covered in detail within this chapter

Disease/phenotype	MIM number	Inheritance	Locus	Gene	Gene/locus MIM number	Protein	Normal protein function
Li–Fraumeni syndrome	151623	AD	17p13	*TP53*	191170	p53	DNA damage response; "guardian of the genome"
BAP1 tumour predisposition syndrome	614327	AD	3p21	*BAP1*	603089	BAP1	A nuclear-localizing deubiquitinating enzyme
Carney complex	160980	AD	17q24	*PRKAR1A*	188830	PRKAR1A	A regulatory subunit of PKA

AD, autosomal dominant.

Table 10.02 Hereditary genetic disorders associated with familial predisposition to particular thoracic neoplasms

Hereditary genetic disorder	Associated thoracic neoplasms
Li–Fraumeni syndrome	Lung carcinoma, mediastinal/cardiac sarcomas, thymic carcinoma
BAP1 tumour predisposition syndrome	Mesothelioma
Carney complex	Atrial myxoma
DICER1 syndrome	Pleuropulmonary blastoma
Tuberous sclerosis	Lymphangioleiomyomatosis, perivascular epithelioid cell tumours (PEComas), cardiac rhabdomyomas
Gorlin syndrome	Cardiac fibromas
Gardner syndrome	Desmoid fibromatosis
Neurofibromatosis type 1	Malignant peripheral nerve sheath tumour, paragangliomas
Neurofibromatosis type 2	Schwannoma
Germline *SMARCB1* or *LZTR1* mutations	Schwannomatosis
Multiple endocrine neoplasia type 2	Paraganglioma
Von Hippel–Lindau syndrome	Paraganglioma
Hereditary paraganglioma-phaeochromocytoma syndrome	Paraganglioma
Carney–Stratakis syndrome	Paraganglioma
Peutz–Jeghers syndrome	Lung carcinoma
Germline *EGFR* p.T790M	Lung carcinoma
ERBB2 germline mutations	Lung carcinoma

Tuberous sclerosis is an autosomal dominant disorder with variable penetrance and expression, characterized by germline loss-of-function mutations in *TSC1* or *TSC2* {1124}. These genes encode the proteins hamartin and tuberin, respectively, which form a protein complex that inhibits the growth-promoting mTOR (mechanistic target of rapamycin) signalling pathway {1124}. Tuberous sclerosis affects multiple organ systems, including the lung, heart, brain, skin, and kidneys. Lymphangioleiomyomatosis (see *Lymphangioleiomyomatosis of the lung*, p. 170) and neoplasms with perivascular epithelioid cell differentiation (formerly known as sugar tumours; see *PEComa of the lung*, p. 172) can occur sporadically or in the setting of tuberous sclerosis {268,849,728}. By contrast, cardiac rhabdomyomas (see *Cardiac rhabdomyoma*, p. 237) occur in the setting of tuberous sclerosis in as many as 70–90% of cases {283,1070,2713,1150}.

Carney complex, an autosomal dominant disorder associated with cardiac and non-cardiac myxomas as well as endocrinopathies and skin pigmentation, should not be confused with Carney triad, a non-hereditary tumour syndrome characterized by gastrointestinal stromal tumours, pulmonary chondromas, and paragangliomas with *SDHC* promoter hypermethylation in the tumours {389,2869,1054}.

It is important for pathologists to have an understanding of the clinicopathological features of tumours potentially related to hereditary tumour predisposition syndromes, in order to increase the opportunity for diagnosis and to optimize patient and family management.

Li–Fraumeni syndrome

Caron O
Thomas DM

Definition
Li–Fraumeni syndrome (LFS) is an autosomal dominant cancer predisposition syndrome caused by germline pathogenic variants of the *TP53* gene {1780}.

MIM numbering
151623 Li–Fraumeni syndrome; LFS

ICD-11 coding
None

Related terminology
Acceptable: SBLA syndrome (sarcoma, breast cancer, brain tumours, leukaemia / lymphoma / lung carcinoma, adrenocortical carcinoma) {1751}.
Not recommended: sarcoma family syndrome of Li and Fraumeni.

Subtype(s)
None

Localization
TP53-associated LFS is associated with cancers of the breast, lung, soft tissue, bone, brain, and adrenal glands.

Clinical features
LFS was historically described in families with paediatric sarcomas and other cancers occurring at a very young age. Several clinical criteria have been defined (see Box 10.01) {1768}. The Chompret criteria take into account the narrow LFS cancer spectrum {294}, but the spectrum is actually broader, especially in adulthood, and cancer can arise at virtually any body site. Nevertheless, penetrance estimates are skewed by ascertainment bias. Lifetime cancer risk is supposed to be 70% in males and 90% in females {1018}, but the identification of pathogenic variants in large gene panels in an unselected population suggests a lower penetrance in some situations, most likely depending on mutation type and genetic modifiers {854}.

Within the core spectrum of cancers associated with LFS, breast cancer (24–39%) and sarcomas (24–31%) are the most common, followed by brain tumours (3.5–14%) and adrenocortical cancers (6.5–10%) {2097,294}. Other tumours are also

Box 10.01 Cancer patients who should be tested for germline disease-causing *TP53* variants[a] {862A}

Recommendation 1

All patients who meet the modified Chompret criteria should be tested for germline *TP53* variants:

- *familial presentation:* proband with a *TP53* core tumour (breast cancer, soft tissue sarcoma, osteosarcoma, CNS tumour, adrenocortical carcinoma) before the age of 46 years AND at least one first-degree or second-degree relative with a core tumour before the age of 56 years; *or*
- *multiple primitive tumours:* proband with multiple tumours, including 2 *TP53* core tumours, the first of which occurred before the age of 46 years, irrespective of family history; *or*
- *rare tumours:* patient with adrenocortical carcinoma, choroid plexus carcinoma, or rhabdomyosarcoma of embryonal anaplastic subtype, irrespective of family history; *or*
- *very early onset breast cancer:* breast cancer before the age of 31 years, irrespective of family history

Recommendation 2

Children and adolescents should be tested for germline *TP53* variants if presenting with:

- hypodiploid acute lymphoblastic leukaemia; *or*
- otherwise unexplained *SHH*-driven[b] medulloblastoma; *or*
- jaw osteosarcoma

Recommendation 3

Patients who develop a second primary tumour within the radiotherapy field of a first core *TP53* tumour that occurred before the age of 46 years should be tested for germline *TP53* variants.

Recommendation 4

- Patients older than 46 years presenting with breast cancer without personal or familial history fulfilling the Chompret criteria should not be tested for germline *TP53* variants.
- Any patient presenting with isolated breast cancer and not fulfilling the Chompret criteria, in whom a disease-causing *TP53* variant has been identified, should be referred to an expert multidisciplinary team for discussion.

Recommendation 5

Children with any cancer from southern and south-eastern Brazilian families should be tested for the p.R337H Brazilian founder germline *TP53* variant.

[a]Testing for disease-causing *TP53* variants should be performed before starting treatment in order to avoid in variant carriers, if possible, radiotherapy and genotoxic chemotherapy and to prioritize surgical treatments. [b]Full approved name of *SHH*: "sonic hedgehog signalling molecule".

observed, with an earlier age of onset than sporadic counterparts remaining a hallmark of LFS {70}.

Thoracic cancers have been reported in LFS patients but are not common. Several recent studies have reported lung adenocarcinomas, predominantly in non-smokers {152}. In the IARC *TP53* Database, thoracic cancers accounted for 75 of 2592 (2.9%) of all cancers reported in individuals carrying *TP53* mutations {1220}. These include adenocarcinomas (23) and squamous cell carcinoma (4), with the remainder not specified. Three individuals with thymic carcinomas have been reported, and another three had sarcomas arising in the mediastinum or heart. In a large prospective screening cohort of LFS patients, lung cancer was the second most frequent new primary cancer (5 of 31 new cancers), occurring mainly in the fifth decade of life {390}.

Epidemiology

The *TP53* carrier rate is estimated at 1 carrier per 20 000 individuals, but it may be as high as 1 carrier per 500 individuals, especially with the widespread use of both tumour and germline profiling {624,2428}. *TP53* pathogenic variants are found in 70% of families fulfilling the classic LFS criteria and 30% fulfilling the broader Chompret criteria.

Most of the pathogenic variants are inherited in an autosomal dominant manner, but de novo mutations occur frequently (in 14% of carriers, in whom one fifth of the cases were mosaic in a recent series) {2467}. Mosaic cases may be mistaken for clonal haematopoiesis of indeterminate potential {3282}.

Etiology

TP53 encodes a transcriptional activator mediating cell responses to DNA damage and oncogenic stress {1882}. It is not required for normal development and appears to have a unique function as a tumour suppressor. Of the 4000 *TP53* mutations reported to date, most comprise missense mutations, although structural variants are also observed. A systematic functional screen of all possible missense substitutions has been reported, greatly enabling interpretation of novel variants {855,2153,1220}.

Pathogenesis

Mutations in *TP53* predominantly affect the DNA-binding core domain, often acting in a dominant negative manner by disrupting a tetrameric complex that is required for binding to regulatory regions in key downstream effector genes such as *CDKN1A* and *BBC3* (*PUMA*) {1882,943}. While a broad spectrum of mutations are observed, the most common mutations occur at codons 175, 248, 249, 273, and 281 {1220} and for the most part closely overlap with those observed to occur somatically in cancers.

Disruption of *TP53* function impairs several key tumour suppressor processes, including cell-cycle arrest and cell death. Because sensing DNA damage is an important function for *TP53*, the tumour spectrum associated with LFS is characterized by genomic instability {2757}. Recent evidence suggests that chromothripsis, the shattering of chromosomes, is frequently present {2439}.

Macroscopic appearance
Not clinically relevant

Histopathology
Histopathological features of thoracic tumours occurring in LFS are the same as those of their sporadic counterparts (see *Tumours of the lung: Introduction*, p. 20).

Cytology
Not clinically relevant

Diagnostic molecular pathology
Germline *TP53* pathogenic variants are the only cause of LFS. Importantly, many germline variants could increasingly be identified through tumour-only sequencing performed for therapeutic purposes, but most of these variants will remain purely somatic. The interpretation of variants of uncertain significance, which are large in number, remains an important challenge for genetic pathology.

Essential and desirable diagnostic criteria
See Box 10.01.

Staging
The staging system for cancers in LFS is the same as for tumours in their sporadic form.

Prognosis and prediction
Overall penetrance is presumed to be very high, with a 90% lifetime risk of cancer for male *TP53* mutation carriers and a nearly 100% risk for female carriers by the age of 70 years, with breast cancer incidence partly responsible for the observed sex difference {2752}; however, these figures may be overestimated due to ascertainment bias. Moreover, some variants might have lower penetrance than others. Mutated *TP53* as seen in LFS confers an elevated risk of radiation-induced secondary malignancies {1122,1138} and possibly increased sensitivity to low-dose radiation exposure from diagnostic procedures such as mammography {2819}. Surveillance strategies for early tumour detection in *TP53* mutation carriers have been reported and are now widely used, with some evidence of reductions in both mortality and treatment-related morbidity in patients who undergo surveillance {3172,1529,152}.

EGFR mutations may be more common in lung adenocarcinomas arising in LFS. In a cohort of 164 carriers of the recurrent *TP53* p.R337H variant in Brazil, 9 people developed lung cancer, with a mean age at diagnosis of 53 years. An *EGFR* activating mutation was found in 8 of 9 tumours, contrasting with the usual 20% rate {158}. This was confirmed by a larger series from France and Spain, in which 19 of 21 lung cancers displayed driver oncogenic alterations (18 *EGFR* mutations and 1 *ROS1* fusion) {1904}. This is in line with LFS breast cancers, in which *ERBB2* is usually amplified. HER-family kinases seem to be frequently activated in LFS tumours.

BAP1 tumour predisposition syndrome

Mandelker D
Ladanyi M
Sauter JL

Definition

BAP1 tumour predisposition syndrome is a hereditary cancer syndrome caused by heterozygous germline pathogenic variants in the *BAP1* (BRCA1 associated protein 1) gene.

MIM numbering

614327 Tumour predisposition syndrome; TPDS

ICD-11 coding

None

Related terminology

None

Subtype(s)

None

Localization

BAP1 tumour predisposition syndrome is associated with peritoneal and pleural mesotheliomas, skin tumours (in particular melanocytic tumours), and clear cell renal cell carcinoma (RCC).

Clinical features

BAP1 germline pathogenic variant carriers have an increased risk of cancers including mesothelioma (more often in the pleura than the peritoneum) {2256}, uveal melanoma, cutaneous melanoma, RCC, cholangiocarcinoma, and basal cell carcinoma {3026,2375,2,3183}. Additionally, many *BAP1* germline pathogenic variant carriers develop benign cutaneous melanocytic neoplasms called melanocytic *BAP1*-mutated atypical intradermal tumours (MBAITs) {3308}. Although penetrance information remains limited because of the small number of cases identified and ascertainment bias, in one study of 324 carriers of *BAP1* loss-of-function germline variants, 84.9% of carriers had developed at least one cancer, with the most common malignancies being uveal melanoma, mesothelioma, and cutaneous melanoma, and with 38 of 40 tested tumours showing loss of expression of BAP1 by immunohistochemistry {3188}. Another study found that 40 of 53 patients (~75%) who underwent total-body skin examinations were found to have MBAITs {1095}.

Although there are no formal diagnostic criteria, testing for *BAP1* tumour predisposition syndrome has been suggested for patients with two or more tumours associated with *BAP1* tumour predisposition syndrome, or one associated tumour and a first- or second-degree relative with one or more associated tumours {2413,462}.

Epidemiology

The prevalence of *BAP1* tumour predisposition syndrome is unknown, but this is considered to be a rare syndrome. *BAP1* loss-of-function germline variants are exceedingly rare in adult populations without cancer: there are only 7 such variants

identified in the Genome Aggregation Database (gnomAD) population database, out of approximately 250 000 chromosomes. Multiple studies have demonstrated that the median age at diagnosis for germline *BAP1*-associated mesothelioma is significantly younger (reported as 55–58 years) than for sporadic mesothelioma (reported as 68–72 years) {178,2156,3188}.

BAP1 tumour predisposition syndrome has been reported in 1–5% of uveal melanoma cases {1037,787,2468} and in a very low proportion of unselected mesothelioma cases {2795,2568, 1166,222}. However, detection of *BAP1* pathogenic variants is

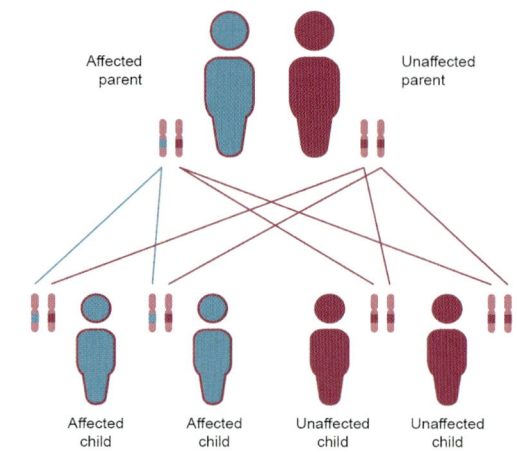

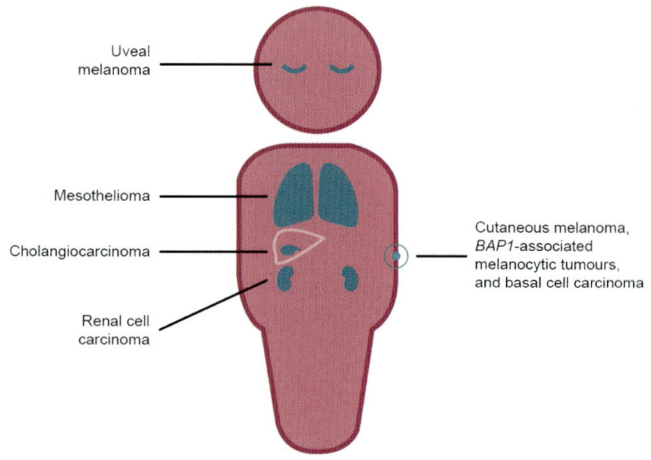

Fig. 10.01 The inheritance of *BAP1* tumour predisposition syndrome. Affected individuals inherit a germline sequence variant in one copy of the *BAP1* gene, leading to melanocytic and mesothelial tumours, lung cancer, renal cell carcinoma, and cholangiocarcinoma. Compiled from {2820A} and {1239A}.

enriched among familial cases of *BAP1*-related tumours such as uveal melanoma, mesothelioma, cholangiocarcinoma, cutaneous melanoma, and RCC {2156,2256,3110}.

Etiology

To date, most individuals diagnosed with *BAP1* tumour predisposition syndrome have inherited the *BAP1* pathogenic germline variant from a parent. The proportion of *BAP1* tumour predisposition syndrome caused by a de novo pathogenic variant arising from a mutation in a germ cell is unknown, although one study found that 2 of 21 probands tested (9.5%) had a probable de novo *BAP1* pathogenic germline variant {462}.

Pathogenesis

BAP1 is located on chromosome 3p21 and encodes a nuclear deubiquitinating enzyme {2116,289}. *BAP1* tumour predisposition syndrome is caused by heterozygous germline variants in *BAP1* that lead to loss of protein function {3026}.

Macroscopic appearance

Not relevant

Histopathology

The histological features of mesothelioma occurring in the setting of *BAP1* tumour predisposition syndrome are the same as those of tumours occurring sporadically.

Cytology

Not relevant

Diagnostic molecular pathology

BAP1 genetic sequencing and deletion/duplication analysis performed on peripheral blood can confirm the diagnosis of *BAP1* tumour predisposition syndrome. The vast majority of reported *BAP1* pathogenic germline variants to date have been sequence variants {2413} as opposed to copy-number changes.

Essential and desirable diagnostic criteria

Essential:
- Demonstration of a germline pathogenic variant in *BAP1*

Staging

Stage as appropriate for tumour type.

Prognosis and prediction

Cancer screening criteria for uveal melanoma, cutaneous melanoma, mesothelioma, cholangiocarcinoma, and RCC have been proposed for carriers of *BAP1* germline pathogenic variants. The recommendations include eye and skin examinations starting in adolescence to screen for melanoma, as well as chest and abdominal imaging to screen for mesothelioma and RCC beginning at the age of 30 years {2839,2413}.

Some studies suggest that individuals with *BAP1* tumour predisposition syndrome who develop mesothelioma have a longer survival than those with sporadic mesothelioma {178,2156, 3474}. However, uveal melanomas in *BAP1* germline pathogenic variant carriers may be more aggressive than sporadic cases {1037,2121}.

Carney complex

Maleszewski JJ
Carney JA

Definition
Carney complex (CNC) is an autosomal dominant syndrome characterized by myxomas, endocrinopathy, and pigmented skin lesions.

MIM numbering
160980 Carney complex, type 1; CNC1

ICD-11 coding
5A70.Y Carney complex

Related terminology
Acceptable: LAMB syndrome (lentigines, atrial myxoma, mucocutaneous myxoma, blue naevus); NAME syndrome (naevi, atrial myxoma, skin myxoma, ephelides); Carney syndrome; myxoma syndrome.

Subtype(s)
None

Localization
The syndrome is characterized by skin pigmentation abnormalities, cardiac myxomas, endocrine tumours or overactivity, and malignant melanotic nerve sheath tumours.

Clinical features
Individuals with CNC most commonly present with pale-brown to black lentigines that increase in number and intensity around puberty. These lesions commonly manifest at the vermillion border of the lips, conjunctiva, and inner and outer canthi. The

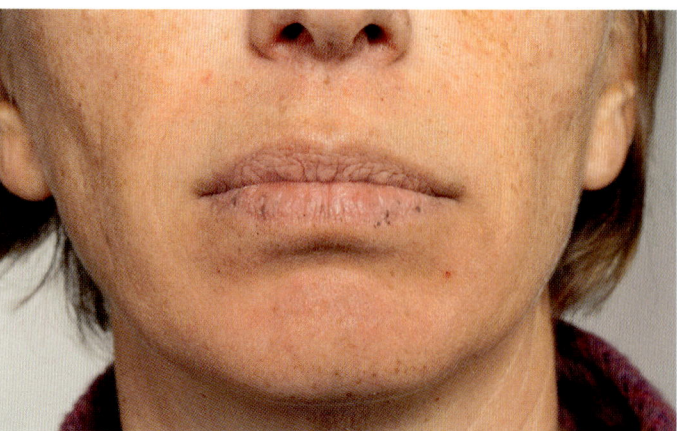

Fig. 10.02 Dermal lentigines. Spotty skin pigmentation of the mucous membranes or about the vermillion border of the lips is a characteristic finding of Carney complex.

vaginal and penile epithelia may also be involved. Development of unusual tumours such as myxomas, large cell calcifying Sertoli cell tumours, thyroid tumours (follicular adenomas or carcinomas), malignant melanotic nerve sheath tumours, blue naevi, ductal adenomas of the breast, pituitary adenomas, and/or osteochondromyxomas is also a feature of the syndrome. Endocrinopathy may result from the pituitary adenomas or primary pigmented nodular adrenocortical disease, which may result in Cushing syndrome.

Cardiac myxomas are the second most common presenting feature, present in more than half of cases. The occurrence of cardiac myxoma is somewhat equally spread across the age spectrum, whereas other manifestations, such as primary pigmented

---

Box 10.02 Diagnosis of Carney complex requires two major criteria or one major criterion plus one supplemental criterion {2870}

Major diagnostic criteria

Spotty skin pigmentation with typical distribution (lips, conjunctiva, inner or outer canthi, vaginal and penile mucosa)

Cardiac myxoma[a]

Myxoma (cutaneous and mucosal)[a]

Breast myxomatosis[a] or fat-suppressed MRI findings suggestive of this diagnosis

Primary pigmented nodular adrenocortical disease[a] or paradoxical positive response of urinary glucocorticoid excretion to dexamethasone administration during the Liddle test

Acromegaly due to growth hormone–producing adenoma[a]

Large cell calcifying Sertoli cell tumour[a] or characteristic calcification on testicular ultrasound

Thyroid follicular adenoma or carcinoma[a] or multiple, hypoechoic nodules on thyroid ultrasound in a young patient

Malignant melanotic nerve sheath tumours[a]

Blue naevus, epithelioid blue naevus (multiple)[a]

Breast ductal adenoma (multiple)[a]

Osteochondromyxoma[a]

Supplemental criteria

Affected first-degree relative

Inactivating mutation of *PRKAR1A*

[a]These tumours all require histological confirmation.

nodular adrenocortical disease, tend to manifest in the second to third decade of life. Large cell calcifying Sertoli cell tumours are seen in approximately a third of boys presenting in the first decade of life and are seen almost universally in men.

Epidemiology

CNC is a relatively rare syndrome, with < 1000 affected individuals having been identified. Cases have been described in various ethnicities around the globe, without a particular ethnic predilection.

Etiology

Approximately two thirds of people diagnosed with CNC have an affected parent, with the remaining third having undergone what appears to be a de novo germline genetic event.

Pathogenesis

Most cases of CNC are caused by mutations in *PRKAR1A*, a gene encoding a regulatory subunit of PKA. Mutations in this subunit lead to constitutive activation of PKA with increased cell proliferation, which causes the various manifestations seen in CNC.

Macroscopic appearance

Not relevant

Histopathology

Cardiac myxoma is described in this volume (see *Cardiac myxoma*, p. 233), other tumours within the relevant volumes of the WHO Classification of Tumours series.

Cytology

Cytology is not relevant for cardiac myxoma, but it may be helpful for thyroid lesions in particular.

Diagnostic molecular pathology

Genetic linkage analysis has implicated two independent loci in CNC: 17q23-q24 and 2p16. Inactivating mutations in the *PRKAR1A* gene located at 17q23-q24, coding for PRKAR1A (protein kinase cAMP-dependent type I regulatory subunit alpha), have been described in two thirds of CNC cases {3169}. The gene at locus 2p16 remains unknown; however, the presence of an activated oncogene at this locus is considered to be responsible for tumorigenesis in at least a subset of patients {1848,3402}.

More than 60% of cases of CNC are caused by mutation in *PRKAR1A* that can be detected by routine DNA sequencing. Another approximately 10–20% are detected by targeted deletion/duplication analysis {2616}. The penetrance of a pathogenic variant in *PRKAR1A* is nearly 100% by the age of 50 years.

A diagnosis of CNC may be suspected when there is demonstration of loss of immunohistochemical expression of *PRKAR1A* in tumour cells, which should then be followed up with germline testing for an underlying mutation in *PRKAR1A* {1777}.

Essential and desirable diagnostic criteria

The diagnosis of CNC requires two major criteria or a combination of one major criterion and one supplemental criterion (see Box 10.02).

Although not formally included in the diagnostic criteria, some conditions have been seen in association with CNC and therefore may raise suspicions for the diagnosis of CNC (see Box 10.03).

Staging

Staging is not relevant for cardiac myxoma, as indicated for other tumour types.

Prognosis and prediction

Because cardiac myxomas are a serious cause of morbidity and mortality in this patient population, people diagnosed with CNC (or first-degree relatives at risk of having CNC) should undergo annual echocardiographic surveillance to evaluate for cardiac myxomas. In addition, annual testicular examinations and thyroid examinations should be considered after puberty in this population. Urinary free cortisol and serum IGF1 levels can also be a consideration in these patients. The finding of any cardiac myxoma should lead to evaluation for CNC, a diagnosis that necessitates follow-up for the patient and their relatives {1777,2232}.

Contributors

AGAIMY, Abbas
Erlangen University Hospital
Krankenhausstraße 8-10
91054 Erlangen

AL-DAYEL, Fouad Hassan
King Faisal Specialist Hospital & Research Centre
Box 3354 Al Maather
Riyadh 11211

AOZASA, Katsuyuki
Osaka University Graduate School of Medicine
2-2 Nakanoshima
Suita, Osaka 565-0871

ASAMURA, Hisao
Keio University School of Medicine
35 Shinanomachi, Shinjuku-ku
Tokyo 160-8582

AUBRY, Marie-Christine*
Mayo Clinic
200 First Street South-West
Rochester MN 55905

BACON, Chris M.
Newcastle University
Herschel Building, Brewery Lane
Newcastle upon Tyne NE1 7RU

BADVE, Sunil*
Indiana University
635 Barnhill Drive, MS A-128
Indianapolis IN 46260

BASSO, Cristina
Pathological Anatomy-Cardiovascular Pathology
University of Padova Medical School
Via Gabelli 61
35121 Padua PD

BEASLEY, Mary Beth*
Icahn School of Medicine at Mount Sinai
1 Gustave L. Levy Place, Annenberg 15-265
New York NY 10025

BILLINGS, Steven D.
Cleveland Clinic
9500 Euclid Avenue, L25
Cleveland OH 44195

BIRONZO, Paolo
Department of Oncology
University of Turin
Regione Gonzole 10
10043 Orbassano TO

BOIS, Melanie C.
Mayo Clinic
200 First Street South-West
Rochester MN 55905

BOLAND, Jennifer M.
Mayo Clinic
200 First Street South-West
Rochester MN 55905

BORCZUK, Alain C.*
Weill Cornell Medicine
1300 York Avenue A607C
New York NY 10065

BOTLING, Johan*
Uppsala University Hospital
Rudbeck Laboratory
75185 Uppsala

BOYER, Daniel Frederick
University of Michigan
2800 Plymouth Road, Building 36
Ann Arbor MI 48109

BRAMBILLA, Elisabeth
University of Grenoble Alpes
Site Santé, Allée des Alpes
38700 La Tronche, Grenoble

BRIDGE, Julia A.
Translational Genomics Research Institute (TGen) / Ashion
445 North Fifth Street
Phoenix AZ 85004

BUBENDORF, Lukas*
Pathology, University Hospital Basel
Schönbeinstrasse 40
4031 Basel

BUENO, Raphael*
Brigham and Women's Hospital and Harvard Medical School
75 Francis Street
Boston MA 02115

BUETTNER, Reinhard*
Institute of Pathology
Kerpener Straße 62
50937 Cologne

BURKE, Allen P.
University of Maryland School of Medicine
21 South Greene Street
Baltimore MD 21201

BUTNOR, Kelly J.
University of Vermont Medical Center
111 Colchester Avenue, ACC Building EP2-120
Burlington VT 05401

CALABRESE, Fiorella
Pathological Anatomy
University of Padova Medical School
Via Gabelli 61
35121 Padua PD

CALONJE, Jaime E.
St John's Institute of Dermatology
St Thomas' Hospital
Westminster Bridge Road
London SE1 7EH

CAMPO, Elias
Hospital Clinic of Barcelona
University of Barcelona
Villarroel 170
08036 Barcelona

CARDONA, Andres F.*
Clínica del Country
Calle 116 #9-72, Carrera 23 #106-84
Bogotá 110111

CARNEIRO, Fátima
Ipatimup/i3S
Rua Júlio Amaral de Carvalho, 45
4200-135 Porto

CARNEY, J. Aidan
Mayo Clinic and Mayo Foundation
200 First Street South-West
Rochester MN 55905

CARON, Olivier
Gustave Roussy
114 Rue Edouard Vaillant
94805 Villejuif

CASTONGUAY, Mathieu C.
Dalhousie University
5788 University Avenue
Halifax NS B3H 1V8

CESARMAN, Ethel*
Weill Cornell Medicine
1300 York Avenue, Room C410
New York NY 10065

CHALABREYSSE, Lara
Groupement Hospitalier Est
59 Boulevard Pinel
69677 Bron Cedex Lyon

---

* Indicates disclosure of interests (see p. 487).

CHAN, John K.C.
Queen Elizabeth Hospital
30 Gascoigne Road
Kowloon, Hong Kong SAR

CHANG, Jason C.
Memorial Sloan Kettering Cancer Center
1275 York Avenue
New York NY 10065

CHANG, Yih-Leong
NTU Cancer Center
NTU College of Medicine
No. 57, Ln. 155, Sec. 3, Keelung Road
Taipei 106

CHEN, Gang
Zhongshan Hospital, Fudan University
180 Fenglin Road
Shanghai 200032

CHEUK, Wah
Queen Elizabeth Hospital
Gascoigne Road
Kowloon, Hong Kong SAR

CHEUNG, Annie Nga-Yin
University of Hong Kong
Queen Mary Hospital
Pok Fu Lam Road
Hong Kong SAR

CHIRIEAC, Lucian R.*
Harvard Medical School
75 Francis Street
Boston MA 02115

CHOU, Teh-Ying
Taipei Veterans General Hospital
201, Section 2, Shi-Pai Road
Taipei 11217

CHUNG, Jin-Haeng
Seoul National University College of Medicine
Seoul National University Bundang Hospital
173 Beon-gil, 82 Gumi-ro, Bundang-gu
Seoul 13620

COHLE, Stephen D.
Spectrum Health Blodgett Hospital
1840 Wealthy Street South-East
Grand Rapids MI 49506

COOK, James R.
Cleveland Clinic
9500 Euclid Avenue, Mail Stop L30
Cleveland OH 44195

COOPER, Wendy A.*
Royal Prince Alfred Hospital
NSW Health Pathology
Missenden Road
Camperdown NSW 2050

CREE, Ian A.
International Agency for Research on Cancer
150 Cours Albert Thomas
69372 Lyon

CREYTENS, David
Ghent University Hospital, Ghent University
Department of Pathology
Corneel Heymanslaan 10
9000 Ghent

DACIC, Sanja*
University of Pittsburgh Medical Center
200 Lothrop Street, PUH C608
Pittsburgh PA 15213

DE LA FOUCHARDIÈRE, Arnaud
Centre Léon Bérard
28 Rue Laennec
69008 Lyon

DE PERROT, Marc*
Princess Margaret Cancer Centre
200 Elizabeth Street, 9N-961
Toronto ON M5G 2C4

DEI TOS, Angelo Paolo
University of Padua School of Medicine /
Azienda Ospedale-Università Padova
(Department of Pathology)
Via Gabelli 61
35121 Padua PD

DEMICCO, Elizabeth G.
University of Toronto
Mount Sinai Hospital, 600 University Avenue
Toronto ON M5G 1X5

DEN BAKKER, Michael A.
Maasstad Hospital
Maasstadweg 21
3079 DZ Rotterdam

DETTERBECK, Frank
Yale School of Medicine
Box 208062
New Haven CT 06520-8062

DEVESA, Susan S.
National Cancer Institute
9609 Medical Center Drive
Bethesda MD 20892

DI TOMMASO, Luca
Humanitas University
Via Manzoni 56
20089 Rozzano MI

DINGEMANS, Anne-Marie
Erasmus Medical Center
Postbus 2040
3000 CA Rotterdam

DOGAN, Ahmet*
Memorial Sloan Kettering Cancer Center
1275 York Avenue
New York NY 10065

DOYLE, Leona A.
Brigham and Women's Hospital and
Harvard Medical School
75 Francis Street
Boston MA 02115

DRY, Sarah M.
University of California, Los Angeles (UCLA)
13-222 CHS, 10833 Le Conte Avenue
Los Angeles CA 90095

DUHIG, Edwina E.
Sullivan Nicolaides Pathology
Box 95
Tugun QLD 4224

EMILE, Jean-François
APHP and Versailles University
9 Avenue Charles de Gaulle
92104 Boulogne

FARAGO, Anna F.*
Massachusetts General Hospital
55 Fruit Street
Boston MA 02114

FARVER, Carol F.
Department of Pathology
University of Michigan
NCRC Building 35, Room 30-1531
2800 Plymouth Road, SPC 2800
Ann Arbor MI 48109-2800

FEND, Falko
University Hospital Tübingen
Liebermeisterstraße 8
72076 Tübingen

FERNANDEZ-CUESTA, Lynnette
International Agency for Research on Cancer
150 Cours Albert Thomas
69372 Lyon

FERRY, Judith A.
Massachusetts General Hospital
55 Fruit Street
Boston MA 02114

FISHBEIN, Gregory Andrew
David Geffen School of Medicine at UCLA
10833 Le Conte Avenue, CHS 27-061
Los Angeles CA 90095

FLIEDER, Douglas B.
Fox Chase Cancer Center
333 Cottman Avenue
Philadelphia PA 19111

FOLPE, Andrew L.
Mayo Clinic
200 First Street South-West
Rochester MN 55905

FRENCH, Christopher A.*
Brigham and Women's Hospital and
Harvard Medical School
New Research Building, Room 630G
77 Avenue Louis Pasteur
Boston MA 02115

FRITCHIE, Karen J.
Mayo Clinic
200 First Street South-West
Rochester MN 55905

GALATEAU-SALLE, Françoise
Centre Léon Bérard
28 Rue Laennec
69008 Lyon

GAULARD, Philippe
Hôpital Henri Mondor
51 Avenue du Maréchal de Lattre de Tassigny
94010 Créteil

GILL, Anthony J.
Royal North Shore Hospital
Pacific Highway
St Leonards NSW 2065

GILL, Ritu R.
Beth Israel Medical Center
330 Brookline Avenue
Boston MA 02112

GIRARD, Nicolas
Institut Curie
26 Rue d'Ulm
75005 Paris

GLASS, Carolyn
Duke University Medical Center
214D Davison Building Box 3712
40 Duke Medicine Circle
Durham NC 27710

GO, Ronald S.
Mayo Clinic
200 First Street South-West
Rochester MN 55905

GUINEE, Donald G.*
Virginia Mason Medical Center
1100 Ninth Avenue, C6-PTH
Seattle WA 98101

HILL, D. Ashley*
Children's National Hospital
111 Michigan Avenue North-West
Washington DC 20010

HIROSHIMA, Kenzo
Chiba University Graduate School of Medicine
1-8-1 Inohana, Chuo-ku
Chiba 260-8670

HORNICK, Jason L.*
Brigham and Women's Hospital
Harvard Medical School
75 Francis Street
Boston MA 02115

HUSAIN, Aliya Noor
University of Chicago
5841 South Maryland Avenue
Room S627, MC6101
Chicago IL 60637

HWANG, David M.*
Sunnybrook Health Sciences Centre
2075 Bayview Avenue
Toronto ON M4N 3M5

INAGAKI, Hiroshi
Nagoya City University
1 Kawasumi, Mizuho-ku
Nagoya 467-8601

ISHII, Genichiro*
National Cancer Center
6-5-1 Kashiwanoha
Kashiwa 277-8577

ISHIKAWA, Yuichi
School of Medicine
International University of Health and Welfare
Mita Hospital, 1-4-3 Mita, Minato-ku
Tokyo 108-8329

JAIN, Deepali
All India Institute of Medical Sciences
Ansari Nagar
New Delhi 110029

JO, Vickie Y.*
Brigham and Women's Hospital and
Harvard Medical School
75 Francis Street
Boston MA 02115

JOUBERT, Philippe
Quebec Heart and Lung Institute
2725 Chemin Sainte-Foy
Québec QC G1V 4G5

KADOTA, Kyuichi
Faculty of Medicine, Kagawa University
1750-1 Ikenobe, Miki-cho
Kagawa 761-0793

KARPATHIOU, Georgia
University Hospital of Saint-Etienne
Cedex 2
42055 Saint-Etienne

KERR, Keith M.*
Department of Pathology
Aberdeen Royal Infirmary
Foresterhill
Aberdeen AB25 2ZD

KHOOR, Andras
Mayo Clinic
4500 San Pablo Road
Jacksonville FL 32224

KLAPPER, Wolfram
University Hospital Schleswig-Holstein
University of Kiel
Arnold-Heller-Straße 3, Haus U33
24105 Kiel

KLEBE, Sonja*
SA Pathology and Flinders University
Flinders Medical Centre, Bedford Park
Adelaide SA 5042

LADANYI, Marc*
Memorial Sloan Kettering Cancer Center
1275 York Avenue
New York NY 10065

LAKHANI, Sunil R.*
University of Queensland and
Pathology Queensland
Royal Brisbane and Women's Hospital
Herston QLD 4029

LANTUEJOUL, Sylvie
Centre Léon Bérard and
Grenoble Alpes University
28 Rue Laennec
69008 Lyon

LARSEN, Brandon T.
Mayo Clinic
13400 East Shea Boulevard
Scottsdale AZ 85259

LAX, Sigurd F.
General Hospital Graz II
Medical University of Graz
Goestingerstrasse 22
8020 Graz

LAZAR, Alexander J.
University of Texas
MD Anderson Cancer Center
1515 Holcombe Boulevard, Unit 85
Houston TX 77030

LE LOARER, François
Université de Bordeaux and
Institut Bergonié
276 Cours de l'Argonne
33000 Bordeaux

LEDUC, Charles
University of Montreal Health Center
1100 Rue Sanguinet, F07
Montréal QC H2X 0C1

LEIGHL, Natasha B.*
Princess Margaret Cancer Centre
7-913 700 University Avenue
Toronto ON M5G 1Z5

LIN, Dong-Mei
Peking University Cancer Hospital and Institute
Key Laboratory of Carcinogenesis and
Translational Research
(Ministry of Education)
52 Fucheng Road
Beijing 100142

LIU, Biao
Suzhou Municipal Hospital
Suzhou Hospital Affiliated to
Nanjing Medical University
16 West Baita Road
Suzhou 215001

LOKUHETTY, Dilani
International Agency for Research on Cancer
150 Cours Albert Thomas
69372 Lyon

LÓPEZ-TERRADA, Dolores H.
Texas Children's Hospital
Baylor College of Medicine
6621 Fannin Street, Suite AB1.195
Houston TX 77030

LU, Shun
Shanghai Chest Hospital
Shanghai Jiaotong University
241 West Huahai Road
Shanghai 200030

MacMAHON, Heber*
University of Chicago
5841 South Maryland Avenue
Chicago IL 60637

MAHAR, Annabelle M.
Royal Prince Alfred Hospital
Missenden Road
Sydney NSW 2050

MALESZEWSKI, Joseph J.
Mayo Clinic
200 First Street South-West
Rochester MN 55905

MANDELKER, Diana
Memorial Sloan Kettering Cancer Center
1275 York Avenue
New York NY 10065

MARCHEVSKY, Alberto Mario*
Cedars-Sinai Medical Center
8700 Beverly Boulevard
Los Angeles CA 90048

MARINO, Mirella
IRCCS Regina Elena National Cancer Institute
Via Elio Chianesi 53
00144 Rome RM

MAROM, Edith Michelle
Chaim Sheba Medical Center, affiliated with
Tel Aviv University
Derech Sheba 2
5265601 Ramat Gan

MARX, Alexander
University Medical Centre Mannheim
Theodor-Kutzer-Ufer 1-3
68167 Mannheim

MASCAUX, Céline*
University Hospital of Strasbourg
1 Place de l'Hôpital
67091 Strasbourg

MATSUBARA, Daisuke
Jichi Medical University
3311-1 Yakushiji, Shimotsuke-shi
Tochigi 329-0498

MATSUNO, Yoshihiro
Hokkaido University Hospital
Kita 14-jo, Nishi 5-chome, Kita-ku
Sapporo 060-8648

MEHRAD, Mitra
Vanderbilt University Medical Center
1161 21st Avenue South, C-3321 A
Medical Center North
Nashville TN 37232

MILLER, Dylan V.
University of Utah and
Intermountain Medical Center
5121 South Intermountain Drive - Pathology
Salt Lake City UT 84157

MINO-KENUDSON, Mari
Massachusetts General Hospital and
Harvard Medical School
55 Fruit Street, Warren 122
Boston MA 02114

MITSUDOMI, Tesuya
Kindai University Faculty of Medicine
377-2 Ohno-Higashi
Osaka-Sayama 589-8511

MOCH, Holger
University of Zurich and
University Hospital Zurich
Schmelzbergstrasse 12
8091 Zurich

MOLINA, Thierry Jo
Hôpital Necker-Enfants Malades
17 bis Boulevard Pasteur
75015 Paris

MOREIRA, Andre L.
New York University Langone Health
560 First Avenue, TH4-15B
New York NY 10016

MOTOI, Noriko
National Cancer Center Hospital
5-1-1 Tsukiji, Chuo-ku
Tokyo 104-0045

MUKAI, Kiyoshi
Keiyu Hospital
3-7-3 Minatomirai, Nishi-ku
Yokohama 250-8521

NABESHIMA, Kazuki
Fukuoka University School of Medicine
7-45-1 Nanakuma, Jonan-ku
Fukuoka 814-0180

NAKAMURA, Shigeo
Nagoya University Hospital
65 Tsurumai-cho, Showa-ku
Nagoya 466-8550

NAKATANI, Yukio
Yokosuka Kyosai Hospital
1-16 Yonegahama-dori
Yokosuka 238-8558

NICHOLSON, Andrew Gordon*
Royal Brompton & Harefield
NHS Foundation Trust
Sydney Street
London SW3 6NP

NOGUCHI, Masayuki
University of Tsukuba
1-1-1 Tennodai
Tsukuba-shi 305-8575

NONAKA, Daisuke
Guy's and St Thomas' NHS Foundation Trust
St Thomas' Hospital, Second Floor
North Wing, Westminster Bridge Road
London SE1 7EH

NOWAK, Anna Katherine*
University of Western Australia
35 Stirling Highway, Crawley
Perth WA 6009

OCHIAI, Atsushi
National Cancer Center
6-5-1 Kashiwanoha
Kashiwa 277-8577

OLIVA, Esther
Massachusetts General Hospital
55 Fruit Street
Boston MA 02114

ORAZI, Attilio
P.L. Foster School of Medicine
Texas Tech Health Sciences Center El Paso
4625 Alberta Avenue
El Paso TX 79905

OSAMURA, Robert Y.
Nippon Koukan Hospital and
Keio University School of Medicine
1-2-1 Koukan-dori, Kawasaki-ku, Kawasaki-shi
Kanagawa 210-0852

OZKAYA, Neval
NIH/National Cancer Institute
10 Center Drive
Building 10, Room 3N248
Bethesda MD 20892-1500

PADERA, Robert F.
Brigham and Women's Hospital
75 Francis Street
Boston MA 02115

PADLEY, Simon P.G.
Royal Brompton Hospital
Sydney Street
London SW3 6NP

PAPOTTI, Mauro
University of Turin
Via Santena 7
10126 Turin TO

PELOSI, Giuseppe
University of Milan
Via Festa del Perdono 7
20122 Milan MI

PERRY, Arie
University of California, San Francisco
505 Parnassus Avenue, M551
San Francisco CA 94143-0102

PILERI, Stefano A.
European Institute of Oncology
Via Ripamonti, 435
20141 Milan MI

PITTALUGA, Stefania
Center for Cancer Research
National Cancer Institute
Building 10, Room 2S235A
Bethesda MD 20892-1500

POLERI, Claudia
Consultant Pathologists Center
Rodríguez Peña 236
C1020ADF Ciudad de Buenos Aires

PORUBSKY, Stefan
University Medical Center of the
Johannes Gutenberg University Mainz
Langenbeckstraße 1
55101 Mainz

QUINTANILLA-MARTINEZ, Leticia
University Hospital Tübingen
Eberhard Karls University of Tübingen
Liebermeisterstraße 8
72076 Tübingen

RAJAN, Arun
National Cancer Institute
National Institutes of Health
10-CRC, Room 4-5330
Bethesda MD 20892

REKHTMAN, Natasha
Memorial Sloan Kettering Cancer Center
1275 York Avenue
New York NY 10065

REMON, Jordi
HM CIOCC - HM Delfos Barcelona
Avinguda de Vallcarca, 151-161
08023 Barcelona

RIEKER, Ralf J.
Institute of Pathology
University Hospital Erlangen
Friedrich-Alexander University Erlangen-Nürnberg
Krankenhausstraße 8-10
91054 Erlangen

RIELY, Gregory*
Memorial Sloan Kettering Cancer Center
1275 York Avenue
New York NY 10065

RODEN, Anja C.
Mayo Clinic Rochester
200 First Street South-West
Rochester MN 55905

ROSENWALD, Andreas
Institute of Pathology
University of Wuerzburg
Josef-Schneider-Straße 2
97080 Würzburg

ROSSI, Giulio*
Azienda USL della Romagna
Ospedale Santa Maria delle Croci
Viale Randi 5
48121 Ravenna RA

ROUS, Brian
Public Health England
Victoria House, Capital Park
Fulbourn, Cambridge CB21 5XA

RUSCH, Valerie Williams*
Memorial Sloan Kettering Cancer Center
1275 York Avenue
New York NY 10065

RUSSELL, Prudence A.
St Vincent's Hospital
41 Victoria Parade
Fitzroy VIC 3065

SAID, Jonathan William
David Geffen School of Medicine
10833 Le Conte Avenue
Los Angeles CA 90095

SAMET, Jonathan M.
Colorado School of Public Health
13001 East 17th Place
Aurora CO 80045

SAUTER, Jennifer L.
Memorial Sloan Kettering Cancer Center
1275 York Avenue
New York NY 10044

SCAGLIOTTI, Giorgio V.*
University of Turin
Regione Gonzole 10
10043 Orbassano TO

SCHMITT, Fernando
IPATIMUP and
Medical Faculty of Porto University
Rua Júlio Amaral de Carvalho 45
4200-135 Porto

SCOLYER, Richard A.
Royal Prince Alfred Hospital,
Melanoma Institute Australia, and
University of Sydney
Missenden Road Camperdown
Sydney NSW 2050

SHEHATA, Bahig M.
Wayne State University School of Medicine
3901 Beaubien Street
Detroit MI 48201

SHEPPARD, Mary Noelle
Clinical and Molecular Science Institute
St George's Medical School
Cranmer Terrace
London SW17 0RE

SHIMADA, Hiroyuki
Stanford University
300 Pasteur Drive
Stanford CA 94305

SHOLL, Lynette M.*
Brigham and Women's Hospital and
Harvard Medical School
75 Francis Street
Boston MA 02115

* Indicates disclosure of interests (see p. 487).

SINGARAVEL, Saranya
Soleil Diagnostics
1, Emgee Green, Antop Hill
Mumbai 400037

SINGH, Rajendra
Mount Sinai School of Medicine
1 Gustave L. Levy Place
New York NY 10029

SMIT, Egbert Frederik
Netherlands Cancer Institute
Plesmanlaan 121
1066 CX Amsterdam

SNEAD, David R.J.*
University Hospitals Coventry and
Warwickshire
NHS Trust
Clifford Bridge Road
Coventry CV2 2DX

SOARES, Fernando Augusto
Rede D'Or Hospitals
Rua das Perobas 266
São Paulo SP 04321-120

SOO, Ross Andrew
National University Cancer Institute
1E Kent Ridge Road
Singapore 119228

SRIGLEY, John R.
Trillium Health Partners
Credit Valley Hospital Site
2200 Eglinton Avenue West
Mississauga ON L5M 2N1

STRÖBEL, Philipp
University Medical Center Göttingen
Robert-Koch-Straße 40
37075 Göttingen

SUURMEIJER, Albert J.H.
University Medical Center Groningen
Hanzeplein 1
9700 RB Groningen

TAKEUCHI, Kengo
Japanese Foundation for Cancer Research
3-8-31 Ariake, Koto
Tokyo 135-8550

TAN, Puay Hoon
Division of Pathology
Singapore General Hospital
20 College Road, Academia, Level 7
Diagnostics Tower
Singapore 169856

TATEYAMA, Hisashi
Kasugai Municipal Hospital
1-1-1 Takagi-cho
Kasugai 486-8510

TAVORA, Fabio
Messejana Heart and Lung Hospital /
Argos Laboratory
Avenida Santos Dumont 5753, #1607
Fortaleza CE 60175-047

TAZELAAR, Henry D.
Mayo Clinic
13400 East Shea Boulevard
Scottsdale AZ 85259

THOMAS, David M.
Garvan Institute of Medical Research
370 Victoria Street
Darlinghurst NSW 2010

THOMAS DE MONTPRÉVILLE, Vincent
Marie Lannelongue Hospital
133 Avenue de la Résistance
92350 Le Plessis-Robinson

THOMPSON, Lester D.R.
Woodland Hills Medical Center
5601 De Soto Avenue
Woodland Hills CA 91365

THWAY, Khin
Royal Marsden Hospital /
Institute of Cancer Research
203 Fulham Road
London SW3 6JJ

TRAVIS, William D.*
Memorial Sloan Kettering Cancer Center
1275 York Avenue
New York NY 10065

TSAO, Ming Sound
University Health Network
200 Elizabeth Street, 11th Floor
Toronto ON M5G 2C4

TSUZUKI, Toyonori
Aichi Medical University Hospital
1-1 Yazakokarimata
Nagakute 480-1195

ULBRIGHT, Thomas M.
Indiana University School of Medicine
350 West 11th Street, Room 4014
Indianapolis IN 46202

VAN SCHIL, Paul E.Y.
Antwerp University Hospital
Wilrijkstraat 10
2650 Edegem (Antwerp)

VARGAS, Sara O.*
Boston Children's Hospital and
Harvard Medical School
300 Longwood Avenue
Boston MA 02115

VEINOT, John P.
University of Ottawa
451 Smyth Road
Ottawa ON K1H 8L6

WANG, En-Hua
College of Basic Medical Sciences and
First Affiliated Hospital
China Medical University
77 Puhe Road
Shenyang 110122

WANG, Jian
Fudan University Shanghai Cancer Center
270 Dong An Road
Shanghai 200032

---

* Indicates disclosure of interests (see p. 487).

WARTH, Arne
Institute of Pathology, Cytopathology and
Molecular Pathology MVZ UEGP
Gießen/Wetzlar/Limburg/Bad Hersfeld
Forsthausstraße 1
35578 Wetzlar

WASHINGTON, Mary K.
Vanderbilt University Medical Center
C-3321 MCN
Nashville TN 37232

WEIS, Cleo-Aron
University Medical Centre Mannheim
Theodor-Kutzer-Ufer 1-3
68167 Mannheim

WEISS, Lawrence M.*
NeoGenomics
31 Columbia
Aliso Viejo CA 92656

WEISSFERDT, Annikka
University of Texas
MD Anderson Cancer Center
1515 Holcombe Boulevard
Houston TX 77030

WHITE, Valerie A.
International Agency for Research on Cancer
150 Cours Albert Thomas
69372 Lyon

WISTUBA, Ignacio*
University of Texas
MD Anderson Cancer Center
1515 Holcome Boulevard
Houston TX 77030

WONG, Maria Pik
University of Hong Kong
Queen Mary Hospital
Pok Fu Lam Road
Hong Kong SAR

YANG, Woo Ick
Yonsei Univesity College of Medicine
50-1 Yonsei-ro, Seodaemun-gu
Seoul 03722

YATABE, Yasushi
National Cancer Center
5-1-1 Tsukiji, Chuo-ku
Tokyo 104-0045

YI, Eunhee S.
Mayo Clinic
200 First Street South-West
Rochester MN 55905

YOKOSE, Tomoyuki
Kanagawa Cancer Center
2-3-2 Nakao, Asahi
Yokohama 241-8515

YOSHIDA, Akihiko
National Cancer Center Hospital
5-1-1 Tsukiji, Chuo-ku
Tokyo 104-0045

YOSHIZAWA, Akihiko
Kyoto University Hospital
54 Shogoin-Kawaharacho, Sakyo-ku
Kyoto 606-8507

ZHANG, Jie
Shanghai Chest Hospital
241 West Huaihai Road
Shanghai 200030

ZNAOR, Ariana
International Agency for Research on Cancer
150 Cours Albert Thomas
69372 Lyon

---

* Indicates disclosure of interests (see p. 487).

Declaration of interests

Dr **Aubry** reports that her unit at Mayo Clinic benefited from research funding from Oncospire Genomics.

Dr **Badve** reports that he and his unit at Indiana University hold patent #10233502, on "Compositions for and methods of detecting, diagnosing, and prognosing thymic cancer".

Dr **Beasley** reports having received personal consultancy fees from various law firms, including Willcox & Savage, DeHay & Elliston, and Kaleo Legal, in connection with expert testimony in relation to litigation regarding causality in mesothelioma cases.

Dr **Borczuk** reports having received personal consultancy fees from Bristol Myers Squibb.

Dr **Botling** reports that his unit at Uppsala University benefits from support for consumables and laboratory personnel from Bristol Myers Squibb.

Dr **Bubendorf** reports receiving personal consultancy fees, in his capacity as an advisory board member, from AstraZeneca, Pfizer, Boehringer Ingelheim, MSD, Bayer, and Eli Lilly, and he reports that his unit at the University Hospital Basel benefited from research funding from Roche and MSD.

Dr **Bueno** reports that his unit at Brigham and Women's Hospital and Harvard Medical School benefits from research funding from Roche, Genentech, Merck, Gritstone, Verastem, and Epizyme; having received support for travel from Intuitive Surgical, Siemens, Novocure, and Johnson & Johnson; and holding patents with Navigation Sciences in his capacity as co-founder.

Dr **Buettner** reports having received personal consultancy fees from AstraZeneca, Bayer, AbbVie, Novartis, Pfizer, MSD, BMS, and Roche; that his unit at the University Hospital Cologne benefited from research funding from the Else Kröner-Fresenius Foundation and Roche; and having a commercial interest in Targos Molecular Pathology GmbH in his capacity as chief scientific officer and co-founder.

Dr **Cardona** reports having received financial research support from Merck Sharp & Dohme, Boehringer Ingelheim, Roche, Bristol Myers Squibb, Foundation Medicine, Roche Diagnostics, Idylla Biocartis, INQBox, Amgen, AstraZeneca, Celldex Therapeutics, Abbie, Merck Serono, and the Foundation for Clinical and Applied Cancer Research (FICMAC); additionally, he was linked to and received honoraria as an advisor from, participated in a speakers' bureau for, and gave expert testimony to Merck Sharp & Dohme, Boehringer Ingelheim, AstraZeneca, Roche, Bristol Myers Squibb, Pfizer, Novartis, Celldex Therapeutics, Foundation Medicine, Eli Lilly, Guardant Health, Rochem Biocare, and FICMAC.

Dr **Cesarman** reports holding patents on "Nucleoside analogue (6-ETI and related structures) for the treatment of cancer" and "Point of care detection method for Kaposi sarcoma".

Dr **Chirieac** reports having provided expert opinion on pathogenetic mechanisms and diagnosis of malignant mesothelioma to several law firms, including Willcox & Savage; Kaleo Legal; O'Connell, Tivin, Miller & Burns; Peter G. Angelos; and Bergman Draper Oslund.

Dr **Cooper** reports having received personal consultancy fees from Pfizer, Merck Sharp & Dohme, and Bristol Myers Squibb.

Dr **Dacic** reports having received personal consultancy fees, in her capacity as an advisory board member, from Bayer Pharmaceuticals, AstraZeneca, and Bristol Myers Squibb.

Dr **de Perrot** reports that his unit at the Toronto General Hospital Foundation benefits from research funding from Bayer.

Dr **Dogan** reports that his unit at Memorial Sloan Kettering Cancer Center benefits from research funding from Roche/Genentech.

Dr **Farago** reports having received personal consultancy fees from several pharmaceutical entities and that her unit at Massachusetts General Hospital benefits from research funding from several pharmaceutical entities.

Dr **French** reports having received personal consultancy fees from GlaxoSmithKline and Boehringer Ingelheim, and that his unit at Harvard Medical School benefited from research funding from GlaxoSmithKline.

Dr **Guinee** reports having received honoraria from AstraZeneca on behalf of his unit at Virginia Mason Medical Center, and holding stocks in Alexion Pharmaceuticals, AstraZeneca, Bristol Myers Squibb, Merck, Novartis, and Pfizer.

Dr **Hill** reports having equity interest in ResourcePath in her capacity as co-owner and medical director.

Dr **Hornick** reports receiving personal consultancy fees from Eli Lilly and Epizyme.

Dr **Hwang** reports having received personal consultancy fees from Merck, Roche, Pfizer, Bayer, and Takeda, and that his unit at Sunnybrook Health Sciences Centre benefits from research funding from Merck, AstraZeneca, Takeda, and Boehringer Ingelheim.

Dr **Ishii** reports that his unit at the National Cancer Center benefits from research funding from Daiichi Sankyo, and receiving personal consultancy fees from Ono Pharmaceutical.

Dr **Jo** reports that her spouse is a salaried employee of Merck & Co.

Dr **Kerr** reports receiving personal consultancy fees from AbbVie, AstraZeneca, Boehringer Ingelheim, Bayer, Bristol Myers Squibb, Lilly, Merck Serono, Merck Sharp & Dohme, Novartis, Pfizer, Roche, and Ventana.

Dr **Klebe** reports having received personal consultancy fees from MSD and Pfizer, having received support for travel from Ventana and MSD, and that her unit at SA Pathology and Flinders University benefited from research funding from Ventana Medical Systems. She reports having provided expert witness reports for courts in Australia, on diagnosis, at the request of lawyers acting on behalf of plaintiffs and defendants.

Dr **Ladanyi** reports having received personal consultancy fees, in his capacity as an advisory board member, from Merck, Lilly Oncology, AstraZeneca, Bristol Myers Squibb, Takeda, Blueprint Medicines, and Bayer, and research support from Loxo Oncology, Helsinn Healthcare, Elevation Oncology, and Merus.

Dr **Lakhani** reports receiving personal consultancy fees from Sullivan Nicolaides Pathology.

Dr **Leighl** reports that her unit at the Princess Margaret Cancer Centre benefits from research funding from Array BioPharma, AstraZeneca, MSD, Pfizer, and Guardant

Health; having received personal consultancy fees from Xcovery, BMS, MSD, Roche, and Novartis; and having received support for travel from AstraZeneca.

Dr MacMahon reports receiving personal consultancy fees from Riverain Technologies, Konica Minolta, and GE Healthcare; that his unit at the University of Chicago benefited from research funding from Bioclinica and Philips Healthcare; and holding stocks in Hologic.

Dr Marchevsky reports providing expert opinion on pathology of mesotheliomas to various law firms, and receiving personal consultancy fees from Roche, Genentech, and Amgen.

Dr Mascaux reports receiving honoraria from Roche, AstraZeneca, Bristol Myers Squibb, Pfizer, and MSD, and holding patents EP19305434.3 and EP19305535.7.

Dr Nicholson reports receiving personal consultancy fees from AbbVie, Pfizer, AstraZeneca, and UpToDate, as well as from law firms in relation to reports on mesothelioma diagnosis, and that his unit at Royal Brompton & Harefield NHS Foundation Trust benefited from research funding from Pfizer.

Dr Nowak reports having received personal consultancy fees from Douglas Pharmaceuticals, Trizell, Boehringer Ingelheim, MSD, PharmAbcine, Atara Biotherapeutics, Bayer, and Roche; that her unit at the National Centre for Asbestos Related Diseases has benefited from research funding from AstraZeneca; and having received support for travel from Boehringer Ingelheim.

Dr Riely reports that his unit at Memorial Sloan Kettering Cancer Center benefits from research funding from Roche, Takeda, Novartis, Mirati, Janssen, and Revolution Medicines, and benefits from non-monetary support from Takeda and Roche.

Dr Rossi reports having received honoraria, in his capacity as a speaker for pharma boards, from Pfizer, Novartis, Eli Lilly, MSD Oncology, Roche, and AstraZeneca.

Dr Rusch reports that her unit at Memorial Sloan Kettering Cancer Center benefits from research support from Genentech and Genelux.

Dr Scagliotti reports receiving honoraria from Lilly, Roche, Pfizer, AstraZeneca, Novartis, and MSD.

Dr Sholl reports receiving personal consultancy fees from EMD Serono and Foghorn Therapeutics, honoraria from AstraZeneca, and fees (in her capacity as an advisory board member) from Loxo Oncology. She reports that her unit at Harvard Medical School benefited from research funding from Roche/Genentech.

Dr Snead reports having provided expert testimony on cases of death from malignant thoracic disease.

Dr Travis reports having received personal consultancy fees, in his capacity as an expert witness for causation of malignant mesothelioma, from Willcox & Savage.

Dr Vargas reports providing medicolegal consultation to various entities.

Dr Weiss reports holding stocks in NeoGenomics in his capacity as chief medical officer, and receiving personal consultancy fees from Roche, Merck, Lilly, Bayer, and Novartis.

Dr Wistuba reports receiving personal consultancy fees, in his capacity as an advisory board member, from Genentech/Roche, Bayer, Bristol Myers Squibb, AstraZeneca/MedImmune, Pfizer, HTG Molecular Diagnostics, Asuragen, Merck, GlaxoSmithKline, Guardant Health, and MSD; having received honoraria from Genentech/Roche; and that his unit at the University of Texas MD Anderson Cancer Center benefits from research funding from Genentech, HTG Molecular Diagnostics, Merck, Bristol Myers Squibb, MedImmune, Adaptive Biotechnologies, Adaptimmune, EMD Serono, Pfizer, Takeda, Amgen, Karus Therapeutics, Johnson & Johnson, Bayer, Iovance Biotherapeutics, 4D Pharma, and Novartis.

IARC/WHO Committee for the International Classification of Diseases for Oncology (ICD-O)

CREE, Ian A.
International Agency for Research on Cancer
150 Cours Albert Thomas
69372 Lyon

FERLAY, Jacques
International Agency for Research on Cancer
150 Cours Albert Thomas
69372 Lyon

JAKOB, Robert
Data Standards and Informatics
World Health Organization (WHO)
20 Avenue Appia
1211 Geneva

ROUS, Brian
Public Health England
Victoria House, Capital Park
Fulbourn, Cambridge CB21 5XA

WATANABE, Reiko
National Cancer Center Hospital East
6-5-1 Kashiwanoha, Kashiwa-shi
Chiba 277-8577

WHITE, Valerie A.
International Agency for Research on Cancer
150 Cours Albert Thomas
69372 Lyon

ZNAOR, Ariana
International Agency for Research on Cancer
150 Cours Albert Thomas
69372 Lyon

Sources

TNM staging tables

Figures

1.01A,B Ferlay J, Ervik M, Lam F, et al. Global Cancer Observatory: Cancer Today [Internet]. Lyon (France): International Agency for Research on Cancer; 2018. Available from: https://gco.iarc.fr/today.
1.02 Devesa SS
1.03 Devesa SS
1.04 Yatabe Y
1.05A,B Travis WD
1.06A,B Travis WD
1.07A,B Travis WD
1.08A,B Travis WD
1.09 Travis WD
1.10A,B Travis WD
1.11A–C Travis WD
1.12A,B Travis WD
1.13A,B Travis WD
1.14 Travis WD
1.15A–C Travis WD
1.16A,B Travis WD
1.17A–D Flieder DB
1.18 Nicholson AG
1.19A,C Travis WD
1.19B Flieder DB
1.20 Flieder DB
1.21 Syed Z. Ali, Division of Cytopathology, Johns Hopkins University School of Medicine, Baltimore (MD)
1.22A–C Wang EH
1.23A,B Wang EH
1.24A–F Wang EH
1.25 Wang EH
1.26 Wang EH
1.27 Travis WD
1.28A–D Sauter JL
1.29A,B Reprinted, with permission, from: Travis WD, Colby TV, Corrin B, et al., editors. Histological typing of lung and pleural tumours. Berlin (Germany): Springer; 1999. Copyright 1999.
1.30 Matsubara D
1.31A Ishikawa Y
1.31B Travis WD
1.31C Yoshida A
1.31D Chang JC
1.32A–C Chang JC
1.33A,B Yoshida A
1.34A,B Reprinted, with permission from Springer Nature, from: Travis WD, Colby TV, Corrin B, et al., editors. Histological typing of lung and pleural tumours. Berlin (Germany): Springer; 1999. Copyright 1999.
1.35A–D Travis WD
1.36A Travis WD
1.36B Adapted with permission from the American Registry of Pathology. Originally published as Figure 4-28 in: Travis WD, Nicholson AG, Geisinger KR, et al. Tumors of the lower respiratory tract. Washington, DC: American Registry of Pathology; 2019. (AFIP atlas of tumor pathology, series 4; fascicle 29).
1.37A,B Travis WD
1.38A Yatabe Y
1.38B © Naidich D
Travis WD, Brambilla E, Burke AP, et al., editors. WHO classification of tumours of the lung, pleura, thymus and heart. Lyon (France): International Agency for Research on Cancer; 2015. (WHO classification of tumours series, 4th ed.; vol. 7). https://publications.iarc.fr/17.
1.39A,B Travis WD
1.40A,B Ishikawa Y
1.41 Travis WD
1.42 Yatabe Y
1.43A–C Travis WD
1.44A–C Travis WD
1.45 Reprinted, with permission, from: Hu X, Fujimoto J, Ying L, et al. Multi-region exome sequencing reveals genomic evolution from preneoplasia to lung adenocarcinoma. Nat Commun. 2019 Jul 5;10(1):2978. PMID:31278276. http://creativecommons.org/licenses/by/4.0/
1.46A,B MacMahon H
1.47 Adapted, with permission, from: Jordan EJ, Kim HR, Arcila ME, et al. Prospective comprehensive molecular characterization of lung adenocarcinomas for efficient patient matching to approved and emerging therapies. Cancer Discov. 2017 Jun;7(6):596–609. PMID:28336552
1.48 Reused, with permission from AME Publishing Company, from: Kohno T, Nakaoku T, Tsuta K, et al. Beyond ALK-RET, ROS1 and other oncogene fusions in lung cancer. Transl Lung Cancer Res. 2015 Apr;4(2):156–64. PMID:25870798

1.49   Adapted, with permission from Nature, from: Cancer Genome Atlas Research Network. Comprehensive molecular profiling of lung adenocarcinoma. Nature. 2014 Jul 31;511(7511):543–50. PMID:2507955

1.50A,B   Aisner DL, Sholl LM, Berry LD, et al. The impact of smoking and TP53 mutations in lung adenocarcinoma patients with targetable mutations-the Lung Cancer Mutation Consortium (LCMC2). Clin Cancer Res. 2018 Mar 1;24(5):1038–47. PMID:29217530

1.51   Cooper WA
1.52A–D   Travis WD
1.53   Cooper WA
1.54   Russell PA
1.55A–D   Travis WD
1.56A,B   Travis WD
1.57A,B   Cooper WA
1.57C   Travis WD
1.58   Chan JKC
1.59   Travis WD
1.60A   Cooper WA
1.60B,C   Bubendorf L
1.61   MacMahon H
1.62   Cooper WA
1.63   Cooper WA
1.64A–D   Yatabe Y
1.65A   Yoshizawa A
1.65B   Travis WD
1.66A,B   Cooper WA
1.67A,B   Cooper WA
1.68A,B   Cooper WA
1.69   Travis WD
1.70A–C   Pelosi G
1.71   Nakatani Y
1.72A,B   Nakatani Y
1.73A,B   Nakatani Y
1.74A,B   Nakatani Y
1.75   Nakatani Y
1.76A,B,D   © Lam S   Travis WD, Brambilla E, Burke AP, et al., editors. WHO classification of tumours of the lung, pleura, thymus and heart. Lyon (France): International Agency for Research on Cancer; 2015. (WHO classification of tumours series, 4th ed.; vol. 7). https://publications.iarc.fr/17.
1.76C   Lantuejoul S
1.77   © Mueller KM, Gerhard-Domagkinstitut für Pathologie, Universitätskliniken Münster (UKM), Münster   Travis WD, Brambilla E, Burke AP, et al., editors. WHO classification of tumours of the lung, pleura, thymus and heart. Lyon (France): International Agency for Research on Cancer; 2015. (WHO classification of tumours series, 4th ed.; vol. 7). https://publications.iarc.fr/17.
1.78   Lantuejoul S
1.79A,B   Travis WD

1.80   Lantuejoul S
1.81   Lantuejoul S
1.82   Travis WD
1.83A   Kerr KM
1.83B   © Fernandez EA, Departamento de Anatomía Patológica, Hospital General Gregorio Marañón, Madrid   Travis WD, Brambilla E, Burke AP, et al., editors. WHO classification of tumours of the lung, pleura, thymus and heart. Lyon (France): International Agency for Research on Cancer; 2015. (WHO classification of tumours series, 4th ed.; vol. 7). https://publications.iarc.fr/17.
1.84   Warth A
1.85A,D   Warth A
1.85B,C   Travis WD
1.86A   Warth A
1.86B   Travis WD
1.86C   Rossi G
1.87   Tsao MS
1.88   Chung JH
1.89   Chung JH
1.90   Chang YL
1.91A,B   Chang YL
1.92A,B   Chang YL
1.92C   Chou TY
1.93   Chan JKC
1.94A,B   Rossi G
1.95A,B   Mino-Kenudson M
1.96A–C   Travis WD
1.97   Kerr KM
1.98A,B   Rossi G
1.99A,B   Rossi G
1.100   Rossi G
1.101   Rossi G
1.102   Modified, with permission, from: Nakatani Y, Hiroshima H, Mark EJ. Sarcomatoid carcinoma and variants. In: Hasleton P, Flieder DB, editors. Spencer's pathology of the lung. 6th ed. Cambridge (UK): Cambridge University Press; 2013. pp. 1186–223. Reproduced with permission of the licensor through PLSclear.
1.103A–F   Nakatani Y
1.104A,B   Nakatani Y
1.105   Nakatani Y
1.106   Borczuk AC
1.107A,B   Borczuk AC
1.107C   Travis WD
1.108A,B   Travis WD
1.109A,B   Rekhtman N
1.110   Chalabreysse L
1.111A–C   Le Loarer F
1.112A,B   Yoshida A
1.113A–E   Yoshida A
1.114A   Rekhtman N
1.114B   Jain D
1.115   Mehrad M
1.116A   Nicholson AG
1.116B   Farver CF
1.117   Farver CF
1.118A,B   Mehrad M
1.119   Kerr KM
1.120A,B   Husain AN

1.121A,B   Kerr KM
1.122A   Travis WD
1.122B,C   Dacic S
1.123A,B   Nicholson AG
1.124   Farver CF
1.125A,B   Farver CF
1.126   Erika Doxtader, Department of Pathology, Cleveland Clinic, Cleveland (OH)
1.127A–C   Hornick JL
1.128A,B   Hornick JL
1.129A,B   MacMahon H
1.130A–C   Rossi G
1.131A,B   Rossi G
1.132A   Papotti M
1.132B   Osamura RY
1.132C   Travis WD
1.133A,B,D   Lantuejoul S
1.133C   Papotti M
1.134A,B   Travis WD
1.135A,B   Papotti M
1.136A   Papotti M
1.136B   Pelosi G
1.137A,B   Papotti M
1.138A,B   Adapted from: Alcala N, Leblay N, Gabriel AAG, et al. Integrative and comparative genomic analyses identify clinically relevant pulmonary carcinoid groups and unveil the supra-carcinoids. Nat Commun. 2019 Aug 20;10(1):3407. PMID:31431620. http://creativecommons.org/licenses/by/4.0/
1.139A   Rekhtman N
1.139B   Osamura RY
1.140   Travis WD
1.141   Beasley MB
1.142   Travis WD
1.143A–C   Beasley MB
1.144A,C   Travis WD
1.144B   Beasley MB
1.145A   Rekhtman N
1.145B   Beasley MB
1.146   Travis WD
1.147A–D   Rekhtman N
1.148A–D   Osamura RY
1.149A–D   Rekhtman N
1.150A,B   Rekhtman N
1.151A–D   Rekhtman N
1.152   Reprinted, with permission, from: Rekhtman N, Pietanza MC, Hellmann MD, et al. Next-generation sequencing of pulmonary large cell neuroendocrine carcinoma reveals small cell carcinoma-like and non-small cell carcinoma-like subsets. Clin Cancer Res. 2016 Jul 15;22(14):3618–29. PMID:26960398
1.153   George J, Walter V, Peifer M, et al. Integrative genomic profiling of large-cell neuroendocrine carcinomas reveals distinct subtypes of high-grade neuroendocrine lung tumors. Nat Commun. 2018 Mar 13;9(1):1048. PMID:29535388.

	http://creativecommons.org/licenses/by/4.0/
1.154A–D	Travis WD
1.155A,C	Travis WD
1.155B	Motoi N
1.156A,B	Travis WD
1.157A,B	Darin White, Division of Thoracic Imaging, Mayo Clinic College of Medicine, Rochester (MN)
1.158	Aubry M-C
1.159A–D	Boland JM
1.160A–D	Aubry M-C
1.161A,B	Yi ES
1.162	Nicholson AG
1.163A–C	Hill DA
1.164A–C	Hill DA
1.165A,B	Nicholson AG
1.166	Mahar AM
1.167A	Travis WD
1.167B	Yi ES
1.167C	Mahar AM
1.168A,B	Travis WD
1.169A–C	Thway K
1.170A	Nicholson AG
1.170B,C	Reprinted from: Thway K, Nicholson AG, Lawson K, et al. Primary pulmonary myxoid sarcoma with EWSR1-CREB1 fusion: a new tumor entity. Am J Surg Pathol. 2011 Nov;35(11):1722–32. PMID:21997693. With permission from Wolters Kluwer Health.
1.171A,B	Padley SPG
1.172A–D	Hornick JL
1.173	Doyle LA
1.174	Doyle LA
1.175	Jain D
1.176	Inagaki H
1.177A–C	Cook JR
1.178A,B	Chan JKC
1.179	Cooper WA
1.180	Quintanilla-Martinez L
1.181A–E	Quintanilla-Martinez L
1.182A–E	Quintanilla-Martinez L
1.183A–C	Pittaluga S
1.184A,B	Pittaluga S
1.185A–D	Pittaluga S
1.186A,B	Pittaluga S
1.187A–C	Pittaluga S
1.188A–D	Takeuchi K
1.189	Robert Vassallo, Department of Pulmonary and Critical Care Medicine, Mayo Clinic, Rochester (MN)
1.190A,C,D	Yi ES
1.190B	Chan JKC
1.191A–D	Jason R. Young, Mayo Clinic, Rochester (MN); Used with permission of Mayo Foundation for Medical Education and Research
1.192A–C	Ozkaya N
1.193	Ozkaya N
2.01	Ferlay J, Ervik M, Lam F, et al. Global Cancer Observatory: Cancer Today [Internet]. Lyon (France): International Agency for Research on Cancer; 2018 [accessed 2020 Mar].

	Available from: https://gco.iarc.fr/today.
2.02A–C	Karpathiou G
2.03A,B	Wang J
2.03C	Butnor KJ
2.04A,B	de Perrot M
2.05A,B	Galateau-Salle F
2.06	Dacic S
2.07A	Klebe S
2.07B	Travis WD
2.08	Bironzo P
2.09A–C	Gill RR
2.10A,B	Sauter JL
2.11A	Galateau-Salle F
2.11B	Travis WD
2.12A–D	Travis WD
2.13A,B,D	Travis WD
2.13C	Sauter JL
2.14A	Sauter JL
2.14B	Galateau-Salle F
2.14C	Travis WD
2.15	Husain AN
2.16	Husain AN
2.17	Nicholson AG
2.18A	Sauter JL
2.18B,C	Travis WD
2.19	Travis WD
2.20A–C	Travis WD
2.21A,B	Husain AN
2.22A	Travis WD
2.22B,C	Galateau-Salle F
2.23	Adapted, with permission from Wolters Kluwer Health, Inc., from: Churg A, Colby TV, Cagle P, et al. The separation of benign and malignant mesothelial proliferations. Am J Surg Pathol. 2000 Sep;24(9):1183–200. PMID:10976692. https://journals.lww.com/ajsp/Abstract/2000/09000/The_Separation_of_Benign_and_Malignant_Mesothelial.1.aspx
2.24	Galateau-Salle F
2.25	Galateau-Salle F
2.26A,B	Travis WD
2.27	Reprinted, with permission from Springer Nature, from: Emoto K, Baine M, Travis W, et al. Histologic features of desmoplastic mesothelioma (DMM) [abstract]. In: Abstracts from USCAP 2020: Pulmonary, mediastinum, pleura, and peritoneum pathology (1869-1980). Mod Pathol. 2020 Mar;33(Suppl 2): 1934–2024. Abstract no. 1896. PMID:32139815
2.28A	Husain AN
2.28B	Travis WD
2.29	Reprinted, with permission from AACR, from: Hmeljak J, Sanchez-Vega F, Hoadley KA, et al. Integrative molecular characterization of malignant pleural mesothelioma. Cancer Discov. 2018 Dec;8(12):1548–65. PMID:30322867
2.30A,B	Françoise Thivolet-Bejui, Centre de Pathologie Est - CHU Lyon Groupement

	Hospitalier Est, Bron
2.30C	Sauter JL
2.31	Travis WD
2.32	Travis WD
2.33	Sean McNair, Cytology Service, Department of Pathology, Memorial Sloan Kettering Cancer Center, New York (NY)
2.34A–C	Chan JKC
2.35A–D	Said JW
2.36A,B	Said JW
2.37	Said JW
2.38	Said JW
2.39	Aozasa K
2.40A	Chan JKC
2.40B	Aozasa K
2.41A–D	Chan JKC
3.01A,B	Maleszewski JJ
3.02A–D	Maleszewski JJ
3.03A,B	Maleszewski JJ
3.04A–D	Maleszewski JJ
3.05A–C	Maleszewski JJ
3.06A–D	Maleszewski JJ
3.07A–D	Maleszewski JJ
3.08A,B	Maleszewski JJ
3.09A	Maleszewski JJ
3.09B	Sheppard MN
3.10	Basso C
3.11A–C	Adapted, with permission, from: Padalino MA, Vida VL, Bhattarai A, et al. Giant intramural left ventricular rhabdomyoma in a newborn. Circulation. 2011 Nov 15;124(20):2275–7. PMID:22083149
3.12A	Maleszewski JJ
3.12B–D	Basso C
3.13A–C	Burke AP
3.14A,C	Maleszewski JJ
3.14B	Burke AP
3.15A,B	Adapted, with permission, from: Basso C, Barbazza R, Thiene G. Images in cardiovascular medicine. Lipomatous hypertrophy of the atrial septum. Circulation. 1998 Apr 14;97(14):1423. PMID:9577955
3.15C	Fritchie KJ
3.16A–C	Bois MC
3.17	Maleszewski JJ
3.18A,B	Maleszewski JJ
3.19A,B	Veinot JP
3.20A–D	Veinot JP
3.21A–C	Veinot JP
3.22A,C	Burke AP
3.22B	Maleszewski JJ
3.23A	Tavora F
3.23B,C	Maleszewski JJ
3.24	Tavora F
3.25	Shehata BM
3.26A,B	Shehata BM
3.27A,B	Shehata BM
3.28A,B	Shehata BM
3.29	Shehata BM
3.30A,B	Cohle SD
3.31	Maleszewski JJ
3.32A,C	Leduc C
3.32B	Cyril Fisher, Department of Musculoskeletal Pathology,

	Robert Aitken Institute for Clinical Research, University of Birmingham, Birmingham
3.33A–C	Leduc C
3.34A	Reprinted from: Mazzola A, Spano JP, Valente M, et al. Leiomyosarcoma of the left atrium mimicking a left atrial myxoma. J Thorac Cardiovasc Surg. 2006 Jan;131(1):224–6. PMID:16399316. Copyright 2006. With permission from Elsevier.
3.34B–D	Basso C
3.35A,B	Burke AP
3.36A,B	Burke AP
3.37A,B	Burke AP
3.38	Burke AP
3.39A,B	Adapted, with permission from Springer Nature, from: Lestuzzi C, Miolo G, De Paoli A. Systemic therapy, radiotherapy, and cardiotoxicity. In: Basso C, Valente M, Thiene G, editors. Cardiac tumor pathology. New York (NY): Springer; 2013. pp. 165–82. Copyright 2013.
3.40A,B	Maleszewski JJ
3.41A–D	Boyer DF
4.01A	Thomas Malfait, Department of Respiratory Medicine, Ghent University Hospital, Ghent
4.01B,C	Travis WD
4.02A	Chan JKC
4.02B	Marx A
4.03	Creytens D
4.04	Creytens D
4.05	Elizabeth Cheek, Mayo Clinic, Rochester (MN)
4.06	Fritchie KJ
4.07	Fritchie KJ
4.08	Calabrese F
4.09A	Demicco EG
4.09B	Travis WD
4.09C	Dacic S
4.10A–C	Mehrad M
4.11	Elizabeth Cheek, Mayo Clinic, Rochester (MN)
4.12A–D	Hornick JL
4.13	Hornick JL
4.14A–C	Hornick JL
4.15	Thway K
4.16	Thway K
4.17A,B	Nicholson AG
4.18A,B	Doyle LA
4.19A,B	Chan JKC
4.20	Doyle LA
4.21A,B	Billings SD
4.22A,B	Billings SD
4.23A–C	Hornick JL
4.24A,B	Hornick JL
4.25A,B	Travis WD
4.26	Borczuk AC
4.27A,B	Perry A
4.28A–D	Boland JM
4.29A,B	Boland JM
4.30A–C	Shimada H
4.31A,B	Shimada H
4.32	Shimada H
4.33	Suurmeijer AJH
4.34	Suurmeijer AJH
4.35	Suurmeijer AJH
4.36A,B	Yoshida A
4.37	Bridge JA
4.38	Yoshida A
5.01A,B	Marx A
5.02	Adapted from: Radovich M, Pickering CR, Felau I, et al. The integrated genomic landscape of thymic epithelial tumors. Cancer Cell. 2018 Feb 12;33(2):244–58.e10. PMID:29438696. Copyright 2018, with permission from Elsevier.
5.03A–D	Adapted from: Radovich M, Pickering CR, Felau I, et al. The integrated genomic landscape of thymic epithelial tumors. Cancer Cell. 2018 Feb 12;33(2):244–58.e10. PMID:29438696. Copyright 2018, with permission from Elsevier.
5.04A	Travis WD
5.04B–D	Ströbel P
5.05A	Ströbel P
5.05B	Travis WD
5.06A–D	Ströbel P
5.07A,B	Ströbel P
5.08A–C	Ströbel P
5.09A,B	Marx A
5.10A,B	Adapted, with permission, from: Marx A, Ströbel P, Badve SS, et al. ITMIG consensus statement on the use of the WHO histological classification of thymoma and thymic carcinoma: refined definitions, histological criteria, and reporting. J Thorac Oncol. 2014 May;9(5):596–611. PMID:24722150. Copyright 2014, with permission from Elsevier.
5.11A,B	Marom EM
5.12	Yang WI
5.13A,B	Chan JKC
5.14A–D	Chan JKC
5.15A–D	Marx A
5.16A–C	Marx A
5.17A,B	Marx A
5.18A,B	Marom EM
5.19A,B	Yang WI
5.20A,B	Marx A
5.21A	Marx A
5.21B	Chan JKC
5.22	Marx A
5.23	Chan JKC
5.24A–C	Marx A
5.25	Marx A
5.26	Marx A
5.27	Chan JKC
5.28	Marx A
5.29A–C	Marom EM
5.30A,B	Yang WI
5.31A	Mukai K
5.31B	Marx A
5.32	Marx A
5.33	Travis WD
5.34	Chan JKC
5.35	Chan JKC
5.36A,C	Marx A
5.36B	Travis WD
5.37	Marx A
5.38A	Travis WD
5.38B,C	Marx A
5.39A,B	Marx A
5.40	Moreira AL
5.41	Travis WD
5.42A,B	Tateyama H
5.43A–C	Tateyama H
5.44A,B	Chan JKC
5.45A–D	Chan JKC
5.46	Roden AC
5.47A,B	Chan JKC
5.48A,B	Chan JKC
5.49A,B	Chan JKC
5.50A–D	Chan JKC
5.51A–C	Chan JKC
5.52	Chan JKC
5.53A–D	Chan JKC
5.54A,B	Chan JKC
5.55A,B	Chan JKC
5.56	Chan JKC
5.57A,B	Papotti M
5.58	Soares FA
5.59	Marx A
5.60	Chan JKC
5.61A,B	Chan JKC
5.62	Chan JKC
5.63	Chan JKC
5.64A,B	Chan JKC
5.65	Chan JKC
5.66	French CA
5.67	French CA
5.68	French CA
5.69A,B	French CA
5.70	French CA
5.71A,B	French CA
5.72A,B	French CA
5.73	French CA
5.74	Porubsky S
5.75A,B	Porubsky S
5.76	Porubsky S
5.77A–C	Marx A
5.78A,B	Marx A
5.79	Roden AC
5.80A,B	Roden AC
5.81	Inagaki H
5.82A,B	Inagaki H
5.83	Porubsky S
5.84	Di Tommaso L
5.85	Di Tommaso L
5.86	Di Tommaso L
5.87	Di Tommaso L
5.88A,B	Di Tommaso L
5.89	Chalabreysse L
5.90A–C	Tateyama H
5.91	Chan JKC
5.92	Chan JKC
5.93	Di Tommaso L
5.94A–C	Di Tommaso L
5.95A,B	Di Tommaso L
5.96A,B	Chan JKC
5.97A–D	Marx A
5.98A–C	Nonaka D
5.99A,B	Marom EM
5.100	Ströbel P
5.101	Adapted from: Dinter H, Bohnenberger H, Beck J, et al. Molecular classification of neuroendocrine tumors of the thymus. J Thorac Oncol. 2019 Aug;14(8):1472–83. PMID:31042566. Copyright

2019, with permission from Elsevier.

5.102A,B	Marom EM
5.103A–F	Ströbel P
5.104A,B	Chan JKC
5.105A,B	Ströbel P
5.106A–D	Ströbel P
5.107A–D	Ströbel P
5.108A,B	Travis WD
5.109A,B	Travis WD
5.110	Marx A
5.111	Borczuk AC
5.112A	Osamura RY
5.112B	Borczuk AC
5.113A–D	Osamura RY
6.01	Roden AC
6.02	Roden AC
6.03	Roden AC
6.04	Marom EM
6.05	Marom EM
6.06A,B	Roden AC
6.06C	Ulbright TM
6.07A–C	Roden AC
6.08A	Roden AC
6.08B	Ulbright TM
6.09A,B	Ulbright TM
6.10A–C	Roden AC
6.11	Marom EM
6.12A–D	Ulbright TM
6.13A–C	Ulbright TM
6.13D	Marx A
6.14A–D	Marx A
6.15	Moreira AL
6.16A,B	Travis WD
6.17A–D	Ulbright TM
6.18	Moreira AL
6.19A–D	Roden AC
6.20A–C	Roden AC
6.21A,B	Roden AC
6.22A–D	Roden AC
6.23A,B	Roden AC
6.24A–C	Orazi A
7.01	Klaus Herfarth, Department of Radiation Oncology, Heidelberg University Hospital, Heidelberg
7.02A,B	Chan JKC
7.03A,B	Chan JKC
7.04A–E	Klapper W
7.05	Klapper W
7.06A,B	Inagaki H
7.07	Inagaki H
7.08A–F	Inagaki H
7.09A–D	Ferry JA
7.10	Ferry JA
7.11A–D	Ferry JA
7.12A,B	Fend F
7.12C	Nakamura S
7.13A,B	Chan JKC
7.14A,B	Travis WD
7.15A,B	Chan JKC
7.16A–E	© Jaffe ES

Swerdlow SH, Campo E, Harris NL, et al., editors. WHO classification of tumours of haematopoietic and lymphoid tissues. Lyon (France): International Agency for Research on Cancer; 2017. (WHO classification of tumours series, 4th rev. ed.; vol. 2).

7.17	https://publications.iarc.fr/556. © Jaffe ES

Swerdlow SH, Campo E, Harris NL, et al., editors. WHO classification of tumours of haematopoietic and lymphoid tissues. Lyon (France): International Agency for Research on Cancer; 2017. (WHO classification of tumours series, 4th rev. ed.; vol. 2). https://publications.iarc.fr/556.

7.18A–C	© Jaffe ES

Swerdlow SH, Campo E, Harris NL, et al., editors. WHO classification of tumours of haematopoietic and lymphoid tissues. Lyon (France): International Agency for Research on Cancer; 2017. (WHO classification of tumours series, 4th rev. ed.; vol. 2). https://publications.iarc.fr/556.

7.19A,B	Pileri SA
7.20A,B	Chan JKC
7.21A	Pileri SA
7.21B	Chan JKC
7.22	Chan JKC
8.01	Weissferdt A
8.02A,B	Weissferdt A
8.03	Weissferdt A
8.04A,B	Weissferdt A
9.01A,B	Hiroshima K
9.02	Travis WD
9.03A–C	Travis WD
9.04A,B	Padera RF
9.05A,B	Joubert P
9.06A–C	Joubert P
9.07A,B	Joubert P
9.08A,B	Padera RF
9.09	Joubert P
9.10	Soares FA
9.11A,B	Travis WD
9.12	Sholl LM
9.13A,B	Sholl LM
9.14A,B	Joubert P
9.15A–C	Joubert P
9.16	Joubert P
9.17A–D	Roden AC
9.18A–D	Travis WD
9.19A,B	Roden AC
9.20A–D	Roden AC
9.21A–D	Padera RF
9.22	Maleszewski JJ
9.23A–D	Padera RF
10.02	Maleszewski JJ

Tables

Table A	Adapted from: WHO Classification of Tumours Editorial Board. Breast tumours. Lyon (France): International Agency for Research on Cancer; 2019. (WHO classification of tumours series, 5th ed.; vol. 2). https://publications.iarc.fr/581.
1.01	Ferlay J, Ervik M, Lam F, et al.

Global Cancer Observatory: Cancer Today [Internet]. Lyon (France): International Agency for Research on Cancer; 2018. Available from: https://gco.iarc.fr/today.

1.02	Adapted from: International Agency for Research on Cancer. List of classifications by cancer sites with sufficient or limited evidence in humans, IARC Monographs Volumes 1–127. Lyon (France): International Agency for Research on Cancer; updated 2020 Oct 9. Available from: https://monographs.iarc.fr/wp-content/uploads/2019/07/Classifications_by_cancer_site.pdf.
1.03	Adapted with permission from the American Registry of Pathology. Originally published as Table 1-1 in: Travis WD, Nicholson AG, Geisinger KR, et al. Tumors of the lower respiratory tract. Washington, DC: American Registry of Pathology; 2019. (AFIP atlas of tumor pathology, series 4; fascicle 29).
1.04	Adapted, with permission, from: Travis WD, Brambilla E, Noguchi M, et al. International Association for the Study of Lung Cancer/American Thoracic Society/European Respiratory Society international multidisciplinary classification of lung adenocarcinoma. J Thorac Oncol. 2011 Feb;6(2):244–85. PMID:21252716. Copyright 2011, with permission from Elsevier. and Travis WD, Brambilla E, Burke AP, et al., editors. WHO classification of tumours of the lung, pleura, thymus and heart. Lyon (France): International Agency for Research on Cancer; 2015. (WHO classification of tumours series, 4th ed.; vol. 7). https://publications.iarc.fr/17. and Adapted with permission from the American Registry of Pathology. Originally published as Table 1.2-2 in: Travis WD, Nicholson AG, Geisinger KR, et al. Tumors of the lower respiratory tract. Washington, DC: American Registry of Pathology; 2019. (AFIP atlas of tumor pathology, series 4; fascicle 29).
1.05	Adapted, with permission, from: Travis WD, Brambilla E, Noguchi M, et al. International

Association for the Study of Lung Cancer/American Thoracic Society/European Respiratory Society international multidisciplinary classification of lung adenocarcinoma. J Thorac Oncol. 2011 Feb;6(2):244–85. PMID:21252716. Copyright 2011, with permission from Elsevier.
and
Travis WD, Brambilla E, Burke AP, et al., editors. WHO classification of tumours of the lung, pleura, thymus and heart. Lyon (France): International Agency for Research on Cancer; 2015. (WHO classification of tumours series, 4th ed.; vol. 7). https://publications.iarc.fr/17.
and
Adapted with permission from the American Registry of Pathology. Originally published as Table 1.2-3 in: Travis WD, Nicholson AG, Geisinger KR, et al. Tumors of the lower respiratory tract. Washington, DC: American Registry of Pathology; 2019. (AFIP atlas of tumor pathology, series 4; fascicle 29).

1.06 Cooper WA
1.07 Cooper WA
1.08 Cooper WA
1.09 Cooper WA
1.10 Travis WD, Brambilla E, Burke AP, et al., editors. WHO classification of tumours of the lung, pleura, thymus and heart. Lyon (France): International Agency for Research on Cancer; 2015. (WHO classification of tumours series, 4th ed.; vol. 7). https://publications.iarc.fr/17.
1.11 Rossi G
1.12 Rossi G
1.13 Kerr KM
1.14 Adapted, with permission, from: Travis WD, Brambilla E, Burke AP, et al., editors. WHO classification of tumours of the lung, pleura, thymus and heart. Lyon (France): International Agency for Research on Cancer; 2015. (WHO classification of tumours series, 4th ed.; vol. 7). https://publications.iarc.fr/17.
1.15 Adapted with permission from the American Registry of Pathology. Originally published as Table 1.7.0.1.1 in: Travis WD, Nicholson AG, Geisinger KR, et al. Tumors of the lower respiratory tract. Washington, DC: American Registry of Pathology; 2019. (AFIP atlas of tumor pathology, series 4; fascicle 29).

1.16 Ozkaya N
2.01 Butnor KJ
2.02 Sauter JL
2.03 Sauter JL
2.04 Adapted, with permission from Wolters Kluwer Health, Inc., from: Churg A, Colby TV, Cagle P, et al. The separation of benign and malignant mesothelial proliferations. Am J Surg Pathol. 2000 Sep;24(9):1183–200. PMID:10976692. https://journals.lww.com/ajsp/Abstract/2000/09000/The_Separation_of_Benign_and_Malignant_Mesothelial.1.aspx
and
Travis WD, Brambilla E, Burke AP, et al., editors. WHO classification of tumours of the lung, pleura, thymus and heart. Lyon (France): International Agency for Research on Cancer; 2015. (WHO classification of tumours series, 4th ed.; vol. 7). https://publications.iarc.fr/17.
2.05 Travis WD, Brambilla E, Burke AP, et al., editors. WHO classification of tumours of the lung, pleura, thymus and heart. Lyon (France): International Agency for Research on Cancer; 2015. (WHO classification of tumours series, 4th ed.; vol. 7). https://publications.iarc.fr/17.
3.01 Boyer DF
4.01 WHO Classification of Tumours Editorial Board. Soft tissue and bone tumours. Lyon (France): International Agency for Research on Cancer; 2020. (WHO classification of tumours series, 5th ed.; vol. 3). https://publications.iarc.fr/588.
5.01 Marx A
Travis WD, Brambilla E, Burke AP, et al., editors. WHO classification of tumours of the lung, pleura, thymus and heart. Lyon (France): International Agency for Research on Cancer; 2015. (WHO classification of tumours series, 4th ed.; vol. 7). https://publications.iarc.fr/17.
5.02 Marx A
5.03 Marx A
5.05 Marx A
5.06 Chan JKC
5.07 Marx A
5.08 Chan JKC
6.01 Roden AC
6.02 Roden AC
6.03 Roden AC
6.04 Reprinted, with permission from Springer Nature, from: Nogales FF, Jimenez RE, editors. Pathology and biology of human germ cell tumors. Berlin (Germany): Springer;

2017. Copyright 2017.
6.05 Roden AC
6.06 Roden AC
7.01 Ferry JA
9.01 Joubert P
9.02 Poleri C
9.03 Modified from: Travis WD, Brambilla E, Burke AP, et al., editors. WHO classification of tumours of the lung, pleura, thymus and heart. Lyon (France): International Agency for Research on Cancer; 2015. (WHO classification of tumours series, 4th ed.; vol. 7). https://publications.iarc.fr/17.
9.04 Nicholson AG
9.05 Roden AC

Boxes

1.01 Adapted, with permission, from:
Travis WD, Brambilla E, Noguchi M, et al. International Association for the Study of Lung Cancer/American Thoracic Society/European Respiratory Society international multidisciplinary classification of lung adenocarcinoma. J Thorac Oncol. 2011 Feb;6(2):244–85. PMID:21252716. Copyright 2011, with permission from Elsevier.
and
Travis WD, Brambilla E, Noguchi M, et al. Diagnosis of lung cancer in small biopsies and cytology: implications of the 2011 International Association for the Study of Lung Cancer/American Thoracic Society/European Respiratory Society classification. Arch Pathol Lab Med. 2013 May;137(5):668–84. PMID:22970842. With permission from Archives of Pathology & Laboratory Medicine. Copyright 2013 College of American Pathologists.
and
Travis WD, Brambilla E, Burke AP, et al., editors. WHO classification of tumours of the lung, pleura, thymus and heart. Lyon (France): International Agency for Research on Cancer; 2015. (WHO classification of tumours series, 4th ed.; vol. 7). https://publications.iarc.fr/17.
1.02 Modified from:
Travis WD, Brambilla E, Noguchi M, et al. Diagnosis of lung adenocarcinoma in resected specimens: implications of the 2011 International Association for

the Study of Lung Cancer/ American Thoracic Society/ European Respiratory Society classification. Arch Pathol Lab Med. 2013 May;137(5):685–705. PMID:22913371. With permission from Archives of Pathology & Laboratory Medicine. Copyright 2013 College of American Pathologists.
and
Travis WD, Brambilla E, Burke AP, et al., editors. WHO classification of tumours of the lung, pleura, thymus and heart. Lyon (France): International Agency for Research on Cancer; 2015. (WHO classification of tumours series, 4th ed.; vol. 7). https://publications.iarc.fr/17.
and
Adapted with permission from the American Registry of Pathology. Originally published as Table 1.3.3.2-2 in: Travis WD, Nicholson AG, Geisinger KR, et al. Tumors of the lower respiratory tract. Washington, DC: American Registry of Pathology; 2019. (AFIP atlas of tumor pathology, series 4; fascicle 29).

1.03 Modified from:
Travis WD, Brambilla E, Noguchi M, et al. Diagnosis of lung adenocarcinoma in resected specimens: implications of the 2011 International Association for the Study of Lung Cancer/ American Thoracic Society/ European Respiratory Society classification. Arch Pathol Lab Med. 2013 May;137(5):685–705. PMID:22913371. With permission from Archives of Pathology & Laboratory Medicine. Copyright 2013 College of American Pathologists.
and
Travis WD, Brambilla E, Burke AP, et al., editors. WHO classification of tumours of the lung, pleura, thymus and heart. Lyon (France): International Agency for Research on Cancer; 2015. (WHO classification of tumours series, 4th ed.; vol. 7). https://publications.iarc.fr/17.
and
Adapted with permission from the American Registry of Pathology. Originally published as Table 1.3.3.2-2 in: Travis WD, Nicholson AG, Geisinger KR, et al. Tumors

of the lower respiratory tract. Washington, DC: American Registry of Pathology; 2019. (AFIP atlas of tumor pathology, series 4; fascicle 29).

1.04 Modified from:
Travis WD, Brambilla E, Noguchi M, et al. Diagnosis of lung adenocarcinoma in resected specimens: implications of the 2011 International Association for the Study of Lung Cancer/ American Thoracic Society/ European Respiratory Society classification. Arch Pathol Lab Med. 2013 May;137(5):685–705. PMID:22913371. With permission from Archives of Pathology & Laboratory Medicine. Copyright 2013 College of American Pathologists.
and
Travis WD, Brambilla E, Burke AP, et al., editors. WHO classification of tumours of the lung, pleura, thymus and heart. Lyon (France): International Agency for Research on Cancer; 2015. (WHO classification of tumours series, 4th ed.; vol. 7). https://publications.iarc.fr/17.
and
Adapted with permission from the American Registry of Pathology. Originally published as Table 1.3.4.3-1 in: Travis WD, Nicholson AG, Geisinger KR, et al. Tumors of the lower respiratory tract. Washington, DC: American Registry of Pathology; 2019. (AFIP atlas of tumor pathology, series 4; fascicle 29).

1.05 Modified from:
Travis WD, Brambilla E, Noguchi M, et al. Diagnosis of lung adenocarcinoma in resected specimens: implications of the 2011 International Association for the Study of Lung Cancer/ American Thoracic Society/ European Respiratory Society classification. Arch Pathol Lab Med. 2013 May;137(5):685–705. PMID:22913371. With permission from Archives of Pathology & Laboratory Medicine. Copyright 2013 College of American Pathologists.
and
Travis WD, Brambilla E, Burke AP, et al., editors. WHO classification of tumours of the lung, pleura, thymus and heart. Lyon (France):

International Agency for Research on Cancer; 2015. (WHO classification of tumours series, 4th ed.; vol. 7). https://publications.iarc.fr/17.
and
Adapted, with permission from the American Registry of Pathology, from: Travis WD, Nicholson AG, Geisinger KR, et al. Tumors of the lower respiratory tract. Washington, DC: American Registry of Pathology; 2019. (AFIP atlas of tumor pathology, series 4; fascicle 29).

1.06 Yatabe Y
1.07 Yatabe Y
1.08 Nicholson AG
1.09 Ozkaya N
2.01 Adapted, with permission, from: Nicholson AG, Sauter JL, Nowak AK, et al. EURACAN/ IASLC proposals for updating the histologic classification of pleural mesothelioma: towards a more multidisciplinary approach. J Thorac Oncol. 2020 Jan;15(1):29–49. PMID:31546041. Copyright 2020, with permission from Elsevier.
2.02 Adapted, with permission, from: Nicholson AG, Sauter JL, Nowak AK, et al. EURACAN/ IASLC proposals for updating the histologic classification of pleural mesothelioma: towards a more multidisciplinary approach. J Thorac Oncol. 2020 Jan;15(1):29–49. PMID:31546041. Copyright 2020, with permission from Elsevier.
10.01 Adapted from: Frebourg T, Bajalica Lagercrantz S, Oliveira C, et al. Guidelines for the Li-Fraumeni and heritable TP53-related cancer syndromes. Eur J Hum Genet. 2020 Oct;28(10):1379–86. PMID:32457520. https://creativecommons.org/ licenses/by/4.0/
10.02 Travis WD, Brambilla E, Burke AP, et al., editors. WHO classification of tumours of the lung, pleura, thymus and heart. Lyon (France): International Agency for Research on Cancer; 2015. (WHO classification of tumours series, 4th ed.; vol. 7). https://publications.iarc.fr/17.
and
Adapted, with permission, from Stratakis CA, Kirschner LS, Carney JA. Clinical and molecular features of the Carney complex: diagnostic

criteria and recommendations for patient evaluation. J Clin Endocrinol Metab. 2001 Sep;86(9):4041–6. PMID:11549623. By permission of Oxford University Press.

10.03   Stratakis CA, Kirschner LS, Carney JA. Clinical and molecular features of the Carney complex: diagnostic criteria and recommendations for patient evaluation. J Clin Endocrinol Metab. 2001 Sep;86(9):4041–6. PMID:11549623. By permission of Oxford University Press.

Images on the cover

Top left	Fig. 1.119: Kerr KM
Middle left	Fig. 1.120B: Husain AN
Bottom left	Fig. 1.121A: Kerr KM
Top centre	Fig. 2.09C: Gill RR
Middle centre	Fig. 2.33: Sean McNair, Cytology Service, Department of Pathology, Memorial Sloan Kettering Cancer Center, New York (NY)
Bottom centre	Fig. 2.30B: Françoise Thivolet-Bejui, Centre de Pathologie Est - CHU Lyon Groupement Hospitalier Est, Bron
Top right	Fig. 5.66: French CA
Middle right	Fig. 5.69A: French CA
Bottom right	Fig. 5.70: French CA

Images on the chapter title pages

Chapter 1	Fig. 1.55B: Travis WD
Chapter 2	Fig. 2.16: Husain AN
Chapter 3	Fig. 3.12C: Basso C
Chapter 4	Fig. 4.31B: Shimada H
Chapter 5	Fig. 5.14C: Chan JKC
Chapter 6	Fig. 6.06C: Ulbright TM
Chapter 7	Fig. 7.11A: Ferry JA
Chapter 8	Fig. 8.03: Weissferdt A
Chapter 9	Fig. 9.23C: Padera RF
Chapter 10	Fig. 10.01: WHO Classification of Tumours Editorial Board. Thoracic tumours. Lyon (France): International Agency for Research on Cancer; 2021. (WHO classification of tumours series, 5th ed.; vol. 5). https://publications.iarc.fr/595.

References

1. Aareleid T, Zimmermann ML, Baburin A, et al. Divergent trends in lung cancer incidence by gender, age and histological type in Estonia: a nationwide population-based study. BMC Cancer. 2017 Aug 30;17(1):596. PMID:28854969

2. Abdel-Rahman MH, Pilarski R, Cebulla CM, et al. Germline BAP1 mutation predisposes to uveal melanoma, lung adenocarcinoma, meningioma, and other cancers. J Med Genet. 2011 Dec;48(12):856–9. PMID:21941004

3. Abdul-Ghafar J, Yong SJ, Kwon W, et al. Primary thymic mucinous adenocarcinoma: a case report. Korean J Pathol. 2012 Aug;46(4):377–81. PMID:23110032

6. Abe A, Sugiyama Y, Furuta R, et al. Usefulness of intraoperative imprint cytology in ovarian germ cell tumors. Acta Cytol. 2013;57(2):171–6. PMID:23406948

7. Abid N, Ltaief R, Sassi A, et al. [Left atrial intimal sarcoma: a rare cause of acute heart failure]. Ann Cardiol Angeiol (Paris). 2019 Oct;68(4):232–5. French. PMID:30290919

8. Abiko K, Mandai M, Hamanishi J, et al. Oct4 expression in immature teratoma of the ovary: relevance to histologic grade and degree of differentiation. Am J Surg Pathol. 2010 Dec;34(12):1842–8. PMID:21107090

9. Abraham KP, Reddy V, Gattuso P. Neoplasms metastatic to the heart: review of 3314 consecutive autopsies. Am J Cardiovasc Pathol. 1990;3(3):195–8. PMID:2095826

10. Abreu G, Salgado A, Bettencourt N, et al. Intimal sarcoma of the left atrium - a rare form of mitral valve obstruction. Rev Port Cardiol. 2018 Jun;37(6):543–4. PMID:29731321

11. Acebo E, Val-Bernal JF, Gómez-Roman JJ. Thrombomodulin, calretinin and c-kit (CD117) expression in cardiac myxoma. Histol Histopathol. 2001 Oct;16(4):1031–6. PMID:11642722

12. Achcar RdeO, Nikiforova MN, Dacic S, et al. Mammalian mastermind like 2 11q21 gene rearrangement in bronchopulmonary mucoepidermoid carcinoma. Hum Pathol. 2009 Jun;40(6):854–60. PMID:19269006

13. Acikel S, Aksoy MM, Kilic H, et al. Cystic and hemorrhagic giant left atrial myxoma in a patient presenting with exertional angina and dyspnea. Cardiovasc Pathol. 2012 Mar-Apr;21(2):e15–8. PMID:21397522

14. Adam P, Hakroush S, Hofmann I, et al. Thymoma with loss of keratin expression (and giant cells): a potential diagnostic pitfall. Virchows Arch. 2014 Sep;465(3):313–20. PMID:24923897

15. Addis BJ, Isaacson PG. Large cell lymphoma of the mediastinum: a B-cell tumour of probable thymic origin. Histopathology. 1986 Apr;10(4):379–90. PMID:2423430

16. Adhikari A, Hafeez A, Halalau A. Cardiac dedifferentiated liposarcoma requiring a mitral valve replacement complicated by severe paravalvular leak: a rare case report with literature review. Case Rep Cardiol. 2018 Sep 4;2018:2506368. PMID:30254766

17. Adriaensen ME, Schaefer-Prokop CM, Duyndam DA, et al. Radiological evidence of lymphangioleiomyomatosis in female and male patients with tuberous sclerosis complex. Clin Radiol. 2011 Jul;66(7):625–8. PMID:21459371

18. Aesif SW, Aubry MC, Yi ES, et al. Loss of p16INK4A expression and homozygous CDKN2A deletion are associated with worse outcome and younger age in thymic carcinomas. J Thorac Oncol. 2017 May;12(5):860–71. PMID:28179162

19. Agacdiken A, Gurbuz Y, Ciftci E, et al. Cardiac lipoma in a patient with proven arrhythmogenic right ventricular dysplasia: a case report. A huge intramyocardial lipoma. Int J Cardiovasc Imaging. 2005 Aug;21(4):463–7. PMID:16047131

19A. Agaimy A, Duell T, Morresi-Hauf AT. EWSR1-fusion-negative, SMARCB1-deficient primary pulmonary myxoid sarcoma. Pol J Pathol. 2017;68(3):261–7. PMID:29363919

20. Agaimy A, Strecker T. Left atrial myxoma with papillary fibroelastoma-like features. Int J Clin Exp Pathol. 2011 Mar;4(3):307–11. PMID:21487526

21. Agaram NP, Chen CL, Zhang L, et al. Recurrent MYOD1 mutations in pediatric and adult sclerosing and spindle cell rhabdomyosarcomas: evidence for a common pathogenesis. Genes Chromosomes Cancer. 2014 Sep;53(9):779–87. PMID:24824843

22. Agaram NP, Chen HW, Zhang L, et al. EWSR1-PBX3: a novel gene fusion in myoepithelial tumors. Genes Chromosomes Cancer. 2015 Feb;54(2):63–71. PMID:25231231

23. Agaram NP, LaQuaglia MP, Alaggio R, et al. MYOD1-mutant spindle cell and sclerosing rhabdomyosarcoma: an aggressive subtype irrespective of age. A reappraisal for molecular classification and risk stratification. Mod Pathol. 2019 Jan;32(1):27–36. PMID:30181563

24. Agaram NP, Prakash S, Antonescu CR. Deep-seated plexiform schwannoma: a pathologic study of 16 cases and comparative analysis with the superficial variety. Am J Surg Pathol. 2005 Aug;29(8):1042–8. PMID:16006798

25. Agaram NP, Sung YS, Zhang L, et al. Dichotomy of genetic abnormalities in PEComas with therapeutic implications. Am J Surg Pathol. 2015 Jun;39(6):813–25. PMID:25651471

26. Aggarwal T, Goyal S, Zaheer S. Pleomorphic rhabdomyosarcoma in left atrium mimicking myxoma. Indian J Pathol Microbiol. 2016 Jul-Sep;59(3):379–81. PMID:27510683

27. Agid R, Sklair-Levy M, Bloom AI, et al. CT-guided biopsy with cutting-edge needle for the diagnosis of malignant lymphoma: experience of 267 biopsies. Clin Radiol. 2003 Feb;58(2):143–7. PMID:12623044

28. Agnihotri S, Jalali S, Wilson MR, et al. The genomic landscape of schwannoma. Nat Genet. 2016 Nov;48(11):1339–48. PMID:27723760

29. Agrawal N, Frederick MJ, Pickering CR, et al. Exome sequencing of head and neck squamous cell carcinoma reveals inactivating mutations in NOTCH1. Science. 2011 Aug 26;333(6046):1154–7. PMID:21798897

30. Agrawal T, Blau AJ, Chwals WJ, et al. A unique case of mediastinal teratoma with mature pancreatic tissue, nesidioblastosis, and aberrant islet differentiation: a case report and literature review. Endocr Pathol. 2016 Mar;27(1):21–4. PMID:26318442

31. Aguayo SM, Miller YE, Waldron JA Jr, et al. Brief report: idiopathic diffuse hyperplasia of pulmonary neuroendocrine cells and airways disease. N Engl J Med. 1992 Oct 29;327(18):1285–8. PMID:1406819

32. Aguilar C, Soca R, Guillen M, et al. Cardiac undifferentiated pleomorphic sarcoma incidentally diagnosed during mitral valve replacement. J Card Surg. 2017 Feb;32(2):91–2. PMID:28127801

33. Ahmad U, Yao X, Detterbeck F, et al. Thymic carcinoma outcomes and prognosis: results of an international analysis. J Thorac Cardiovasc Surg. 2015 Jan;149(1):95–100, 101.e1–2. PMID:25524678

34. Ahn D, Lee GJ, Sohn JH, et al. Fine-needle aspiration cytology versus core-needle biopsy for the diagnosis of extracranial head and neck schwannoma. Head Neck. 2018 Dec;40(12):2695–700. PMID:30457183

35. Ahn S, Lee JJ, Ha SY, et al. Clinicopathological analysis of 21 thymic neuroendocrine tumors. Korean J Pathol. 2012 Jun;46(3):221–5. PMID:23110006

36. Aisner DL, Sholl LM, Berry LD, et al. The impact of smoking and TP53 mutations in lung adenocarcinoma patients with targetable mutations-the Lung Cancer Mutation Consortium (LCMC2). Clin Cancer Res. 2018 Mar 1;24(5):1038–47. PMID:29217530

37. Akahori H. A case of mediastinal teratoma with pancreatic islets accompanied by discontinuation of insulin treatment in insulin-dependent diabetes mellitus. Diabetol Int. 2019 Jul 2;10(4):295–9. PMID:31592406

38. Akata S, Okada S, Maeda J, et al. Computed tomographic findings of large cell neuroendocrine carcinoma of the lung. Clin Imaging. 2007 Nov-Dec;31(6):379–84. PMID:17996599

39. Akeno N, Reece AL, Callahan M, et al. TRP53 mutants drive neuroendocrine lung cancer through loss-of-function mechanisms with gain-of-function effects on chemotherapy response. Mol Cancer Ther. 2017 Dec;16(12):2913–26. PMID:28847987

40. Akkaya Z, Gursoy A, Erden A. The disastrous "sun ray" sign in cardiac magnetic resonance: an indicator of angiosarcoma. Cardiol Young. 2014 Oct;24(5):929–31. PMID:24702744

41. Aktoz M, Tatli E, Ege T, et al. Cardiac rhabdomyoma in an adult patient presenting with right ventricular outflow tract obstruction. Int J Cardiol. 2008 Nov 28;130(3):e105–7. PMID:17727983

42. Al-Abbadi MA, Almasri NM, Al-Quran S, et al. Cytokeratin and epithelial membrane antigen expression in angiosarcomas: an immunohistochemical study of 33 cases. Arch Pathol Lab Med. 2007 Feb;131(2):288–92. PMID:17284115

43. Alaggio R, Coffin CM, Weiss SW, et al. Liposarcomas in young patients: a study of 82 cases occurring in patients younger than 22 years of age. Am J Surg Pathol. 2009 May;33(5):645–58. PMID:19194281

44. Alaggio R, Zhang L, Sung YS, et al. A molecular study of pediatric spindle and sclerosing rhabdomyosarcoma: identification of novel and recurrent VGLL2-related fusions in infantile cases. Am J Surg Pathol. 2016 Feb;40(2):224–35. PMID:26501226

45. Alam N, Gustafson KS, Ladanyi M, et al. Small-cell carcinoma with an epidermal growth factor receptor mutation in a never-smoker with gefitinib-responsive adenocarcinoma of the lung. Clin Lung Cancer. 2010 Sep 1;11(5):E1–4. PMID:20837450

46. Alassiri AH, Ali RH, Shen Y, et al. ETV6-NTRK3 is expressed in a subset of ALK-negative inflammatory myofibroblastic tumors. Am J Surg Pathol. 2016 Aug;40(8):1051–61. PMID:27259007

47. Al-Azizi KM, Hamandi M, Baxter R, et al. Papillary fibroelastoma of the ascending aorta. J Investig Med High Impact Case Rep. 2019 Jan-Dec;7:2324709619840377. PMID:31010309

48. Alberg AJ, Brock MV, Ford JG, et al. Epidemiology of lung cancer: diagnosis and management of lung cancer, 3rd ed: American College of Chest Physicians evidence-based clinical practice guidelines. Chest. 2013 May;143(5 Suppl):e1S–29S. PMID:23649439

49. Albergo JI, Gaston CL, Laitinen M, et al. Ewing's sarcoma: only patients with 100% of necrosis after chemotherapy should be classified as having a good response. Bone Joint J. 2016 Aug;98-B(8):1138–44. PMID:27482030

50. Alcala N, Leblay N, Gabriel AAG, et al. Integrative and comparative genomic analyses identify clinically relevant pulmonary carcinoid groups and unveil the supra-carcinoids. Nat Commun. 2019 Aug 20;10(1):3407. PMID:31431620

51. Alcala N, Mangiante L, Le-Stang N, et al. Redefining malignant pleural mesothelioma types as a continuum uncovers immune-vascular interactions. EBioMedicine. 2019 Oct;48:191–202. PMID:31648983

52. Alchami FS, Attanoos RL, Bamber AR. Myxoid variant epithelioid pleural mesothelioma defines a favourable prognosis group: an analysis of 191 patients with pleural malignant mesothelioma. J Clin Pathol. 2017 Feb;70(2):179–82. PMID:27798081

53. Alekseyenko AA, Walsh EM, Wang X, et al. The oncogenic BRD4-NUT chromatin regulator drives aberrant transcription within large topological domains. Genes Dev. 2015 Jul 15;29(14):1507–23. PMID:26220994

54. Alekseyenko AA, Walsh EM, Zee BM, et al. Ectopic protein interactions within BRD4-chromatin complexes drive oncogenic megadomain formation in NUT midline carcinoma. Proc Natl Acad Sci U S A. 2017 May 23;114(21):E4184–92. PMID:28484033

55. Alexandrov LB, Nik-Zainal S, Wedge DC, et al. Signatures of mutational processes in human cancer. Nature. 2013 Aug 22;500(7463):415–21. PMID:23945592

56. Alexanian S, Said J, Lones M, et al. KSHV/HHV8-negative effusion-based lymphoma, a distinct entity associated with fluid overload states. Am J Surg Pathol. 2013 Feb;37(2):241–9. PMID:23282971

57. Alexiev BA, Drachenberg CB, Burke AP. Thymomas: a cytological and immunohistochemical study, with emphasis on lymphoid and neuroendocrine markers. Diagn Pathol. 2007 May 11;2:13. PMID:17498299

58. Ali SZ, Smilari TF, Teichberg S, et al. Pleomorphic rhabdomyosarcoma of the heart metastatic to bone. Report of a case with fine needle aspiration biopsy findings. Acta Cytol. 1995 May-Jun;39(3):555–8. PMID:7762352

59. Allan BJ, Thorson CM, Davis JS, et al. An analysis of 73 cases of pediatric malignant tumors of the thymus. J Surg Res. 2013 Sep;184(1):397–403. PMID:23570972

60. Allen BC, Mohammed TL, Tan CD, et al. Metastatic melanoma to the heart. Curr Probl Diagn Radiol. 2012 Sep-Oct;41(5):159–64. PMID:22818836

61. Allen CT, Lee S, Norberg SM, et al. Safety and clinical activity of PD-L1 blockade in patients with aggressive recurrent respiratory papillomatosis. J Immunother Cancer. 2019 May 3;7(1):119. PMID:31053174

62. Allen MS Jr, Drash EC. Primary melanoma of the lung. Cancer. 1968 Jan;21(1):154–9. PMID:5634845

63. Allen TC, Cagle PT, Churg AM, et al. Localized malignant mesothelioma. Am J Surg Pathol. 2005 Jul;29(7):866–73. PMID:15958850

64. Al-Mamgani A, Baartman L, Baaijens M, et al. Cardiac metastases. Int J Clin Oncol. 2008 Aug;13(4):369–72. PMID:18704641

64A. Alobeid B, Beneck D, Sreekantaiah C, et al. Congenital pulmonary myofibroblastic tumor: a case report with cytogenetic analysis and review of the literature. Am J Surg Pathol. 1997 May;21(5):610–4. PMID:9158688

65. Alper F, Kaynar H, Kantarci M, et al. Trichoptysis caused by intrapulmonary teratoma: computed tomography and magnetic resonance imaging findings. Australas Radiol. 2005 Feb;49(1):53–6. PMID:15727610

66. Alqahtani A, Nguyen LT, Flageole H, et al. 25 years' experience with lymphangiomas in children. J Pediatr Surg. 1999 Jul;34(7):1164–8. PMID:10442614

67. Altinay S, Metovic J, Massa F, et al. Spread through air spaces (STAS) is a predictor of poor outcome in atypical carcinoids of the lung. Virchows Arch. 2019 Sep;475(3):325–34. PMID:31201506

68. Al-Toubah T, Strosberg J, Halfdanarson TR, et al. Somatostatin analogs improve respiratory symptoms in patients with diffuse idiopathic neuroendocrine cell hyperplasia. Chest. 2020 Jul;158(1):401–5. PMID:32059961

69. Aly RG, Rekhtman N, Li X, et al. Spread through air spaces (STAS) is prognostic in atypical carcinoid, large cell neuroendocrine carcinoma, and small cell carcinoma of the lung. J Thorac Oncol. 2019 Sep;14(9):1583–93. PMID:31121325

70. Amadou A, Achatz MIW, Hainaut P. Revisiting tumor patterns and penetrance in germline TP53 mutation carriers: temporal phases of Li-Fraumeni syndrome. Curr Opin Oncol. 2018 Jan;30(1):23–9. PMID:29076966

71. Amar L, Baudin E, Burnichon N, et al. Succinate dehydrogenase B gene mutations predict survival in patients with malignant pheochromocytomas or paragangliomas. J Clin Endocrinol Metab. 2007 Oct;92(10):3822–8. PMID:17652212

72. Amar L, Bertherat J, Baudin E, et al. Genetic testing in pheochromocytoma or functional paraganglioma. J Clin Oncol. 2005 Dec 1;23(34):8812–8. PMID:16314641

73. Amato E, Molin MD, Mafficini A, et al. Targeted next-generation sequencing of cancer genes dissects the molecular profiles of intraductal papillary neoplasms of the pancreas. J Pathol. 2014 Jul;233(3):217–27. PMID:24604757

74. Amer W, Toth C, Vassella E, et al. Evolution analysis of heterogeneous non-small cell lung carcinoma by ultra-deep sequencing of the mitochondrial genome. Sci Rep. 2017 Sep 11;7(1):11069. PMID:28894165

75. Amin MB, Edge S, Greene F, et al., editors. AJCC cancer staging manual. 8th ed. New York (NY): Springer; 2017.

76. Anagnostopoulos I, Hansmann ML, Franssila K, et al. European Task Force on Lymphoma project on lymphocyte predominance Hodgkin disease: histologic and immunohistologic analysis of submitted cases reveals 2 types of Hodgkin disease with a nodular growth pattern and abundant lymphocytes. Blood. 2000 Sep 1;96(5):1889–99. PMID:10961891

77. Anderson CD, Hashimi S, Brown T, et al. Primary benign interatrial schwannoma encountered during aortic valve replacement. J Card Surg. 2011 Jan;26(1):63–5. PMID:21073532

78. Anderson T, Zhang L, Hameed M, et al. Thoracic epithelioid malignant vascular tumors: a clinicopathologic study of 52 cases with emphasis on pathologic grading and molecular studies of WWTR1-CAMTA1 fusions. Am J Surg Pathol. 2015 Jan;39(1):132–9. PMID:25353289

79. Andino L, Cagle PT, Murer B, et al. Pleuropulmonary desmoid tumors: immunohistochemical comparison with solitary fibrous tumors and assessment of beta-catenin and cyclin D1 expression. Arch Pathol Lab Med. 2006 Oct;130(10):1503–9. PMID:17090192

80. Ando M, Sato Y, Takata K, et al. A20 (TNFAIP3) deletion in Epstein-Barr virus-associated lymphoproliferative disorders/lymphomas. PLoS One. 2013;8(2):e56741. PMID:23418597

81. Andrade FM, Abou-Mourad OM, Judice LF, et al. Endotracheal inflammatory pseudotumor: the role of interventional bronchoscopy. Ann Thorac Surg. 2010 Sep;90(3):e36–7. PMID:20732473

82. Andrici J, Sheen A, Sioson L, et al. Loss of expression of BAP1 is a useful adjunct, which strongly supports the diagnosis of mesothelioma in effusion cytology. Mod Pathol. 2015 Oct;28(10):1360–8. PMID:26226841

83. Andujar P, Lacourt A, Brochard P, et al. Five years update on relationships between malignant pleural mesothelioma and exposure to asbestos and other elongated mineral particles. J Toxicol Environ Health B Crit Rev. 2016;19(5-6):151–72. PMID:27705546

83A. Ang PP, Tan GC, Karim N, er al. Diagnostic value of the EZH2 immunomarker in malignant effusion cytology. Acta Cytol. 2020;64(3):248–55. PMID:31352449

84. Antic T, Kapur U, Vigneswaran WT, et al. Inflammatory sarcomatoid carcinoma: a case report and discussion of a malignant tumor with benign appearance. Arch Pathol Lab Med. 2005 Oct;129(10):1334–7. PMID:16196527

85. Antoch G, Stattaus J, Nemat AT, et al. Non-small cell lung cancer: dual-modality PET/CT in preoperative staging. Radiology. 2003 Nov;229(2):526–33. PMID:14512512

86. Antonescu CR, Katabi N, Zhang L, et al. EWSR1-ATF1 fusion is a novel and consistent finding in hyalinizing clear-cell carcinoma of salivary gland. Genes Chromosomes Cancer. 2011 Jul;50(7):559–70. PMID:21484932

87. Antonescu CR, Le Loarer F, Mosquera JM, et al. Novel YAP1-TFE3 fusion defines a distinct subset of epithelioid hemangioendothelioma. Genes Chromosomes Cancer. 2013 Aug;52(8):775–84. PMID:23737213

88. Antonescu CR, Owosho AA, Zhang L, et al. Sarcomas with CIC-rearrangements are a distinct pathologic entity with aggressive outcome: a clinicopathologic and molecular study of 115 cases. Am J Surg Pathol. 2017 Jul;41(7):941–9. PMID:28346326

89. Antonescu CR, Suurmeijer AJ, Zhang L, et al. Molecular characterization of inflammatory myofibroblastic tumors with frequent ALK and ROS1 gene fusions and rare novel RET rearrangement. Am J Surg Pathol. 2015 Jul;39(7):957–67. PMID:25723109

90. Antonescu CR, Yoshida A, Guo T, et al. KDR activating mutations in human angiosarcomas are sensitive to specific kinase inhibitors. Cancer Res. 2009 Sep 15;69(18):7175–9. PMID:19723655

91. Antonescu CR, Zhang L, Chang NE, et al. EWSR1-POU5F1 fusion in soft tissue myoepithelial tumors. A molecular analysis of sixty-six cases, including soft tissue, bone, and visceral lesions, showing common involvement of the EWSR1 gene. Genes Chromosomes Cancer. 2010 Dec;49(12):1114–24. PMID:20815032

92. Aozasa K, Ohsawa M, Iuchi K, et al. Artificial pneumothorax as a risk factor for development of pleural lymphoma. Jpn J Cancer Res. 1993 Jan;84(1):55–7. PMID:8449828

93. Aozasa K, Ohsawa M, Iuchi K, et al. Prognostic factors for pleural lymphoma patients. Jpn J Clin Oncol. 1991 Dec;21(6):417–21. PMID:1805046

94. Aozasa K, Takakuwa T, Nakatsuka S. Pyothorax-associated lymphoma: a lymphoma developing in chronic inflammation. Adv Anat Pathol. 2005 Nov;12(6):324–31. PMID:16330929

95. Arbour KC, Naidoo J, Steele KE, et al. Expression of PD-L1 and other immunotherapeutic targets in thymic epithelial tumors. PLoS One. 2017 Aug 3;12(8):e0182665. PMID:28771603

96. Archie PH, Beasley MB, Ross HJ. Biphasic pulmonary blastoma with germ cell differentiation in a 36-year-old man. J Thorac Oncol. 2008 Oct;3(10):1185–7. PMID:18827617

97. Arcila ME, Chaft JE, Nafa K, et al. Prevalence, clinicopathologic associations, and molecular spectrum of ERBB2 (HER2) tyrosine kinase mutations in lung adenocarcinomas. Clin Cancer Res. 2012 Sep 15;18(18):4910–8. PMID:22761469

98. Arcila ME, Drilon A, Sylvester BE, et al. MAP2K1 (MEK1) mutations define a distinct subset of lung adenocarcinoma associated with smoking. Clin Cancer Res. 2015 Apr 15;21(8):1935–43. PMID:25351745

99. Argani P, Aulmann S, Illei PB, et al. A distinctive subset of PEComas harbors TFE3 gene fusions. Am J Surg Pathol. 2010 Oct;34(10):1395–406. PMID:20871214

100. Argani P, Erlandson RA, Rosai J. Thymic neuroblastoma in adults: report of three cases with special emphasis on its association with the syndrome of inappropriate secretion of antidiuretic hormone. Am J Clin Pathol. 1997 Nov;108(5):537–43. PMID:9353092

101. Argani P, Rosai J. Hyperplastic mesothelial cells in lymph nodes: report of six cases of a benign process that can stimulate metastatic involvement by mesothelioma or carcinoma. Hum Pathol. 1998 Apr;29(4):339–46. PMID:9563782

102. Arlotta P, Tai AK, Manfioletti G, et al. Transgenic mice expressing a truncated form of the high mobility group I-C protein develop adiposity and an abnormally high prevalence of lipomas. J Biol Chem. 2000 May 12;275(19):14394–400. PMID:10747931

103. Armbruster C, Bernhardt K, Setinek U. Pulmonary tumorlet: a case report of a diagnostic pitfall in cytology. Acta Cytol. 2008 Mar-Apr;52(2):223–7. PMID:18500000

105. Arnaud L, Gorochov G, Charlotte F, et al. Systemic perturbation of cytokine and chemokine networks in Erdheim-Chester disease: a single-center series of 37 patients. Blood. 2011 Mar 10;117(10):2783–90. PMID:21205927

106. Arnaud L, Hervier B, Néel A, et al. CNS involvement and treatment with interferon-α are independent prognostic factors in Erdheim-Chester disease: a multicenter survival analysis of 53 patients. Blood. 2011 Mar 10;117(10):2778–82. PMID:21239701

107. Arnaud L, Pierre I, Beigelman-Aubry C, et al. Pulmonary involvement in Erdheim-Chester disease: a single-center study of thirty-four patients and a review of the literature. Arthritis Rheum. 2010 Nov;62(11):3504–12. PMID:20662053

108. Arnold DT, De Fonseka D, Perry S, et al. Investigating unilateral pleural effusions: the role of cytology. Eur Respir J. 2018 Nov 8;52(5):1801254. PMID:30262573

109. Arriola E, Paredes-Lario A, García-Gomez R, et al. Comparison of plasma ctDNA and tissue/cytology-based techniques for the detection of EGFR mutation status in advanced NSCLC: Spanish data subset from ASSESS. Clin Transl Oncol. 2018 Oct;20(10):1261–7. PMID:29623586

110. Asada Y, Marutsuka K, Mitsukawa T, et al. Ganglioneuroblastoma of the thymus: an adult case with the syndrome of inappropriate secretion of antidiuretic hormone. Hum Pathol. 1996 May;27(5):506–9. PMID:8621190

111. Asakura K, Izumi Y, Ikeda T, et al. Mediastinal germ cell tumor with somatic-type malignancy: report of 5 stage I/II cases. Ann Thorac Surg. 2010 Sep;90(3):1014–6. PMID:20732540

112. Asamura H. Multiple primary cancers or multiple metastases, that is the question. J Thorac Oncol. 2010 Jul;5(7):930–1. PMID:20581574

113. Asamura H, Chansky K, Crowley J, et al. The International Association for the Study of Lung Cancer Lung Cancer Staging Project: proposals for the revision of the N descriptors in the forthcoming 8th edition of the TNM classification for lung cancer. J Thorac Oncol. 2015 Dec;10(12):1675–84. PMID:26709477

114. Ascani S, Carloni A, Agostinelli C, et al. Thymoma arising in the wall of a thymic cyst. Pathologica. 2008 Dec;100(6):476–7. PMID:19475891

115. Ascani S, Piccioli M, Poggi S, et al. Pyothorax-associated lymphoma: description of the first two cases detected in Italy. Ann Oncol. 1997 Nov;8(11):1133–8. PMID:9426333

116. Ashby MA, Williams CJ, Buchanan RB, et al. Mediastinal germ cell tumour associated with malignant histiocytosis and high rubella titres. Hematol Oncol. 1986 Jul-Sep;4(3):183–94. PMID:3770648

117. Asirvatham JR, Esposito MJ, Bhuiya TA. Role of PAX-8, CD5, and CD117 in distinguishing thymic carcinoma from poorly differentiated lung carcinoma. Appl Immunohistochem Mol Morphol. 2014 May-Jun;22(5):372–6. PMID:23958552

118. Aslan DL, Gulbahce HE, Pambuccian SE, et al. Ki-67 immunoreactivity in the differential diagnosis of pulmonary neuroendocrine neoplasms in specimens with extensive crush artifact. Am J Clin Pathol. 2005 Jun;123(6):874–8. PMID:15899778

119. Attanoos RL, Churg A, Galateau-Salle F, et al. Malignant mesothelioma and its non-asbestos causes. Arch Pathol Lab Med. 2018 Jun;142(6):753–60. PMID:29480760

120. Attanoos RL, Dojcinov SD, Webb R, et al. Anti-mesothelial markers in sarcomatoid mesothelioma and other spindle cell neoplasms. Histopathology. 2000 Sep;37(3):224–31. PMID:10971698

121. Attanoos RL, Galateau-Salle F, Gibbs AR, et al. Primary thymic epithelial tumours of the pleura mimicking malignant mesothelioma. Histopathology. 2002 Jul;41(1):42–9. PMID:12121236

122. Attanoos RL, Gibbs AR. 'Pseudomesotheliomatous' carcinomas of the pleura: a 10-year analysis of cases from the Environmental Lung Disease Research Group, Cardiff. Histopathology. 2003 Nov;43(5):444–52. PMID:14636270

123. Attanoos RL, Thomas DH, Gibbs AR. Synchronous diffuse malignant mesothelioma and carcinomas in asbestos-exposed individuals. Histopathology. 2003 Oct;43(4):387–92. PMID:14511258

124. Aubry MC, Heinrich MC, Molina J, et al. Primary adenoid cystic carcinoma of the lung:

absence of KIT mutations. Cancer. 2007 Dec 1;110(11):2507–10. PMID:17932891
125. Aubry MC, Thomas CF Jr, Jett JR, et al. Significance of multiple carcinoid tumors and tumorlets in surgical lung specimens: analysis of 28 patients. Chest. 2007 Jun;131(6):1635–43. PMID:17400673
126. Auger D, Pressacco J, Marcotte F, et al. Cardiac masses: an integrative approach using echocardiography and other imaging modalities. Heart. 2011 Jul;97(13):1101–9. PMID:21642661
127. Auger M, Katz RL, Johnston DA. Differentiating cytological features of bronchioloalveolar carcinoma from adenocarcinoma of the lung in fine-needle aspirations: a statistical analysis of 27 cases. Diagn Cytopathol. 1997 Mar;16(3):253–7. PMID:9099548
128. Austin JH, Garg K, Aberle D, et al. Radiologic implications of the 2011 classification of adenocarcinoma of the lung. Radiology. 2013 Jan;266(1):62–71. PMID:23070271
129. Aviel-Ronen S, Coe BP, Lau SK, et al. Genomic markers for malignant progression in pulmonary adenocarcinoma with bronchioloalveolar features. Proc Natl Acad Sci U S A. 2008 Jul 22;105(29):10155–60. PMID:18632575
130. Awad MM, Oxnard GR, Jackman DM, et al. MET exon 14 mutations in non-small-cell lung cancer are associated with advanced age and stage-dependent MET genomic amplification and c-Met overexpression. J Clin Oncol. 2016 Mar 1;34(7):721–30. PMID:26729443
131. Ayadi L, Chaabouni S, Chabchoub I, et al. [Primary rhabdomyosarcoma of the pleura presenting as recurrent pneumothorax]. Rev Mal Respir. 2009 Mar;26(3):333–7. French. PMID:19367209
132. Aygun C, Slawson RG, Bajaj K, et al. Primary mediastinal seminoma. Urology. 1984 Feb;23(2):109–17. PMID:6364524
133. Baba M, Iyoda A, Nomoto Y, et al. Cytological findings of pre-invasive bronchial lesions detected by light-induced fluorescence endoscopy in a lung cancer screening system. Oncol Rep. 2007 Mar;17(3):579–83. PMID:17273736
134. Badalian-Very G, Vergilio JA, Degar BA, et al. Recurrent BRAF mutations in Langerhans cell histiocytosis. Blood. 2010 Sep 16;116(11):1919–23. PMID:20519626
135. Bae SY, Kim HS, Jang HJ, et al. Primary pulmonary chordoid meningioma. Korean J Thorac Cardiovasc Surg. 2018 Dec;51(6):410–4. PMID:30588452
136. Baghai-Wadji M, Sianati M, Nikpour H, et al. Pleomorphic adenoma of the trachea in an 8-year-old boy: a case report. J Pediatr Surg. 2006 Aug;41(8):e23–6. PMID:16863832
137. Bagwan IN, Desai S, Wotherspoon A, et al. Unusual presentation of primary cardiac lymphoma. Interact Cardiovasc Thorac Surg. 2009 Jul;9(1):127–9. PMID:19351686
138. Bagwan IN, Sheppard MN. Cardiac lipoma causing sudden cardiac death. Eur J Cardiothorac Surg. 2009 Apr;35(4):727. PMID:19211255
139. Bahrami A, Lee S, Schaefer IM, et al. TERT promoter mutations and prognosis in solitary fibrous tumor. Mod Pathol. 2016 Dec;29(12):1511–22. PMID:27562490
140. Bahrami A, Ro JY, Ayala AG. An overview of testicular germ cell tumors. Arch Pathol Lab Med. 2007 Aug;131(8):1267–80. PMID:17683189
141. Bai S, Wei S, Pasha TL, et al. Immunohistochemical studies of metastatic germ-cell tumors in retroperitoneal dissection specimens: a sensitive and specific panel. Int J Surg Pathol. 2013 Aug;21(4):342–51. PMID:23893437
142. Bailey P, Chang DK, Nones K, et al. Genomic analyses identify molecular subtypes of pancreatic cancer. Nature. 2016 Mar 3;531(7592):47–52. PMID:26909576
143. Bailey-Wilson JE, Amos CI, Pinney SM, et al. A major lung cancer susceptibility locus maps to chromosome 6q23-25. Am J Hum Genet. 2004 Sep;75(3):460–74. PMID:15272417
143A. Baine MK, Hsieh MS, Lai WV, et al. SCLC subtypes defined by ASCL1, NEUROD1, POU2F3, and YAP1: a comprehensive immunohistochemical and histopathologic characterization. J Thorac Oncol. 2020 Dec;15(12):1823–35. PMID:33011388
144. Baine MK, Rekhtman N. Multiple faces of pulmonary large cell neuroendocrine carcinoma: update with a focus on practical approach to diagnosis. Transl Lung Cancer Res. 2020 Jun;9(3):860–78. PMID:32676352
145. Baine MK, Sinard JH, Cai G, et al. A semiquantitative scoring system may allow biopsy diagnosis of pulmonary large cell neuroendocrine carcinoma. Am J Clin Pathol. 2020 Jan 2;153(2):165–74. PMID:31593583
146. Bains S, Eguchi T, Warth A, et al. Procedure-specific risk prediction for recurrence in patients undergoing lobectomy or sublobar resection for small (≤2 cm) lung adenocarcinoma: an international cohort analysis. J Thorac Oncol. 2019 Jan;14(1):72–86. PMID:30253972
147. Baird C, Blalock S, Bengur R, et al. Right atrial hemangioma in the newborn: utility of fetal imaging. Ann Pediatr Cardiol. 2012 Jan;5(1):81–4. PMID:22529610
148. Bakaeen FG, Reardon MJ, Coselli JS, et al. Surgical outcome in 85 patients with primary cardiac tumors. Am J Surg. 2003 Dec;186(6):641–7, discussion 647. PMID:14672772
149. Balbach ST, Makarova O, Bonn BR, et al. Proposal of a genetic classifier for risk group stratification in pediatric T-cell lymphoblastic lymphoma reveals differences from adult T-cell lymphoblastic leukemia. Leukemia. 2016 Apr;30(4):970–3. PMID:26216196
150. Baldovini C, Rossi G, Ciarrocchi A. Approaches to tumor classification in pulmonary sarcomatoid carcinoma. Lung Cancer (Auckl). 2019 Dec 5;10:131–49. PMID:31824199
151. Ball A, Bromley A, Glaze S, et al. A rare case of NUT midline carcinoma. Gynecol Oncol Case Rep. 2012 Oct 8;3:1–3. PMID:24371650
152. Ballinger ML, Best A, Mai PL, et al. Baseline surveillance in Li-Fraumeni syndrome using whole-body magnetic resonance imaging: a meta-analysis. JAMA Oncol. 2017 Dec 1;3(12):1634–9. PMID:28772291
153. Banerjee SS, Eyden B. Divergent differentiation in malignant melanomas: a review. Histopathology. 2008 Jan;52(2):119–29. PMID:17825057
154. Banito A, Li X, Laporte AN, et al. The SS18-SSX oncoprotein hijacks KDM2B-PRC1.1 to drive synovial sarcoma. Cancer Cell. 2018 Mar 12;33(3):527–541.e8. PMID:29502955
155. Banki F, Khalil K, Kott MM, et al. Adenoid cystic carcinoma of the thymus gland: a rare tumor. Ann Thorac Surg. 2010 Oct;90(4):e56–8. PMID:20868782
156. Barahona ML, Dueñas VP, Sánchez MT, et al. Case report. Primary mucosa-associated lymphoid tissue lymphoma as a pleural mass. Br J Radiol. 2011 Dec;84(1008):e229–31. PMID:22101588
157. Barbareschi M, Cantaloni C, Del Vescovo V, et al. Heterogeneity of large cell carcinoma of the lung: an immunophenotypic and miRNA-based analysis. Am J Clin Pathol. 2011 Nov;136(5):773–82. PMID:22031317
158. Barbosa MVR, Cordeiro de Lima VC, Formiga MN, et al. High prevalence of EGFR mutations in lung adenocarcinomas from Brazilian patients harboring the TP53 p.R337H variant. Clin Lung Cancer. 2020 Mar;21(2):e37–44. PMID:31889631
159. Barker N. The canonical Wnt/beta-catenin signalling pathway. Methods Mol Biol. 2008;468:5–15. PMID:19089242
160. Barksdale EM Jr, Obokhare I. Teratomas in infants and children. Curr Opin Pediatr. 2009 Jun;21(3):344–9. PMID:19417664
161. Barnaś E, Książek M, Raś R, et al. Benign metastasizing leiomyoma: a review of current literature in respect to the time and type of previous gynecological surgery. PLoS One. 2017 Apr 20;12(4):e0175875. PMID:28426767
162. Barr FG, Qualman SJ, Macris MH, et al. Genetic heterogeneity in the alveolar rhabdomyosarcoma subset without typical gene fusions. Cancer Res. 2002 Aug 15;62(16):4704–10. PMID:12183429
163. Barta JA, Powell CA, Wisnivesky JP. Global epidemiology of lung cancer. Ann Glob Health. 2019 Jan 22;85(1):8. PMID:30741509
164. Basile A, Gregoris A, Antoci B, et al. Malignant change in a benign pulmonary hamartoma. Thorax. 1989 Mar;44(3):232–3. PMID:2705156
165. Bass AJ, Watanabe H, Mermel CH, et al. SOX2 is an amplified lineage-survival oncogene in lung and esophageal squamous cell carcinomas. Nat Genet. 2009 Nov;41(11):1238–42. PMID:19801978
166. Bassan R, Maino E, Cortelazzo S. Lymphoblastic lymphoma: an updated review on biology, diagnosis, and treatment. Eur J Haematol. 2016 May;96(5):447–60. PMID:26679753
167. Basso C, Barbazza R, Thiene G. Images in cardiovascular medicine. Lipomatous hypertrophy of the atrial septum. Circulation. 1998 Apr 14;97(14):1423. PMID:9577955
168. Basso C, Rizzo S, Valente M, et al. Cardiac masses and tumours. Heart. 2016 Aug 1;102(15):1230–45. PMID:27277840
169. Basso C, Valente M, Casarotto D, et al. Cardiac lithomyxoma. Am J Cardiol. 1997 Nov 1;80(9):1249–51. PMID:9359568
170. Basso C, Valente M, Poletti A, et al. Surgical pathology of primary cardiac and pericardial tumors. Eur J Cardiothorac Surg. 1997 Nov;12(5):730–7, discussion 737–8. PMID:9458144
171. Basso C, Valente M, Thiene G, editors. Cardiac tumor pathology. New York (NY): Springer Humana Press; 2013.
172. Basu A, Moreira AL, Simms A, et al. Sarcomatoid carcinoma in cytology: report of a rare entity presenting in pleural and pericardial fluid preparations. Diagn Cytopathol. 2019 Aug;47(8):813–6. PMID:30908904
173. Baudin E, Hayes AR, Scoazec JY, et al. Unmet medical needs in pulmonary neuroendocrine (carcinoid) neoplasms. Neuroendocrinology. 2019;108(1):7–17. PMID:30248673
174. Bauer AJ, Stewart DR, Kamihara J, et al. DICER1 and associated conditions: identification of at-risk individuals and recommended surveillance strategies-response. Clin Cancer Res. 2019 Mar 1;25(5):1689–90. PMID:30824630
175. Bauer DE, Mitchell CM, Strait KM, et al. Clinicopathologic features and long-term outcomes of NUT midline carcinoma. Clin Cancer Res. 2012 Oct 15;18(20):5773–9. PMID:22896655
176. Baumann F, Buck BJ, Metcalf RV, et al. Reply to "No increased risk for mesothelioma in relation to natural-occurring asbestos in southern Nevada". J Thorac Oncol. 2015 Jul;10(7):e64–5. PMID:26134238
177. Baumann F, Buck BJ, Metcalf RV, et al. The presence of asbestos in the natural environment is likely related to mesothelioma in young individuals and women from southern Nevada. J Thorac Oncol. 2015 May;10(5):731–7. PMID:25668121
178. Baumann F, Flores E, Napolitano A, et al. Mesothelioma patients with germline BAP1 mutations have 7-fold improved long-term survival. Carcinogenesis. 2015 Jan;36(1):76–81. PMID:25380601
179. Baysal BE. Hereditary paraganglioma targets diverse paraganglia. J Med Genet. 2002 Sep;39(9):617–22. PMID:12205103
180. Beasley MB, Dembitzer FR, Flores RM. Surgical pathology of early stage non-small cell lung carcinoma. Ann Transl Med. 2016 Jun;4(12):238. PMID:27429964
181. Beasley MB, Lantuejoul S, Abbondanzo S, et al. The P16/cyclin D1/Rb pathway in neuroendocrine tumors of the lung. Hum Pathol. 2003 Feb;34(2):136–42. PMID:12612881
182. Beasley MB, Thunnissen FB, Brambilla E, et al. Pulmonary atypical carcinoid: predictors of survival in 106 cases. Hum Pathol. 2000 Oct;31(10):1255–65. PMID:11070119
183. Beasley SW, Tiedemann K, Howat A, et al. Precocious puberty associated with malignant thoracic teratoma and malignant histiocytosis in a child with Klinefelter's syndrome. Med Pediatr Oncol. 1987;15(5):277–80. PMID:2443827
184. Becker AB, Roth RA. Insulin receptor structure and function in normal and pathological conditions. Annu Rev Med. 1990;41:99–115. PMID:2184752
185. Becker AE. Primary heart tumors in the pediatric age group: a review of salient pathologic features relevant for clinicians. Pediatr Cardiol. 2000 Jul-Aug;21(4):317–23. PMID:10865004
186. Beckles MA, Spiro SG, Colice GL, et al. Initial evaluation of the patient with lung cancer: symptoms, signs, laboratory tests, and paraneoplastic syndromes. Chest. 2003 Jan;123(1 Suppl):97S–104S. PMID:12527569
187. Beckwith C, Butera J, Sadaniantz A, et al. Diagnosis in oncology. Case 1: primary transmural cardiac lymphoma. J Clin Oncol. 2000 May;18(9):1996–7. PMID:10784641
188. Beert E, Brems H, Daniëls B, et al. Atypical neurofibromas in neurofibromatosis type 1 are premalignant tumors. Genes Chromosomes Cancer. 2011 Dec;50(12):1021–32. PMID:21987445
189. Beghetti M, Gow RM, Haney I, et al. Pediatric primary benign cardiac tumors: a 15-year review. Am Heart J. 1997 Dec;134(6):1107–14. PMID:9424072
190. Bégin LR, Eskandari J, Joncas J, et al. Epstein-Barr virus related lymphoepithelioma-like carcinoma of lung. J Surg Oncol. 1987 Dec;36(4):280–3. PMID:2826922
191. Bégueret H, Galateau-Salle F, Guillou L, et al. Primary intrathoracic synovial sarcoma: a clinicopathologic study of 40 t(X;18)-positive cases from the French Sarcoma Group and the Mesopath Group. Am J Surg Pathol. 2005 Mar;29(3):339–46. PMID:15725802
192. Bégueret H, Vergier B, Parrens M, et al. Primary lung small B-cell lymphoma versus lymphoid hyperplasia: evaluation of diagnostic criteria in 26 cases. Am J Surg Pathol. 2002 Jan;26(1):76–81. PMID:11756772
193. Behboudi A, Enlund F, Winnes M, et al. Molecular classification of mucoepidermoid carcinomas-prognostic significance of the MECT1-MAML2 fusion oncogene. Genes Chromosomes Cancer. 2006 May;45(5):470–81. PMID:16444749
194. Behjati S, Tarpey PS, Sheldon H, et al. Recurrent PTPRB and PLCG1 mutations in angiosarcoma. Nat Genet. 2014 Apr;46(4):376–9. PMID:24633157
195. Behrens C, Feng L, Kadara H, et al. Expression of interleukin-1 receptor-associated kinase-1 in non-small cell lung carcinoma and preneoplastic lesions. Clin Cancer Res. 2010 Jan 1;16(1):34–44. PMID:20028769
196. Bell C, Domingo F, Miller AD, et al. Traumatic rupture of a posterior mediastinal

teratoma following motor-vehicle accident. Case Rep Surg. 2016;2016:7172062. PMID:27660731
197. Bell DA, Greco MA. Cardiac myxoma with chondroid features: a light and electron microscopic study. Hum Pathol. 1981 Apr;12(4):370–4. PMID:7239503
198. Bell DW, Gore I, Okimoto RA, et al. Inherited susceptibility to lung cancer may be associated with the T790M drug resistance mutation in EGFR. Nat Genet. 2005 Dec;37(12):1315–6. PMID:16258541
199. Bell DW, Lynch TJ, Haserlat SM, et al. Epidermal growth factor receptor mutations and gene amplification in non-small-cell lung cancer: molecular analysis of the IDEAL/INTACT gefitinib trials. J Clin Oncol. 2005 Nov 1;23(31):8081–92. PMID:16204011
200. Beller JP, Maddalo S, Zamuco R, et al. Right ventricular undifferentiated pleomorphic sarcoma: a case report. J Cardiol Cases. 2015 Nov 26;13(2):60–2. PMID:30524557
201. Bellini C, Rutigliani M, Boccardo FM, et al. Nuchal translucency and lymphatic system maldevelopment. J Perinat Med. 2009;37(6):673–6. PMID:19591554
202. Bellizzi AM, Bruzzi C, French CA, et al. The cytologic features of NUT midline carcinoma. Cancer. 2009 Dec 25;117(6):508–15. PMID:19795508
203. Benayed R, Offin M, Mullaney K, et al. High yield of RNA sequencing for targetable kinase fusions in lung adenocarcinomas with no mitogenic driver alteration detected by DNA sequencing and low tumor mutation burden. Clin Cancer Res. 2019 Aug 1;25(15):4712–22. PMID:31028088
204. Bene MC, Castoldi G, Knapp W, et al. Proposals for the immunological classification of acute leukemias. Leukemia. 1995 Oct;9(10):1783–6. PMID:7564526
205. Benn DE, Gimenez-Roqueplo AP, Reilly JR, et al. Clinical presentation and penetrance of pheochromocytoma/paraganglioma syndromes. J Clin Endocrinol Metab. 2006 Mar;91(3):827–36. PMID:16317055
206. Benn DE, Robinson BG, Clifton-Bligh RJ. 15 years of paraganglioma: clinical manifestations of paraganglioma syndromes types 1-5. Endocr Relat Cancer. 2015 Aug;22(4):T91–103. PMID:26273102
207. Bennett JA, Braga AC, Pinto A, et al. Uterine PEComas: a morphologic, immunohistochemical, and molecular analysis of 32 tumors. Am J Surg Pathol. 2018 Oct;42(10):1370–83. PMID:30001237
208. Bennett WP, Colby TV, Travis WD, et al. p53 protein accumulates frequently in early bronchial neoplasia. Cancer Res. 1993 Oct 15;53(20):4817–22. PMID:8402667
209. Bentz M, Barth TF, Brüderlein S, et al. Gain of chromosome arm 9p is characteristic of primary mediastinal B-cell lymphoma (MBL): comprehensive molecular cytogenetic analysis and presentation of a novel MBL cell line. Genes Chromosomes Cancer. 2001 Apr;30(4):393–401. PMID:11241792
210. Benveniste MF, Moran CA, Mawlawi O, et al. FDG PET-CT aids in the preoperative assessment of patients with newly diagnosed thymic epithelial malignancies. J Thorac Oncol. 2013 Apr;8(4):502–10. PMID:23446204
211. Beresford L, Fernandez CV, Cummings E, et al. Mediastinal polyembryoma associated with Klinefelter syndrome. J Pediatr Hematol Oncol. 2003 Apr;25(4):321–3. PMID:12679648
212. Berezowski K, Grimes MM, Gal A, et al. CD5 immunoreactivity of epithelial cells in thymic carcinoma and CASTLE using paraffin-embedded tissue. Am J Clin Pathol. 1996 Oct;106(4):483–6. PMID:8853036
213. Berg KB, Churg A. GATA3 immunohistochemistry for distinguishing sarcomatoid and desmoplastic mesothelioma from sarcomatoid carcinoma of the lung. Am J Surg Pathol. 2017 Sep;41(9):1221–5. PMID:28614203
214. Berg KB, Churg AM, Cheung S, et al. Usefulness of methylthioadenosine phosphorylase and BRCA-associated protein 1 immunohistochemistry in the diagnosis of malignant mesothelioma in effusion cytology specimens. Cancer Cytopathol. 2020 Feb;128(2):126–32. PMID:31821740
215. Berg KB, Dacic S, Miller C, et al. Utility of methylthioadenosine phosphorylase compared with BAP1 immunohistochemistry, and CDKN2A and NF2 fluorescence in situ hybridization in separating reactive mesothelial proliferations from epithelioid malignant mesotheliomas. Arch Pathol Lab Med. 2018 Dec;142(12):1549–53. PMID:30059257
216. Bergh P, Meis-Kindblom JM, Gherlinzoni F, et al. Synovial sarcoma: identification of low and high risk groups. Cancer. 1999 Jun 15;85(12):2596–607. PMID:10375108
217. Bernheim A, Toujani S, Saulnier P, et al. High-resolution array comparative genomic hybridization analysis of human bronchial and salivary adenoid cystic carcinoma. Lab Invest. 2008 May;88(5):464–73. PMID:18332873
218. Bernstein E, Caudy AA, Hammond SM, et al. Role for a bidentate ribonuclease in the initiation step of RNA interference. Nature. 2001 Jan 18;409(6818):363–6. PMID:11201747
219. Bertario L, Russo A, Sala P, et al. Genotype and phenotype factors as determinants of desmoid tumors in patients with familial adenomatous polyposis. Int J Cancer. 2001 Mar 20;95(2):102–7. PMID:11241320
220. Best SR, Mohr M, Zur KB. Systemic bevacizumab for recurrent respiratory papillomatosis: a national survey. Laryngoscope. 2017 Oct;127(10):2225–9. PMID:28657692
221. Betancourt B, Defendini EA, Johnson C, et al. Severe right ventricular outflow tract obstruction caused by an intracavitary cardiac neurilemoma: succesful surgical removal and postoperative diagnosis. Chest. 1979 Apr;75(4):522–4. PMID:446150
222. Betti M, Casalone E, Ferrante D, et al. Inference on germline BAP1 mutations and asbestos exposure from the analysis of familial and sporadic mesothelioma in a high-risk area. Genes Chromosomes Cancer. 2015 Jan;54(1):51–62. PMID:25231345
223. Bhagat P, Bal A, Das A, et al. Pulmonary inflammatory myofibroblastic tumor and IgG4-related inflammatory pseudotumor: a diagnostic dilemma. Virchows Arch. 2013 Dec;463(6):743–7. PMID:24100523
224. Bhat SP, Gowda GS, Chikkatur R, et al. Lipomatous hamartoma of mitral valve. Asian Cardiovasc Thorac Ann. 2016 Jan;24(1):34–5. PMID:24821963
225. Bi Y, Deng Y, Li S, et al. Immunophenotypic and prognostic analysis of PAX8 and TTF-1 expressions in neuroendocrine carcinomas of thymic origin: a comparative study with their pulmonary counterparts. J Surg Oncol. 2016 Nov;114(6):697–702. PMID:27761900
226. Bi Y, Qu Y, Liang Z, et al. Clinicopathological analysis of large cell lung carcinomas definitely diagnosed according to the new World Health Organization criteria. Pathol Res Pract. 2018 Apr;214(4):555–9. PMID:29525405
227. Bian T, Zhao J, Feng J, et al. Combination of cadherin-17 and SATB homeobox 2 serves as potential optimal makers for the differential diagnosis of pulmonary enteric adenocarcinoma and metastatic colorectal adenocarcinoma. Oncotarget. 2017 Jun 28;8(38):63442–52. PMID:28969003
228. Bianchi C, Bianchi T. Global mesothelioma epidemic: trend and features. Indian J Occup Environ Med. 2014 May;18(2):82–8. PMID:25568603
229. Bianchi C, Bianchi T. Non-Hodgkin lymphoma and pleural mesothelioma in a person exposed to asbestos. Turk Patoloji Derg. 2018;34(2):190–3. PMID:28272659
230. Bianchi G, Ferrarini M, Matteucci M, et al. Giant solitary fibrous tumor of the epicardium causing reversible heart failure. Ann Thorac Surg. 2013 Aug;96(2):e49–51. PMID:23910146
230A. Biermann K, Klingmüller D, Koch A, et al. Diagnostic value of markers M2A, OCT3/4, AP-2gamma, PLAP and c-KIT in the detection of extragonadal seminomas. Histopathology. 2006 Sep;49(3):290–7. PMID:16918976
231. Bigi R, Landis JT, An H, et al. Epstein-Barr virus enhances genome maintenance of Kaposi sarcoma-associated herpesvirus. Proc Natl Acad Sci U S A. 2018 Nov 27;115(48):E11379–87. PMID:30429324
232. Billeret Lebranchu V. [Granular cell tumor. Epidemiology of 263 cases]. Arch Anat Cytol Pathol. 1999;47(1):26–30. French. PMID:10089680
233. Binh MB, Sastre-Garau X, Guillou L, et al. MDM2 and CDK4 immunostainings are useful adjuncts in diagnosing well-differentiated and dedifferentiated liposarcoma subtypes: a comparative analysis of 559 soft tissue neoplasms with genetic data. Am J Surg Pathol. 2005 Oct;29(10):1340–7. PMID:16160477
234. Bird LM, Krous HF, Eichenfield LF, et al. Female infant with oncocytic cardiomyopathy and microphthalmia with linear skin defects (MLS): a clue to the pathogenesis of oncocytic cardiomyopathy? Am J Med Genet. 1994 Nov 1;53(2):141–8. PMID:7856638
235. Bireta C, Popov AF, Schotola H, et al. Carney-complex: multiple resections of recurrent cardiac myxoma. J Cardiothorac Surg. 2011 Feb 3;6:12. PMID:21291531
236. Birkbak NJ, McGranahan N. Cancer genome evolutionary trajectories in metastasis. Cancer Cell. 2020 Jan 13;37(1):8–19. PMID:31935374
237. Bishop JA, French CA, Ali SZ. Cytopathologic features of NUT midline carcinoma: a series of 26 specimens from 13 patients. Cancer Cytopathol. 2016 Dec;124(12):901–8. PMID:27400194
238. Bishop JA, Ogawa T, Chang X, et al. HPV analysis in distinguishing second primary tumors from lung metastases in patients with head and neck squamous cell carcinoma. Am J Surg Pathol. 2012 Jan;36(1):142–8. PMID:22173119
239. Bishop JA, Teruya-Feldstein J, Westra WH, et al. p40 (ΔNp63) is superior to p63 for the diagnosis of pulmonary squamous cell carcinoma. Mod Pathol. 2012 Mar;25(3):405–15. PMID:22056955
240. Björnsson J, McLeod RA, Unni KK, et al. Primary chondrosarcoma of long bones and limb girdles. Cancer. 1998 Nov 15;83(10):2105–19. PMID:9827715
241. Black M, Wei XJ, Sun W, et al. Adult rhabdomyoma presenting as thyroid nodule on fine-needle aspiration in patient with Birt-Hogg-Dubé syndrome: case report and literature review. Diagn Cytopathol. 2020 Jun;48(6):576–80. PMID:32187885
242. Blanco LZ, Heagley DE, Montebelli F, et al. Cytologic features of sclerosing hemangioma of the lung on crush preparations. Diagn Cytopathol. 2013 Mar;41(3):242–6. PMID:21710650
243. Blank A, Schmitt AM, Korpershoek E, et al. SDHB loss predicts malignancy in pheochromocytomas/sympathethic paragangliomas, but not through hypoxia signalling. Endocr Relat Cancer. 2010 Oct 5;17(4):919–28. PMID:20702724
244. Blaukovitsch M, Halbwedl I, Kothmaier H, et al. Sarcomatoid carcinomas of the lung–Are these histogenetically heterogeneous tumors? Virchows Arch. 2006 Oct;449(4):455–61. PMID:16941152
245. Blum Y, Meiller C, Quetel L, et al. Dissecting heterogeneity in malignant pleural mesothelioma through histo-molecular gradients for clinical applications. Nat Commun. 2019 Mar 22;10(1):1333. PMID:30902996
246. Bo N, Wang D, Wu B, et al. Analysis of β-catenin expression and exon 3 mutations in pediatric sporadic aggressive fibromatosis. Pediatr Dev Pathol. 2012 May-Jun;15(3):173–8. PMID:21323417
247. Bocklage TJ, Dail D, Colby TV. Primary lung tumors infiltrated by osteoclast-like giant cells. Ann Diagn Pathol. 1998 Aug;2(4):229–40. PMID:9845743
248. Bode-Lesniewska B, Zhao J, Speel EJ, et al. Gains of 12q13-14 and overexpression of mdm2 are frequent findings in intimal sarcomas of the pulmonary artery. Virchows Arch. 2001 Jan;438(1):57–65. PMID:11213836
249. Bodner SM, Koss MN. Mutations in the p53 gene in pulmonary blastomas: immunohistochemical and molecular studies. Hum Pathol. 1996 Nov;27(11):1117–23. PMID:8912818
250. Boers JE, ten Velde GP, Thunnissen FB. p53 in squamous metaplasia: a marker for risk of respiratory tract carcinoma. Am J Respir Crit Care Med. 1996 Jan;153(1):411–6. PMID:8542151
251. Boffetta P, Malvezzi M, Pira E, et al. International analysis of age-specific mortality rates from mesothelioma on the basis of the International Classification of Diseases, 10th revision. J Glob Oncol. 2018 Sep;4:1–15. PMID:30241199
252. Boffetta P, Pershagen G, Jöckel KH, et al. Cigar and pipe smoking and lung cancer risk: a multicenter study from Europe. J Natl Cancer Inst. 1999 Apr 21;91(8):697–701. PMID:10218507
253. Bofill M, Janossy G, Willcox N, et al. Microenvironments in the normal thymus and the thymus in myasthenia gravis. Am J Pathol. 1985 Jun;119(3):462–73. PMID:3874554
254. Böhle A, Studer UE, Sonntag RW, et al. Primary or secondary extragonadal germ cell tumors? J Urol. 1986 May;135(5):939–43. PMID:3007784
255. Bois MC, Bois JP, Anavekar NS, et al. Benign lipomatous masses of the heart: a comprehensive series of 47 cases with cytogenetic evaluation. Hum Pathol. 2014 Sep;45(9):1859–65. PMID:24996689
256. Bois MC, May AM, Vassallo R, et al. Morphometric study of pulmonary arterial changes in pulmonary Langerhans cell histiocytosis. Arch Pathol Lab Med. 2018 Aug;142(8):929–37. PMID:30040456
257. Bois MC, Milosevic D, Kipp BR, et al. KRAS mutations in papillary fibroelastomas: a study of 50 cases with etiologic and diagnostic implications. Am J Surg Pathol. 2020 May;44(5):626–32. PMID:32141886
258. Bokemeyer C, Nichols CR, Droz JP, et al. Extragonadal germ cell tumors of the mediastinum and retroperitoneum: results from an international analysis. J Clin Oncol. 2002 Apr 1;20(7):1864–73. PMID:11919246
259. Boland JM, Colby TV, Folpe AL. Intrathoracic peripheral nerve sheath tumors-a clinicopathological study of 75 cases. Hum Pathol. 2015 Mar;46(3):419–25. PMID:25595633
260. Boland JM, Colby TV, Folpe AL. Liposarcomas of the mediastinum and thorax: a clinicopathologic and molecular cytogenetic study of 24 cases, emphasizing unusual and diverse histologic features. Am J Surg Pathol. 2012 Sep;36(9):1395–403. PMID:22895273
261. Boland JM, Fritchie KJ, Erickson-Johnson MR, et al. Endobronchial lipomatous tumors:

clinicopathologic analysis of 12 cases with molecular cytogenetic evidence supporting classification as "lipoma". Am J Surg Pathol. 2013 Nov;37(11):1715–21. PMID:24121172

262. Boland JM, Froemming AT, Wampfler JA, et al. Adenocarcinoma in situ, minimally invasive adenocarcinoma, and invasive pulmonary adenocarcinoma–analysis of interobserver agreement, survival, radiographic characteristics, and gross pathology in 296 nodules. Hum Pathol. 2016 May;51:41–50. PMID:27067781

262A. Boland JM, Lee HE, Barr Fritcher EG, et al. Molecular genetic landscape of sclerosing pneumocytomas. Am J Clin Pathol. 2021 Feb 11;155(3):397–404. PMID:33145590

263. Boland JM, Maleszewski JJ, Wampfler JA, et al. Pulmonary invasive mucinous adenocarcinoma and mixed invasive mucinous/nonmucinous adenocarcinoma-a clinicopathological and molecular genetic study with survival analysis. Hum Pathol. 2018 Jan;71:8–19. PMID:28823574

264. Boland JM, Tazelaar HD, Colby TV, et al. Diffuse pulmonary lymphatic disease presenting as interstitial lung disease in adulthood: report of 3 cases. Am J Surg Pathol. 2012 Oct;36(10):1548–54. PMID:22982897

265. Boland JM, Wampfler JA, Jang JS, et al. Pulmonary adenocarcinoma with signet ring cell features: a comprehensive study from 3 distinct patient cohorts. Am J Surg Pathol. 2014 Dec;38(12):1681–8. PMID:25007143

266. Boland JM, Wampfler JA, Yang P, et al. Growth pattern-based grading of pulmonary adenocarcinoma-Analysis of 534 cases with comparison between observers and survival analysis. Lung Cancer. 2017 Jul;109:14–20. PMID:28577944

267. Bond J, Graux C, Lhermitte L, et al. Early response-based therapy stratification improves survival in adult early thymic precursor acute lymphoblastic leukemia: a Group for Research on Adult Acute Lymphoblastic Leukemia study. J Clin Oncol. 2017 Aug 10;35(23):2683–91. PMID:28605290

268. Bonetti F, Martignoni G, Colato C, et al. Abdominopelvic sarcoma of perivascular epithelioid cells. Report of four cases in young women, one with tuberous sclerosis. Mod Pathol. 2001 Jun;14(6):563–8. PMID:11406657

269. Bonetti F, Pea M, Martignoni G, et al. PEC and sugar. Am J Surg Pathol. 1992 Mar;16(3):307–8. PMID:1599021

270. Bongiovanni D, Saccomani V, Piovan E. Aberrant signaling pathways in T-cell acute lymphoblastic leukemia. Int J Mol Sci. 2017 Sep 5;18(9):E1904. PMID:28872614

271. Bonnet P, Chasset F, Moguelet P, et al. Erdheim-Chester disease associated with chronic myelomonocytic leukemia harboring the same clonal mutation. Haematologica. 2019 Nov;104(11):e530–3. PMID:31221777

272. Bonnichsen CR, Dearani JA, Maleszewski JJ, et al. Recurrent Ebstein-Barr virus-associated diffuse large B-cell lymphoma in an ascending aorta graft. Circulation. 2013 Sep 24;128(13):1481–3. PMID:24060945

273. Borczuk AC. Uncommon types of lung carcinoma with mixed histology: sarcomatoid carcinoma, adenosquamous carcinoma, and mucoepidermoid carcinoma. Arch Pathol Lab Med. 2018 Aug;142(8):914–21. PMID:30040455

274. Borczuk AC, Kim HK, Yegen HA, et al. Lung adenocarcinoma global profiling identifies type II transforming growth factor-beta receptor as a repressor of invasiveness. Am J Respir Crit Care Med. 2005 Sep 15;172(6):729–37. PMID:15976377

275. Borczuk AC, Qian F, Kazeros A, et al. Invasive size is an independent predictor of survival in pulmonary adenocarcinoma. Am J Surg

Pathol. 2009 Mar;33(3):462–9. PMID:19092635

276. Bordalo AD, Alves I, Nobre AL, et al. [New clinical aspects of cardiac myxomas: a clinical and pathological reappraisal]. Rev Port Cardiol. 2012 Sep;31(9):567–75. Portuguese. PMID:22832502

277. Borden EC, Baker LH, Bell RS, et al. Soft tissue sarcomas of adults: state of the translational science. Clin Cancer Res. 2003 Jun;9(6):1941–56. PMID:12796356

278. Borghaei H, Paz-Ares L, Horn L, et al. Nivolumab versus docetaxel in advanced nonsquamous non-small-cell lung cancer. N Engl J Med. 2015 Oct 22;373(17):1627–39. PMID:26412456

279. Borie R, Wislez M, Antoine M, et al. Clonality and phenotyping analysis of alveolar lymphocytes is suggestive of pulmonary MALT lymphoma. Respir Med. 2011 Aug;105(8):1231–7. PMID:21481576

280. Borie R, Wislez M, Antoine M, et al. Lymphoproliferative disorders of the lung. Respiration. 2017;94(2):157–75. PMID:28609772

281. Borie R, Wislez M, Thabut G, et al. Clinical characteristics and prognostic factors of pulmonary MALT lymphoma. Eur Respir J. 2009 Dec;34(6):1408–16. PMID:19541720

282. Boroumand N, Ly TL, Sonstein J, et al. Microscopic diffuse large B-cell lymphoma (DLBCL) occurring in pseudocysts: Do these tumors belong to the category of DLBCL associated with chronic inflammation? Am J Surg Pathol. 2012 Jul;36(7):1074–80. PMID:22472958

283. Bosi G, Lintermans JP, Pellegrino PA, et al. The natural history of cardiac rhabdomyoma with and without tuberous sclerosis. Acta Paediatr. 1996 Aug;85(8):928–31. PMID:8863873

284. Bossé Y, Amos CI. A decade of GWAS results in lung cancer. Cancer Epidemiol Biomarkers Prev. 2018 Apr;27(4):363–79. PMID:28615365

285. Bossert T, Gummert JF, Battellini R, et al. Surgical experience with 77 primary cardiac tumors. Interact Cardiovasc Thorac Surg. 2005 Aug;4(4):311–5. PMID:17670419

286. Bossert T, Walther T, Vondrys D, et al. Cardiac fibroma as an inherited manifestation of nevoid basal-cell carcinoma syndrome. Tex Heart Inst J. 2006;33(1):88–90. PMID:16572881

287. Bota S, Auliac JB, Paris C, et al. Follow-up of bronchial precancerous lesions and carcinoma in situ using fluorescence endoscopy. Am J Respir Crit Care Med. 2001 Nov 1;164(9):1688–93. PMID:11719311

288. Bothe W, Goebel H, Kunze M, et al. Right atrial solitary fibrous tumor - a new cardiac neoplasm? Interact Cardiovasc Thorac Surg. 2005 Oct;4(5):396–7. PMID:17670440

289. Bott M, Brevet M, Taylor BS, et al. The nuclear deubiquitinase BAP1 is commonly inactivated by somatic mutations and 3p21.1 losses in malignant pleural mesothelioma. Nat Genet. 2011 Jun 5;43(7):668–72. PMID:21642991

290. Bott MJ, James B, Collins BT, et al. A prospective clinical trial of telecytopathology for rapid interpretation of specimens obtained during endobronchial ultrasound-fine needle aspiration. Ann Thorac Surg. 2015 Jul;100(1):201–5, discussion 205–6. PMID:26002445

291. Bott MJ, Wang H, Travis W, et al. Management and outcomes of relapse after treatment for thymoma and thymic carcinoma. Ann Thorac Surg. 2011 Dec;92(6):1984–91, discussion 1991–2. PMID:22115206

292. Bottillo I, Ahlquist T, Brekke H, et al. Germline and somatic NF1 mutations in sporadic and NF1-associated malignant peripheral nerve sheath tumours. J Pathol. 2009 Apr;217(5):693–701. PMID:19142971

293. Bouabdallaoui N, Juthier F, Mouquet F, et

al. Cardiac rhabomyoma in a young adult presenting with junctional tachycardia. Eur Heart J Cardiovasc Imaging. 2013 Jul;14(7):719. PMID:23329642

294. Bougeard G, Renaux-Petel M, Flaman JM, et al. Revisiting Li-Fraumeni syndrome from TP53 mutation carriers. J Clin Oncol. 2015 Jul 20;33(21):2345–52. PMID:26014290

295. Boulanger E, Hermine O, Fermand JP, et al. Human herpesvirus 8 (HHV-8)-associated peritoneal primary effusion lymphoma (PEL) in two HIV-negative elderly patients. Am J Hematol. 2004 May;76(1):88–91. PMID:15114607

296. Boyer DF, McKelvie PA, de Leval L, et al. Fibrin-associated EBV-positive large B-cell lymphoma: an indolent neoplasm with features distinct from diffuse large B-cell lymphoma associated with chronic inflammation. Am J Surg Pathol. 2017 Mar;41(3):299–312. PMID:28195879

297. Boylan E, Wyers M, Jaffar R. A rare case of thymoma in a 15-month-old girl. Pediatr Radiol. 2011 Nov;41(11):1469–71. PMID:21556822

298. Bradshaw SH, Hendry P, Boodhwani M, et al. Left ventricular mesenchymal hamartoma, a new hamartoma of the heart. Cardiovasc Pathol. 2011 Sep-Oct;20(5):307–14. PMID:20850353

299. Braham E, Ben Rejeb H, Aouadi S, et al. Pulmonary carcinosarcoma with heterologous component: report of two cases with literature review. Ann Transl Med. 2014 Apr;2(4):41. PMID:25333016

300. Brahmer J, Reckamp KL, Baas P, et al. Nivolumab versus docetaxel in advanced squamous-cell non-small-cell lung cancer. N Engl J Med. 2015 Jul 9;373(2):123–35. PMID:26028407

301. Brambilla C, Laffaire J, Lantuejoul S, et al. Lung squamous cell carcinomas with basaloid histology represent a specific molecular entity. Clin Cancer Res. 2014 Nov 15;20(22):5777–86. PMID:25189482

302. Brambilla E, Gazdar A. Pathogenesis of lung cancer signalling pathways: roadmap for therapies. Eur Respir J. 2009 Jun;33(6):1485–97. PMID:19483050

303. Brambilla E, Gazzeri S, Lantuejoul S, et al. p53 mutant immunophenotype and deregulation of p53 transcription pathway (Bcl2, Bax, and Waf1) in precursor bronchial lesions of lung cancer. Clin Cancer Res. 1998 Jul;4(7):1609–18. PMID:9676834

304. Brambilla E, Gazzeri S, Moro D, et al. Alterations of Rb pathway (Rb-p16INK4-cyclin D1) in preinvasive bronchial lesions. Clin Cancer Res. 1999 Feb;5(2):243–50. PMID:10037171

305. Brambilla E, Moro D, Gazzeri S, et al. Cytotoxic chemotherapy induces cell differentiation in small-cell lung carcinoma. J Clin Oncol. 1991 Jan;9(1):50–61. PMID:1702146

306. Braverman RM, Lipshultz SE, McCarten KM, et al. Pediatric case of the day. Cardiac hemangioma. Radiographics. 1991 Sep;11(5):932–4. PMID:1947327

307. Bravo-Balado A, Torres Castellanos L, Carrillo Rodríguez A, et al. Primary mediastinal pure seminomatous germ cell tumor (germinoma) as a rare cause of precocious puberty in a 9-year-old patient. Urology. 2017 Dec;110:216–9. PMID:28888750

308. Bray F, Colombet M, Mery L, et al., editors. Cancer incidence in five continents. Volume XI. Lyon (France): International Agency for Research on Cancer; 2017. (IARC Scientific Publication No. 166). http://ci5.iarc.fr/CI5-XI.

309. Bray F, Ferlay J, Soerjomataram I, et al. Global cancer statistics 2018: GLOBOCAN estimates of incidence and mortality worldwide for 36 cancers in 185 countries. CA Cancer J Clin. 2018 Nov;68(6):394–424. PMID:30207593

310. Brčić L, Jakopović M, Brčić I, et al.

Reproducibility of histological subtyping of malignant pleural mesothelioma. Virchows Arch. 2014 Dec;465(6):679–85. PMID:25300229

311. Brennan MF, Antonescu CR, Moraco N, et al. Lessons learned from the study of 10,000 patients with soft tissue sarcoma. Ann Surg. 2014 Sep;260(3):416–21, discussion 421–2. PMID:25115417

312. Brenneman M, Field A, Yang J, et al. Temporal order of RNase IIIb and loss-of-function mutations during development determines phenotype in pleuropulmonary blastoma / DICER1 syndrome: a unique variant of the two-hit tumor suppression model. F1000Res. 2015 Jul 10;4:214. PMID:26925222

313. Breuer RH, Pasic A, Smit EF, et al. The natural course of preneoplastic lesions in bronchial epithelium. Clin Cancer Res. 2005 Jan 15;11(2 Pt 1):537–43. PMID:15701838

314. Bridge JA, Sumegi J, Druta M, et al. Clinical, pathological, and genomic features of EWSR1-PATZ1 fusion sarcoma. Mod Pathol. 2019 Nov;32(11):1593–604. PMID:31189996

315. Brierley JD, Gospodarowicz MK, Wittekind C, editors. TNM classification of malignant tumours. 8th ed. Oxford (UK): Wiley-Blackwell; 2017.

316. Brobeil A, Wagenlehner F, Gattenlöhner S. Expression of terminal deoxynucleotidyl transferase (TdT) in classical seminoma: a potential diagnostic pitfall. Virchows Arch. 2018 Mar;472(3):433–40. PMID:29455318

317. Brodeur GM, Hogarty MD, Moose YP, et al. Neuroblastoma. In: Pizzo PA, Poplack DG, editors. Principles and practice of pediatric oncology. 6th ed. Philadelphia (PA): Lippincott Williams & Wilkins; 2011. pp. 886–922.

318. Brodeur GM, Pritchard J, Berthold F, et al. Revisions of the international criteria for neuroblastoma diagnosis, staging, and response to treatment. J Clin Oncol. 1993 Aug;11(8):1466–77. PMID:8336186

319. Brodeur GM, Seeger RC, Schwab M, et al. Amplification of N-myc in untreated human neuroblastomas correlates with advanced disease stage. Science. 1984 Jun 8;224(4653):1121–4. PMID:6719137

320. Brose MS, Volpe P, Feldman M, et al. BRAF and RAS mutations in human lung cancer and melanoma. Cancer Res. 2002 Dec 1;62(23):6997–7000. PMID:12460918

321. Brown JG, Familiari U, Papotti M, et al. Thymic basaloid carcinoma: a clinicopathologic study of 12 cases, with a general discussion of basaloid carcinoma and its relationship with adenoid cystic carcinoma. Am J Surg Pathol. 2009 Aug;33(8):1113–24. PMID:19461509

322. Brown K, Collins JD, Batra P, et al. Mediastinal germ cell tumor in a young woman. Med Pediatr Oncol. 1989;17(2):164–7. PMID:2704337

323. Brown LR, Reiman HM, Rosenow EC 3rd, et al. Intrathoracic lymphangioma. Mayo Clin Proc. 1986 Nov;61(11):882–92. PMID:3762227

324. Brown ML, Zayas GE, Abel MD, et al. Mediastinal paragangliomas: the mayo clinic experience. Ann Thorac Surg. 2008 Sep;86(3):946–51. PMID:18721588

325. Bruce CJ. Cardiac tumours: diagnosis and management. Heart. 2011 Jan;97(2):151–60. PMID:21163893

326. Brun C, Gay P, Cottier M, et al. Comparison of cytology, chest computed and positron emission tomography findings in malignant pleural effusion from lung cancer. J Thorac Dis. 2018 Dec;10(12):6903–11. PMID:30746236

327. Bruzzi JF, Komaki R, Walsh GL, et al. Imaging of non-small cell lung cancer of the superior sulcus: part 2: initial staging and assessment of resectability and therapeutic response. Radiographics. 2008 Mar-Apr;28(2):561–72.

PMID:18349458

328. Buckley C, Douek D, Newsom-Davis J, et al. Mature, long-lived CD4+ and CD8+ T cells are generated by the thymoma in myasthenia gravis. Ann Neurol. 2001 Jul;50(1):64–72. PMID:11456312

329. Buckley O, Madan R, Kwong R, et al. Cardiac masses, part 1: imaging strategies and technical considerations. AJR Am J Roentgenol. 2011 Nov;197(5):W837–41. PMID:22021530

330. Bueno R, Stawiski EW, Goldstein LD, et al. Comprehensive genomic analysis of malignant pleural mesothelioma identifies recurrent mutations, gene fusions and splicing alterations. Nat Genet. 2016 Apr;48(4):407–16. PMID:26928227

331. Buero A, Quadrelli S, Pankl LG, et al. Two-year disease remission of an unresectable basaloid thymic carcinoma with second line chemotherapy drugs: report of a case. Pan Afr Med J. 2019 May 24;33:53. PMID:31448016

332. Buksa M, Gerc V, Dilic M, et al. Clinical, echocardiographic and echophonocardiographic characteristics of the atrial myxomas in 22 years period. Med Arh. 2009;63(6):320–2. PMID:20380110

333. Bull JC Jr, Grimes OF. Pulmonary carcinosarcoma. Chest. 1974 Jan;65(1):9–12. PMID:4809344

334. Bulman W, Saqi A, Powell CA. Acquisition and processing of endobronchial ultrasound-guided transbronchial needle aspiration specimens in the era of targeted lung cancer chemotherapy. Am J Respir Crit Care Med. 2012 Mar 15;185(6):606–11. PMID:22071327

335. Bumber Z, Jurlina M, Manojlović S, et al. Inflammatory pseudotumor of the trachea. J Pediatr Surg. 2001 Apr;36(4):631–4. PMID:11283894

336. Buonocore DJ, Konno F, Jungbluth AA, et al. CytoLyt fixation significantly inhibits MIB1 immunoreactivity whereas alternative Ki-67 clone 30-9 is not susceptible to the inhibition: critical diagnostic implications. Cancer Cytopathol. 2019 Oct;127(10):643–9. PMID:31398281

337. Burack WR, Laughlin TS, Friedberg JW, et al. PCR assays detect B-lymphocyte clonality in formalin-fixed, paraffin-embedded specimens of classical Hodgkin lymphoma without microdissection. Am J Clin Pathol. 2010 Jul;134(1):104–11. PMID:20551274

338. Bürger T, Schaefer IM, Küffer S, et al. Metastatic type A thymoma: morphological and genetic correlation. Histopathology. 2017 Apr;70(5):704–10. PMID:27926794

339. Burke A. Primary malignant cardiac tumors. Semin Diagn Pathol. 2008 Feb;25(1):39–46. PMID:18350921

340. Burke A, Johns JP, Virmani R. Hemangiomas of the heart. A clinicopathologic study of ten cases. Am J Cardiovasc Pathol. 1990;3(4):283–90. PMID:2129569

341. Burke A, Tavora F. The 2015 WHO classification of tumors of the heart and pericardium. J Thorac Oncol. 2016 Apr;11(4):441–52. PMID:26725181

342. Burke AP, Cowan D, Virmani R. Primary sarcomas of the heart. Cancer. 1992 Jan 15;69(2):387–95. PMID:1728367

343. Burke AP, Gatto-Weis C, Griego JE, et al. Adult cellular rhabdomyoma of the heart: a report of 3 cases. Hum Pathol. 2002 Nov;33(11):1092–7. PMID:12454813

344. Burke AP, Ribe JK, Bajaj AK, et al. Hamartoma of mature cardiac myocytes. Hum Pathol. 1998 Sep;29(9):904–9. PMID:9744305

345. Burke AP, Rosado-de-Christenson M, Templeton PA, et al. Cardiac fibroma: clinicopathologic correlates and surgical treatment. J Thorac Cardiovasc Surg. 1994 Nov;108(5):862–70. PMID:7967668

346. Burke AP, Virmani R. Cardiac myxoma. A clinicopathologic study. Am J Clin Pathol. 1993 Dec;100(6):671–80. PMID:8249916

347. Burke AP, Virmani R. Sarcomas of the great vessels. A clinicopathologic study. Cancer. 1993 Mar 1;71(5):1761–73. PMID:8448740

348. Burke LM, Rush WI, Khoor A, et al. Alveolar adenoma: a histochemical, immunohistochemical, and ultrastructural analysis of 17 cases. Hum Pathol. 1999 Feb;30(2):158–67. PMID:10029443

349. Burkhardt B, Mueller S, Khanam T, et al. Current status and future directions of T-lymphoblastic lymphoma in children and adolescents. Br J Haematol. 2016 May;173(4):545–59. PMID:26991119

350. Burkhardt B, Zimmermann M, Oschlies I, et al. The impact of age and gender on biology, clinical features and treatment outcome of non-Hodgkin lymphoma in childhood and adolescence. Br J Haematol. 2005 Oct;131(1):39–49. PMID:16173961

351. Burt BM, Lee HS, Lenge De Rosen V, et al. Soluble mesothelin-related peptides to monitor recurrence after resection of pleural mesothelioma. Ann Thorac Surg. 2017 Nov;104(5):1679–87. PMID:28964420

352. Bussani R, De-Giorgio F, Abbate A, et al. Cardiac metastases. J Clin Pathol. 2007 Jan;60(1):27–34. PMID:17098886

353. Busuttil A. Dendritic pigmented cells within human laryngeal mucosa. Arch Otolaryngol. 1976 Jan;102(1):43–4. PMID:1247414

354. Butany J, Leong SW, Carmichael K, et al. A 30-year analysis of cardiac neoplasms at autopsy. Can J Cardiol. 2005 Jun;21(8):675–80. PMID:16003450

355. Butany J, Nair V, Naseemuddin A, et al. Cardiac tumours: diagnosis and management. Lancet Oncol. 2005 Apr;6(4):219–28. PMID:15811617

356. Butany J, Yu W. Cardiac angiosarcoma: two cases and a review of the literature. Can J Cardiol. 2000 Feb;16(2):197–205. PMID:10694590

356A. Butnor KJ, Burchette JL, Sporn TA, et al. The spectrum of Kit (CD117) immunoreactivity in lung and pleural tumors: a study of 96 cases using a single-source antibody with a review of the literature. Arch Pathol Lab Med. 2004 May;128(5):538–43. PMID:15086281

357. Butnor KJ, Sporn TA, Hammar SP, et al. Well-differentiated papillary mesothelioma. Am J Surg Pathol. 2001 Oct;25(10):1304–9. PMID:11688466

358. Byrne J, Blanc WA, Warburton D, et al. The significance of cystic hygroma in fetuses. Hum Pathol. 1984 Jan;15(1):61–7. PMID:6693110

359. Cabibi D, Lo Iacono G, Raffaele F, et al. Nodular histiocytic/mesothelial hyperplasia as consequence of chronic mesothelium irritation by subphrenic abscess. Future Oncol. 2015;11(24 Suppl):51–5. PMID:26638925

360. Cagle PT, Wessels R, Greenberg SD. Concurrent mesothelioma and adenocarcinoma of the lung in a patient with asbestosis. Mod Pathol. 1993 Jul;6(4):438–41. PMID:8415588

361. Cai D, Li H, Wang R, et al. Comparison of clinical features, molecular alterations, and prognosis in morphological subgroups of lung invasive mucinous adenocarcinoma. Onco Targets Ther. 2014 Nov 18;7:2127–32. PMID:25429229

362. Calaminici M, Piper K, Lee AM, et al. CD23 expression in mediastinal large B-cell lymphomas. Histopathology. 2004 Dec;45(6):619–24. PMID:15569053

363. Calvete O, Garcia-Pavia P, Domínguez F, et al. POT1 and damage response malfunction trigger acquisition of somatic activating mutations in the VEGF pathway in cardiac angiosarcomas. J Am Heart Assoc. 2019 Sep 17;8(18):e012875. PMID:31510873

364. Calvete O, Martinez P, Garcia-Pavia P, et al. A mutation in the POT1 gene is responsible for cardiac angiosarcoma in TP53-negative Li-Fraumeni-like families. Nat Commun. 2015 Sep 25;6:8383. PMID:26403419

365. Camidge DR, Doebele RC, Kerr KM. Comparing and contrasting predictive biomarkers for immunotherapy and targeted therapy of NSCLC. Nat Rev Clin Oncol. 2019 Jun;16(6):341–55. PMID:30718843

366. Campana D, Walter T, Pusceddu S, et al. Correlation between MGMT promoter methylation and response to temozolomide-based therapy in neuroendocrine neoplasms: an observational retrospective multicenter study. Endocrine. 2018 Jun;60(3):490–8. PMID:29150792

367. Campbell JD, Alexandrov A, Kim J, et al. Distinct patterns of somatic genome alterations in lung adenocarcinomas and squamous cell carcinomas. Nat Genet. 2016 Jun;48(6):607–16. PMID:27158780

368. Campbell JD, Yau C, Bowlby R, et al. Genomic, pathway network, and immunologic features distinguishing squamous carcinomas. Cell Rep. 2018 Apr 3;23(1):194–212.e6. PMID:29617660

368A. Campobasso O, Andrion A, Ribotta M, et al. The value of the 1981 WHO histological classification in inter-observer reproducibility and changing pattern of lung cancer. Int J Cancer. 1993 Jan 21;53(2):205–8. PMID:8381110

368B. Canadian Cancer Statistics Advisory Committee. Canadian Cancer Statistics: a 2020 special report on lung cancer. Toronto (ON): Canadian Cancer Society; 2020 Sep [cited 2020 Oct 13]. Available from: https://www.cancer.ca/Canadian-Cancer-Statistics-2020-EN.

369. Cancer Genome Atlas Research Network. Comprehensive genomic characterization of squamous cell lung cancers. Nature. 2012 Sep 27;489(7417):519–25. PMID:22960745

370. Cancer Genome Atlas Research Network. Comprehensive molecular profiling of lung adenocarcinoma. Nature. 2014 Jul 31;511(7511):543–50. PMID:25079552

371. Cancer Genome Atlas Research Network. Comprehensive and integrated genomic characterization of adult soft tissue sarcomas. Cell. 2017 Nov 2;171(4):950–965.e28. PMID:29100075

372. Candes FP, Ajinkya MS. Primary mediastinal choriocarcinoma (a case report). J Postgrad Med. 1987 Oct;33(4):219–21. PMID:3449627

373. Cañizares MA, Matilla JM, Cueto A, et al. Atypical carcinoid tumours of the lung: prognostic factors and patterns of recurrence. Thorax. 2014 Jul;69(7):648–53. PMID:24603194

374. Cantley RL, Kapur U, Truong L, et al. Fine-needle aspiration diagnosis of metastatic urothelial carcinoma: a review. Diagn Cytopathol. 2012 Feb;40(2):173–8. PMID:22246936

375. Cao D, Allan RW, Cheng L, et al. RNA-binding protein LIN28 is a marker for testicular germ cell tumors. Hum Pathol. 2011 May;42(5):710–8. PMID:21288558

376. Cao D, Humphrey PA, Allan RW. SALL4 is a novel sensitive and specific marker for metastatic germ cell tumors, with particular utility in detection of metastatic yolk sac tumors. Cancer. 2009 Jun 15;115(12):2640–51. PMID:19365862

377. Cao D, Li J, Guo CC, et al. SALL4 is a novel diagnostic marker for testicular germ cell tumors. Am J Surg Pathol. 2009 Jul;33(7):1065–77. PMID:19390421

378. Cao D, Liu A, Wang F, et al. RNA-binding protein LIN28 is a marker for primary extragonadal germ cell tumors: an immunohistochemical study of 131 cases. Mod Pathol. 2011 Feb;24(2):288–96. PMID:21057460

379. Caplin ME, Baudin E, Ferolla P, et al. Pulmonary neuroendocrine (carcinoid) tumors: European Neuroendocrine Tumor Society expert consensus and recommendations for best practice for typical and atypical pulmonary carcinoids. Ann Oncol. 2015 Aug;26(8):1604–20. PMID:25646366

380. Cappell MS, Lapin S, Rose M. Large right atrial myxoma containing gastric heterotopia presenting with dyspnea and bilateral leg edema due to pulmonary emboli and cardiovascular obstruction: the first known report of gastric heterotopia in the cardiovascular system. Dig Dis Sci. 2008 Feb;53(2):405–9. PMID:17592776

381. Carbone A, Gloghini A. PEL and HHV8-unrelated effusion lymphomas: classification and diagnosis. Cancer. 2008 Aug 25;114(4):225–7. PMID:18473348

382. Carbone M, Baris YI, Bertino P, et al. Erionite exposure in North Dakota and Turkish villages with mesothelioma. Proc Natl Acad Sci U S A. 2011 Aug 16;108(33):13618–23. PMID:21788493

383. Carbone M, Ferris LK, Baumann F, et al. BAP1 cancer syndrome: malignant mesothelioma, uveal and cutaneous melanoma, and MBAITs. J Transl Med. 2012 Aug 30;10:179. PMID:22935333

384. Carbone M, Flores EG, Emi M, et al. Combined genetic and genealogic studies uncover a large BAP1 cancer syndrome kindred tracing back nine generations to a common ancestor from the 1700s. PLoS Genet. 2015 Dec 18;11(12):e1005633. PMID:26683624

385. Carbone M, Kanodia S, Chao A, et al. Consensus report of the 2015 Weinman International Conference on Mesothelioma. J Thorac Oncol. 2016 Aug;11(8):1246–62. PMID:27453164

386. Cardenas-Garcia J, Talwar A, Shah R, et al. Update in primary pulmonary lymphomas. Curr Opin Pulm Med. 2015 Jul;21(4):333–7. PMID:25978630

387. Cardillo G, Rea F, Lucchi M, et al. Primary neuroendocrine tumors of the thymus: a multicenter experience of 35 patients. Ann Thorac Surg. 2012 Jul;94(1):241–5, discussion 245–6. PMID:22632882

388. Carlson JW, Fletcher CD. Immunohistochemistry for beta-catenin in the differential diagnosis of spindle cell lesions: analysis of a series and review of the literature. Histopathology. 2007 Oct;51(4):509–14. PMID:17711447

389. Carney JA. Carney triad: a syndrome featuring paraganglionic, adrenocortical, and possibly other endocrine tumors. J Clin Endocrinol Metab. 2009 Oct;94(10):3656–62. PMID:19723753

390. Caron O, Frebourg T, Benusiglio PR, et al. Lung adenocarcinoma as part of the Li-Fraumeni syndrome spectrum: preliminary data of the LIFSCREEN randomized clinical trial. JAMA Oncol. 2017 Dec 1;3(12):1736–7. PMID:28772306

391. Carras S, Berger F, Chalabreysse L, et al. Primary cardiac lymphoma: diagnosis, treatment and outcome in a modern series. Hematol Oncol. 2017 Dec;35(4):510–9. PMID:27140394

392. Carrero N, Salazar G, Guerrero AF, et al. Recurrent undifferentiated pleomorphic sarcoma in the left atrium. CASE (Phila). 2018 Jan 12;2(2):38–41. PMID:30062306

393. Carretta A, Libretti L, Taccagni G, et al. Salivary gland-type mixed tumor (pleomorphic adenoma) of the lung. Interact Cardiovasc Thorac Surg. 2004 Dec;3(4):663–5. PMID:17670335

394. Carretto E, Inserra A, Ferrari A, et al. Epithelial thymic tumours in paediatric age: a report from the TREP project. Orphanet J Rare Dis. 2011 May 21;6:28. PMID:21600006

395. Carsillo T, Astrinidis A, Henske EP. Mutations in the tuberous sclerosis complex gene TSC2 are a cause of sporadic pulmonary lymphangioleiomyomatosis. Proc Natl Acad Sci U S A. 2000 May 23;97(11):6085–90. PMID:10823953
396. Carter BW, Benveniste MF, Truong MT, et al. State of the art: MR imaging of thymoma. Magn Reson Imaging Clin N Am. 2015 May;23(2):165–77. PMID:25952513
397. Carter BW, Erasmus JJ. Chapter 8: Current concepts in the diagnosis and staging of lung cancer. 2019 Feb 20. In: Hodler J, Kubik-Huch RA, von Schulthess GK, editors. Diseases of the chest, breast, heart and vessels 2019-2022: diagnostic and interventional imaging [Internet]. Cham (Switzerland): Springer; 2019. PMID:32096949
398. Carter BW, Marom EM, Detterbeck FC. Approaching the patient with an anterior mediastinal mass: a guide for clinicians. J Thorac Oncol. 2014 Sep;9(9 Suppl 2):S102–9. PMID:25396306
399. Casal RF, Vial MR, Miller R, et al. What exactly is a centrally located lung tumor? Results of an online survey. Ann Am Thorac Soc. 2017 Jan;14(1):118–23. PMID:27854541
400. Casella M, Carbucicchio C, Dello Russo A, et al. Radiofrequency catheter ablation of life-threatening ventricular arrhythmias caused by left ventricular metastatic infiltration. Circ Arrhythm Electrophysiol. 2011 Apr;4(2):e7–10. PMID:21505171
401. Casha AR, Davidson LA, Roberts P, et al. Familial angiosarcoma of the heart. J Thorac Cardiovasc Surg. 2002 Aug;124(2):392–4. PMID:12167801
402. Casiraghi M, De Pas T, Maisonneuve P, et al. A 10-year single-center experience on 708 lung metastasectomies: the evidence of the "International Registry of Lung Metastases". J Thorac Oncol. 2011 Aug;6(8):1373–8. PMID:21642869
403. Caso R, Jones GD, Bains MS, et al. Outcomes after multidisciplinary management of primary mediastinal germ cell tumors. Ann Surg. 2020 Jan 21 [Epub ahead of print]. PMID:31977510
404. Cassidy A, 't Mannetje A, van Tongeren M, et al. Occupational exposure to crystalline silica and risk of lung cancer: a multicenter case-control study in Europe. Epidemiology. 2007 Jan;18(1):36–43. PMID:17149143
405. Castillo JJ, Winer ES, Olszewski AJ. Sites of extranodal involvement are prognostic in patients with diffuse large B-cell lymphoma in the rituximab era: an analysis of the Surveillance, Epidemiology and End Results database. Am J Hematol. 2014 Mar;89(3):310–4. PMID:24273125
406. Castorino F, Masiello P, Quattrocchi E, et al. Primary cardiac rhabdomyosarcoma of the left atrium: an unusual presentation. Tex Heart Inst J. 2000;27(2):206–8. PMID:10928510
407. Caswell DR, Swanton C. The role of tumour heterogeneity and clonal cooperativity in metastasis, immune evasion and clinical outcome. BMC Med. 2017 Jul 18;15(1):133. PMID:28716075
408. Cavalli G, Guglielmi B, Berti A, et al. The multifaceted clinical presentations and manifestations of Erdheim-Chester disease: comprehensive review of the literature and of 10 new cases. Ann Rheum Dis. 2013 Oct;72(10):1691–5. PMID:23396641
409. Cavazza A, Colby TV, Tsokos M, et al. Lung tumors with a rhabdoid phenotype. Am J Clin Pathol. 1996 Feb;105(2):182–8. PMID:8607442
410. Cavazza A, Paci M, De Marco L, et al. Alveolar adenoma of the lung: a clinicopathologic, immunohistochemical, and molecular study of an unusual case. Int J Surg Pathol. 2004 Apr;12(2):155–9. PMID:15173924
411. Cazals-Hatem D, Lepage E, Brice P, et al. Primary mediastinal large B-cell lymphoma. A clinicopathologic study of 141 cases compared with 916 nonmediastinal large B-cell lymphomas, a GELA ("Groupe d'Etude des Lymphomes de l'Adulte") study. Am J Surg Pathol. 1996 Jul;20(7):877–88. PMID:8669537
412. Cedrés S, Ponce-Aix S, Zugazagoitia J, et al. Analysis of expression of programmed cell death 1 ligand 1 (PD-L1) in malignant pleural mesothelioma (MPM). PLoS One. 2015 Mar 16;10(3):e0121071. PMID:25774992
413. Celik B, Bulut T, Khoor A. Subtyping of non-small cell lung cancer by cytology specimens: a proposal for resource-poor hospitals. Cytojournal. 2019 Apr 22;16:8. PMID:31080486
414. Cellerin L, Marcq M, Sagan C, et al. [Malignant pleural effusion as the presenting site of cancer: comparison with metastatic pleural effusions from known cancers]. Rev Mal Respir. 2008 Nov;25(9):1104–9. French. PMID:19106906
415. Centeno I, Blay P, Santamaría I, et al. Germ-line mutations in epidermal growth factor receptor (EGFR) are rare but may contribute to oncogenesis: a novel germ-line mutation in EGFR detected in a patient with lung adenocarcinoma. BMC Cancer. 2011 May 16;11:172. PMID:21575252
416. Ceresa F, Calarco G, Franzì E, et al. Right atrial lipoma in patient with Cowden syndrome. Interact Cardiovasc Thorac Surg. 2010 Dec;11(6):803–4. PMID:20852328
417. Ceresoli GL, Ferreri AJ, Bucci E, et al. Primary cardiac lymphoma in immunocompetent patients: diagnostic and therapeutic management. Cancer. 1997 Oct 15;80(8):1497–506. PMID:9338475
418. Cerfolio RJ, Allen MS, Nascimento AG, et al. Inflammatory pseudotumors of the lung. Ann Thorac Surg. 1999 Apr;67(4):933–6. PMID:10320231
419. Cesarman E, Chang Y, Moore PS, et al. Kaposi's sarcoma-associated herpesvirus-like DNA sequences in AIDS-related body-cavity-based lymphomas. N Engl J Med. 1995 May 4;332(18):1186–91. PMID:7700311
420. Cesarman E, Damania B, Krown SE, et al. Kaposi sarcoma. Nat Rev Dis Primers. 2019 Jan 31;5(1):9. PMID:30705286
421. Cesarman E, Knowles DM. Kaposi's sarcoma-associated herpesvirus: a lymphotropic human herpesvirus associated with Kaposi's sarcoma, primary effusion lymphoma, and multicentric Castleman's disease. Semin Diagn Pathol. 1997 Feb;14(1):54–66. PMID:9044510
422. Cesarman E, Nador RG, Aozasa K, et al. Kaposi's sarcoma-associated herpesvirus in non-AIDS related lymphomas occurring in body cavities. Am J Pathol. 1996 Jul;149(1):53–7. PMID:8686762
423. Cessna MH, Zhou H, Sanger WG, et al. Expression of ALK1 and p80 in inflammatory myofibroblastic tumor and its mesenchymal mimics: a study of 135 cases. Mod Pathol. 2002 Sep;15(9):931–8. PMID:12218210
424. Cha MJ, Lee HY, Lee KS, et al. Micropapillary and solid subtypes of invasive lung adenocarcinoma: clinical predictors of histopathology and outcome. J Thorac Cardiovasc Surg. 2014 Mar;147(3):921–928.e2. PMID:24199757
425. Cha YJ, Han J, Kim J, et al. A rare case of mixed type a thymoma and micronodular thymoma with lymphoid stroma. J Pathol Transl Med. 2015 Jan;49(1):75–7. PMID:25812662
426. Chaari Z, Charfi S, Hentati A, et al. Primary Burkitt lymphoma in the posterior mediastinum. Asian Cardiovasc Thorac Ann. 2015 Nov;23(9):1110–2. PMID:26038605
427. Chabchoub Ben Abdallah R, Maalej B, Abdelmoulla S, et al. [Thymoma in children: a report of one case]. Arch Pediatr. 2011 Jul;18(7):745–9. French. PMID:21596536
428. Chadburn A, Hyjek E, Mathew S, et al. KSHV-positive solid lymphomas represent an extra-cavitary variant of primary effusion lymphoma. Am J Surg Pathol. 2004 Nov;28(11):1401–16. PMID:15489644
429. Chaft JE, Rekhtman N, Ladanyi M, et al. ALK-rearranged lung cancer: adenosquamous lung cancer masquerading as pure squamous carcinoma. J Thorac Oncol. 2012 Apr;7(4):768–9. PMID:22425930
430. Chaganti RS, Ladanyi M, Samaniego F, et al. Leukemic differentiation of a mediastinal germ cell tumor. Genes Chromosomes Cancer. 1989 Sep;1(1):83–7. PMID:2562115
431. Chaganti RS, Rodriguez E, Mathew S. Origin of adult male mediastinal germ-cell tumours. Lancet. 1994 May 7;343(8906):1130–2. PMID:7910232
431A. Chakrabarti A, Bandyopadhyay M, Purkayastha B. Malignant perivascular epitheloid cell tumour (PEComa) of the lung - a rare entity. Innov Surg Sci. 2017 Feb 23;2(1):39–42. PMID:31579733
432. Chakraborty R, Burke TM, Hampton OA, et al. Alternative genetic mechanisms of BRAF activation in Langerhans cell histiocytosis. Blood. 2016 Nov 24;128(21):2533–7. PMID:27729324
433. Chalabreysse L, Berger F, Loire R, et al. Primary cardiac lymphoma in immunocompetent patients: a report of three cases and review of the literature. Virchows Arch. 2002 Nov;441(5):456–61. PMID:12447675
434. Chalabreysse L, Etienne-Mastroianni B, Adeleine P, et al. Thymic carcinoma: a clinicopathological and immunohistological study of 19 cases. Histopathology. 2004 Apr;44(4):367–74. PMID:15049903
435. Chalabreysse L, Gengler C, Sefiani S, et al. [Thymic neuroendocrine tumors: report on 6 cases]. Ann Pathol. 2005 Jun;25(3):205–10. French. PMID:16230946
436. Chalabreysse L, Roy P, Cordier JF, et al. Correlation of the WHO schema for the classification of thymic epithelial neoplasms with prognosis: a retrospective study of 90 tumors. Am J Surg Pathol. 2002 Dec;26(12):1605–11. PMID:12459627
437. Chan AC, Chan JK. Can pulmonary sclerosing haemangioma be accurately diagnosed by intra-operative frozen section? Histopathology. 2002 Nov;41(5):392–403. PMID:12405907
438. Chan AC, Chan JK. Pulmonary sclerosing hemangioma consistently expresses thyroid transcription factor-1 (TTF-1): a new clue to its histogenesis. Am J Surg Pathol. 2000 Nov;24(11):1531–6. PMID:11075855
439. Chan AC, Chan JK, Yan KW, et al. Anaplastic large cell lymphoma presenting as a pleural effusion and mimicking primary effusion lymphoma. A report of 2 cases. Acta Cytol. 2003 Sep-Oct;47(5):809–16. PMID:14526684
440. Chan AC, Serrano-Olmo J, Erlandson RA, et al. Cytokeratin-positive malignant tumors with reticulum cell morphology: a subtype of fibroblastic reticulum cell neoplasm? Am J Surg Pathol. 2000 Jan;24(1):107–16. PMID:10632494
441. Chan AW, Chau SL, Tong JH, et al. The landscape of actionable molecular alterations in immunomarker-defined large-cell carcinoma of the lung. J Thorac Oncol. 2019 Jul;14(7):1213–22. PMID:30978501
442. Chan JK, Hui PK, Tsang WY, et al. Primary lymphoepithelioma-like carcinoma of the lung. A clinicopathologic study of 11 cases. Cancer. 1995 Aug 1;76(3):413–22. PMID:8625122
442A. Chan LP, Chiang FY, Lee KW, et al. Carcinoma showing thymus-like differentiation (CASTLE) of thyroid: a case report and literature review. Kaohsiung J Med Sci. 2008 Nov;24(11):591–7. PMID:19239992
442B. Chang C, Hung LY, Thanh TT, et al. Congenital peribronchial myofibroblastic tumour with features of maturation in the older infant: report of two cases with a literature review. Histopathology. 2014 Apr;64(5):755–7. PMID:24117734
443. Chang JC, Alex D, Bott M, et al. Comprehensive next-generation sequencing unambiguously distinguishes separate primary lung carcinomas from intrapulmonary metastases: comparison with standard histopathologic approach. Clin Cancer Res. 2019 Dec 1;25(23):7113–25. PMID:31471310
444. Chang JC, Montecalvo J, Borsu L, et al. Bronchiolar adenoma: expansion of the concept of ciliated muconodular papillary tumors with proposal for revised terminology based on morphologic, immunophenotypic, and genomic analysis of 25 cases. Am J Surg Pathol. 2018 Aug;42(8):1010–26. PMID:29846186
445. Chang JC, Zhang L, Drilon AE, et al. Expanding the molecular characterization of thoracic inflammatory myofibroblastic tumors beyond ALK gene rearrangements. J Thorac Oncol. 2019 May;14(5):825–34. PMID:30550870
446. Chang YL, Lee YC, Shih JY, et al. Pulmonary pleomorphic (spindle) cell carcinoma: peculiar clinicopathologic manifestations different from ordinary non-small cell carcinoma. Lung Cancer. 2001 Oct;34(1):91–7. PMID:11557118
447. Chang YL, Wu CT, Lee YC. Mediastinal and retroperitoneal teratoma with focal gastrointestinal adenocarcinoma. J Thorac Oncol. 2006 Sep;1(7):729–31. PMID:17409945
448. Chang YL, Wu CT, Shih JY, et al. New aspects in clinicopathologic and oncogene studies of 23 pulmonary lymphoepithelioma-like carcinomas. Am J Surg Pathol. 2002 Jun;26(6):715–23. PMID:12023575
449. Chang YL, Wu CT, Shih JY, et al. Unique p53 and epidermal growth factor receptor gene mutation status in 46 pulmonary lymphoepithelioma-like carcinomas. Cancer Sci. 2011 Jan;102(1):282–7. PMID:21070477
450. Chang YL, Yang CY, Lin MW, et al. PD-L1 is highly expressed in lung lymphoepithelioma-like carcinoma: a potential rationale for immunotherapy. Lung Cancer. 2015 Jun;88(3):254–9. PMID:25862146
451. Chansky K, Detterbeck FC, Nicholson AG, et al. The IASLC Lung Cancer Staging Project: external validation of the revision of the TNM stage groupings in the eighth edition of the TNM classification of lung cancer. J Thorac Oncol. 2017 Jul;12(7):1109–21. PMID:28461257
452. Chapel DB, Schulte JJ, Berg K, et al. MTAP immunohistochemistry is an accurate and reproducible surrogate for CDKN2A fluorescence in situ hybridization in diagnosis of malignant pleural mesothelioma. Mod Pathol. 2020 Feb;33(2):245–54. PMID:31231127
452A. Chapel DB, Schulte JJ, Husain AN, et al. Application of immunohistochemistry in diagnosis and management of malignant mesothelioma. Transl Lung Cancer Res. 2020 Feb;9(Suppl 1):S3–27. PMID:32206567
453. Chapman AD, Kerr KM. The association between atypical adenomatous hyperplasia and primary lung cancer. Br J Cancer. 2000 Sep;83(5):632–6. PMID:10944604
454. Chapman E, Skalova A, Ptakova N, et al. Molecular profiling of hyalinizing clear cell carcinomas revealed a subset of tumors harboring a novel EWSR1-CREM fusion: report of 3 cases. Am J Surg Pathol. 2018 Sep;42(9):1182–9. PMID:29975250
455. Chapuy B, Stewart C, Dunford AJ, et al.

Genomic analyses of PMBL reveal new drivers and mechanisms of sensitivity to PD-1 blockade. Blood. 2019 Dec 26;134(26):2369–82. PMID:31697821
456. Chapuy B, Stewart C, Dunford AJ, et al. Molecular subtypes of diffuse large B cell lymphoma are associated with distinct pathogenic mechanisms and outcomes. Nat Med. 2018 May;24(5):679–90. PMID:29713087
457. Chariot P, Monnet I, Gaulard P, et al. Systemic mastocytosis following mediastinal germ cell tumor: an association confirmed. Hum Pathol. 1993 Jan;24(1):111–2. PMID:8380274
458. Charruau L, Parrens M, Jougon J, et al. Mediastinal lymphangioma in adults: CT and MR imaging features. Eur Radiol. 2000;10(8):1310–4. PMID:10939497
459. Chassagnon G, Favelle O, Marchand-Adam S, et al. DIPNECH: when to suggest this diagnosis on CT. Clin Radiol. 2015 Mar;70(3):317–25. PMID:25465294
460. Chatziandreou I, Tsioli P, Sakellariou S, et al. Comprehensive molecular analysis of NSCLC; clinicopathological associations. PLoS One. 2015 Jul 24;10(7):e0133859. PMID:26208325
461. Chatzopoulos K, Fritchie KJ, Aubry MC, et al. Loss of succinate dehydrogenase B immunohistochemical expression distinguishes pulmonary chondromas from hamartomas. Histopathology. 2019 Dec;75(6):825–32. PMID:31236950
462. Chau C, van Doorn R, van Poppelen NM, et al. Families with BAP1-tumor predisposition syndrome in the Netherlands: path to identification and a proposal for genetic screening guidelines. Cancers (Basel). 2019 Aug 4;11(8):E1114. PMID:31382694
463. Chau NG, Hurwitz S, Mitchell CM, et al. Intensive treatment and survival outcomes in NUT midline carcinoma of the head and neck. Cancer. 2016 Dec 1;122(23):3632–40. PMID:27509377
464. Chau NG, Ma C, Danga K, et al. An anatomical site and genetic-based prognostic model for patients with nuclear protein in testis (NUT) midline carcinoma: analysis of 124 patients. JNCI Cancer Spectr. 2019 Nov 6;4(2):pkz094. PMID:32328562
465. Chavez JC, Sandoval-Sus J, Horna P, et al. Lymphomatoid granulomatosis: a single institution experience and review of the literature. Clin Lymphoma Myeloma Leuk. 2016 Aug;16 Suppl:S170–4. PMID:27521314
466. Chebib I, Hornicek FJ, Nielsen GP, et al. Cytomorphologic features that distinguish schwannoma from other low-grade spindle cell lesions. Cancer Cytopathol. 2015 Mar;123(3):171–9. PMID:25641870
467. Chemi F, Rothwell DG, McGranahan N, et al. Pulmonary venous circulating tumor cell dissemination before tumor resection and disease relapse. Nat Med. 2019 Oct;25(10):1534–9. PMID:31591595
468. Chen B, Gao J, Chen H, et al. Pulmonary sclerosing hemangioma: a unique epithelial neoplasm of the lung (report of 26 cases). World J Surg Oncol. 2013 Apr 15;11:85. PMID:23587094
469. Chen BJ, Chapuy B, Ouyang J, et al. PD-L1 expression is characteristic of a subset of aggressive B-cell lymphomas and virus-associated malignancies. Clin Cancer Res. 2013 Jul 1;19(13):3462–73. PMID:23674495
470. Chen CC, Yang SF, Lin PC, et al. Pulmonary blastoma in children: report of a rare case and review of the literature. Int J Surg Pathol. 2017 Dec;25(8):721–6. PMID:28675947
471. Chen D, Mao Y, Wen J, et al. Tumor spread through air spaces in non-small cell lung cancer: a systematic review and meta-analysis. Ann Thorac Surg. 2019 Sep;108(3):945–54. PMID:30914285
472. Chen G, Marx A, Chen WH, et al. New WHO histologic classification predicts prognosis of thymic epithelial tumors: a clinicopathologic study of 200 thymoma cases from China. Cancer. 2002 Jul 15;95(2):420–9. PMID:12124843
473. Chen H, Carrot-Zhang J, Zhao Y, et al. Genomic and immune profiling of pre-invasive lung adenocarcinoma. Nat Commun. 2019 Nov 29;10(1):5472. PMID:31784532
474. Chen JJ, Lin YC, Yao PL, et al. Tumor-associated macrophages: the double-edged sword in cancer progression. J Clin Oncol. 2005 Feb 10;23(5):953–64. PMID:15598976
475. Chen KT. Familial peritoneal multifocal calcifying fibrous tumor. Am J Clin Pathol. 2003 Jun;119(6):811–5. PMID:12817428
476. Chen M, Liu P, Yan F, et al. Distinctive features of immunostaining and mutational load in primary pulmonary enteric adenocarcinoma: implications for differential diagnosis and immunotherapy. J Transl Med. 2018 Mar 27;16(1):81. PMID:29587865
477. Chen M, Yang J, Zhu L, et al. Primary intrathoracic liposarcoma: a clinicopathologic study and prognostic analysis of 23 cases. J Cardiothorac Surg. 2014 Jul 4;9:119. PMID:24993036
478. Chen PC, Pan CC, Yang AH, et al. Detection of Epstein-Barr virus genome within thymic epithelial tumours in Taiwanese patients by nested PCR, PCR in situ hybridization, and RNA in situ hybridization. J Pathol. 2002 Aug;197(5):684–8. PMID:12210090
479. Chen S, Zheng Y, Chen L, et al. A broad ligament solitary fibrous tumor with Doege-Potter syndrome. Medicine (Baltimore). 2018 Sep;97(39):e12564. PMID:30278559
480. Chen TW, Loong HH, Srikanthan A, et al. Primary cardiac sarcomas: a multi-national retrospective review. Cancer Med. 2019 Jan;8(1):104–10. PMID:30575309
481. Chen W, Lau SK, Fong D, et al. High frequency of clonal immunoglobulin receptor gene rearrangements in sporadic histiocytic/dendritic cell sarcomas. Am J Surg Pathol. 2009 Jun;33(6):863–73. PMID:19145200
482. Chen X, Pang Z, Wang Y, et al. The role of surgery for atypical bronchopulmonary carcinoid tumor: development and validation of a model based on Surveillance, Epidemiology, and End Results (SEER) database. Lung Cancer. 2020 Jan;139:94–102. PMID:31759223
483. Chen X, Sheng W, Wang J. Well-differentiated papillary mesothelioma: a clinicopathological and immunohistochemical study of 18 cases with additional observation. Histopathology. 2013 Apr;62(5):805–13. PMID:23530588
484. Chen Y, Chen A, Jiang H, et al. HRCT in primary pulmonary lymphoma: Can CT imaging phenotypes differentiate histological subtypes between mucosa-associated lymphoid tissue (MALT) lymphoma and non-MALT lymphoma? J Thorac Dis. 2018 Nov;10(11):6040–9. PMID:30622775
485. Chen Y, Shen D, Sun K, et al. Epithelioid angiosarcoma of bone and soft tissue: a report of seven cases with emphasis on morphologic diversity, immunohistochemical features and clinical outcome. Tumori. 2011 Sep-Oct;97(5):585–9. PMID:22158488
486. Chen Y, Takita J, Choi YL, et al. Oncogenic mutations of ALK kinase in neuroblastoma. Nature. 2008 Oct 16;455(7215):971–4. PMID:18923524
487. Chen YB, Guo LC, Huang JA, et al. Clear cell tumor of the lung: a retrospective analysis. Am J Med Sci. 2014 Jan;347(1):50–3. PMID:23744522
488. Cheng DL, Hu YX, Hu PQ, et al. Clinicopathological and multisection CT features of primary pulmonary mucoepidermoid carcinoma. Clin Radiol. 2017 Jul;72(7):610.e1–7. PMID:28292512
489. Cheng I, Le GM, Noone AM, et al. Lung cancer incidence trends by histology type among Asian American, Native Hawaiian, and Pacific Islander populations in the United States, 1990-2010. Cancer Epidemiol Biomarkers Prev. 2014 Nov;23(11):2250–65. PMID:25368400
490. Chernow B, Sahn SA. Carcinomatous involvement of the pleura: an analysis of 96 patients. Am J Med. 1977 Nov;63(5):695–702. PMID:930945
491. Chervenak FA, Isaacson G, Blakemore KJ, et al. Fetal cystic hygroma. Cause and natural history. N Engl J Med. 1983 Oct 6;309(14):822–5. PMID:6888468
492. Cheson BD, Fisher RI, Barrington SF, et al. Recommendations for initial evaluation, staging, and response assessment of Hodgkin and non-Hodgkin lymphoma: the Lugano classification. J Clin Oncol. 2014 Sep 20;32(27):3059–68. PMID:25113753
493. Cheuk W, Chan AC, Chan JK, et al. Metallic implant-associated lymphoma: a distinct subgroup of large B-cell lymphoma related to pyothorax-associated lymphoma? Am J Surg Pathol. 2005 Jun;29(6):832–6. PMID:15897752
494. Cheuk W, Kwan MY, Suster S, et al. Immunostaining for thyroid transcription factor 1 and cytokeratin 20 aids the distinction of small cell carcinoma from Merkel cell carcinoma, but not pulmonary from extrapulmonary small cell carcinomas. Arch Pathol Lab Med. 2001 Feb;125(2):228–31. PMID:11175640
495. Cheuk W, Tsang WY, Chan JK. Microthymoma: definition of the entity and distinction from nodular hyperplasia of the thymic epithelium (so-called microscopic thymoma). Am J Surg Pathol. 2005 Mar;29(3):415–9. PMID:15725813
496. Cheung F, Alam N, Wright G. Pulmonary metastasectomy: analysis of survival and prognostic factors in 243 patients. ANZ J Surg. 2018 Dec;88(12):1316–21. PMID:30211472
497. Cheung NK, Zhang J, Lu C, et al. Association of age at diagnosis and genetic mutations in patients with neuroblastoma. JAMA. 2012 Mar 14;307(10):1062–71. PMID:22416102
497A. Chevrier M, Monaco SE, Jerome JA, et al. Testing for BAP1 loss and CDKN2A/p16 homozygous deletion improves the accurate diagnosis of mesothelial proliferations in effusion cytology. Cancer Cytopathol. 2020 Dec;128(12):939–47. PMID:32678499
498. Chhieng DC, Rose D, Ludwig ME, et al. Cytology of thymomas: emphasis on morphology and correlation with histologic subtypes. Cancer. 2000 Feb 25;90(1):24–32. PMID:10692213
499. Chiariello GA, Colizzi C, Pavone N, et al. Left ventricular rhabdomyoma in an adult patient: a rare disease successfully treated. Int J Cardiol. 2014 Oct 20;176(3):e107–9. PMID:25127964
500. Chibon F, Lagarde P, Salas S, et al. Validated prediction of clinical outcome in sarcomas and multiple types of cancer on the basis of a gene expression signature related to genome complexity. Nat Med. 2010 Jul;16(7):781–7. PMID:20581836
501. Chilosi M, Zamò A, Brighenti A, et al. Constitutive expression of DeltaN-p63alpha isoform in human thymus and thymic epithelial tumours. Virchows Arch. 2003 Aug;443(2):175–83. PMID:12851817
502. Chim CS, Chan AC, Kwong YL, et al. Primary cardiac lymphoma. Am J Hematol. 1997 Jan;54(1):79–83. PMID:8980266
503. Chinen K, Izumo T. Cardiac involvement by malignant lymphoma: a clinicopathologic study of 25 autopsy cases based on the WHO classification. Ann Hematol. 2005 Aug;84(8):498–505. PMID:15782345
504. Chiosea SI, Dacic S, Nikiforova MN, et al. Prospective testing of mucoepidermoid carcinoma for the MAML2 translocation: clinical implications. Laryngoscope. 2012 Aug;122(8):1690–4. PMID:22833306
505. Chirieac LR, Barletta JA, Yeap BY, et al. Clinicopathologic characteristics of malignant mesotheliomas arising in patients with a history of radiation for Hodgkin and non-Hodgkin lymphoma. J Clin Oncol. 2013 Dec 20;31(36):4544–9. PMID:24248693
506. Chirieac LR, Pinkus GS, Pinkus JL, et al. The immunohistochemical characterization of sarcomatoid malignant mesothelioma of the pleura. Am J Cancer Res. 2011;1(1):14–24. PMID:21969119
507. Chmielecki J, Crago AM, Rosenberg M, et al. Whole-exome sequencing identifies a recurrent NAB2-STAT6 fusion in solitary fibrous tumors. Nat Genet. 2013 Feb;45(2):131–2. PMID:23313954
508. Chng WJ, Remstein ED, Fonseca R, et al. Gene expression profiling of pulmonary mucosa-associated lymphoid tissue lymphoma identifies new biologic insights with potential diagnostic and therapeutic applications. Blood. 2009 Jan 15;113(3):635–45. PMID:18974375
509. Cho HJ, Lee JH, Lee GK, et al. Case of sclerosing pneumocytoma combined with a typical carcinoid and pulmonary adenocarcinoma in different lobes. Thorac Cancer. 2017 Jul;8(4):372–5. PMID:28474862
510. Cho JH, Kim S, Namgung M, et al. The prognostic importance of the number of metastases in pulmonary metastasectomy of colorectal cancer. World J Surg Oncol. 2015 Jul 25;13:222. PMID:26205014
511. Cho JM, Danielson GK, Puga FJ, et al. Surgical resection of ventricular cardiac fibromas: early and late results. Ann Thorac Surg. 2003 Dec;76(6):1929–34. PMID:14667615
512. Choi CH, Park CH, Kim JS, et al. Giant biatrial myxoma nearly obstructing the orifice of the inferior vena cava. J Cardiothorac Surg. 2013 Jun 10;8:148. PMID:23758983
513. Choi HS, Seol H, Heo IY, et al. Fine-needle aspiration cytology of pleomorphic carcinomas of the lung. Korean J Pathol. 2012 Dec;46(6):576–82. PMID:23323109
513A. Choi SM, Furth EE, Zhang PJ. Unexpected TTF-1 positivity in a subset of gastric adenocarcinomas. Appl Immunohistochem Mol Morphol. 2016 Sep;24(8):603–7. PMID:26469324
514. Choi WW, Lui YH, Lau WH, et al. Adenocarcinoma of the thymus: report of two cases, including a previously undescribed mucinous subtype. Am J Surg Pathol. 2003 Jan;27(1):124–30. PMID:12502935
515. Chong CR, Wirth LJ, Nishino M, et al. Chemotherapy for locally advanced and metastatic pulmonary carcinoid tumors. Lung Cancer. 2014 Nov;86(2):241–6. PMID:25218177
516. Chou ST, Arkles LB, Gill GD, et al. Primary lymphoma of the heart. A case report. Cancer. 1983 Aug 15;52(4):744–7. PMID:6305485
517. Chougule A, Taylor MS, Nardi V, et al. Spindle and round cell sarcoma with EWSR1-PATZ1 gene fusion: a sarcoma with polyphenotypic differentiation. Am J Surg Pathol. 2019 Feb;43(2):220–8. PMID:30379650
518. Christakis I, Qiu W, Silva Figueroa AM, et al. Clinical features, treatments, and outcomes of patients with thymic carcinoids and multiple endocrine neoplasia type 1 syndrome at MD Anderson Cancer Center. Horm Cancer. 2016 Aug;7(4):279–87. PMID:27311764
519. Christie B 3rd, Moremen JR. Thymic carcinoma: incidence, classification and treatment

strategies of a rare tumor. Am Surg. 2012 Jul;78(7):E335–7. PMID:22748521
520. Christodoulou J, Schoch C, Schnittger S, et al. Myelodysplastic syndrome (RARS) with +i(12p) abnormality in a patient 10 months after diagnosis and successful treatment of a mediastinal germ cell tumor (MGCT). Ann Hematol. 2004 Jun;83(6):386–9. PMID:14615911
521. Christopoulos P, Dopfer EP, Malkovsky M, et al. A novel thymoma-associated immunodeficiency with increased naive T cells and reduced CD247 expression. J Immunol. 2015 Apr 1;194(7):3045–53. PMID:25732729
522. Chu P, Wu E, Weiss LM. Cytokeratin 7 and cytokeratin 20 expression in epithelial neoplasms: a survey of 435 cases. Mod Pathol. 2000 Sep;13(9):962–72. PMID:11007036
522A. Chu PG, Arber DA, Weiss LM. Expression of T/NK-cell and plasma cell antigens in nonhematopoietic epithelioid neoplasms. An immunohistochemical study of 447 cases. Am J Clin Pathol. 2003 Jul;120(1):64–70. PMID:12866374
523. Chu PG, Chung L, Weiss LM, et al. Determining the site of origin of mucinous adenocarcinoma: an immunohistochemical study of 175 cases. Am J Surg Pathol. 2011 Dec;35(12):1830–6. PMID:21881489
524. Chu PH, Yeh HI, Jung SM, et al. Irregular connexin43 expressed in a rare cardiac hamartoma containing adipose tissue in the crista terminalis. Virchows Arch. 2004 Apr;444(4):383–6. PMID:15067542
525. Chubachi A, Miura I, Takahashi N, et al. Acute myelogenous leukemia associated with a mediastinal tumor. Leuk Lymphoma. 1993 Dec;12(1-2):143–6. PMID:8161930
526. Chun YS, Wang L, Nascimento AG, et al. Pediatric inflammatory myofibroblastic tumor: anaplastic lymphoma kinase (ALK) expression and prognosis. Pediatr Blood Cancer. 2005 Nov;45(6):796–801. PMID:15602716
527. Chung HC, Piha-Paul SA, Lopez-Martin J, et al. Pembrolizumab after two or more lines of previous therapy in patients with recurrent or metastatic SCLC: results from the KEYNOTE-028 and KEYNOTE-158 studies. J Thorac Oncol. 2020 Apr;15(4):618–27. PMID:31870883
528. Churg A, Allen T, Borczuk AC, et al. Well-differentiated papillary mesothelioma with invasive foci. Am J Surg Pathol. 2014 Jul;38(7):990–8. PMID:24618613
529. Churg A, Cagle P, Colby TV, et al. The fake fat phenomenon in organizing pleuritis: a source of confusion with desmoplastic malignant mesotheliomas. Am J Surg Pathol. 2011 Dec;35(12):1823–9. PMID:21959310
530. Churg A, Cagle PT, Roggli VL. Tumors of the serosal membranes. Washington, DC: American Registry of Pathology; 2006. (AFIP atlas of tumor pathology, series 4; fascicle 3).
531. Churg A, Colby TV, Cagle P, et al. The separation of benign and malignant mesothelial proliferations. Am J Surg Pathol. 2000 Sep;24(9):1183–200. PMID:10976692
532. Churg A, Galateau-Salle F. The separation of benign and malignant mesothelial proliferations. Arch Pathol Lab Med. 2012 Oct;136(10):1217–26. PMID:23020727
533. Churg A, Galateau-Salle F, Roden AC, et al. Malignant mesothelioma in situ: morphologic features and clinical outcome. Mod Pathol. 2020 Feb;33(2):297–302. PMID:31375770
534. Churg A, Hwang H, Tan L, et al. Malignant mesothelioma in situ. Histopathology. 2018 May;72(6):1033–8. PMID:29350783
535. Churg A, Nabeshima K, Ali G, et al. Highlights of the 14th International Mesothelioma Interest Group Meeting: pathologic separation of benign from malignant mesothelial proliferations and histologic/molecular analysis of malignant mesothelioma subtypes. Lung Cancer. 2018 Oct;124:95–101. PMID:30268487
536. Chute DJ, Cousar JB, Mahadevan MS, et al. Detection of immunoglobulin heavy chain gene rearrangements in classic Hodgkin lymphoma using commercially available BIOMED-2 primers. Diagn Mol Pathol. 2008 Jun;17(2):65–72. PMID:18382369
537. Cianciulli TF, Soumoulou JB, Lax JA, et al. Papillary fibroelastoma: clinical and echocardiographic features and initial approach in 54 cases. Echocardiography. 2016 Dec;33(12):1811–7. PMID:27566126
538. Cipriani NA, Lusardi JJ, McElherne J, et al. Mucoepidermoid carcinoma: a comparison of histologic grading systems and relationship to MAML2 rearrangement and prognosis. Am J Surg Pathol. 2019 Jul;43(7):885–97. PMID:31021855
539. Claerhout H, Van Aelst S, Melis C, et al. Clinicopathological characteristics of de novo and secondary myeloid sarcoma: a monocentric retrospective study. Eur J Haematol. 2018 Jun;100(6):603–12. PMID:29532520
540. Clay MR, Martinez AP, Weiss SW, et al. MDM2 amplification in problematic lipomatous tumors: analysis of FISH testing criteria. Am J Surg Pathol. 2015 Oct;39(10):1433–9. PMID:26146760
541. Clayton F. Bronchioloalveolar carcinomas. Cell types, patterns of growth, and prognostic correlates. Cancer. 1986 Apr 15;57(8):1555–64. PMID:3004694
542. Clement PB, Young RH, Scully RE. Endometrioid-like variant of ovarian yolk sac tumor. A clinicopathological analysis of eight cases. Am J Surg Pathol. 1987 Oct;11(10):767–78. PMID:3661822
543. Clinical Lung Cancer Genome Project (CLCGP), Network Genomic Medicine (NGM). A genomics-based classification of human lung tumors. Sci Transl Med. 2013 Oct 30;5(209):209ra153. PMID:24174329
544. ClinicalTrials.gov [Internet]. Bethesda (MD): U.S. National Library of Medicine; 2020. Identifier NCT01225601, Prospective evaluation of adult pulmonary Langerhans cell histiocytosis (LCHA1); first posted 2010 Oct 21 [updated 2016 Apr 18]. Available from: https://clinicaltrials.gov/ct2/show/NCT01225601.
545. ClinicalTrials.gov [Internet]. Bethesda (MD): U.S. National Library of Medicine; 2020. Identifier NCT01473797, Evaluation of efficacy and tolerance of cladribine in symptomatic pulmonary Langerhans cell histiocytosis (ECLA); first posted 2011 Nov 17 [updated 2020 Jan 7]. Available from: https://clinicaltrials.gov/ct2/show/NCT01473797.
546. ClinicalTrials.gov [Internet]. Bethesda (MD): U.S. National Library of Medicine; 2020. Identifier NCT02516553, BI 894999 First in human dose finding study in advanced malignancies; first posted 2015 Aug 6 [updated 2020 Aug 12]. Available from: https://clinicaltrials.gov/ct2/show/NCT02516553.
547. Cobb CJ, Wynn J, Cobb SR, et al. Cytologic findings in an effusion caused by rupture of a benign cystic teratoma of the mediastinum into a serous cavity. Acta Cytol. 1985 Nov-Dec;29(6):1015–20. PMID:3866453
548. Coca-Pelaz A, Rodrigo JP, Bradley PJ, et al. Adenoid cystic carcinoma of the head and neck–An update. Oral Oncol. 2015 Jul;51(7):652–61. PMID:25943783
549. Coffin CM, Hornick JL, Fletcher CD. Inflammatory myofibroblastic tumor: comparison of clinicopathologic, histologic, and immunohistochemical features including ALK expression in atypical and aggressive cases. Am J Surg Pathol. 2007 Apr;31(4):509–20. PMID:17414097
550. Cohen AJ, Sbaschnig RJ, Hochholzer L, et al. Mediastinal hemangiomas. Ann Thorac Surg. 1987 Jun;43(6):656–9. PMID:3592837
551. Cohen AJ, Thompson L, Edwards FH, et al. Primary cysts and tumors of the mediastinum. Ann Thorac Surg. 1991 Mar;51(3):378–84, discussion 385–6. PMID:1998414
552. Cohen Aubart F, Emile JF, Carrat F, et al. Targeted therapies in 54 patients with Erdheim-Chester disease, including follow-up after interruption (the LOVE study). Blood. 2017 Sep 14;130(11):1377–80. PMID:28667012
553. Cohen MB, Friend DS, Molnar JJ, et al. Gonadal endodermal sinus (yolk sac) tumor with pure intestinal differentiation: a new histologic type. Pathol Res Pract. 1987 Oct;182(5):609–16. PMID:2446292
554. Cohen RE, Weaver MG, Montenegro HD, et al. Pulmonary blastoma with malignant melanoma component. Arch Pathol Lab Med. 1990 Oct;114(10):1076–8. PMID:2222150
555. Cohen-Aubart F, Emile JF, Carrat F, et al. Phenotypes and survival in Erdheim-Chester disease: results from a 165-patient cohort. Am J Hematol. 2018 May;93(5):E114–7. PMID:29396850
556. Cohle SD. Cystic tumour of the atrioventricular node: case report and literature review. Forensic Sci Res. 2019 May 16;4(3):287–9. PMID:31489395
557. Cohn SL, Pearson AD, London WB, et al. The International Neuroblastoma Risk Group (INRG) classification system: an INRG Task Force report. J Clin Oncol. 2009 Jan 10;27(2):289–97. PMID:19047291
558. Coindre JM. Grading of soft tissue sarcomas: review and update. Arch Pathol Lab Med. 2006 Oct;130(10):1448–53. PMID:17090186
559. Colby TV. Benign mesothelial cells in lymph node. Adv Anat Pathol. 1999 Jan;6(1):41–8. PMID:10197237
560. Colby TV. Malignancies in the lung and pleura mimicking benign processes. Semin Diagn Pathol. 1995 Feb;12(1):30–44. PMID:7770673
561. Colby TV. The diagnosis of desmoplastic malignant mesothelioma. Am J Clin Pathol. 1998 Aug;110(2):135–6. PMID:9704609
562. Colin GC, Gerber BL, Amzulescu M, et al. Cardiac myxoma: a contemporary multimodality imaging review. Int J Cardiovasc Imaging. 2018 Nov;34(11):1789–808. PMID:29974293
563. Colin GC, Symons R, Dymarkowski S, et al. Value of CMR to differentiate cardiac angiosarcoma from cardiac lymphoma. JACC Cardiovasc Imaging. 2015 Jun;8(6):744–6. PMID:25459304
564. Collins BT, Cramer HM. Fine needle aspiration cytology of carcinoid tumors. Acta Cytol. 1996 Jul-Aug;40(4):695–707. PMID:8693889
565. Colombo C, Bolshakov S, Hajibashi S, et al. 'Difficult to diagnose' desmoid tumours: a potential role for CTNNB1 mutational analysis. Histopathology. 2011 Aug;59(2):336–40. PMID:21884214
566. Colombo C, Miceli R, Lazar AJ, et al. CTNNB1 45F mutation is a molecular prognosticator of increased postoperative primary desmoid tumor recurrence: an independent, multicenter validation study. Cancer. 2013 Oct 15;119(20):3696–702. PMID:23913621
567. Combaz-Lair C, Galateau-Sallé F, McLeer-Florin A, et al. Immune biomarkers PD-1/PD-L1 and TLR3 in malignant pleural mesotheliomas. Hum Pathol. 2016 Jun;52:9–18. PMID:26980049
568. Cook AG, Viswanath O, D'Mello J. Papillary fibroelastoma found with transesophageal echocardiography after a normal transthoracic echocardiography. Semin Cardiothorac Vasc Anesth. 2017 Sep;21(3):217–20. PMID:28758563
569. Cooke DT, Nguyen DV, Yang Y, et al. Survival comparison of adenosquamous, squamous cell, and adenocarcinoma of the lung after lobectomy. Ann Thorac Surg. 2010 Sep;90(3):943–8. PMID:20732522
570. Cope O. Surgery of hyperparathyroidism: the occurrence of parathyroids in the anterior mediastinum and the division of the operation into two stages. Ann Surg. 1941 Oct;114(4):706–33. PMID:17857905
571. Copie-Bergman C, Gaulard P, Maouche-Chrétien L, et al. The MAL gene is expressed in primary mediastinal large B-cell lymphoma. Blood. 1999 Nov 15;94(10):3567–75. PMID:10552968
572. Copie-Bergman C, Niedobitek G, Mangham DC, et al. Epstein-Barr virus in B-cell lymphomas associated with chronic suppurative inflammation. J Pathol. 1997 Nov;183(3):287–92. PMID:9422983
573. Coppage L, Shaw C, Curtis AM. Metastatic disease to the chest in patients with extrathoracic malignancy. J Thorac Imaging. 1987 Oct;2(4):24–37. PMID:3316682
574. Corgnati G, Drago S, Bonamini R, et al. Solitary fibrous tumor of the pericardium presenting itself as a pericardial effusion and right ventricular obstruction. J Cardiovasc Surg (Torino). 2004 Aug;45(4):393–4. PMID:15365524
575. Cornejo KM, Shi M, Akalin A, et al. Pulmonary papillary adenoma: a case report and review of the literature. J Bronchology Interv Pulmonol. 2013 Jan;20(1):52–7. PMID:23328145
576. Cortelazzo S, Ferreri A, Hoelzer D, et al. Lymphoblastic lymphoma. Crit Rev Oncol Hematol. 2017 May;113:304–17. PMID:28427520
577. Cosgrove MM, Chandrasoma PT, Martin SE. Diagnosis of pulmonary blastoma by fine-needle aspiration biopsy: cytologic and immunocytochemical findings. Diagn Cytopathol. 1991;7(1):83–7. PMID:1709089
578. Cosío BG, Villena V, Echave-Sustaeta J, et al. Endobronchial hamartoma. Chest. 2002 Jul;122(1):202–5. PMID:12114359
579. Costanzo L, Scarlata S, Perrone G, et al. Malignant transformation of well-differentiated papillary mesothelioma 13 years after the diagnosis: a case report. Clin Respir J. 2014 Jan;8(1):124–9. PMID:24118858
580. Courtiol P, Maussion C, Moarii M, et al. Deep learning-based classification of mesothelioma improves prediction of patient outcome. Nat Med. 2019 Oct;25(10):1519–25. PMID:31591589
581. Coustan-Smith E, Mullighan CG, Onciu M, et al. Early T-cell precursor leukaemia: a subtype of very high-risk acute lymphoblastic leukaemia. Lancet Oncol. 2009 Feb;10(2):147–56. PMID:19147408
582. Cozzi D, Dini C, Mungai F, et al. Primary pulmonary lymphoma: imaging findings in 30 cases. Radiol Med. 2019 Dec;124(12):1262–9. PMID:31583557
583. Crago AM, Chmielecki J, Rosenberg M, et al. Near universal detection of alterations in CTNNB1 and Wnt pathway regulators in desmoid-type fibromatosis by whole-exome sequencing and genomic analysis. Genes Chromosomes Cancer. 2015 Oct;54(10):606–15. PMID:26171757
584. Cree IA, Foss AJ, Luthert PJ. Undefined high-power fields. Lancet. 1996 Jan 27;347(8996):273–4. PMID:8551926
585. Creytens D. A contemporary review of myxoid adipocytic tumors. Semin Diagn Pathol. 2019 Mar;36(2):129–41. PMID:30853315
586. Creytens D. SATB2 and TLE1 expression in BCOR-CCNB3 (Ewing-like) sarcoma, mimicking small cell osteosarcoma and poorly differentiated synovial sarcoma.

Appl Immunohistochem Mol Morphol. 2020 Jan;28(1):e10–2. PMID:29084055

587. Creytens D. What's new in adipocytic neoplasia? Virchows Arch. 2020 Jan;476(1):29–39. PMID:31501988

588. Crombé A, Alberti N, Villard N, et al. Imaging features of SMARCA4-deficient thoracic sarcomas: a multi-centric study of 21 patients. Eur Radiol. 2019 Sep;29(9):4730–41. PMID:30762113

589. Crombé A, Lintingre PF, Le Loarer F, et al. Multiple skeletal muscle metastases revealing a cardiac intimal sarcoma. Skeletal Radiol. 2018 Jan;47(1):125–30. PMID:28887581

590. Crona J, Björklund P, Welin S, et al. Treatment, prognostic markers and survival in thymic neuroendocrine tumours. a study from a single tertiary referral centre. Lung Cancer. 2013 Mar;79(3):289–93. PMID:23286964

591. Croti UA, Braile DM, Moscardini AC, et al. [Solitary fibrous tumor in a child's heart]. Rev Bras Cir Cardiovasc. 2008 Jan-Mar;23(1):139–41. Portuguese. PMID:18719844

592. Crotty EJ, McAdams HP, Erasmus JJ, et al. Epithelioid hemangioendothelioma of the pleura: clinical and radiologic features. AJR Am J Roentgenol. 2000 Dec;175(6):1545–9. PMID:11090371

593. Crotty TB, Edwards WD, Oh JK, et al. Lipomatous hamartoma of the tricuspid valve: echocardiographic-pathologic correlations. Clin Cardiol. 1991 Mar;14(3):262–6. PMID:2013183

594. Crotty TB, Myers JL, Katzenstein AL, et al. Localized malignant mesothelioma. A clinicopathologic and flow cytometric study. Am J Surg Pathol. 1994 Apr;18(4):357–63. PMID:7511353

595. Crow J, Slavin G, Kreel L. Pulmonary metastasis: a pathologic and radiologic study. Cancer. 1981 Jun 1;47(11):2595–602. PMID:7260854

596. Cui A, Jin XG, Zhai K, et al. Diagnostic values of soluble mesothelin-related peptides for malignant pleural mesothelioma: updated meta-analysis. BMJ Open. 2014 Feb 24;4(2):e004145. PMID:24566531

597. Cui M, Augert A, Rongione M, et al. PTEN is a potent suppressor of small cell lung cancer. Mol Cancer Res. 2014 May;12(5):654–9. PMID:24482365

598. Curry WA, McKay CE, Richardson RL, et al. Klinefelter's syndrome and mediastinal germ cell neoplasms. J Urol. 1981 Jan;125(1):127–9. PMID:7193252

599. Cusumano G, Fournel L, Strano S, et al. Surgical resection for pulmonary carcinoid: long-term results of multicentric study-the importance of pathological N status, more than we thought. Lung. 2017 Dec;195(6):789–98. PMID:29022070

600. Dacic S, Finkelstein SD, Sasatomi E, et al. Molecular pathogenesis of pulmonary carcinosarcoma as determined by microdissection-based allelotyping. Am J Surg Pathol. 2002 Apr;26(4):510–6. PMID:11914631

601. Dacic S, Le Stang N, Husain A, et al. Interobserver variation in the assessment of the sarcomatoid and transitional components in biphasic mesotheliomas. Mod Pathol. 2020 Feb;33(2):255–62. PMID:31273316

601A. Dacic S, Roy S, Lyons MA, et al. Whole exome sequencing reveals BAP1 somatic abnormalities in mesothelioma in situ. Lung Cancer. 2020 Nov;149:1–4. PMID:32932212

602. Dagogo-Jack I, Schrock AB, Kem M, et al. Clinicopathologic characteristics of BRG1-deficient NSCLC. J Thorac Oncol. 2020 May;15(5):766–76. PMID:31988001

603. Daher T, Tur MK, Brobeil A, et al. Combined human papillomavirus typing and TP53 mutation analysis in distinguishing second primary tumors from lung metastases in patients with head and neck squamous cell carcinoma. Head Neck. 2018 Jun;40(6):1109–19. PMID:29522268

604. Dail DH, Liebow AA, Gmelich JT, et al. Intravascular, bronchiolar, and alveolar tumor of the lung (IVBAT). An analysis of twenty cases of a peculiar sclerosing endothelial tumor. Cancer. 1983 Feb 1;51(3):452–64. PMID:6295602

605. Dainese E, Pozzi B, Milani M, et al. Primary pleural epithelioid angiosarcoma. A case report and review of the literature. Pathol Res Pract. 2010 Jun 15;206(6):415–9. PMID:20089367

606. Dal Cin P, De Wolf-Peeters C, Deneffe G, et al. Thymoma with a t(15;22)(p11;q11). Cancer Genet Cytogenet. 1996 Jul 15;89(2):181–3. PMID:8697431

607. Dal Cin P, Kools P, De Jonge I, et al. Rearrangement of 12q14-15 in pulmonary chondroid hamartoma. Genes Chromosomes Cancer. 1993 Oct;8(2):131–3. PMID:7504517

608. Dalia S, Jaglal M, Chervenick P, et al. Clinicopathologic characteristics and outcomes of histiocytic and dendritic cell neoplasms: the Moffitt Cancer Center experience over the last twenty five years. Cancers (Basel). 2014 Nov 14;6(4):2275–95. PMID:25405526

609. Dalia S, Shao H, Sagatys E, et al. Dendritic cell and histiocytic neoplasms: biology, diagnosis, and treatment. Cancer Control. 2014 Oct;21(4):290–300. PMID:25310210

610. Dalsgaard SB, Würtz ET, Hansen J, et al. Environmental asbestos exposure in childhood and risk of mesothelioma later in life: a long-term follow-up register-based cohort study. Occup Environ Med. 2019 Jun;76(6):407–13. PMID:30804166

611. Damadoglu E, Salturk C, Takir HB, et al. Mediastinal thymolipoma: an analysis of 10 cases. Respirology. 2007 Nov;12(6):924–7. PMID:17986126

612. Danel C, Israel-Biet D, Costabel U, et al. The clinical role of BAL in pulmonary histiocytosis X. Eur Respir J. 1990 Sep;3(8):949–50, 961–9. PMID:2292298

613. Daniels JM, Sutedja TG. Detection and minimally invasive treatment of early squamous lung cancer. Ther Adv Med Oncol. 2013 Jul;5(4):235–48. PMID:23858332

614. Das DK. Serous effusions in malignant lymphomas: a review. Diagn Cytopathol. 2006 May;34(5):335–47. PMID:16604559

615. Dasanu CA, Shimanovsky A, Jain K, et al. Mediastinal choriocarcinoma presenting with syncope. Conn Med. 2013 Sep;77(8):473–5. PMID:24156175

616. Dasgupta S, Bose D, Bhattacharyya NK, et al. A clinicopathological study of mediastinal masses operated in a tertiary care hospital in Eastern India in 3 years with special reference to thymoma. Indian J Pathol Microbiol. 2016 Jan-Mar;59(1):20–4. PMID:26960629

617. Dashiell TG, Payne WS, Hepper NG, et al. Desmoid tumors of the chest wall. Chest. 1978 Aug;74(2):157–62. PMID:679743

618. Datta D, Gerardi DA, Lahiri B. Mediastinal angiosarcoma presenting as diffuse alveolar hemorrhage. Respir Med Case Rep. 2018 Feb 3;23:115–7. PMID:29719795

619. Davies SJ, Gosney JR, Hansell DM, et al. Diffuse idiopathic pulmonary neuroendocrine cell hyperplasia: an under-recognised spectrum of disease. Thorax. 2007 Mar;62(3):248–52. PMID:17099078

620. Davis MP, Eagan RT, Weiland LH, et al. Carcinosarcoma of the lung: Mayo Clinic experience and response to chemotherapy. Mayo Clin Proc. 1984 Sep;59(9):598–603. PMID:6381913

621. Davis R, Deak K, Glass CH. Pulmonary granular cell tumors: a study of 4 cases including a malignant phenotype. Am J Surg Pathol. 2019 Oct;43(10):1397–402. PMID:31180915

622. Davis SD. CT evaluation for pulmonary metastases in patients with extrathoracic malignancy. Radiology. 1991 Jul;180(1):1–12. PMID:2052672

623. Daya SK, Gowda RM, Gowda MR, et al. Thoracic cystic lymphangioma (cystic hygroma): a chest pain syndrome–a case report. Angiology. 2004 Sep-Oct;55(5):561–4. PMID:15378120

624. de Andrade KC, Mirabello L, Stewart DR, et al. Higher-than-expected population prevalence of potentially pathogenic germline TP53 variants in individuals unselected for cancer history. Hum Mutat. 2017 Dec;38(12):1723–30. PMID:28861920

625. De Backer A, Madern GC, Pieters R, et al. Influence of tumor site and histology on long-term survival in 193 children with extracranial germ cell tumors. Eur J Pediatr Surg. 2008 Feb;18(1):1–6. PMID:18302061

626. de Bruin EC, McGranahan N, Mitter R, et al. Spatial and temporal diversity in genomic instability processes defines lung cancer evolution. Science. 2014 Oct 10;346(6206):251–6. PMID:25301630

627. de Hoop B, Schaefer-Prokop C, Gietema HA, et al. Screening for lung cancer with digital chest radiography: sensitivity and number of secondary work-up CT examinations. Radiology. 2010 May;255(2):629–37. PMID:20413773

628. de Jong WK, Blaauwgeers JL, Schaapveld M, et al. Thymic epithelial tumours: a population-based study of the incidence, diagnostic procedures and therapy. Eur J Cancer. 2008 Jan;44(1):123–30. PMID:18068351

629. de Kock L, Bah I, Brunet J, et al. Somatic DICER1 mutations in adult-onset pulmonary blastoma. Eur Respir J. 2016 Jun;47(6):1879–82. PMID:27126690

630. de Kock L, Bah I, Wu Y, et al. Germline and somatic DICER1 mutations in a well-differentiated fetal adenocarcinoma of the lung. J Thorac Oncol. 2016 Mar;11(3):e31–3. PMID:26886166

631. de Koning HJ, van der Aalst CM, de Jong PA, et al. Reduced lung-cancer mortality with volume CT screening in a randomized trial. N Engl J Med. 2020 Feb 6;382(6):503–13. PMID:31995683

632. de Leval L, Ferry JA, Falini B, et al. Expression of bcl-6 and CD10 in primary mediastinal large B-cell lymphoma: evidence for derivation from germinal center B cells? Am J Surg Pathol. 2001 Oct;25(10):1277–82. PMID:11688462

633. de Los Santos-Aguilar RG, Chávez-Villa M, Contreras AG, et al. Successful multimodal treatment of an IGF2-producing solitary fibrous tumor with acromegaloid changes and hypoglycemia. J Endocr Soc. 2019 Jan 8;3(3):537–43. PMID:30788455

633A. de Noronha L, Cecílio WA, da Silva TF, et al. Congenital peribronchial myofibroblastic tumor: a case report. Pediatr Dev Pathol. 2010 May-Jun;13(3):243–6. PMID:20064015

634. De Pas TM, Giovannini M, Manzotti M, et al. Large-cell neuroendocrine carcinoma of the lung harboring EGFR mutation and responding to gefitinib. J Clin Oncol. 2011 Dec 1;29(34):e819–22. PMID:22042963

635. De Pasquale MD, Crocoli A, Conte M, et al. Mediastinal germ cell tumors in pediatric patients: a report from the Italian Association of Pediatric Hematology and Oncology. Pediatr Blood Cancer. 2016 May;63(5):808–12. PMID:26766550

636. de Perrot M, Spiliopoulos A, Fischer S, et al. Neuroendocrine carcinoma (carcinoid) of the thymus associated with Cushing's syndrome. Ann Thorac Surg. 2002 Feb;73(2):675–81. PMID:11845907

637. de Queiroga EM, Chikota H, Bacchi CE, et al. Rhabdomyomatous carcinoma of the thymus. Am J Surg Pathol. 2004

Sep;28(9):1245–50. PMID:15316327

638. De Raedt T, Beert E, Pasmant E, et al. PRC2 loss amplifies Ras-driven transcription and confers sensitivity to BRD4-based therapies. Nature. 2014 Oct 9;514(7521):247–51. PMID:25119042

639. De Rosa N, Maiorino A, De Rosa I, et al. CD34 expression in the stromal cells of alveolar adenoma. Case Rep Med. 2012;2012:913517. PMID:23118769

640. de Vilhena AF, das Neves Pereira JC, Parra ER, et al. Histomorphometric evaluation of the Ki-67 proliferation rate and CD34 microvascular and D2-40 lymphovascular densities drives the pulmonary typical carcinoid outcome. Hum Pathol. 2018 Nov;81:201–10. PMID:30031097

641. de Wilt JH, Farmer SE, Scolyer RA, et al. Isolated melanoma in the lung where there is no known primary site: metastatic disease or primary lung tumour? Melanoma Res. 2005 Dec;15(6):531–7. PMID:16314739

642. Dear RF, Kelly PJ, Wright GM, et al. Pulmonary metastasectomy for bone and soft tissue sarcoma in Australia: 114 patients from 1978 to 2008. Asia Pac J Clin Oncol. 2012 Sep;8(3):292–302. PMID:22897801

643. Deavers M, Guinee D, Koss MN, et al. Granular cell tumors of the lung. Clinicopathologic study of 20 cases. Am J Surg Pathol. 1995 Jun;19(6):627–35. PMID:7755149

644. Debelenko LV, Brambilla E, Agarwal SK, et al. Identification of MEN1 gene mutations in sporadic carcinoid tumors of the lung. Hum Mol Genet. 1997 Dec;6(13):2285–90. PMID:9361035

645. Debelenko LV, Swalwell JI, Kelley MJ, et al. MEN1 gene mutation analysis of high-grade neuroendocrine lung carcinoma. Genes Chromosomes Cancer. 2000 May;28(1):58–65. PMID:10738303

646. Deepak J, Babu MN, Gowrishankar BC, et al. Mediastinal hemangioma: masquerading as pleural effusion. J Indian Assoc Pediatr Surg. 2013 Oct;18(4):162–4. PMID:24347874

647. Delas A, Gaulard P, Plat G, et al. Follicular variant of peripheral T cell lymphoma with mediastinal involvement in a child: a case report. Virchows Arch. 2015 Mar;466(3):351–5. PMID:25604350

648. Delisle V, Perron J, Lafrenière-Bessi V, et al. Neonatal cardiac arrest from left ventricular cardiac hemangioma: a surprising presentation. Can J Cardiol. 2019 Apr;35(4):544.e3–5. PMID:30935649

649. Dell'Amore A, Lanzanova G, Silenzi A, et al. Hamartoma of mature cardiac myocytes: case report and review of the literature. Heart Lung Circ. 2011 May;20(5):336–40. PMID:21354369

650. DeMent SH, Eggleston JC, Spivak JL. Association between mediastinal germ cell tumors and hematologic malignancies. Report of two cases and review of the literature. Am J Surg Pathol. 1985 Jan;9(1):23–30. PMID:3855613

651. Demicco EG, Harms PW, Patel RM, et al. Extensive survey of STAT6 expression in a large series of mesenchymal tumors. Am J Clin Pathol. 2015 May;143(5):672–82. PMID:25873501

652. Demicco EG, Park MS, Araujo DM, et al. Solitary fibrous tumor: a clinicopathological study of 110 cases and proposed risk assessment model. Mod Pathol. 2012 Sep;25(9):1298–306. PMID:22575866

653. Demicco EG, Wagner MJ, Maki RG, et al. Risk assessment in solitary fibrous tumors: validation and refinement of a risk stratification model. Mod Pathol. 2017 Oct;30(10):1433–42. PMID:28731041

654. Demir HA, Ekici F, Yazal Erdem A, et al.

Everolimus: a challenging drug in the treatment of multifocal inoperable cardiac rhabdomyoma. Pediatrics. 2012 Jul;130(1):e243–7. PMID:22732179
655. Demir HA, Yalçin B, Büyükpamukçu N, et al. Thoracic neuroblastic tumors in childhood. Pediatr Blood Cancer. 2010 Jul 1;54(7):885–9. PMID:20049935
656. de Montpréville VT, Macchiarini P, Dulmet E. Thymic neuroendocrine carcinoma (carcinoid): a clinicopathologic study of fourteen cases. J Thorac Cardiovasc Surg. 1996 Jan;111(1):134–41. PMID:8551758
657. den Bakker MA, Beverloo BH, van den Heuvel-Eibrink MM, et al. NUT midline carcinoma of the parotid gland with mesenchymal differentiation. Am J Surg Pathol. 2009 Aug;33(8):1253–8. PMID:19561446
658. den Bakker MA, Marx A, Mukai K, et al. Mesenchymal tumours of the mediastinum–part I. Virchows Arch. 2015 Nov;467(5):487–500. PMID:26358059
659. den Bakker MA, Oosterhuis JW. Tumours and tumour-like conditions of the thymus other than thymoma; a practical approach. Histopathology. 2009 Jan;54(1):69–89. PMID:19054157
659A. den Bakker MA, Willemsen S, Grünberg K, et al. Small cell carcinoma of the lung and large cell neuroendocrine carcinoma interobserver variability. Histopathology. 2010 Feb;56(3):356–63. PMID:20459535
660. Deng C, Wu SG, Tian Y. Lung large cell neuroendocrine carcinoma: an analysis of patients from the Surveillance, Epidemiology, and End-Results (SEER) database. Med Sci Monit. 2019 May 16;25:3636–46. PMID:31095532
661. De Oliveira Duarte Achcar R, Nikiforova MN, Yousem SA. Micropapillary lung adenocarcinoma: EGFR, K-ras, and BRAF mutational profile. Am J Clin Pathol. 2009 May;131(5):694–700. PMID:19369630
662. Deora S, Gurmukhani S, Shah S, et al. Cardiac epithelioid leiomyosarcoma as both intracardiac and pericardial mass with massive pericardial effusion: a rare presentation. J Am Coll Cardiol. 2013 Sep 24;62(13):e25. PMID:23916929
663. Derenoncourt AN, Castro-Magana M, Jones KL. Mediastinal teratoma and precocious puberty in a boy with mosaic Klinefelter syndrome. Am J Med Genet. 1995 Jan 2;55(1):38–42. PMID:7535510
664. Derkay CS, Wiatrak B. Recurrent respiratory papillomatosis: a review. Laryngoscope. 2008 Jul;118(7):1236–47. PMID:18496162
665. Derks JL, Dingemans AC, van Suylen RJ, et al. Is the sum of positive neuroendocrine immunohistochemical stains useful for diagnosis of large cell neuroendocrine carcinoma (LCNEC) on biopsy specimens? Histopathology. 2019 Mar;74(4):555–66. PMID:30485478
666. Derks JL, Hendriks LE, Buikhuisen WA, et al. Clinical features of large cell neuroendocrine carcinoma: a population-based overview. Eur Respir J. 2016 Feb;47(2):615–24. PMID:26541538
667. Derks JL, Leblay N, Lantuejoul S, et al. New insights into the molecular characteristics of pulmonary carcinoids and large cell neuroendocrine carcinomas, and the impact on their clinical management. J Thorac Oncol. 2018 Jun;13(6):752–66. PMID:29454048
668. Derks JL, Leblay N, Thunnissen E, et al. Molecular subtypes of pulmonary large-cell neuroendocrine carcinoma predict chemotherapy treatment outcome. Clin Cancer Res. 2018 Jan 1;24(1):33–42. PMID:29066508
669. Dermawan JK, Doxtader E, Chute DJ, et al. Cytologic findings of an adult rhabdomyoma in the parapharyngeal space: a report of a case and review of the literature. Diagn Cytopathol. 2018 May;46(5):419–24. PMID:29131558
670. Dermawan JK, Farver CF. The prognostic significance of the 8th edition TNM staging of pulmonary carcinoid tumors: a single institution study with long-term follow-up. Am J Surg Pathol. 2019 Sep;43(9):1291–6. PMID:31094922
671. Dermawan JKT, Farver CF. The role of histologic grading and Ki-67 index in predicting outcomes in pulmonary carcinoid tumors. Am J Surg Pathol. 2020 Feb;44(2):224–31. PMID:31490236
672. Dermawan JKT, Policarpio-Nicolas ML. Malignancies in pleural, peritoneal, and pericardial effusions. Arch Pathol Lab Med. 2020 Sep 1;144(9):1086–91. PMID31913661
673. Desai NR, Lee HJ. Diagnosis and management of malignant pleural effusions: state of the art in 2017. J Thorac Dis. 2017 Sep;9(Suppl 10):S1111–22. PMID:29214068
674. de Saint Aubain Somerhausen N, Rubin BP, Fletcher CD. Myxoid solitary fibrous tumor: a study of seven cases with emphasis on differential diagnosis. Mod Pathol. 1999 May;12(5):463–71. PMID:10349983
675. Desmeules P, Joubert P, Zhang L, et al. A subset of malignant mesotheliomas in young adults are associated with recurrent EWSR1/FUS-ATF1 fusions. Am J Surg Pathol. 2017 Jul;41(7):980–8. PMID:28505004
676. Dessy E, Braidotti P, Del Curto B, et al. Peripheral papillary tumor of type-II pneumocytes: a rare neoplasm of undetermined malignant potential. Virchows Arch. 2000 Mar;436(3):289–95. PMID:10782889
677. Detterbeck F, Decker RH, Tanaoue L, et al. Non-small cell lung cancer. In: DeVita VT, Lawrence TS, Rosenberg SA, editors. DeVita, Hellman, and Rosenberg's cancer: principles and practice of oncology. 10th ed. Philadelphia (PA): Wolters Kluwer; 2015. pp. 495–535.
678. Detterbeck F, Youssef S, Ruffini E, et al. A review of prognostic factors in thymic malignancies. J Thorac Oncol. 2011 Jul;6(7 Suppl 3):S1698–704. PMID:21847050
679. Detterbeck FC. Clinical value of the WHO classification system of thymoma. Ann Thorac Surg. 2006 Jun;81(6):2328–34. PMID:16731193
680. Detterbeck FC, Bolejack V, Arenberg DA, et al. The IASLC Lung Cancer Staging Project: background data and proposals for the classification of lung cancer with separate tumor nodules in the forthcoming eighth edition of the TNM classification for lung cancer. J Thorac Oncol. 2016 May;11(5):681–92. PMID:26940530
681. Detterbeck FC, Chansky K, Groome P, et al. The IASLC Lung Cancer Staging Project: methodology and validation used in the development of proposals for revision of the stage classification of NSCLC in the forthcoming (eighth) edition of the TNM classification of lung cancer. J Thorac Oncol. 2016 Sep;11(9):1433–46. PMID:27448762
682. Detterbeck FC, Franklin WA, Nicholson AG, et al. The IASLC Lung Cancer Staging Project: background data and proposed criteria to distinguish separate primary lung cancers from metastatic foci in patients with two lung tumors in the forthcoming eighth edition of the TNM classification for lung cancer. J Thorac Oncol. 2016 May;11(5):651–65. PMID:26944304
683. Detterbeck FC, Marom EM, Arenberg DA, et al. The IASLC Lung Cancer Staging Project: background data and proposals for the application of TNM staging rules to lung cancer presenting as multiple nodules with ground glass or lepidic features or a pneumonic type of involvement in the forthcoming eighth edition of the TNM classification. J Thorac Oncol. 2016 May;11(5):666–80. PMID:26940527
684. Detterbeck FC, Nicholson AG, Franklin WA, et al. The IASLC Lung Cancer Staging Project: summary of proposals for revisions of the classification of lung cancers with multiple pulmonary sites of involvement in the forthcoming eighth edition of the TNM classification. J Thorac Oncol. 2016 May;11(5):639–50. PMID:26940528
685. Detterbeck FC, Nicholson AG, Kondo K, et al. The Masaoka-Koga stage classification for thymic malignancies: clarification and definition of terms. J Thorac Oncol. 2011 Jul;6(7 Suppl 3):S1710–6. PMID:21847052
686. Detterbeck FC, Parsons AM. Thymic tumors. Ann Thorac Surg. 2004 May;77(5):1860–9. PMID:15111216
687. Detterbeck FC, Stratton K, Giroux D, et al. The IASLC/ITMIG Thymic Epithelial Tumors Staging Project: proposal for an evidence-based stage classification system for the forthcoming (8th) edition of the TNM classification of malignant tumors. J Thorac Oncol. 2014 Sep;9(9 Suppl 2):S65–72. PMID:25396314
688. Devouassoux-Shisheboran M, de la Fouchardière A, Thivolet-Béjui F, et al. Endobronchial variant of sclerosing hemangioma of the lung: histological and cytological features on endobronchial material. Mod Pathol. 2004 Feb;17(2):252–7. PMID:14704717
689. Devouassoux-Shisheboran M, Hayashi T, Linnoila RI, et al. A clinicopathologic study of 100 cases of pulmonary sclerosing hemangioma with immunohistochemical studies: TTF-1 is expressed in both round and surface cells, suggesting an origin from primitive respiratory epithelium. Am J Surg Pathol. 2000 Jul;24(7):906–16. PMID:10895813
690. Dewaele B, Floris G, Finalet-Ferreiro J, et al. Coactivated platelet-derived growth factor receptor alpha and epidermal growth factor receptor are potential therapeutic targets in intimal sarcoma. Cancer Res. 2010 Sep 15;70(18):7304–14. PMID:20685895
691. Dexeus FH, Logothetis CJ, Chong C, et al. Genetic abnormalities in men with germ cell tumors. J Urol. 1988 Jul;140(1):80–4. PMID:2837589
692. Deyrup AT, Lee VK, Hill CE, et al. Epstein-Barr virus-associated smooth muscle tumors are distinctive mesenchymal tumors reflecting multiple infection events: a clinicopathologic and molecular analysis of 29 tumors from 19 patients. Am J Surg Pathol. 2006 Jan;30(1):75–82. PMID:16330945
693. Deyrup AT, Miettinen M, North PE, et al. Angiosarcomas arising in the viscera and soft tissue of children and young adults: a clinicopathologic study of 15 cases. Am J Surg Pathol. 2009 Feb;33(2):264–9. PMID:18987547
694. Deyrup AT, Tighiouart M, Montag AG, et al. Epithelioid hemangioendothelioma of soft tissue: a proposal for risk stratification based on 49 cases. Am J Surg Pathol. 2008 Jun;32(6):924–7. PMID:18551749
695. Di Tommaso L, Kuhn E, Kurrer M, et al. Thymic tumor with adenoid cystic carcinomalike features: a clinicopathologic study of 4 cases. Am J Surg Pathol. 2007 Aug;31(8):1161–7. PMID:17667537
696. Diamond EL, Dagna L, Hyman DM, et al. Consensus guidelines for the diagnosis and clinical management of Erdheim-Chester disease. Blood. 2014 Jul 24;124(4):483–92. PMID:24850756
697. Diamond EL, Durham BH, Haroche J, et al. Diverse and targetable kinase alterations drive histiocytic neoplasms. Cancer Discov. 2016 Feb;6(2):154–65. PMID:26566875
698. Diamond EL, Durham BH, Ulaner GA, et al. Efficacy of MEK inhibition in patients with histiocytic neoplasms. Nature. 2019 Mar;567(7749):521–4. PMID:30867592
699. Diamond EL, Subbiah V, Lockhart AC, et al. Vemurafenib for BRAF V600-mutant Erdheim-Chester disease and Langerhans cell histiocytosis: analysis of data from the histology-independent, phase 2, open-label VE-BASKET study. JAMA Oncol. 2018 Mar 1;4(3):384–8. PMID:29188284
700. Dias P, Chen B, Dilday B, et al. Strong immunostaining for myogenin in rhabdomyosarcoma is significantly associated with tumors of the alveolar subclass. Am J Pathol. 2000 Feb;156(2):399–408. PMID:10666368
701. Diaz-Perez JA, Nielsen GP, Antonescu C, et al. EWSR1/FUS-NFATc2 rearranged round cell sarcoma: clinicopathological series of 4 cases and literature review. Hum Pathol. 2019 Aug;90:45–53. PMID:31078563
702. DiBardino DM, Rawson DW, Saqi A, et al. Next-generation sequencing of non-small cell lung cancer using a customized, targeted sequencing panel: emphasis on small biopsy and cytology. Cytojournal. 2017 Mar 20;14:7. PMID:28413430
703. Dickson BC, Sung YS, Rosenblum MK, et al. NUTM1 gene fusions characterize a subset of undifferentiated soft tissue and visceral tumors. Am J Surg Pathol. 2018 May;42(5):636–45. PMID:29356724
704. Digumarthy SR, Mendoza DP, Zhang EW, et al. Clinicopathologic and imaging features of non-small-cell lung cancer with MET exon 14 skipping mutations. Cancers (Basel). 2019 Dec 17;11(12):E2033. PMID:31861060
705. Dijkhuizen T, de Jong B, Meuzelaar JJ, et al. No cytogenetic evidence for involvement of gene(s) at 2p16 in sporadic cardiac myxomas: cytogenetic changes in ten sporadic cardiac myxomas. Cancer Genet Cytogenet. 2001 Apr 15;126(2):162–5. PMID:11376810
706. Dillon KM, Hill CM, Cameron CH, et al. Mediastinal mixed dendritic cell sarcoma with hybrid features. J Clin Pathol. 2002 Oct;55(10):791–4. PMID:12354813
707. Dimitriades VR, Devlin V, Pittaluga S, et al. DOCK 8 deficiency, EBV+ lymphomatoid granulomatosis, and intrafamilial variation in presentation. Front Pediatr. 2017 Feb 28;5:38. PMID:28293550
708. Ding L, Getz G, Wheeler DA, et al. Somatic mutations affect key pathways in lung adenocarcinoma. Nature. 2008 Oct 23;455(7216):1069–75. PMID:18948947
709. Dinmohamed AG, Visser O, Doorduijn JK, et al. Treatment and survival of patients with primary effusion lymphoma in the Netherlands: a population-based analysis, 2002-2015. Hemasphere. 2018 Oct;2(5):e143. PMID:30887007
710. Dinter H, Bohnenberger H, Beck J, et al. Molecular classification of neuroendocrine tumors of the thymus. J Thorac Oncol. 2019 Aug;14(8):1472–83. PMID:31042566
711. Diolaiti D, Dela Cruz FS, Gundem G, et al. A recurrent novel MGA-NUTM1 fusion identifies a new subtype of high-grade spindle cell sarcoma. Cold Spring Harb Mol Case Stud. 2018 Dec 17;4(6):a003194. PMID:30552129
712. Di Sant'Agnese PA, Knowles DM 2nd. Extracardiac rhabdomyoma: a clinicopathologic study and review of the literature. Cancer. 1980 Aug 15;46(4):780–9. PMID:7397640
713. Dishop MK, McKay EM, Kreiger PA, et al. Fetal lung interstitial tumor (FLIT): a proposed newly recognized lung tumor of infancy to be differentiated from cystic pleuropulmonary blastoma and other developmental pulmonary lesions. Am J Surg Pathol. 2010 Dec;34(12):1762–72. PMID:21107081
714. Disibio G, French SW. Metastatic patterns of cancers: results from a large autopsy study. Arch Pathol Lab Med. 2008 Jun;132(6):931–9. PMID:18517275

715. Di Vito A, Mignogna C, Donato G. The mysterious pathways of cardiac myxomas: a review of histogenesis, pathogenesis and pathology. Histopathology. 2015 Feb;66(3):321–32. PMID:25297937

716. Dojcinov SD, Fend F, Quintanilla-Martinez L. EBV-positive lymphoproliferations of B- T- and NK-cell derivation in non-immunocompromised hosts. Pathogens. 2018 Mar 7;7(1):E28. PMID:29518976

717. Dojcinov SD, Venkataraman G, Pittaluga S, et al. Age-related EBV-associated lymphoproliferative disorders in the Western population: a spectrum of reactive lymphoid hyperplasia and lymphoma. Blood. 2011 May 5;117(18):4726–35. PMID:21385849

718. Dômont J, Salas S, Lacroix L, et al. High frequency of beta-catenin heterozygous mutations in extra-abdominal fibromatosis: a potential molecular tool for disease management. Br J Cancer. 2010 Mar 16;102(6):1032–6. PMID:20197769

719. Dorfman DM, Shahsafaei A, Chan JK. Thymic carcinomas, but not thymomas and carcinomas of other sites, show CD5 immunoreactivity. Am J Surg Pathol. 1997 Aug;21(8):936–40. PMID:9255257

720. Doroshow DB, Sanmamed MF, Hastings K, et al. Immunotherapy in non-small cell lung cancer: facts and hopes. Clin Cancer Res. 2019 Aug 1;25(15):4592–602. PMID:30824587

721. dos Santos CL, Fernandes LR, Meruje M, et al. Primary pulmonary melanoma: the unexpected tumour. BMJ Case Rep. 2013 Oct 9;2013:bcr2013200706. PMID:24108769

722. Dosios TJ, Angouras DC, Floros DG. Primary desmoid tumor of the posterior mediastinum. Ann Thorac Surg. 1998 Dec;66(6):2098–9. PMID:9930504

723. Dotto GP, Rustgi AK. Squamous cell cancers: a unified perspective on biology and genetics. Cancer Cell. 2016 May 9;29(5):622–37. PMID:27165741

724. Dotto J, Pelosi G, Rosai J. Expression of p63 in thymomas and normal thymus. Am J Clin Pathol. 2007 Mar;127(3):415–20. PMID:17276940

725. Downie PA, Vogelzang NJ, Moldwin RL, et al. Establishment of a leukemia cell line with i(12p) from a patient with a mediastinal germ cell tumor and acute lymphoblastic leukemia. Cancer Res. 1994 Sep 15;54(18):4999–5004. PMID:8069867

726. Doxtader EE, Shah AA, Zhang Y, et al. Primary salivary gland-type tumors of the tracheobronchial tree diagnosed by transbronchial fine needle aspiration: clinical and cytomorphologic features with histopathologic correlation. Diagn Cytopathol. 2019 Nov;47(11):1168–76. PMID:31343850

727. Doyle LA, Fletcher CD, Hornick JL. Nuclear expression of CAMTA1 distinguishes epithelioid hemangioendothelioma from histologic mimics. Am J Surg Pathol. 2016 Jan;40(1):94–102. PMID:26414223

728. Doyle LA, Hornick JL, Fletcher CD. PEComa of the gastrointestinal tract: clinicopathologic study of 35 cases with evaluation of prognostic parameters. Am J Surg Pathol. 2013 Dec;37(12):1769–82. PMID:24061520

729. Doyle LA, Vivero M, Fletcher CD, et al. Nuclear expression of STAT6 distinguishes solitary fibrous tumor from histologic mimics. Mod Pathol. 2014 Mar;27(3):390–5. PMID:24030747

730. Dragoescu EA, Liu L. Pericardial fluid cytology: an analysis of 128 specimens over a 6-year period. Cancer Cytopathol. 2013 May;121(5):242–51. PMID:23362233

730A. Drilon A, Oxnard GR, Tan DSW, et al. Efficacy of selpercatinib in RET fusion-positive non-small-cell lung cancer. N Engl J Med. 2020 Aug 27;383(9):813–24. PMID:32846060

731. Driver BR, Portier BP, Mody DR, et al. Next-generation sequencing of a cohort of pulmonary large cell carcinomas reclassified by World Health Organization 2015 criteria. Arch Pathol Lab Med. 2016 Apr;140(4):312–7. PMID:26430808

732. Du EZ, Goldstraw P, Zacharias J, et al. TTF-1 expression is specific for lung primary in typical and atypical carcinoids: TTF-1-positive carcinoids are predominantly in peripheral location. Hum Pathol. 2004 Jul;35(7):825–31. PMID:15257545

733. Du M, Thompson J, Fisher H, et al. Genomic alterations of plasma cell-free DNAs in small cell lung cancer and their clinical relevance. Lung Cancer. 2018 Jun;120:113–21. PMID:29748005

734. Du MJ, Shen Q, Yin H, et al. Diagnostic roles of MUC1 and GLUT1 in differentiating thymic carcinoma from type B3 thymoma. Pathol Res Pract. 2016 Nov;212(11):1048–51. PMID:27688088

735. Duan F, Smith LM, Gustafson DM, et al. Genomic and clinical analysis of fusion gene amplification in rhabdomyosarcoma: a report from the Children's Oncology Group. Genes Chromosomes Cancer. 2012 Jul;51(7):662–74. PMID:22447499

736. Duan XF, Zhao Q. TERT-mediated and ATRX-mediated telomere maintenance and neuroblastoma. J Pediatr Hematol Oncol. 2018 Jan;40(1):1–6. PMID:28452859

737. Duarte IG, Bufkin BL, Pennington MF, et al. Angiogenesis as a predictor of survival after surgical resection for stage I non-small-cell lung cancer. J Thorac Cardiovasc Surg. 1998 Mar;115(3):652–8, discussion 658–9. PMID:9535454

738. Dubois S, Viailly PJ, Mareschal S, et al. Next-generation sequencing in diffuse large B-cell lymphoma highlights molecular divergence and therapeutic opportunities: a LYSA study. Clin Cancer Res. 2016 Jun 15;22(12):2919–28. PMID:26819451

739. Dubois SG, London WB, Zhang Y, et al. Lung metastases in neuroblastoma at initial diagnosis: a report from the International Neuroblastoma Risk Group (INRG) project. Pediatr Blood Cancer. 2008 Nov;51(5):589–92. PMID:18649370

740. Ducassou S, Seyrig F, Thomas C, et al. Thymus and mediastinal node involvement in childhood Langerhans cell histiocytosis: long-term follow-up from the French national cohort. Pediatr Blood Cancer. 2013 Nov;60(11):1759–65. PMID:23813854

741. Ducatman BS, Scheithauer BW, Piepgras DG, et al. Malignant peripheral nerve sheath tumors. A clinicopathologic study of 120 cases. Cancer. 1986 May 15;57(10):2006–21. PMID:3082508

742. Dulmet EM, Macchiarini P, Suc B, et al. Germ cell tumors of the mediastinum. A 30-year experience. Cancer. 1993 Sep 15;72(6):1894–901. PMID:7689921

743. Dunleavy K, Grant C, Eberle FC, et al. Gray zone lymphoma: better treated like Hodgkin lymphoma or mediastinal large B-cell lymphoma? Curr Hematol Malig Rep. 2012 Sep;7(3):241–7. PMID:22833351

744. Duran-Moreno J, Kokkali S, Ramfidis V, et al. Primary sarcoma of the lung - prognostic value of clinicopathological characteristics of 26 cases. Anticancer Res. 2020 Mar;40(3):1697–703. PMID:32132077

745. Durham BH, Lopez Rodrigo E, Picarsic J, et al. Activating mutations in CSF1R and additional receptor tyrosine kinases in histiocytic neoplasms. Nat Med. 2019 Dec;25(12):1839–42. PMID:31768065

746. Durham BH, Roos-Weil D, Baillou C, et al. Functional evidence for derivation of systemic histiocytic neoplasms from hematopoietic stem/progenitor cells. Blood. 2017 Jul 13;130(2):176–80. PMID:28566492

747. Duwe BV, Sterman DH, Musani AI. Tumors of the mediastinum. Chest. 2005 Oct;128(4):2893–909. PMID:16236967

748. Eberhardt WE, Mitchell A, Crowley J, et al. The IASLC Lung Cancer Staging Project: proposals for the revision of the M descriptors in the forthcoming eighth edition of the TNM classification of lung cancer. J Thorac Oncol. 2015 Nov;10(11):1515–22. PMID:26536193

749. Eberle FC, Mani H, Jaffe ES. Histopathology of Hodgkin's lymphoma. Cancer J. 2009 Mar-Apr;15(2):129–37. PMID:19390308

750. Eberle FC, Rodriguez-Canales J, Wei L, et al. Methylation profiling of mediastinal gray zone lymphoma reveals a distinctive signature with elements shared by classical Hodgkin's lymphoma and primary mediastinal large B-cell lymphoma. Haematologica. 2011 Apr;96(4):558–66. PMID:21454882

751. Eberle FC, Salaverria I, Steidl C, et al. Gray zone lymphoma: chromosomal aberrations with immunophenotypic and clinical correlations. Mod Pathol. 2011 Dec;24(12):1586–97. PMID:21822207

752. Economopoulos GC, Lewis JW Jr, Lee MW, et al. Carcinoid tumors of the thymus. Ann Thorac Surg. 1990 Jul;50(1):58–61. PMID:2196019

753. Egan AJ, Boardman LA, Tazelaar HD, et al. Erdheim-Chester disease: clinical, radiologic, and histopathologic findings in five patients with interstitial lung disease. Am J Surg Pathol. 1999 Jan;23(1):17–26. PMID:9888700

754. Egan AM, McPhillips D, Sarkar S, et al. Malignant pleural effusion. QJM. 2014 Mar;107(3):179–84. PMID:24368856

755. Eguchi T, Kameda K, Lu S, et al. Lobectomy is associated with better outcomes than sublobar resection in spread through air spaces (STAS)-positive T1 lung adenocarcinoma: a propensity score-matched analysis. J Thorac Oncol. 2019 Jan;14(1):87–98. PMID:30244070

756. Eichhorn F, Harms A, Warth A, et al. PD-L1 expression in large cell neuroendocrine carcinoma of the lung. Lung Cancer. 2018 Apr;118:76–82. PMID:29572007

757. Eimoto T, Kitaoka M, Ogawa H, et al. Thymic sarcomatoid carcinoma with skeletal muscle differentiation: report of two cases, one with cytogenetic analysis. Histopathology. 2002 Jan;40(1):46–57. PMID:11903597

758. El Hag M, Schmidt L, Roh M, et al. Utility of TTF-1 and napsin-A in the work-up of malignant effusions. Diagn Cytopathol. 2016 Apr;44(4):299–304. PMID:26799356

759. Elbardissi AW, Dearani JA, Daly RC, et al. Survival after resection of primary cardiac tumors: a 48-year experience. Circulation. 2008 Sep 30;118(14 Suppl):S7–15. PMID:18824772

760. el-Domeiri AA, Hutter RV, Pool JL, et al. Primary seminoma of the anterior mediastinum. Ann Thorac Surg. 1968 Dec;6(6):513–21. PMID:5747337

761. Elmes PC, Simpson JC. The clinical aspects of mesothelioma. Q J Med. 1976 Jul;45(179):427–49. PMID:948545

762. Elnayal A, Moran CA, Fox PS, et al. Primary salivary gland-type lung cancer: imaging and clinical predictors of outcome. AJR Am J Roentgenol. 2013 Jul;201(1):W57–63. PMID:23789697

763. Emerson LL, Layfield LJ. Solitary peripheral pulmonary papilloma evaluation on frozen section: a potential pitfall for the pathologist. Pathol Res Pract. 2012 Dec 15;208(12):726–9. PMID:23131661

764. Emerson RE, Ulbright TM. The use of immunohistochemistry in the differential diagnosis of tumors of the testis and paratestis. Semin Diagn Pathol. 2005 Feb;22(1):33–50. PMID:16512598

765. Emile JF, Abla O, Fraitag S, et al. Revised classification of histiocytoses and neoplasms of the macrophage-dendritic cell lineages. Blood. 2016 Jun 2;127(22):2672–81. PMID:26966089

766. Emile JF, Diamond EL, Hélias-Rodzewicz Z, et al. Recurrent RAS and PIK3CA mutations in Erdheim-Chester disease. Blood. 2014 Nov 6;124(19):3016–9. PMID:25150293

767. Emoto K, Eguchi T, Tan KS, et al. Expansion of the concept of micropapillary adenocarcinoma to include a newly recognized filigree pattern as well as the classical pattern based on 1468 stage I lung adenocarcinomas. J Thorac Oncol. 2019 Nov;14(11):1948–61. PMID:31352072

768. Endo A, Ohtahara A, Kinugawa T, et al. Characteristics of cardiac myxoma with constitutional signs: a multicenter study in Japan. Clin Cardiol. 2002 Aug;25(8):367–70. PMID:12173903

769. Engels EA. Epidemiology of thymoma and associated malignancies. J Thorac Oncol. 2010 Oct;5(10 Suppl 4):S260–5. PMID:20859116

770. Engels EA, Shen M, Chapman RS, et al. Tuberculosis and subsequent risk of lung cancer in Xuanwei, China. Int J Cancer. 2009 Mar 1;124(5):1183–7. PMID:19058197

771. England DM, Hochholzer L. Truly benign "bronchial adenoma". Report of 10 cases of mucous gland adenoma with immunohistochemical and ultrastructural findings. Am J Surg Pathol. 1995 Aug;19(8):887–99. PMID:7611535

772. England DM, Hochholzer L, McCarthy MJ. Localized benign and malignant fibrous tumors of the pleura. A clinicopathologic review of 223 cases. Am J Surg Pathol. 1989 Aug;13(8):640–58. PMID:2665534

773. Engleson J, Soller M, Panagopoulos I, et al. Midline carcinoma with t(15;19) and BRD4-NUT fusion oncogene in a 30-year-old female with response to docetaxel and radiotherapy. BMC Cancer. 2006 Mar 16;6:69. PMID:16542442

774. Enkner F, Pichlhöfer B, Zaharie AT, et al. Molecular profiling of thymoma and thymic carcinoma: genetic differences and potential novel therapeutic targets. Pathol Oncol Res. 2017 Jul;23(3):551–64. PMID:27844328

775. Enzan N, Kitadate A, Tanaka A, et al. Incisional random skin biopsy, not punch biopsy, is an appropriate method for diagnosis of intravascular large B-cell lymphoma: a clinicopathological study of 25 patients. Br J Dermatol. 2019 Jul;181(1):200–1. PMID:30609011

776. Epler GR, McLoud TC, Munn CS, et al. Pleural lipoma. Diagnosis by computed tomography. Chest. 1986 Aug;90(2):265–8. PMID:3731900

777. Erber R, Warth A, Muley T, et al. BAP1 loss is a useful adjunct to distinguish malignant mesothelioma including the adenomatoid-like variant from benign adenomatoid tumors. Appl Immunohistochem Mol Morphol. 2020 Jan;28(1):67–73. PMID:30640754

778. Erickson LA, Mete O. Immunohistochemistry in diagnostic parathyroid pathology. Endocr Pathol. 2018 Jun;29(2):113–29. PMID:29626276

779. Errani C, Sung YS, Zhang L, et al. Monoclonality of multifocal epithelioid hemangioendothelioma of the liver by analysis of WWTR1-CAMTA1 breakpoints. Cancer Genet. 2012 Jan-Feb;205(1-2):12–7. PMID:22429593

780. Errani C, Zhang L, Sung YS, et al. A novel WWTR1-CAMTA1 gene fusion is a consistent abnormality in epithelioid hemangioendothelioma of different anatomic sites. Genes Chromosomes Cancer. 2011 Aug;50(8):644–53. PMID:21584898

781. Ersek JL, Symanowski JT, Han Y, et al.

Pulmonary carcinosarcoma: a Surveillance, Epidemiology, and End Results (SEER) analysis. Clin Lung Cancer. 2020 Mar;21(2):160–70. PMID:31455596
782. Ertel V, Früh M, Guenther A, et al. Thymoma with molecularly verified "conversion" to T lymphoblastic leukemia/lymphoma over 9 years. Leuk Lymphoma. 2013 Dec;54(12):2765–8. PMID:23566161
783. Ertuğrul T, Dindar A, Elmaci TT, et al. An intrapericardial teratoma with endocrine function. J Cardiovasc Surg (Torino). 2001 Dec;42(6):781–3. PMID:11698946
784. Essary LR, Vargas SO, Fletcher CD. Primary pleuropulmonary synovial sarcoma: reappraisal of a recently described anatomic subset. Cancer. 2002 Jan 15;94(2):459–69. PMID:11905413
785. Estrada-Veras JI, O'Brien KJ, Boyd LC, et al. The clinical spectrum of Erdheim-Chester disease: an observational cohort study. Blood Adv. 2017 Feb 14;1(6):357–66. PMID:28553668
786. Evans AG, French CA, Cameron MJ, et al. Pathologic characteristics of NUT midline carcinoma arising in the mediastinum. Am J Surg Pathol. 2012 Aug;36(8):1222–7. PMID:22790861
787. Ewens KG, Lalonde E, Richards-Yutz J, et al. Comparison of germline versus somatic BAP1 mutations for risk of metastasis in uveal melanoma. BMC Cancer. 2018 Nov 26;18(1):1172. PMID:30477459
788. Exarchos GD, Attanoos RL. Pseudomesotheliomatous small-cell neuroendocrine carcinoma of the lung with calretinin expression. Histopathology. 2015 May;66(6):895–6. PMID:25040312
789. Fabbri A, Cossa M, Sonzogni A, et al. Thymus neuroendocrine tumors with CTNNB1 gene mutations, disarrayed ß-catenin expression, and dual intra-tumor Ki-67 labeling index compartmentalization challenge the concept of secondary high-grade neuroendocrine tumor: a paradigm shift. Virchows Arch. 2017 Jul;471(1):31–47. PMID:28451756
790. Facchetti F, Pileri SA, Lorenzi L, et al. Histiocytic and dendritic cell neoplasms: what have we learnt by studying 67 cases. Virchows Arch. 2017 Oct;471(4):467–89. PMID:28695297
791. Faggiano A, Ferolla P, Grimaldi F, et al. Natural history of gastro-entero-pancreatic and thoracic neuroendocrine tumors. Data from a large prospective and retrospective Italian epidemiological study: the NET management study. J Endocrinol Invest. 2012 Oct;35(9):817–23. PMID:22080849
792. Faivre-Finn C, Snee M, Ashcroft L, et al. Concurrent once-daily versus twice-daily chemoradiotherapy in patients with limited-stage small-cell lung cancer (CONVERT): an open-label, phase 3, randomised, superiority trial. Lancet Oncol. 2017 Aug;18(8):1116–25. PMID:28642008
793. Falconieri G, Bussani R, Mirra M, et al. Pseudomesotheliomatous angiosarcoma: a pleuropulmonary lesion simulating malignant pleural mesothelioma. Histopathology. 1997 May;30(5):419–24. PMID:9181362
794. Falk N, Weissferdt A, Kalhor N, et al. Primary pulmonary salivary gland-type tumors: a review and update. Adv Anat Pathol. 2016 Jan;23(1):13–23. PMID:26645458
795. Fallet V, Saffroy R, Girard N, et al. High-throughput somatic mutation profiling in pulmonary sarcomatoid carcinomas using the LungCarta™ Panel: exploring therapeutic targets. Ann Oncol. 2015 Aug;26(8):1748–53. PMID:25969368
796. Fanburg-Smith JC, Majidi M, Miettinen M. Keratin expression in schwannoma; a study of 115 retroperitoneal and 22 peripheral schwannomas. Mod Pathol. 2006 Jan;19(1):115–21. PMID:16357842
797. Fanburg-Smith JC, Meis-Kindblom JM, Fante R, et al. Malignant granular cell tumor of soft tissue: diagnostic criteria and clinicopathologic correlation. Am J Surg Pathol. 1998 Jul;22(7):779–94. PMID:9669341
798. Fang L, He L, Chen Y, et al. Infiltrating lipoma of the right ventricle involving the interventricular septum and tricuspid valve: report of a rare case and literature review. Medicine (Baltimore). 2016 Jan;95(3):e2561. PMID:26817909
799. Fantone JC, Geisinger KR, Appelman HD. Papillary adenoma of the lung with lamellar and electron dense granules. An ultrastructural study. Cancer. 1982 Dec 15;50(12):2839–44. PMID:7139574
800. Farago AF, Taylor MS, Doebele RC, et al. Clinicopathologic features of non-small-cell lung cancer harboring an NTRK gene fusion. JCO Precis Oncol. 2018;2018:PO.18.00037. PMID:30215037
801. Farioli A, Ottone M, Morganti AG, et al. Radiation-induced mesothelioma among long-term solid cancer survivors: a longitudinal analysis of SEER database. Cancer Med. 2016 May;5(5):950–9. PMID:26860323
802. Fatima J, Duncan AA, Maleszewski JJ, et al. Primary angiosarcoma of the aorta, great vessels, and the heart. J Vasc Surg. 2013 Mar;57(3):756–64. PMID:23312835
803. Faure Conter C, Fresneau B, Thebaud E, et al. Two tumors in 1: What should be the therapeutic target? Pediatric germ cell tumor with somatic malignant transformation. J Pediatr Hematol Oncol. 2017 Jul;39(5):388–94. PMID:28375941
804. Fealey ME, Edwards WD, Miller DV, et al. Hamartomas of mature cardiac myocytes: report of 7 new cases and review of literature. Hum Pathol. 2008 Jul;39(7):1064–71. PMID:18508110
805. Fedoriw A, Rajapurkar SR, O'Brien S, et al. Anti-tumor activity of the type I PRMT inhibitor, GSK3368715, synergizes with PRMT5 inhibition through MTAP loss. Cancer Cell. 2019 Jul 8;36(1):100–114.e25. PMID:31257072
806. Fedyanin M, Tryakin A, Mosyakova Y, et al. Prognostic factors and efficacy of different chemotherapeutic regimens in patients with mediastinal nonseminomatous germ cell tumors. J Cancer Res Clin Oncol. 2014 Feb;140(2):311–8. PMID:24337455
807. Fehrenbacher L, Spira A, Ballinger M, et al. Atezolizumab versus docetaxel for patients with previously treated non-small-cell lung cancer (POPLAR): a multicentre, open-label, phase 2 randomised controlled trial. Lancet. 2016 Apr 30;387(10030):1837–46. PMID:26970723
808. Feng Y, Lei Y, Wu X, et al. GTF2I mutation frequently occurs in more indolent thymic epithelial tumors and predicts better prognosis. Lung Cancer. 2017 Aug;110:48–52. PMID:28676218
809. Fenoglio JJ Jr, McAllister HA Jr, Ferrans VJ. Cardiac rhabdomyoma: a clinicopathologic and electron microscopic study. Am J Cardiol. 1976 Aug;38(2):241–51. PMID:952267
810. Ferguson MK, DeMeester TR, DesLauriers J, et al. Diagnosis and management of synchronous lung cancers. J Thorac Cardiovasc Surg. 1985 Mar;89(3):378–85. PMID:3974273
811. Ferlay J, Colombet M, Bray F. Cancer Incidence in Five Continents, CI5plus: IARC CancerBase No. 9 [Internet]. Lyon (France): International Agency for Research on Cancer; 2018. Available from: http://ci5.iarc.fr.
812. Ferlay J, Ervik M, Lam F, et al. Global Cancer Observatory: Cancer Today [Internet]. Lyon (France): International Agency for Research on Cancer; 2018. Available from: https://gco.iarc.fr/today.
813. Fernández AL, Vega M, El-Diasty MM, et al. Myxoma of the aortic valve. Interact Cardiovasc Thorac Surg. 2012 Sep;15(3):560–2. PMID:22617509
814. Fernandez AP, Sun Y, Tubbs RR, et al. FISH for MYC amplification and anti-MYC immunohistochemistry: useful diagnostic tools in the assessment of secondary angiosarcoma and atypical vascular proliferations. J Cutan Pathol. 2012 Feb;39(2):234–42. PMID:22121953
815. Fernandez FG, Battafarano RJ. Large-cell neuroendocrine carcinoma of the lung. Cancer Control. 2006 Oct;13(4):270–5. PMID:17075564
816. Fernandez-Cuesta L, Peifer M, Lu X, et al. Frequent mutations in chromatin-remodelling genes in pulmonary carcinoids. Nat Commun. 2014 Mar 27;5:3518. PMID:24670920
817. Fernandez-Cuesta L, Plenker D, Osada H, et al. CD74-NRG1 fusions in lung adenocarcinoma. Cancer Discov. 2014 Apr;4(4):415–22. PMID:24469108
818. Fernández-Trujillo L, Bolaños JE, Velásquez M, et al. Primary effusion lymphoma in a human immunodeficiency virus-negative patient with unexpected unusual complications: a case report. J Med Case Rep. 2019 Sep 23;13(1):301. PMID:31543075
819. Ferolla P, Daddi N, Urbani M, et al. Tumorlets, multicentric carcinoids, lymph-nodal metastases, and long-term behavior in bronchial carcinoids. J Thorac Oncol. 2009 Mar;4(3):383–7. PMID:19247084
820. Ferolla P, Falchetti A, Filosso P, et al. Thymic neuroendocrine carcinoma (carcinoid) in multiple endocrine neoplasia type 1 syndrome: the Italian series. J Clin Endocrinol Metab. 2005 May;90(5):2603–9. PMID:15713725
821. Ferrara R, Mezquita L, Besse B. Progress in the management of advanced thoracic malignancies in 2017. J Thorac Oncol. 2018 Mar;13(3):301–22. PMID:29331646
822. Ferraro P, Trastek VF, Adlakha H, et al. Primary non-Hodgkin's lymphoma of the lung. Ann Thorac Surg. 2000 Apr;69(4):993–7. PMID:10800781
823. Ferreri AJ, Campo E, Seymour JF, et al. Intravascular lymphoma: clinical presentation, natural history, management and prognostic factors in a series of 38 cases, with special emphasis on the 'cutaneous variant'. Br J Haematol. 2004 Oct;127(2):173–83. PMID:15461623
824. Ferreri AJ, Dognini GP, Bairey O, et al. The addition of rituximab to anthracycline-based chemotherapy significantly improves outcome in 'Western' patients with intravascular large B-cell lymphoma. Br J Haematol. 2008 Oct;143(2):253–7. PMID:18699850
825. Ferreri AJ, Dognini GP, Govi S, et al. Can rituximab change the usually dismal prognosis of patients with intravascular large B-cell lymphoma? J Clin Oncol. 2008 Nov 1;26(31):5134–6, author reply 5136–7. PMID:18838697
826. Fetsch PA, Fetsch JF, Marincola FM, et al. Comparison of melanoma antigen recognized by T cells (MART-1) to HMB-45: additional evidence to support a common lineage for angiomyolipoma, lymphangiomyomatosis, and clear cell sugar tumor. Mod Pathol. 1998 Aug;11(8):699–703. PMID:9720495
827. Feuerhake F, Kutok JL, Monti S, et al. NFkappaB activity, function, and target-gene signatures in primary mediastinal large B-cell lymphoma and diffuse large B-cell lymphoma subtypes. Blood. 2005 Aug 15;106(4):1392–9. PMID:15870177
828. Filippini A, Zorzi F, Bna' C, et al. Dark sputum: an atypical presentation of primary pulmonary malignant melanoma. Respir Med Case Rep. 2015 May 14;15:118–20. PMID:26236620
829. Filosso PL, Evangelista A, Ruffini E, et al. Does myasthenia gravis influence overall survival and cumulative incidence of recurrence in thymoma patients? A retrospective clinicopathological multicentre analysis on 797 patients. Lung Cancer. 2015 Jun;88(3):338–43. PMID:25819383
830. Filosso PL, Guerrera F, Evangelista A, et al. Adjuvant chemotherapy for large-cell neuroendocrine lung carcinoma: results from the European Society for Thoracic Surgeons Lung Neuroendocrine Tumours retrospective database. Eur J Cardiothorac Surg. 2017 Aug 1;52(2):339–45. PMID:28459956
831. Filosso PL, Guerrera F, Evangelista A, et al. Prognostic model of survival for typical bronchial carcinoid tumours: analysis of 1109 patients on behalf of the European Association of Thoracic Surgeons (ESTS) Neuroendocrine Tumours Working Group. Eur J Cardiothorac Surg. 2015 Sep;48(3):441–7, discussion 447. PMID:25564217
832. Filosso PL, Rena O, Donati G, et al. Bronchial carcinoid tumors: surgical management and long-term outcome. J Thorac Cardiovasc Surg. 2002 Feb;123(2):303–9. PMID:11828290
833. Filosso PL, Rena O, Guerrera F, et al. Clinical management of atypical carcinoid and large-cell neuroendocrine carcinoma: a multicentre study on behalf of the European Association of Thoracic Surgeons (ESTS) Neuroendocrine Tumours of the Lung Working Group†. Eur J Cardiothorac Surg. 2015 Jul;48(1):55–64. PMID:25406425
834. Filosso PL, Yao X, Ahmad U, et al. Outcome of primary neuroendocrine tumors of the thymus: a joint analysis of the International Thymic Malignancy Interest Group and the European Society of Thoracic Surgeons databases. J Thorac Cardiovasc Surg. 2015 Jan;149(1):103–9.e2. PMID:25308116
835. Filosso PL, Yao X, Ruffini E, et al. Comparison of outcomes between neuroendocrine thymic tumours and other subtypes of thymic carcinomas: a joint analysis of the European Society of Thoracic Surgeons and the International Thymic Malignancy Interest Group. Eur J Cardiothorac Surg. 2016 Oct;50(4):766–71. PMID:27032473
836. Fine NM, Foley DA, Breen JF, et al. Multimodality imaging of a giant aortic valve papillary fibroelastoma. Case Rep Med. 2013;2013:705101. PMID:23983711
837. Fine SW, Whitney KD. Multiple cavernous hemangiomas of the lung: a case report and review of the literature. Arch Pathol Lab Med. 2004 Dec;128(12):1439–41. PMID:15578892
838. Finn RS, Brims FJH, Gandhi A, et al. Postmortem findings of malignant pleural mesothelioma: a two-center study of 318 patients. Chest. 2012 Nov;142(5):1267–73. PMID:22576637
839. Fishback NF, Travis WD, Moran CA, et al. Pleomorphic (spindle/giant cell) carcinoma of the lung. A clinicopathologic correlation of 78 cases. Cancer. 1994 Jun 15;73(12):2936–45. PMID:8199991
840. Fite JJ, Maleki Z. Paraganglioma: cytomorphologic features, radiologic and clinical findings in 12 cases. Diagn Cytopathol. 2018 Jun;46(6):473–81. PMID:29575826
841. Fletcher CD, Beham A, Bekir S, et al. Epithelioid angiosarcoma of deep soft tissue: a distinctive tumor readily mistaken for an epithelial neoplasm. Am J Surg Pathol. 1991 Oct;15(10):915–24. PMID:1718176
842. Fletcher JA, Longtine J, Wallace K, et al. Cytogenetic and histologic findings in 17 pulmonary chondroid hamartomas: evidence for a pathogenetic relationship with lipomas and

leiomyomas. Genes Chromosomes Cancer. 1995 Mar;12(3):220–3. PMID:7536462
843. Flieder DB. Screen-detected adenocarcinoma of the lung. Practical points for surgical pathologists. Am J Clin Pathol. 2003 Jun;119 Suppl:S39–57. PMID:12951843
844. Flieder DB, Koss MN, Nicholson A, et al. Solitary pulmonary papillomas in adults: a clinicopathologic and in situ hybridization study of 14 cases combined with 27 cases in the literature. Am J Surg Pathol. 1998 Nov;22(11):1328–42. PMID:9808125
845. Flores RM, Routledge T, Seshan VE, et al. The impact of lymph node station on survival in 348 patients with surgically resected malignant pleural mesothelioma: implications for revision of the American Joint Committee on Cancer staging system. J Thorac Cardiovasc Surg. 2008 Sep;136(3):605–10. PMID:18805259
846. Flucke U, Requena L, Mentzel T. Radiation-induced vascular lesions of the skin: an overview. Adv Anat Pathol. 2013 Nov;20(6):407–15. PMID:24113311
847. Flucke U, Vogels RJ, de Saint Aubain Somerhausen N, et al. Epithelioid hemangioendothelioma: clinicopathologic, immunhistochemical, and molecular genetic analysis of 39 cases. Diagn Pathol. 2014 Jul 1;9:131. PMID:24986479
848. Folpe AL, Chand EM, Goldblum JR, et al. Expression of Fli-1, a nuclear transcription factor, distinguishes vascular neoplasms from potential mimics. Am J Surg Pathol. 2001 Aug;25(8):1061–6. PMID:11474291
849. Folpe AL, Mentzel T, Lehr HA, et al. Perivascular epithelioid cell neoplasms of soft tissue and gynecologic origin: a clinicopathologic study of 26 cases and review of the literature. Am J Surg Pathol. 2005 Dec;29(12):1558–75. PMID:16327428
850. Folpe AL, Weiss SW. Lipoleiomyosarcoma (well-differentiated liposarcoma with leiomyosarcomatous differentiation): a clinicopathologic study of nine cases including one with dedifferentiation. Am J Surg Pathol. 2002 Jun;26(6):742–9. PMID:12023578
851. Fonseca AL, Ozgediz DE, Christison-Lagay ER, et al. Pediatric thymomas: report of two cases and comprehensive review of the literature. Pediatr Surg Int. 2014 Mar;30(3):275–86. PMID:24322668
852. Fontanini G, Calcinai A, Boldrini L, et al. Modulation of neoangiogenesis in bronchial preneoplastic lesions. Oncol Rep. 1999 Jul-Aug;6(4):813–7. PMID:10373662
852A. Forbes SA, Beare D, Gunasekaran P, et al. COSMIC: exploring the world's knowledge of somatic mutations in human cancer. Nucleic Acids Res. 2015 Jan;43(Database issue):D805–11. PMID:25355519
853. Fortes HR, von Ranke FM, Escuissato DL, et al. Recurrent respiratory papillomatosis: a state-of-the-art review. Respir Med. 2017 May;126:116–21. PMID:28427542
854. Fortuno C, James PA, Spurdle AB. Current review of TP53 pathogenic germline variants in breast cancer patients outside Li-Fraumeni syndrome. Hum Mutat. 2018 Dec;39(12):1764–73. PMID:30240537
855. Fortuno C, James PA, Young EL, et al. Improved, ACMG-compliant, in silico prediction of pathogenicity for missense substitutions encoded by TP53 variants. Hum Mutat. 2018 Aug;39(8):1061–9. PMID:29775997
856. Fotouhi Ghiam A, Dawson LA, Abuzeid W, et al. Role of palliative radiotherapy in the management of mural cardiac metastases: Who, when and how to treat? A case series of 10 patients. Cancer Med. 2016 Jun;5(6):989–96. PMID:26880683
856A. Fraire AE, Johnson EH, Yesner R, et al. Prognostic significance of histopathologic subtype and stage in small cell lung cancer. Hum Pathol. 1992 May;23(5):520–8. PMID:1314777
857. Francischetti IMB, Cajigas A, Suhrland M, et al. Incidental primary mediastinal choriocarcinoma diagnosed by endobronchial ultrasound-guided fine needle aspiration in a patient presenting with transient ischemic attack and stroke. Diagn Cytopathol. 2017 Aug;45(8):738–43. PMID:28397369
858. Francisco A, Gouveia R, Anjos R. Mitral valve lipomatous hamartoma: a rare entity. Cardiol Young. 2014 Oct;24(5):923–5. PMID:24044592
859. Franke A, Ströbel P, Fackeldey V, et al. Hepatoid thymic carcinoma: report of a case. Am J Surg Pathol. 2004 Feb;28(2):250–6. PMID:15043316
860. Franklin WA, Gazdar AF, Haney J, et al. Widely dispersed p53 mutation in respiratory epithelium. A novel mechanism for field carcinogenesis. J Clin Invest. 1997 Oct 15;100(8):2133–7. PMID:9329980
861. Fraternali Orcioni G, Ravetti JL, Gaggero G, et al. Primary embryonal spindle cell cardiac rhabdomyosarcoma: case report. Pathol Res Pract. 2010 May 15;206(5):325–30. PMID:19577381
862. Frazier AL, Weldon C, Amatruda J. Fetal and neonatal germ cell tumors. Semin Fetal Neonatal Med. 2012 Aug;17(4):222–30. PMID:22647545
862A. Frebourg T, Bajalica Lagercrantz S, Oliveira C, et al. Guidelines for the Li-Fraumeni and heritable TP53-related cancer syndromes. Eur J Hum Genet. 2020 Oct;28(10):1379–86. PMID:32457520
863. Freedom RM, Lee KJ, MacDonald C, et al. Selected aspects of cardiac tumors in infancy and childhood. Pediatr Cardiol. 2000 Jul-Aug;21(4):299–316. PMID:10865003
864. Freeman C, Berg JW, Cutler SJ. Occurrence and prognosis of extranodal lymphomas. Cancer. 1972 Jan;29(1):252–60. PMID:5007387
865. French CA. NUT carcinoma: clinicopathologic features, pathogenesis, and treatment. Pathol Int. 2018 Nov;68(11):583–95. PMID:30362654
866. French CA. Pathogenesis of NUT midline carcinoma. Annu Rev Pathol. 2012;7:247–65. PMID:22017582
867. French CA, Kutok JL, Faquin WC, et al. Midline carcinoma of children and young adults with NUT rearrangement. J Clin Oncol. 2004 Oct 15;22(20):4135–9. PMID:15483023
868. French CA, Miyoshi I, Kubonishi I, et al. BRD4-NUT fusion oncogene: a novel mechanism in aggressive carcinoma. Cancer Res. 2003 Jan 15;63(2):304–7. PMID:12543779
869. French CA, Rahman S, Walsh EM, et al. NSD3-NUT fusion oncoprotein in NUT midline carcinoma: implications for a novel oncogenic mechanism. Cancer Discov. 2014 Aug;4(8):928–41. PMID:24875858
870. French CA, Ramirez CL, Kolmakova J, et al. BRD-NUT oncoproteins: a family of closely related nuclear proteins that block epithelial differentiation and maintain the growth of carcinoma cells. Oncogene. 2008 Apr 3;27(15):2237–42. PMID:17934517
871. Frey A, Alatassi H, Wiese TA, et al. Cytomorphologic findings and differential diagnosis of pulmonary papillary adenoma: a case report and literature review. Diagn Cytopathol. 2016 Jun;44(6):543–7. PMID:27040894
872. Fritz A, Percy C, Jack A, et al., editors. International classification of diseases for oncology (ICD-O). 3rd ed. 1st rev. Geneva (Switzerland): World Health Organization; 2013.
873. Fu B, Yu H, Yang J. Primary intimal (spindle cell) sarcoma of the left atrium. Echocardiography. 2015 Jan;32(1):192–4. PMID:25196496
874. Fu F, She X. Mature cardiac myocytohamartoma: a case report and review of literature. Int J Clin Exp Pathol. 2019 Apr 1;12(4):1424–8. PMID:31933959
875. Fu H, Gu ZT, Fang WT, et al. Long-term survival after surgical treatment of thymic carcinoma: a retrospective analysis from the Chinese Alliance for Research of Thymoma database. Ann Surg Oncol. 2016 Feb;23(2):619–25. PMID:26474558
876. Fu Y, Wu Q, Su F, et al. Novel gene mutations in well-differentiated fetal adenocarcinoma of the lung in the next generation sequencing era. Lung Cancer. 2018 Oct;124:1–5. PMID:30268445
877. Fu Z, Yang K, Yang X, et al. Primary intrathoracic liposarcoma: a clinical analysis of 31 cases. Cancer Commun (Lond). 2019 Apr 2;39(1):15. PMID:30940199
878. Fuchs J, Urla C, Sparber-Sauer M, et al. Treatment and outcome of patients with localized intrathoracic and chest wall rhabdomyosarcoma: a report of the Cooperative Weichteilsarkom Studiengruppe (CWS). J Cancer Res Clin Oncol. 2018 May;144(5):925–34. PMID:29464349
879. Fujimoto K, Müller NL, Sadohara J, et al. Alveolar adenoma of the lung: computed tomography and magnetic resonance imaging findings. J Thorac Imaging. 2002 Apr;17(2):163–6. PMID:11956369
880. Fujimoto M, Haga H, Okamoto M, et al. EBV-associated diffuse large B-cell lymphoma arising in the chest wall with surgical mesh implant. Pathol Int. 2008 Oct;58(10):668–71. PMID:18801089
881. Fujino K, Motooka Y, Hassan WA, et al. Insulinoma-associated protein 1 is a crucial regulator of neuroendocrine differentiation in lung cancer. Am J Pathol. 2015 Dec;185(12):3164–77. PMID:26482608
882. Fujioka S, Nakamura H, Miwa K, et al. Thymic metastasis of breast cancer 22 years after surgery: a case report. Asian J Endosc Surg. 2013 Nov;6(4):330–2. PMID:24308597
883. Fujiwara A, Tsushima K, Sugiyama S, et al. Histological types and localizations of lung cancers in patients with combined pulmonary fibrosis and emphysema. Thorac Cancer. 2013 Nov;4(4):354–60. PMID:28920226
884. Fukai I, Masaoka A, Fujii Y, et al. Thymic neuroendocrine tumor (thymic carcinoid): a clinicopathologic study in 15 patients. Ann Thorac Surg. 1999 Jan;67(1):208–11. PMID:10086551
885. Fukai I, Masaoka A, Hashimoto T, et al. The distribution of epithelial membrane antigen in thymic epithelial neoplasms. Cancer. 1992 Oct 15;70(8):2077–81. PMID:1394038
886. Fukano R, Sunami S, Sekimizu M, et al. Clinical features and prognosis according to immunophenotypic subtypes including the early T-cell precursor subtype of T-lymphoblastic lymphoma in the Japanese Pediatric Leukemia/Lymphoma Study Group ALB-NHL03 study. J Pediatr Hematol Oncol. 2018 Jan;40(1):e34–7. PMID:28538509
887. Fukuda T, Ohnishi Y, Kanai I, et al. Papillary adenoma of the lung. Histological and ultrastructural findings in two cases. Acta Pathol Jpn. 1992 Jan;42(1):56–61. PMID:1557989
888. Fukunaga A, Sasamura Y, Takada A, et al. Solitary thymic metastasis of breast cancer 13 years after surgery. Asian Cardiovasc Thorac Ann. 2017 Jul;25(6):469–71. PMID:28605955
889. Fukunaga M, Naganuma H, Nikaido T, et al. Extrapleural solitary fibrous tumor: a report of seven cases. Mod Pathol. 1997 May;10(5):443–50. PMID:9160308
890. Fukushima T, Noguchi T, Kobayashi T, et al. Late and rapid relapse in mediastinum from testicular germ cell tumor stage I over 13 years after surgery. Case Rep Oncol. 2019 Jun 26;12(2):500–5. PMID:31320874
891. Fulford LG, Kamata Y, Okudera K, et al. Epithelial-myoepithelial carcinomas of the bronchus. Am J Surg Pathol. 2001 Dec;25(12):1508–14. PMID:11717540
892. Furlong MA, Mentzel T, Fanburg-Smith JC. Pleomorphic rhabdomyosarcoma in adults: a clinicopathologic study of 38 cases with emphasis on morphologic variants and recent skeletal muscle-specific markers. Mod Pathol. 2001 Jun;14(6):595–603. PMID:11406662
893. Furtado A, Nogueira R, Ferreira D, et al. Papillary adenocarcinoma of the thymus: case report and review of the literature. Int J Surg Pathol. 2010 Dec;18(6):530–3. PMID:18611939
894. Furukawa S, Haruta M, Arai Y, et al. Yolk sac tumor but not seminoma or teratoma is associated with abnormal epigenetic reprogramming pathway and shows frequent hypermethylation of various tumor suppressor genes. Cancer Sci. 2009 Apr;100(4):698–708. PMID:19245437
895. Furukawa T, Watanabe S, Kodama T, et al. T-zone histiocytes in adenocarcinoma of the lung in relation to postoperative prognosis. Cancer. 1985 Dec 1;56(11):2651–6. PMID:3902198
896. Furuya K, Murayama S, Soeda H, et al. New classification of small pulmonary nodules by margin characteristics on high-resolution CT. Acta Radiol. 1999 Sep;40(5):496–504. PMID:10485238
897. Gaensler EA, Carrington CB. Open biopsy for chronic diffuse infiltrative lung disease: clinical, roentgenographic, and physiological correlations in 502 patients. Ann Thorac Surg. 1980 Nov;30(5):411–26. PMID:7436611
898. Gaffey MJ, Mills SE, Askin FB. Minute pulmonary meningothelial-like nodules. A clinicopathologic study of so-called minute pulmonary chemodectoma. Am J Surg Pathol. 1988 Mar;12(3):167–75. PMID:2830799
899. Gaffney EF, Dervan PA, Fletcher CD. Pleomorphic rhabdomyosarcoma in adulthood. Analysis of 11 cases with definition of diagnostic criteria. Am J Surg Pathol. 1993 Jun;17(6):601–9. PMID:8333559
900. Gainor JF, Varghese AM, Ou SH, et al. ALK rearrangements are mutually exclusive with mutations in EGFR or KRAS: an analysis of 1,683 patients with non-small cell lung cancer. Clin Cancer Res. 2013 Aug 1;19(15):4273–81. PMID:23729361
901. Gal AA, Kornstein MJ, Cohen C, et al. Neuroendocrine tumors of the thymus: a clinicopathological and prognostic study. Ann Thorac Surg. 2001 Oct;72(4):1179–82. PMID:11603433
902. Galateau Salle F, Le Stang N, Nicholson AG, et al. New insights on diagnostic reproducibility of biphasic mesotheliomas: a multi-institutional evaluation by the International Mesothelioma Panel from the MESOPATH Reference Center. J Thorac Oncol. 2018 Aug;13(8):1189–203. PMID:29723687
902A. Galateau Salle F, Le Stang N, Tirode F, et al. Comprehensive molecular and pathologic evaluation of transitional mesothelioma assisted by deep learning approach: a multi-institutional study of the International Mesothelioma Panel from the MESOPATH Reference Center. J Thorac Oncol. 2020 Jun;15(6):1037–53. PMID:32165206
903. Galateau-Sallé F, Attanoos R, Gibbs AR, et al. Lymphohistiocytoid variant of malignant mesothelioma of the pleura: a series of 22 cases. Am J Surg Pathol. 2007 May;31(5):711–6. PMID:17460454
904. Galateau-Sallé F, Vignaud JM, Burke L, et al. Well-differentiated papillary mesothelioma of the pleura: a series of 24 cases.

Am J Surg Pathol. 2004 Apr;28(4):534–40. PMID:15087673
905. Galluzzi L, Chan TA, Kroemer G, et al. The hallmarks of successful anticancer immunotherapy. Sci Transl Med. 2018 Sep 19;10(459):eaat7807. PMID:30232229
906. Gandotra S, Dotson T, Lamar Z, et al. Endobronchial ultrasound transbronchial needle aspiration for the diagnosis of lymphoma. J Bronchology Interv Pulmonol. 2018 Apr;25(2):97–102. PMID:29076937
907. Gao S, Stein S, Petre EN, et al. Micropapillary and/or solid histologic subtype based on pre-treatment biopsy predicts local recurrence after thermal ablation of lung adenocarcinoma. Cardiovasc Intervent Radiol. 2018 Feb;41(2):253–9. PMID:28770314
908. Gao Y, Jiang J, Liu Q. Extragonadal malignant germ cell tumors: a clinicopathological and immunohistochemical analysis of 48 cases at a single Chinese institution. Int J Clin Exp Pathol. 2015 May 1;8(5):5650–7. PMID:26191277
909. Gao ZH, Urbanski SJ. The spectrum of pulmonary mucinous cystic neoplasia : a clinicopathologic and immunohistochemical study of ten cases and review of literature. Am J Clin Pathol. 2005 Jul;124(1):62–70. PMID:15923171
910. García JF, Mollejo M, Fraga M, et al. Large B-cell lymphoma with Hodgkin's features. Histopathology. 2005 Jul;47(1):101–10. PMID:15982329
911. Garcia JJ, Jin L, Jackson SB, et al. Primary pulmonary hyalinizing clear cell carcinoma of bronchial submucosal gland origin. Hum Pathol. 2015 Mar;46(3):471–5. PMID:25543160
912. Garcia JM, Gonzalez R, Silva JM, et al. Mutational status of K-ras and TP53 genes in primary sarcomas of the heart. Br J Cancer. 2000 Mar;82(6):1183–5. PMID:10735503
913. García-Escudero A, González-Cámpora R, Villar-Rodríguez JL, et al. Thyroid transcription factor-1 expression in pulmonary blastoma. Histopathology. 2004 May;44(5):507–8. PMID:15140003
914. Garfield DH, Cadranel J. The importance of distinguishing mucinous and nonmucinous bronchioloalveolar carcinomas. Lung. 2009 May-Jun;187(3):207–8. PMID:19408043
915. Garg N, Moorthy N, Agrawal SK, et al. Delayed cardiac metastasis from phyllodes breast tumor presenting as cardiogenic shock. Tex Heart Inst J. 2011;38(4):441–4. PMID:21841880
916. Garg PK, Sharma G, Rai S, et al. Primary salivary gland-type tumors of the lung: a systematic review and pooled analysis. Lung India. 2019 Mar-Apr;36(2):118–22. PMID:30829245
917. Garg R, Bal A, Das A, et al. Proliferation marker (Ki67) in sub-categorization of neuroendocrine tumours of the lung. Turk Patoloji Derg. 2019;35(1):15–21. PMID:30070306
918. Garnick MB, Griffin JD. Idiopathic thrombocytopenia in association with extragonadal germ cell cancer. Ann Intern Med. 1983 Jun;98(6):926–7. PMID:6305246
919. Gartner LA, Voorhess ML. Adrenocorticotropic hormone–producing thymic carcinoid in a teenager. Cancer. 1993 Jan 1;71(1):106–11. PMID:8380112
920. Gaspar LE, McNamara EJ, Gay EG, et al. Small-cell lung cancer: prognostic factors and changing treatment over 15 years. Clin Lung Cancer. 2012 Mar;13(2):115–22. PMID:22000695
921. Gatta G, van der Zwan JM, Casali PG, et al. Rare cancers are not so rare: the rare cancer burden in Europe. Eur J Cancer. 2011 Nov;47(17):2493–511. PMID:22033323
922. Gaude GS, Patil P, Malur PR, et al. Primary mediastinal choriocarcinoma. South Asian J Cancer. 2013 Apr;2(2):79. PMID:24455559
923. Gaur P, Leary C, Yao JC. Thymic neuroendocrine tumors: a SEER database analysis of 160 patients. Ann Surg. 2010 Jun;251(6):1117–21. PMID:20485130
924. Gawrychowski J, Bruliński K, Malinowski E, et al. Prognosis and survival after radical resection of primary adenosquamous lung carcinoma. Eur J Cardiothorac Surg. 2005 Apr;27(4):686–92. PMID:15784375
925. Gazdar A, Robinson L, Oliver D, et al. Hereditary lung cancer syndrome targets never smokers with germline EGFR gene T790M mutations. J Thorac Oncol. 2014 Apr;9(4):456–63. PMID:24736066
926. Gazdar AF, Savage TK, Johnson JE, et al. The comparative pathology of genetically engineered mouse models for neuroendocrine carcinomas of the lung. J Thorac Oncol. 2015 Apr;10(4):553–64. PMID:25675280
927. Gazzeri S, Brambilla E, Jacrot M, et al. Activation of myc gene family in human lung carcinomas and during heterotransplantation into nude mice. Cancer Res. 1991 May 15;51(10):2566–71. PMID:1850659
928. GBD 2017 Risk Factor Collaborators. Global, regional, and national comparative risk assessment of 84 behavioural, environmental and occupational, and metabolic risks or clusters of risks for 195 countries and territories, 1990-2017: a systematic analysis for the Global Burden of Disease Study 2017. Lancet. 2018 Nov 10;392(10159):1923–94. PMID:30496105
929. Ge Y, Ro JY, Kim D, et al. Clinicopathologic and immunohistochemical characteristics of adult primary cardiac angiosarcomas: analysis of 10 cases. Ann Diagn Pathol. 2011 Aug;15(4):262–7. PMID:21546292
930. Geha AS, Weidman WH, Soule EH, et al. Intramural ventricular cardiac fibroma. Successful removal in two cases and review of the literature. Circulation. 1967 Sep;36(3):427–40. PMID:6033170
931. Gehrmann J, Kehl HG, Diallo R, et al. Cardiac leiomyosarcoma of the right atrium in a teenager: unusual manifestation with a lifetime history of atrial ectopic tachycardia. Pacing Clin Electrophysiol. 2001 Jul;24(7):1161–4. PMID:11475835
932. Geisinger KR, Stanley MW, Raab SS, et al. Modern cytopathology. Bethesda (MD): Churchill Livingstone; 2003.
933. Geisinger KR, Travis WD, Perkins LA, et al. Aspiration cytomorphology of fetal adenocarcinoma of the lung. Am J Clin Pathol. 2010 Dec;134(6):894–902. PMID:21088152
934. Geles A, Gruber-Moesenbacher U, Quehenberger F, et al. Pulmonary mucinous adenocarcinomas: architectural patterns in correlation with genetic changes, prognosis and survival. Virchows Arch. 2015 Dec;467(6):675–86. PMID:26450556
935. Gélinas JF, Manoukian J, Côté A. Lung involvement in juvenile onset recurrent respiratory papillomatosis: a systematic review of the literature. Int J Pediatr Otorhinolaryngol. 2008 Apr;72(4):433–52. PMID:18281102
936. Geller RL, Hookim K, Sullivan HC, et al. Cytologic features of angiosarcoma: a review of 26 cases diagnosed on FNA. Cancer Cytopathol. 2016 Sep;124(9):659–68. PMID:27088896
936A. Gelvez-Zapata SM, Gaffney D, Scarci M, et al. What is the survival after surgery for localized malignant pleural mesothelioma? Interact Cardiovasc Thorac Surg. 2013 Apr;16(4):533–7. PMID:23328002
937. George J, Lim JS, Jang SJ, et al. Comprehensive genomic profiles of small cell lung cancer. Nature. 2015 Aug 6;524(7563):47–53. PMID:26168399
938. George J, Walter V, Peifer M, et al. Integrative genomic profiling of large-cell neuroendocrine carcinomas reveals distinct subtypes of high-grade neuroendocrine lung tumors. Nat Commun. 2018 Mar 13;9(1):1048. PMID:29535388
939. Georgescu SR, Mitran CI, Mitran MI, et al. New insights in the pathogenesis of HPV infection and the associated carcinogenic processes: the role of chronic inflammation and oxidative stress. J Immunol Res. 2018 Aug 27;2018:5315816. PMID:30225270
940. Gerbaudo VH, Britz-Cunningham S, Sugarbaker DJ, et al. Metabolic significance of the pattern, intensity and kinetics of 18F-FDG uptake in malignant pleural mesothelioma. Thorax. 2003 Dec;58(12):1077–82. PMID:14645979
941. Ghosh M, Islam N, Saha H, et al. Cytodiagnosis of inflammatory myofibroblastic tumor: a report of three cases in infants. Diagn Cytopathol. 2018 Sep;46(9):776–81. PMID:29673102
942. Giaccone G, Kim C, Thompson J, et al. Pembrolizumab in patients with thymic carcinoma: a single-arm, single-centre, phase 2 study. Lancet Oncol. 2018 Mar;19(3):347–55. PMID:29395863
943. Giacomelli AO, Yang X, Lintner RE, et al. Mutational processes shape the landscape of TP53 mutations in human cancer. Nat Genet. 2018 Oct;50(10):1381–7. PMID:30224644
944. Giaj Levra M, Novello S, Scagliotti GV, et al. Primary pleuropulmonary sarcoma: a rare disease entity. Clin Lung Cancer. 2012 Nov;13(6):399–407. PMID:22673623
945. Gibas Z, Miettinen M. Recurrent parapharyngeal rhabdomyoma. Evidence of neoplastic nature of the tumor from cytogenetic study. Am J Surg Pathol. 1992 Jul;16(7):721–8. PMID:1530111
946. Gibbons D, Leitch M, Coscia J, et al. Fine needle aspiration cytology and histologic findings of granular cell tumor of the breast: review of 19 cases with clinical/radiologic correlation. Breast J. 2000 Jan;6(1):27–30. PMID:11348331
947. Gibril F, Chen YJ, Schrump DS, et al. Prospective study of thymic carcinoids in patients with multiple endocrine neoplasia type 1. J Clin Endocrinol Metab. 2003 Mar;88(3):1066–81. PMID:12629087
948. Gilg Soit Ilg A, Audignon S. Chamming's S, et al. Programme national de surveillance du mésothéliome pleural (PNSM) : vingt années de surveillance (1998-2017) des cas de mésothéliome, de leurs expositions et des processus d'indemnisation. Saint-Maurice (France): Santé publique France; 2019. Available from: https://www.santepubliquefrance.fr/maladies-et-traumatismes/cancers/mesotheliomes/documents/rapport-synthese/programme-national-de-surveillance-du-mesotheliome-pleural-pnsm-vingt-annees-de-surveillance-1998-2017-des-cas-de-mesotheliome-de-leurs-expo. French.
949. Gilham C, Rake C, Hodgson J, et al. Past and current asbestos exposure and future mesothelioma risks in Britain: The Inhaled Particles Study (TIPS). Int J Epidemiol. 2018 Dec 1;47(6):1745–56. PMID:29534192
950. Gill AJ, Benn DE, Chou A, et al. Immunohistochemistry for SDHB triages genetic testing of SDHB, SDHC, and SDHD in paraganglioma-pheochromocytoma syndromes. Hum Pathol. 2010 Jun;41(6):805–14. PMID:20236688
951. Gill PS, Chandraratna PA, Meyer PR, et al. Malignant lymphoma: cardiac involvement at initial presentation. J Clin Oncol. 1987 Feb;5(2):216–24. PMID:3543244
952. Gill RR. Imaging of mesothelioma. Recent Results Cancer Res. 2011;189:27–43. PMID:21479894
953. Gill RR, Gerbaudo VH, Sugarbaker DJ, et al. Current trends in radiologic management of malignant pleural mesothelioma. Semin Thorac Cardiovasc Surg. 2009 Summer;21(2):111–20. PMID:19822282
954. Gill RR, Richards WG, Yeap BY, et al. Epithelial malignant pleural mesothelioma after extrapleural pneumonectomy: stratification of survival with CT-derived tumor volume. AJR Am J Roentgenol. 2012 Feb;198(2):359–63. PMID:22268178
955. Gill RR, Tsao AS, Kindler HL, et al. Radiologic considerations and standardization of malignant pleural mesothelioma imaging within clinical trials: consensus statement from the NCI Thoracic Malignancy Steering Committee - International Association for the Study of Lung Cancer - Mesothelioma Applied Research Foundation Clinical Trials Planning Meeting. J Thorac Oncol. 2019 Oct;14(10):1718–31. PMID:31470129
956. Gill RR, Umeoka S, Mamata H, et al. Diffusion-weighted MRI of malignant pleural mesothelioma: preliminary assessment of apparent diffusion coefficient in histologic subtypes. AJR Am J Roentgenol. 2010 Aug;195(2):W125–30. PMID:20651171
957. Gill RR, Yeap BY, Bueno R, et al. Quantitative clinical staging for patients with malignant pleural mesothelioma. J Natl Cancer Inst. 2018 Mar 1;110(3):258–64. PMID:29931180
958. Gillis AJ, Stoop H, Biermann K, et al. Expression and interdependencies of pluripotency factors LIN28, OCT3/4, NANOG and SOX2 in human testicular germ cells and tumours of the testis. Int J Androl. 2011 Aug;34(4 Pt 2):e160–74. PMID:21631526
959. Gilman G, Wright RS, Glockner JF, et al. Ventricular septal hamartoma mimicking hypertrophic cardiomyopathy in a 41-year-old woman presenting with paroxysmal supraventricular tachycardia. J Am Soc Echocardiogr. 2005 Mar;18(3):272–4. PMID:15746719
960. Gimenez-Roqueplo AP, Dahia PL, Robledo M. An update on the genetics of paraganglioma, pheochromocytoma, and associated hereditary syndromes. Horm Metab Res. 2012 May;44(5):328–33. PMID:22328163
961. Girard N. Chemotherapy and targeted agents for thymic malignancies. Expert Rev Anticancer Ther. 2012 May;12(5):685–95. PMID:22594902
962. Girard N, Deshpande C, Lau C, et al. Comprehensive histologic assessment helps to differentiate multiple lung primary nonsmall cell carcinomas from metastases. Am J Surg Pathol. 2009 Dec;33(12):1752–64. PMID:19773638
963. Girard N, Ostrovnaya I, Lau C, et al. Genomic and mutational profiling to assess clonal relationships between multiple non-small cell lung cancers. Clin Cancer Res. 2009 Aug 15;15(16):5184–90. PMID:19671847
964. Girard N, Ruffini E, Marx A, et al. Thymic epithelial tumours: ESMO Clinical Practice Guidelines for diagnosis, treatment and follow-up. Ann Oncol. 2015 Sep;26 Suppl 5:v40–55. PMID:26314779
965. Girard N, Shen R, Guo T, et al. Comprehensive genomic analysis reveals clinically relevant molecular distinctions between thymic carcinomas and thymomas. Clin Cancer Res. 2009 Nov 15;15(22):6790–9. PMID:19861435
966. Giusca S, Mereles D, Ochs A, et al. Incremental value of cardiac magnetic resonance for the evaluation of cardiac tumors in adults: experience of a high volume tertiary cardiology centre. Int J Cardiovasc Imaging. 2017 Jun;33(6):879–88. PMID:28138817
967. Gkampeta A, Tziola TS, Tragiannidis A, et al. Primary posterior mediastinal germ cell tumor in a child. Turk Pediatri Ars. 2019 Sep

25;54(3):185–8. PMID:31619931

968. Gladdy RA, Qin LX, Moraco N, et al. Do radiation-associated soft tissue sarcomas have the same prognosis as sporadic soft tissue sarcomas? J Clin Oncol. 2010 Apr 20;28(12):2064–9. PMID:20308666

969. Glaser SL, Jarrett RF. The epidemiology of Hodgkin's disease. Baillieres Clin Haematol. 1996 Sep;9(3):401–16. PMID:8922237

970. Gleason BC, Fletcher CD. Myoepithelial carcinoma of soft tissue in children: an aggressive neoplasm analyzed in a series of 29 cases. Am J Surg Pathol. 2007 Dec;31(12):1813–24. PMID:18043035

971. Gleeson M, Hawkes EA, Cunningham D, et al. Rituximab, cyclophosphamide, doxorubicin, vincristine and prednisolone (R-CHOP) in the management of primary mediastinal B-cell lymphoma: a subgroup analysis of the UK NCRI R-CHOP 14 versus 21 trial. Br J Haematol. 2016 Nov;175(4):668–72. PMID:27477167

972. Gleeson T, Thiessen R, Hannigan A, et al. Pulmonary hamartomas: CT pixel analysis for fat attenuation using radiologic-pathologic correlation. J Med Imaging Radiat Oncol. 2013 Oct;57(5):534–43. PMID:24119266

973. Go C, Schwartz MR, Donovan DT. Molecular transformation of recurrent respiratory papillomatosis: viral typing and p53 overexpression. Ann Otol Rhinol Laryngol. 2003 Apr;112(4):298–302. PMID:12731623

974. Go H, Cho HJ, Paik JH, et al. Thymic extranodal marginal zone B-cell lymphoma of mucosa-associated lymphoid tissue: a clinicopathological and genetic analysis of six cases. Leuk Lymphoma. 2011 Dec;52(12):2276–83. PMID:21745165

975. Go H, Jeon YK, Huh J, et al. Frequent detection of BRAF(V600E) mutations in histiocytic and dendritic cell neoplasms. Histopathology. 2014 Aug;65(2):261–72. PMID:24720374

976. Göbel U, Schneider DT, Teske C, et al. Brain metastases in children and adolescents with extracranial germ cell tumor - data of the MAHO/MAKEI-registry. Klin Padiatr. 2010 May;222(3):140–4. PMID:20514616

977. Göbel U, von Kries R, Teske C, et al. Brain metastases during follow-up of children and adolescents with extracranial malignant germ cell tumors: risk adapted management decision tree analysis based on data of the MAHO/MAKEI-registry. Pediatr Blood Cancer. 2013 Feb;60(2):217–23. PMID:22693072

978. Gökmen-Polar Y, Cano OD, Kesler KA, et al. NUT midline carcinomas in the thymic region. Mod Pathol. 2014 Dec;27(12):1649–56. PMID:24851833

979. Gökmen-Polar Y, Cook RW, Goswami CP, et al. A gene signature to determine metastatic behavior in thymomas. PLoS One. 2013 Jul 24;8(7):e66047. PMID:23894276

980. Gökmen-Polar Y, Kesler K, Loehrer PJ Sr, et al. NUT midline carcinoma masquerading as a thymic carcinoma. J Clin Oncol. 2016 May 10;34(14):e126–9. PMID:24733790

981. Gökmen-Polar Y, Sanders KL, Goswami CP, et al. Establishment and characterization of a novel cell line derived from human thymoma AB tumor. Lab Invest. 2012 Nov;92(11):1564–73. PMID:22926645

982. Goldberg AD, Blankstein R, Padera RF. Tumors metastatic to the heart. Circulation. 2013 Oct 15;128(16):1790–4. PMID:24126323

983. Goldblum JR, Rice TW. Epithelioid angiosarcoma of the pulmonary artery. Hum Pathol. 1995 Nov;26(11):1275–7. PMID:7590704

984. Goldstein MG, Siegel R. Thymoma developing 30 years after mantle radiation for Hodgkin's lymphoma. Conn Med. 2009 Oct;73(9):521–3. PMID:19860271

985. Goldstraw P, Chansky K, Crowley J, et al. The IASLC Lung Cancer Staging Project: proposals for revision of the TNM stage groupings in the forthcoming (eighth) edition of the TNM classification for lung cancer. J Thorac Oncol. 2016 Jan;11(1):39–51. PMID:26762738

986. Gomez-Aracil V, Mayayo E, Alvira R, et al. Fine needle aspiration cytology of primary pulmonary meningioma associated with minute meningotheliallike nodules. Report of a case with histologic, immunohistochemical and ultrastructural studies. Acta Cytol. 2002 Sep-Oct;46(5):899–903. PMID:12365227

987. Gonzalez-Vela JL, Savage PD, Manivel JC, et al. Poor prognosis of mediastinal germ cell cancers containing sarcomatous components. Cancer. 1990 Sep 15;66(6):1114–6. PMID:1698114

988. Goode B, Joseph NM, Stevers M, et al. Adenomatoid tumors of the male and female genital tract are defined by TRAF7 mutations that drive aberrant NF-kB pathway activation. Mod Pathol. 2018 Apr;31(4):660–73. PMID:29148537

989. Gopaldas RR, Atluri PV, Blaustein AS, et al. Papillary fibroelastoma of the aortic valve: operative approaches upon incidental discovery. Tex Heart Inst J. 2009;36(2):160–3. PMID:19436815

990. Gorshtein A, Gross DJ, Barak D, et al. Diffuse idiopathic pulmonary neuroendocrine cell hyperplasia and the associated lung neuroendocrine tumors: clinical experience with a rare entity. Cancer. 2012 Feb 1;118(3):612–9. PMID:21751183

991. Gošev I, Paić F, Durić Z, et al. Cardiac myxoma the great imitators: comprehensive histopathological and molecular approach. Int J Cardiol. 2013 Mar 20;164(1):7–20. PMID:22243936

992. Gosney JR, Williams IJ, Dodson AR, et al. Morphology and antigen expression profile of pulmonary neuroendocrine cells in reactive proliferations and diffuse idiopathic pulmonary neuroendocrine cell hyperplasia (DIPNECH). Histopathology. 2011 Oct;59(4):751–62. PMID:22014055

993. Goto K, Kodama T, Matsuno Y, et al. Clinicopathologic and DNA cytometric analysis of carcinoid tumors of the thymus. Mod Pathol. 2001 Oct;14(10):985–94. PMID:11598168

994. Goudet P, Murat A, Cardot-Bauters C, et al. Thymic neuroendocrine tumors in multiple endocrine neoplasia type 1: a comparative study on 21 cases among a series of 761 MEN1 from the GTE (Groupe des Tumeurs Endocrines). World J Surg. 2009 Jun;33(6):1197–207. PMID:19294466

995. Govender D, Pillay SV. Mediastinal immature teratoma with yolk sac tumor and myelomonocytic leukemia associated with Klinefelter's syndrome. Int J Surg Pathol. 2002 Apr;10(2):157–62. PMID:12075411

996. Gowda RM, Khan IA. Clinical perspectives of primary cardiac lymphoma. Angiology. 2003 Sep-Oct;54(5):599–604. PMID:14565636

997. Gowda RM, Khan IA, Nair CK, et al. Cardiac papillary fibroelastoma: a comprehensive analysis of 725 cases. Am Heart J. 2003 Sep;146(3):404–10. PMID:12947356

997A. Goyal G, Heaney ML, Collin M, et al. Erdheim-Chester disease: consensus recommendations for evaluation, diagnosis, and treatment in the molecular era. Blood. 2020 May 28;135(22):1929–45. PMID 32187362

998. Goyal G, Liu Y, Ravindran A, et al. Concomitant Erdheim-Chester disease and chronic myelomonocytic leukaemia: genomic insights into a common clonal origin. Br J Haematol. 2019 Oct;187(2):e51–4. PMID:31475353

999. Goyal G, Ravindran A, Liu Y, et al. Bone marrow findings in Erdheim-Chester disease: increased prevalence of chronic myeloid neoplasms. Haematologica. 2020 Jan 31;105(2):e84–6. PMID:31624111

1000. Goyal G, Young JR, Koster MJ, et al. The Mayo Clinic Histiocytosis Working Group consensus statement for the diagnosis and evaluation of adult patients with histiocytic neoplasms: Erdheim-Chester disease, Langerhans cell histiocytosis, and Rosai-Dorfman disease. Mayo Clin Proc. 2019 Oct;94(10):2054–71. PMID:31472931

1001. Graeme-Cook F, Mark EJ. Pulmonary mucinous cystic tumors of borderline malignancy. Hum Pathol. 1991 Feb;22(2):185–90. PMID:2001880

1002. Grajkowska W, Matyja E, Kunicki J, et al. AB thymoma with atypical type A component with delayed multiple lung and brain metastases. J Thorac Dis. 2017 Sep;9(9):E808–14. PMID:29221349

1003. Grande AM, Ragni T, Viganò M. Primary cardiac tumors. A clinical experience of 12 years. Tex Heart Inst J. 1993;20(3):223–30. PMID:8219826

1004. Gray N. The consequences of the unregulated cigarette. Tob Control. 2006 Oct;15(5):405–8. PMID:16998176

1005. Grayson AR, Walsh EM, Cameron MJ, et al. MYC, a downstream target of BRD-NUT, is necessary and sufficient for the blockade of differentiation in NUT midline carcinoma. Oncogene. 2014 Mar 27;33(13):1736–42. PMID:23604113

1006. Green AC, Marx A, Ströbel P, et al. Type A and AB thymomas: histological features associated with increased stage. Histopathology. 2015 May;66(6):884–91. PMID:25382290

1007. Green MR, Monti S, Rodig SJ, et al. Integrative analysis reveals selective 9p24.1 amplification, increased PD-1 ligand expression, and further induction via JAK2 in nodular sclerosing Hodgkin lymphoma and primary mediastinal large B-cell lymphoma. Blood. 2010 Oct 28;116(17):3268–77. PMID:20628145

1008. Grewal RG, Austin JH. CT demonstration of calcification in carcinoma of the lung. J Comput Assist Tomogr. 1994 Nov-Dec;18(6):867–71. PMID:7962791

1009. Griffin GK, Sholl LM, Lindeman NI, et al. Targeted genomic sequencing of follicular dendritic cell sarcoma reveals recurrent alterations in NF-κB regulatory genes. Mod Pathol. 2016 Jan;29(1):67–74. PMID:26564005

1010. Grosfeld JL, Skinner MA, Rescorla FJ, et al. Mediastinal tumors in children: experience with 196 cases. Ann Surg Oncol. 1994 Mar;1(2):121–7. PMID:7834436

1011. Grosu HB, Iliesiu M, Caraway NP, et al. Endobronchial ultrasound-guided transbronchial needle aspiration for the diagnosis and subtyping of lymphoma. Ann Am Thorac Soc. 2015 Sep;12(9):1336–44. PMID:26146788

1011A. Gruver AM, Amin MB, Luthringer DJ, et al. Selective immunohistochemical markers to distinguish between metastatic high-grade urothelial carcinoma and primary poorly differentiated invasive squamous cell carcinoma of the lung. Arch Pathol Lab Med. 2012 Nov;136(11):1339–46. PMID:23106579

1012. Gruver AM, Huba MA, Dogan A, et al. Fibrin-associated large B-cell lymphoma: part of the spectrum of cardiac lymphomas. Am J Surg Pathol. 2012 Oct;36(10):1527–37. PMID:22982895

1013. Grzegorczyk F, Dybowska M, Kuca P, et al. Pulmonary artery stenosis due to embryonal carcinoma with primary mediastinal location. Pneumonol Alergol Pol. 2015;83(2):151–6. PMID:25754058

1014. Gu L, Xu Y, Chen Z, et al. Clinical analysis of 95 cases of pulmonary sarcomatoid carcinoma. Biomed Pharmacother. 2015 Dec;76:134–40. PMID:26653560

1015. Gu L, Zhang L, Hou N, et al. Clinical and radiographic characterization of primary seminomas and nonseminomatous germ cell tumors. Niger J Clin Pract. 2019 Mar;22(3):342–9. PMID:30837421

1016. Gualis J, Carrascal Y, de la Fuente L, et al. Heart transplantation treatment for a malignant cardiac granular cell tumor: 33 months of survival. Interact Cardiovasc Thorac Surg. 2007 Oct;6(5):679–81. PMID:17670739

1017. Guardiola T, Horton E, Lopez-Camarillo L, et al. Cardiac myxoma: a cytogenetic study of two cases. Cancer Genet Cytogenet. 2004 Jan 15;148(2):145–7. PMID:14734227

1018. Guha T, Malkin D. Inherited TP53 mutations and the Li-Fraumeni syndrome. Cold Spring Harb Perspect Med. 2017 Apr 3;7(4):a026187. PMID:28270529

1019. Guibert N, Attias D, Pontier S, et al. Mediastinal teratoma and trichoptysis. Ann Thorac Surg. 2011 Jul;92(1):351–3. PMID:21718876

1020. Guibert N, Brouchet L, Rouquette I, et al. Thymoma and solid-organ transplantation. Lung Cancer. 2012 Jul;77(1):232–4. PMID:22487431

1021. Guillet S, Gérard L, Meignin V, et al. Classic and extracavitary primary effusion lymphoma in 51 HIV-infected patients from a single institution. Am J Hematol. 2016 Feb;91(2):233–7. PMID:26799611

1022. Guillou L, Aurias A. Soft tissue sarcomas with complex genomic profiles. Virchows Arch. 2010 Feb;456(2):201–17. PMID:20217954

1023. Guillou L, Benhattar J, Bonichon F, et al. Histologic grade, but not SYT-SSX fusion type, is an important prognostic factor in patients with synovial sarcoma: a multicenter, retrospective analysis. J Clin Oncol. 2004 Oct 15;22(20):4040–50. PMID:15364967

1024. Guillou L, Coindre JM, Bonichon F, et al. Comparative study of the National Cancer Institute and French Federation of Cancer Centers Sarcoma Group grading systems in a population of 410 adult patients with soft tissue sarcoma. J Clin Oncol. 1997 Jan;15(1):350–62. PMID:8996162

1025. Guimaraes AR, Wain JC, Mark EJ, et al. Mucinous cystadenoma of the lung. AJR Am J Roentgenol. 2004 Aug;183(2):282. PMID:15269012

1026. Guimarães MD, Benveniste MF, Bitencourt AG, et al. Thymoma originating in a giant thymolipoma: a rare intrathoracic lesion. Ann Thorac Surg. 2013 Sep;96(3):1083–5. PMID:23992709

1027. Guinee DG Jr, Perkins SL, Travis WD, et al. Proliferation and cellular phenotype in lymphomatoid granulomatosis: implications of a higher proliferation index in B cells. Am J Surg Pathol. 1998 Sep;22(9):1093–100. PMID:9737242

1028. Guinee DG Jr, Thornberry DS, Azumi N, et al. Unique pulmonary presentation of an angiomyolipoma. Analysis of clinical, radiographic, and histopathologic features. Am J Surg Pathol. 1995 Apr;19(4):476–80. PMID:7694950

1029. Gunawardana J, Chan FC, Telenius A, et al. Recurrent somatic mutations of PTPN1 in primary mediastinal B cell lymphoma and Hodgkin lymphoma. Nat Genet. 2014 Apr;46(4):329–35. PMID:24531327

1030. Guo LR, Myers ML, Kirk ME. Incidental malignancy in internal thoracic artery lymph nodes. Ann Thorac Surg. 2001 Aug;72(2):625–7. PMID:11515920

1031. Guo M, Tomoshige K, Meister M, et al. Gene signature driving invasive mucinous adenocarcinoma of the lung. EMBO Mol Med. 2017 Apr;9(4):462–81. PMID:28255028

1032. Guo T, Zhang L, Chang NE, et al. Consistent MYC and FLT4 gene amplification in radiation-induced angiosarcoma but not in other radiation-associated atypical vascular lesions. Genes Chromosomes Cancer. 2011 Jan;50(1):25–33. PMID:20949568

1033. Guo X, Zhang Y, Zheng L, et al. Global characterization of T cells in non-small-cell lung cancer by single-cell sequencing. Nat Med. 2018 Jul;24(7):978–85. PMID:29942094

1034. Gupta A, Harris K, Dhillon SS. Role of bronchoscopy in management of central squamous cell lung carcinoma in situ. Ann Transl Med. 2019 Aug;7(15):354. PMID:31516900

1035. Gupta GK, Jaffe ES, Pittaluga S. A study of PD-L1 expression in intravascular large B cell lymphoma: correlation with clinical and pathological features. Histopathology. 2019 Aug;75(2):282–6. PMID:30938862

1036. Gupta GP, Nguyen DX, Chiang AC, et al. Mediators of vascular remodelling co-opted for sequential steps in lung metastasis. Nature. 2007 Apr 12;446(7137):765–70. PMID:17429393

1037. Gupta MP, Lane AM, DeAngelis MM, et al. Clinical characteristics of uveal melanoma in patients with germline BAP1 mutations. JAMA Ophthalmol. 2015 Aug;133(8):881–7. PMID:25974357

1038. Gupta N, Henske EP. Pulmonary manifestations in tuberous sclerosis complex. Am J Med Genet C Semin Med Genet. 2018 Sep;178(3):326–37. PMID:30055039

1039. Gupta P, Singh S, Yadava K, et al. Typical carcinoid arising in mature teratoma of anterior mediastinum. Asian Cardiovasc Thorac Ann. 2012 Feb;20(1):80–2. PMID:22371952

1040. Gupta R, Marchevsky AM, McKenna RJ, et al. Evidence-based pathology and the pathologic evaluation of thymomas: transcapsular invasion is not a significant prognostic feature. Arch Pathol Lab Med. 2008 Jun;132(6):926–30. PMID:18517274

1041. Gupta R, Verma S, Bansal K, et al. Thymolipoma in child: a case diagnosed by correlation of ultrasound-guided fine needle aspiration (EUS-FNA) cytology and computed tomography with histological confirmation. Cytopathology. 2014 Aug;25(4):278–9. PMID:23902624

1042. Gurbuz AK, Giardiello FM, Petersen GM, et al. Desmoid tumours in familial adenomatous polyposis. Gut. 1994 Mar;35(3):377–81. PMID:8150351

1043. Gurel B, Ali TZ, Montgomery EA, et al. NKX3.1 as a marker of prostatic origin in metastatic tumors. Am J Surg Pathol. 2010 Aug;34(8):1097–105. PMID:20588175

1044. Gurney JG, Davis S, Severson RK, et al. Trends in cancer incidence among children in the U.S. Cancer. 1996 Aug 1;78(3):532–41. PMID:8697401

1045. Gurney JG, Ross JA, Wall DA, et al. Infant cancer in the U.S.: histology-specific incidence and trends, 1973 to 1992. J Pediatr Hematol Oncol. 1997 Sep-Oct;19(5):428–32. PMID:9329464

1046. Gustafson P. Soft tissue sarcoma. Epidemiology and prognosis in 508 patients. Acta Orthop Scand Suppl. 1994 Jun;259:1–31. PMID:8042499

1047. Gustafsson BI, Kidd M, Chan A, et al. Bronchopulmonary neuroendocrine tumors. Cancer. 2008 Jul 1;113(1):5–21. PMID:18473355

1048. Haack H, Johnson LA, Fry CJ, et al. Diagnosis of NUT midline carcinoma using a NUT-specific monoclonal antibody. Am J Surg Pathol. 2009 Jul;33(7):984–91. PMID:19363441

1049. Habougit C, Yvorel V, Sulaiman A, et al. Mediastinal mature teratoma with malignant carcinomatous transformation (somatic-type malignancy) with metastatic course. Int J Surg Pathol. 2015 Dec;23(8):682–4. PMID:26113666

1050. Hahn HP, Fletcher CD. Primary mediastinal liposarcoma: clinicopathologic analysis of 24 cases. Am J Surg Pathol. 2007 Dec;31(12):1868–74. PMID:18043041

1051. Hajar R, Roberts WC, Folger GM Jr. Embryonal botryoid rhabdomyosarcoma of the mitral valve. Am J Cardiol. 1986 Feb 1;57(4):376. PMID:3946244

1052. Hajdu M, Singer S, Maki RG, et al. IGF2 over-expression in solitary fibrous tumours is independent of anatomical location and is related to loss of imprinting. J Pathol. 2010 Jul;221(3):300–7. PMID:20527023

1053. Hakiri S, Fukui T, Mori S, et al. Clinicopathologic features of thymoma with the expression of programmed death ligand 1. Ann Thorac Surg. 2019 Feb;107(2):418–24. PMID:30312607

1054. Haller F, Moskalev EA, Faucz FR, et al. Aberrant DNA hypermethylation of SDHC: a novel mechanism of tumor development in Carney triad. Endocr Relat Cancer. 2014 Aug;21(4):567–77. PMID:24859990

1055. Halperin DM, Shen C, Dasari A, et al. Frequency of carcinoid syndrome at neuroendocrine tumour diagnosis: a population-based study. Lancet Oncol. 2017 Apr;18(4):525–34. PMID:28238592

1056. Hamidi M, Moody JS, Weigel TL, et al. Primary cardiac sarcoma. Ann Thorac Surg. 2010 Jul;90(1):176–81. PMID:20609770

1057. Hamza A, Vouyoukas E, Anderson IJ, et al. Thymic teratoma presenting as non-immune hydrops fetalis. Autops Case Rep. 2018 Feb 27;8(1):e2018004. PMID:29515979

1058. Hamza A, Younes AI, Kalhor N. Thymic mucoepidermoid carcinoma: a systematic review and meta-analysis. Adv Anat Pathol. 2019 Nov;26(6):341–5. PMID:31593977

1059. Han AJ, Xiong M, Zong YS. Association of Epstein-Barr virus with lymphoepithelioma-like carcinoma of the lung in southern China. Am J Clin Pathol. 2000 Aug;114(2):220–6. PMID:10941337

1060. Han W, Wang HM. Refractory diarrhea: a paraneoplastic syndrome of neuroblastoma. World J Gastroenterol. 2015 Jul 7;21(25):7929–32. PMID:26167095

1061. Han X, Li F, Fang Z, et al. Transdifferentiation of lung adenocarcinoma in mice with Lkb1 deficiency to squamous cell carcinoma. Nat Commun. 2014;5:3261. PMID:24531128

1062. Hancock BJ, Di Lorenzo M, Youssef S, et al. Childhood primary pulmonary neoplasms. J Pediatr Surg. 1993 Sep;28(9):1133–6. PMID:8308677

1063. Handra-Luca A, Couvelard A, Abd Alsamad I, et al. [Adenomatoid tumor of the pleura. Case report]. Ann Pathol. 2000 Sep;20(4):369–72. French. PMID:11015658

1064. Hanley KZ, Dureau ZJ, Cohen C, et al. Orthopedia homeobox is preferentially expressed in typical carcinoids of the lung. Cancer Cytopathol. 2018 Apr;126(4):236–42. PMID:29316326

1065. Hao X, Feng R, Bi Y, et al. Dramatic efficacy of dabrafenib in Erdheim-Chester disease (ECD): a pediatric patient with multiple large intracranial ECD lesions hidden by refractory Langerhans cell histiocytosis. J Neurosurg Pediatr. 2018 Sep 28;23(1):48–53. PMID:30265230

1066. Haque AK, Myers JL, Hudnall SD, et al. Pulmonary lymphomatoid granulomatosis in acquired immunodeficiency syndrome: lesions with Epstein-Barr virus infection. Mod Pathol. 1998 Apr;11(4):347–56. PMID:9578085

1067. Hara M, Sato Y, Kitase M, et al. CT and MR findings of a pleomorphic adenoma in the peripheral lung. Radiat Med. 2001 Mar-Apr;19(2):111–4. PMID:11383642

1068. Harada H, Miura K, Tsutsui Y, et al. Solitary squamous cell papilloma of the lung in a 40-year-old woman with recurrent laryngeal papillomatosis. Pathol Int. 2000 May;50(5):431–9. PMID:10849335

1069. Harbhajanka A, Dahoud W, Michael CW, et al. Cytohistological correlation, immunohistochemistry and murine double minute clone 2 amplification of pulmonary artery intimal sarcoma: a case report with review of literature. Diagn Cytopathol. 2019 May;47(5):494–7. PMID:30552756

1070. Harding CO, Pagon RA. Incidence of tuberous sclerosis in patients with cardiac rhabdomyoma. Am J Med Genet. 1990 Dec;37(4):443–6. PMID:2260584

1071. Hardy JD, Snavely JR, Langford HG. Low intrathoracic parathyroid adenoma: large functioning tumor representing fifth parathyroid, opposite eighth dorsal vertebra with independent arterial supply and opacified at operation with arteriogram. Ann Surg. 1964 Feb;159:310–5. PMID:14119197

1072. Hare SS, Souza CA, Bain G, et al. The radiological spectrum of pulmonary lymphoproliferative disease. Br J Radiol. 2012 Jul;85(1015):848–64. PMID:22745203

1073. Harigae H, Ichinohasama R, Miura I, et al. Primary marginal zone lymphoma of the thymus accompanied by chromosomal anomaly 46,X,dup(X)(p11p22). Cancer Genet Cytogenet. 2002 Mar;133(2):142–7. PMID:11943341

1074. Harnath T, Marx A, Ströbel P, et al. Thymoma-a clinico-pathological long-term study with emphasis on histology and adjuvant radiotherapy dose. J Thorac Oncol. 2012 Dec;7(12):1867–71. PMID:23154559

1075. Haroche J, Charlotte F, Arnaud L, et al. High prevalence of BRAF V600E mutations in Erdheim-Chester disease but not in other non-Langerhans cell histiocytoses. Blood. 2012 Sep 27;120(13):2700–3. PMID:22879539

1076. Haroutunian SG, O'Brien KJ, Estrada-Veras JI, et al. Clinical and histopathologic features of interstitial lung disease in Erdheim-Chester disease. J Clin Med. 2018 Aug 28;7(9):E243. PMID:30154360

1077. Harris NL. Shades of gray between large B-cell lymphomas and Hodgkin lymphomas: differential diagnosis and biological implications. Mod Pathol. 2013 Jan;26 Suppl 1:S57–70. PMID:23281436

1078. Harris NL, Jaffe ES, Stein H, et al. A revised European-American classification of lymphoid neoplasms: a proposal from the International Lymphoma Study Group. Blood. 1994 Sep 1;84(5):1361–92. PMID:8068936

1079. Hartel PH, Fanburg-Smith JC, Frazier AA, et al. Primary pulmonary and mediastinal synovial sarcoma: a clinicopathologic study of 60 cases and comparison with five prior series. Mod Pathol. 2007 Jul;20(7):760–9. PMID:17464314

1080. Hartmann CA, Roth C, Minck C, et al. Thymic carcinoma. Report of five cases and review of the literature. J Cancer Res Clin Oncol. 1990;116(1):69–82. PMID:2179229

1081. Hartmann JT, Fossa SD, Nichols CR, et al. Incidence of metachronous testicular cancer in patients with extragonadal germ cell tumors. J Natl Cancer Inst. 2001 Nov 21;93(22):1733–8. PMID:11717334

1082. Hartmann JT, Nichols CR, Droz JP, et al. Hematologic disorders associated with primary mediastinal nonseminomatous germ cell tumors. J Natl Cancer Inst. 2000 Jan 5;92(1):54–61. PMID:10620634

1083. Hartmann JT, Nichols CR, Droz JP, et al. Prognostic variables for response and outcome in patients with extragonadal germ-cell tumors. Ann Oncol. 2002 Jul;13(7):1017–28. PMID:12176779

1084. Haruki T, Nakamura H, Taniguchi Y, et al. Pulmonary mucinous cystadenoma: a rare benign tumor of the lung. Gen Thorac Cardiovasc Surg. 2010 Jun;58(6):287–90. PMID:20549459

1085. Harvey KF, Zhang X, Thomas DM. The Hippo pathway and human cancer. Nat Rev Cancer. 2013 Apr;13(4):246–57. PMID:23467301

1086. Hasegawa T, Matsuno Y, Shimoda T, et al. Proximal-type epithelioid sarcoma: a clinicopathologic study of 20 cases. Mod Pathol. 2001 Jul;14(7):655–63. PMID:11454997

1087. Hashimoto K, Okuma Y, Hosomi Y, et al. Malignant mesothelioma of the pleura with desmoplastic histology: a case series and literature review. BMC Cancer. 2016 Sep 6;16:718. PMID:27599565

1088. Hasle H, Jacobsen BB, Asschenfeldt P, et al. Mediastinal germ cell tumour associated with Klinefelter syndrome. A report of case and review of the literature. Eur J Pediatr. 1992 Oct;151(10):735–9. PMID:1425792

1089. Hasle H, Mellemgaard A, Nielsen J, et al. Cancer incidence in men with Klinefelter syndrome. Br J Cancer. 1995 Feb;71(2):416–20. PMID:7841064

1090. Hassan MM, Phan A, Li D, et al. Risk factors associated with neuroendocrine tumors: a U.S.-based case-control study. Int J Cancer. 2008 Aug 15;123(4):867–73. PMID:18491401

1091. Hassan R, Alexander R. Nonpleural mesotheliomas: mesothelioma of the peritoneum, tunica vaginalis, and pericardium. Hematol Oncol Clin North Am. 2005 Dec;19(6):1067–87, vi. PMID:16325124

1092. Hasserjian RP, Klimstra DS, Rosai J. Carcinoma of the thymus with clear-cell features. Report of eight cases and review of the literature. Am J Surg Pathol. 1995 Jul;19(7):835–41. PMID:7793482

1093. Hata A, Katakami N, Fujita S, et al. Frequency of EGFR and KRAS mutations in Japanese patients with lung adenocarcinoma with features of the mucinous subtype of bronchioloalveolar carcinoma. J Thorac Oncol. 2010 Aug;5(8):1197–200. PMID:20661086

1094. Hattab EM, Tu PH, Wilson JD, et al. OCT4 immunohistochemistry is superior to placental alkaline phosphatase (PLAP) in the diagnosis of central nervous system germinoma. Am J Surg Pathol. 2005 Mar;29(3):368–71. PMID:15725806

1095. Haugh AM, Njauw CN, Bubley JA, et al. Genotypic and phenotypic features of BAP1 cancer syndrome: a report of 8 new families and review of cases in the literature. JAMA Dermatol. 2017 Oct 1;153(10):999–1006. PMID:28793149

1096. Håvik AL, Bruland O, Myrseth E, et al. Genetic landscape of sporadic vestibular schwannoma. J Neurosurg. 2018 Mar;128(3):911–22. PMID:28409725

1097. Hawkins DS, Gupta AA, Rudzinski ER. What is new in the biology and treatment of pediatric rhabdomyosarcoma? Curr Opin Pediatr. 2014 Feb;26(1):50–6. PMID:24326270

1098. Hayashi A, Fumon T, Miki Y, et al. The evaluation of immunohistochemical markers and thymic cortical microenvironmental cells in distinguishing thymic carcinoma from type B3 thymoma or lung squamous cell carcinoma. J Clin Exp Hematop. 2013;53(1):9–19. PMID:23801129

1099. Hayashi A, Takamori S, Tayama K, et al. Thymolipoma: clinical and pathological features–report of three cases and review of literature. Kurume Med J. 1997;44(2):141–6. PMID:9255058

1100. Hayashi N, Fujita A, Saikai T, et al. Large cell neuroendocrine carcinoma harboring an anaplastic lymphoma kinase (ALK) rearrangement with response to alectinib. Intern Med. 2018 Mar 1;57(5):713–6. PMID:29151522

1101. Hayashi T, Haba R, Kushida Y, et al. Cytopathologic findings and differential diagnostic considerations of primary clear cell carcinoma of the lung. Diagn Cytopathol. 2013 Jun;41(6):550–4. PMID:21987503
1102. Hayashi T, Haba R, Tanizawa J, et al. Cytopathologic features and differential diagnostic considerations of primary lymphoepithelioma-like carcinoma of the lung. Diagn Cytopathol. 2012 Sep;40(9):820–5. PMID:21433005
1103. Hayashi T, Takamochi K, Yanai Y, et al. Non-small cell lung carcinoma with diffuse coexpression of thyroid transcription factor-1 and ΔNp63/p40. Hum Pathol. 2018 Aug;78:177–81. PMID:29410129
1103A. Hazim AZ, Ruan GJ, Ravindran A, et al. Efficacy of BRAF-inhibitor therapy in BRAFV600E -mutated adult Langerhans cell histiocytosis. Oncologist. 2020 Dec;25(12):1001–4. PMID:32985015
1104. He D, Chen M, Chen H, et al. Primary cardiac dedifferentiated liposarcoma with homologous and heterologous differentiation: a case report. Int J Clin Exp Pathol. 2015 Aug 1;8(8):9662–6. PMID:26464734
1105. He J, Shen J, Pan H, et al. Pulmonary lymphoepithelioma-like carcinoma: a Surveillance, Epidemiology, and End Results database analysis. J Thorac Dis. 2015 Dec;7(12):2330–8. PMID:26793355
1106. Heard BE, Corrin B, Dewar A. Pathology of seven mucous cell adenomas of the bronchial glands with particular reference to ultrastructure. Histopathology. 1985 Jul;9(7):687–701. PMID:4043932
1107. Hecht SS. Tobacco smoke carcinogens and lung cancer. J Natl Cancer Inst. 1999 Jul 21;91(14):1194–210. PMID:10413421
1108. Hecht SS, Szabo E. Fifty years of tobacco carcinogenesis research: from mechanisms to early detection and prevention of lung cancer. Cancer Prev Res (Phila). 2014 Jan;7(1):1–8. PMID:24403288
1109. Heelan R. Staging and response to therapy of malignant pleural mesothelioma. Lung Cancer. 2004 Aug;45 Suppl 1:S59–61. PMID:15261435
1110. Hegg CA, Flint A, Singh G. Papillary adenoma of the lung. Am J Clin Pathol. 1992 Mar;97(3):393–7. PMID:1543163
1111. Heide S, Masliah-Planchon J, Isidor B, et al. Oncologic phenotype of peripheral neuroblastic tumors associated with PHOX2B non-polyalanine repeat expansion mutations. Pediatr Blood Cancer. 2016 Jan;63(1):71–7. PMID:26375764
1112. Heitzer E, Sunitsch S, Gilg MM, et al. Expanded molecular profiling of myxofibrosarcoma reveals potentially actionable targets. Mod Pathol. 2017 Dec;30(12):1698–709. PMID:28776571
1113. Hekimgil M, Hamulu F, Cagirici U, et al. Small cell neuroendocrine carcinoma of the thymus complicated by Cushing's syndrome. Report of a 58-year-old woman with a 3-year history of hypertension. Pathol Res Pract. 2001;197(2):129–33. PMID:11261817
1114. Hellmann MD, Callahan MK, Awad MM, et al. Tumor mutational burden and efficacy of nivolumab monotherapy and in combination with ipilimumab in small-cell lung cancer. Cancer Cell. 2018 May 14;33(5):853–861.e4. PMID:29731394
1115. Hellmann MD, Ciuleanu TE, Pluzanski A, et al. Nivolumab plus ipilimumab in lung cancer with a high tumor mutational burden. N Engl J Med. 2018 May 31;378(22):2093–104. PMID:29658845
1116. Hemachandran M, Kakkar N, Khandelwal N. Giant-cell-rich myxoma of right atrium. An ultrastructural analysis. Cardiovasc Pathol. 2003 Sep-Oct;12(5):287–9. PMID:14507579
1117. Henderson DW, Attwood HD, Constance TJ, et al. Lymphohistiocytoid mesothelioma: a rare lymphomatoid variant of predominantly sarcomatoid mesothelioma. Ultrastruct Pathol. 1988;12(4):367–84. PMID:2458647
1118. Hendriksen BS, Hollenbeak CS, Reed MF, et al. Perioperative chemotherapy is not associated with improved survival in stage I pleomorphic lung cancer. J Thorac Cardiovasc Surg. 2019 Aug;158(2):581–591.e11. PMID:31122617
1119. Henley JD, Cummings OW, Loehrer PJ Sr. Tyrosine kinase receptor expression in thymomas. J Cancer Res Clin Oncol. 2004 Apr;130(4):222–4. PMID:14762710
1120. Henley SJ, Larson TC, Wu M, et al. Mesothelioma incidence in 50 states and the District of Columbia, United States, 2003-2008. Int J Occup Environ Health. 2013 Jan-Mar;19(1):1–10. PMID:23582609
1121. Henon C, Blay JY, Massard C, et al. Long lasting major response to pembrolizumab in a thoracic malignant rhabdoid-like SMARCA4-deficient tumor. Ann Oncol. 2019 Aug 1;30(8):1401–3. PMID:31114851
1122. Henry E, Villalobos V, Million L, et al. Chest wall leiomyosarcoma after breast-conservative therapy for early-stage breast cancer in a young woman with Li-Fraumeni syndrome. J Natl Compr Canc Netw. 2012 Aug;10(8):939–42. PMID:22878818
1123. Henschke CI, Yip R, Smith JP, et al. CT screening for lung cancer: part-solid nodules in baseline and annual repeat rounds. AJR Am J Roentgenol. 2016 Dec;207(6):1176–84. PMID:27726410
1124. Henske EP, Jóźwiak S, Kingswood JC, et al. Tuberous sclerosis complex. Nat Rev Dis Primers. 2016 May 26;2:16035. PMID:27226234
1125. Heravi-Moussavi A, Anglesio MS, Cheng SW, et al. Recurrent somatic DICER1 mutations in nonepithelial ovarian cancers. N Engl J Med. 2012 Jan 19;366(3):234–42. PMID:22187960
1126. Herbst H, Dallenbach F, Hummel M, et al. Epstein-Barr virus latent membrane protein expression in Hodgkin and Reed-Sternberg cells. Proc Natl Acad Sci U S A. 1991 Jun 1;88(11):4766–70. PMID:1647016
1127. Herbst RS, Baas P, Kim DW, et al. Pembrolizumab versus docetaxel for previously treated, PD-L1-positive, advanced non-small-cell lung cancer (KEYNOTE-010): a randomised controlled trial. Lancet. 2016 Apr 9;387(10027):1540–50. PMID:26712084
1128. Herbst RS, Heymach JV, Lippman SM. Lung cancer. N Engl J Med. 2008 Sep 25;359(13):1367–80. PMID:18815398
1129. Herman TE, McAlister WH, Dehner LP. Posterior mediastinal capillary hemangioma with extradural extension resembling neuroblastoma. Pediatr Radiol. 1999 Jul;29(7):517–9. PMID:10398787
1130. Hermans BCM, Derks JL, Thunnissen E, et al. Prevalence and prognostic value of PD-L1 expression in molecular subtypes of metastatic large cell neuroendocrine carcinoma (LCNEC). Lung Cancer. 2019 Apr;130:179–86. PMID:30885341
1131. Herpel E, Rieker RJ, Dienemann H, et al. SMARCA4 and SMARCA2 deficiency in non-small cell lung cancer: immunohistochemical survey of 316 consecutive specimens. Ann Diagn Pathol. 2017 Feb;26:47–51. PMID:28038711
1132. Herrmann MA, Shankerman RA, Edwards WD, et al. Primary cardiac angiosarcoma: a clinicopathologic study of six cases. J Thorac Cardiovasc Surg. 1992 Apr;103(4):655–64. PMID:1548908
1133. Herth FJ, Eberhardt R, Anantham D, et al. Narrow-band imaging bronchoscopy increases the specificity of bronchoscopic early lung cancer detection. J Thorac Oncol. 2009 Sep;4(9):1060–5. PMID:19704335
1134. Hertwig F, Peifer M, Fischer M. Telomere maintenance is pivotal for high-risk neuroblastoma. Cell Cycle. 2016;15(3):311–2. PMID:26653081
1135. Hervier B, Arnaud L, Charlotte F, et al. Treatment of Erdheim-Chester disease with long-term high-dose interferon-α. Semin Arthritis Rheum. 2012 Jun;41(6):907–13. PMID:22300602
1136. Hervier B, Haroche J, Arnaud L, et al. Association of both Langerhans cell histiocytosis and Erdheim-Chester disease linked to the BRAFV600E mutation. Blood. 2014 Aug 14;124(7):1119–26. PMID:24894769
1137. Hes O, Perez-Montiel DM, Alvarado Cabrero I, et al. Thread-like bridging strands: a morphologic feature present in all adenomatoid tumors. Ann Diagn Pathol. 2003 Oct;7(5):273–7. PMID:14571427
1138. Heymann S, Delaloge S, Rahal A, et al. Radio-induced malignancies after breast cancer postoperative radiotherapy in patients with Li-Fraumeni syndrome. Radiat Oncol. 2010 Nov 8;5:104. PMID:21059199
1139. Hibbitts E, Chi YY, Hawkins DS, et al. Refinement of risk stratification for childhood rhabdomyosarcoma using FOXO1 fusion status in addition to established clinical outcome predictors: a report from the Children's Oncology Group. Cancer Med. 2019 Oct;8(14):6437–48. PMID:31456361
1140. Hibiya T, Tanaka M, Matsumura M, et al. An NRAS mutation in primary malignant melanoma of the lung: a case report. Diagn Pathol. 2020 Feb 7;15(1):11. PMID:32028967
1141. Hida T, Hamasaki M, Matsumoto S, et al. Immunohistochemical detection of MTAP and BAP1 protein loss for mesothelioma diagnosis: comparison with 9p21 FISH and BAP1 immunohistochemistry. Lung Cancer. 2017 Feb;104:98–105. PMID:28213009
1142. Higashi H, Inaba S, Izutani H, et al. An unusual cause of life-threatening right-sided heart failure: undifferentiated pleomorphic sarcoma in the right ventricular outflow tract. Eur Heart J. 2016 Mar 21;37(12):1002. PMID:26670651
1143. Higashiyama M, Doi O, Kodama K, et al. Lymphoepithelioma-like carcinoma of the lung: analysis of two cases for Epstein-Barr virus infection. Hum Pathol. 1995 Nov;26(11):1278–82. PMID:7590705
1144. Higgins JP, Warnke RA. CD30 expression is common in mediastinal large B-cell lymphoma. Am J Clin Pathol. 1999 Aug;112(2):241–7. PMID:10439805
1145. Higuchi T, Matsuo K, Hashida Y, et al. Epstein-Barr virus-positive pyothorax-associated lymphoma expresses CCL17 and CCL22 chemokines that attract CCR4-expressing regulatory T cells. Cancer Lett. 2019 Jul 1;453:184–92. PMID:30953706
1146. Hill DA, Ivanovich J, Priest JR, et al. DICER1 mutations in familial pleuropulmonary blastoma. Science. 2009 Aug 21;325(5943):965. PMID:19556464
1147. Hill DA, Jarzembowski JA, Priest JR, et al. Type I pleuropulmonary blastoma: pathology and biology study of 51 cases from the international pleuropulmonary blastoma registry. Am J Surg Pathol. 2008 Feb;32(2):282–95. PMID:18223332
1148. Hillerdal G. Malignant mesothelioma 1982: review of 4710 published cases. Br J Dis Chest. 1983 Oct;77(4):321–43. PMID:6357260
1149. Hinterberger M, Reineke T, Storz M, et al. D2-40 and calretinin - a tissue microarray analysis of 341 malignant mesotheliomas with emphasis on sarcomatoid differentiation. Mod Pathol. 2007 Feb;20(2):248–55. PMID:17361207
1150. Hinton RB, Prakash A, Romp RL, et al. Cardiovascular manifestations of tuberous sclerosis complex and summary of the revised diagnostic criteria and surveillance and management recommendations from the International Tuberous Sclerosis Consensus Group. J Am Heart Assoc. 2014 Nov 25;3(6):e001493. PMID:25424575
1151. Hirabayashi H, Fujii Y, Sakaguchi M, et al. p16INK4, pRB, p53 and cyclin D1 expression and hypermethylation of CDKN2 gene in thymoma and thymic carcinoma. Int J Cancer. 1997 Nov 27;73(5):639–44. PMID:9398039
1152. Hirai I, Tanese K, Obata S, et al. A case of primary malignant melanoma of the lung responded to anti-PD-1 antibody therapy. Indian J Thorac Cardiovasc Surg. 2017 Jun;33:173–5. doi:10.1007/s12055-017-0488-z.
1153. Hirakata K, Nakata H, Nakagawa T. CT of pulmonary metastases with pathological correlation. Semin Ultrasound CT MR. 1995 Oct;16(5):379–94. PMID:8527171
1154. Hirano H, Maeda H, Takeuchi Y, et al. Primary pulmonary Ewing sarcoma. Pathol Int. 2016 Apr;66(4):239–41. PMID:26698372
1155. Hirano H, Maeda T, Tsuji M, et al. Malignant mesothelioma of the pericardium: case reports and immunohistochemical studies including Ki-67 expression. Pathol Int. 2002 Oct;52(10):669–76. PMID:12445141
1156. Hirooka K, Oonuki M, Manabe S, et al. Radiation therapy for recurrent cardiac undifferentiated pleomorphic sarcoma after three operations. Gen Thorac Cardiovasc Surg. 2018 Mar;66(3):168–71. PMID:28434140
1157. Hiroshima K, Mino-Kenudson M. Update on large cell neuroendocrine carcinoma. Transl Lung Cancer Res. 2017 Oct;6(5):530–9. PMID:29114469
1158. Hirsch FR, Bunn PA Jr. Progress in research on screening and genetics in lung cancer. Lancet Respir Med. 2014 Jan;2(1):19–21. PMID:24461890
1159. Hirsch FR, Franklin WA, Gazdar AF, et al. Early detection of lung cancer: clinical perspectives of recent advances in biology and radiology. Clin Cancer Res. 2001 Jan;7(1):5–22. PMID:11205917
1159A. Hirsch FR, Matthews MJ, Yesner R. Histopathologic classification of small cell carcinoma of the lung: comments based on an interobserver examination. Cancer. 1982 Oct 1;50(7):1360–6. PMID:6286092
1160. Hirsch FR, Prindiville SA, Miller YE, et al. Fluorescence versus white-light bronchoscopy for detection of preneoplastic lesions: a randomized study. J Natl Cancer Inst. 2001 Sep 19;93(18):1385–91. PMID:11562389
1161. Hirsch FR, Suda K, Wiens J, et al. New and emerging targeted treatments in advanced non-small-cell lung cancer. Lancet. 2016 Sep 3;388(10048):1012–24. PMID:27598681
1162. Hishida T, Nomura S, Yano M, et al. Long-term outcome and prognostic factors of surgically treated thymic carcinoma: results of 306 cases from a Japanese nationwide database study. Eur J Cardiothorac Surg. 2016 Mar;49(3):835–41. PMID:26116920
1163. Hishima T, Fukayama M, Fujisawa M, et al. CD5 expression in thymic carcinoma. Am J Pathol. 1994 Aug;145(2):268–75. PMID:7519823
1164. Hishima T, Fukayama M, Hayashi Y, et al. Neuroendocrine differentiation in thymic epithelial tumors with special reference to thymic carcinoma and atypical thymoma. Hum Pathol. 1998 Apr;29(4):330–8. PMID:9563781
1165. Hissong E, Rao R. Pneumocytoma (sclerosing hemangioma), a potential pitfall. Diagn Cytopathol. 2017 Aug;45(8):744–9.

PMID:28398699
1166. Hmeljak J, Sanchez-Vega F, Hoadley KA, et al. Integrative molecular characterization of malignant pleural mesothelioma. Cancer Discov. 2018 Dec;8(12):1548–65. PMID:30322867
1167. Ho FC, Ho JC. Pigmented carcinoid tumour of the thymus. Histopathology. 1977 Sep;1(5):363–9. PMID:615841
1168. Hochhegger B, Nin CS, Alves GR, et al. Multidetector computed tomography findings in pulmonary hamartomas: a new fat detection threshold. J Thorac Imaging. 2016 Jan;31(1):11–4. PMID:26447871
1169. Hochstenbag MM, Twijnstra A, Wilmink JT, et al. Asymptomatic brain metastases (BM) in small cell lung cancer (SCLC): MR-imaging is useful at initial diagnosis. J Neurooncol. 2000 Jul;48(3):243–8. PMID:11100822
1170. Hoffman OA, Gillespie DJ, Aughenbaugh GL, et al. Primary mediastinal neoplasms (other than thymoma). Mayo Clin Proc. 1993 Sep;68(9):880–91. PMID:8396701
1171. Hofscheier A, Ponciano A, Bonzheim I, et al. Geographic variation in the prevalence of Epstein-Barr virus-positive diffuse large B-cell lymphoma of the elderly: a comparative analysis of a Mexican and a German population. Mod Pathol. 2011 Aug;24(8):1046–54. PMID:21499229
1172. Holladay AO, Siegel RJ, Schwartz DA. Cardiac malignant lymphoma in acquired immune deficiency syndrome. Cancer. 1992 Oct 15;70(8):2203–7. PMID:1394052
1173. Holley DG, Martin GR, Brenner JI, et al. Diagnosis and management of fetal cardiac tumors: a multicenter experience and review of published reports. J Am Coll Cardiol. 1995 Aug;26(2):516–20. PMID:7608458
1174. Holst VA, Finkelstein S, Colby TV, et al. p53 and K-ras mutational genotyping in pulmonary carcinosarcoma, spindle cell carcinoma, and pulmonary blastoma: implications for histogenesis. Am J Surg Pathol. 1997 Jul;21(7):801–11. PMID:9236836
1175. Holzhauser L, Heymer J, Kasner M, et al. Rare case of a multilocular primary cardiac intimal sarcoma presenting as left atrial mass with new onset atrial fibrillation. Eur Heart J. 2015 Sep 14;36(35):2402. PMID:26040800
1176. Homma T, Yamamoto Y, Imura J, et al. Spontaneous hemothorax caused by pulmonary micro-venous hemangioma. Ann Thorac Surg. 2015 Jul;100(1):299–301. PMID:26140771
1177. Hongyo T, Kurooka M, Taniguchi E, et al. Frequent p53 mutations at dipyrimidine sites in patients with pyothorax-associated lymphoma. Cancer Res. 1998 Mar 15;58(6):1105–7. PMID:9515788
1178. Horn L, Mansfield AS, Szczęsna A, et al. First-line atezolizumab plus chemotherapy in extensive-stage small-cell lung cancer. N Engl J Med. 2018 Dec 6;379(23):2220–9. PMID:30280641
1179. Hornick JL, Fletcher CD. Myoepithelial tumors of soft tissue: a clinicopathologic and immunohistochemical study of 101 cases with evaluation of prognostic parameters. Am J Surg Pathol. 2003 Sep;27(9):1183–96. PMID:12960802
1180. Hornick JL, Fletcher CD. PEComa: What do we know so far? Histopathology. 2006 Jan;48(1):75–82. PMID:16359539
1181. Hosaka Y, Tsuchida M, Umezu H, et al. Primary thymic adenocarcinoma coexisting with type AB thymoma: a rare case with long-term survival. Gen Thorac Cardiovasc Surg. 2010 Sep;58(9):488–91, discussion 491–2. PMID:20859731
1182. Hoshino A, Costa-Silva B, Shen TL, et al. Tumour exosome integrins determine organotropic metastasis. Nature. 2015 Nov 19;527(7578):329–35. PMID:26524530
1183. Hosler GA, Steinberg DM, Sheth S, et al. Inflammatory pseudotumor: a diagnostic dilemma in cytopathology. Diagn Cytopathol. 2004 Oct;31(4):267–70. PMID:15452903
1184. Hostein I, Andraud-Fregeville M, Guillou L, et al. Rhabdomyosarcoma: value of myogenin expression analysis and molecular testing in diagnosing the alveolar subtype: an analysis of 109 paraffin-embedded specimens. Cancer. 2004 Dec 15;101(12):2817–24. PMID:15536621
1184A. Hotokebuchi Y, Kohashi K, Toyoshima S, et al. Congenital peribronchial myofibroblastic tumor. Pathol Int. 2014 Apr;64(4):189–91. PMID:24750190
1185. Hottenrott G, Mentzel T, Peters A, et al. Intravascular ("intimal") epithelioid angiosarcoma: clinicopathological and immunohistochemical analysis of three cases. Virchows Arch. 1999 Nov;435(5):473–8. PMID:10592050
1186. Houston KA, Henley SJ, Li J, et al. Patterns in lung cancer incidence rates and trends by histologic type in the United States, 2004-2009. Lung Cancer. 2014 Oct;86(1):22–8. PMID:25172266
1187. Houston KA, Mitchell KA, King J, et al. Histologic lung cancer incidence rates and trends vary by race/ethnicity and residential county. J Thorac Oncol. 2018 Apr;13(4):497–509. PMID:29360512
1188. Hsieh MS, Wu CT, Chang YL. Unusual presentation of lymphoepithelioma-like carcinoma of lung as a thin-walled cavity. Ann Thorac Surg. 2013 Nov;96(5):1857–9. PMID:24182474
1189. Hsu C. Cytologic detection of malignancy in pleural effusion: a review of 5,255 samples from 3,811 patients. Diagn Cytopathol. 1987 Mar;3(1):8–12. PMID:3568976
1190. Hsu CH, Chan JK, Yin CH, et al. Trends in the incidence of thymoma, thymic carcinoma, and thymic neuroendocrine tumor in the United States. PLoS One. 2019 Dec 31;14(12):e0227197. PMID:31891634
1191. Hsueh C, Kuo TT, Tsang NM, et al. Thymic lymphoepitheliomalike carcinoma in children: clinicopathologic features and molecular analysis. J Pediatr Hematol Oncol. 2006 Dec;28(12):785–90. PMID:17164646
1192. Hu J, Schuster AE, Fritsch MK, et al. Deletion mapping of 6q21-26 and frequency of 1p36 deletion in childhood endodermal sinus tumors by microsatellite analysis. Oncogene. 2001 Nov 29;20(55):8042–4. PMID:11753688
1193. Hu MM, Hu Y, He JB, et al. Primary adenoid cystic carcinoma of the lung: clinicopathological features, treatment and results. Oncol Lett. 2015 Mar;9(3):1475–81. PMID:25663934
1194. Hu WM, Jin JT, Wu CY, et al. Expression of p63 and its correlation with prognosis in diffuse large B-cell lymphoma: a single center experience. Diagn Pathol. 2019 Nov 11;14(1):128. PMID:31711519
1195. Hu X, Fujimoto J, Ying L, et al. Multi-region exome sequencing reveals genomic evolution from preneoplasia to lung adenocarcinoma. Nat Commun. 2019 Jul 5;10(1):2978. PMID:31278276
1196. Huang CC, Collins BT, Flint A, et al. Pulmonary neuroendocrine tumors: an entity in search of cytologic criteria. Diagn Cytopathol. 2013 Aug;41(8):689–96. PMID:23166111
1197. Huang CC, Michael CW. Deciduoid mesothelioma: cytologic presentation and diagnostic pitfalls. Diagn Cytopathol. 2013 Jul;41(7):629–35. PMID:23008275
1198. Huang HY, Lal P, Qin J, et al. Low-grade myxofibrosarcoma: a clinicopathologic analysis of 49 cases treated at a single institution with simultaneous assessment of the efficacy of 3-tier and 4-tier grading systems. Hum Pathol. 2004 May;35(5):612–21. PMID:15138937
1199. Huang J, Ahmad U, Antonicelli A, et al. Development of the International Thymic Malignancy Interest Group international database: an unprecedented resource for the study of a rare group of tumors. J Thorac Oncol. 2014 Oct;9(10):1573–8. PMID:25521402
1200. Huang M, Zeki J, Sumarsono N, et al. Epigenetic targeting of TERT-associated gene expression signature in human neuroblastoma with TERT overexpression. Cancer Res. 2020 Mar 1;80(5):1024–35. PMID:31900258
1201. Huang SC, Chen HW, Zhang L, et al. Novel FUS-KLF17 and EWSR1-KLF17 fusions in myoepithelial tumors. Genes Chromosomes Cancer. 2015 May;54(5):267–75. PMID:25706482
1202. Huang SC, Zhang L, Sung YS, et al. Recurrent CIC gene abnormalities in angiosarcomas: a molecular study of 120 cases with concurrent investigation of PLCG1, KDR, MYC, and FLT4 gene alterations. Am J Surg Pathol. 2016 May;40(5):645–55. PMID:26735859
1203. Huang Y, Yang X, Lu T, et al. Assessment of the prognostic factors in patients with pulmonary carcinoid tumor: a population-based study. Cancer Med. 2018 Jun;7(6):2434–41. PMID:29733505
1204. Hudacko R, Aviv H, Langenfeld J, et al. Thymolipoma: clues to pathogenesis revealed by cytogenetics. Ann Diagn Pathol. 2009 Jun;13(3):185–8. PMID:19433298
1205. Hughes JH, Young NA, Wilbur DC, et al. Fine-needle aspiration of pulmonary hamartoma: a common source of false-positive diagnoses in the College of American Pathologists Interlaboratory Comparison Program in Nongynecologic Cytology. Arch Pathol Lab Med. 2005 Jan;129(1):19–22. PMID:15628903
1206. Hui KS, Green LK, Schmidt WA. Primary cardiac rhabdomyosarcoma: definition of a rare entity. Am J Cardiovasc Pathol. 1988;2(1):19–29. PMID:3207486
1207. Hui M, Paul TR, Uppin SG, et al. Lipofibroadenoma with B1 thymoma: a case report of a rare thymic tumor. Indian J Pathol Microbiol. 2018 Oct-Dec;61(4):630–2. PMID:30303172
1208. Hummel P, Cangiarella JF, Cohen JM, et al. Transthoracic fine-needle aspiration biopsy of pulmonary spindle cell and mesenchymal lesions: a study of 61 cases. Cancer. 2001 Jun 25;93(3):187–98. PMID:11391606
1209. Hung YP, Dong F, Dubuc AM, et al. Molecular characterization of localized pleural mesothelioma. Mod Pathol. 2020 Feb;33(2):271–80. PMID:31371807
1210. Hung YP, Dong F, Watkins JC, et al. Identification of ALK rearrangements in malignant peritoneal mesothelioma. JAMA Oncol. 2018 Feb 1;4(2):235–8. PMID:28910456
1211. Hung YP, Fletcher CD, Hornick JL. Evaluation of ETV4 and WT1 expression in CIC-rearranged sarcomas and histologic mimics. Mod Pathol. 2016 Nov;29(11):1324–34. PMID:27443513
1212. Huo Z, Wu H, Li J, et al. Primary pulmonary mucoepidermoid carcinoma: histopathological and moleculargenetic studies of 26 cases. PLoS One. 2015 Nov 17;10(11):e0143169. PMID:26575266
1212A. Huppmann AR, Coffin CM, Hoot AC, et al. Congenital peribronchial myofibroblastic tumor: comparison of fetal and postnatal morphology. Pediatr Dev Pathol. 2011 Mar-Apr;14(2):124–9. PMID:20367454
1213. Husain AN, Colby TV, Ordóñez NG, et al. Guidelines for pathologic diagnosis of malignant mesothelioma 2017 update of the consensus statement from the International Mesothelioma Interest Group. Arch Pathol Lab Med. 2018 Jan;142(1):89–108. PMID:28686500
1214. Hussein-Jelen T, Bankier AA, Eisenberg RL. Solid pleural lesions. AJR Am J Roentgenol. 2012 Jun;198(6):W512–20. PMID:22623565
1215. Hüttmann A, Rekowski J, Müller SP, et al. Six versus eight doses of rituximab in patients with aggressive B cell lymphoma receiving six cycles of CHOP: results from the "Positron Emission Tomography-Guided Therapy of Aggressive Non-Hodgkin Lymphomas" (PETAL) trial. Ann Hematol. 2019 Apr;98(4):897–907. PMID:30610279
1216. Hwang DH, Sholl LM, Rojas-Rudilla V, et al. KRAS and NKX2-1 mutations in invasive mucinous adenocarcinoma of the lung. J Thorac Oncol. 2016 Apr;11(4):496–503. PMID:26829311
1217. Hwang EJ, Park CM, Ryu Y, et al. Pulmonary adenocarcinomas appearing as part-solid ground-glass nodules: Is measuring solid component size a better prognostic indicator? Eur Radiol. 2015 Feb;25(2):558–67. PMID:25274618
1218. Hwang HC, Pyott S, Rodriguez S, et al. BAP1 immunohistochemistry and p16 FISH in the diagnosis of sarcomatous and desmoplastic mesotheliomas. Am J Surg Pathol. 2016 May;40(5):714–8. PMID:26900815
1219. Iacobone M, Mondi I, Viel G, et al. The results of surgery for mediastinal parathyroid tumors: a comparative study of 63 patients. Langenbecks Arch Surg. 2010 Sep;395(7):947–53. PMID:20623135
1220. IARC TP53 Database [Internet]. Lyon (France): International Agency for Research on Cancer; 2019. Version R20, July 2019. Available from: https://p53.iarc.fr/.
1220A. IARC Working Group on the Evaluation of Carcinogenic Risks to Humans. Arsenic, metals, fibres, and dusts. IARC Monogr Eval Carcinog Risks Hum. 2012;100(Pt C):11–465. PMID:23189751
1221. IARC Working Group on the Evaluation of Carcinogenic Risks to Humans. Household use of solid fuels and high-temperature frying. IARC Monogr Eval Carcinog Risks Hum. 2010;95:1–430. PMID:20701241
1222. Ibi T, Hirai K, Takeuchi S, et al. Mature teratoma of the posterior mediastinum: report of a case. Gen Thorac Cardiovasc Surg. 2013 Nov;61(11):655–8. PMID:23104458
1223. Ibrahim A, Luk A, Singhal P, et al. Primary intimal (spindle cell) sarcoma of the heart: a case report and review of the literature. Case Rep Med. 2013;2013:461815. PMID:23424592
1224. Icard B, Grider DJ, Aziz S, et al. Primary tracheal hyalinizing clear cell carcinoma. Lung Cancer. 2018 Nov;125:100–2. PMID:30429005
1225. Ichinohasama R, Miura I, Kobayashi N, et al. Herpes virus type 8-negative primary effusion lymphoma associated with PAX-5 gene rearrangement and hepatitis C virus: a case report and review of the literature. Am J Surg Pathol. 1998 Dec;22(12):1528–37. PMID:9850179
1226. Iczkowski KA, Butler SL, Shanks JH, et al. Trials of new germ cell immunohistochemical stains in 93 extragonadal and metastatic germ cell tumors. Hum Pathol. 2008 Feb;39(2):275–81. PMID:18045648
1227. Ide T, Miyoshi T, Katsuragi S, et al. Prediction of postnatal arrhythmia in fetuses with cardiac rhabdomyoma. J Matern Fetal Neonatal Med. 2019 Aug;32(15):2463–8. PMID:29415597
1228. Idowu MO, Powers CN. Lung cancer cytology: potential pitfalls and mimics - a review. Int J Clin Exp Pathol. 2010 Mar 25;3(4):367–85. PMID:20490328
1229. Iezzoni JC, Gaffey MJ, Weiss LM. The role of Epstein-Barr virus in lymphoepithelioma-like carcinomas. Am J Clin Pathol. 1995 Mar;103(3):308–15. PMID:7872253
1230. Iezzoni JC, Nass LB. Thymic basaloid carcinoma: a case report and review of the

literature. Mod Pathol. 1996 Jan;9(1):21–5. PMID:8821951

1231. Iftikhar IH, Musani AI. Narrow-band imaging bronchoscopy in the detection of pre-malignant airway lesions: a meta-analysis of diagnostic test accuracy. Ther Adv Respir Dis. 2015 Oct;9(5):207–16. PMID:26085510

1232. Iida T, Nomori H, Shiba M, et al. Prognostic factors after pulmonary metastasectomy for colorectal cancer and rationale for determining surgical indications: a retrospective analysis. Ann Surg. 2013 Jun;257(6):1059–64. PMID:23001087

1233. Ikdahl T, Josefsen D, Jakobsen E, et al. Concurrent mediastinal germ-cell tumour and haematological malignancy: case report and short review of literature. Acta Oncol. 2008;47(3):466–9. PMID:18348004

1234. Ikeda K, Tate G, Suzuki T, et al. Cytomorphologic features of immature ovarian teratoma in peritoneal effusion: a case report. Diagn Cytopathol. 2005 Jul;33(1):39–42. PMID:15945092

1235. Ikeda N, Usuda J, Kato H, et al. New aspects of photodynamic therapy for central type early stage lung cancer. Lasers Surg Med. 2011 Sep;43(7):749–54. PMID:22057502

1236. Ikegaki N, Shimada H, International Neuroblastoma Pathology Committee. Subgrouping of unfavorable histology neuroblastomas with immunohistochemistry toward precision prognosis and therapy stratification. JCO Precis Oncol. 2019;3:PO.18.00312. PMID:31840131

1237. Ikuta N, Tano M, Iwata M, et al. [A case of adenomatoid mesothelioma of the pleura]. Nihon Kyobu Shikkan Gakkai Zasshi. 1989 Dec;27(12):1540–4. Japanese. PMID:2630775

1238. Ilhan I, Kutluk T, Göğüş S, et al. Hypertrophic pulmonary osteoarthropathy in a child with thymic carcinoma: an unusual presentation in childhood. Med Pediatr Oncol. 1994;23(2):140–3. PMID:8202038

1239. Illei PB, Rosai J, Klimstra DS. Expression of thyroid transcription factor-1 and other markers in sclerosing hemangioma of the lung. Arch Pathol Lab Med. 2001 Oct;125(10):1335–9. PMID:11570910

1239A. Impact Genetics [Internet]. Brampton (ON): Impact Genetics; 2020. What is BAP1-TPDS: info for patients & clinicians. Available from: https://impact-genetics.com/testing-services/bap1-tumor-predisposition-syndrome-bap1-tpds/bap1-tpds-info-patients-clinicians/.

1240. Inafuku K, Yokose T, Ito H, et al. Two cases of lung neuroendocrine carcinoma with carcinoid morphology. Diagn Pathol. 2019 Sep 12;14(1):104. PMID:31511024

1241. Inagaki H, Chan JK, Ng JW, et al. Primary thymic extranodal marginal-zone B-cell lymphoma of mucosa-associated lymphoid tissue type exhibits distinctive clinicopathological and molecular features. Am J Pathol. 2002 Apr;160(4):1435–43. PMID:11943727

1242. Inage T, Nakajima T, Fujiwara T, et al. Pathological diagnosis of pulmonary large cell neuroendocrine carcinoma by endobronchial ultrasound-guided transbronchial needle aspiration. Thorac Cancer. 2018 Feb;9(2):273–7. PMID:29271588

1243. Inage T, Nakajima T, Yoshino I, et al. Early lung cancer detection. Clin Chest Med. 2018 Mar;39(1):45–55. PMID:29433724

1244. Inaguma S, Wang Z, Lasota J, et al. Comprehensive immunohistochemical study of programmed cell death ligand 1 (PD-L1): analysis in 5536 cases revealed consistent expression in trophoblastic tumors. Am J Surg Pathol. 2016 Aug;40(8):1133–42. PMID:27158757

1245. Inamura K, Kumasaka T, Furuta R, et al. Mixed squamous cell and glandular papilloma of the lung: a case study and literature review. Pathol Int. 2011 Apr;61(4):252–8. PMID:21418399

1246. Inamura K, Satoh Y, Okumura S, et al. Pulmonary adenocarcinomas with enteric differentiation: histologic and immunohistochemical characteristics compared with metastatic colorectal cancers and usual pulmonary adenocarcinomas. Am J Surg Pathol. 2005 May;29(5):660–5. PMID:15832091

1247. Incarbone M, Ceresoli GL, Di Tommaso L, et al. Primary pulmonary meningioma: report of a case and review of the literature. Lung Cancer. 2008 Dec;62(3):401–7. PMID:18486986

1248. Inci I, Soltermann A, Schneiter D, et al. Pulmonary malignant peripheral nerve sheath tumour. Eur J Cardiothorac Surg. 2014 Aug;46(2):331–2. PMID:24282191

1249. Inoki K, Corradetti MN, Guan KL. Dysregulation of the TSC-mTOR pathway in human disease. Nat Genet. 2005 Jan;37(1):19–24. PMID:15624019

1250. Inoue A, Tomiyama N, Fujimoto K, et al. MR imaging of thymic epithelial tumors: correlation with World Health Organization classification. Radiat Med. 2006 Apr;24(3):171–81. PMID:16875304

1251. Inoue M, Marx A, Zettl A, et al. Chromosome 6 suffers frequent and multiple aberrations in thymoma. Am J Pathol. 2002 Oct;161(4):1507–13. PMID:12368223

1252. Inoue M, Nakajima T, Tsujimura H, et al. Mediastinal follicular lymphoma diagnosed with multidirectional analysis using tissue samples obtained by EBUS-TBNA. Intern Med. 2010;49(19):2147–9. PMID:20930445

1253. Inoue M, Starostik P, Zettl A, et al. Correlating genetic aberrations with World Health Organization-defined histology and stage across the spectrum of thymomas. Cancer Res. 2003 Jul 1;63(13):3708–15. PMID:12839963

1254. Inoue T, Owada Y, Watanabe Y, et al. Recurrent intrapulmonary solitary fibrous tumor with malignant transformation. Ann Thorac Surg. 2016 Jul;102(1):e43–5. PMID:27343529

1255. International Agency for Research on Cancer. List of classifications by cancer sites with sufficient or limited evidence in humans, Volumes 1 to 127. Lyon (France): International Agency for Research on Cancer; updated 2020 Jun 26. Available from: https://monographs.iarc.fr/wp-content/uploads/2019/07/Classifications_by_cancer_site_127.pdf.

1256. International Association of Cancer Registries (IACR) [Internet]. Lyon (France): International Agency for Research on Cancer; 2019. ICD-O-3.2; updated 2019 Apr 23. Available from: http://www.iacr.com.fr/index.php?option=com_content&view=article&id=149:icd-o-3-2&catid=80&Itemid=545.

1257. International Germ Cell Cancer Collaborative Group. International Germ Cell Consensus Classification: a prognostic factor-based staging system for metastatic germ cell cancers. J Clin Oncol. 1997 Feb;15(2):594–603. PMID:9053482

1258. Ionescu DN, Sasatomi E, Aldeeb D, et al. Pulmonary meningothelial-like nodules: a genotypic comparison with meningiomas. Am J Surg Pathol. 2004 Feb;28(2):207–14. PMID:15043310

1259. Ionescu DN, Treaba D, Gilks CB, et al. Nonsmall cell lung carcinoma with neuroendocrine differentiation–an entity of no clinical or prognostic significance. Am J Surg Pathol. 2007 Jan;31(1):26–32. PMID:17197916

1260. Isaacs H Jr. Fetal and neonatal cardiac tumors. Pediatr Cardiol. 2004 May-Jun;25(3):252–73. PMID:15360117

1261. Isaacs H Jr. Perinatal (fetal and neonatal) germ cell tumors. J Pediatr Surg. 2004 Jul;39(7):1003–13. PMID:15213888

1262. Isaka M, Nakagawa K, Maniwa T, et al. Disseminated calcifying tumor of the pleura: review of the literature and a case report with immunohistochemical study of its histogenesis. Gen Thorac Cardiovasc Surg. 2011 Aug;59(8):579–82. PMID:21850588

1263. Ishida H, Shimizu Y, Sakaguchi H, et al. Distinctive clinicopathological features of adenocarcinoma in situ and minimally invasive adenocarcinoma of the lung: a retrospective study. Lung Cancer. 2019 Mar;129:16–21. PMID:30797486

1264. Ishikawa M, Sumitomo S, Imamura N, et al. Ciliated muconodular papillary tumor of the lung: report of five cases. J Surg Case Rep. 2016 Aug 25;2016(8):rjw144. PMID:27562578

1265. Ishikawa Y, Kato K, Taniguchi T, et al. Imaging of a case of metaplastic thymoma on 18F-FDG PET/CT. Clin Nucl Med. 2013 Dec;38(12):e463–4. PMID:24212449

1266. Ishikawa Y, Tateyama H, Yoshida M, et al. Micronodular thymoma with lymphoid stroma: an immunohistochemical study of the distribution of Langerhans cells and mature dendritic cells in six patients. Histopathology. 2015 Jan;66(2):300–7. PMID:24702632

1267. Ishizumi T, McWilliams A, MacAulay C, et al. Natural history of bronchial preinvasive lesions. Cancer Metastasis Rev. 2010 Mar;29(1):5–14. PMID:20112052

1268. Ismail S, Haydar M, Ghanem A, et al. Pediatric mediastinal ALK- negative anaplastic large cell lymphoma (Hodgkin-like pattern) in a 13-year-old girl: a case report and review of literature. Oxf Med Case Reports. 2019 Aug 28;2019(8):omz077. PMID:31772744

1269. Itakura E, Yamamoto H, Oda Y, et al. Detection and characterization of vascular endothelial growth factors and their receptors in a series of angiosarcomas. J Surg Oncol. 2008 Jan 1;97(1):74–81. PMID:18041747

1270. Italiano A, Chen CL, Thomas R, et al. Alterations of the p53 and PIK3CA/AKT/mTOR pathways in angiosarcomas: a pattern distinct from other sarcomas with complex genomics. Cancer. 2012 Dec 1;118(23):5878–87. PMID:22648906

1271. Ito M, Ishii G, Nagai K, et al. Prognostic impact of cancer-associated stromal cells in patients with stage I lung adenocarcinoma. Chest. 2012 Jul;142(1):151–8. PMID:22302300

1272. Ito Y, Maeda D, Yoshida M, et al. Cardiac intimal sarcoma with PDGFRβ mutation and co-amplification of PDGFRα and MDM2: an autopsy case analyzed by whole-exome sequencing. Virchows Arch. 2017 Sep;471(3):423–8. PMID:28474091

1273. Iuchi K, Aozasa K, Yamamoto S, et al. Non-Hodgkin's lymphoma of the pleural cavity developing from long-standing pyothorax. Summary of clinical and pathological findings in thirty-seven cases. Jpn J Clin Oncol. 1989 Sep;19(3):249–57. PMID:2681886

1274. Ivancic R, Iqbal H, deSilva B, et al. Current and future management of recurrent respiratory papillomatosis. Laryngoscope Investig Otolaryngol. 2018 Jan 14;3(1):22–34. PMID:29492465

1275. Iwa N, Yutani C. Cytology of cardiac myxomas: presence of Ulex europaeus agglutinin-I (UEA-I) lectin by immunoperoxidase staining. Diagn Cytopathol. 1993 Dec;9(6):661–4. PMID:8143540

1276. Iwamoto N, Ishida M, Yoshida K, et al. Mediastinal seminoma: a case report with special emphasis on SALL4 as a new immunocytochemical marker. Diagn Cytopathol. 2013 Sep;41(9):821–4. PMID:22298374

1276A. Iyamu I, Wachsmann J, Truelson J, et al. Detection of widespread metastasis in a case of aggressive carcinoma showing thymuslike differentiation (CASTLE disease) using 18F-FDG PET/CT. Clin Nucl Med. 2015

Aug;40(8):689–91. PMID:25899588

1277. Iyoda A, Hiroshima K, Nakatani Y, et al. Pulmonary large cell neuroendocrine carcinoma: its place in the spectrum of pulmonary carcinoma. Ann Thorac Surg. 2007 Aug;84(2):702–7. PMID:17643676

1278. Iyoda A, Hiroshima K, Toyozaki T, et al. Clinical characterization of pulmonary large cell neuroendocrine carcinoma and large cell carcinoma with neuroendocrine morphology. Cancer. 2001 Jun 1;91(11):1992–2000. PMID:11391577

1279. Izumchenko E, Chang X, Brait M, et al. Targeted sequencing reveals clonal genetic changes in the progression of early lung neoplasms and paired circulating DNA. Nat Commun. 2015 Sep 16;6:8258. PMID:26374070

1280. Izumi N, Nishiyama N, Iwata T, et al. Primary pulmonary meningioma presenting with hemoptysis on exertion. Ann Thorac Surg. 2009 Aug;88(2):647–8. PMID:19632430

1281. Jackett LA, Scolyer RA, Bishop JF, et al. Chapter 17: Primary melanoma of the lung. In: Raghavan D, Ahluwalia MS, Blanke CD, et al., editors. Textbook of uncommon cancer. 5th ed. Hoboken (NJ): John Wiley & Sons; 2017. pp. 287–92.

1282. Jackson MW, Palma DA, Camidge DR, et al. The impact of postoperative radiotherapy for thymoma and thymic carcinoma. J Thorac Oncol. 2017 Apr;12(4):734–44. PMID:28126540

1283. Jacoby LB, MacCollin M, Barone R, et al. Frequency and distribution of NF2 mutations in schwannomas. Genes Chromosomes Cancer. 1996 Sep;17(1):45–55. PMID:8889506

1284. Jaconi M, Magni F, Raimondo F, et al. TdT expression in germ cell tumours: a possible immunohistochemical cross-reaction and diagnostic pitfall. J Clin Pathol. 2019 Aug;72(8):536–41. PMID:31055472

1285. Jain D, Maleszewski JJ, Halushka MK. Benign cardiac tumors and tumorlike conditions. Ann Diagn Pathol. 2010 Jun;14(3):215–30. PMID:20471569

1286. Jain P, Kantarjian H, Jain N, et al. Clinical characteristics and outcomes of previously untreated patients with adult onset T-acute lymphoblastic leukemia and T-lymphoblastic lymphoma with hyper-CVAD based regimens. Am J Hematol. 2017 Oct;92(10):E595–7. PMID:28646517

1287. Jain RK, Mehta RJ, Henley JD, et al. WHO types A and AB thymomas: not always benign. Mod Pathol. 2010 Dec;23(12):1641–9. PMID:20834239

1288. Jain S, Maleszewski JJ, Stephenson CR, et al. Current diagnosis and management of cardiac myxomas. Expert Rev Cardiovasc Ther. 2015 Apr;13(4):369–75. PMID:25797902

1289. Jäkel J, Ramaswamy A, Köhler U, et al. Massive pulmonary tumor microembolism from a hepatocellular carcinoma. Pathol Res Pract. 2006;202(5):395–9. PMID:16488087

1290. Jamal-Hanjani M, Wilson GA, McGranahan N, et al. Tracking the evolution of non-small-cell lung cancer. N Engl J Med. 2017 Jun 1;376(22):2109–21. PMID:28445112

1291. Janigan DT, Husain A, Robinson NA. Cardiac angiosarcomas. A review and a case report. Cancer. 1986 Feb 15;57(4):852–9. PMID:3510706

1292. Jansson JO, Svensson J, Bengtsson BA, et al. Acromegaly and Cushing's syndrome due to ectopic production of GHRH and ACTH by a thymic carcinoid tumour: in vitro responses to GHRH and GHRP-6. Clin Endocrinol (Oxf). 1998 Feb;48(2):243–50. PMID:9579239

1293. Jardin F, Pujals A, Pelletier L, et al. Recurrent mutations of the exportin 1 gene (XPO1) and their impact on selective inhibitor of nuclear export compounds sensitivity in primary mediastinal B-cell lymphoma. Am J Hematol. 2016 Sep;91(9):923–30. PMID:27312795

1294. Jarrett AF, Armstrong AA, Alexander E. Epidemiology of EBV and Hodgkin's lymphoma. Ann Oncol. 1996;7 Suppl 4:5–10. PMID:8836402

1295. Jaso J, Chen L, Li S, et al. CD5-positive mucosa-associated lymphoid tissue (MALT) lymphoma: a clinicopathologic study of 14 cases. Hum Pathol. 2012 Sep;43(9):1436–43. PMID:22406370

1296. Jean WC, Walski-Easton SM, Nussbaum ES. Multiple intracranial aneurysms as delayed complications of an atrial myxoma: case report. Neurosurgery. 2001 Jul;49(1):200–2, discussion 202–3. PMID:11440443

1297. Jeanmart M, Lantuejoul S, Fievet F, et al. Value of immunohistochemical markers in preinvasive bronchial lesions in risk assessment of lung cancer. Clin Cancer Res. 2003 Jun;9(6):2195–203. PMID:12796386

1298. Jeffus SK, Gardner JM, Steliga MA, et al. Hyalinizing clear cell carcinoma of the lung: case report and review of the literature. Am J Clin Pathol. 2017 Jul 1;148(1):73–80. PMID:28927164

1299. Jeffus SK, Joiner AK, Siegel ER, et al. Rapid on-site evaluation of EBUS-TBNA specimens of lymph nodes: comparative analysis and recommendations for standardization. Cancer Cytopathol. 2015 Jun;123(6):362–72. PMID:25931443

1300. Jegalian AG, Bodo J, Hsi ED. NOTCH1 intracellular domain immunohistochemistry as a diagnostic tool to distinguish T-lymphoblastic lymphoma from thymoma. Am J Surg Pathol. 2015 Apr;39(4):565–72. PMID:25517959

1301. Jemal A, Ma J, Siegel RL. Incidence of lung cancer among young women. N Engl J Med. 2018 Sep 6;379(10):990–1. PMID:30184458

1302. Jenkins TM, Morrissette JJD, Kucharczuk JC, et al. ROS1 rearrangement in a case of classic biphasic pulmonary blastoma. Int J Surg Pathol. 2018 Jun;26(4):360–3. PMID:29295663

1303. Jennings TA, Peterson L, Axiotis CA, et al. Angiosarcoma associated with foreign body material. A report of three cases. Cancer. 1988 Dec 1;62(11):2436–44. PMID:3052791

1304. Jeon YK, Moon KC, Park SH, et al. Primary pulmonary myxoid sarcomas with EWSR1-CREB1 translocation might originate from primitive peribronchial mesenchymal cells undergoing (myo)fibroblastic differentiation. Virchows Arch. 2014 Oct;465(4):453–61. PMID:25134518

1305. Jeremy George P, Banerjee AK, Read CA, et al. Surveillance for the detection of early lung cancer in patients with bronchial dysplasia. Thorax. 2007 Jan;62(1):43–50. PMID:16825337

1306. Jeudy J, Burke AP, Frazier AA. Cardiac lymphoma. Radiol Clin North Am. 2016 Jul;54(4):689–710. PMID:27265603

1307. Jeudy J, Kirsch J, Tavora F, et al. From the radiologic pathology archives: cardiac lymphoma: radiologic-pathologic correlation. Radiographics. 2012 Sep-Oct;32(5):1369–80. PMID:22977025

1308. Jeung MY, Gasser B, Gangi A, et al. Bronchial carcinoid tumors of the thorax: spectrum of radiologic findings. Radiographics. 2002 Mar-Apr;22(2):351–65. PMID:11896225

1308A. Jha V, Sharma P, Mandal AK. Utility of cluster of differentiation 5 and cluster of differentiation 117 immunoprofile in distinguishing thymic carcinoma from pulmonary squamous cell carcinoma: a study on 1800 nonsmall cell lung cancer cases. Indian J Med Paediatr Oncol. 2017 Oct-Dec;38(4):430–3. PMID:29333007

1309. Jiang G, Zhang M, Tan Q, et al.

Identification of the BRAF V600E mutation in a patient with sclerosing pneumocytoma: a case report. Lung Cancer. 2019 Nov;137:52–5. PMID:31546071

1310. Jiang K, Nie J, Wang J, et al. Multiple calcifying fibrous pseudotumor of the bilateral pleura. Jpn J Clin Oncol. 2011 Jan;41(1):130–3. PMID:20621934

1311. Jiang L, Huang Y, Tang Q, et al. 18F-FDG PET/CT characteristics of pulmonary sclerosing hemangioma vs. pulmonary hamartoma. Oncol Lett. 2018 Jul;16(1):660–5. PMID:29930720

1312. Jiang L, Mino-Kenudson M, Roden AC, et al. Association between the novel classification of lung adenocarcinoma subtypes and EGFR/KRAS mutation status: a systematic literature review and pooled-data analysis. Eur J Surg Oncol. 2019 May;45(5):870–6. PMID:30833014

1313. Jiang X, Liu Y, Chen C, et al. The value of biomarkers in patients with sarcomatoid carcinoma of the lung: molecular analysis of 33 cases. Clin Lung Cancer. 2012 Jul;13(4):288–96. PMID:22169481

1314. Jiang Y, Hou G, Cheng W. The utility of 18F-FDG and 68Ga-DOTA-peptide PET/CT in the evaluation of primary pulmonary carcinoid: a systematic review and meta-analysis. Medicine (Baltimore). 2019 Mar;98(10):e14769. PMID:30855482

1315. Jimbo N, Komatsu M, Itoh T, et al. MDM2 dual-color in situ hybridization (DISH) aids the diagnosis of intimal sarcomas. Cardiovasc Pathol. 2019 Nov-Dec;43:107142. PMID:31442826

1316. Jiménez Heffernan JA, Salas C, Tejerina E, et al. Gamna-Gandy bodies from cardiac myxoma on intraoperative cytology. Cytopathology. 2010 Jun;21(3):203–5. PMID:19744188

1317. Jimenez-Heffernan JA, Lopez-Ferrer P, Vicandi B, et al. Fine-needle aspiration cytology of large cell neuroendocrine carcinoma of the lung: a cytohistologic correlation study of 11 cases. Cancer. 2008 Jun 25;114(3):180–6. PMID:18433011

1318. Jo VY, Cibas ES, Pinkus GS. Claudin-4 immunohistochemistry is highly effective in distinguishing adenocarcinoma from malignant mesothelioma in effusion cytology. Cancer Cytopathol. 2014 Apr;122(4):299–306. PMID:24421209

1319. Jo VY, Fletcher CDM. SMARCB1/INI1 loss in epithelioid schwannoma: a clinicopathologic and immunohistochemical study of 65 cases. Am J Surg Pathol. 2017 Aug;41(8):1013–22. PMID:28368924

1320. Johnen G, Gawrych K, Raiko I, et al. Calretinin as a blood-based biomarker for mesothelioma. BMC Cancer. 2017 May 30;17(1):386. PMID:28558669

1321. Johnson DE, Appelt G, Samuels ML, et al. Metastases from testicular carcinoma. Study of 78 autopsied cases. Urology. 1976 Sep;8(3):234–9. PMID:987634

1321A. Johnson DH, Fehrenbacher L, Novotny WF, et al. Randomized phase II trial comparing bevacizumab plus carboplatin and paclitaxel with carboplatin and paclitaxel alone in previously untreated locally advanced or metastatic non-small-cell lung cancer. J Clin Oncol. 2004 Jun 1;22(11):2184–91. PMID:15169807

1322. Johnson SR, Taveira-DaSilva AM, Moss J. Lymphangioleiomyomatosis. Clin Chest Med. 2016 Sep;37(3):389–403. PMID:27514586

1323. Johnston WW. The malignant pleural effusion. A review of cytopathologic diagnoses of 584 specimens from 472 consecutive patients. Cancer. 1985 Aug 15;56(4):905–9. PMID:4016683

1324. Jones TD, Ulbright TM, Eble JN, et al. OCT4 staining in testicular tumors: a sensitive and specific marker for seminoma and embryonal carcinoma. Am J Surg Pathol. 2004

Jul;28(7):935–40. PMID:15223965

1325. Joos S, Otaño-Joos MI, Ziegler S, et al. Primary mediastinal (thymic) B-cell lymphoma is characterized by gains of chromosomal material including 9p and amplification of the REL gene. Blood. 1996 Feb 15;87(4):1571–8. PMID:8608249

1325A. Jordan EJ, Kim HR, Arcila ME, et al. Prospective comprehensive molecular characterization of lung adenocarcinomas for efficient patient matching to approved and emerging therapies. Cancer Discov. 2017 Jun;7(6):596–609. PMID:28336552

1326. Jorge C, Almeida AG, Mendes M, et al. Multiple 'crumbled' cardiac myxomas presenting as gait ataxia. Int J Cardiol. 2013 Aug 20;167(4):e104–5. PMID:23639462

1327. Joseph MG, Shibani A, Panjwani N, et al. Usefulness of Ki-67, mitoses, and tumor size for predicting metastasis in carcinoid tumors of the lung: a study of 48 cases at a tertiary care centre in Canada. Lung Cancer Int. 2015;2015:545601. PMID:26770831

1328. Joseph NM, Chen YY, Nasr A, et al. Genomic profiling of malignant peritoneal mesothelioma reveals recurrent alterations in epigenetic regulatory genes BAP1, SETD2, and DDX3X. Mod Pathol. 2017 Feb;30(2):246–54. PMID:27813512

1329. Joshi K, de Massy MR, Ismail M, et al. Spatial heterogeneity of the T cell receptor repertoire reflects the mutational landscape in lung cancer. Nat Med. 2019 Oct;25(10):1549–59. PMID:31591606

1330. Le Stang N, Burke L, Blaizot G, et al. Differential diagnosis of epithelioid malignant mesothelioma with lung and breast pleural metastasis: a systematic review compared with a standardized panel of antibodies-a new proposal that may influence pathologic practice. Arch Pathol Lab Med. 2020 Apr;144(4):446–56. PMID:31389715

1331. Jung M, Kim S, Lee JK, et al. Clinicopathological and preclinical findings of NUT carcinoma: a multicenter study. Oncologist. 2019 Aug;24(8):e740–8. PMID:30696721

1332. Jung SH, Kim MS, Lee SH, et al. Whole-exome sequencing identifies recurrent AKT1 mutations in sclerosing hemangioma of lung. Proc Natl Acad Sci U S A. 2016 Sep 20;113(38):10672–7. PMID:27601661

1333. Jung SM, Chu PH, Shiu TF, et al. Expression of OCT4 in the primary germ cell tumors and thymoma in the mediastinum. Appl Immunohistochem Mol Morphol. 2006 Sep;14(3):273–5. PMID:16932017

1334. Jurmeister P, Schöler A, Arnold A, et al. DNA methylation profiling reliably distinguishes pulmonary enteric adenocarcinoma from metastatic colorectal cancer. Mod Pathol. 2019 Jun;32(6):855–65. PMID:30723296

1335. Jurmeister P, Vollbrecht C, Behnke A, et al. Next generation sequencing of lung adenocarcinoma subtypes with intestinal differentiation reveals distinct molecular signatures associated with histomorphology and therapeutic options. Lung Cancer. 2019 Dec;138:43–51. PMID:31634654

1336. Kadakia KC, Patel SM, Yi ES, et al. Diffuse pulmonary lymphangiomatosis. Can Respir J. 2013 Jan-Feb;20(1):52–4. PMID:23457676

1337. Kadara H, Scheet P, Wistuba II, et al. Early events in the molecular pathogenesis of lung cancer. Cancer Prev Res (Phila). 2016 Jul;9(7):518–27. PMID:27006378

1338. Kadota K, Haba R, Katsuki N, et al. Cytological findings of mixed squamous cell and glandular papilloma in the lung. Diagn Cytopathol. 2010 Dec;38(12):913–7. PMID:20301213

1339. Kadota K, Kushida Y, Kagawa S, et al.

Cribriform subtype is an independent predictor of recurrence and survival after adjustment for the eighth edition of TNM staging system in patients with resected lung adenocarcinoma. J Thorac Oncol. 2019 Feb;14(2):245–54. PMID:30336325

1340. Kadota K, Kushida Y, Kagawa S, et al. Limited resection is associated with a higher risk of locoregional recurrence than lobectomy in stage I lung adenocarcinoma with tumor spread through air spaces. Am J Surg Pathol. 2019 Aug;43(8):1033–41. PMID:31107717

1341. Kadota K, Nitadori J, Rekhtman N, et al. Reevaluation and reclassification of resected lung carcinomas originally diagnosed as squamous cell carcinoma using immunohistochemical analysis. Am J Surg Pathol. 2015 Sep;39(9):1170–80. PMID:25871623

1342. Kadota K, Nitadori JI, Sima CS, et al. Tumor spread through air spaces is an important pattern of invasion and impacts the frequency and location of recurrences after limited resection for small stage I lung adenocarcinomas. J Thorac Oncol. 2015 May;10(5):806–14. PMID:25629637

1343. Kadota K, Suzuki K, Colovos C, et al. A nuclear grading system is a strong predictor of survival in epitheloid diffuse malignant pleural mesothelioma. Mod Pathol. 2012 Feb;25(2):260–71. PMID:21983936

1344. Kadota K, Suzuki K, Sima CS, et al. Pleomorphic epithelioid diffuse malignant pleural mesothelioma: a clinicopathological review and conceptual proposal to reclassify as biphasic or sarcomatoid mesothelioma. J Thorac Oncol. 2011 May;6(5):896–904. PMID:21358344

1345. Kadota K, Villena-Vargas J, Yoshizawa A, et al. Prognostic significance of adenocarcinoma in situ, minimally invasive adenocarcinoma, and nonmucinous lepidic predominant invasive adenocarcinoma of the lung in patients with stage I disease. Am J Surg Pathol. 2014 Apr;38(4):448–60. PMID:24472852

1346. Kadota K, Yeh YC, Sima CS, et al. The cribriform pattern identifies a subset of acinar predominant tumors with poor prognosis in patients with stage I lung adenocarcinoma: a conceptual proposal to classify cribriform predominant tumors as a distinct histologic subtype. Mod Pathol. 2014 May;27(5):690–700. PMID:24186133

1347. Kaira K, Endo M, Abe M, et al. Biologic correlation of 2-[18F]-fluoro-2-deoxy-D-glucose uptake on positron emission tomography in thymic epithelial tumors. J Clin Oncol. 2010 Aug 10;28(23):3746–53. PMID:20625125

1348. Kaira K, Murakami H, Serizawa M, et al. MUC1 expression in thymic epithelial tumors: MUC1 may be useful marker as differential diagnosis between type B3 thymoma and thymic carcinoma. Virchows Arch. 2011 May;458(5):615–20. PMID:21253760

1349. Kakinuma R, Noguchi M, Ashizawa K, et al. Natural history of pulmonary subsolid nodules: a prospective multicenter study. J Thorac Oncol. 2016 Jul;11(7):1012–28. PMID:27089851

1350. Kakuta N, Sumitani M, Sugitani A, et al. Mediastinal peripheral T-cell lymphoma diagnosed by repeated biopsies after an initial diagnosis of fibrosing mediastinitis. Respirol Case Rep. 2017 Sep 18;5(6):e00272. PMID:28932400

1351. Kalemkerian GP, Loo BW, Akerley W, et al. NCCN Guidelines Insights: Small Cell Lung Cancer, Version 2.2018. J Natl Compr Canc Netw. 2018 Oct;16(10):1171–82. PMID:30323087

1352. Kalhor N, Moran CA. Primary thymic adenocarcinomas: a clinicopathological and immunohistochemical study of 16 cases with emphasis on the morphological spectrum of

differentiation. Hum Pathol. 2018 Apr;74:73–82. PMID:29339175
1353. Kalhor N, Moran CA. Thymic epithelial neoplasms with rhabdomyomatous component: a clinicopathological and immunohistochemical study of 7 cases. Hum Pathol. 2019 Jan;83:100–5. PMID:30217623
1354. Kalhor N, Moran CA. Thymic epithelial neoplasms with sebaceous differentiation: a clinicopathological and immunohistochemical study of 8 cases. Hum Pathol. 2019 Apr;86:124–8. PMID:30537491
1355. Kalhor N, Staerkel GA, Moran CA. So-called sclerosing hemangioma of lung: current concept. Ann Diagn Pathol. 2010 Feb;14(1):60–7. PMID:20123460
1356. Kalhor N, Suster S, Moran CA. Primary pulmonary chondrosarcomas: a clinicopathologic study of 4 cases. Hum Pathol. 2011 Nov;42(11):1629–34. PMID:21496864
1357. Kalhor N, Suster S, Moran CA. Spindle cell thymomas (WHO type A) with prominent papillary and pseudopapillary features: a clinicopathologic and immunohistochemical study of 10 cases. Am J Surg Pathol. 2011 Mar;35(3):372–7. PMID:21317709
1358. Kalhor N, Weissferdt A, Moran CA. Primary salivary gland type tumors of the thymus. Adv Anat Pathol. 2017 Jan;24(1):15–23. PMID:27941539
1359. Kamata T, Sunami K, Yoshida A, et al. Frequent BRAF or EGFR mutations in ciliated muconodular papillary tumors of the lung. J Thorac Oncol. 2016 Feb;11(2):261–5. PMID:26718882
1360. Kamata T, Yoshida A, Kosuge T, et al. Ciliated muconodular papillary tumors of the lung: a clinicopathologic analysis of 10 cases. Am J Surg Pathol. 2015 Jun;39(6):753–60. PMID:25803171
1361. Kameda K, Eguchi T, Lu S, et al. Implications of the eighth edition of the TNM proposal: invasive versus total tumor size for the T descriptor in pathologic stage I-IIA lung adenocarcinoma. J Thorac Oncol. 2018 Dec;13(12):1919–29. PMID:30195703
1362. Kameda K, Shono T, Takagishi S, et al. Epstein-Barr virus-positive diffuse large B-cell primary central nervous system lymphoma associated with organized chronic subdural hematoma: a case report and review of the literature. Pathol Int. 2015 Mar;65(3):138–43. PMID:25597523
1363. Kamel OW, Gocke CD, Kell DL, et al. True histiocytic lymphoma: a study of 12 cases based on current definition. Leuk Lymphoma. 1995 Jun;18(1-2):81–6. PMID:8580833
1364. Kaminuma Y, Tanahashi M, Yukiue H, et al. Micronodular thymoma with lymphoid stroma diagnosed 10 years after the first operation: a case report. J Med Case Rep. 2019 Mar 16;13(1):69. PMID:30876482
1365. Kamiya H, Yasuda T, Nagamine H, et al. Surgical treatment of primary cardiac tumors: 28 years' experience in Kanazawa University Hospital. Jpn Circ J. 2001 Apr;65(4):315–9. PMID:11316130
1366. Kamran SC, Shinagare AB, Howard SA, et al. Intrathoracic malignant peripheral nerve sheath tumors: imaging features and implications for management. Radiol Oncol. 2013 Jul 30;47(3):230–8. PMID:24133387
1367. Kanavaros P, Gaulard P, Charlotte F, et al. Discordant expression of immunoglobulin and its associated molecule mb-1/CD79a is frequently found in mediastinal large B cell lymphomas. Am J Pathol. 1995 Mar;146(3):735–41. PMID:7887454
1368. Kane A, Thorpe MP, Morse MA, et al. Predictors of survival in 211 patients with stage IV pulmonary and gastroenteropancreatic MIBG-positive neuroendocrine tumors treated with 131I-MIBG. J Nucl Med. 2018 11;59(11):1708–13. PMID:29777005
1369. Kang CH, Kim YT, Jheon SH, et al. Surgical treatment of malignant mediastinal nonseminomatous germ cell tumor. Ann Thorac Surg. 2008 Feb;85(2):379–84. PMID:18222229
1370. Kang G, Yoon N, Han J, et al. Metaplastic thymoma: report of 4 cases. Korean J Pathol. 2012 Feb;46(1):92–5. PMID:23109986
1371. Kanno H, Naka N, Yasunaga Y, et al. Production of the immunosuppressive cytokine interleukin-10 by Epstein-Barr-virus-expressing pyothorax-associated lymphoma: possible role in the development of overt lymphoma in immunocompetent hosts. Am J Pathol. 1997 Jan;150(1):349–57. PMID:9006350
1372. Kanno H, Nakatsuka S, Iuchi K, et al. Sequences of cytotoxic T-lymphocyte epitopes in the Epstein-Barr virus (EBV) nuclear antigen-3B gene in a Japanese population with or without EBV-positive lymphoid malignancies. Int J Cancer. 2000 Nov 15;88(4):626–32. PMID:11058881
1373. Kanno H, Ohsawa M, Hashimoto M, et al. HLA-A alleles of patients with pyothorax-associated lymphoma: anti-Epstein-Barr virus (EBV) host immune responses during the development of EBV latent antigen-positive lymphomas. Int J Cancer. 1999 Aug 27;82(5):630–4. PMID:10417757
1374. Kanno H, Yasunaga Y, Iuchi K, et al. Interleukin-6-mediated growth enhancement of cell lines derived from pyothorax-associated lymphoma. Lab Invest. 1996 Aug;75(2):167–73. PMID:8765317
1375. Kanzaki R, Ikeda N, Okura E, et al. Thymic carcinoma with adenoid cystic carcinomalike features with distant metastases. Ann Thorac Cardiovasc Surg. 2012;18(6):544–7. PMID:22572229
1376. Kao CS, Bangs CD, Aldrete G, et al. A clinicopathologic and molecular analysis of 34 mediastinal germ cell tumors suggesting different modes of teratoma development. Am J Surg Pathol. 2018 Dec;42(12):1662–73. PMID:30256256
1377. Kao CS, Idrees MT, Young RH, et al. Solid pattern yolk sac tumor: a morphologic and immunohistochemical study of 52 cases. Am J Surg Pathol. 2012 Mar;36(3):360–7. PMID:22261704
1378. Kao YC, Sung YS, Zhang L, et al. BCOR overexpression is a highly sensitive marker in round cell sarcomas with BCOR genetic abnormalities. Am J Surg Pathol. 2016 Dec;40(12):1670–8. PMID:27428733
1379. Kao YC, Sung YS, Zhang L, et al. EWSR1 fusions with CREB family transcription factors define a novel myxoid mesenchymal tumor with predilection for intracranial location. Am J Surg Pathol. 2017 Apr;41(4):482–90. PMID:28009602
1380. Kao YC, Sung YS, Zhang L, et al. Recurrent BCOR internal tandem duplication and YWHAE-NUTM2B fusions in soft tissue undifferentiated round cell sarcoma of infancy: overlapping genetic features with clear cell sarcoma of kidney. Am J Surg Pathol. 2016 Aug;40(8):1009–20. PMID:26945340
1381. Kapatia G, Gupta P, Rohilla M, et al. The spectrum of malignant melanoma on cytology: a tertiary care center study. Diagn Cytopathol. 2019 Oct;47(10):1018–23. PMID:31260174
1382. Kapila K, Pathan SK, Amir T, et al. Mucoepidermoid thymic carcinoma: a challenging mediastinal aspirate. Diagn Cytopathol. 2009 Jun;37(6):433–6. PMID:19217053
1383. Kaplan J, Davidson T. Intrathoracic desmoids: report of two cases. Thorax. 1986 Nov;41(11):894–5. PMID:3824278
1384. Kaplan MA, Tazelaar HD, Hayashi T, et al. Adenomatoid tumors of the pleura. Am J Surg Pathol. 1996 Oct;20(10):1219–23. PMID:8827028
1385. Karamchandani JR, Nielsen TO, van de Rijn M, et al. Sox10 and S100 in the diagnosis of soft-tissue neoplasms. Appl Immunohistochem Mol Morphol. 2012 Oct;20(5):445–50. PMID:22495377
1386. Karasu BB, Yeter E, Yilmazer D, et al. Primary valvular lipomatous hamartoma: a case report and a collective review of the literature. Cardiovasc Pathol. 2011 Nov-Dec;20(6):377–80. PMID:21036628
1387. Karlsson A, Brunnström H, Lindquist KE, et al. Mutational and gene fusion analyses of primary large cell and large cell neuroendocrine lung cancer. Oncotarget. 2015 Sep 8;6(26):22028–37. PMID:26124082
1388. Karpathiou G, Mobarki M, Stachowicz ML, et al. Pericardial and pleural metastases: clinical, histologic, and molecular differences. Ann Thorac Surg. 2018 Sep;106(3):872–9. PMID:29852147
1389. Karpathiou G, Sivridis E, Mikroulis D, et al. Pulmonary mucus gland adenomas: Are they always of endobronchial localization? Case Rep Pathol. 2013;2013:239173. PMID:23533890
1390. Kasagi Y, Yamazaki K, Nakashima A, et al. Chondroblastic osteosarcoma arising from the pleura: report of a case. Surg Today. 2009;39(12):1064–7. PMID:19997802
1391. Kasajima A, Konukiewitz B, Oka N, et al. Clinicopathological profiling of lung carcinoids with a Ki67 index > 20. Neuroendocrinology. 2019;108(2):109–20. PMID:30485860
1392. Kasper B, Baumgarten C, Garcia J, et al. An update on the management of sporadic desmoid-type fibromatosis: a European Consensus Initiative between Sarcoma PAtients EuroNet (SPAEN) and European Organization for Research and Treatment of Cancer (EORTC)/Soft Tissue and Bone Sarcoma Group (STBSG). Ann Oncol. 2017 Oct 1;28(10):2399–408. PMID:28961825
1393. Katabi N, Xu B, Jungbluth AA, et al. PLAG1 immunohistochemistry is a sensitive marker for pleomorphic adenoma: a comparative study with PLAG1 genetic abnormalities. Histopathology. 2018 Jan;72(2):285–93. PMID:28796899
1394. Kathuria S, Jablokow VR. Primary choriocarcinoma of mediastinum with immunohistochemical study and review of the literature. J Surg Oncol. 1987 Jan;34(1):39–42. PMID:2433543
1395. Katsuya Y, Fujita Y, Horinouchi H, et al. Immunohistochemical status of PD-L1 in thymoma and thymic carcinoma. Lung Cancer. 2015 May;88(2):154–9. PMID:25799277
1396. Katz SL, Das P, Ngan BY, et al. Remote intrapulmonary spread of recurrent respiratory papillomatosis with malignant transformation. Pediatr Pulmonol. 2005 Feb;39(2):185–8. PMID:15532092
1397. Katzenstein AL, Doxtader E, Narendra S. Lymphomatoid granulomatosis: insights gained over 4 decades. Am J Surg Pathol. 2010 Dec;34(12):e35–48. PMID:21107080
1398. Kaufmann O, Dietel M. Expression of thyroid transcription factor-1 in pulmonary and extrapulmonary small cell carcinomas and other neuroendocrine carcinomas of various primary sites. Histopathology. 2000 May;36(5):415–20. PMID:10792482
1399. Kaul TK, Fields BL, Kahn DR. Primary malignant pericardial mesothelioma: a case report and review. J Cardiovasc Surg (Torino). 1994 Jun;35(3):261–7. PMID:8040178
1400. Kawabe M, Sasaki K, Shinoda T, et al. [Yolk sac tumor of the anterior mediastinum and pulmonary metastases; report of a case]. Kyobu Geka. 2005 Nov;58(12):1102–5. Japanese. PMID:16281866
1401. Kawachi K, Murakami A, Sasaki T, et al. Blastomatoid carcinosarcoma of the lung. Pathol Int. 2013 Jul;63(7):377–9. PMID:23865578
1402. Kawagishi S, Ose N, Minami M, et al. Total thymectomy for thymic lymphoepithelioma-like carcinoma-report of two cases. Surg Case Rep. 2019 Oct 26;5(1):158. PMID:31655916
1403. Kawaguchi K, Kishida S, Okeda R, et al. Encephalomyeloneuritis with mediastinal germ cell tumor. A paraneoplastic condition? Acta Pathol Jpn. 1988 Mar;38(3):351–9. PMID:2839954
1404. Kawaguchi T, Takada M, Kubo A, et al. Performance status and smoking status are independent favorable prognostic factors for survival in non-small cell lung cancer: a comprehensive analysis of 26,957 patients with NSCLC. J Thorac Oncol. 2010 May;5(5):620–30. PMID:20354456
1405. Kawahara K, Miyawaki M, Anami K, et al. A patient with mediastinal mature teratoma presenting with paraneoplastic limbic encephalitis. J Thorac Oncol. 2012 Jan;7(1):258–9. PMID:22173664
1406. Kawahara K, Sasada S, Nagano T, et al. Pleural MALT lymphoma diagnosed on thoracoscopic resection under local anesthesia using an insulation-tipped diathermic knife. Pathol Int. 2008 Apr;58(4):253–6. PMID:18324920
1407. Kawai O, Ishii G, Kubota K, et al. Predominant infiltration of macrophages and CD8(+) T cells in cancer nests is a significant predictor of survival in stage IV nonsmall cell lung cancer. Cancer. 2008 Sep 15;113(6):1387–95. PMID:18671239
1408. Kawai T, Hiroi S, Nakanishi K, et al. Lymphohistiocytoid mesothelioma of the pleura. Pathol Int. 2010 Aug;60(8):566–74. PMID:20618734
1409. Kawamoto K, Miyoshi H, Yoshida N, et al. Clinicopathological, cytogenetic, and prognostic analysis of 131 myeloid sarcoma patients. Am J Surg Pathol. 2016 Nov;40(11):1473–83. PMID:27631510
1410. Kawanami K, Wakao N, Kamiya M, et al. A case of mediastinal embryonal carcinoma successfully treated by integrative therapy. Nagoya J Med Sci. 2014 Feb;76(1-2):225–33. PMID:25130010
1411. Kawase A, Ishii G, Nagai K, et al. Podoplanin expression by cancer associated fibroblasts predicts poor prognosis of lung adenocarcinoma. Int J Cancer. 2008 Sep 1;123(5):1053–9. PMID:18546264
1412. Kayani I, Conry BG, Groves AM, et al. A comparison of 68Ga-DOTATATE and 18F-FDG PET/CT in pulmonary neuroendocrine tumors. J Nucl Med. 2009 Dec;50(12):1927–32. PMID:19910422
1413. Kazerooni EA, Bhalla M, Shepard JA, et al. Adenosquamous carcinoma of the lung: radiologic appearance. AJR Am J Roentgenol. 1994 Aug;163(2):301–6. PMID:8037019
1414. Kazmierczak B, Wanschura S, Rosigkeit J, et al. Molecular characterization of 12q14-15 rearrangements in three pulmonary chondroid hamartomas. Cancer Res. 1995 Jun 15;55(12):2497–9. PMID:7780955
1415. Kearney DL, Titus JL, Hawkins EP, et al. Pathologic features of myocardial hamartomas causing childhood tachyarrhythmias. Circulation. 1987 Apr;75(4):705–10. PMID:3829332
1416. Keeling IM, Ploner F, Rigler B. Familial cardiac angiosarcoma. Ann Thorac Surg. 2006 Oct;82(4):1576. PMID:16996998
1417. Kehrer-Sawatzki H, Farschtschi S, Mautner VF, et al. The molecular pathogenesis of schwannomatosis, a paradigm for the co-involvement of multiple tumour suppressor genes in tumorigenesis. Hum Genet. 2017

Feb;136(2):129–48. PMID:27921248

1418. Keith RL, Miller YE, Gemmill RM, et al. Angiogenic squamous dysplasia in bronchi of individuals at high risk for lung cancer. Clin Cancer Res. 2000 May;6(5):1616–25. PMID:10815878

1419. Kelly RJ, Sharon E, Hassan R. Chemotherapy and targeted therapies for unresectable malignant mesothelioma. Lung Cancer. 2011 Sep;73(3):256–63. PMID:21620512

1420. Kelly S. European drug regulation. Lancet. 1991 Jul 27;338(8761):257. PMID:1676811

1422. Kerr KM, Popper HH. The differential diagnosis of pulmonary pre-invasive lesions. In: Timens W, Popper HH, editors. Pathology of the lung. Sheffield (UK): European Respiratory Society Journals; 2007. pp. 37–62. (European Respiratory Monograph No. 39).

1423. Keshava HB, Tang A, Siddiqui HU, et al. Largely unchanged annual incidence and overall survival of pleural mesothelioma in the USA. World J Surg. 2019 Dec;43(12):3239–47. PMID:31428834

1424. Kesler KA, Brooks JA, Rieger KM, et al. Mediastinal metastases from testicular nonseminomatous germ cell tumors: patterns of dissemination and predictors of long-term survival with surgery. J Thorac Cardiovasc Surg. 2003 Apr;125(4):913–23. PMID:12698156

1425. Kesler KA, Rieger KM, Ganjoo KN, et al. Primary mediastinal nonseminomatous germ cell tumors: the influence of postchemotherapy pathology on long-term survival after surgery. J Thorac Cardiovasc Surg. 1999 Oct;118(4):692–700. PMID:10504636

1426. Kesler KA, Rieger KM, Hammoud ZT, et al. A 25-year single institution experience with surgery for primary mediastinal nonseminomatous germ cell tumors. Ann Thorac Surg. 2008 Feb;85(2):371–8. PMID:18222228

1427. Khan NE, Bauer AJ, Schultz KAP, et al. Quantification of thyroid cancer and multinodular goiter risk in the DICER1 syndrome: a family-based cohort study. J Clin Endocrinol Metab. 2017 May 1;102(5):1614–22. PMID:28323992

1428. Khanna A, Alshabani K, Mukhopadhyay S, et al. Sclerosing pneumocytoma: case report of a rare endobronchial presentation. Medicine (Baltimore). 2019 Apr;98(15):e15038. PMID:30985653

1429. Khawaja MR, Nelson RP Jr, Miller N, et al. Immune-mediated diseases and immunodeficiencies associated with thymic epithelial neoplasms. J Clin Immunol. 2012 Jun;32(3):430–7. PMID:22228568

1430. Khoury T, Chandrasekhar R, Wilding G, et al. Tumour eosinophilia combined with an immunohistochemistry panel is useful in the differentiation of type B3 thymoma from thymic carcinoma. Int J Exp Pathol. 2011 Apr;92(2):87–96. PMID:21044186

1431. Khuder SA. Effect of cigarette smoking on major histological types of lung cancer: a meta-analysis. Lung Cancer. 2001 Feb-Mar;31(2-3):139–48. PMID:11165392

1432. Kiffer JD, Sandeman TF. Primary malignant mediastinal germ cell tumors: a study of eleven cases and a review of the literature. Int J Radiat Oncol Biol Phys. 1989 Oct;17(4):835–41. PMID:2550400

1433. Kiffer JD, Sandeman TF. Primary malignant mediastinal germ cell tumours: a literature review and a study of 18 cases. Australas Radiol. 1999 Feb;43(1):58–68. PMID:10901872

1434. Kiliś-Pstrusińska K, Medyńska A, Zwolińska D, et al. Lymphoepithelioma-like thymic carcinoma in a 16-year-old boy with nephrotic syndrome–a case report. Pediatr Nephrol. 2008 Jun;23(6):1001–3. PMID:18046582

1435. Killion MJ, Brodovsky HS, Schwarting R. Pericardial angiosarcoma after mediastinal

irradiation for seminoma. A case report and a review of the literature. Cancer. 1996 Aug 15;78(4):912–7. PMID:8756389

1435A. Kim BR, Van de Laar E, Cabanero M, et al. SOX2 and PI3K cooperate to induce and stabilize a squamous-committed stem cell injury state during lung squamous cell carcinoma pathogenesis. PLoS Biol. 2016 Nov 23;14(11):e1002581. PMID:27880766

1436. Kim BS, Kim JK, Kang CH, et al. An immunohistochemical panel consisting of EZH2, C-KIT, and CD205 is useful for distinguishing thymic squamous cell carcinoma from type B3 thymoma. Pathol Res Pract. 2018 Mar;214(3):343–9. PMID:29487009

1437. Kim C, Kim MY, Kang JW, et al. Pulmonary artery intimal sarcoma versus pulmonary artery thromboembolism: CT and clinical findings. Korean J Radiol. 2018 Jul-Aug;19(4):792–802. PMID:29962886

1438. Kim CH, Dancer JY, Coffey D, et al. Clinicopathologic study of 24 patients with primary cardiac sarcomas: a 10-year single institution experience. Hum Pathol. 2008 Jun;39(6):933–8. PMID:18538171

1439. Kim CH, Lee YC, Hung RJ, et al. Exposure to secondhand tobacco smoke and lung cancer by histological type: a pooled analysis of the International Lung Cancer Consortium (ILCCO). Int J Cancer. 2014 Oct 15;135(8):1918–30. PMID:24615328

1440. Kim DJ, Yang WI, Choi SS, et al. Prognostic and clinical relevance of the World Health Organization schema for the classification of thymic epithelial tumors: a clinicopathologic study of 108 patients and literature review. Chest. 2005 Mar;127(3):755–61. PMID:15764754

1441. Kim E, Choi SW, Min D, et al. A case of a resected benign myxoma-like hemorrhagic cyst, which later recurred as undifferentiated pleomorphic sarcoma in the left atrium. Medicine (Baltimore). 2017 Apr;96(16):e6353. PMID:28422827

1442. Kim EE, Wallace S, Abello R, et al. Malignant cardiac fibrous histiocytomas and angiosarcomas: MR features. J Comput Assist Tomogr. 1989 Jul-Aug;13(4):627–32. PMID:2545752

1443. Kim GH, Kim MY, Koo HJ, et al. Primary pulmonary synovial sarcoma in a tertiary referral center: clinical characteristics, CT, and 18F-FDG PET findings, with pathologic correlations. Medicine (Baltimore). 2015 Aug;94(34):e1392. PMID:26313782

1444. Kim GY, Kim J, Kim TS, et al. Pulmonary adenocarcinoma with heterotopic ossification. J Korean Med Sci. 2009 Jun;24(3):504–10. PMID:19543517

1445. Kim J, Field A, Schultz KAP, et al. The prevalence of DICER1 pathogenic variation in population databases. Int J Cancer. 2017 Nov 15;141(10):2030–6. PMID:28748527

1446. Kim JH, Lee SH, Park J, et al. Primary pulmonary non-Hodgkin's lymphoma. Jpn J Clin Oncol. 2004 Sep;34(9):510–4. PMID:15466823

1447. Kim JY, Lee CH, Park WY, et al. Adenocarcinoma with sarcomatous dedifferentiation arising from mature cystic teratoma of the anterior mediastinum. Pathol Res Pract. 2012 Dec 15;208(12):741–5. PMID:23089288

1448. Kim KI, Flint JD, Müller NL. Pulmonary carcinosarcoma: radiologic and pathologic findings in three patients. AJR Am J Roentgenol. 1997 Sep;169(3):691–4. PMID:9275879

1449. Kim NR, Lee JI, Ha SY. Micronodular thymoma with lymphoid stroma in a multilocular thymic cyst: a case study. Korean J Pathol. 2013 Aug;47(4):392–4. PMID:24009637

1450. Kim S, Kim MY, Koh J, et al. Programmed death-1 ligand 1 and 2 are highly expressed in pleomorphic carcinomas of the lung:

comparison of sarcomatous and carcinomatous areas. Eur J Cancer. 2015 Nov;51(17):2698–707. PMID:26329973

1451. Kim S, Lee M, Shin HJ, et al. Coexistence of intracranial Langerhans cell histiocytosis and Erdheim-Chester disease in a pediatric patient: a case report. Childs Nerv Syst. 2016 May;32(5):893–6. PMID:26466952

1452. Kim SH, Koh IS, Minn YK. Pathologic finding of thymic carcinoma accompanied by myasthenia gravis. J Clin Neurol. 2015 Oct;11(4):372–5. PMID:26320843

1453. Kim TH, Kim SJ, Ryu YH, et al. Pleomorphic carcinoma of lung: comparison of CT features and pathologic findings. Radiology. 2004 Aug;232(2):554–9. PMID:15215543

1454. Kim TS, Han J, Lee KS, et al. CT findings of surgically resected pleomorphic carcinoma of the lung in 30 patients. AJR Am J Roentgenol. 2005 Jul;185(1):120–5. PMID:15972411

1455. Kim Y, Hammerman PS, Kim J, et al. Integrative and comparative genomic analysis of lung squamous cell carcinomas in East Asian patients. J Clin Oncol. 2014 Jan 10;32(2):121–8. PMID:24323028

1456. Kimura A, Tsuji M, Isogai T, et al. A mass filling the right atrium: primary cardiac rhabdomyosarcoma. Intern Med. 2018 Dec 15;57(24):3575–80. PMID:30101906

1457. Kimura M, Ito H, Furuta T, et al. Pyothorax-associated angiosarcoma of the pleura with metastasis to the brain. Pathol Int. 2003 Aug;53(8):547–51. PMID:12895234

1458. Kimura N, Watanabe T, Noshiro T, et al. Histological grading of adrenal and extra-adrenal pheochromocytomas and relationship to prognosis: a clinicopathological analysis of 116 adrenal pheochromocytomas and 30 extra-adrenal sympathetic paragangliomas including 38 malignant tumors. Endocr Pathol. 2005 Spring;16(1):23–32. PMID:16000843

1459. Kindler HL, Ismaila N, Armato SG 3rd, et al. Treatment of malignant pleural mesothelioma: American Society of Clinical Oncology clinical practice guideline. J Clin Oncol. 2018 May 1;36(13):1343–73. PMID:29346042

1460. King LJ, Padley SP, Wotherspoon AC, et al. Pulmonary MALT lymphoma: imaging findings in 24 cases. Eur Radiol. 2000;10(12):1932–8. PMID:11305574

1461. King RL, Goodlad JR, Calaminici M, et al. Lymphomas arising in immune-privileged sites: insights into biology, diagnosis, and pathogenesis. Virchows Arch. 2020 May;476(5):647–65. PMID:31863183

1462. King RL, Howard MT, Bagg A. Hodgkin lymphoma: pathology, pathogenesis, and a plethora of potential prognostic predictors. Adv Anat Pathol. 2014 Jan;21(1):12–25. PMID:24316907

1463. Kinno T, Tsuta K, Shiraishi K, et al. Clinicopathological features of nonsmall cell lung carcinomas with BRAF mutations. Ann Oncol. 2014 Jan;25(1):138–42. PMID:24297085

1464. Kinoshita T, Muramatsu R, Fujita T, et al. Prognostic value of tumor-infiltrating lymphocytes differs depending on histological type and smoking habit in completely resected non-small-cell lung cancer. Ann Oncol. 2016 Nov;27(11):2117–23. PMID:27502728

1465. Kinoshita Y, Hamasaki M, Yoshimura M, et al. A combination of MTAP and BAP1 immunohistochemistry is effective for distinguishing sarcomatoid mesothelioma from fibrous pleuritis. Lung Cancer. 2018 Nov;125:198–204. PMID:30429020

1466. Kinoshita Y, Hida T, Hamasaki M, et al. A combination of MTAP and BAP1 immunohistochemistry in pleural effusion cytology for the diagnosis of mesothelioma. Cancer Cytopathol. 2018 Jan;126(1):54–63. PMID:29053210

1467. Kinslow CJ, May MS, Saqi A, et al.

Large-cell neuroendocrine carcinoma of the lung: a population-based study. Clin Lung Cancer. 2020 Mar;21(2):e99–113. PMID:31601526

1468. Kirk GD, Merlo C, O' Driscoll P, et al. HIV infection is associated with an increased risk for lung cancer, independent of smoking. Clin Infect Dis. 2007 Jul 1;45(1):103–10. PMID:17554710

1469. Kisand K, Bøe Wolff AS, Podkrajsek KT, et al. Chronic mucocutaneous candidiasis in APECED or thymoma patients correlates with autoimmunity to Th17-associated cytokines. J Exp Med. 2010 Feb 15;207(2):299–308. PMID:20123959

1470. Kishibuchi R, Kondo K, Soejima S, et al. DNA methylation of GHSR, GNG4, HOXD9 and SALL3 is a common epigenetic alteration in thymic carcinoma. Int J Oncol. 2020 Jan;56(1):315–26. PMID:31746370

1471. Kitamura H, Kameda Y, Ito T, et al. Atypical adenomatous hyperplasia of the lung. Implications for the pathogenesis of peripheral lung adenocarcinoma. Am J Clin Pathol. 1999 May;111(5):610–22. PMID:10230351

1472. Kitamura H, Kameda Y, Ito T, et al. Cytodifferentiation of atypical adenomatous hyperplasia and bronchioloalveolar lung carcinoma: immunohistochemical and ultrastructural studies. Virchows Arch. 1997 Dec;431(6):415–24. PMID:9428929

1473. Kitazawa R, Kitazawa S, Nishimura Y, et al. Lung carcinosarcoma with liposarcoma element: autopsy case. Pathol Int. 2006 Aug;56(8):449–52. PMID:16872439

1474. Klang E, Rozendorn N, Raskin S, et al. CT measurement of breast glandular tissue and its association with testicular cancer. Eur Radiol. 2017 Feb;27(2):536–42. PMID:27229339

1475. Klebe S, Brownlee NA, Mahar A, et al. Sarcomatoid mesothelioma: a clinical-pathologic correlation of 326 cases. Mod Pathol. 2010 Mar;23(3):470–9. PMID:20081811

1476. Klebe S, Mahar A, Henderson DW, et al. Malignant mesothelioma with heterologous elements: clinicopathological correlation of 27 cases and literature review. Mod Pathol. 2008 Sep;21(9):1084–94. PMID:18587319

1477. Klebe S, Prabhakaran S, Hocking A, et al. Pleural malignant mesothelioma versus pleuropulmonary synovial sarcoma: a clinicopathological study of 22 cases with molecular analysis and survival data. Pathology. 2018 Oct;50(6):629–34. PMID:30170702

1478. Klein R, Marx A, Ströbel P, et al. Autoimmune associations and autoantibody screening show focused recognition in patient subgroups with generalized myasthenia gravis. Hum Immunol. 2013 Sep;74(9):1184–93. PMID:23792059

1479. Klemm KM, Moran CA, Suster S. Pigmented thymic carcinoids: a clinicopathological and immunohistochemical study of two cases. Mod Pathol. 1999 Oct;12(10):946–8. PMID:10530558

1480. Kligerman SJ, Franks TJ, Galvin JR. Primary extranodal lymphoma of the thorax. Radiol Clin North Am. 2016 Jul;54(4):673–87. PMID:27265602

1481. Klimstra DS, Moran CA, Perino G, et al. Liposarcoma of the anterior mediastinum and thymus. A clinicopathologic study of 28 cases. Am J Surg Pathol. 1995 Jul;19(7):782–91. PMID:7793476

1482. Knapp RH, Hurt RD, Payne WS, et al. Malignant germ cell tumors of the mediastinum. J Thorac Cardiovasc Surg. 1985 Jan;89(1):82–9. PMID:2981374

1483. Kneuertz PJ, Kamel MK, Stiles BM, et al. Incidence and prognostic significance of carcinoid lymph node metastases. Ann Thorac Surg. 2018 Oct;106(4):981–8. PMID:29908980

1484. Knight JK, Marshall MB. Minimally

invasive management of complex recurrent lymphangioma of the thorax and abdomen. Ann Thorac Surg. 2016 Jun;101(6):e195–7. PMID:27211980
1485. Knösel T, Heretsch S, Altendorf-Hofmann A, et al. TLE1 is a robust diagnostic biomarker for synovial sarcomas and correlates with t(X;18): analysis of 319 cases. Eur J Cancer. 2010 Apr;46(6):1170–6. PMID:20189377
1486. Knowles JW, Elliott AB, Brody J. A case of complete heart block reverting to normal sinus rhythm after treatment for cardiac invasive Burkitt's lymphoma. Ann Hematol. 2007 Sep;86(9):687–90. PMID:17410366
1487. Ko HM, Geddie WR, Boerner SL, et al. Cytomorphological and clinicopathological spectrum of pulmonary marginal zone lymphoma: the utility of immunophenotyping, PCR and FISH studies. Cytopathology. 2014 Aug;25(4):250–8. PMID:24261323
1488. Ko JM, Jung JI, Park SH, et al. Benign tumors of the tracheobronchial tree: CT-pathologic correlation. AJR Am J Roentgenol. 2006 May;186(5):1304–13. PMID:16632723
1489. Ko JS, Billings SD, Lanigan CP, et al. Fully automated dual-color dual-hapten silver in situ hybridization staining for MYC amplification: a diagnostic tool for discriminating secondary angiosarcoma. J Cutan Pathol. 2014 Mar;41(3):286–92. PMID:24329959
1490. Koba H, Kimura H, Nishikawa S, et al. Next-generation sequencing analysis identifies genomic alterations in pathological morphologies: a case of pulmonary carcinosarcoma harboring EGFR mutations. Lung Cancer. 2018 Aug;122:146–50. PMID:30032823
1491. Kobayashi N, Koizumi T, Eguchi T, et al. A mediastinal somatic-type germ cell tumor with hepatic metastasis successfully treated by multiple modalities. Anticancer Res. 2010 Dec;30(12):5117–20. PMID:21187499
1492. Kobayashi Y, Ambrogio C, Mitsudomi T. Ground-glass nodules of the lung in never-smokers and smokers: clinical and genetic insights. Transl Lung Cancer Res. 2018 Aug;7(4):487–97. PMID:30225212
1493. Kobayashi Y, Kamitsuji Y, Kuroda J, et al. Comparison of human herpes virus 8 related primary effusion lymphoma with human herpes virus 8 unrelated primary effusion lymphoma-like lymphoma on the basis of HIV: report of 2 cases and review of 212 cases in the literature. Acta Haematol. 2007;117(3):132–44. PMID:17135726
1494. Kobayashi Y, Mitsudomi T, Sakao Y, et al. Genetic features of pulmonary adenocarcinoma presenting with ground-glass nodules: the differences between nodules with and without growth. Ann Oncol. 2015 Jan;26(1):156–61. PMID:25361983
1495. Kodama H, Hirotani T, Suzuki Y, et al. Cardiomyogenic differentiation in cardiac myxoma expressing lineage-specific transcription factors. Am J Pathol. 2002 Aug;161(2):381–9. PMID:12163362
1496. Koelsche C, Schweizer L, Renner M, et al. Nuclear relocation of STAT6 reliably predicts NAB2-STAT6 fusion for the diagnosis of solitary fibrous tumour. Histopathology. 2014 Nov;65(5):613–22. PMID:24702701
1497. Koelsche C, Tavernar L, Neumann O, et al. Primary pulmonary myxoid sarcoma with an unusual gene fusion between exon 7 of EWSR1 and exon 5 of CREB1. Virchows Arch. 2020 May;476(5):787–91. PMID:31776646
1498. Koga K, Matsuno Y, Noguchi M, et al. A review of 79 thymomas: modification of staging system and reappraisal of conventional division into invasive and non-invasive thymoma. Pathol Int. 1994 May;44(5):359–67. PMID:8044305
1499. Koga T, Hashimoto S, Sugio K, et al. Lung adenocarcinoma with bronchioloalveolar carcinoma component is frequently associated with foci of high-grade atypical adenomatous hyperplasia. Am J Clin Pathol. 2002 Mar;117(3):464–70. PMID:11888087
1500. Kogo M, Shimizu R, Uehara K, et al. Transformation to large cell neuroendocrine carcinoma as acquired resistance mechanism of EGFR tyrosine kinase inhibitor. Lung Cancer. 2015 Nov;90(2):364–8. PMID:26384434
1501. Kohno T, Kakinuma R, Iwasaki M, et al. Association of CYP19A1 polymorphisms with risks for atypical adenomatous hyperplasia and bronchioloalveolar carcinoma in the lungs. Carcinogenesis. 2010 Oct;31(10):1794–9. PMID:20688833
1501A. Kohno T, Nakaoku T, Tsuta K, et al. Beyond ALK-RET, ROS1 and other oncogene fusions in lung cancer. Transl Lung Cancer Res. 2015 Apr;4(2):156–64. PMID:25870798
1502. Koivunen JP, Kim J, Lee J, et al. Mutations in the LKB1 tumour suppressor are frequently detected in tumours from Caucasian but not Asian lung cancer patients. Br J Cancer. 2008 Jul 22;99(2):245–52. PMID:18594528
1503. Koizumi JH, Schron DS. Cytologic features of colonic adenocarcinoma. Differences between primary and metastatic neoplasms. Acta Cytol. 1997 Mar-Apr;41(2):419–26. PMID:9100776
1504. Kojika M, Ishii G, Yoshida J, et al. Immunohistochemical differential diagnosis between thymic carcinoma and type B3 thymoma: diagnostic utility of hypoxic marker, GLUT-1, in thymic epithelial neoplasms. Mod Pathol. 2009 Oct;22(10):1341–50. PMID:19648882
1505. Kollmannsberger C, Beyer J, Droz JP, et al. Secondary leukemia following high cumulative doses of etoposide in patients treated for advanced germ cell tumors. J Clin Oncol. 1998 Oct;16(10):3386–91. PMID:9779717
1506. Kominato S, Nakayama T, Sato F, et al. Characterization of chromosomal aberrations in thymic MALT lymphoma. Pathol Int. 2012 Feb;62(2):93–8. PMID:22243778
1507. Komiya K, Nakashima C, Nakamura T, et al. Current status and problems of T790M detection, a molecular biomarker of acquired resistance to EGFR tyrosine kinase inhibitors, with liquid biopsy and re-biopsy. Anticancer Res. 2018 Jun;38(6):3559–66. PMID:29848710
1508. Kondo K, Monden Y. Therapy for thymic epithelial tumors: a clinical study of 1,320 patients from Japan. Ann Thorac Surg. 2003 Sep;76(3):878–84, discussion 884–5. PMID:12963221
1509. Kondo K, Van Schil P, Detterbeck FC, et al. The IASLC/ITMIG Thymic Epithelial Tumors Staging Project: proposals for the N and M components for the forthcoming (8th) edition of the TNM classification of malignant tumors. J Thorac Oncol. 2014 Sep;9(9 Suppl 2):S81–7. PMID:25396316
1510. Kondo K, Yoshizawa K, Tsuyuguchi M, et al. WHO histologic classification is a prognostic indicator in thymoma. Ann Thorac Surg. 2004 Apr;77(4):1183–8. PMID:15063231
1511. Kong M, Sung JY, Lee SH. Osimertinib for secondary T790M-mutation-positive squamous cell carcinoma transformation after afatinib failure. J Thorac Oncol. 2018 Dec;13(12):e252–4. PMID:30467047
1512. Konno S, Shigemura M, Ogi T, et al. Clinical course of histologically proven multifocal micronodular pneumocyte hyperplasia in tuberous sclerosis complex: a case series and comparison with lymphangiomyomatosis. Respiration. 2018;95(5):310–6. PMID:29393256
1513. Konstanty-Kalandyk J, Wierzbicki K, Bartuś K, et al. [Acute myocardial infarction due to coronary embolisation as the first manifestation of left atrial myxoma]. Kardiol Pol. 2013;71(4):403–5. Polish. PMID:23788348
1514. Koo CW, Baliff JP, Torigian DA, et al. Spectrum of pulmonary neuroendocrine cell proliferation: diffuse idiopathic pulmonary neuroendocrine cell hyperplasia, tumorlet, and carcinoids. AJR Am J Roentgenol. 2010 Sep;195(3):661–8. PMID:20729444
1515. Kooijman CD. Immature teratomas in children. Histopathology. 1988 May;12(5):491–502. PMID:3397045
1516. Koppula BR, Pipavath S, Lewis DH. Epstein-Barr virus (EBV) associated lymphoepithelioma-like thymic carcinoma associated with paraneoplastic syndrome of polymyositis: a rare tumor with rare association. Clin Nucl Med. 2009 Oct;34(10):686–8. PMID:19893401
1517. Kornstein MJ, Rosai J. CD5 labeling of thymic carcinomas and other nonlymphoid neoplasms. Am J Clin Pathol. 1998 Jun;109(6):722–6. PMID:9620029
1518. Korpershoek E, Favier J, Gaal J, et al. SDHA immunohistochemistry detects germline SDHA gene mutations in apparently sporadic paragangliomas and pheochromocytomas. J Clin Endocrinol Metab. 2011 Sep;96(9):E1472–6. PMID:21752896
1519. Kosemehmetoglu K, Vrana JA, Folpe AL. TLE1 expression is not specific for synovial sarcoma: a whole section study of 163 soft tissue and bone neoplasms. Mod Pathol. 2009 Jul;22(7):872–8. PMID:19363472
1520. Koshiol J, Rotunno M, Gillison ML, et al. Assessment of human papillomavirus in lung tumor tissue. J Natl Cancer Inst. 2011 Mar 16;103(6):501–7. PMID:21293027
1521. Koss MN, Hochholzer L, Frommelt RA. Carcinosarcomas of the lung: a clinicopathologic study of 66 patients. Am J Surg Pathol. 1999 Dec;23(12):1514–26. PMID:10584705
1522. Koss MN, Hochholzer L, Langloss JM, et al. Lymphomatoid granulomatosis: a clinicopathologic study of 42 patients. Pathology. 1986 Jul;18(3):283–8. PMID:3785978
1523. Koss MN, Hochholzer L, O'Leary T. Pulmonary blastomas. Cancer. 1991 May 1;67(9):2368–81. PMID:1849449
1524. Kossakowski CA, Morresi-Hauf A, Schnabel PA, et al. Preparation of cell blocks for lung cancer diagnosis and prediction: protocol and experience of a high-volume center. Respiration. 2014;87(5):432–8. PMID:24457174
1525. Kotiligam D, Lazar AJ, Pollock RE, et al. Desmoid tumor: a disease opportune for molecular insights. Histol Histopathol. 2008 Jan;23(1):117–26. PMID:17952864
1526. Kozu Y, Maniwa T, Ohde Y, et al. A solitary mixed squamous cell and glandular papilloma of the lung. Ann Thorac Cardiovasc Surg. 2014;20 Suppl:625–8. PMID:23995347
1527. Kragel PJ, Devaney KO, Meth BM, et al. Mucinous cystadenoma of the lung. A report of two cases with immunohistochemical and ultrastructural analysis. Arch Pathol Lab Med. 1990 Oct;114(10):1053–6. PMID:1699507
1528. Krasinskas AM, Chiosea SI, Pal T, et al. KRAS mutational analysis and immunohistochemical studies can help distinguish pancreatic metastases from primary lung adenocarcinomas. Mod Pathol. 2014 Feb;27(2):262–70. PMID:23887294
1529. Kratz CP, Achatz MI, Brugières L, et al. Cancer screening recommendations for individuals with Li-Fraumeni syndrome. Clin Cancer Res. 2017 Jun 1;23(11):e38–45. PMID:28572266
1530. Krema H, Navajas E, Simpson ER, et al. Choroidal metastasis from a mediastinal choriocarcinoma in a male. Can J Ophthalmol. 2011 Dec;46(6):551–2. PMID:22153647
1531. Krewski D, Lubin JH, Zielinski JM, et al. A combined analysis of North American case-control studies of residential radon and lung cancer. J Toxicol Environ Health A. 2006 Apr;69(7):533–97. PMID:16608828
1532. Krieg AH, Hefti F, Speth BM, et al. Synovial sarcomas usually metastasize after >5 years: a multicenter retrospective analysis with minimum follow-up of 10 years for survivors. Ann Oncol. 2011 Feb;22(2):458–67. PMID:20716627
1533. Kriegsmann K, Zgorzelski C, Kazdal D, et al. Insulinoma-associated protein 1 (INSM1) in thoracic tumors is less sensitive but more specific compared with synaptophysin, chromogranin A, and CD56. Appl Immunohistochem Mol Morphol. 2020 Mar;28(3):237–42. PMID:30358615
1534. Kriegsmann M, Harms A, Longuespée R, et al. Role of conventional immunomarkers, HNF4-α and SATB2, in the differential diagnosis of pulmonary and colorectal adenocarcinomas. Histopathology. 2018 May;72(6):997–1006. PMID:29243296
1535. Kriegsmann M, Muley T, Harms A, et al. Differential diagnostic value of CD5 and CD117 expression in thoracic tumors: a large scale study of 1465 non-small cell lung cancer cases. Diagn Pathol. 2015 Dec 8;10:210. PMID:26643918
1536. Kriekard P, Garcia JA, Nardi-Korver L, et al. Tumor melt: primary effusion lymphoma of the heart. Am J Med. 2012 Sep;125(9):e5–6. PMID:22682793
1537. Krier JB, Kalia SS, Green RC. Genomic sequencing in clinical practice: applications, challenges, and opportunities. Dialogues Clin Neurosci. 2016 Sep;18(3):299–312. PMID:27757064
1538. Krimsky W, Muganlinskaya N, Sarkar S, et al. The changing anatomic position of squamous cell carcinoma of the lung - a new conundrum. J Community Hosp Intern Med Perspect. 2016 Dec 15;6(6):33299. PMID:27987285
1539. Kris MG, Johnson BE, Berry LD, et al. Using multiplexed assays of oncogenic drivers in lung cancers to select targeted drugs. JAMA. 2014 May 21;311(19):1998–2006. PMID:24846037
1540. Kristoffersson U, Heim S, Mandahl N, et al. Multiple clonal chromosome aberrations in two thymomas. Cancer Genet Cytogenet. 1989 Aug;41(1):93–8. PMID:2766255
1541. Krüger S, Buck AK, Blumstein NM, et al. Use of integrated FDG PET/CT imaging in pulmonary carcinoid tumours. J Intern Med. 2006 Dec;260(6):545–50. PMID:17116005
1542. Krugmann J, Feichtinger H, Greil R, et al. Thymic Hodgkin's disease–a histological and immunohistochemical study of three cases. Pathol Res Pract. 1999;195(10):681–7. PMID:10549032
1543. Kuang M, Shen X, Yuan C, et al. Clinical significance of complex glandular patterns in lung adenocarcinoma: clinicopathologic and molecular study in a large series of cases. Am J Clin Pathol. 2018 May 31;150(1):65–73. PMID:29746612
1544. Kuhn E, Wistuba II. Molecular pathology of thymic epithelial neoplasms. Hematol Oncol Clin North Am. 2008 Jun;22(3):443–55. PMID:18514126
1545. Kukuyan AM, Sementino E, Kadariya Y, et al. Inactivation of Bap1 cooperates with losses of Nf2 and Cdkn2a to drive the development of pleural malignant mesothelioma in conditional mouse models. Cancer Res. 2019 Aug 15;79(16):4113–23. PMID:31151962
1546. Kum JB, Ulbright TM, Williamson SR, et al. Molecular genetic evidence supporting the origin of somatic-type malignancy and teratoma from the same progenitor cell. Am J Surg Pathol. 2012 Dec;36(12):1849–56. PMID:23154771
1547. Kumar G, Macdonald RJ, Sorajja P, et al. Papillary fibroelastomas in 19 patients with

hypertrophic cardiomyopathy undergoing septal myectomy. J Am Soc Echocardiogr. 2010 Jun;23(6):595–8. PMID:20497859

1548. Kumar N, Chaudhary N, Prabhu AJ, et al. Undifferentiated thymic carcinoma with intracranial metastasis in a two-year-old. Asian Cardiovasc Thorac Ann. 2018 Mar;26(3):239–41. PMID:29411634

1549. Kumar RV, Devi MG, Biswas S. Cytology of cardiac angiosarcoma in fine needle aspirates. Acta Cytol. 2001 Sep-Oct;45(5):891–3. PMID:11575669

1550. Kumar S, Kumar S, Kumar S, et al. Dumbbell-shaped lymphangioma of neck and thorax. Natl J Maxillofac Surg. 2014 Jan;5(1):90–2. PMID:25298728

1551. Kumar V, Soni P, Garg M, et al. A comparative study of primary adenoid cystic and mucoepidermoid carcinoma of lung. Front Oncol. 2018 May 15;8:153. PMID:29868475

1552. Kunii R, Jiang S, Hasegawa G, et al. The predominant expression of hepatocyte nuclear factor 4α (HNF4α) in thyroid transcription factor-1 (TTF-1)-negative pulmonary adenocarcinoma. Histopathology. 2011 Feb;58(3):467–76. PMID:21348892

1553. Kunze K, Spieker T, Gamerdinger U, et al. A recurrent activating PLCG1 mutation in cardiac angiosarcomas increases apoptosis resistance and invasiveness of endothelial cells. Cancer Res. 2014 Nov 1;74(21):6173–83. PMID:25252913

1554. Kuo KT, Hsu WH, Wu YC, et al. Sclerosing hemangioma of the lung: an analysis of 44 cases. J Chin Med Assoc. 2003 Jan;66(1):33–8. PMID:12728972

1555. Kuo T. Sclerosing thymoma–a possible phenomenon of regression. Histopathology. 1994 Sep;25(3):289–91. PMID:7821901

1556. Kuo T, Shih LY. Histologic types of thymoma associated with pure red cell aplasia: a study of five cases including a composite tumor of organoid thymoma associated with an unusual lipofibroadenoma. Int J Surg Pathol. 2001 Jan;9(1):29–35. PMID:11469342

1557. Kuo TT. Carcinoid tumor of the thymus with divergent sarcomatoid differentiation: report of a case with histogenetic consideration. Hum Pathol. 1994 Mar;25(3):319–23. PMID:7908657

1558. Kuo TT. Cytokeratin profiles of the thymus and thymomas: histogenetic correlations and proposal for a histological classification of thymomas. Histopathology. 2000 May;36(5):403–14. PMID:10792481

1559. Kuo TT, Chan JK. Thymic carcinoma arising in thymoma is associated with alterations in immunohistochemical profile. Am J Surg Pathol. 1998 Dec;22(12):1474–81. PMID:9850173

1560. Kuo TT, Chang JP, Lin FJ, et al. Thymic carcinomas: histopathological varieties and immunohistochemical study. Am J Surg Pathol. 1990 Jan;14(1):24–34. PMID:2294778

1561. Kuo TT, Lo SK. Thymoma: a study of the pathologic classification of 71 cases with evaluation of the Muller-Hermelink system. Hum Pathol. 1993 Jul;24(7):766–71. PMID:8319955

1562. Kure K, Lingamfelter D, Taboada E. Large multifocal cardiac myxoma causing the sudden unexpected death of a 2-month-old infant–a rapidly growing, acquired lesion versus a congenital process?: A case report. Am J Forensic Med Pathol. 2011 Jun;32(2):166–8. PMID:21512386

1563. Kurihara N, Saito H, Nanjo H, et al. Thymic carcinoma with myasthenia gravis: two case reports. Int J Surg Case Rep. 2016;27:110–2. PMID:27591911

1564. Kuroda N, Ohara M, Mizuno K, et al. Imprint cytologic and immunocytochemical findings of sclerosing pneumocytoma. Diagn Cytopathol. 2017 Mar;45(3):274–8. PMID:27902879

1565. Kuroda N, Toi M, Hiroi M, et al. Diagnostic pitfall of D2-40 in adenomatosid tumour. Histopathology. 2007 Nov;51(5):719–21. PMID:17927601

1566. Kurtin PJ, Myers JL, Adlakha H, et al. Pathologic and clinical features of primary pulmonary extranodal marginal zone B-cell lymphoma of MALT type. Am J Surg Pathol. 2001 Aug;25(8):997–1008. PMID:11474283

1567. Kurup AN, Tazelaar HD, Edwards WD, et al. Iatrogenic cardiac papillary fibroelastoma: a study of 12 cases (1990 to 2000). Hum Pathol. 2002 Dec;33(12):1165–9. PMID:12514783

1567A. Kushitani K, Amatya VJ, Okada Y, et al. Utility and pitfalls of immunohistochemistry in the differential diagnosis between epithelioid mesothelioma and poorly differentiated lung squamous cell carcinoma. Histopathology. 2017 Feb;70(3):375–84. PMID:27589012

1568. Kushner BH, Khakoo Y. Enigmatic entities: opsoclonus myoclonus ataxia syndrome linked to neuroblastoma. Lancet Child Adolesc Health. 2018 Jan;2(1):3–5. PMID:30169194

1569. Kuwahara M, Nagafuchi M, Rikimaru T, et al. Pulmonary papillary adenoma. Gen Thorac Cardiovasc Surg. 2010 Oct;58(10):542–5. PMID:20941571

1570. Kwon AY, Han J, Cho HY, et al. Cytologic characteristics of thymic adenocarcinoma with enteric differentiation: a study of four fine-needle aspiration specimens. J Pathol Transl Med. 2017 Sep;51(5):509–12. PMID:28772352

1571. Kwon AY, Han J, Chu J, et al. Histologic characteristics of thymic adenocarcinomas: clinicopathologic study of a nine-case series and a review of the literature. Pathol Res Pract. 2017 Feb;213(2):106–12. PMID:28038793

1572. Kwon D, Koh J, Kim S, et al. MET exon 14 skipping mutation in triple-negative pulmonary adenocarcinomas and pleomorphic carcinomas: an analysis of intratumoral MET status heterogeneity and clinicopathological characteristics. Lung Cancer. 2017 Apr;106:131–7. PMID:28285687

1573. Kwon JW, Goo JM, Seo JB, et al. Mucous gland adenoma of the bronchus: CT findings in two patients. J Comput Assist Tomogr. 1999 Sep-Oct;23(5):758–60. PMID:10524862

1574. Kwon MS. Aspiration cytology of mediastinal seminoma: report of a case with emphasis on the diagnostic role of aspiration cytology, cell block and immunocytochemistry. Acta Cytol. 2005 Nov-Dec;49(6):669–72. PMID:16450911

1575. Kyriakopoulos C, Zarkavelis G, Andrianopoulou A, et al. Primary pulmonary malignant melanoma: report of an important entity and literature review. Case Rep Oncol Med. 2017;2017:8654326. PMID:28352484

1576. Lack EE, Worsham GF, Callihan MD, et al. Granular cell tumor: a clinicopathologic study of 110 patients. J Surg Oncol. 1980;13(4):301–16. PMID:6246310

1577. Lacourt A, Gramond C, Rolland P, et al. Occupational and non-occupational attributable risk of asbestos exposure for malignant pleural mesothelioma. Thorax. 2014 Jun;69(6):532–9. PMID:24508707

1578. Lacronique J, Roth C, Battesti JP, et al. Chest radiological features of pulmonary histiocytosis X: a report based on 50 adult cases. Thorax. 1982 Feb;37(2):104–9. PMID:6979115

1579. Ladanyi M, Roy I. Mediastinal germ cell tumors and histiocytosis. Hum Pathol. 1988 May;19(5):586–90. PMID:2453444

1580. Ladanyi M, Samaniego F, Reuter VE, et al. Cytogenetic and immunohistochemical evidence for the germ cell origin of a subset of acute leukemias associated with mediastinal germ cell tumors. J Natl Cancer Inst. 1990 Feb 7;82(3):221–7. PMID:2153216

1581. Ladanyi M, Sanchez Vega F, Zauderer M. Loss of BAP1 as a candidate predictive biomarker for immunotherapy of mesothelioma. Genome Med. 2019 Mar 26;11(1):18. PMID:30914057

1582. Laddha SV, da Silva EM, Robzyk K, et al. Integrative genomic characterization identifies molecular subtypes of lung carcinoids. Cancer Res. 2019 Sep 1;79(17):4339–47. PMID:31300474

1583. Lagana SM, Hanna RF, Borczuk AC. Pleomorphic (spindle and squamous cell) carcinoma arising in a peripheral mixed squamous and glandular papilloma in a 70-year-old man. Arch Pathol Lab Med. 2011 Oct;135(10):1353–6. PMID:21970492

1584. Laginestra MA, Tripodo C, Agostinelli C, et al. Distinctive histogenesis and immunological microenvironment based on transcriptional profiles of follicular dendritic cell sarcomas. Mol Cancer Res. 2017 May;15(5):541–52. PMID:28130401

1585. Lagrange W, Dahm HH, Karstens J, et al. Melanocytic neuroendocrine carcinoma of the thymus. Cancer. 1987 Feb 1;59(3):484–8. PMID:3024805

1586. Lale SA, Tiscornia-Wasserman PG, Aziz M. Diagnosis of thymic clear cell carcinoma by cytology. Case Rep Pathol. 2013;2013:617810. PMID:24175107

1587. Lam HC, Nijmeh J, Henske EP. New developments in the genetics and pathogenesis of tumours in tuberous sclerosis complex. J Pathol. 2017 Jan;241(2):219–25. PMID:27753446

1588. Lam S, leRiche JC, Zheng Y, et al. Sex-related differences in bronchial epithelial changes associated with tobacco smoking. J Natl Cancer Inst. 1999 Apr 21;91(8):691–6. PMID:10218506

1589. Lam S, Standish B, Baldwin C, et al. In vivo optical coherence tomography imaging of preinvasive bronchial lesions. Clin Cancer Res. 2008 Apr 1;14(7):2006–11. PMID:18381938

1590. Lamba G, Frishman WH. Cardiac and pericardial tumors. Cardiol Rev. 2012 Sep-Oct;20(5):237–52. PMID:22447042

1591. Lan T, Chen H, Xiong B, et al. Primary pleuropulmonary and mediastinal synovial sarcoma: a clinicopathologic and molecular study of 26 genetically confirmed cases in the largest institution of southwest China. Diagn Pathol. 2016 Jul 11;11(1):62. PMID:27401493

1592. Landa I, Ibrahimpasic T, Boucai L, et al. Genomic and transcriptomic hallmarks of poorly differentiated and anaplastic thyroid cancers. J Clin Invest. 2016 Mar 1;126(3):1052–66. PMID:26878173

1593. Lang TU, Khalbuss WE, Monaco SE, et al. Solitary tracheobronchial papilloma: cytomorphology and ancillary studies with histologic correlation. Cytojournal. 2011 Mar 3;8:6. PMID:21383960

1594. Lanphear BP, Buncher CR. Latent period for malignant mesothelioma of occupational origin. J Occup Med. 1992 Jul;34(7):718–21. PMID:1494965

1595. Lantuéjoul S, Constantin B, Drabkin H, et al. Expression of VEGF, semaphorin SEMA3F, and their common receptors neuropilins NP1 and NP2 in preinvasive bronchial lesions, lung tumours, and cell lines. J Pathol. 2003 Jul;200(3):336–47. PMID:12845630

1596. Lantuejoul S, Sound-Tsao M, Cooper WA, et al. PD-L1 testing for lung cancer in 2019: perspective from the IASLC Pathology Committee. J Thorac Oncol. 2020 Apr;15(4):499–519. PMID:31870882

1597. Larsen BT, Klein JR, Hornychová H, et al. Diffuse intrapulmonary malignant mesothelioma masquerading as interstitial lung disease: a distinctive variant of mesothelioma. Am J Surg Pathol. 2013 Oct;37(10):1555–64. PMID:23797722

1598. Larsen M, Evans WK, Shepherd FA, et al. Acute lymphoblastic leukemia. Possible origin from a mediastinal germ cell tumor. Cancer. 1984 Feb 1;53(3):441–4. PMID:6318949

1599. Larson DA, Derkay CS. Epidemiology of recurrent respiratory papillomatosis. APMIS. 2010 Jun;118(6-7):450–4. PMID:20553527

1600. Lassaletta L, Torres-Martín M, Peña-Granero C, et al. NF2 genetic alterations in sporadic vestibular schwannomas: clinical implications. Otol Neurotol. 2013 Sep;34(7):1355–61. PMID:23921927

1601. Latimer KM. Lung cancer: clinical presentation and diagnosis. FP Essent. 2018 Jan;464:23–6. PMID:29313654

1602. Lau K, Massad M, Pollak C, et al. Clinical patterns and outcome in epithelioid hemangioendothelioma with or without pulmonary involvement: insights from an internet registry in the study of a rare cancer. Chest. 2011 Nov;140(5):1312–8. PMID:21546438

1603. Lau SK, Desrochers MJ, Luthringer DJ. Expression of thyroid transcription factor-1, cytokeratin 7, and cytokeratin 20 in bronchioloalveolar carcinomas: an immunohistochemical evaluation of 67 cases. Mod Pathol. 2002 May;15(5):538–42. PMID:12011259

1604. Lau SK, Weiss LM, Chu PG. D2-40 immunohistochemistry in the differential diagnosis of seminoma and embryonal carcinoma: a comparative immunohistochemical study with KIT (CD117) and CD30. Mod Pathol. 2007 Mar;20(3):320–5. PMID:17277761

1605. Laurent E, Begueret H, Bonhomme B, et al. SOX10, GATA3, GCDFP15, androgen receptor, and mammaglobin for the differential diagnosis between triple-negative breast cancer and TTF1-negative lung adenocarcinoma. Am J Surg Pathol. 2019 Mar;43(3):293–302. PMID:30628926

1606. Lauriola L, Erlandson RA, Rosai J. Neuroendocrine differentiation is a common feature of thymic carcinoma. Am J Surg Pathol. 1998 Sep;22(9):1059–66. PMID:9737237

1607. Lawson K, Maher TM, Hansell DM, et al. Successful treatment of progressive diffuse PEComatosis. Eur Respir J. 2012 Dec;40(6):1578–80. PMID:23204027

1608. Layfield LJ, Baloch Z, Elsheikh T, et al. Standardized terminology and nomenclature for respiratory cytology: the Papanicolaou Society of Cytopathology guidelines. Diagn Cytopathol. 2016 May;44(5):399–409. PMID:26990836

1609. Lazar AJ, Tuvin D, Hajibashi S, et al. Specific mutations in the beta-catenin gene (CTNNB1) correlate with local recurrence in sporadic desmoid tumors. Am J Pathol. 2008 Nov;173(5):1518–27. PMID:18832571

1610. Lázaro S, Pérez-Crespo M, Lorz C, et al. Differential development of large-cell neuroendocrine or small-cell lung carcinoma upon inactivation of 4 tumor suppressor genes. Proc Natl Acad Sci U S A. 2019 Oct 29;116(44):22300–6. PMID:31611390

1611. Lazzarino M, Orlandi E, Paulli M, et al. Primary mediastinal B-cell lymphoma with sclerosis: an aggressive tumor with distinctive clinical and pathologic features. J Clin Oncol. 1993 Dec;11(12):2306–13. PMID:8246020

1612. Lazzarino M, Orlandi E, Paulli M, et al. Treatment outcome and prognostic factors for primary mediastinal (thymic) B-cell lymphoma: a multicenter study of 106 patients. J Clin Oncol. 1997 Apr;15(4):1646–53. PMID:9193365

1613. Lazzarotto D, Candoni A, Filì C, et al. Clinical outcome of myeloid sarcoma in adult patients and effect of allogeneic stem cell transplantation. Results from a multicenter survey. Leuk Res. 2017 Feb;53:74–81. PMID:28056398

1614. Le Calvez F, Mukeria A, Hunt JD, et al. TP53 and KRAS mutation load and types in lung

cancers in relation to tobacco smoke: distinct patterns in never, former, and current smokers. Cancer Res. 2005 Jun 15;65(12):5076–83. PMID:15958551
1615. Le Guellec S, Decouvelaere AV, Filleron T, et al. Malignant peripheral nerve sheath tumor is a challenging diagnosis: a systematic pathology review, immunohistochemistry, and molecular analysis in 160 patients from the French Sarcoma Group database. Am J Surg Pathol. 2016 Jul;40(7):896–908. PMID:27158754
1616. Le Guellec S, Soubeyran I, Rochaix P, et al. CTNNB1 mutation analysis is a useful tool for the diagnosis of desmoid tumors: a study of 260 desmoid tumors and 191 potential morphologic mimics. Mod Pathol. 2012 Dec;25(12):1551–8. PMID:22766794
1617. Le Loarer F, Watson S, Pierron G, et al. SMARCA4 inactivation defines a group of undifferentiated thoracic malignancies transcriptionally related to BAF-deficient sarcomas. Nat Genet. 2015 Oct;47(10):1200–5. PMID:26343384
1618. Le Loarer F, Zhang L, Fletcher CD, et al. Consistent SMARCB1 homozygous deletions in epithelioid sarcoma and in a subset of myoepithelial carcinomas can be reliably detected by FISH in archival material. Genes Chromosomes Cancer. 2014 Jun;53(6):475–86. PMID:24585572
1619. Le Pavec J, Lorillon G, Jaïs X, et al. Pulmonary Langerhans cell histiocytosis-associated pulmonary hypertension: clinical characteristics and impact of pulmonary arterial hypertension therapies. Chest. 2012 Nov;142(5):1150–7. PMID:22459770
1620. Le Stang N, Burke L, Blaizot G, et al. Differential diagnosis of epithelioid malignant mesothelioma with lung and breast pleural metastasis: a systematic review compared with a standardized panel of antibodies-a new proposal that may influence pathologic practice. Arch Pathol Lab Med. 2020 Apr;144(4):446–56. PMID:31389715
1620A. Leal JL, Peters G, Szaumkessel M, et al. NTRK and ALK rearrangements in malignant pleural mesothelioma, pulmonary neuroendocrine tumours and non-small cell lung cancer. Lung Cancer. 2020 Aug;146:154–9. PMID:32540558
1621. Leathers CA, Azar MM, Badve SS, et al. Opportunistic infections in a patient with HIV and thymoma. J Allergy Clin Immunol Pract. 2013 Jul-Aug;1(4):413–5. PMID:24565551
1622. Leduc C, Jenkins SM, Sukov WR, et al. Cardiac angiosarcoma: histopathologic, immunohistochemical, and cytogenetic analysis of 10 cases. Hum Pathol. 2017 Feb;60:199–207. PMID:27818284
1623. Leduc C, Zhang L, Öz B, et al. Thoracic myoepithelial tumors: a pathologic and molecular study of 8 cases with review of the literature. Am J Surg Pathol. 2016 Feb;40(2):212–23. PMID:26645726
1624. Lee AC, Kwong YI, Fu KH, et al. Disseminated mediastinal carcinoma with chromosomal translocation (15;19). A distinctive clinicopathologic syndrome. Cancer. 1993 Oct 1;72(7):2273–6. PMID:8374886
1625. Lee AY, Agaram NP, Qin LX, et al. Optimal percent myxoid component to predict outcome in high-grade myxofibrosarcoma and undifferentiated pleomorphic sarcoma. Ann Surg Oncol. 2016 Mar;23(3):818–25. PMID:26759307
1626. Lee B, Sir JJ, Park SW, et al. Right-sided myxomas with extramedullary hematopoiesis and ossification in Carney complex. Int J Cardiol. 2008 Nov 12;130(2):e63–5. PMID:18230408
1627. Lee GJ, Lee H, Woo IS, et al. High expression level of SOX2 is significantly associated with shorter survival in patients with thymic epithelial tumors. Lung Cancer. 2019 Jun;132:9–16. PMID:31097100
1628. Lee GY, Kim WS, Ko YH, et al. Primary cardiac lymphoma mimicking infiltrative cardiomyopathy. Eur J Heart Fail. 2013 May;15(5):589–91. PMID:23248217
1629. Lee GY, Yang WI, Jeung HC, et al. Genome-wide genetic aberrations of thymoma using cDNA microarray based comparative genomic hybridization. BMC Genomics. 2007 Sep 3;8:305. PMID:17764580
1630. Lee HE, Molina JR, Sukov WR, et al. BAP1 loss is unusual in well-differentiated papillary mesothelioma and may predict development of malignant mesothelioma. Hum Pathol. 2018 Sep;79:168–76. PMID:29763720
1631. Lee HI, Jang IS, Jeon KN, et al. Thymoma and synchronous primary mediastinal seminomas with florid follicular lymphoid hyperplasia in the anterior mediastinum: a case report and review of the literature. J Pathol Transl Med. 2017 Mar;51(2):165–70. PMID:28147469
1632. Lee HS, Jang HJ, Shah R, et al. Genomic analysis of thymic epithelial tumors identifies novel subtypes associated with distinct clinical features. Clin Cancer Res. 2017 Aug 15;23(16):4855–64. PMID:28400429
1633. Lee HY, Cha MJ, Lee KS, et al. Prognosis in resected invasive mucinous adenocarcinomas of the lung: related factors and comparison with resected nonmucinous adenocarcinomas. J Thorac Oncol. 2016 Jul;11(7):1064–73. PMID:27016260
1634. Lee HY, Lee KS, Han J, et al. Mucinous versus nonmucinous solitary pulmonary nodular bronchioloalveolar carcinoma: CT and FDG PET findings and pathologic comparisons. Lung Cancer. 2009 Aug;65(2):170–5. PMID:19111932
1635. Lee HY, Lee SH, Won JK, et al. Analysis of fifty hotspot mutations of lung squamous cell carcinoma in never-smokers. J Korean Med Sci. 2017 Mar;32(3):415–20. PMID:28145643
1636. Lee JC, Li CF, Huang HY, et al. ALK oncoproteins in atypical inflammatory myofibroblastic tumours: novel RRBP1-ALK fusions in epithelioid inflammatory myofibroblastic sarcoma. J Pathol. 2017 Feb;241(3):316–23. PMID:27874193
1637. Lee JH, Jeong JS, Kim SR, et al. Mediastinal desmoid tumor with remarkably rapid growth: a case report. Medicine (Baltimore). 2015 Dec;94(52):e2370. PMID:26717381
1638. Lee JK, Louzada S, An Y, et al. Complex chromosomal rearrangements by single catastrophic pathogenesis in NUT midline carcinoma. Ann Oncol. 2017 Apr 1;28(4):890–7. PMID:28203693
1639. Lee JM, Song HN, Kang Y, et al. Isolated mediastinal myeloid sarcoma successfully treated with chemoradiotherapy followed by unrelated allogeneic stem cell transplantation. Intern Med. 2011;50(24):3003–7. PMID:22185993
1640. Lee KC, Yeung K, Welsh C, et al. Angiosarcoma following treatment of testicular seminoma: case report and literature review. J Urol. 1995 Mar;153(3 Pt 2):1055–6. PMID:7853561
1641. Lee KW, Lee Y, Oh SW, et al. Large cell neuroendocrine carcinoma of the lung: CT and FDG PET findings. Eur J Radiol. 2015 Nov;84(11):2332–8. PMID:26279139
1642. Lee MW, Stephens RL. Klinefelter's syndrome and extragonadal germ cell tumors. Cancer. 1987 Sep 1;60(5):1053–5. PMID:3038295
1643. Lee SY, Jo YM, Lee J, et al. Neuroendocrine carcinoma arising in a mediastinal teratoma with pulmonary metastasis: a case report and the chemotherapy response. Intern Med. 2015;54(10):1277–80. PMID:25986270
1644. Lee T, Seo Y, Han J, et al. Analysis of chromosome 12p over-representation and clinicopathological features in mediastinal teratomas. Pathology. 2019 Jan;51(1):62–6. PMID:30470411
1645. Lee W, Teckie S, Wiesner T, et al. PRC2 is recurrently inactivated through EED or SUZ12 loss in malignant peripheral nerve sheath tumors. Nat Genet. 2014 Nov;46(11):1227–32. PMID:25240281
1646. Lee Y, Chung JH, Kim SE, et al. Adenosquamous carcinoma of the lung: CT, FDG PET, and clinicopathologic findings. Clin Nucl Med. 2014 Feb;39(2):107–12. PMID:23751831
1647. Lee Y, Park S, Lee SH, et al. Characterization of genetic aberrations in a single case of metastatic thymic adenocarcinoma. BMC Cancer. 2017 May 15;17(1):330. PMID:28506304
1648. Leeman JE, Rimner A, Montecalvo J, et al. Histologic subtype in core lung biopsies of early-stage lung adenocarcinoma is a prognostic factor for treatment response and failure patterns after stereotactic body radiation therapy. Int J Radiat Oncol Biol Phys. 2017 Jan 1;97(1):138–45. PMID:27839909
1649. Legault S, Couture C, Bourgault C, et al. Primary cardiac Burkitt-like lymphoma of the right atrium. Can J Cardiol. 2009 Mar;25(3):163–5. PMID:19279985
1650. Lehrke HD, Johnson CK, Zapolanski A, et al. Intracardiac juvenile xanthogranuloma with presentation in adulthood. Cardiovasc Pathol. 2014 Jan-Feb;23(1):54–6. PMID:24012116
1651. Leithäuser F, Bäuerle M, Huynh MQ, et al. Isotype-switched immunoglobulin genes with a high load of somatic hypermutation and lack of ongoing mutational activity are prevalent in mediastinal B-cell lymphoma. Blood. 2001 Nov 1;98(9):2762–70. PMID:11675349
1652. Leone O, Veinot JP, Angelini A, et al. 2011 consensus statement on endomyocardial biopsy from the Association for European Cardiovascular Pathology and the Society for Cardiovascular Pathology. Cardiovasc Pathol. 2012 Jul-Aug;21(4):245–74. PMID:22137237
1653. Lepanto D, Maffini F, Petrella F, et al. Atypical primary pulmonary meningioma: a report of a case suspected of being a lung metastasis. Ecancermedicalscience. 2014 Mar 31;8:414. PMID:24761155
1654. Lepus CM, Vivero M. Updates in effusion cytology. Surg Pathol Clin. 2018 Sep;11(3):523–44. PMID:30190139
1655. Leroy X, Augusto D, Leteurtre E, et al. CD30 and CD117 (c-kit) used in combination are useful for distinguishing embryonal carcinoma from seminoma. J Histochem Cytochem. 2002 Feb;50(2):283–5. PMID:11799147
1656. Lesluyes T, Pérot G, Largeau MR, et al. RNA sequencing validation of the Complexity INdex in SARComas prognostic signature. Eur J Cancer. 2016 Apr;57:104–11. PMID:26916546
1657. Levine GD, Rosai J. A spindle cell varient of thymic carcinoid tumor. A clinical, histologic, and fine structural study with emphasis on its distinction from spindle cell thymoma. Arch Pathol Lab Med. 1976 Jun;100(6):293–300. PMID:946757
1658. Levine GD, Rosai J. Thymic hyperplasia and neoplasia: a review of current concepts. Hum Pathol. 1978 Sep;9(5):495–515. PMID:361541
1659. Lewis BD, Hurt RD, Payne WS, et al. Benign teratomas of the mediastinum. J Thorac Cardiovasc Surg. 1983 Nov;86(5):727–31. PMID:6632945
1660. Lewis DR, Check DP, Caporaso NE, et al. US lung cancer trends by histologic type. Cancer. 2014 Sep 15;120(18):2883–92. PMID:25113306
1661. Lewis MA, Hendrickson AW, Moynihan TJ. Oncologic emergencies: pathophysiology, presentation, diagnosis, and treatment. CA Cancer J Clin. 2011 Sep-Oct;61(5):287–314. PMID:21858793
1662. Li AY, McCusker MG, Russo A, et al. RET fusions in solid tumors. Cancer Treat Rev. 2019 Dec;81:101911. PMID:31715421
1663. Li CF, Fang FM, Lan J, et al. AMACR amplification in myxofibrosarcomas: a mechanism of overexpression that promotes cell proliferation with therapeutic relevance. Clin Cancer Res. 2014 Dec 1;20(23):6141–52. PMID:25384383
1664. Li CF, Wang JM, Kang HY, et al. Characterization of gene amplification-driven SKP2 overexpression in myxofibrosarcoma: potential implications in tumor progression and therapeutics. Clin Cancer Res. 2012 Mar 15;18(6):1598–610. PMID:22322669
1665. Li F, He M, Li F, et al. Histologic characteristics and prognosis of lung mixed squamous cell and glandular papilloma: six case reports. Int J Clin Exp Pathol. 2019 Sep 1;12(9):3542–8. PMID:31934202
1666. Li G, Hansmann ML, Zwingers T, et al. Primary lymphomas of the lung: morphological, immunohistochemical and clinical features. Histopathology. 1990 Jun;16(6):519–31. PMID:2198222
1667. Li G, Ogose A, Kawashima H, et al. Cytogenetic and real-time quantitative reverse-transcriptase polymerase chain reaction analyses in pleomorphic rhabdomyosarcoma. Cancer Genet Cytogenet. 2009 Jul;192(1):1–9. PMID:19480930
1668. Li Q, Su YL, Shen WX. A novel prognostic signature of seven genes for the prediction in patients with thymoma. J Cancer Res Clin Oncol. 2019 Jan;145(1):109–16. PMID:30328513
1669. Li S, Yuan Y, Xiao H, et al. Discovery and validation of DNA methylation markers for overall survival prognosis in patients with thymic epithelial tumors. Clin Epigenetics. 2019 Mar 4;11(1):38. PMID:30832724
1670. Li VD, Li KH, Li JT. TP53 mutations as potential prognostic markers for specific cancers: analysis of data from The Cancer Genome Atlas and the International Agency for Research on Cancer TP53 Database. J Cancer Res Clin Oncol. 2019 Mar;145(3):625–36. PMID:30542790
1671. Li X, Chen Y, Liu J, et al. Cardiac magnetic resonance imaging of primary cardiac tumors. Quant Imaging Med Surg. 2020 Jan;10(1):294–313. PMID:31956550
1672. Liang X, Lovell MA, Capocelli KE, et al. Thymoma in children: report of 2 cases and review of the literature. Pediatr Dev Pathol. 2010 May-Jun;13(3):202–8. PMID:20055684
1673. Liang Y, Wang L, Zhu Y, et al. Primary pulmonary lymphoepithelioma-like carcinoma: fifty-two patients with long-term follow-up. Cancer. 2012 Oct 1;118(19):4748–58. PMID:22359203
1674. Libshitz HI, North LB. Pulmonary metastases. Radiol Clin North Am. 1982 Sep;20(3):437–51. PMID:7111701
1675. Lichtenberger JP 3rd, Biko DM, Carter BW, et al. Primary lung tumors in children: radiologic-pathologic correlation from the radiologic pathology archives. Radiographics. 2018 Nov-Dec;38(7):2151–72. PMID:30422774
1676. Lie CH, Chao TY, Chung YH, et al. Primary pulmonary malignant melanoma presenting with haemoptysis. Melanoma Res. 2005 Jun;15(3):219–21. PMID:15917706
1677. Liegl B, Bennett MW, Fletcher CD. Microcystic/reticular schwannoma: a distinct variant with predilection for visceral locations. Am J Surg Pathol. 2008 Jul;32(7):1080–7. PMID:18520439

1678. Ligon AH, Moore SD, Parisi MA, et al. Constitutional rearrangement of the architectural factor HMGA2: a novel human phenotype including overgrowth and lipomas. Am J Hum Genet. 2005 Feb;76(2):340–8. PMID:15593017
1679. Lim LC, Tan MH, Eng C, et al. Thymic carcinoid in multiple endocrine neoplasia 1: genotype-phenotype correlation and prevention. J Intern Med. 2006 Apr;259(4):428–32. PMID:16594911
1680. Lim ZF, Ma PC. Emerging insights of tumor heterogeneity and drug resistance mechanisms in lung cancer targeted therapy. J Hematol Oncol. 2019 Dec 9;12(1):134. PMID:31815659
1681. Lima RdeC, Mendes A, Bezerra E, et al. Surgical treatment of primary cardiac rhabdomyosarcoma. Rev Bras Cir Cardiovasc. 2009 Apr-Jun;24(2):242–4. PMID:19768306
1682. Lin CY, Chen YJ, Hsieh MH, et al. Advanced primary pulmonary lymphoepithelioma-like carcinoma: clinical manifestations, treatment, and outcome. J Thorac Dis. 2017 Jan;9(1):123–8. PMID:28203414
1683. Lin H, Tong ZH, Xu QQ, et al. Interplay of Th1 and Th17 cells in murine models of malignant pleural effusion. Am J Respir Crit Care Med. 2014 Mar 15;189(6):697–706. PMID:24410406
1684. Lin KL, Chen CY, Hsu HH, et al. Ectopic ACTH syndrome due to thymic carcinoid tumor in a girl. J Pediatr Endocrinol Metab. 1999 Jul-Aug;12(4):573–8. PMID:10417976
1685. Lin LI, Xu CW, Zhang BO, et al. Clinicopathological observation of primary lung enteric adenocarcinoma and its response to chemotherapy: a case report and review of the literature. Exp Ther Med. 2016 Jan;11(1):201–7. PMID:26889240
1686. Lin MW, Huang YL, Yang CY, et al. The differences in clinicopathologic and prognostic characteristics between surgically resected peripheral and central lung squamous cell carcinoma. Ann Surg Oncol. 2019 Jan;26(1):217–29. PMID:30456676
1687. Lin O, Olgac S, Green I, et al. Immunohistochemical staining of cytologic smears with MIB-1 helps distinguish low-grade from high-grade neuroendocrine neoplasms. Am J Clin Pathol. 2003 Aug;120(2):209–16. PMID:12931551
1688. Lin XY, Han Q, Wang EH, et al. Pulmonary papillary adenoma presenting in central portion: a case report. Diagn Pathol. 2015 Oct 17;10:190. PMID:26474555
1689. Lin XY, Wang Y, Fan CF, et al. Pulmonary sclerosing hemangioma presenting with dense spindle stroma cells: a potential diagnostic pitfall. Diagn Pathol. 2012 Dec 10;7:174. PMID:23227905
1690. Linares I, Molina-Portillo E, Expósito J, et al. Trends in lung cancer incidence by histologic subtype in the south of Spain, 1985-2012: a population-based study. Clin Transl Oncol. 2016 May;18(5):489–96. PMID:26329296
1691. Lindeman NI, Cagle PT, Aisner DL, et al. Updated molecular testing guideline for the selection of lung cancer patients for treatment with targeted tyrosine kinase inhibitors: guideline from the College of American Pathologists, the International Association for the Study of Lung Cancer, and the Association for Molecular Pathology. Arch Pathol Lab Med. 2018 Mar;142(3):321–46. PMID:29355391
1692. Lindeman NI, Cagle PT, Aisner DL, et al. Updated molecular testing guideline for the selection of lung cancer patients for treatment with targeted tyrosine kinase inhibitors: guideline from the College of American Pathologists, the International Association for the Study of Lung Cancer, and the Association for Molecular Pathology. J Thorac Oncol. 2018 Mar;13(3):323–58. PMID:29396253
1693. Lindeman NI, Cagle PT, Beasley MB, et al. Molecular testing guideline for selection of lung cancer patients for EGFR and ALK tyrosine kinase inhibitors: guideline from the College of American Pathologists, International Association for the Study of Lung Cancer, and Association for Molecular Pathology. J Thorac Oncol. 2013 Jul;8(7):823–59. PMID:23552377
1694. Lindfors KK, Meyer JE, Dedrick CG, et al. Thymic cysts in mediastinal Hodgkin disease. Radiology. 1985 Jul;156(1):37–41. PMID:4001419
1695. Lindner LH, Litière S, Sleijfer S, et al. Prognostic factors for soft tissue sarcoma patients with lung metastases only who are receiving first-line chemotherapy: an exploratory, retrospective analysis of the European Organization for Research and Treatment of Cancer-Soft Tissue and Bone Sarcoma Group (EORTC-STBSG). Int J Cancer. 2018 Jun 15;142(12):2610–20. PMID:29383713
1696. Linfeng Q, Xingjie X, Henry D, et al. Cardiac angiosarcoma: a case report and review of current treatment. Medicine (Baltimore). 2019 Dec;98(49):e18193. PMID:31804339
1697. Linke-Serinsöz E, Fend F, Quintanilla-Martinez L. Human immunodeficiency virus (HIV) and Epstein-Barr virus (EBV) related lymphomas, pathology view point. Semin Diagn Pathol. 2017 Jul;34(4):352–63. PMID:28506687
1698. Linnoila RI, Keiser HR, Steinberg SM, et al. Histopathology of benign versus malignant sympathoadrenal paragangliomas: clinicopathologic study of 120 cases including unusual histologic features. Hum Pathol. 1990 Nov;21(11):1168–80. PMID:2172151
1699. Lipson D, Capelletti M, Yelensky R, et al. Identification of new ALK and RET gene fusions from colorectal and lung cancer biopsies. Nat Med. 2012 Feb 12;18(3):382–4. PMID:22327622
1700. Lissowska J, Bardin-Mikolajczak A, Fletcher T, et al. Lung cancer and indoor pollution from heating and cooking with solid fuels: the IARC international multicentre case-control study in Eastern/Central Europe and the United Kingdom. Am J Epidemiol. 2005 Aug 15;162(4):326–33. PMID:16014775
1701. Littman CD. Metastatic melanoma mimicking primary bronchial melanoma. Histopathology. 1991 Jun;18(6):561–3. PMID:1879817
1702. Liu A, Cheng L, Du J, et al. Diagnostic utility of novel stem cell markers SALL4, OCT4, NANOG, SOX2, UTF1, and TCL1 in primary mediastinal germ cell tumors. Am J Surg Pathol. 2010 May;34(5):697–706. PMID:20410807
1704. Liu B, Rao Q, Zhu Y, et al. Metaplastic thymoma of the mediastinum. A clinicopathologic, immunohistochemical, and genetic analysis. Am J Clin Pathol. 2012 Feb;137(2):261–9. PMID:22261452
1705. Liu CH, Peng YJ, Wang HH, et al. Spontaneous rupture of a cystic mediastinal teratoma complicated by superior vena cava syndrome. Ann Thorac Surg. 2014 Feb;97(2):689–91. PMID:24484811
1706. Liu H, Yin Q, Yang G, et al. Prognostic impact of tumor spread through air spaces in non-small cell lung cancers: a meta-analysis including 3564 patients. Pathol Oncol Res. 2019 Oct;25(4):1303–10. PMID:30767114
1707. Liu HC, Hsu WH, Chen YJ, et al. Primary thymic carcinoma. Ann Thorac Surg. 2002 Apr;73(4):1076–81. PMID:11996244
1708. Liu J, Guzman MA, Pezanowski D, et al. FOXO1-FGFR1 fusion and amplification in a solid variant of alveolar rhabdomyosarcoma. Mod Pathol. 2011 Oct;24(10):1327–35. PMID:21666686
1709. Liu L, Jentoft ME, Boland JM. Glioblastoma arising within a mediastinal mature teratoma. Hum Pathol. 2016 Oct;56:109–13. PMID:27327191
1710. Liu L, Qin C, Guo Y. Rare case of left ventricular mesenchymal hamartoma. J Thorac Cardiovasc Surg. 2018 Jan;155(1):346–50. PMID:29103814
1711. Liu M, Chen G, Fu Z, et al. Occult mediastinal yolk sac tumor producing α-fetoprotein detected by 18F-FDG PET/CT. Clin Nucl Med. 2016 Jul;41(7):585–6. PMID:27088388
1712. Liu R, Liu J, Shi T, et al. Clinicopathological and genetic characteristics of pulmonary large cell carcinoma under 2015 WHO classification: a pilot study. Oncotarget. 2017 Oct 11;8(59):100754–63. PMID:29246019
1713. Liu W, Tian XY, Li Y, et al. Coexistence of pulmonary sclerosing hemangioma and primary adenocarcinoma in the same nodule of lung. Diagn Pathol. 2011 May 20;6:41. PMID:21599956
1714. Liu X, Jia Y, Stoopler MB, et al. Next-generation sequencing of pulmonary sarcomatoid carcinoma reveals high frequency of actionable MET gene mutations. J Clin Oncol. 2016 Mar 10;34(8):794–802. PMID:26215952
1715. Liu Y, Sui X, Chen K, et al. Thoracic lymphangiomatosis: report of 3 patients with different presentations. Ann Thorac Surg. 2012 Dec;94(6):2111–3. PMID:23176925
1716. Liu YG, Sun KK, Sui XZ, et al. Thymic carcinosarcoma consisting of sarcomatous and adenosquamous carcinomatous component. Chin Med J (Engl). 2012 Nov;125(22):4154–5. PMID:23158163
1717. Llombart-Cussac A, Pivot X, Contesso G, et al. Adjuvant chemotherapy for primary cardiac sarcomas: the IGR experience. Br J Cancer. 1998 Dec;78(12):1624–8. PMID:9862574
1718. Lloyd RV, Osamura RY, Klöppel G, et al., editors. WHO classification of tumours of endocrine organs. Lyon (France): International Agency for Research on Cancer; 2017. (WHO classification of tumours series, 4th ed.; vol. 10). https://publications.iarc.fr/554.
1719. Lo Curto M, D'Angelo P, Cecchetto G, et al. Mature and immature teratomas: results of the first paediatric Italian study. Pediatr Surg Int. 2007 Apr;23(4):315–22. PMID:17333214
1720. Lococo F, Cafarotti S, Treglia G. Is 18F-FDG-PET/CT really able to differentiate between malignant and benign solitary fibrous tumor of the pleura? Clin Imaging. 2013 Sep-Oct;37(5):976. PMID:23834904
1721. Lococo F, Cusumano G, Margaritora S, et al. Tapias score for predicting recurrences in resected solitary fibrous tumor of the pleura: controversial points and future perspectives emerging from an external validation. Chest. 2015 Mar;147(3):e115–6. PMID:25732461
1722. Lococo F, Rapicetta C, Cardillo G, et al. Pathologic findings and long-term results after surgical treatment for pulmonary sarcomatoid tumors: a multicenter analysis. Ann Thorac Surg. 2017 Apr;103(4):1142–50. PMID:28027731
1723. Lococo F, Rapicetta C, Filice A, et al. The role of 68Ga-DOTATOC PET/CT in the detection of relapsed malignant solitary fibrous tumor of the pleura. Rev Esp Med Nucl Imagen Mol. 2018 Jul-Aug;37(4):257–8. PMID:29636234
1724. Lococo F, Torricelli F, Rossi G, et al. Inter-relationship between PD-L1 expression and clinic-pathological features and driver gene mutations in pulmonary sarcomatoid carcinomas. Lung Cancer. 2017 Nov;113:93–101. PMID:29110857
1725. Loddenkemper C, Anagnostopoulos I, Hummel M, et al. Differential Emu enhancer activity and expression of BOB.1/OBF.1, Oct2, PU.1, and immunoglobulin in reactive B-cell populations, B-cell non-Hodgkin lymphomas, and Hodgkin lymphomas. J Pathol. 2004 Jan;202(1):60–9. PMID:14694522
1726. Lohmann DR, Gillessen-Kaesbach G. Multiple subcutaneous granular-cell tumours in a patient with Noonan syndrome. Clin Dysmorphol. 2000 Oct;9(4):301–2. PMID:11045593
1727. Long KB, Srivastava A, Hirsch MS, et al. PAX8 expression in well-differentiated pancreatic endocrine tumors: correlation with clinicopathologic features and comparison with gastrointestinal and pulmonary carcinoid tumors. Am J Surg Pathol. 2010 May;34(5):723–9. PMID:20414099
1728. Looijenga LH, Gillis AJ, Stoop HJ, et al. Chromosomes and expression in human testicular germ-cell tumors: insight into their cell of origin and pathogenesis. Ann N Y Acad Sci. 2007 Dec;1120:187–214. PMID:17911410
1729. Looijenga LH, Stoop H, de Leeuw HP, et al. POU5F1 (OCT3/4) identifies cells with pluripotent potential in human germ cell tumors. Cancer Res. 2003 May 1;63(9):2244–50. PMID:12727846
1730. Look AT, Hayes FA, Nitschke R, et al. Cellular DNA content as a predictor of response to chemotherapy in infants with unresectable neuroblastoma. N Engl J Med. 1984 Jul 26;311(4):231–5. PMID:6738617
1731. Look Hong NJ, Pandalai PK, Hornick JL, et al. Cardiac angiosarcoma management and outcomes: 20-year single-institution experience. Ann Surg Oncol. 2012 Aug;19(8):2707–15. PMID:22476752
1732. Loomis D, Huang W, Chen G. The International Agency for Research on Cancer (IARC) evaluation of the carcinogenicity of outdoor air pollution: focus on China. Chin J Cancer. 2014 Apr;33(4):189–96. PMID:24694836
1733. Loong F, Chan AC, Ho BC, et al. Diffuse large B-cell lymphoma associated with chronic inflammation as an incidental finding and new clinical scenarios. Mod Pathol. 2010 Apr;23(4):493–501. PMID:20062008
1734. Loong HH, Raymond VM, Shiotsu Y, et al. Clinical application of genomic profiling with circulating tumor DNA for management of advanced non-small-cell lung cancer in Asia. Clin Lung Cancer. 2018 Sep;19(5):e601–8. PMID:29807856
1735. Lorenzi L, Döring C, Rausch T, et al. Identification of novel follicular dendritic cell sarcoma markers, FDCSP and SRGN, by whole transcriptome sequencing. Oncotarget. 2017 Mar 7;8(10):16463–72. PMID:28145886
1736. Lorenzo Bermejo J, Hemminki K. Familial lung cancer and aggregation of smoking habits: a simulation of the effect of shared environmental factors on the familial risk of cancer. Cancer Epidemiol Biomarkers Prev. 2005 Jul;14(7):1738–40. PMID:16030110
1737. Lorillon G, Tazi A. How I manage pulmonary Langerhans cell histiocytosis. Eur Respir Rev. 2017 Sep 6;26(145):170070. PMID:28877978
1738. Lortet-Tieulent J, Renteria E, Sharp L, et al. Convergence of decreasing male and increasing female incidence rates in major tobacco-related cancers in Europe in 1988-2010. Eur J Cancer. 2015 Jun;51(9):1144–63. PMID:24269041
1739. Lortet-Tieulent J, Soerjomataram I, Ferlay J, et al. International trends in lung cancer incidence by histological subtype: adenocarcinoma stabilizing in men but still increasing in women. Lung Cancer. 2014 Apr;84(1):13–22. PMID:24524818
1740. Louis DN, Ohgaki H, Wiestler OD, et al., editors. WHO classification of tumours of the central nervous system. Lyon (France): International Agency for Research on Cancer; 2016. (WHO classification of tumours series, 4th rev. ed.; vol. 1). https://publications.iarc.fr/543.

1741. Lovly CM, Gupta A, Lipson D, et al. Inflammatory myofibroblastic tumors harbor multiple potentially actionable kinase fusions. Cancer Discov. 2014 Aug;4(8):889–95. PMID:24875859

1742. Lovrenski A, Vasilijević M, Panjković M, et al. Sclerosing pneumocytoma: a ten-year experience at a western Balkan university hospital. Medicina (Kaunas). 2019 Jan 25;55(2):E27. PMID:30691016

1743. Lozano R, Naghavi M, Foreman K, et al. Global and regional mortality from 235 causes of death for 20 age groups in 1990 and 2010: a systematic analysis for the Global Burden of Disease Study 2010. Lancet. 2012 Dec 15;380(9859):2095–128. PMID:23245604

1744. Lu HS, Gan MF, Zhou T, et al. Sarcomatoid thymic carcinoma arising in metaplastic thymoma: a case report. Int J Surg Pathol. 2011 Oct;19(5):677–80. PMID:20034984

1745. Lu S, Stein JE, Rimm DL, et al. Comparison of biomarker modalities for predicting response to PD-1/PD-L1 checkpoint blockade: a systematic review and meta-analysis. JAMA Oncol. 2019 Jul 18;5(8):1195–204. PMID:31318407

1745A. Lu S, Yu Y, Li Z, et al. EGFR and ERBB2 germline mutations in Chinese lung cancer patients and their roles in genetic susceptibility to cancer. J Thorac Oncol. 2019 Apr;14(4):732–6. PMID:30610926

1746. Luc JGY, Phan K, Tchantchaleishvili V. Cystic tumor of the atrioventricular node: a review of the literature. J Thorac Dis. 2017 Sep;9(9):3313–8. PMID:29221317

1747. Lugli A, Forster Y, Haas P, et al. Calretinin expression in human normal and neoplastic tissues: a tissue microarray analysis on 5233 tissue samples. Hum Pathol. 2003 Oct;34(10):994–1000. PMID:14608532

1748. Luks VL, Kamitaki N, Vivero MP, et al. Lymphatic and other vascular malformative/overgrowth disorders are caused by somatic mutations in PIK3CA. J Pediatr. 2015 Apr;166(4):1048–54.e1, 5. PMID:25681199

1750. Lurain K, Polizzotto MN, Aleman K, et al. Viral, immunologic, and clinical features of primary effusion lymphoma. Blood. 2019 Apr 18;133(16):1753–61. PMID:30782610

1751. Lynch HT, Radford B, Lynch JF. SBLA syndrome revisited. Oncology. 1990;47(1):75–9. PMID:2300390

1752. Lynch TJ, Bell DW, Sordella R, et al. Activating mutations in the epidermal growth factor receptor underlying responsiveness of non-small-cell lung cancer to gefitinib. N Engl J Med. 2004 May 20;350(21):2129–39. PMID:15118073

1753. Mabuchi T, Shimizu M, Ino H, et al. PRKAR1A gene mutation in patients with cardiac myxoma. Int J Cardiol. 2005 Jul 10;102(2):273–7. PMID:15982496

1754. Machado Medeiros T, Altmayer S, Watte G, et al. 18F-FDG PET/CT and whole-body MRI diagnostic performance in M staging for non-small cell lung cancer: a systematic review and meta-analysis. Eur Radiol. 2020 Jul;30(7):3641–9. PMID:32125513

1755. Macher-Goeppinger S, Penzel R, Roth W, et al. Expression and mutation analysis of EGFR, c-KIT, and β-catenin in pulmonary blastoma. J Clin Pathol. 2011 Apr;64(4):349–53. PMID:21292787

1756. Machida E, Haniuda M, Eguchi T, et al. Granular cell tumor of the mediastinum. Intern Med. 2003 Feb;42(2):178–81. PMID:12636238

1757. Mackie AS, Kozakewich HP, Geva T, et al. Vascular tumors of the heart in infants and children: case series and review of the literature. Pediatr Cardiol. 2005 Jul-Aug;26(4):344–9. PMID:15549621

1758. MacMahon H, Naidich DP, Goo JM, et al. Guidelines for management of incidental pulmonary nodules detected on CT images: from the Fleischner Society 2017. Radiology. 2017 Jul;284(1):228–43. PMID:28240562

1759. Maeda D, Ota S, Ikeda S, et al. Mucinous adenocarcinoma of the thymus: a distinct variant of thymic carcinoma. Lung Cancer. 2009 Apr;64(1):22–7. PMID:18722686

1760. Maeda H, Matsumura A, Kawabata T, et al. Adenosquamous carcinoma of the lung: surgical results as compared with squamous cell and adenocarcinoma cases. Eur J Cardiothorac Surg. 2012 Feb;41(2):357–61. PMID:21737295

1761. Maeshima AM, Tochigi N, Yoshida A, et al. Histological scoring for small lung adenocarcinomas 2 cm or less in diameter: a reliable prognostic indicator. J Thorac Oncol. 2010 Mar;5(3):333–9. PMID:20125041

1762. Maeyashiki T, Suzuki K, Hattori A, et al. The size of consolidation on thin-section computed tomography is a better predictor of survival than the maximum tumour dimension in resectable lung cancer. Eur J Cardiothorac Surg. 2013 May;43(5):915–8. PMID:23024235

1763. Maghbool M, Ramzi M, Nagel I, et al. Primary adenocarcinoma of the thymus: an immunohistochemical and molecular study with review of the literature. BMC Clin Pathol. 2013 May 31;13(1):17. PMID:23725376

1764. Mahmud T, Mal G, Majeed FA, et al. A massive pleural-based desmoid tumour. Respirol Case Rep. 2016 Dec 1;5(1):e00205. PMID:28031839

1765. Mahon BM, Placido JB, Gattuso P. Fine-needle aspiration of classic biphasic pulmonary blastoma. Diagn Cytopathol. 2010 Jun;38(6):427–9. PMID:19937760

1766. Mahoney MC, Shipley RT, Corcoran HL, et al. CT demonstration of calcification in carcinoma of the lung. AJR Am J Roentgenol. 1990 Feb;154(2):255–8. PMID:2153329

1767. Mahoney NR, Liu GT, Menacker SJ, et al. Pediatric horner syndrome: etiologies and roles of imaging and urine studies to detect neuroblastoma and other responsible mass lesions. Am J Ophthalmol. 2006 Oct;142(4):651–9. PMID:17011859

1768. Mai PL, Malkin D, Garber JE, et al. Li-Fraumeni syndrome: report of a clinical research workshop and creation of a research consortium. Cancer Genet. 2012 Oct;205(10):479–87. PMID:22939227

1769. Majak BM, Bock G. Pulmonary sclerosing haemangioma diagnosed by frozen section. Histopathology. 2003 Jun;42(6):621–2. PMID:12786904

1770. Makdisi G, Roden AC, Shen KR. Successful resection of giant mediastinal lipofibroadenoma of the thymus by video-assisted thoracoscopic surgery. Ann Thorac Surg. 2015 Aug;100(2):698–700. PMID:26234840

1771. Makhlouf HR, Ishak KG, Goodman ZD. Epithelioid hemangioendothelioma of the liver: a clinicopathologic study of 137 cases. Cancer. 1999 Feb 1;85(3):562–82. PMID:10091730

1772. Malagón HD, Valdez AM, Moran CA, et al. Germ cell tumors with sarcomatous components: a clinicopathologic and immunohistochemical study of 46 cases. Am J Surg Pathol. 2007 Sep;31(9):1356–62. PMID:17721191

1773. Maleki Z, Muller S, Layfield L, et al. Pulmonary sclerosing pneumocytoma: cytomorphology and immunoprofile. Cancer Cytopathol. 2020 Jun;128(6):414–23. PMID:32022435

1774. Maleszewski JJ, Anavekar NS, Moynihan TJ, et al. Pathology, imaging, and treatment of cardiac tumours. Nat Rev Cardiol. 2017 Sep;14(9):536–49. PMID:28436488

1775. Maleszewski JJ, Bois MC, Bois JP, et al. Neoplasia and the heart: pathological review of effects with clinical and radiological correlation. J Am Coll Cardiol. 2018 Jul 10;72(2):202–27. PMID:29976295

1776. Maleszewski JJ, Hristov AC, Halushka MK, et al. Extranodal Rosai-Dorfman disease involving the heart: report of two cases. Cardiovasc Pathol. 2010 Nov-Dec;19(6):380–4. PMID:19819734

1777. Maleszewski JJ, Larsen BT, Kip NS, et al. PRKAR1A in the development of cardiac myxoma: a study of 110 cases including isolated and syndromic tumors. Am J Surg Pathol. 2014 Aug;38(8):1079–87. PMID:24618615

1778. Malhotra J, Malvezzi M, Negri E, et al. Risk factors for lung cancer worldwide. Eur Respir J. 2016 Sep;48(3):889–902. PMID:27174888

1779. Malinowska I, Kwiatkowski DJ, Weiss S, et al. Perivascular epithelioid cell tumors (PEComas) harboring TFE3 gene rearrangements lack the TSC2 alterations characteristic of conventional PEComas: further evidence for a biological distinction. Am J Surg Pathol. 2012 May;36(5):783–4. PMID:22456611

1780. Malkin D, Li FP, Strong LC, et al. Germ line p53 mutations in a familial syndrome of breast cancer, sarcomas, and other neoplasms. Science. 1990 Nov 30;250(4985):1233–8. PMID:1978757

1781. Maneenil K, Xue Z, Liu M, et al. Sarcomatoid carcinoma of the lung: the Mayo Clinic experience in 127 patients. Clin Lung Cancer. 2018 May;19(3):e323–33. PMID:29454534

1782. Mangano WE, Cagle PT, Churg A, et al. The diagnosis of desmoplastic malignant mesothelioma and its distinction from fibrous pleurisy: a histologic and immunohistochemical analysis of 31 cases including p53 immunostaining. Am J Clin Pathol. 1998 Aug;110(2):191–9. PMID:9704618

1783. Manivel C, Wick MR, Abenoza P, et al. The occurrence of sarcomatous components in primary mediastinal germ cell tumors. Am J Surg Pathol. 1986 Oct;10(10):711–7. PMID:3021008

1784. Manivel JC, Priest JR, Watterson J, et al. Pleuropulmonary blastoma. The so-called pulmonary blastoma of childhood. Cancer. 1988 Oct 15;62(8):1516–26. PMID:3048630

1785. Mann S, Khawar S, Moran C, et al. Revisiting localized malignant mesothelioma. Ann Diagn Pathol. 2019 Apr;39:74–7. PMID:30798074

1786. Manner J, Radlwimmer B, Hohenberger P, et al. MYC high level gene amplification is a distinctive feature of angiosarcomas after irradiation or chronic lymphedema. Am J Pathol. 2010 Jan;176(1):34–9. PMID:20008140

1787. Mansencal N, Revault-d'Allonnes L, Pelage JP, et al. Usefulness of contrast echocardiography for assessment of intracardiac masses. Arch Cardiovasc Dis. 2009 Mar;102(3):177–83. PMID:19375671

1788. Mansuet-Lupo A, Barritault M, Alifano M, et al. Proposal for a combined histomolecular algorithm to distinguish multiple primary adenocarcinomas from intrapulmonary metastasis in patients with multiple lung tumors. J Thorac Oncol. 2019 May;14(5):844–56. PMID:30721797

1789. Manthri S, Rehman HH, Costello PN, et al. Thymic basaloid carcinoma: a rare clinical entity. BMJ Case Rep. 2019 Nov 28;12(11):e231980. PMID:31780620

1790. Mantovani G, Bondioni S, Corbetta S, et al. Analysis of GNAS1 and PRKAR1A gene mutations in human cardiac myxomas not associated with multiple endocrine disorders. J Endocrinol Invest. 2009 Jun;32(6):501–4. PMID:19494712

1791. Manucha V, Hansen JT, Gonzalez MF, et al. Role of cytology and immunochemistry in diagnosis of metastatic malignancies in the lung: a critical appraisal. Diagn Cytopathol. 2018 Nov;46(11):936–44. PMID:30353676

1792. Manzotti G, Torricelli F, Benedetta D, et al. An epithelial-to-mesenchymal transcriptional switch triggers evolution of pulmonary sarcomatoid carcinoma (PSC) and identifies dasatinib as new therapeutic option. Clin Cancer Res. 2019 Apr 1;25(7):2348–60. PMID:30587547

1793. Mao L, Lee JS, Kurie JM, et al. Clonal genetic alterations in the lungs of current and former smokers. J Natl Cancer Inst. 1997 Jun 18;89(12):857–62. PMID:9196251

1794. Marchevsky A, Marx A, Ströbel P, et al. Policies and reporting guidelines for small biopsy specimens of mediastinal masses. J Thorac Oncol. 2011 Jul;6(7 Suppl 3):S1724–9. PMID:21847054

1795. Marchevsky A, Nieburgs HE, Olenko E, et al. Pulmonary tumorlets in cases of "tuberculoma" of the lung with malignant cells in brush biopsy. Acta Cytol. 1982 Jul-Aug;26(4):491–4. PMID:6957103

1796. Marchevsky AM, Gupta R, Balzer B. Diagnosis of metastatic neoplasms: a clinicopathologic and morphologic approach. Arch Pathol Lab Med. 2010 Feb;134(2):194–206. PMID:20121607

1797. Marchevsky AM, Gupta R, Casadio C, et al. World Health Organization classification of thymomas provides significant prognostic information for selected stage III patients: evidence from an international thymoma study group. Hum Pathol. 2010 Oct;41(10):1413–21. PMID:20573368

1798. Marchevsky AM, Gupta R, McKenna RJ, et al. Evidence-based pathology and the pathologic evaluation of thymomas: the World Health Organization classification can be simplified into only 3 categories other than thymic carcinoma. Cancer. 2008 Jun 15;112(12):2780–8. PMID:18442102

1799. Marchevsky AM, Hendifar A, Walts AE. The use of Ki-67 labeling index to grade pulmonary well-differentiated neuroendocrine neoplasms: current best evidence. Mod Pathol. 2018 Oct;31(10):1523–31. PMID:29802361

1800. Marchevsky AM, Khoor A, Walts AE, et al. Localized malignant mesothelioma, an unusual and poorly characterized neoplasm of serosal origin: best current evidence from the literature and the International Mesothelioma Panel. Mod Pathol. 2020 Feb;33(2):281–96. PMID:31485011

1801. Marchevsky AM, LeStang N, Hiroshima K, et al. The differential diagnosis between pleural sarcomatoid mesothelioma and spindle cell/pleomorphic (sarcomatoid) carcinomas of the lung: evidence-based guidelines from the International Mesothelioma Panel and the MESOPATH National Reference Center. Hum Pathol. 2017 Sep;67:160–8. PMID:28782639

1802. Marchevsky AM, McKenna RJ Jr, Gupta R. Thymic epithelial neoplasms: a review of current concepts using an evidence-based pathology approach. Hematol Oncol Clin North Am. 2008 Jun;22(3):543–62. PMID:18514132

1803. Marchevsky AM, Walts AE. Diffuse idiopathic pulmonary neuroendocrine cell hyperplasia (DIPNECH). Semin Diagn Pathol. 2015 Nov;32(6):438–44. PMID:26472691

1804. Marchevsky AM, Walts AE. PD-L1, PD-1, CD4, and CD8 expression in neoplastic and nonneoplastic thymus. Hum Pathol. 2017 Feb;60:16–23. PMID:27746267

1805. Marchevsky AM, Wirtschafter E, Walts AE. The spectrum of changes in adults with multifocal pulmonary neuroendocrine proliferations: What is the minimum set of pathologic criteria to diagnose DIPNECH? Hum Pathol. 2015 Feb;46(2):176–81. PMID:25532694

1806. Marchiò C, Gatti G, Massa F, et al. Distinctive pathological and clinical features of lung carcinoids with high proliferation index.

Virchows Arch. 2017 Dec;471(6):713–20. PMID:28631159
1807. Marciello F, Mercier O, Ferolla P, et al. Natural history of localized and locally advanced atypical lung carcinoids after complete resection: a joined French-Italian retrospective multicenter study. Neuroendocrinology. 2018;106(3):264–73. PMID:28813709
1808. Marcoux N, Gettinger SN, O'Kane G, et al. EGFR-mutant adenocarcinomas that transform to small-cell lung cancer and other neuroendocrine carcinomas: clinical outcomes. J Clin Oncol. 2019 Feb 1;37(4):278–85. PMID:30550363
1809. Margolin K, Traweek T. The unique association of malignant histiocytosis and a primary gonadal germ cell tumor. Med Pediatr Oncol. 1992;20(2):162–4. PMID:1734222
1810. Marina NM, Cushing B, Giller R, et al. Complete surgical excision is effective treatment for children with immature teratomas with or without malignant elements: a Pediatric Oncology Group/Children's Cancer Group Intergroup study. J Clin Oncol. 1999 Jul;17(7):2137–43. PMID:10561269
1811. Mariño-Enríquez A, Fletcher CD. Round cell sarcomas - biologically important refinements in subclassification. Int J Biochem Cell Biol. 2014 Aug;53:493–504. PMID:24801613
1812. Marmor S, Koren R, Halpern M, et al. Transthoracic needle biopsy in the diagnosis of large-cell neuroendocrine carcinoma of the lung. Diagn Cytopathol. 2005 Oct;33(4):238–43. PMID:16138368
1813. Marom EM. Advances in thymoma imaging. J Thorac Imaging. 2013 Mar;28(2):69–80, quiz 81–3. PMID:23422781
1814. Marom EM, Milito MA, Moran CA, et al. Computed tomography findings predicting invasiveness of thymoma. J Thorac Oncol. 2011 Jul;6(7):1274–81. PMID:21623235
1815. Marques Mendes E, Ferreira A, Felgueiras P, et al. Primary intimal sarcoma of the left atrium presenting with constitutional symptoms. Oxf Med Case Reports. 2017 Jul 5;2017(7):omx031. PMID:28694971
1816. Martin B, Verdebout JM, Mascaux C, et al. Expression of p53 in preneoplastic and early neoplastic bronchial lesions. Oncol Rep. 2002 Mar-Apr;9(2):223–9. PMID:11836584
1817. Maruyama H, Seyama K, Sobajima J, et al. Multifocal micronodular pneumocyte hyperplasia and lymphangioleiomyomatosis in tuberous sclerosis with a TSC2 gene. Mod Pathol. 2001 Jun;14(6):609–14. PMID:11406664
1818. Marx A, Ströbel P, Badve SS, et al. ITMIG consensus statement on the use of the WHO histological classification of thymoma and thymic carcinoma: refined definitions, histological criteria, and reporting. J Thorac Oncol. 2014 May;9(5):596–611. PMID:24722150
1819. Marx A, Willcox N, Leite MI, et al. Thymoma and paraneoplastic myasthenia gravis. Autoimmunity. 2010 Aug;43(5-6):413–27. PMID:20380583
1820. Mas C, Penny DJ, Menahem S. Pre-excitation syndrome secondary to cardiac rhabdomyomas in tuberous sclerosis. J Paediatr Child Health. 2000 Feb;36(1):84–6. PMID:10723700
1821. Masai K, Sakurai H, Suzuki S, et al. Clinicopathological features of colloid adenocarcinoma of the lung: a report of six cases. J Surg Oncol. 2016 Aug;114(2):211–5. PMID:27220284
1822. Mascaux C, Angelova M, Vasaturo A, et al. Immune evasion before tumour invasion in early lung squamous carcinogenesis. Nature. 2019 Jul;571(7766):570–5. PMID:31243362
1823. Mascaux C, Bex F, Martin B, et al. The role of NPM, p14arf and MDM2 in precursors of bronchial squamous cell carcinoma. Eur Respir J. 2008 Sep;32(3):678–86. PMID:18480108
1824. Masciari S, Dillon DA, Rath M, et al. Breast cancer phenotype in women with TP53 germline mutations: a Li-Fraumeni syndrome consortium effort. Breast Cancer Res Treat. 2012 Jun;133(3):1125–30. PMID:22392042
1824A. Massoth LR, Hung YP, Dias-Santagata D, et al. Pan-cancer landscape analysis reveals recurrent KMT2A-MAML2 gene fusion in aggressive histologic subtypes of thymoma. JCO Precis Oncol. 2020 Feb 26;4:PO.19.00288. PMID:32923872
1825. Massoth LR, Selig MK, Little BP, et al. Multiple calcifying fibrous pseudotumors of the pleura: ultrastructural analysis provides insight on mechanism of dissemination. Ultrastruct Pathol. 2019;43(4-5):154–61. PMID:31746679
1826. Mastrangelo G, Coindre JM, Ducimetière F, et al. Incidence of soft tissue sarcoma and beyond: a population-based prospective study in 3 European regions. Cancer. 2012 Nov 1;118(21):5339–48. PMID:22517534
1827. Masunaga A, Nagashio R, Iwamoto S, et al. A case of pulmonary papillary adenoma: possible relationship between tumor histogenesis/tumorigenesis and fibroblast growth factor receptor 2 IIIb. Pathol Int. 2012 Sep;62(9):640–5. PMID:22924850
1828. Masunaga A, Oide T, Kamata T, et al. GLUT-1 expression of pulmonary mixed squamous cell and glandular papilloma may be associated with high SUVmax on fluorodeoxyglucose-positron emission tomography. Pathol Int. 2017 Jul;67(7):373–4. PMID:28590021
1829. Mathas S, Hartmann S, Küppers R. Hodgkin lymphoma: pathology and biology. Semin Hematol. 2016 Jul;53(3):139–47. PMID:27496304
1830. Mather JP, Roberts PE, Pan Z, et al. Isolation of cancer stem like cells from human adenosquamous carcinoma of the lung supports a monoclonal origin from a multipotential tissue stem cell. PLoS One. 2013 Dec 4;8(12):e79456. PMID:24324581
1831. Matoso A, Singh K, Jacob R, et al. Comparison of thyroid transcription factor-1 expression by 2 monoclonal antibodies in pulmonary and nonpulmonary primary tumors. Appl Immunohistochem Mol Morphol. 2010 Mar;18(2):142–9. PMID:19887917
1832. Matsuba K, Saito T, Ando K, et al. Atypical lipoma of the lung. Thorax. 1991 Sep;46(9):685. PMID:1948801
1833. Matsubara D, Kishaba Y, Ishikawa S, et al. Lung cancer with loss of BRG1/BRM, shows epithelial mesenchymal transition phenotype and distinct histologic and genetic features. Cancer Sci. 2013 Feb;104(2):266–73. PMID:23163725
1834. Matsubara D, Morikawa T, Goto A, et al. Subepithelial myofibroblast in lung adenocarcinoma: a histological indicator of excellent prognosis. Mod Pathol. 2009 Jun;22(6):776–85. PMID:19329939
1835. Matsubara D, Soda M, Yoshimoto T, et al. Inactivating mutations and hypermethylation of the NKX2-1/TTF-1 gene in non-terminal respiratory unit-type lung adenocarcinomas. Cancer Sci. 2017 Sep;108(9):1888–96. PMID:28677170
1836. Matsubayashi H, Yamashita R, Sasaki K, et al. Retroperitoneal choriocarcinoma diagnosed by endoscopic ultrasonography-guided fine needle aspiration biopsy. Arab J Gastroenterol. 2018 Sep;19(3):130–3. PMID:30262237
1837. Matsubayashi J, Miyake S, Kudo Y, et al. Cytological differences between invasive and noninvasive or minimally invasive lung adenocarcinomas diagnosed in Japanese patients using needle biopsy specimens of pulmonary lesions ≤3 cm in diameter. Diagn Cytopathol. 2019 Jul;47(7):688–94. PMID:30968597
1838. Matsue K, Abe Y, Kitadate A, et al. Sensitivity and specificity of incisional random skin biopsy for diagnosis of intravascular large B-cell lymphoma. Blood. 2019 Mar 14;133(11):1257–9. PMID:30647028
1839. Matsui K, Beasley MB, Nelson WK, et al. Prognostic significance of pulmonary lymphangioleiomyomatosis histologic score. Am J Surg Pathol. 2001 Apr;25(4):479–84. PMID:11257622
1839A. Matsui K, Tatsuguchi A, Valencia J, et al. Extrapulmonary lymphangioleiomyomatosis (LAM): clinicopathologic features in 22 cases. Hum Pathol. 2000 Oct;31(10):1242–8. PMID:11070117
1840. Matsuno Y, Morozumi N, Hirohashi S, et al. Papillary carcinoma of the thymus: report of four cases of a new microscopic type of thymic carcinoma. Am J Surg Pathol. 1998 Jul;22(7):873–80. PMID:9669349
1841. Matsuo T, Hayashida R, Kobayashi K, et al. Thymic basaloid carcinoma with hepatic metastasis. Ann Thorac Surg. 2002 Aug;74(2):579–82. PMID:12173853
1842. Matsushima J, Yazawa T, Suzuki M, et al. Clinicopathological, immunohistochemical, and mutational analyses of pulmonary enteric adenocarcinoma: usefulness of SATB2 and β-catenin immunostaining for differentiation from metastatic colorectal carcinoma. Hum Pathol. 2017 Jun;64:179–85. PMID:28438615
1843. Matsushita M, Kuwamoto S. Cytologic features of SMARCA4-deficient thoracic sarcoma: a case report and comparison with other SWI/SNF complex-deficient tumors. Acta Cytol. 2018;62(5-6):456–62. PMID:30286456
1844. Matsuyama A, Hisaoka M, Iwasaki M, et al. TLE1 expression in malignant mesothelioma. Virchows Arch. 2010 Nov;457(5):577–83. PMID:20857142
1845. Matsuyama A, Shiba E, Umekita Y, et al. Clinicopathologic diversity of undifferentiated sarcoma with BCOR-CCNB3 fusion: analysis of 11 cases with a reappraisal of the utility of immunohistochemistry for BCOR and CCNB3. Am J Surg Pathol. 2017 Dec;41(12):1713–21. PMID:28877060
1847. Mattson ME, Pollack ES, Cullen JW. What are the odds that smoking will kill you? Am J Public Health. 1987 Apr;77(4):425–31. PMID:3826460
1848. Matyakhina L, Pack S, Kirschner LS, et al. Chromosome 2 (2p16) abnormalities in Carney complex tumours. J Med Genet. 2003 Apr;40(4):268–77. PMID:12676898
1849. Mauclet C, Duplaquet F, Pirard L, et al. Complete tumor response of a locally advanced lung large-cell neuroendocrine carcinoma after palliative thoracic radiotherapy and immunotherapy with nivolumab. Lung Cancer. 2019 Feb;128:53–6. PMID:30642453
1850. Maurac A, Debray MP, Crestani B, et al. Thoracic involvement of diffuse lymphangiomatosis successfully treated with sildenafil. BMJ Case Rep. 2019 Apr 23;12(4):e228523. PMID:31015245
1851. Mavrakis KJ, McDonald ER 3rd, Schlabach MR, et al. Disordered methionine metabolism in MTAP/CDKN2A-deleted cancers leads to dependence on PRMT5. Science. 2016 Mar 11;351(6278):1208–13. PMID:26912361
1852. Mayall FG, Gibbs AR. The histology and immunohistochemistry of small cell mesothelioma. Histopathology. 1992 Jan;20(1):47–51. PMID:1310669
1853. Mazzola A, Spano JP, Valente M, et al. Leiomyosarcoma of the left atrium mimicking a left atrial myxoma. J Thorac Cardiovasc Surg. 2006 Jan;131(1):224–6. PMID:16399316
1854. McAllister HA Jr, Hall RJ, Cooley DA. Tumors of the heart and pericardium. Curr Probl Cardiol. 1999 Feb;24(2):57–116. PMID:10028128
1855. McBride MJ, Pulice JL, Beird HC, et al. The SS18-SSX fusion oncoprotein hijacks BAF complex targeting and function to drive synovial sarcoma. Cancer Cell. 2018 Jun 11;33(6):1128–1141.e7. PMID:29861296
1856. McCaughan BC, Martini N, Bains MS. Bronchial carcinoids. Review of 124 cases. J Thorac Cardiovasc Surg. 1985 Jan;89(1):8–17. PMID:2981373
1857. McCleary AJ. Massive haemothorax secondary to angiosarcoma. Thorax. 1994 Oct;49(10):1036–7. PMID:7974301
1858. McCormack FX, Gupta N, Finlay GR, et al. Official American Thoracic Society/Japanese Respiratory Society clinical practice guidelines: lymphangioleiomyomatosis diagnosis and management. Am J Respir Crit Care Med. 2016 Sep 15;194(6):748–61. PMID:27628078
1859. McCormack FX, Inoue Y, Moss J, et al. Efficacy and safety of sirolimus in lymphangioleiomyomatosis. N Engl J Med. 2011 Apr 28;364(17):1595–606. PMID:21410393
1860. McDonald M, McLean T, Belhorn T, et al. Thymic carcinoma in a child with HIV infection. Pediatr Blood Cancer. 2007 Dec;49(7):1004–7. PMID:16317759
1860A. McGinnis M, Jacobs G, el-Naggar A, et al. Congenital peribronchial myofibroblastic tumor (so-called "congenital leiomyosarcoma"). A distinct neonatal lung lesion associated with nonimmune hydrops fetalis. Mod Pathol. 1993 Jul;6(4):487–92. PMID:8415597
1861. McGranahan N, Rosenthal R, Hiley CT, et al. Allele-specific HLA loss and immune escape in lung cancer evolution. Cell. 2017 Nov 30;171(6):1259–1271.e11. PMID:29107330
1862. McGregor SM, Dunning R, Hyjek E, et al. BAP1 facilitates diagnostic objectivity, classification, and prognostication in malignant pleural mesothelioma. Hum Pathol. 2015 Nov;46(11):1670–8. PMID:26376834
1863. McKenney JK, Heerema-McKenney A, Rouse RV. Extragonadal germ cell tumors: a review with emphasis on pathologic features, clinical prognostic variables, and differential diagnostic considerations. Adv Anat Pathol. 2007 Mar;14(2):69–92. PMID:17471115
1864. McLeer-Florin A, Moro-Sibilot D, Melis A, et al. Dual IHC and FISH testing for ALK gene rearrangement in lung adenocarcinomas in a routine practice: a French study. J Thorac Oncol. 2012 Feb;7(2):348–54. PMID:22071784
1865. McMenamin ME, Fletcher CD. Expanding the spectrum of malignant change in schwannomas: epithelioid malignant change, epithelioid malignant peripheral nerve sheath tumor, and epithelioid angiosarcoma: a study of 17 cases. Am J Surg Pathol. 2001 Jan;25(1):13–25. PMID:11145248
1866. McMillan RR, Sima CS, Moraco NH, et al. Recurrence patterns after resection of soft tissue sarcomas of the chest wall. Ann Thorac Surg. 2013 Oct;96(4):1223–8. PMID:23891404
1867. McNamee CJ, Lien D, Puttagunta L, et al. Solitary squamous papillomas of the bronchus: a case report and literature review. J Thorac Cardiovasc Surg. 2003 Sep;126(3):861–3. PMID:14502170
1868. McWilliams A, Shaipanich T, Lam S. Fluorescence and navigational bronchoscopy. Thorac Surg Clin. 2013 May;23(2):153–61. PMID:23566967
1869. Mechtersheimer G, Otaño-Joos M, Ohl S, et al. Analysis of chromosomal imbalances in sporadic and NF1-associated peripheral nerve sheath tumors by comparative genomic hybridization. Genes Chromosomes Cancer. 1999 Aug;25(4):362–9. PMID:10398430
1870. Meder L, König K, Ozretić L, et al. NOTCH, ASCL1, p53 and RB alterations define an alternative pathway driving neuroendocrine and small cell lung carcinomas. Int J Cancer.

2016 Feb 15;138(4):927–38. PMID:26340530
1871. Meert AP, Feoli F, Martin B, et al. Ki67 expression in bronchial preneoplastic lesions and carcinoma in situ defined according to the new 1999 WHO/IASLC criteria: a preliminary study. Histopathology. 2004 Jan;44(1):47–53. PMID:14717669
1872. Mehrad M, LaFramboise WA, Lyons MA, et al. Whole-exome sequencing identifies unique mutations and copy number losses in calcifying fibrous tumor of the pleura: report of 3 cases and review of the literature. Hum Pathol. 2018 Aug;78:36–43. PMID:29689243
1873. Mehta A, Sriramanakoppa NN, Agarwal P, et al. Predictive biomarkers in nonsmall cell carcinoma and their clinico-pathological association. South Asian J Cancer. 2019 Oct-Dec;8(4):250–4. PMID:31807491
1874. Mei L, Alikhan M, Mujacic I, et al. Genomic alterations in undifferentiated malignant tumors with rhabdoid phenotype and loss of BRG1 immunoexpression identified by fine needle aspirates. Acta Cytol. 2019;63(5):438–44. PMID:31230044
1875. Meijerink JP. Genetic rearrangements in relation to immunophenotype and outcome in T-cell acute lymphoblastic leukaemia. Best Pract Res Clin Haematol. 2010 Sep;23(3):307–18. PMID:21112032
1876. Meir K, Maly A, Doviner V, et al. Intraoperative cytologic diagnosis of unsuspected cardiac myxoma: a case report. Acta Cytol. 2004 Jul-Aug;48(4):565–8. PMID:15296348
1877. Meisinger QC, Klein JS, Butnor KJ, et al. CT features of peripheral pulmonary carcinoid tumors. AJR Am J Roentgenol. 2011 Nov;197(5):1073–80. PMID:22021498
1878. Meis-Kindblom JM, Kindblom LG. Angiosarcoma of soft tissue: a study of 80 cases. Am J Surg Pathol. 1998 Jun;22(6):683–97. PMID:9630175
1879. Meister M, Schirmacher P, Dienemann H, et al. Mutational status of the epidermal growth factor receptor (EGFR) gene in thymomas and thymic carcinomas. Cancer Lett. 2007 Apr 18;248(2):186–91. PMID:16919868
1880. Melani C, Advani R, Roschewski M, et al. End-of-treatment and serial PET imaging in primary mediastinal B-cell lymphoma following dose-adjusted EPOCH-R: a paradigm shift in clinical decision making. Haematologica. 2018 Aug;103(8):1337–44. PMID:29748435
1881. Melani C, Jaffe ES, Wilson WH. Pathobiology and treatment of lymphomatoid granulomatosis, a rare EBV-driven disorder. Blood. 2020 Apr 16;135(16):1344–52. PMID:32107539
1882. Mello SS, Attardi LD. Deciphering p53 signaling in tumor suppression. Curr Opin Cell Biol. 2018 Apr;51:65–72. PMID:29195118
1883. Mende S, Moschopulos M, Marx A, et al. Ectopic micronodular thymoma with lymphoid stroma. Virchows Arch. 2004 Apr;444(4):397–9. PMID:15067545
1884. Mendlick MR, Nelson M, Pickering D, et al. Translocation t(1;3)(p36.3;q25) is a nonrandom aberration in epithelioid hemangioendothelioma. Am J Surg Pathol. 2001 May;25(5):684–7. PMID:11342784
1885. Menestrina F, Chilosi M, Bonetti F, et al. Mediastinal large-cell lymphoma of B-type, with sclerosis: histopathological and immunohistochemical study of eight cases. Histopathology. 1986 Jun;10(6):589–600. PMID:3525372
1886. Mengoli MC, Longo FR, Fraggetta F, et al. The 2015 World Health Organization classification of lung tumors: new entities since the 2004 classification. Pathologica. 2018 Mar;110(1):39–67. PMID:30259912
1887. Mengoli MC, Rossi G, Cavazza A, et al. Diffuse idiopathic pulmonary neuroendocrine cell hyperplasia (DIPNECH) syndrome and carcinoid tumors with/without NECH: a clinicopathologic, radiologic, and immunomolecular comparison study. Am J Surg Pathol. 2018 May;42(5):646–55. PMID:29438170
1888. Mensi C, Giacomini S, Sieno C, et al. Pericardial mesothelioma and asbestos exposure. Int J Hyg Environ Health. 2011 Jun;214(3):276–9. PMID:21156353
1889. Mentzel T, Beham A, Calonje E, et al. Epithelioid hemangioendothelioma of skin and soft tissues: clinicopathologic and immunohistochemical study of 30 cases. Am J Surg Pathol. 1997 Apr;21(4):363–74. PMID:9130982
1890. Mentzel T, Calonje E, Wadden C, et al. Myxofibrosarcoma. Clinicopathologic analysis of 75 cases with emphasis on the low-grade variant. Am J Surg Pathol. 1996 Apr;20(4):391–405. PMID:8604805
1891. Mentzel T, Katenkamp D. Intraneural angiosarcoma and angiosarcoma arising in benign and malignant peripheral nerve sheath tumours: clinicopathological and immunohistochemical analysis of four cases. Histopathology. 1999 Aug;35(2):114–20. PMID:10460655
1892. Mentzel T, Schildhaus HU, Palmedo G, et al. Postradiation cutaneous angiosarcoma after treatment of breast carcinoma is characterized by MYC amplification in contrast to atypical vascular lesions after radiotherapy and control cases: clinicopathological, immunohistochemical and molecular analysis of 66 cases. Mod Pathol. 2012 Jan;25(1):75–85. PMID:21909081
1893. Meraj R, Wikenheiser-Brokamp KA, Young LR, et al. Lymphangioleiomyomatosis: new concepts in pathogenesis, diagnosis, and treatment. Semin Respir Crit Care Med. 2012 Oct;33(5):486–97. PMID:23001803
1894. Merchant AM, Hedrick HL, Johnson MP, et al. Management of fetal mediastinal teratoma. J Pediatr Surg. 2005 Jan;40(1):228–31. PMID:15868589
1895. Merrick DT, Edwards MG, Franklin WA, et al. Altered cell-cycle control, inflammation, and adhesion in high-risk persistent bronchial dysplasia. Cancer Res. 2018 Sep 1;78(17):4971–83. PMID:29997230
1896. Merrick DT, Kittelson J, Winterhalder R, et al. Analysis of c-ErbB1/epidermal growth factor receptor and c-ErbB2/HER-2 expression in bronchial dysplasia: evaluation of potential targets for chemoprevention of lung cancer. Clin Cancer Res. 2006 Apr 1;12(7 Pt 1):2281–8. PMID:16609045
1897. Mertens F, Wiebe T, Adlercreutz C, et al. Successful treatment of a child with t(15;19)-positive tumor. Pediatr Blood Cancer. 2007 Dec;49(7):1015–7. PMID:16435379
1898. Messinger YH, Stewart DR, Priest JR, et al. Pleuropulmonary blastoma: a report on 350 central pathology-confirmed pleuropulmonary blastoma cases by the International Pleuropulmonary Blastoma Registry. Cancer. 2015 Jan 15;121(2):276–85. PMID:25209242
1899. Metaxas Y, Rivalland G, Mauti LA, et al. Pembrolizumab as palliative immunotherapy in malignant pleural mesothelioma. J Thorac Oncol. 2018 Nov;13(11):1784–91. PMID:30142389
1900. Meyer PC. Metastatic carcinoma of the pleura. Thorax. 1966 Sep;21(5):437–43. PMID:5969243
1901. Meyer PN, Fu K, Greiner TC, et al. Immunohistochemical methods for predicting cell of origin and survival in patients with diffuse large B-cell lymphoma treated with rituximab. J Clin Oncol. 2011 Jan 10;29(2):200–7. PMID:21135273
1902. Meyer WH, Spunt SL. Soft tissue sarcomas of childhood. Cancer Treat Rev. 2004 May;30(3):269–80. PMID:15059650
1903. Meza R, Meernik C, Jeon J, et al. Lung cancer incidence trends by gender, race and histology in the United States, 1973-2010. PLoS One. 2015 Mar 30;10(3):e0121323. PMID:25822850
1904. Mezquita L, Jové M, Nadal E, et al. High prevalence of somatic oncogenic driver alterations in patients with NSCLC and Li-Fraumeni syndrome. J Thorac Oncol. 2020 Jul;15(7):1232–9. PMID:32179180
1905. Mian I, Abdullaev Z, Morrow B, et al. Anaplastic lymphoma kinase gene rearrangement in children and young adults with mesothelioma. J Thorac Oncol. 2020 Mar;15(3):457–61. PMID:31783178
1905A. Michalova K, Tretiakova M, Pivovarcikova K, et al. Expanding the morphologic spectrum of chromophobe renal cell carcinoma: a study of 8 cases with papillary architecture. Ann Diagn Pathol. 2020 Feb;44:151448. PMID:31918172
1906. Michel M, Pratt JW. Anterior mediastinal nonseminomatous germ cell tumor with malignant transformation: a case report. Curr Surg. 2004 Nov-Dec;61(6):576–9. PMID:15590027
1907. Micke P, Botling J, Mattsson JSM, et al. Mucin staining is of limited value in addition to basic immunohistochemical analyses in the diagnostics of non-small cell lung cancer. Sci Rep. 2019 Feb 4;9(1):1319. PMID:30718697
1908. Micke P, Mattsson JS, Djureinovic D, et al. The impact of the fourth edition of the WHO classification of lung tumours on histological classification of resected pulmonary NSCCs. J Thorac Oncol. 2016 Jun;11(6):862–72. PMID:26872818
1909. Midha A, Dearden S, McCormack R. EGFR mutation incidence in non-small-cell lung cancer of adenocarcinoma histology: a systematic review and global map by ethnicity (mutMapII). Am J Cancer Res. 2015 Aug 15;5(9):2892–911. PMID:26609494
1910. Miettinen M, Fetsch JF. Distribution of keratins in normal endothelial cells and a spectrum of vascular tumors: implications in tumor diagnosis. Hum Pathol. 2000 Sep;31(9):1062–7. PMID:11014572
1911. Miettinen M, Limon J, Niezabitowski A, et al. Calretinin and other mesothelioma markers in synovial sarcoma: analysis of antigenic similarities and differences with malignant mesothelioma. Am J Surg Pathol. 2001 May;25(5):610–7. PMID:11342772
1912. Miettinen M, Lindenmayer AE, Chaubal A. Endothelial cell markers CD31, CD34, and BNH9 antibody to H- and Y-antigens–evaluation of their specificity and sensitivity in the diagnosis of vascular tumors and comparison with von Willebrand factor. Mod Pathol. 1994 Jan;7(1):82–90. PMID:7512718
1913. Miettinen M, McCue PA, Sarlomo-Rikala M, et al. GATA3: a multispecific but potentially useful marker in surgical pathology: a systematic analysis of 2500 epithelial and nonepithelial tumors. Am J Surg Pathol. 2014 Jan;38(1):13–22. PMID:24145643
1914. Miettinen M, Wang Z, McCue PA, et al. SALL4 expression in germ cell and non-germ cell tumors: a systematic immunohistochemical study of 3215 cases. Am J Surg Pathol. 2014 Mar;38(3):410–20. PMID:24525512
1915. Miettinen M, Wang ZF, Paetau A, et al. ERG transcription factor as an immunohistochemical marker for vascular endothelial tumors and prostatic carcinoma. Am J Surg Pathol. 2011 Mar;35(3):432–41. PMID:21317715
1916. Mignarri A, Gentili F, Masia F, et al. Imaging of the thymus in myotonic dystrophy type 1. Neurol Sci. 2018 Feb;39(2):347–51. PMID:29177794
1917. Miki M, Ball DW, Linnoila RI. Insights into the achaete-scute homolog-1 gene (hASH1) in normal and neoplastic human lung. Lung Cancer. 2012 Jan;75(1):58–65. PMID:21684625
1918. Mikubo M, Maruyama R, Kakinuma H, et al. Ciliated muconodular papillary tumors of the lung: cytologic features and diagnostic pitfalls in intraoperative examinations. Diagn Cytopathol. 2019 Jul;47(7):716–9. PMID:30848550
1919. Millar AC, Mete O, Cusimano RJ, et al. Functional cardiac paraganglioma associated with a rare SDHC mutation. Endocr Pathol. 2014 Sep;25(3):315–20. PMID:24402737
1920. Miller BS, Rusinko RY, Fowler L. Synchronous thymoma and thymic carcinoid in a woman with multiple endocrine neoplasia type 1: case report and review. Endocr Pract. 2008 Sep;14(6):713–6. PMID:18996790
1921. Miller DL, Allen MS. Rare pulmonary neoplasms. Mayo Clin Proc. 1993 May;68(5):492–8. PMID:8386792
1922. Miller DV, Firchau DJ, McClure RF, et al. Epstein-Barr virus-associated diffuse large B-cell lymphoma arising on cardiac prostheses. Am J Surg Pathol. 2010 Mar;34(3):377–84. PMID:20139760
1923. Miller DV, Tazelaar HD, Handy JR, et al. Thymoma arising within cardiac myxoma. Am J Surg Pathol. 2005 Sep;29(9):1208–13. PMID:16096411
1924. Miller RR. Bronchioloalveolar cell adenomas. Am J Surg Pathol. 1990 Oct;14(10):904–12. PMID:2403196
1925. Miller RR, Müller NL. Neuroendocrine cell hyperplasia and obliterative bronchiolitis in patients with peripheral carcinoid tumors. Am J Surg Pathol. 1995 Jun;19(6):653–8. PMID:7755151
1926. Milne P, Bigley V, Bacon CM, et al. Hematopoietic origin of Langerhans cell histiocytosis and Erdheim-Chester disease in adults. Blood. 2017 Jul 13;130(2):167–75. PMID:28512190
1927. Min KW. Two different types of carcinoid tumors of the lung: immunohistochemical and ultrastructural investigation and their histogenetic consideration. Ultrastruct Pathol. 2013 Feb;37(1):23–35. PMID:23383615
1928. Minami K, Jimbo N, Tanaka Y, et al. Malignant mesothelioma in situ diagnosed by methylthioadenosine phosphorylase loss and homozygous deletion of CDKN2A: a case report. Virchows Arch. 2020 Mar;476(3):469–73. PMID:31667596
1929. Minami Y, Matsuno Y, Iijima T, et al. Prognostication of small-sized primary pulmonary adenocarcinomas by histopathological and karyometric analysis. Lung Cancer. 2005 Jun;48(3):339–48. PMID:15893002
1930. Minato H, Nojima T, Kurose N, et al. Adenomatoid tumor of the pleura. Pathol Int. 2009 Aug;59(8):567–71. PMID:19627540
1931. Miranda-Filho A, Piñeros M, Bray F. The descriptive epidemiology of lung cancer and tobacco control: a global overview 2018. Salud Publica Mex. 2019 May-Jun;61(3):219–29. PMID:31276337
1932. Mirza I, Kazimi SN, Ligi R, et al. Cytogenetic profile of a thymoma. A case report and review of the literature. Arch Pathol Lab Med. 2000 Nov;124(11):1714–6. PMID:11079034
1933. Mishriki YY, Lane BP, Lozowski MS, et al. Hürthle-cell tumor arising in the mediastinal ectopic thyroid and diagnosed by fine needle aspiration. Light microscopic and ultrastructural features. Acta Cytol. 1983 Mar-Apr;27(2):188–92. PMID:6573091
1934. Mitchell A, Meunier C, Ouellette D, et al. Extranodal marginal zone lymphoma of mucosa-associated lymphoid tissue with initial presentation in the pleura. Chest. 2006 Mar;129(3):791–4. PMID:16537883
1935. Mito K, Kashima K, Daa T, et al. Multiple calcifying fibrous tumors of the pleura. Virchows Arch. 2005 Jan;446(1):78–81. PMID:15660285
1936. Mittal V. Epithelial mesenchymal transition in tumor metastasis. Annu Rev Pathol.

2018 Jan 24;13:395–412. PMID:29414248
1937. Miura K, Hamanaka K, Matsuoka S, et al. Primary mediastinal dedifferentiated liposarcoma: five case reports and a review. Thorac Cancer. 2018 Dec;9(12):1733–40. PMID:30329218
1938. Miura S, Kagamu H, Sakai T, et al. Advanced thymic cancer treated with carboplatin and paclitaxel in a patient undergoing hemodialysis. Intern Med. 2015;54(1):55–8. PMID:25742894
1939. Miwa H, Takakuwa T, Nakatsuka S, et al. DNA sequences of the immunoglobulin heavy chain variable region gene in pyothorax-associated lymphoma. Oncology. 2002;62(3):241–50. PMID:12065872
1939A. Miyagawa-Hayashino A, Tazelaar HD, Langel DJ, et al. Pulmonary sclerosing hemangioma with lymph node metastases: report of 4 cases. Arch Pathol Lab Med. 2003 Mar;127(3):321–5. PMID:12653576
1940. Miyagi J, Tsuhako K, Kinjo T, et al. Rhabdoid tumour of the lung is a dedifferentiated phenotype of pulmonary adenocarcinoma. Histopathology. 2000 Jul;37(1):37–44. PMID:10931217
1941. Miyahara N, Nii K, Benazzo A, et al. Solid predominant subtype in lung adenocarcinoma is related to poor prognosis after surgical resection: a systematic review and meta-analysis. Eur J Surg Oncol. 2019 Jul;45(7):1156–62. PMID:30772108
1942. Miyahara S, Hamasaki M, Hamatake D, et al. Clinicopathological analysis of pleomorphic carcinoma of the lung: diffuse ZEB1 expression predicts poor survival. Lung Cancer. 2015 Jan;87(1):39–44. PMID:25479687
1943. Miyanaga A, Masuda M, Tsuta K, et al. Hippo pathway gene mutations in malignant mesothelioma: revealed by RNA and targeted exon sequencing. J Thorac Oncol. 2015 May;10(5):844–51. PMID:25902174
1944. Miyazaki H, Goto A, Hino R, et al. Pleural cavity angiosarcoma arising in chronic expanding hematoma after pneumonectomy. Hum Pathol. 2011 Oct;42(10):1576–9. PMID:21497371
1945. Miyoshi T, Umemura S, Matsumura Y, et al. Genomic profiling of large-cell neuroendocrine carcinoma of the lung. Clin Cancer Res. 2017 Feb 1;23(3):757–65. PMID:27507618
1946. Mizuuchi H, Suda K, Kitahara H, et al. Solitary pulmonary metastasis from malignant melanoma of the bulbar conjunctiva presenting as a pulmonary ground glass nodule: report of a case. Thorac Cancer. 2015 Jan;6(1):97–100. PMID:26273342
1947. Mneimneh WS, Gökmen-Polar Y, Kesler KA, et al. Micronodular thymic neoplasms: case series and literature review with emphasis on the spectrum of differentiation. Mod Pathol. 2015 Nov;28(11):1415–27. PMID:26360499
1948. Mochizuki T, Ishii G, Nagai K, et al. Pleomorphic carcinoma of the lung: clinicopathologic characteristics of 70 cases. Am J Surg Pathol. 2008 Nov;32(11):1727–35. PMID:18769330
1949. Moding EJ, Diehn M, Wakelee HA. Circulating tumor DNA testing in advanced non-small cell lung cancer. Lung Cancer. 2018 May;119:42–7. PMID:29656751
1950. Modlin IM, Lye KD, Kidd M. A 5-decade analysis of 13,715 carcinoid tumors. Cancer. 2003 Feb 15;97(4):934–59. PMID:12569593
1951. Moeller KH, Rosado-de-Christenson ML, Templeton PA. Mediastinal mature teratoma: imaging features. AJR Am J Roentgenol. 1997 Oct;169(4):985–90. PMID:9308448
1952. Mok TS, Wu YL, Thongprasert S, et al. Gefitinib or carboplatin-paclitaxel in pulmonary adenocarcinoma. N Engl J Med. 2009 Sep 3;361(10):947–57. PMID:19692680
1953. Molajo AO, McWilliam L, Ward C, et al. Cardiac lymphoma: an unusual case of myocardial perforation–clinical, echocardiographic, haemodynamic and pathological features. Eur Heart J. 1987 May;8(5):549–52. PMID:3609049
1954. Molina JR, Aubry MC, Lewis JE, et al. Primary salivary gland-type lung cancer: spectrum of clinical presentation, histopathologic and prognostic factors. Cancer. 2007 Nov 15;110(10):2253–9. PMID:17918258
1955. Molina JR, Yang P, Cassivi SD, et al. Non-small cell lung cancer: epidemiology, risk factors, treatment, and survivorship. Mayo Clin Proc. 2008 May;83(5):584–94. PMID:18452692
1956. Molina-Arcas M, Moore C, Rana S, et al. Development of combination therapies to maximize the impact of KRAS-G12C inhibitors in lung cancer. Sci Transl Med. 2019 Sep 18;11(510):eaaw7999. PMID:31534020
1957. Mollaoglu G, Guthrie MR, Böhm S, et al. MYC Drives progression of small cell lung cancer to a variant neuroendocrine subtype with vulnerability to Aurora kinase inhibition. Cancer Cell. 2017 Feb 13;31(2):270–85. PMID:28089889
1958. Möller P, Lämmler B, Herrmann B, et al. The primary mediastinal clear cell lymphoma of B-cell type has variable defects in MHC antigen expression. Immunology. 1986 Nov;59(3):411–7. PMID:3491784
1959. Möller P, Moldenhauer G, Momburg F, et al. Mediastinal lymphoma of clear cell type is a tumor corresponding to terminal steps of B cell differentiation. Blood. 1987 Apr;69(4):1087–95. PMID:3103712
1960. Momoi A, Nagai K, Isahai N, et al. Thymic extranodal marginal zone lymphoma of mucosa-associated lymphoid tissue with 8q24 abnormality. Intern Med. 2016;55(7):799–803. PMID:27041168
1961. Monaco S, Mehrad M, Dacic S. Recent advances in the diagnosis of malignant mesothelioma: focus on approach in challenging cases and in limited tissue and cytologic samples. Adv Anat Pathol. 2018 Jan;25(1):24–30. PMID:29227332
1962. Monappa V, Valiathan M, Bhat SS, et al. Metastatic immature teratoma: a diagnostic challenge on fine-needle aspiration cytology. Indian J Pathol Microbiol. 2011 Apr-Jun;54(2):402–4. PMID:21623106
1963. Monclair T, Brodeur GM, Ambros PF, et al. The International Neuroblastoma Risk Group (INRG) staging system: an INRG Task Force report. J Clin Oncol. 2009 Jan 10;27(2):298–303. PMID:19047290
1964. Moonen L, Derks J, Dingemans AM, et al. Orthopedia homeobox (OTP) in pulmonary neuroendocrine tumors: the diagnostic value and possible molecular interactions. Cancers (Basel). 2019 Oct 8;11(10):E1508. PMID:31597385
1965. Moore DA, Sereno M, Das M, et al. In situ growth in early lung adenocarcinoma may represent precursor growth or invasive clone outgrowth-a clinically relevant distinction. Mod Pathol. 2019 Jul;32(8):1095–105. PMID:30932019
1966. Moran CA, Hochholzer L, Fishback N, et al. Mucinous (so-called colloid) carcinomas of lung. Mod Pathol. 1992 Nov;5(6):634–8. PMID:1369799
1967. Moran CA, Hochholzer L, Rush W, et al. Primary intrapulmonary meningiomas. A clinicopathologic and immunohistochemical study of ten cases. Cancer. 1996 Dec 1;78(11):2328–33. PMID:8941002
1968. Moran CA, Kalhor N, Suster S. Invasive spindle cell thymomas (WHO type A): a clinicopathologic correlation of 41 cases. Am J Clin Pathol. 2010 Nov;134(5):793–8. PMID:20959663
1969. Moran CA, Rosado-de-Christenson M, Suster S. Thymolipoma: clinicopathologic review of 33 cases. Mod Pathol. 1995 Sep;8(7):741–4. PMID:8539231
1970. Moran CA, Suster S. "Ancient" (sclerosing) thymomas: a clinicopathologic study of 10 cases. Am J Clin Pathol. 2004 Jun;121(6):867–71. PMID:15198359
1971. Moran CA, Suster S. Angiomatoid neuroendocrine carcinoma of the thymus: report of a distinctive morphological variant of neuroendocrine tumor of the thymus resembling a vascular neoplasm. Hum Pathol. 1999 Jun;30(6):635–9. PMID:10374770
1972. Moran CA, Suster S. Hepatoid yolk sac tumors of the mediastinum: a clinicopathologic and immunohistochemical study of four cases. Am J Surg Pathol. 1997 Oct;21(10):1210–4. PMID:9331294
1973. Moran CA, Suster S. Mediastinal hemangiomas: a study of 18 cases with emphasis on the spectrum of morphological features. Hum Pathol. 1995 Apr;26(4):416–21. PMID:7705821
1974. Moran CA, Suster S. Mediastinal seminomas with prominent cystic changes. A clinicopathologic study of 10 cases. Am J Surg Pathol. 1995 Sep;19(9):1047–53. PMID:7661278
1975. Moran CA, Suster S. Mucoepidermoid carcinomas of the thymus. A clinicopathologic study of six cases. Am J Surg Pathol. 1995 Jul;19(7):826–34. PMID:7793481
1976. Moran CA, Suster S. Neuroendocrine carcinomas (carcinoid tumor) of the thymus. A clinicopathologic analysis of 80 cases. Am J Clin Pathol. 2000 Jul;114(1):100–10. PMID:10884805
1977. Moran CA, Suster S. On the histologic heterogeneity of thymic epithelial neoplasms. Impact of sampling in subtyping and classification of thymomas. Am J Clin Pathol. 2000 Nov;114(5):760–6. PMID:11068551
1978. Moran CA, Suster S. Primary germ cell tumors of the mediastinum: I. Analysis of 322 cases with special emphasis on teratomatous lesions and a proposal for histopathologic classification and clinical staging. Cancer. 1997 Aug 15;80(4):681–90. PMID:9264351
1979. Moran CA, Suster S. Primary mediastinal choriocarcinomas: a clinicopathologic and immunohistochemical study of eight cases. Am J Surg Pathol. 1997 Sep;21(9):1007–12. PMID:9298876
1980. Moran CA, Suster S. Primary neuroendocrine carcinoma (thymic carcinoid) of the thymus with prominent oncocytic features: a clinicopathologic study of 22 cases. Mod Pathol. 2000 May;13(5):489–94. PMID:10824919
1981. Moran CA, Suster S. Primary parathyroid tumors of the mediastinum: a clinicopathologic and immunohistochemical study of 17 cases. Am J Clin Pathol. 2005 Nov;124(5):749–54. PMID:16203274
1982. Moran CA, Suster S. Spindle-cell neuroendocrine carcinomas of the thymus (spindle-cell thymic carcinoid): a clinicopathologic and immunohistochemical study of seven cases. Mod Pathol. 1999 Jun;12(6):587–91. PMID:10392634
1983. Moran CA, Suster S. Thymic neuroendocrine carcinomas with combined features ranging from well-differentiated (carcinoid) to small cell carcinoma. A clinicopathologic and immunohistochemical study of 11 cases. Am J Clin Pathol. 2000 Mar;113(3):345–50. PMID:10705813
1984. Moran CA, Suster S. Thymoma with prominent cystic and hemorrhagic changes and areas of necrosis and infarction: a clinicopathologic study of 25 cases. Am J Surg Pathol. 2001 Aug;25(8):1086–90. PMID:11474295
1985. Moran CA, Suster S, Koss MN. Endobronchial lipomas: a clinicopathologic study of four cases. Mod Pathol. 1994 Feb;7(2):212–4. PMID:8008745
1986. Moran CA, Suster S, Koss MN. Primary germ cell tumors of the mediastinum: III. Yolk sac tumor, embryonal carcinoma, choriocarcinoma, and combined nonteratomatous germ cell tumors of the mediastinum–a clinicopathologic and immunohistochemical study of 64 cases. Cancer. 1997 Aug 15;80(4):699–707. PMID:9264353
1987. Moran CA, Suster S, Przygodzki RM, et al. Primary germ cell tumors of the mediastinum: II. Mediastinal seminomas–a clinicopathologic and immunohistochemical study of 120 cases. Cancer. 1997 Aug 15;80(4):691–8. PMID:9264352
1988. Moran CA, Weissferdt A, Kalhor N, et al. Thymomas I: a clinicopathologic correlation of 250 cases with emphasis on the World Health Organization schema. Am J Clin Pathol. 2012 Mar;137(3):444–50. PMID:22338057
1989. Moran CA, Zeren H, Koss MN. Thymofibrolipoma. A histologic variant of thymolipoma. Arch Pathol Lab Med. 1994 Mar;118(3):281–2. PMID:8135632
1990. Mordant P, Grand B, Cazes A, et al. Adenosquamous carcinoma of the lung: surgical management, pathologic characteristics, and prognostic implications. Ann Thorac Surg. 2013 Apr;95(4):1189–95. PMID:23473060
1990A. Moreira AL, Ocampo PSS, Xia Y, et al. A grading system for invasive pulmonary adenocarcinoma: a proposal from the International Association for the Study of Lung Cancer Pathology Committee. J Thorac Oncol. 2020 Oct;15(10):1599–1610. PMID:32562873
1991. Moreira AL, Joubert P, Downey RJ, et al. Cribriform and fused glands are patterns of high-grade pulmonary adenocarcinoma. Hum Pathol. 2014 Feb;45(2):213–20. PMID:24439219
1991A. Moreira LF, Maino MM, Garbin HI, et al. CD117 expression in squamous cell carcinoma of the oesophagus. Anticancer Res. 2018 Jul;38(7):3929–33. PMID:29970514
1992. Morency E, Rodriguez Urrego PA, Szporn AH, et al. The "drunken honeycomb" feature of pulmonary mucinous adenocarcinoma: a diagnostic pitfall of bronchial brushing cytology. Diagn Cytopathol. 2013 Jan;41(1):63–6. PMID:21563323
1993. Mori M, Hanagiri T, Nakanishi R, et al. Primary epithelial-myoepithelial carcinoma of the lung with cavitary lesion: a case report. Mol Clin Oncol. 2018 Sep;9(3):315–7. PMID:30155254
1994. Mori M, Rao SK, Popper HH, et al. Atypical adenomatous hyperplasia of the lung: a probable forerunner in the development of adenocarcinoma of the lung. Mod Pathol. 2001 Feb;14(2):72–84. PMID:11235908
1995. Mori T, Nomori H, Ikeda K, et al. Three cases of multiple thymoma with a review of the literature. Jpn J Clin Oncol. 2007 Feb;37(2):146–9. PMID:17337514
1996. Mori T, Yamada T, Ohba Y, et al. A case of desmoid-type fibromatosis arising after thoracotomy for lung cancer with a review of the english and Japanese literature. Ann Thorac Cardiovasc Surg. 2014;20 Suppl:465–9. PMID:23558226
1997. Moriguchi S, Uruga H, Fujii T, et al. Transformation of epidermal growth factor receptor T790M mutation-positive adenosquamous carcinoma of the lung to small cell carcinoma and large-cell neuroendocrine carcinoma following osimertinib therapy: an autopsy case report. Respirol Case Rep. 2019 Feb 21;7(3):e00402. PMID:30828454
1998. Morikawa H, Tanaka T, Hamaji M, et al. Papillary adenocarcinoma developed in a thymic cyst. Gen Thorac Cardiovasc Surg. 2010 Jun;58(6):295–7. PMID:20549461

1999. Morinaga S, Nomori H, Kobayashi R, et al. Well-differentiated adenocarcinoma arising from mature cystic teratoma of the mediastinum (teratoma with malignant transformation). Report of a surgical case. Am J Clin Pathol. 1994 Apr;101(4):531–4. PMID:8160647
2000. Morita S, Goto A, Sakatani T, et al. Multicystic mesothelioma of the pericardium. Pathol Int. 2011 May;61(5):319–21. PMID:21501299
2001. Morita S, Yoshida A, Goto A, et al. High-grade lung adenocarcinoma with fetal lung-like morphology: clinicopathologic, immunohistochemical, and molecular analyses of 17 cases. Am J Surg Pathol. 2013 Jun;37(6):924–32. PMID:23629442
2002. Moritani S, Ichihara S, Mukai K, et al. Sarcomatoid carcinoma of the thymus arising in metaplastic thymoma. Histopathology. 2008 Feb;52(3):409–11. PMID:18269593
2003. Morley JE, Jacobson RJ, Melamed J, et al. Choriocarcinoma as a cause of thyrotoxicosis. Am J Med. 1976 Jun;60(7):1036–40. PMID:945690
2004. Morodomi Y, Okamoto T, Takenoyama M, et al. Clinical significance of detecting somatic gene mutations in surgically resected adenosquamous cell carcinoma of the lung in Japanese patients. Ann Surg Oncol. 2015 Aug;22(8):2593–8. PMID:25373537
2005. Moro-Sibilot D, Jeanmart M, Lantuejoul S, et al. Cigarette smoking, preinvasive bronchial lesions, and autofluorescence bronchoscopy. Chest. 2002 Dec;122(6):1902–8. PMID:12475824
2006. Morotti RA, Nicol KK, Parham DM, et al. An immunohistochemical algorithm to facilitate diagnosis and subtyping of rhabdomyosarcoma: the Children's Oncology Group experience. Am J Surg Pathol. 2006 Aug;30(8):962–8. PMID:16861966
2007. Morris-Stiff G, Falk GA, El-Hayek K, et al. Jejunal cavernous lymphangioma. BMJ Case Rep. 2011 May 12;2011:bcr0320114022. PMID:22696733
2008. Moser B, Schiefer AI, Janik S, et al. Adenocarcinoma of the thymus, enteric type: report of 2 cases, and proposal for a novel subtype of thymic carcinoma. Am J Surg Pathol. 2015 Apr;39(4):541–8. PMID:25517960
2009. Mosquera JM, Fletcher CD. Expanding the spectrum of malignant progression in solitary fibrous tumors: a study of 8 cases with a discrete anaplastic component–Is this dedifferentiated SFT? Am J Surg Pathol. 2009 Sep;33(9):1314–21. PMID:19718788
2010. Mosquera JM, Sboner A, Zhang L, et al. Recurrent NCOA2 gene rearrangements in congenital/infantile spindle cell rhabdomyosarcoma. Genes Chromosomes Cancer. 2013 Jun;52(6):538–50. PMID:23463663
2011. Mossé YP. Anaplastic lymphoma kinase as a cancer target in pediatric malignancies. Clin Cancer Res. 2016 Feb 1;22(3):546–52. PMID:26503946
2012. Motoi N, Szoke J, Riely GJ, et al. Lung adenocarcinoma: modification of the 2004 WHO mixed subtype to include the major histologic subtype suggests correlations between papillary and micropapillary adenocarcinoma subtypes, EGFR mutations and gene expression analysis. Am J Surg Pathol. 2008 Jun;32(6):810–27. PMID:18391747
2013. Motta G, Conticello C, Amato G, et al. Pleuric presentation of extranodal marginal zone lymphoma of mucosa-associated lymphoid tissue: a case report and a review of the literature. Int J Hematol. 2010 Sep;92(2):369–73. PMID:20725816
2014. Mottok A, Hung SS, Chavez EA, et al. Integrative genomic analysis identifies key pathogenic mechanisms in primary mediastinal large B-cell lymphoma. Blood. 2019 Sep 5;134(10):802–13. PMID:31292115
2015. Mottok A, Woolcock B, Chan FC, et al. Genomic alterations in CIITA are frequent in primary mediastinal large B cell lymphoma and are associated with diminished MHC class II expression. Cell Rep. 2015 Nov 17;13(7):1418–31. PMID:26549456
2016. Mottok A, Wright G, Rosenwald A, et al. Molecular classification of primary mediastinal large B-cell lymphoma using routinely available tissue specimens. Blood. 2018 Nov 29;132(22):2401–5. PMID:30257882
2017. Motzer RJ, Amsterdam A, Prieto V, et al. Teratoma with malignant transformation: diverse malignant histologies arising in men with germ cell tumors. J Urol. 1998 Jan;159(1):133–8. PMID:9400455
2018. Mousavi N, Cheezum MK, Aghayev A, et al. Assessment of cardiac masses by cardiac magnetic resonance imaging: histological correlation and clinical outcomes. J Am Heart Assoc. 2019 Jan 8;8(1):e007829. PMID:30616453
2019. Movahedi N, Boroumand MA, Sotoudeh Anvari M, et al. Mature cardiac myocyte hamartoma in the right atrium. Asian Cardiovasc Thorac Ann. 2008 Oct;16(5):e47–8. PMID:18812338
2020. Mukherjee S, Ibrahimi S, John S, et al. Non-seminomatous mediastinal germ cell tumor and acute megakaryoblastic leukemia. Ann Hematol. 2017 Sep;96(9):1435–9. PMID:28578457
2021. Mukherjee S, Ibrahimi S, Scordino T, et al. Granulocytic sarcoma and mediastinal germ cell tumor: a common cell of origin? Hematol Oncol Stem Cell Ther. 2019 Dec;12(4):228–9. PMID:29913128
2022. Mukhopadhyay S, Dermawan JK, Lanigan CP, et al. Insulinoma-associated protein 1 (INSM1) is a sensitive and highly specific marker of neuroendocrine differentiation in primary lung neoplasms: an immunohistochemical study of 345 cases, including 292 whole-tissue sections. Mod Pathol. 2019 Jan;32(1):100–9. PMID:30154579
2022A. Mukhopadhyay S, Katzenstein AL. Subclassification of non-small cell lung carcinomas lacking morphologic differentiation on biopsy specimens: utility of an immunohistochemical panel containing TTF-1, napsin A, p63, and CK5/6. Am J Surg Pathol. 2011 Jan;35(1):15–25. PMID:21164283
2023. Muller S, Victoria Lai W, Adusumilli PS, et al. V-domain Ig-containing suppressor of T-cell activation (VISTA), a potentially targetable immune checkpoint molecule, is highly expressed in epithelioid malignant pleural mesothelioma. Mod Pathol. 2020 Feb;33(2):303–11. PMID:31537897
2024. Müller-Hermelink HK, Marx A. Pathological aspects of malignant and benign thymic disorders. Ann Med. 1999 Oct;31 Suppl 2:5–14. PMID:10574149
2025. Mulliken JB, Marler JJ, Burrows PE, et al. Reticular infantile hemangioma of the limb can be associated with ventral-caudal anomalies, refractory ulceration, and cardiac overload. Pediatr Dermatol. 2007 Jul-Aug;24(4):356–62. PMID:17845155
2026. Multani A, Gomez CA, Montoya JG. Prevention of infectious diseases in patients with Good syndrome. Curr Opin Infect Dis. 2018 Aug;31(4):267–77. PMID:29878906
2027. Munin MA, Goerner MS, Raggio I, et al. A rare cause of dyspnea: undifferentiated pleomorphic sarcoma in the left atrium. Cardiol Res. 2017 Oct;8(5):241–5. PMID:29118888
2028. Munker R, Hasenclever D, Brosteanu O, et al. Bone marrow involvement in Hodgkin's disease: an analysis of 135 consecutive cases. J Clin Oncol. 1995 Feb;13(2):403–9. PMID:7844601
2029. Murakawa Y, Satake N, Kato S, et al. Alpha-FP normalization as a prognostic factor for mediastinal origin embryonal carcinoma: report of five cases. Intern Med. 2002 Oct;41(10):883–8. PMID:12413016
2030. Murali R, Doubrovsky A, Watson GF, et al. Diagnosis of metastatic melanoma by fine-needle biopsy: analysis of 2,204 cases. Am J Clin Pathol. 2007 Mar;127(3):385–97. PMID:17276948
2031. Muraoka M, Oka T, Akamine S, et al. Endobronchial lipoma: review of 64 cases reported in Japan. Chest. 2003 Jan;123(1):293–6. PMID:12527636
2032. Murase T, Yamaguchi M, Suzuki R, et al. Intravascular large B-cell lymphoma (IVL-BCL): a clinicopathologic study of 96 cases with special reference to the immunophenotypic heterogeneity of CD5. Blood. 2007 Jan 15;109(2):478–85. PMID:16985183
2033. Murphy MC, Sweeney MS, Putnam JB Jr, et al. Surgical treatment of cardiac tumors: a 25-year experience. Ann Thorac Surg. 1990 Apr;49(4):612–7, discussion 617–8. PMID:2322057
2034. Murphy SB. Classification, staging and end results of treatment of childhood non-Hodgkin's lymphomas: dissimilarities from lymphomas in adults. Semin Oncol. 1980 Sep;7(3):332–9. PMID:7414342
2035. Murphy SJ, Aubry MC, Harris FR, et al. Identification of independent primary tumors and intrapulmonary metastases using DNA rearrangements in non-small-cell lung cancer. J Clin Oncol. 2014 Dec 20;32(36):4050–8. PMID:25385739
2036. Murphy SJ, Harris FR, Kosari F, et al. Using genomics to differentiate multiple primaries from metastatic lung cancer. J Thorac Oncol. 2019 Sep;14(9):1567–82. PMID:31103780
2037. Murray PG, Young LS. An etiological role for the Epstein-Barr virus in the pathogenesis of classical Hodgkin lymphoma. Blood. 2019 Aug 15;134(7):591–6. PMID:31186275
2038. Mushtaque M, Naqash SH, Malik AA, et al. Papillary carcinoma thyroid with metastasis to ectopic cervical thymus. World J Surg Oncol. 2011 Feb 18;9:22. PMID:21332990
2039. Musk ABW, de Klerk N, Brims FJ. Mesothelioma in Australia: a review. Med J Aust. 2017 Nov 20;207(10):449–52. PMID:29129162
2040. Myhre-Jensen O. A consecutive 7-year series of 1331 benign soft tissue tumours. Clinicopathologic data. Comparison with sarcomas. Acta Orthop Scand. 1981 Jun;52(3):287–93. PMID:7282321
2041. Myint ZW, McCormick J, Chauhan A, et al. Management of diffuse idiopathic pulmonary neuroendocrine cell hyperplasia: review and a single center experience. Lung. 2018 Oct;196(5):577–81. PMID:30167840
2042. Naeini YB, Arcega R, Hirschowitz S, et al. Post-irradiation pericardial malignant mesothelioma with deletion of p16: a case report. Cancer Biol Med. 2018 Feb;15(1):97–102. PMID:29545973
2043. Nagata K, Irie K, Morimatsu M, et al. Rhabdomyosarcoma of the right ventricle. Acta Pathol Jpn. 1982 Sep;32(5):843–9. PMID:7136697
2044. Nagayoshi Y, Yamamoto K, Hashimoto S, et al. An autopsy case of lepidic pulmonary metastasis from cholangiocarcinoma. Intern Med. 2016;55(19):2849–53. PMID:27725547
2044A. Nagi DK, Jones WG, Belchetz PE. Gynaecomastia caused by a primary mediastinal seminoma. Clin Endocrinol (Oxf). 1994 Apr;40(4):545–8; discussion 548–9. PMID:7514514
2045. Naidoo J, Santos-Zabala ML, Iyriboz T, et al. Large cell neuroendocrine carcinoma of the lung: clinico-pathologic features, treatment, and outcomes. Clin Lung Cancer. 2016 Sep;17(5):e121–9. PMID:26898325
2046. Naito M, Tamiya A, Takeda M, et al. A high PD-L1 expression in pulmonary pleomorphic carcinoma correlates with parietal-pleural invasion and might predict a poor prognosis. Intern Med. 2019 Apr 1;58(7):921–7. PMID:30568128
2047. Naka N, Tomita Y, Nakanishi H, et al. Mutations of p53 tumor-suppressor gene in angiosarcoma. Int J Cancer. 1997 Jun 11;71(6):952–5. PMID:9185695
2048. Nakagawa K, Matsuno Y, Kunitoh H, et al. Immunohistochemical KIT (CD117) expression in thymic epithelial tumors. Chest. 2005 Jul;128(1):140–4. PMID:16002927
2049. Nakagawa M, Hara M, Shibamoto Y, et al. CT findings of bronchial glandular papilloma. J Thorac Imaging. 2008 Aug;23(3):210–2. PMID:18728552
2050. Nakajima N, Yoshizawa A, Nakajima T, et al. GATA6-positive lung adenocarcinomas are associated with invasive mucinous adenocarcinoma morphology, hepatocyte nuclear factor 4α expression, and KRAS mutations. Histopathology. 2018 Jul;73(1):38–48. PMID:29469192
2051. Nakajima Y, Waku M, Kojima A, et al. [Prognosis of the surgical treatment for non-Hodgkin lymphoma originating from chronic tuberculous empyema–analysis of 11 cases with pleuropneumonectomy]. Nihon Kyobu Geka Gakkai Zasshi. 1996 Apr;44(4):484–92. Japanese. PMID:8666866
2052. Nakamura H, Tsuta K, Nakagawa T, et al. Human herpes virus 8-unrelated primary effusion lymphoma-like lymphoma in the pericardium: a case with latency type III Epstein-Barr virus infection showing good prognosis without chemotherapy. Pathol Res Pract. 2015 Dec;211(12):1010–3. PMID:26384578
2053. Nakamura H, Tsuta K, Tsuda H, et al. NUT midline carcinoma of the mediastinum showing two types of poorly differentiated tumor cells: a case report and a literature review. Pathol Res Pract. 2015 Jan;211(1):92–8. PMID:25433996
2054. Nakamura S, Fukui T, Taniguchi T, et al. Prognostic impact of tumor size eliminating the ground glass opacity component: modified clinical T descriptors of the tumor, node, metastasis classification of lung cancer. J Thorac Oncol. 2013 Dec;8(12):1551–7. PMID:24389437
2055. Nakamura S, Tateyama H, Taniguchi T, et al. Multilocular thymic cyst associated with thymoma: a clinicopathologic study of 20 cases with an emphasis on the pathogenesis of cyst formation. Am J Surg Pathol. 2012 Dec;36(12):1857–64. PMID:23026930
2056. Nakanishi K. Alveolar epithelial hyperplasia and adenocarcinoma of the lung. Arch Pathol Lab Med. 1990 Apr;114(4):363–8. PMID:2322096
2057. Nakanishi K, Kawai T, Kumaki F, et al. Expression of human telomerase RNA component and telomerase reverse transcriptase mRNA in atypical adenomatous hyperplasia of the lung. Hum Pathol. 2002 Jul;33(7):697–702. PMID:12196920
2058. Nakanishi K, Sakakura N, Matsui T, et al. Clinicopathological features, surgical outcomes, oncogenic status and PD-L1 expression of pulmonary pleomorphic carcinoma. Anticancer Res. 2019 Oct;39(10):5789–95. PMID:31570483
2059. Nakaoku T, Tsuta K, Ichikawa H, et al. Druggable oncogene fusions in invasive mucinous lung adenocarcinoma. Clin Cancer Res. 2014 Jun 15;20(12):3087–93. PMID:24727320
2060. Nakas A, Martin-Ucar AE, Edwards JG, et al. Localised malignant pleural mesothelioma: a separate clinical entity requiring aggressive local surgery. Eur J Cardiothorac Surg. 2008

Feb;33(2):303–6. PMID:18155556
2061. Nakashima Y, Morita R, Ui A, et al. Epithelial-myoepithelial carcinoma of the lung: a case report. Surg Case Rep. 2018 Jul 9;4(1):74. PMID:29987577
2062. Nakatani Y, Dickersin GR, Mark EJ. Pulmonary endodermal tumor resembling fetal lung: a clinicopathologic study of five cases with immunohistochemical and ultrastructural characterization. Hum Pathol. 1990 Nov;21(11):1097–107. PMID:2172150
2063. Nakatani Y, Kitamura H, Inayama Y, et al. Pulmonary adenocarcinomas of the fetal lung type: a clinicopathologic study indicating differences in histology, epidemiology, and natural history of low-grade and high-grade forms. Am J Surg Pathol. 1998 Apr;22(4):399–411. PMID:9537466
2064. Nakatani Y, Masudo K, Miyagi Y, et al. Aberrant nuclear localization and gene mutation of beta-catenin in low-grade adenocarcinoma of fetal lung type: up-regulation of the Wnt signaling pathway may be a common denominator for the development of tumors that form morules. Mod Pathol. 2002 Jun;15(6):617–24. PMID:12065775
2065. Nakatani Y, Miyagi Y, Takemura T, et al. Aberrant nuclear/cytoplasmic localization and gene mutation of beta-catenin in classic pulmonary blastoma: beta-catenin immunostaining is useful for distinguishing between classic pulmonary blastoma and a blastomatoid variant of carcinosarcoma. Am J Surg Pathol. 2004 Jul;28(7):921–7. PMID:15223963
2066. Nakatsuka S, Yao M, Hoshida Y, et al. Pyothorax-associated lymphoma: a review of 106 cases. J Clin Oncol. 2002 Oct 15;20(20):4255–60. PMID:12377970
2067. Nakayama H, Noguchi M, Tsuchiya R, et al. Clonal growth of atypical adenomatous hyperplasia of the lung: cytofluorometric analysis of nuclear DNA content. Mod Pathol. 1990 May;3(3):314–20. PMID:2362938
2068. Nakayama T, Ohtsuka T, Kazama A, et al. Classic pulmonary blastoma: a subtype of biphasic pulmonary blastoma. Ann Thorac Cardiovasc Surg. 2012;18(2):125–7. PMID:22001215
2069. Nam JE, Ryu YH, Cho SH, et al. Air-trapping zone surrounding sclerosing hemangioma of the lung. J Comput Assist Tomogr. 2002 May-Jun;26(3):358–61. PMID:12016362
2070. Nambirajan A, Parshad R, Goyal A, et al. Innocuous clinical presentation of a SMARCA4-deficient thoracic sarcoma arising in a patient with chronic empyema thoracis. Pathology. 2019 Oct;51(6):657–9. PMID:31470991
2071. Nambirajan A, Singh V, Bhardwaj N, et al. SMARCA4/BRG1-deficient non-small cell lung carcinomas: a case series and review of the literature. Arch Pathol Lab Med. 2020 Apr 9 [Epub ahead of print]. PMID:32271611
2072. Napieralska A, Majewski W, Osewski W, et al. Primary mediastinal seminoma. J Thorac Dis. 2018 Jul;10(7):4335–41. PMID:30174881
2073. Napolitano A, Antoine DJ, Pellegrini L, et al. HMGB1 and its hyperacetylated isoform are sensitive and specific serum biomarkers to detect asbestos exposure and to identify mesothelioma patients. Clin Cancer Res. 2016 Jun 15;22(12):3087–96. PMID:26733616
2074. Naranjo A, Irwin MS, Hogarty MD, et al. Statistical framework in support of a revised Children's Oncology Group neuroblastoma risk classification system. JCO Clin Cancer Inform. 2018 Dec;2:1–15. PMID:30652588
2075. Narimatsu H, Ota Y, Kami M, et al. Clinicopathological features of pyothorax-associated lymphoma; a retrospective survey involving 98 patients. Ann Oncol. 2007 Jan;18(1):122–8. PMID:17043091
2076. Nascimento AF, Bertoni F, Fletcher CD. Epithelioid variant of myxofibrosarcoma: expanding the clinicomorphologic spectrum of myxofibrosarcoma in a series of 17 cases. Am J Surg Pathol. 2007 Jan;31(1):99–105. PMID:17197925
2077. Nascimento AF, Fletcher CD. The controversial nosology of benign nerve sheath tumors: neurofilament protein staining demonstrates intratumoral axons in many sporadic schwannomas. Am J Surg Pathol. 2007 Sep;31(9):1363–70. PMID:17721192
2078. Nassar AA, Jaroszewski DE, Helmers RA, et al. Diffuse idiopathic pulmonary neuroendocrine cell hyperplasia: a systematic overview. Am J Respir Crit Care Med. 2011 Jul 1;184(1):8–16. PMID:21471097
2079. Nassr AA, Shazly SA, Morris SA, et al. Prenatal management of fetal intrapericardial teratoma: a systematic review. Prenat Diagn. 2017 Sep;37(9):849–63. PMID:28695637
2080. Nathaniels EK, Nathaniels AM, Wang CA. Mediastinal parathyroid tumors: a clinical and pathological study of 84 cases. Ann Surg. 1970 Feb;171(2):165–70. PMID:5413453
2081. Church TR, Black WC, Aberle DR, et al. Results of initial low-dose computed tomographic screening for lung cancer. N Engl J Med. 2013 May 23;368(21):1980–91. PMID:23697514
2082. Neiman RS, Orazi A. Mediastinal non-seminomatous germ cell tumours: their association with non-germ cell malignancies. Pathol Res Pract. 1999;195(8):589–94. PMID:10483591
2083. Nelson BA, Lee EY, French CA, et al. BRD4-NUT carcinoma of the mediastinum in a pediatric patient: multidetector computed tomography imaging findings. J Thorac Imaging. 2010 Aug;25(3):W93-6. PMID:20395873
2084. Nelson ER, Sharma R, Argani P, et al. Utility of Sox10 labeling in metastatic breast carcinomas. Hum Pathol. 2017 Sep;67:205–10. PMID:28843711
2085. Neri M, Di Donato S, Maglietta R, et al. Sudden death as presenting symptom caused by cardiac primary multicentric left ventricle rhabdomyoma, in an 11-month-old baby. An immunohistochemical study. Diagn Pathol. 2012 Dec 3;7:169. PMID:23206573
2086. Neri N, Jesús Nambo M, Avilés A. Diffuse large B-cell lymphoma primary of lung. Hematology. 2011 Mar;16(2):110–2. PMID:21418743
2087. Neumann HP, Bausch B, McWhinney SR, et al. Germ-line mutations in nonsyndromic pheochromocytoma. N Engl J Med. 2002 May 9;346(19):1459–66. PMID:12000816
2088. Neuville A, Chibon F, Coindre JM. Grading of soft tissue sarcomas: from histological to molecular assessment. Pathology. 2014 Feb;46(2):113–20. PMID:24378389
2089. Neuville A, Collin F, Bruneval P, et al. Intimal sarcoma is the most frequent primary cardiac sarcoma: clinicopathologic and molecular retrospective analysis of 100 primary cardiac sarcomas. Am J Surg Pathol. 2014 Apr;38(4):461–9. PMID:24625414
2090. Newman E, Shaha AR. Substernal goiter. J Surg Oncol. 1995 Nov;60(3):207–12. PMID:7475073
2091. Ngaage DL, Mullany CJ, Daly RC, et al. Surgical treatment of cardiac papillary fibroelastoma: a single center experience with eighty-eight patients. Ann Thorac Surg. 2005 Nov;80(5):1712–8. PMID:16242444
2092. Nguyen TH, Barr FG. Therapeutic approaches targeting PAX3-FOXO1 and its regulatory and transcriptional pathways in rhabdomyosarcoma. Molecules. 2018 Oct 28;23(11):E2798. PMID:30373318
2093. Nichols CR, Heerema NA, Palmer C, et al. Klinefelter's syndrome associated with mediastinal germ cell neoplasms. J Clin Oncol. 1987 Aug;5(8):1290–4. PMID:3040921
2094. Nichols CR, Hoffman R, Einhorn LH, et al. Hematologic malignancies associated with primary mediastinal germ-cell tumors. Ann Intern Med. 1985 May;102(5):603–9. PMID:2984971
2095. Nichols CR, Hoffman R, Glant MD, et al. Malignant disorders of megakaryocytes associated with primary mediastinal germ cell tumors. Prog Clin Biol Res. 1986;215:347–53. PMID:3014553
2096. Nichols CR, Roth BJ, Heerema N, et al. Hematologic neoplasia associated with primary mediastinal germ-cell tumors. N Engl J Med. 1990 May 17;322(20):1425–9. PMID:2158625
2097. Nichols KE, Malkin D, Garber JE, et al. Germ-line p53 mutations predispose to a wide spectrum of early-onset cancers. Cancer Epidemiol Biomarkers Prev. 2001 Feb;10(2):83–7. PMID:11219776
2098. Nicholson AG, Baandrup U, Florio R, et al. Malignant myxoid endobronchial tumour: a report of two cases with a unique histological pattern. Histopathology. 1999 Oct;35(4):313–8. PMID:10564385
2099. Nicholson AG, Chansky K, Crowley J, et al. The International Association for the Study of Lung Cancer Lung Cancer Staging Project: proposals for the revision of the clinical and pathologic staging of small cell lung cancer in the forthcoming eighth edition of the TNM classification for lung cancer. J Thorac Oncol. 2016 Mar;11(3):300–11. PMID:26723244
2100. Nicholson AG, Detterbeck FC, Marino M, et al. The IASLC/ITMIG Thymic Epithelial Tumors Staging Project: proposals for the T component for the forthcoming (8th) edition of the TNM classification of malignant tumors. J Thorac Oncol. 2014 Sep;9(9 Suppl 2):S73–80. PMID:25396315
2101. Nicholson AG, Magkou C, Snead D, et al. Unusual sclerosing haemangiomas and sclerosing haemangioma-like lesions, and the value of TTF-1 in making the diagnosis. Histopathology. 2002 Nov;41(5):404–13. PMID:12405908
2102. Nicholson AG, Perry LJ, Cury PM, et al. Reproducibility of the WHO/IASLC grading system for pre-invasive squamous lesions of the bronchus: a study of inter-observer and intra-observer variation. Histopathology. 2001 Mar;38(3):202–8. PMID:11260299
2103. Nicholson AG, Sauter JL, Nowak AK, et al. EURACAN/IASLC proposals for updating the histologic classification of pleural mesothelioma: towards a more multidisciplinary approach. J Thorac Oncol. 2020 Jan;15(1):29–49. PMID:31546041
2104. Nicholson AG, Torkko K, Viola P, et al. Interobserver variation among pathologists and refinement of criteria in distinguishing separate primary tumors from intrapulmonary metastases in lung. J Thorac Oncol. 2018 Feb;13(2):205–17. PMID:29127023
2105. Nicholson AG, Tsao MS, Travis WD, et al. Eighth edition staging of thoracic malignancies: implications for the reporting pathologist. Arch Pathol Lab Med. 2018 May;142(5):645–61. PMID:29480761
2106. Nicholson AG, Wotherspoon AC, Diss TC, et al. Pulmonary B-cell non-Hodgkin's lymphomas. The value of immunohistochemistry and gene analysis in diagnosis. Histopathology. 1995 May;26(5):395–403. PMID:7544760
2107. Nicholson AG, Wotherspoon AC, Jones AL, et al. Pulmonary B-cell non-Hodgkin's lymphoma associated with autoimmune disorders: a clinicopathological review of six cases. Eur Respir J. 1996 Oct;9(10):2022–5. PMID:8902461
2108. Nicholson SA, Beasley MB, Brambilla E, et al. Small cell lung carcinoma (SCLC): a clinicopathologic study of 100 cases with surgical specimens. Am J Surg Pathol. 2002 Sep;26(9):1184–97. PMID:12218575
2109. Nicol KK, Geisinger KR. The cytomorphology of pleuropulmonary blastoma. Arch Pathol Lab Med. 2000 Mar;124(3):416–8. PMID:10705397
2110. Nicolae A, Pittaluga S, Abdullah S, et al. EBV-positive large B-cell lymphomas in young patients: a nodal lymphoma with evidence for a tolerogenic immune environment. Blood. 2015 Aug 13;126(7):863–72. PMID:25999451
2111. Nicolini A, Perazzo A, Lanata S. Desmoplastic malignant mesothelioma of the pericardium: description of a case and review of the literature. Lung India. 2011 Jul;28(3):219–21. PMID:21886962
2112. Niederkohr RD, Cameron MJ, French CA. FDG PET/CT imaging of NUT midline carcinoma. Clin Nucl Med. 2011 Sep;36(9):e124–6. PMID:21825839
2113. Niehues T, Harms D, Jürgens H, et al. Treatment of pediatric malignant thymoma: long-term remission in a 14-year-old boy with EBV-associated thymic carcinoma by aggressive, combined modality treatment. Med Pediatr Oncol. 1996 Jun;26(6):419–24. PMID:8614381
2114. Nield LE, Mendelson M, Ahmad N, et al. Clinical review of obstructive primary cardiac tumors in childhood. Congenit Heart Dis. 2014 May-Jun;9(3):244–51. PMID:23962026
2115. Nikanne E, Sopanen J, Seppä A. Inflammatory pseudotumor of the trachea. Otolaryngol Head Neck Surg. 2004 Feb;130(2):274–6. PMID:14990929
2116. Nishikawa H, Wu W, Koike A, et al. BRCA1-associated protein 1 interferes with BRCA1/BARD1 RING heterodimer activity. Cancer Res. 2009 Jan 1;69(1):111–9. PMID:19117993
2117. Nishimura M, Kodama T, Nishiyama H, et al. A case of sarcomatoid carcinoma of the thymus. Pathol Int. 1997 Apr;47(4):260–3. PMID:9103218
2118. Nishioka Y, Tane S, Nishio W, et al. A rare resected case of pulmonary rhabdomyosarcoma. Gen Thorac Cardiovasc Surg. 2019 Dec;67(12):1089–92. PMID:30806970
2119. Nishiu M, Tomita Y, Nakatsuka S, et al. Distinct pattern of gene expression in pyothorax-associated lymphoma (PAL), a lymphoma developing in long-standing inflammation. Cancer Sci. 2004 Oct;95(10):828–34. PMID:15504251
2120. Nitadori J, Bograd AJ, Kadota K, et al. Impact of micropapillary histologic subtype in selecting limited resection vs lobectomy for lung adenocarcinoma of 2cm or smaller. J Natl Cancer Inst. 2013 Aug 21;105(16):1212–20. PMID:23926067
2121. Njauw CN, Kim I, Piris A, et al. Germline BAP1 inactivation is preferentially associated with metastatic ocular melanoma and cutaneous-ocular melanoma families. PLoS One. 2012;7(4):e35295. PMID:22545102
2122. Noda T, Higashiyama M, Oda K, et al. Mucoepidermoid carcinoma of the thymus treated by multimodality therapy: a case report. Ann Thorac Cardiovasc Surg. 2006 Aug;12(4):273–8. PMID:16977299
2123. Nogales FF, Jimenez RE, editors. Pathology and biology of human germ cell tumors. Berlin (Germany): Springer; 2017.
2124. Nogales FF, Quiñonez E, López-Marín L, et al. A diagnostic immunohistochemical panel for yolk sac (primitive endodermal) tumours based on an immunohistochemical comparison with the human yolk sac. Histopathology. 2014 Jul;65(1):51–9. PMID:24444105
2125. Noguchi M, Kodama T, Shimosato Y, et al. Papillary adenoma of type 2 pneumocytes. Am J Surg Pathol. 1986 Feb;10(2):134–9. PMID:3006525

2126. Noguchi M, Morikawa A, Kawasaki M, et al. Small adenocarcinoma of the lung. Histologic characteristics and prognosis. Cancer. 1995 Jun 15;75(12):2844–52. PMID:7773933

2127. Noh TW, Kim SH, Lim BJ, et al. Thymoma with pseudosarcomatous stroma. Yonsei Med J. 2001 Oct;42(5):571–5. PMID:11675689

2128. Nolte DA, Larsen BT, Sobonya RE, et al. Recurrent intracardiac juvenile xanthogranuloma in an adult. Ann Thorac Surg. 2019 Apr;107(4):e285. PMID:30447189

2129. Noma D, Morohoshi T, Adachi H, et al. A resected case of combined small cell lung carcinoma with carcinosarcoma. Pathol Int. 2015 Jun;65(6):332–4. PMID:25721926

2130. Nonaka D. Differential expression of SOX2 and SOX17 in testicular germ cell tumors. Am J Clin Pathol. 2009 May;131(5):731–6. PMID:19369635

2131. Nonaka D, Chiriboga L, Rubin BP. Sox10: a pan-schwannian and melanocytic marker. Am J Surg Pathol. 2008 Sep;32(9):1291–8. PMID:18636017

2132. Nonaka D, Henley JD, Chiriboga L, et al. Diagnostic utility of thymic epithelial markers CD205 (DEC205) and Foxn1 in thymic epithelial neoplasms. Am J Surg Pathol. 2007 Jul;31(7):1038–44. PMID:17592270

2133. Nonaka D, Klimstra D, Rosai J. Thymic mucoepidermoid carcinomas: a clinicopathologic study of 10 cases and review of the literature. Am J Surg Pathol. 2004 Nov;28(11):1526–31. PMID:15489658

2134. Nonaka D, Papaxoinis G, Mansoor W. Diagnostic utility of orthopedia homeobox (OTP) in pulmonary carcinoid tumors. Am J Surg Pathol. 2016 Jun;40(6):738–44. PMID:26927888

2135. Nonaka D, Rodriguez J, Rollo JL, et al. Undifferentiated large cell carcinoma of the thymus associated with Castleman disease-like reaction: a distinctive type of thymic neoplasm characterized by an indolent behavior. Am J Surg Pathol. 2005 Apr;29(4):490–5. PMID:15767803

2136. Nonaka D, Rosai J. Is there a spectrum of cytologic atypia in type A thymomas analogous to that seen in type B thymomas? A pilot study of 13 cases. Am J Surg Pathol. 2012 Jun;36(6):889–94. PMID:22472953

2137. Nonami Y, Moriki T. Synchronous independent bifocal orthotopic thymomas. A case report. J Cardiovasc Surg (Torino). 2004 Dec;45(6):585–7. PMID:15746641

2138. Nonomura A, Kurumaya H, Kono N, et al. Primary pulmonary artery sarcoma. Report of two autopsy cases studied by immunohistochemistry and electron microscopy, and review of 110 cases reported in the literature. Acta Pathol Jpn. 1988 Jul;38(7):883–96. PMID:3055809

2139. Noone AM, Cronin KA, Altekruse SF, et al. Cancer incidence and survival trends by subtype using data from the Surveillance Epidemiology and End Results Program, 1992-2013. Cancer Epidemiol Biomarkers Prev. 2017 Apr;26(4):632–41. PMID:27956436

2140. Nora JD, Hallett JW Jr, O'Brien PC, et al. Surgical resection of carotid body tumors: long-term survival, recurrence, and metastasis. Mayo Clin Proc. 1988 Apr;63(4):348–52. PMID:3352318

2140A. North JP, McCalmont TH, Fehr A, et al. Detection of MYB alterations and other immunohistochemical markers in primary cutaneous adenoid cystic carcinoma. Am J Surg Pathol. 2015 Oct;39(10):1347–56. PMID:26076064

2141. Nosotti M, Mendogni P, Rosso L, et al. Alveolar adenoma of the lung: unusual diagnosis of a lesion positive on PET scan. A case report. J Cardiothorac Surg. 2012 Jan 3;7:1. PMID:22214375

2142. Nottegar A, Tabbò F, Luchini C, et al. Pulmonary adenocarcinoma with enteric differentiation: dissecting oncogenic genes alterations with DNA sequencing and FISH analysis. Exp Mol Pathol. 2017 Apr;102(2):276–9. PMID:28237660

2143. Nottegar A, Tabbò F, Luchini C, et al. Pulmonary adenocarcinoma with enteric differentiation: immunohistochemistry and molecular morphology. Appl Immunohistochem Mol Morphol. 2018 Jul;26(6):383–7. PMID:27753661

2144. Noujaim J, Thway K, Jones RL, et al. Adult pleomorphic rhabdomyosarcoma: a multicentre retrospective study. Anticancer Res. 2015 Nov;35(11):6213–7. PMID:26504053

2145. Nowak AK, Chansky K, Rice DC, et al. The IASLC Mesothelioma Staging Project: proposals for revisions of the T descriptors in the forthcoming eighth edition of the TNM classification for pleural mesothelioma. J Thorac Oncol. 2016 Dec;11(12):2089–99. PMID:27687963

2146. Nusse R, Clevers H. Wnt/β-catenin signaling, disease, and emerging therapeutic modalities. Cell. 2017 Jun 1;169(6):985–99. PMID:28575679

2146A. O'Brien TD, Jia P, Aldrich MC, et al. Lung cancer: one disease or many. Hum Hered. 2018;83(2):65–70. PMID:29864749

2147. Ocal N, Yildiz B, Karadurmus N, et al. Comparison of the clinical features and hematopoietic stem cell transplantation outcomes of mediastinal malignant germ cell tumors with nonmediastinal extragonadal placements. Onco Targets Ther. 2016 Dec 9;9:7445–50. PMID:28003760

2148. O'Connor S, Recavarren R, Nichols LC, et al. Lipomatous hypertrophy of the interatrial septum: an overview. Arch Pathol Lab Med. 2006 Mar;130(3):397–9. PMID:16519573

2149. Odim J, Reehal V, Laks H, et al. Surgical pathology of cardiac tumors. Two decades at an urban institution. Cardiovasc Pathol. 2003 Sep-Oct;12(5):267–70. PMID:14507576

2150. Oechsle K, Bokemeyer C, Kollmannsberger C, et al. Bone metastases in germ cell tumor patients. J Cancer Res Clin Oncol. 2012 Jun;138(6):947–52. PMID:22350540

2151. Ogawa F, Amano H, Iyoda A, et al. Thymic neuroblastoma with the syndrome of inappropriate secretion of antidiuretic hormone. Interact Cardiovasc Thorac Surg. 2009 Nov;9(5):903–5. PMID:19661118

2152. Ogawa K, Toita T, Uno T, et al. Treatment and prognosis of thymic carcinoma: a retrospective analysis of 40 cases. Cancer. 2002 Jun 15;94(12):3115–9. PMID:12115342

2153. Ognjanovic S, Olivier M, Bergemann TL, et al. Sarcomas in TP53 germline mutation carriers: a review of the IARC TP53 Database. Cancer. 2012 Mar 1;118(5):1387–96. PMID:21837677

2154. Ogura K, Hosoda F, Arai Y, et al. Integrated genetic and epigenetic analysis of myxofibrosarcoma. Nat Commun. 2018 Jul 17;9(1):2765. PMID:30018380

2155. Oh JE, Ohta T, Satomi K, et al. Alterations in the NF2/LATS1/LATS2/YAP pathway in schwannomas. J Neuropathol Exp Neurol. 2015 Oct;74(10):952–9. PMID:26360373

2156. Ohar JA, Cheung M, Talarchek J, et al. Germline BAP1 mutational landscape of asbestos-exposed malignant mesothelioma patients with family history of cancer. Cancer Res. 2016 Jan 15;76(2):206–15. PMID:26719535

2157. Ohashi K, Sequist LV, Arcila ME, et al. Characteristics of lung cancers harboring NRAS mutations. Clin Cancer Res. 2013 May 1;19(9):2584–91. PMID:23515407

2158. Ohashi-Nakatani K, Shibuki Y, Fujima M, et al. Primary pulmonary meningioma: a rare case report of aspiration cytological features and immunohistochemical assessment. Diagn Cytopathol. 2019 Apr;47(4):330–3. PMID:30548187

2159. Ohchi T, Tanaka H, Shibuya Y, et al. Thymic carcinoid with mucinous stroma: a case report. Respir Med. 1998 Jun;92(6):880–2. PMID:9850376

2160. Ohe M, Yokose T, Sakuma Y, et al. Stromal micropapillary component as a novel unfavorable prognostic factor of lung adenocarcinoma. Diagn Pathol. 2012 Jan 6;7:3. PMID:22225786

2161. Ohgami RS, Arber DA, Zehnder JL, et al. Indolent T-lymphoblastic proliferation (iT-LBP): a review of clinical and pathologic features and distinction from malignant T-lymphoblastic lymphoma. Adv Anat Pathol. 2013 May;20(3):137–40. PMID:23574769

2162. Ohgami RS, Sendamarai AK, Atwater SK, et al. Indolent T-lymphoblastic proliferation with disseminated multinodal involvement and partial CD33 expression. Am J Surg Pathol. 2014 Sep;38(9):1298–304. PMID:24618611

2163. Ohgami RS, Zhao S, Ohgami JK, et al. TdT+ T-lymphoblastic populations are increased in Castleman disease, in Castleman disease in association with follicular dendritic cell tumors, and in angioimmunoblastic T-cell lymphoma. Am J Surg Pathol. 2012 Nov;36(11):1619–28. PMID:23060347

2164. Ohori NP, Santa Maria EL. Cytopathologic diagnosis of bronchioloalveolar carcinoma: Does it correlate with the 1999 World Health Organization definition? Am J Clin Pathol. 2004 Jul;122(1):44–50. PMID:15272529

2165. Ohsawa M, Tomita Y, Kanno H, et al. Role of Epstein-Barr virus in pleural lymphomagenesis. Mod Pathol. 1995 Oct;8(8):848–53. PMID:8552574

2166. Ohtahara A, Hattori K, Fukuki M, et al. Cardiac angiosarcoma. Intern Med. 1996 Oct;35(10):795–8. PMID:8933189

2167. Ohtake H, Yamakawa M. Interdigitating dendritic cell sarcoma and follicular dendritic cell sarcoma: histopathological findings for differential diagnosis. J Clin Exp Hematop. 2013;53(3):179–84. PMID:24369219

2168. Ohtaki Y, Shimizu K, Kawabata-Iwakawa R, et al. Carbonic anhydrase 9 expression is associated with poor prognosis, tumor proliferation, and radiosensitivity of thymic carcinomas. Oncotarget. 2019 Feb 12;10(13):1306–19. PMID:30863491

2169. Ohtsuka K, Ohnishi H, Kurai D, et al. Familial lung adenocarcinoma caused by the EGFR V843I germ-line mutation. J Clin Oncol. 2011 Mar 10;29(8):e191–2. PMID:21172876

2170. Ohue Y, Matsuoka S, Kumeda H, et al. Development of combined thymic carcinoma and thymoma in an extrathymic lesion during long follow-up for recurrent thymoma. Mol Clin Oncol. 2016 Feb;4(2):139–42. PMID:26893849

2171. Oike T, Ogiwara H, Tominaga Y, et al. A synthetic lethality-based strategy to treat cancers harboring a genetic deficiency in the chromatin remodeling factor BRG1. Cancer Res. 2013 Sep 1;73(17):5508–18. PMID:23872584

2172. Oikonomou A, Giatromanolaki A, Margaritis D, et al. Primary pleural lymphoma: plaque-like thickening of the pleura. Jpn J Radiol. 2010 Jan;28(1):62–5. PMID:20112096

2173. Oka N, Kasajima A, Konukiewitz B, et al. Classification and prognostic stratification of bronchopulmonary neuroendocrine neoplasms. Neuroendocrinology. 2020;110(5):393–403. PMID:31422400

2174. Oka S, Inoue M, Honda Y, et al. Thymic papillary adenocarcinoma coexisting with type A thymoma: a case report. Int J Surg Case Rep. 2019;57:142–4. PMID:30959362

2175. Oka S, Taira A, Shinohara S, et al. Complete resection of thymic sarcomatoid carcinoma through total aortic arch replacement. Ann Thorac Surg. 2016 Dec;102(6):e557–9. PMID:27847081

2176. Okabe M, Inagaki H, Ohshima K, et al. API2-MALT1 fusion defines a distinctive clinicopathologic subtype in pulmonary extranodal marginal zone B-cell lymphoma of mucosa-associated lymphoid tissue. Am J Pathol. 2003 Apr;162(4):1113–22. PMID:12651604

2177. Okada S, Itoh K, Ishihara S, et al. Significance of PD-L1 expression in pulmonary metastases from head and neck squamous cell carcinoma. Surg Oncol. 2018 Jun;27(2):259–65. PMID:29937180

2178. Okada S, Ohshima K, Mori M. The Cushing syndrome induced by atrial natriuretic peptide-producing thymic carcinoid. Ann Intern Med. 1994 Jul 1;121(1):75–6. PMID:8198356

2179. Okada T, Lee AY, Qin LX, et al. Integrin-α10 dependency identifies RAC and RICTOR as therapeutic targets in high-grade myxofibrosarcoma. Cancer Discov. 2016 Oct;6(10):1148–65. PMID:27577794

2180. Okami J, Shintani Y, Okumura M, et al. Demographics, safety and quality, and prognostic information in both the seventh and eighth editions of the TNM classification in 18,973 surgical cases of the Japanese Joint Committee of Lung Cancer Registry database in 2010. J Thorac Oncol. 2019 Feb;14(2):212–22. PMID:30316011

2181. Okereke IC, Kesler KA, Freeman RK, et al. Thymic carcinoma: outcomes after surgical resection. Ann Thorac Surg. 2012 May;93(5):1668–72, discussion 1672–3. PMID:22421590

2182. Okuda K, Watanabe T, Oda R, et al. Pulmonary inflammatory myofibroblastic tumor with TPM4-ALK translocation. J Thorac Dis. 2017 Nov;9(11):E1013–7. PMID:29268561

2183. Okuda M, Huang CL, Haba R, et al. Clear cell carcinoma originating from ectopic thymus. Gen Thorac Cardiovasc Surg. 2009 May;57(5):269–71. PMID:19440827

2184. Okumura M, Ohta M, Tateyama H, et al. The World Health Organization histologic classification system reflects the oncologic behavior of thymoma: a clinical study of 273 patients. Cancer. 2002 Feb 1;94(3):624–32. PMID:11857293

2185. Okumura M, Yoshino I, Yano M, et al. Tumour size determines both recurrence-free survival and disease-specific survival after surgical treatment for thymoma. Eur J Cardiothorac Surg. 2019 Jul 1;56(1):174–81. PMID:30783650

2186. Okumura T, Asamura H, Suzuki K, et al. Intrapulmonary metastasis of non-small cell lung cancer: a prognostic assessment. J Thorac Cardiovasc Surg. 2001 Jul;122(1):24–8. PMID:11436033

2187. Oldridge DA, Truong B, Russ D, et al. Differences in genomic profiles and outcomes between thoracic and adrenal neuroblastoma. J Natl Cancer Inst. 2019 Nov 1;111(11):1192–201. PMID:30793172

2188. Oliaro A, Filosso PL, Cavallo A, et al. The significance of intrapulmonary metastasis in non-small cell lung cancer: upstaging or downstaging? A re-appraisal for the next TNM staging system. Eur J Cardiothorac Surg. 2008 Aug;34(2):438–43, discussion 443. PMID:18502660

2189. Oliveira P, Moura Nunes JF, Clode AL, et al. Alveolar adenoma of the lung: further characterization of this uncommon tumour. Virchows Arch. 1996 Oct;429(2-3):101–8. PMID:8917711

2190. Oliveira R, Branco L, Galrinho A, et al. Cardiac myxoma: a 13-year experience in echocardiographic diagnosis. Rev Port Cardiol. 2010 Jul-Aug;29(7-8):1087–100.

PMID:21066964
2191. Oliveira RC, Carvalho L, Ferreira AJ, et al. Bronchial mucous gland adenoma: a rare tumor. Rev Port Pneumol (2006). 2017 Jul-Aug;23(4):241–2. PMID:28558921
2192. O'Mahony D, Debnath I, Janik J, et al. Cardiac involvement with human T-cell lymphotrophic virus type-1-associated adult T-cell leukemia/lymphoma: the NIH experience. Leuk Lymphoma. 2008 Mar;49(3):439–46. PMID:18297519
2192A. Ongkeko WM, Altuna X, Weisman RA, et al. Expression of protein tyrosine kinases in head and neck squamous cell carcinomas. Am J Clin Pathol. 2005 Jul;124(1):71–6. PMID:15923166
2192B. Onoda T, Kanno M, Sato H, et al. Identification of novel ALK rearrangement A2M-ALK in a neonate with fetal lung interstitial tumor. Genes Chromosomes Cancer. 2014 Oct;53(10):865–74. PMID:24965693
2193. Onozato ML, Kovach AE, Yeap BY, et al. Tumor islands in resected early-stage lung adenocarcinomas are associated with unique clinicopathologic and molecular characteristics and worse prognosis. Am J Surg Pathol. 2013 Feb;37(2):287–94. PMID:23095504
2194. Onuki N, Wistuba II, Travis WD, et al. Genetic changes in the spectrum of neuroendocrine lung tumors. Cancer. 1999 Feb 1;85(3):600–7. PMID:10091733
2195. Onuki T, Iguchi K, Inagaki M, et al. [Lipofibroadenoma of the thymus]. Kyobu Geka. 2009 May;62(5):395–8. Japanese. PMID:19425382
2196. Onyeforo E, Barnett A, Zagami D, et al. Diffuse pulmonary lymphangiomatosis treated with bevacizumab. Respirol Case Rep. 2018 Nov 28;7(1):e00384. PMID:30510764
2197. Oomman A, Santhosham R, Vijayakumar C, et al. Anterior mediastinal teratoma presenting as cardiac tamponade. Indian Heart J. 2004 Jan-Feb;56(1):64–6. PMID:15129796
2198. Oosterhuis JW, Looijenga LH. Testicular germ-cell tumours in a broader perspective. Nat Rev Cancer. 2005 Mar;5(3):210–22. PMID:15738984
2199. Oosterhuis JW, Stoop H, Honecker F, et al. Why human extragonadal germ cell tumours occur in the midline of the body: old concepts, new perspectives. Int J Androl. 2007 Aug;30(4):256–63, discussion 263–4. PMID:17705807
2200. Opitz I, Lauk O, Schneiter D, et al. Intraluminal EWSR1-CREB1 gene rearranged, low-grade myxoid sarcoma of the pulmonary artery resembling extraskeletal myxoid chondrosarcoma (EMC). Histopathology. 2019 Feb;74(3):526–30. PMID:30326150
2201. Oprescu N, McCormack FX, Byrnes S, et al. Clinical predictors of mortality and cause of death in lymphangioleiomyomatosis: a population-based registry. Lung. 2013 Feb;191(1):35–42. PMID:23007140
2202. Orazi A, Neiman RS, Ulbright TM, et al. Hematopoietic precursor cells within the yolk sac tumor component are the source of secondary hematopoietic malignancies in patients with mediastinal germ cell tumors. Cancer. 1993 Jun 15;71(12):3873–81. PMID:8389653
2203. Ordóñez NG. Application of immunohistochemistry in the diagnosis of epithelioid mesothelioma: a review and update. Hum Pathol. 2013 Jan;44(1):1–19. PMID:22963903
2204. Ordóñez NG. D2-40 and podoplanin are highly specific and sensitive immunohistochemical markers of epithelioid malignant mesothelioma. Hum Pathol. 2005 Apr;36(4):372–80. PMID:15891998
2205. Ordóñez NG. Deciduoid mesothelioma: report of 21 cases with review of the literature. Mod Pathol. 2012 Nov;25(11):1481–95. PMID:22684220
2206. Ordóñez NG. Epithelial mesothelioma with deciduoid features: report of four cases. Am J Surg Pathol. 2000 Jun;24(6):816–23. PMID:10843283
2207. Ordóñez NG. Mesothelioma with rhabdoid features: an ultrastructural and immunohistochemical study of 10 cases. Mod Pathol. 2006 Mar;19(3):373–83. PMID:16400322
2207A. Ordóñez NG. Mesothelioma with signet-ring cell features: report of 23 cases. Mod Pathol. 2013 Mar;26(3):370–84. PMID:23041828
2208. Ordóñez NG. Mesotheliomas with small cell features: report of eight cases. Mod Pathol. 2012 May;25(5):689–98. PMID:22222641
2209. Ordóñez NG. Napsin A expression in lung and kidney neoplasia: a review and update. Adv Anat Pathol. 2012 Jan;19(1):66–73. PMID:22156835
2210. Ordóñez NG. Pleomorphic mesothelioma: report of 10 cases. Mod Pathol. 2012 Jul;25(7):1011–22. PMID:22388762
2211. Ordóñez NG. Value of PAX8, PAX2, napsin A, carbonic anhydrase IX, and claudin-4 immunostaining in distinguishing pleural epithelioid mesothelioma from metastatic renal cell carcinoma. Mod Pathol. 2013 Aug;26(8):1132–43. PMID:23503645
2212. Ordóñez NG, Sahin AA. Diagnostic utility of immunohistochemistry in distinguishing between epithelioid pleural mesotheliomas and breast carcinomas: a comparative study. Hum Pathol. 2014 Jul;45(7):1529–40. PMID:24816068
2213. Orlandi A, Ciucci A, Ferlosio A, et al. Cardiac myxoma cells exhibit embryonic endocardial stem cell features. J Pathol. 2006 Jun;209(2):231–9. PMID:16508920
2214. Orlandi A, Ciucci A, Ferlosio A, et al. Increased expression and activity of matrix metalloproteinases characterize embolic cardiac myxomas. Am J Pathol. 2005 Jun;166(6):1619–28. PMID:15920147
2215. Ortega P, Suster D, Falconieri G, et al. Liposarcomas of the posterior mediastinum: clinicopathologic study of 18 cases. Mod Pathol. 2015 May;28(5):721–31. PMID:25475695
2216. Ortega-Guerrero MA, Carrasco-Núñez G, Barragán-Campos H, et al. High incidence of lung cancer and malignant mesothelioma linked to erionite fibre exposure in a rural community in Central Mexico. Occup Environ Med. 2015 Mar;72(3):216–8. PMID:25231672
2217. Osborn M, Mandys V, Beddow E, et al. Cystic fibrohistiocytic tumours presenting in the lung: primary or metastatic disease? Histopathology. 2003 Dec;43(6):556–62. PMID:14636256
2218. Ose N, Maeda H, Inoue M, et al. Results of treatment for thymic neuroendocrine tumours: multicentre clinicopathological study. Interact Cardiovasc Thorac Surg. 2018 Jan 1;26(1):18–24. PMID:29049806
2219. Oser MG, Niederst MJ, Sequist LV, et al. Transformation from non-small-cell lung cancer to small-cell lung cancer: molecular drivers and cells of origin. Lancet Oncol. 2015 Apr;16(4):e165–72. PMID:25846096
2220. Oshiro Y, Kusumoto M, Matsuno Y, et al. CT findings of surgically resected large cell neuroendocrine carcinoma of the lung in 38 patients. AJR Am J Roentgenol. 2004 Jan;182(1):87–91. PMID:14684518
2221. Osterlind K, Andersen PK. Prognostic factors in small cell lung cancer: multivariate model based on 778 patients treated with chemotherapy with or without irradiation. Cancer Res. 1986 Aug;46(8):4189–94. PMID:3015384
2222. Ote EL, Oriuchi N, Miyashita G, et al. Pulmonary artery intimal sarcoma: the role of ^{18}F-fluorodeoxyglucose positron emission tomography in monitoring response to treatment. Jpn J Radiol. 2011 May;29(4):279–82. PMID:21607843
2223. Otto HF, Löning T, Lachenmayer L, et al. Thymolipoma in association with myasthenia gravis. Cancer. 1982 Oct 15;50(8):1623–8. PMID:7116295
2224. Ovrum E, Birkeland S. Mediastinal tumours and cysts. A review of 91 cases. Scand J Thorac Cardiovasc Surg. 1979;13(2):161–8. PMID:224452
2225. Owen D, Chu B, Lehman AM, et al. Expression patterns, prognostic value, and intratumoral heterogeneity of PD-L1 and PD-1 in thymoma and thymic carcinoma. J Thorac Oncol. 2018 Aug;13(8):1204–12. PMID:29702286
2226. Oxnard GR, Miller VA, Robson ME, et al. Screening for germline EGFR T790M mutations through lung cancer genotyping. J Thorac Oncol. 2012 Jun;7(6):1049–52. PMID:22588155
2227. Oyama T, Yamamoto K, Asano N, et al. Age-related EBV-associated B-cell lymphoproliferative disorders constitute a distinct clinicopathologic group: a study of 96 patients. Clin Cancer Res. 2007 Sep 1;13(17):5124–32. PMID:17785567
2227A. Ozcan A, Shen SS, Hamilton C, et al. PAX 8 expression in non-neoplastic tissues, primary tumors, and metastatic tumors: a comprehensive immunohistochemical study. Mod Pathol. 2011 Jun;24(6):751–64. PMID:21317881
2228. Ozkaya N, Rosenblum MK, Durham BH, et al. The histopathology of Erdheim-Chester disease: a comprehensive review of a molecularly characterized cohort. Mod Pathol. 2018 Apr;31(4):581–97. PMID:29192649
2229. Pacak K, Wimalawansa SJ. Pheochromocytoma and paraganglioma. Endocr Pract. 2015 Apr;21(4):406–12. PMID:25716634
2230. Pachter MR, Lattes R. Mesenchymal tumors of the mediastinum. I. Tumors of fibrous tissue, adipose tissue, smooth muscle, and striated muscle. Cancer. 1963 Jan;16:74–94. PMID:13940960
2231. Pachter MR, Lattes R. Uncommon mediastinal tumors. Report of two parathyroid adenomas, one nonfunctional parathyroid carcinoma and one "bronchial-type-adenoma". Dis Chest. 1963 May;43:519–28. PMID:13940962
2232. Pacini D, Careddu L, Pantaleo A, et al. Primary benign cardiac tumours: long-term results. Eur J Cardiothorac Surg. 2012 Apr;41(4):812–9. PMID:22219403
2233. Pacini G, Cavalli G, Tomelleri A, et al. The fibrogenic chemokine CCL18 is associated with disease severity in Erdheim-Chester disease. Oncoimmunology. 2018 Mar 15;7(7):e1440929. PMID:29900045
2234. Padalino MA, Vida VL, Bhattarai A, et al. Giant intramural left ventricular rhabdomyoma in a newborn. Circulation. 2011 Nov 15;124(20):2275–7. PMID:22083149
2235. Padalino MA, Vida VL, Boccuzzo G, et al. Surgery for primary cardiac tumors in children: early and late results in a multicenter European Congenital Heart Surgeons Association study. Circulation. 2012 Jul 3;126(1):22–30. PMID:22626745
2236. Padda SK, Riess JW, Schwartz EJ, et al. Diffuse high intensity PD-L1 staining in thymic epithelial tumors. J Thorac Oncol. 2015 Mar;10(3):500–8. PMID:25402569
2237. Padda SK, Yao X, Antonicelli A, et al. Paraneoplastic syndromes and thymic malignancies: an examination of the International Thymic Malignancy Interest Group retrospective database. J Thorac Oncol. 2018 Mar;13(3):436–46. PMID:29191778
2238. Padgett DM, Cathro HP, Wick MR, et al. Podoplanin is a better immunohistochemical marker for sarcomatoid mesothelioma than calretinin. Am J Surg Pathol. 2008 Jan;32(1):123–7. PMID:18162779
2239. Paez JG, Jänne PA, Lee JC, et al. EGFR mutations in lung cancer: correlation with clinical response to gefitinib therapy. Science. 2004 Jun 4;304(5676):1497–500. PMID:15118125
2240. Pai S, Eng HL, Lee SY, et al. Correction: pleuropulmonary blastoma, not rhabdomyosarcoma in a congenital lung cyst. Pediatr Blood Cancer. 2007 Mar;48(3):370–1. PMID:16856157
2241. Paik PK, Arcila ME, Fara M, et al. Clinical characteristics of patients with lung adenocarcinomas harboring BRAF mutations. J Clin Oncol. 2011 May 20;29(15):2046–51. PMID:21483012
2242. Paik PK, Drilon A, Fan PD, et al. Response to MET inhibitors in patients with stage IV lung adenocarcinomas harboring MET mutations causing exon 14 skipping. Cancer Discov. 2015 Aug;5(8):842–9. PMID:25971939
2242A. Paik PK, Felip E, Veillon R, et al. Tepotinib in non-small-cell lung cancer with MET exon 14 skipping mutations. N Engl J Med. 2020 Sep 3;383(10):931–43. PMID:32469185
2243. Pairon JC, Laurent F, Rinaldo M, et al. Pleural plaques and the risk of pleural mesothelioma. J Natl Cancer Inst. 2013 Feb 20;105(4):293–301. PMID:23355760
2244. Paliwal N, Gupta K, Dewan RK, et al. Adenocarcinoma (somatic-type malignancy) in mature teratoma of anterior mediastinum. Indian J Chest Dis Allied Sci. 2013 Jan-Mar;55(1):39–41. PMID:23798089
2245. Palmer RD, Barbosa-Morais NL, Gooding EL, et al. Pediatric malignant germ cell tumors show characteristic transcriptome profiles. Cancer Res. 2008 Jun 1;68(11):4239–47. PMID:18519683
2246. Palmieri G, Marino M, Buonerba C, et al. Imatinib mesylate in thymic epithelial malignancies. Cancer Chemother Pharmacol. 2012 Feb;69(2):309–15. PMID:21710245
2247. Pan CC, Chen PC, Chiang H. KIT (CD117) is frequently overexpressed in thymic carcinomas but is absent in thymomas. J Pathol. 2004 Mar;202(3):375–81. PMID:14991904
2248. Pan CC, Chen PC, Chou TY, et al. Expression of calretinin and other mesothelioma-related markers in thymic carcinoma and thymoma. Hum Pathol. 2003 Nov;34(11):1155–62. PMID:14652817
2249. Pan CC, Chen WY, Chiang H. Spindle cell and mixed spindle/lymphocytic thymomas: an integrated clinicopathologic and immunohistochemical study of 81 cases. Am J Surg Pathol. 2001 Jan;25(1):111–20. PMID:11145245
2250. Pan CC, Jong YJ, Chen YJ. Comparative genomic hybridization analysis of thymic neuroendocrine tumors. Mod Pathol. 2005 Mar;18(3):358–64. PMID:15272285
2251. Pan CH, Chiang CY, Chen SS. Thymolipoma in patients with myasthenia gravis: report of two cases and review. Acta Neurol Scand. 1988 Jul;78(1):16–21. PMID:3051856
2252. Pan Y, Wang R, Ye T, et al. Comprehensive analysis of oncogenic mutations in lung squamous cell carcinoma with minor glandular component. Chest. 2014 Mar 1;145(3):473–9. PMID:24158231
2253. Pan Y, Zhang Y, Li Y, et al. ALK, ROS1 and RET fusions in 1139 lung adenocarcinomas: a comprehensive study of common and fusion pattern-specific clinicopathologic, histologic and cytologic features. Lung Cancer. 2014 May;84(2):121–6. PMID:24629636
2254. Panagopoulos I, Thorsen J, Gorunova L, et al. RNA sequencing identifies fusion of the EWSR1 and YY1 genes in mesothelioma with t(14;22)(q32;q12). Genes

Chromosomes Cancer. 2013 Aug;52(8):733–40. PMID:23630070
2255. Pande M, Wei C, Chen J, et al. Cancer spectrum in DNA mismatch repair gene mutation carriers: results from a hospital based Lynch syndrome registry. Fam Cancer. 2012 Sep;11(3):441–7. PMID:22714864
2256. Panou V, Gadiraju M, Wolin A, et al. Frequency of germline mutations in cancer susceptibility genes in malignant mesothelioma. J Clin Oncol. 2018 Oct 1;36(28):2863–71. PMID:30113886
2257. Pao W, Girard N. New driver mutations in non-small-cell lung cancer. Lancet Oncol. 2011 Feb;12(2):175–80. PMID:21277552
2258. Pao W, Miller V, Zakowski M, et al. EGF receptor gene mutations are common in lung cancers from "never smokers" and are associated with sensitivity of tumors to gefitinib and erlotinib. Proc Natl Acad Sci U S A. 2004 Sep 7;101(36):13306–11. PMID:15329413
2259. Papachristos IC, Laoutides G, Papaefthimiou O, et al. Gigantic primary lipoma of the diaphragm presenting with respiratory failure. Eur J Cardiothorac Surg. 1998 May;13(5):609–11. PMID:9663548
2260. Papaxoinis G, Lamarca A, Quinn AM, et al. Clinical and pathologic characteristics of pulmonary carcinoid tumors in central and peripheral locations. Endocr Pathol. 2018 Sep;29(3):259–68. PMID:29770932
2261. Papaxoinis G, Nonaka D, O'Brien C, et al. Prognostic significance of CD44 and orthopedia homeobox protein (OTP) expression in pulmonary carcinoid tumours. Endocr Pathol. 2017 Mar;28(1):60–70. PMID:27873160
2262. Papla B. Papillary adenoma of the lung. Pol J Pathol. 2009;60(1):49–51. PMID:19670704
2262A. Papo M, Cohen-Aubart F, Trefond L, et al. Systemic histiocytosis (Langerhans cell histiocytosis, Erdheim-Chester disease, Destombes-Rosai-Dorfman disease): from oncogenic mutations to inflammatory disorders. Curr Oncol Rep. 2019 May 21;21(7):62. PMID:31115724
2263. Papo M, Diamond EL, Cohen-Aubart F, et al. High prevalence of myeloid neoplasms in adults with non-Langerhans cell histiocytosis. Blood. 2017 Aug 24;130(8):1007–13. PMID:28679734
2264. Paquette M, Truong PT, Hart J, et al. Primary sarcoma of the mediastinum: a report of 16 cases referred to the British Columbia Cancer Agency. J Thorac Oncol. 2010 Jun;5(6):898–906. PMID:20521357
2265. Pareja F, Brandes AH, Basili T, et al. Loss-of-function mutations in ATP6AP1 and ATP6AP2 in granular cell tumors. Nat Commun. 2018 Aug 30;9(1):3533. PMID:30166553
2266. Paris C, Benichou J, Bota S, et al. Occupational and nonoccupational factors associated with high grade bronchial pre-invasive lesions. Eur Respir J. 2003 Feb;21(2):332–41. PMID:12608450
2267. Paris C, Clement-Duchene C, Vignaud JM, et al. Relationships between lung adenocarcinoma and gender, age, smoking and occupational risk factors: a case-case study. Lung Cancer. 2010 May;68(2):146–53. PMID:19586681
2268. Parish JM, Rosenow EC 3rd, Swensen SJ, et al. Pulmonary artery sarcoma. Clinical features. Chest. 1996 Dec;110(6):1480–8. PMID:8989065
2269. Park CK, Cho YA, Kim M, et al. Malignant lymphoma arising in cardiac myxoma, presenting with peripheral arterial emboli. Cardiovasc Pathol. 2018 Jan-Feb;32:26–9. PMID:29153872
2270. Park E, Ahn S, Kim H, et al. Targeted sequencing analysis of pulmonary adenocarcinoma with multiple synchronous ground-glass/lepidic nodules. J Thorac Oncol. 2018 Nov;13(11):1776–83. PMID:30121391
2271. Park J, Song JM, Shin E, et al. Cystic cardiac mass in the left atrium: hemorrhage in myxoma. Circulation. 2011 Mar 15;123(10):e368–9. PMID:21403117
2272. Park JR, Bagatell R, London WB, et al. Children's Oncology Group's 2013 blueprint for research: neuroblastoma. Pediatr Blood Cancer. 2013 Jun;60(6):985–93. PMID:23255319
2273. Park MS, Chung KY, Kim KD, et al. Prognosis of thymic epithelial tumors according to the new World Health Organization histologic classification. Ann Thorac Surg. 2004 Sep;78(3):992–7, discussion 997–8. PMID:15337034
2274. Park SB, Kim HH, Shin HJ, et al. Thymic metastasis in breast cancer: a case report. Korean J Radiol. 2007 Jul-Aug;8(4):360–3. PMID:17673850
2275. Park SH, Kim TJ, Chi JG. Congenital granular cell tumor with systemic involvement. Immunohistochemical and ultrastructural study. Arch Pathol Lab Med. 1991 Sep;115(9):934–8. PMID:1929790
2276. Parra ER, Behrens C, Rodriguez-Canales J, et al. Image analysis-based assessment of PD-L1 and tumor-associated immune cells density supports distinct intratumoral microenvironment groups in non-small cell lung carcinoma patients. Clin Cancer Res. 2016 Dec 15;22(24):6278–89. PMID:27252415
2277. Parwani AV, Sheth S, Ali SZ. Recurrent respiratory papillomatosis: cytopathological findings in an unusual case. Diagn Cytopathol. 2004 Dec;31(6):407–12. PMID:15540180
2278. Pass H, Giroux D, Kennedy C, et al. The IASLC Mesothelioma Staging Project: improving staging of a rare disease through international participation. J Thorac Oncol. 2016 Dec;11(12):2082–8. PMID:27670823
2279. Pass HI, Levin SM, Harbut MR, et al. Fibulin-3 as a blood and effusion biomarker for pleural mesothelioma. N Engl J Med. 2012 Oct 11;367(15):1417–27. PMID:23050525
2280. Passiglia F, Calandri M, Guerrera F, et al. Lung cancer in Italy. J Thorac Oncol. 2019 Dec;14(12):2046–52. PMID:31757374
2281. Patankar T, Prasad S, Shenoy A, et al. Pulmonary inflammatory pseudotumour in children. Australas Radiol. 2000 Aug;44(3):318–20. PMID:10974727
2282. Patel A, Borczuk AC, Siddiqui MT. Utility of claudin-4 versus BerEP4 and B72.3 in pleural fluids with metastatic lung adenocarcinoma. J Am Soc Cytopathol. 2020 May-Jun;9(3):146–51. PMID:32184064
2283. Patel IJ, Hsiao E, Ahmad AH, et al. AIRP best cases in radiologic-pathologic correlation: mediastinal mature cystic teratoma. Radiographics. 2013 May;33(3):797–801. PMID:23674775
2284. Patel J, Sheppard MN. Pathological study of primary cardiac and pericardial tumours in a specialist UK centre: surgical and autopsy series. Cardiovasc Pathol. 2010 Nov-Dec;19(6):343–52. PMID:19747857
2285. Patel J, Sheppard MN. Primary malignant mesothelioma of the pericardium. Cardiovasc Pathol. 2011 Mar-Apr;20(2):107–9. PMID:20117025
2286. Patel R, Lynn KC. Masquerading myxoma. Am J Med Sci. 2009 Aug;338(2):161–3. PMID:19680024
2287. Patel SB, Kadi W, Walts AE, et al. Next-generation sequencing: a novel approach to distinguish multifocal primary lung adenocarcinomas from intrapulmonary metastases. J Mol Diagn. 2017 Nov;19(6):870–80. PMID:28866070
2288. Patel SD, Peterson A, Bartczak A, et al. Primary cardiac angiosarcoma - a review. Med Sci Monit. 2014 Jan 23;20:103–9. PMID:24452054
2289. Paties C, Zangrandi A, Vassallo G, et al. Multidirectional carcinoma of the thymus with neuroendocrine and sarcomatoid components and carcinoid syndrome. Pathol Res Pract. 1991 Mar;187(2-3):170–7. PMID:2067996
2290. Patnana M, Sevrukov AB, Elsayes KM, et al. Inflammatory pseudotumor: the great mimicker. AJR Am J Roentgenol. 2012 Mar;198(3):W217–27. PMID:22358018
2291. Paulli M, Sträter J, Gianelli U, et al. Mediastinal B-cell lymphoma: a study of its histomorphologic spectrum based on 109 cases. Hum Pathol. 1999 Feb;30(2):178–87. PMID:10029446
2292. Pawlak Cieślik A, Szturmowicz M, Fijałkowska A, et al. Diagnosis of malignant pericarditis: a single centre experience. Kardiol Pol. 2012;70(11):1147–53. PMID:23180523
2293. Paz-Ares L, Dvorkin M, Chen Y, et al. Durvalumab plus platinum-etoposide versus platinum-etoposide in first-line treatment of extensive-stage small-cell lung cancer (CASPIAN): a randomised, controlled, open-label, phase 3 trial. Lancet. 2019 Nov 23;394(10212):1929–39. PMID:31590988
2293A. PDQ Pediatric Treatment Editorial Board. Rare Cancers of Childhood Treatment (PDQ®): Health Professional Version. In: PDQ Cancer Information Summaries [Internet]. Bethesda (MD): National Cancer Institute (US); 2020 May 21. PMID:26389315
2294. Peachell M, Mayo J, Kalloger S, et al. Calcifying fibrous pseudotumour of the lung. Thorax. 2003 Dec;58(12):1018–9. PMID:14645962
2295. Pei G, Han Y, Zhou S, et al. Giant mediastinal thymolipoma in a patient with Gardner's syndrome. Thorac Cancer. 2015 Nov;6(6):808–11. PMID:26557924
2296. Pei J, Flieder DB, Patchefsky A, et al. Detecting MYB and MYBL1 fusion genes in tracheobronchial adenoid cystic carcinoma by targeted RNA-sequencing. Mod Pathol. 2019 Oct;32(10):1416–20. PMID:31028361
2297. Peifer M, Fernández-Cuesta L, Sos ML, et al. Integrative genome analyses identify key somatic driver mutations of small-cell lung cancer. Nat Genet. 2012 Oct;44(10):1104–10. PMID:22941188
2298. Peiró JL, Sbragia L, Scorletti F, et al. Management of fetal teratomas. Pediatr Surg Int. 2016 Jul;32(7):635–47. PMID:27112491
2299. Pekmezci M, Reuss DE, Hirbe AC, et al. Morphologic and immunohistochemical features of malignant peripheral nerve sheath tumors and cellular schwannomas. Mod Pathol. 2015 Feb;28(2):187–200. PMID:25189642
2299A. Pelkey TJ, Frierson HF Jr, Mills SE, et al. Detection of the alpha-subunit of inhibin in trophoblastic neoplasia. Hum Pathol. 1999 Jan;30(1):26–31. PMID:9923923
2300. Pellegrino M, Gianotti L, Cassibba S, et al. Neuroblastoma in the elderly and SIADH: case report and review of the literature. Case Rep Med. 2012;2012:952645. PMID:22956963
2301. Pelosi G, Barbareschi M, Cavazza A, et al. Large cell carcinoma of the lung: a tumor in search of an author. A clinically oriented critical reappraisal. Lung Cancer. 2015 Mar;87(3):226–31. PMID:25620799
2302. Pelosi G, Fabbri A, Cossa M, et al. What clinicians are asking pathologists when dealing with lung neuroendocrine neoplasms? Semin Diagn Pathol. 2015 Nov;32(6):469–79. PMID:26561395
2303. Pelosi G, Fabbri A, Papotti M, et al. Dissecting pulmonary large-cell carcinoma by targeted next generation sequencing of several cancer genes pushes genotypic-phenotypic correlations to emerge. J Thorac Oncol. 2015 Nov;10(11):1560–9. PMID:26317919
2304. Pelosi G, Fabbri A, Tamborini E, et al. Challenging lung carcinoma with coexistent ΔNp63/p40 and thyroid transcription factor-1 labeling within the same individual tumor cells. J Thorac Oncol. 2015 Oct;10(10):1500–2. PMID:26398824
2305. Pelosi G, Fraggetta F, Nappi O, et al. Pleomorphic carcinomas of the lung show a selective distribution of gene products involved in cell differentiation, cell cycle control, tumor growth, and tumor cell motility: a clinicopathologic and immunohistochemical study of 31 cases. Am J Surg Pathol. 2003 Sep;27(9):1203–15. PMID:12960804
2306. Pelosi G, Gasparini P, Cavazza A, et al. Multiparametric molecular characterization of pulmonary sarcomatoid carcinoma reveals a nonrandom amplification of anaplastic lymphoma kinase (ALK) gene. Lung Cancer. 2012 Sep;77(3):507–14. PMID:22705117
2307. Pelosi G, Gasparini P, Conte D, et al. Synergistic activation upon MET and ALK coamplification sustains targeted therapy in sarcomatoid carcinoma, a deadly subtype of lung cancer. J Thorac Oncol. 2016 May;11(5):718–28. PMID:26804638
2308. Pelosi G, Haspinger ER, Bimbatti M, et al. Does immunohistochemistry affect response to therapy and survival of inoperable non-small cell lung carcinoma patients? A survey of 145 stage III-IV consecutive cases. Int J Surg Pathol. 2014 Apr;22(2):136–48. PMID:24326823
2309. Pelosi G, Massa F, Gatti G, et al. Ki-67 evaluation for clinical decision in metastatic lung carcinoids: a proof of concept. Clin Pathol. 2019 Feb 19;12:X19829259. PMID:31041430
2310. Pelosi G, Melotti F, Cavazza A, et al. A modified vimentin histological score helps recognize pulmonary sarcomatoid carcinoma in small biopsy samples. Anticancer Res. 2012 Apr;32(4):1463–73. PMID:22493387
2311. Pelosi G, Rindi G, Travis WD, et al. Ki-67 antigen in lung neuroendocrine tumors: unraveling a role in clinical practice. J Thorac Oncol. 2014 Mar;9(3):273–84. PMID:24518085
2312. Pelosi G, Rodriguez J, Viale G, et al. Typical and atypical pulmonary carcinoid tumor overdiagnosed as small-cell carcinoma on biopsy specimens: a major pitfall in the management of lung cancer patients. Am J Surg Pathol. 2005 Feb;29(2):179–87. PMID:15644774
2313. Pelosi G, Rossi G, Bianchi F, et al. Immunhistochemistry by means of widely agreed-upon markers (cytokeratins 5/6 and 7, p63, thyroid transcription factor-1, and vimentin) on small biopsies of non-small cell lung cancer effectively parallels the corresponding profiling and eventual diagnoses on surgical specimens. J Thorac Oncol. 2011 Jun;6(6):1039–49. PMID:21512408
2314. Pelosi G, Rossi G, Cavazza A, et al. ΔNp63 (p40) distribution inside lung cancer: a driver biomarker approach to tumor characterization. Int J Surg Pathol. 2013 Jun;21(3):229–39. PMID:23486764
2315. Pelosi G, Scarpa A, Forest F, et al. The impact of immunohistochemistry on the classification of lung tumors. Expert Rev Respir Med. 2016 Oct;10(10):1105–21. PMID:27617475
2316. Pelosi G, Sonzogni A, De Pas T, et al. Review article: pulmonary sarcomatoid carcinomas: a practical overview. Int J Surg Pathol. 2010 Apr;18(2):103–20. PMID:19124452
2317. Pelosi G, Sonzogni A, Harari S, et al. Classification of pulmonary neuroendocrine tumors: new insights. Transl Lung Cancer Res. 2017 Oct;6(5):513–29. PMID:29114468
2318. Pelosi G, Zancanaro C, Sbabo L, et al. Development of innumerable neuroendocrine tumorlets in pulmonary lobe scarred by

intralobar sequestration. Immunohistochemical and ultrastructural study of an unusual case. Arch Pathol Lab Med. 1992 Nov;116(11):1167–74. PMID:1280078
2319. Pemov A, Hansen NF, Sindiri S, et al. Low mutation burden and frequent loss of CDKN2A/B and SMARCA2, but not PRC2, define pre-malignant neurofibromatosis type 1-associated atypical neurofibromas. Neuro Oncol. 2019 Feb 5;21(8):981–92. PMID:30722027
2319A. Penel N, Chibon F, Salas S. Adult desmoid tumors: biology, management and ongoing trials. Curr Opin Oncol. 2017 Jul;29(4):268–74. PMID:28489620
2320. Penel N, Taieb S, Ceugnart L, et al. Report of eight recent cases of locally advanced primary pulmonary artery sarcomas: failure of doxorubicin-based chemotherapy. J Thorac Oncol. 2008 Aug;3(8):907–11. PMID:18670310
2321. Penzel R, Hoegel J, Schmitz W, et al. Clusters of chromosomal imbalances in thymic epithelial tumours are associated with the WHO classification and the staging system according to Masaoka. Int J Cancer. 2003 Jul 1;105(4):494–8. PMID:12712440
2322. Perazzolo Marra M, Thiene G, De Lazzari M, et al. Concealed metastatic lung carcinoma presenting as acute coronary syndrome with progressive conduction abnormalities. Circulation. 2012 Mar 27;125(12):e499–502. PMID:22451611
2323. Perez EA, Koniaris LG, Snell SE, et al. 7201 carcinoids: increasing incidence overall and disproportionate mortality in the elderly. World J Surg. 2007 May;31(5):1022–30. PMID:17429568
2323A. Perkins SM, Shinohara ET. Interdigitating and follicular dendritic cell sarcomas: a SEER analysis. Am J Clin Oncol. 2013 Aug;36(4):395–8. PMID:22772431
2324. Perret R, Chalabreysse L, Watson S, et al. SMARCA4-deficient thoracic sarcomas: clinicopathologic study of 30 cases with an emphasis on their nosology and differential diagnoses. Am J Surg Pathol. 2019 Apr;43(4):455–65. PMID:30451731
2325. Perry AM, Nelson M, Sanger WG, et al. Cytogenetic abnormalities in follicular dendritic cell sarcoma: report of two cases and literature review. In Vivo. 2013 Mar-Apr;27(2):211–4. PMID:23422480
2326. Persson M, Andrén Y, Mark J, et al. Recurrent fusion of MYB and NFIB transcription factor genes in carcinomas of the breast and head and neck. Proc Natl Acad Sci U S A. 2009 Nov 3;106(44):18740–4. PMID:19841262
2327. Pessotto R, Silvestre G, Luciani GB, et al. Primary cardiac leiomyosarcoma: seven-year survival with combined surgical and adjuvant therapy. Int J Cardiol. 1997 Jun 27;60(1):91–4. PMID:9209944
2328. Peters HC, Liu X, Iqbal A, et al. Colorectal cancer metastasis to the thymus gland: rare presentation of colorectal cancer as anterior mediastinal mass. Case Rep Surg. 2017;2017:6581965. PMID:28116210
2329. Peters S, Camidge DR, Shaw AT, et al. Alectinib versus crizotinib in untreated ALK-positive non-small-cell lung cancer. N Engl J Med. 2017 Aug 31;377(9):829–38. PMID:28586279
2330. Peterson CM, Buckley C, Holley S, et al. Teratomas: a multimodality review. Curr Probl Diagn Radiol. 2012 Nov-Dec;41(6):210–9. PMID:23009771
2331. Petit A, Trinquand A, Chevret S, et al. Oncogenetic mutations combined with MRD improve outcome prediction in pediatric T-cell acute lymphoblastic leukemia. Blood. 2018 Jan 18;131(3):289–300. PMID:29051182
2332. Petitjean B, Jardin F, Joly B, et al. Pyothorax-associated lymphoma: a peculiar clinicopathologic entity derived from B cells at late stage of differentiation and with occasional aberrant dual B- and T-cell phenotype. Am J Surg Pathol. 2002 Jun;26(6):724–32. PMID:12023576
2333. Petrich A, Cho SI, Billett H. Primary cardiac lymphoma: an analysis of presentation, treatment, and outcome patterns. Cancer. 2011 Feb 1;117(3):581–9. PMID:20922788
2334. Petrini I, Meltzer PS, Kim IK, et al. A specific missense mutation in GTF2I occurs at high frequency in thymic epithelial tumors. Nat Genet. 2014 Aug;46(8):844–9. PMID:24974848
2335. Petrini I, Meltzer PS, Zucali PA, et al. Copy number aberrations of BCL2 and CDKN2A/B identified by array-CGH in thymic epithelial tumors. Cell Death Dis. 2012 Jul 19;3:e351. PMID:22825469
2336. Petrini I, Rajan A, Pham T, et al. Whole genome and transcriptome sequencing of a B3 thymoma. PLoS One. 2013;8(4):e60572. PMID:23577124
2337. Petrini I, Wang Y, Zucali PA, et al. Copy number aberrations of genes regulating normal thymus development in thymic epithelial tumors. Clin Cancer Res. 2013 Apr 15;19(8):1960–71. PMID:23444221
2338. Petrini I, Zucali PA, Lee HS, et al. Expression and mutational status of c-kit in thymic epithelial tumors. J Thorac Oncol. 2010 Sep;5(9):1447–53. PMID:20651610
2339. Petrini P, French CA, Rajan A, et al. NUT rearrangement is uncommon in human thymic epithelial tumors. J Thorac Oncol. 2012 Apr;7(4):744–50. PMID:22425924
2340. Petscavage JM, Richardson ML, Nett M, et al. Primary chordoid meningioma of the lung. J Thorac Imaging. 2011 Feb;26(1):W14–6. PMID:20634760
2341. Peuchmaur M, d'Amore ES, Joshi VV, et al. Revision of the International Neuroblastoma Pathology Classification: confirmation of favorable and unfavorable prognostic subsets in ganglioneuroblastoma, nodular. Cancer. 2003 Nov 15;98(10):2274–81. PMID:14601099
2342. Pfannschmidt J, Egerer G, Bischof M, et al. Surgical intervention for pulmonary metastases. Dtsch Arztebl Int. 2012 Oct;109(40):645–51. PMID:23094000
2343. Pfeifer GP, Denissenko MF, Olivier M, et al. Tobacco smoke carcinogens, DNA damage and p53 mutations in smoking-associated cancers. Oncogene. 2002 Oct 21;21(48):7435–51. PMID:12379884
2344. Piciu D, Piciu A, Irimie A. Papillary thyroid microcarcinoma and ectopic papillary thyroid carcinoma in mediastinum: a case report. Clin Nucl Med. 2012 Feb;37(2):214–5. PMID:22228358
2345. Pietanza MC, Krug L, Wu AJ, et al. Small cell and neuroendocrine tumors of the lung. In: DeVita VT, Lawrence TS, Rosenberg SA, editors. DeVita, Hellman, and Rosenberg's cancer: principles and practice of oncology. 10th ed. Philadelphia (PA): Wolters Kluwer; 2015. pp. 536–59.
2346. Pileri SA, Ascani S, Cox MC, et al. Myeloid sarcoma: clinico-pathologic, phenotypic and cytogenetic analysis of 92 adult patients. Leukemia. 2007 Feb;21(2):340–50. PMID:17170724
2347. Pileri SA, Cavazza A, Schiavina M, et al. Clear-cell proliferation of the lung with lymphangioleiomyomatosis-like change. Histopathology. 2004 Feb;44(2):156–63. PMID:14764059
2348. Pileri SA, Gaidano G, Zinzani PL, et al. Primary mediastinal B-cell lymphoma: high frequency of BCL-6 mutations and consistent expression of the transcription factors OCT-2, BOB.1, and PU.1 in the absence of immunoglobulins. Am J Pathol. 2003 Jan;162(1):243–53. PMID:12507907
2349. Pileri SA, Grogan TM, Harris NL, et al. Tumours of histiocytes and accessory dendritic cells: an immunohistochemical approach to classification from the International Lymphoma Study Group based on 61 cases. Histopathology. 2002 Jul;41(1):1–29. PMID:12121233
2350. Pilichowska M, Pittaluga S, Ferry JA, et al. Clinicopathologic consensus study of gray zone lymphoma with features intermediate between DLBCL and classical HL. Blood Adv. 2017 Dec 11;1(26):2600–9. PMID:29296913
2351. Pillon M, Aricò M, Mussolin L, et al. Mediastinal Burkitt lymphoma in childhood. Pediatr Blood Cancer. 2014 Nov;61(11):2127–8. PMID:25053233
2352. Pilozzi E, Cacchi C, Di Napoli A, et al. Primary malignant tumour of the lung with neuroendocrine and melanoma differentiation. Virchows Arch. 2011 Aug;459(2):239–43. PMID:21735167
2353. Pilozzi E, Müller-Hermelink HK, Falini B, et al. Gene rearrangements in T-cell lymphoblastic lymphoma. J Pathol. 1999 Jul;188(3):267–70. PMID:10419594
2354. Piña-Oviedo S, Moran CA. Primary mediastinal classical Hodgkin lymphoma. Adv Anat Pathol. 2016 Sep;23(5):285–309. PMID:27441757
2355. Piña-Oviedo S, Moran CA. Primary mediastinal nodal and extranodal non-Hodgkin lymphomas: current concepts, historical evolution, and useful diagnostic approach: part 2. Adv Anat Pathol. 2019 Nov;26(6):371–89. PMID:31567129
2356. Piña-Oviedo S, Weissferdt A, Kalhor N, et al. Primary pulmonary lymphomas. Adv Anat Pathol. 2015 Nov;22(6):355–75. PMID:26452211
2357. Pinede L, Duhaut P, Loire R. Clinical presentation of left atrial cardiac myxoma. A series of 112 consecutive cases. Medicine (Baltimore). 2001 May;80(3):159–72. PMID:11388092
2358. Pinheiro PS, Jin H. No increased risk for mesothelioma in relation to natural-occurring asbestos in southern Nevada. J Thorac Oncol. 2015 Jul;10(7):e62–3. PMID:26134237
2359. Pinkard NB, Wilson RW, Lawless N, et al. Calcifying fibrous pseudotumor of pleura. A report of three cases of a newly described entity involving the pleura. Am J Clin Pathol. 1996 Feb;105(2):189–94. PMID:8607443
2360. Piotrowska Z, Isozaki H, Lennerz JK, et al. Landscape of acquired resistance to osimertinib in EGFR-mutant NSCLC and clinical validation of combined EGFR and RET inhibition with osimertinib and BLU-667 for acquired RET fusion. Cancer Discov. 2018 Dec;8(12):1529–39. PMID:30257958
2361. Pisapia P, Malapelle U, Roma G, et al. Consistency and reproducibility of next-generation sequencing in cytopathology: a second worldwide ring trial study on improved cytological molecular reference specimens. Cancer Cytopathol. 2019 May;127(5):285–96. PMID:31021538
2362. Planchard D, Besse B, Groen HJM, et al. Dabrafenib plus trametinib in patients with previously treated BRAF(V600E)-mutant metastatic non-small cell lung cancer: an open-label, multicentre phase 2 trial. Lancet Oncol. 2016 Jul;17(7):984–93. PMID:27283860
2363. Planchard D, Popat S, Kerr K, et al. Metastatic non-small cell lung cancer: ESMO Clinical Practice Guidelines for diagnosis, treatment and follow-up. Ann Oncol. 2018 Oct 1;29(Suppl 4):iv192–237. PMID:30285222
2364. Planchard D, Popat S, Kerr K, et al. Correction to: "Metastatic non-small cell lung cancer: ESMO Clinical Practice Guidelines for diagnosis, treatment and follow-up". Ann Oncol. 2019 May;30(5):863–70. PMID:31987360
2365. Plathow C, Staab A, Schmaehl A, et al. Computed tomography, positron emission tomography, positron emission tomography/computed tomography, and magnetic resonance imaging for staging of limited pleural mesothelioma: initial results. Invest Radiol. 2008 Oct;43(10):737–44. PMID:18791416
2366. Plaza JA, Wakely PE Jr, Moran C, et al. Sclerosing paraganglioma: report of 19 cases of an unusual variant of neuroendocrine tumor that may be mistaken for an aggressive malignant neoplasm. Am J Surg Pathol. 2006 Jan;30(1):7–12. PMID:16330936
2366A. Pocrnich CE, Ramalingam P, Euscher ED, et al. Neuroendocrine carcinoma of the endometrium: a clinicopathologic study of 25 cases. Am J Surg Pathol. 2016 May;40(5):577–86. PMID:26945341
2367. Poirier JT, George J, Owonikoko TK, et al. New approaches to SCLC therapy: from the laboratory to the clinic. J Thorac Oncol. 2020 Apr;15(4):520–40. PMID:32018053
2368. Polansky SM, Barwick KW, Ravin CE. Primary mediastinal seminoma. AJR Am J Roentgenol. 1979 Jan;132(1):17–21. PMID:103398
2369. Policarpio-Nicolas ML, Covell J, Bregman S, et al. Fine needle aspiration cytology of clear cell "sugar" tumor (PEComa) of the lung: report of a case. Diagn Cytopathol. 2008 Feb;36(2):89–93. PMID:18181192
2370. Pollefliet C, Peters K, Janssens A, et al. Endobronchial lipomas: rare benign lung tumors, two case reports. J Thorac Oncol. 2009 May;4(5):658–60. PMID:19395910
2371. Polsani A, Braithwaite KA, Alazraki AL, et al. NUT midline carcinoma: an imaging case series and review of literature. Pediatr Radiol. 2012 Feb;42(2):205–10. PMID:22033856
2372. Ponzoni M, Arrigoni G, Gould VE, et al. Lack of CD 29 (beta1 integrin) and CD 54 (ICAM-1) adhesion molecules in intravascular lymphomatosis. Hum Pathol. 2000 Feb;31(2):220–6. PMID:10685637
2373. Poorabdollah M, Mehdizadeh E, Mohammadi F, et al. Metaplastic thymoma: report of an unusual thymic epithelial neoplasm arising in the wall of a thymic cyst. Int J Surg Pathol. 2009 Feb;17(1):51–4. PMID:18397900
2374. Popat N, Raghavan N, McIvor RA. Severe bronchorrhea in a patient with bronchioloalveolar carcinoma. Chest. 2012 Feb;141(2):513–4. PMID:22315118
2375. Popova T, Hebert L, Jacquemin V, et al. Germline BAP1 mutations predispose to renal cell carcinomas. Am J Hum Genet. 2013 Jun 6;92(6):974–80. PMID:23684012
2376. Popper HH, el-Shabrawi Y, Wöckel W, et al. Prognostic importance of human papilloma virus typing in squamous cell papilloma of the bronchus: comparison of in situ hybridization and the polymerase chain reaction. Hum Pathol. 1994 Nov;25(11):1191–7. PMID:7959664
2377. Popper HH, Wirnsberger G, Jüttner-Smolle FM, et al. The predictive value of human papilloma virus (HPV) typing in the prognosis of bronchial squamous cell papillomas. Histopathology. 1992 Oct;21(4):323–30. PMID:1328017
2378. Porcel JM, Gasol A, Bielsa S, et al. Clinical features and survival of lung cancer patients with pleural effusions. Respirology. 2015 May;20(4):654–9. PMID:25706291
2379. Porcel JM, Hernández P, Martínez-Alonso M, et al. Accuracy of fluorodeoxyglucose-PET imaging for differentiating benign from malignant pleural effusions: a meta-analysis. Chest. 2015 Feb;147(2):502–12. PMID:25188411
2380. Porubsky S, Jessup P, Kee D, et al. Potentially actionable FGFR2 high-level amplification in thymic sebaceous carcinoma. Virchows Arch. 2020 Feb;476(2):323–7.

PMID:31401665
2380A. Porubsky S, Popovic ZV, Badve S, et al. Thymic hyperplasia with lymphoepithelial sialadenitis (LESA)-like features: strong association with lymphomas and non-myasthenic autoimmune diseases. Cancers (Basel). 2021 Jan 16;13(2):E315. PMID:33467055
2381. Porubsky S, Rudolph B, Rückert JC, et al. EWSR1 translocation in primary hyalinising clear cell carcinoma of the thymus. Histopathology. 2019 Sep;75(3):431–6. PMID:31050844
2382. Posligua L, Ylagan L. Fine-needle aspiration cytology of thymic basaloid carcinoma: case studies and review of the literature. Diagn Cytopathol. 2006 May;34(5):358–66. PMID:16604555
2383. Prat J, Bhan AK, Dickersin GR, et al. Hepatoid yolk sac tumor of the ovary (endodermal sinus tumor with hepatoid differentiation): a light microscopic, ultrastructural and immunohistochemical study of seven cases. Cancer. 1982 Dec 1;50(11):2355–68. PMID:7139531
2384. Prayson RA, Farver CF. Primary pulmonary malignant meningioma. Am J Surg Pathol. 1999 Jun;23(6):722–6. PMID:10366156
2385. Preusser M, Berghoff AS, Berger W, et al. High rate of FGFR1 amplifications in brain metastases of squamous and non-squamous lung cancer. Lung Cancer. 2014 Jan;83(1):83–9. PMID:24183471
2386. Priest JR, McDermott MB, Bhatia S, et al. Pleuropulmonary blastoma: a clinicopathologic study of 50 cases. Cancer. 1997 Jul 1;80(1):147–61. PMID:9210721
2387. Priest JR, Watterson J, Strong L, et al. Pleuropulmonary blastoma: a marker for familial disease. J Pediatr. 1996 Feb;128(2):220–4. PMID:8636815
2388. Prieto-Granada CN, Ganim RB, Zhang L, et al. Primary pulmonary myxoid sarcoma: a newly described entity-report of a case and review of the literature. Int J Surg Pathol. 2017 Sep;25(6):518–25. PMID:28449608
2389. Prieto-Granada CN, Inagaki H, Mueller J. Thymic mucoepidermoid carcinoma: report of a case with CTRC1/3-MALM2 molecular studies. Int J Surg Pathol. 2015 Jun;23(4):277–83. PMID:25782731
2390. Prieto-Granada CN, Wiesner T, Messina JL, et al. Loss of H3K27me3 expression is a highly sensitive marker for sporadic and radiation-induced MPNST. Am J Surg Pathol. 2016 Apr;40(4):479–89. PMID:26645727
2391. Prim N, Legrain M, Guerin E, et al. Germ-line exon 21 EGFR mutations, V843I and P848L, in nonsmall cell lung cancer patients. Eur Respir Rev. 2014 Sep;23(133):390–2. PMID:25176975
2392. Przygodzki RM, Hubbs AE, Zhao FQ, et al. Primary mediastinal seminomas: evidence of single and multiple KIT mutations. Lab Invest. 2002 Oct;82(10):1369–75. PMID:12379771
2393. Przygodzki RM, Moran CA, Suster S, et al. Primary mediastinal and testicular seminomas: a comparison of K-ras-2 gene sequence and p53 immunoperoxidase analysis of 26 cases. Hum Pathol. 1996 Sep;27(9):975–9. PMID:8816895
2394. Pugh TJ, Yu W, Yang J, et al. Exome sequencing of pleuropulmonary blastoma reveals frequent biallelic loss of TP53 and two hits in DICER1 resulting in retention of 5p-derived miRNA hairpin loop sequences. Oncogene. 2014 Nov 6;33(45):5295–302. PMID:24909177
2395. Pulford E, Huilgol K, Moffat D, et al. Malignant mesothelioma, BAP1 immunohistochemistry, and VEGFA: Does BAP1 have potential for early diagnosis and assessment of prognosis? Dis Markers. 2017;2017:1310478. PMID:29085180
2396. Puliyel MM, Mascarenhas L, Zhou S, et al. Nuclear protein in testis midline carcinoma misdiagnosed as adamantinoma. J Clin Oncol. 2014 May 20;32(15):e57–60. PMID:24470009
2397. Puskarz-Thomas S, Dettrick A, Pohlner PG. Cardiac myxoma with oncocytic change–cardiac oncocytoma? Cardiovasc Pathol. 2012 Mar-Apr;21(2):e11–3. PMID:22104003
2398. Pyo JS, Kim JH. Clinicopathological significance of micropapillary pattern in lung adenocarcinoma. Pathol Oncol Res. 2018 Jul;24(3):547–55. PMID:28685219
2399. Qi J, Yu J, Zhang M, et al. Multicentric granular cell tumors with heart involvement: a case report. J Clin Oncol. 2012 Feb 20;30(6):e79–82. PMID:22215746
2400. Qian J, Zhao S, Zou Y, et al. Genomic underpinnings of tumor behavior in in situ and early lung adenocarcinoma. Am J Respir Crit Care Med. 2020 Mar 15;201(6):697–706. PMID:31747302
2401. Qian Y, Jiang T, Liu S. Sclerosing hemangioma of the lung manifesting as a cystic lesion with an air-fluid level. Respiration. 2012;84(2):142–3. PMID:22832056
2402. Qin BD, Jiao XD, Liu K, et al. Clinical, pathological and treatment factors associated with the survival of patients with primary pulmonary salivary gland-type tumors. Lung Cancer. 2018 Dec;126:174–81. PMID:30527184
2403. Qu G, Yu G, Zhang Q, et al. Lipofibroadenoma of the thymus: a case report. Diagn Pathol. 2013 Jul 15;8:117. PMID:23856156
2404. Qu L, Xiong Y, Yao Q, et al. Micronodular thymoma with lymphoid stroma: two cases, one in a multilocular thymic cyst, and literature review. Thorac Cancer. 2017 Nov;8(6):734–40. PMID:28941195
2405. Quinn AM, Chaturvedi A, Nonaka D. High-grade neuroendocrine carcinoma of the lung with carcinoid morphology: a study of 12 cases. Am J Surg Pathol. 2017 Feb;41(2):263–70. PMID:27879513
2406. Quintanilla-Martinez L, Wilkins EW Jr, Choi N, et al. Thymoma. Histologic subclassification is an independent prognostic factor. Cancer. 1994 Jul 15;74(2):606–17. PMID:8033040
2407. Ra SH, Fishbein MC, Baruch-Oren T, et al. Mucinous adenocarcinomas of the thymus: report of 2 cases and review of the literature. Am J Surg Pathol. 2007 Sep;31(9):1330–6. PMID:17721187
2408. Raab SS, Silverman JF, McLeod DL, et al. Fine needle aspiration biopsy of fibromatoses. Acta Cytol. 1993 May-Jun;37(3):323–8. PMID:8498134
2409. Radovich M, Pickering CR, Felau I, et al. The integrated genomic landscape of thymic epithelial tumors. Cancer Cell. 2018 Feb 12;33(2):244–258.e10. PMID:29438696
2410. Radovich M, Solzak JP, Hancock BA, et al. A large microRNA cluster on chromosome 19 is a transcriptional hallmark of WHO type A and AB thymomas. Br J Cancer. 2016 Feb 16;114(4):477–84. PMID:26766736
2411. Raffa GM, Malvindi PG, Settepani F, et al. Hamartoma of mature cardiac myocytes in adults and young: case report and literature review. Int J Cardiol. 2013 Feb 20;163(2):e28–30. PMID:23041004
2412. Rahouma M, Kamel M, Narula N, et al. Role of wedge resection in bronchial carcinoid (BC) tumors: SEER database analysis. J Thorac Dis. 2019 Apr;11(4):1355–62. PMID:31179077
2413. Rai K, Pilarski R, Cebulla CM, et al. Comprehensive review of BAP1 tumor predisposition syndrome with report of two new cases. Clin Genet. 2016 Mar;89(3):285–94. PMID:26096145
2414. Rajan A, Heery CR, Thomas A, et al. Efficacy and tolerability of anti-programmed death-ligand 1 (PD-L1) antibody (avelumab) treatment in advanced thymoma. J Immunother Cancer. 2019 Oct 21;7(1):269. PMID:31639039
2415. Rajan A, Zhao C. Deciphering the biology of thymic epithelial tumors. Mediastinum. 2019 Sep;3:36. PMID:31608319
2416. Rajiah P, To AC, Tan CD, et al. Multimodality imaging of an unusual case of right ventricular lipoma. Circulation. 2011 Oct 25;124(17):1897–8. PMID:22025640
2417. Ramalingam P, Teague D, Reid-Nicholson M. Imprint cytology of high-grade immature ovarian teratoma: a case report, literature review, and distinction from other ovarian small round cell tumors. Diagn Cytopathol. 2008 Aug;36(8):595–9. PMID:18618728
2418. Ramasamy K, Lim Z, Pagliuca A, et al. Acute myeloid leukaemia presenting with mediastinal myeloid sarcoma: report of three cases and review of literature. Leuk Lymphoma. 2007 Feb;48(2):290–4. PMID:17325888
2419. Ramaswami R, Chia G, Dalla Pria A, et al. Evolution of HIV-associated lymphoma over 3 decades. J Acquir Immune Defic Syndr. 2016 Jun 1;72(2):177–83. PMID:26859827
2420. Ramaswamy PV, Storm CA, Filiano JJ, et al. Multiple granular cell tumors in a child with Noonan syndrome. Pediatr Dermatol. 2010 Mar-Apr;27(2):209–11. PMID:20537083
2421. Rami-Porta R, Asamura H, Travis WD, et al. Lung cancer - major changes in the American Joint Committee on Cancer eighth edition cancer staging manual. CA Cancer J Clin. 2017 Mar;67(2):138–55. PMID:28140453
2422. Rami-Porta R, Bolejack V, Crowley J, et al. The IASLC Lung Cancer Staging Project: proposals for the revisions of the T descriptors in the forthcoming eighth edition of the TNM classification for lung cancer. J Thorac Oncol. 2015 Jul;10(7):990–1003. PMID:26134221
2423. Rami-Porta R, Bolejack V, Giroux DJ, et al. The IASLC Lung Cancer Staging Project: the new database to inform the eighth edition of the TNM classification of lung cancer. J Thorac Oncol. 2014 Nov;9(11):1618–24. PMID:25436796
2424. Ramlawi B, Leja MJ, Abu Saleh WK, et al. Surgical treatment of primary cardiac sarcomas: review of a single-institution experience. Ann Thorac Surg. 2016 Feb;101(2):698–702. PMID:26476808
2425. Rammos KS, Ketikoglou DG, Hatzibougias IG. Large left ventricular capillary hemangioma with cavernous areas. Tex Heart Inst J. 2007;34(1):128–9. PMID:17420812
2426. Ramos SG, Rezende GG, Faccio AA. A rare presentation of biphasic pulmonary blastoma. Arch Pathol Lab Med. 2002 Jul;126(7):875–6. PMID:12125652
2427. Rampisela D, Zreik R, Donner LR. Thymic tumor with adenoid cystic carcinoma-like features: a study of a clinically favorable case followed for 9 years. Int J Surg Pathol. 2015 Oct;23(7):557–60. PMID:26194601
2428. Rana HQ, Gelman R, LaDuca H, et al. Differences in TP53 mutation carrier phenotypes emerge from panel-based testing. J Natl Cancer Inst. 2018 Aug 1;110(8):863–70. PMID:29529297
2429. Randhawa JS, Budd GT, Randhawa M, et al. Primary cardiac sarcoma: 25-year Cleveland Clinic experience. Am J Clin Oncol. 2016 Dec;39(6):593–9. PMID:25036471
2430. Rao N. Adenosquamous carcinoma. Semin Diagn Pathol. 2014 Jul;31(4):271–7. PMID:25002356
2431. Rao N, Colby TV, Falconieri G, et al. Intrapulmonary solitary fibrous tumors: clinicopathologic and immunohistochemical study of 24 cases. Am J Surg Pathol. 2013 Feb;37(2):155–66. PMID:23108019
2432. Rao Q, Shen Q, Xia QY, et al. PSF/SFPQ is a very common gene fusion partner in TFE3 rearrangement-associated perivascular epithelioid cell tumors (PEComas) and melanotic Xp11 translocation renal cancers: clinicopathologic, immunohistochemical, and molecular characteristics suggesting classification as a distinct entity. Am J Surg Pathol. 2015 Sep;39(9):1181–96. PMID:26274027
2433. Raoufi M, Herrak L, Benali A, et al. Mediastinal mature teratoma revealed by empyema. Case Rep Pulmonol. 2016;2016:7869476. PMID:27144046
2434. Raphael KL, Martinez AP, Clements SD, et al. Role of multimodal cardiac imaging in diagnosing a primary intimal sarcoma of the left atrial appendage. Tex Heart Inst J. 2019 Feb 1;46(1):28–31. PMID:30833834
2435. Rapicetta C, Lococo F, Stefani A, et al. Primary sarcomatoid carcinoma of the lung: radiometabolic ((18)F-FDG PET/CT) findings and correlation with clinico-pathological and survival results. Lung. 2016 Aug;194(4):653–7. PMID:27300448
2436. Rapisarda V, Salemi R, Marconi A, et al. Fluoro-edenite induces fibulin-3 overexpression in non-malignant human mesothelial cells. Oncol Lett. 2016 Nov;12(5):3363–7. PMID:27900005
2437. Rathore KS, Hussenbocus S, Stuklis R, et al. Novel strategies for recurrent cardiac myxoma. Ann Thorac Surg. 2008 Jun;85(6):2125–6. PMID:18498840
2438. Ratschiller D, Heighway J, Gugger M, et al. Cyclin D1 overexpression in bronchial epithelia of patients with lung cancer is associated with smoking and predicts survival. J Clin Oncol. 2003 Jun 1;21(11):2085–93. PMID:12775733
2439. Rausch T, Jones DT, Zapatka M, et al. Genome sequencing of pediatric medulloblastoma links catastrophic DNA rearrangements with TP53 mutations. Cell. 2012 Jan 20;148(1-2):59–71. PMID:22265402
2440. Raut CP, Miceli R, Strauss DC, et al. External validation of a multi-institutional retroperitoneal sarcoma nomogram. Cancer. 2016 May 1;122(9):1417–24. PMID:26916507
2441. Ravandi-Kashani F, Cortes J, Giles FJ. Myelodysplasia presenting as granulocytic sarcoma of mediastinum causing superior vena cava syndrome. Leuk Lymphoma. 2000 Feb;36(5-6):631–7. PMID:10784409
2442. Raz DJ, Nelson RA, Grannis FW, et al. Natural history of typical pulmonary carcinoid tumors: a comparison of nonsurgical and surgical treatment. Chest. 2015 Apr;147(4):1111–7. PMID:25539082
2443. Razanamahery J, Diamond EL, Cohen-Aubart F, et al. Erdheim-Chester disease with concomitant Rosai-Dorfman like lesions: a distinct entity mainly driven by MAP2K1. Haematologica. 2020 Jan;105(1):e5–8. PMID:31123032
2444. Rea G, Homfray T, Till J, et al. Histiocytoid cardiomyopathy and microphthalmia with linear skin defects syndrome: phenotypes linked by truncating variants in NDUFB11. Cold Spring Harb Mol Case Stud. 2017 Jan;3(1):a001271. PMID:28050600
2445. Reck M, Rodríguez-Abreu D, Robinson AG, et al. Pembrolizumab versus chemotherapy for PD-L1-positive non-small-cell lung cancer. N Engl J Med. 2016 Nov 10;375(19):1823–33. PMID:27718847
2446. Reck M, Schenker M, Lee KH, et al. Nivolumab plus ipilimumab versus chemotherapy as first-line treatment in advanced non-small-cell lung cancer with high tumour mutational burden: patient-reported outcomes results from the randomised, open-label, phase III CheckMate 227 trial. Eur J Cancer. 2019 Jul;116:137–47. PMID:31195357
2447. Reece IJ, Cooley DA, Frazier OH, et al. Cardiac tumors. Clinical spectrum and

prognosis of lesions other than classical benign myxoma in 20 patients. J Thorac Cardiovasc Surg. 1984 Sep;88(3):439–46. PMID:6381889
2448. Reid A, Franklin P, Berry G, et al. Are children more vulnerable to mesothelioma than adults? A comparison of mesothelioma risk among children and adults exposed non-occupationally to blue asbestos at Wittenoom. Occup Environ Med. 2018 Dec;75(12):898–903. PMID:30158318
2449. Reisenauer JS, Mneimneh W, Jenkins S, et al. Comparison of risk stratification models to predict recurrence and survival in pleuropulmonary solitary fibrous tumor. J Thorac Oncol. 2018 Sep;13(9):1349–62. PMID:29935303
2450. Reis-Filho JS, Pope LZ, Milanezi F, et al. Primary epithelial malignant mesothelioma of the pericardium with deciduoid features: cytohistologic and immunohistochemical study. Diagn Cytopathol. 2002 Feb;26(2):117–22. PMID:11813331
2451. Reiter A, Schrappe M, Ludwig WD, et al. Intensive ALL-type therapy without local radiotherapy provides a 90% event-free survival for children with T-cell lymphoblastic lymphoma: a BFM group report. Blood. 2000 Jan 15;95(2):416–21. PMID:10627444
2452. Rekhi B, Gupta C, Chinnaswamy G, et al. Clinicopathologic features of 300 rhabdomyosarcomas with emphasis upon differential expression of skeletal muscle specific markers in the various subtypes: a single institutional experience. Ann Diagn Pathol. 2018 Oct;36:50–60. PMID:30098515
2453. Rekhi B, Upadhyay P, Ramteke MP, et al. MYOD1 (L122R) mutations are associated with spindle cell and sclerosing rhabdomyosarcomas with aggressive clinical outcomes. Mod Pathol. 2016 Dec;29(12):1532–40. PMID:27562493
2454. Rekhtman N. Neuroendocrine tumors of the lung: an update. Arch Pathol Lab Med. 2010 Nov;134(11):1628–38. PMID:21043816
2455. Rekhtman N, Ang DC, Riely GJ, et al. KRAS mutations are associated with solid growth pattern and tumor-infiltrating leukocytes in lung adenocarcinoma. Mod Pathol. 2013 Oct;26(10):1307–19. PMID:23619604
2456. Rekhtman N, Ang DC, Sima CS, et al. Immunohistochemical algorithm for differentiation of lung adenocarcinoma and squamous cell carcinoma based on large series of whole-tissue sections with validation in small specimens. Mod Pathol. 2011 Oct;24(10):1348–59. PMID:21623384
2457. Rekhtman N, Brandt SM, Sigel CS, et al. Suitability of thoracic cytology for new therapeutic paradigms in non-small cell lung carcinoma: high accuracy of tumor subtyping and feasibility of EGFR and KRAS molecular testing. J Thorac Oncol. 2011 Mar;6(3):451–8. PMID:21266922
2458. Rekhtman N, Desmeules P, Litvak AM, et al. Stage IV lung carcinoids: spectrum and evolution of proliferation rate, focusing on variants with elevated proliferation indices. Mod Pathol. 2019 Jul;32(8):1106–22. PMID:30923345
2459. Rekhtman N, Kazi S. Nonspecific reactivity of polyclonal napsin a antibody in mucinous adenocarcinomas of various sites: a word of caution. Arch Pathol Lab Med. 2015 Apr;139(4):434–6. PMID:25521803
2460. Rekhtman N, Montecalvo J, Chang JC, et al. SMARCA4-deficient thoracic sarcomatoid tumors represent primarily smoking-related undifferentiated carcinomas rather than primary thoracic sarcomas. J Thorac Oncol. 2020 Feb;15(2):231–47. PMID:31751681
2461. Rekhtman N, Paik PK, Arcila ME, et al. Clarifying the spectrum of driver oncogene mutations in biomarker-verified squamous carcinoma of lung: lack of EGFR/KRAS and presence of PIK3CA/AKT1 mutations. Clin Cancer Res. 2012 Feb 15;18(4):1167–76. PMID:22228640
2462. Rekhtman N, Pietanza CM, Sabari J, et al. Pulmonary large cell neuroendocrine carcinoma with adenocarcinoma-like features: napsin A expression and genomic alterations. Mod Pathol. 2018 Jan;31(1):111–21. PMID:28884744
2463. Rekhtman N, Pietanza MC, Hellmann MD, et al. Next-generation sequencing of pulmonary large cell neuroendocrine carcinoma reveals small cell carcinoma-like and non-small cell carcinoma-like subsets. Clin Cancer Res. 2016 Jul 15;22(14):3618–29. PMID:26960398
2464. Rekhtman N, Tafe LJ, Chaft JE, et al. Distinct profile of driver mutations and clinical features in immunomarker-defined subsets of pulmonary large-cell carcinoma. Mod Pathol. 2013 Apr;26(4):511–22. PMID:23196793
2465. Rekhtman N, Travis WD. Large no more: the journey of pulmonary large cell carcinoma from common to rare entity. J Thorac Oncol. 2019 Jul;14(7):1125–7. PMID:31235033
2466. Remstein ED, Kurtin PJ, Einerson RR, et al. Primary pulmonary MALT lymphomas show frequent and heterogeneous cytogenetic abnormalities, including aneuploidy and translocations involving API2 and MALT1 and IGH and MALT1. Leukemia. 2004 Jan;18(1):156–60. PMID:14574335
2467. Renaux-Petel M, Charbonnier F, Théry JC, et al. Contribution of de novo and mosaic TP53 mutations to Li-Fraumeni syndrome. J Med Genet. 2018 Mar;55(3):173–80. PMID:29070607
2468. Repo P, Järvinen RS, Jäntti JE, et al. Population-based analysis of BAP1 germline variations in patients with uveal melanoma. Hum Mol Genet. 2019 Jul 15;28(14):2415–26. PMID:31058963
2469. Reuling EMBP, Dickhoff C, Plaisier PW, et al. Endobronchial and surgical treatment of pulmonary carcinoid tumors: a systematic literature review. Lung Cancer. 2019 Aug;134:85–95. PMID:31320001
2470. Reuter VE. The pre and post chemotherapy pathologic spectrum of germ cell tumors. Chest Surg Clin N Am. 2002 Nov;12(4):673–94. PMID:12471871
2471. Reynen K, Köckeritz U, Strasser RH. Metastases to the heart. Ann Oncol. 2004 Mar;15(3):375–81. PMID:14998838
2472. Reynoird N, Schwartz BE, Delvecchio M, et al. Oncogenesis by sequestration of CBP/p300 in transcriptionally inactive hyperacetylated chromatin domains. EMBO J. 2010 Sep 1;29(17):2943–52. PMID:20676058
2473. Reynolds CJ, Minelli C, Darnton A, et al. Mesothelioma mortality in Great Britain: How much longer will dockyards dominate? Occup Environ Med. 2019 Dec;76(12):908–12. PMID:31662422
2474. Ribeiro C, Campelos S, Moura CS, et al. Well-differentiated papillary mesothelioma: clustering in a Portuguese family with a germline BAP1 mutation. Ann Oncol. 2013 Aug;24(8):2147–50. PMID:23585512
2475. Ricaurte LM, Arrieta O, Zatarain-Barrón ZL, et al. Comprehensive review of fetal adenocarcinoma of the lung. Lung Cancer (Auckl). 2018 Aug 23;9:57–63. PMID:30197546
2476. Rice D, Chansky K, Nowak A, et al. The IASLC Mesothelioma Staging Project: proposals for revisions of the N descriptors in the forthcoming eighth edition of the TNM classification for pleural mesothelioma. J Thorac Oncol. 2016 Dec;11(12):2100–11. PMID:27687964
2477. Richardson SE, Sudak J, Warbey V, et al. Routine bone marrow biopsy is not necessary in the staging of patients with classical Hodgkin lymphoma in the 18F-fluoro-2-deoxyglucose positron emission tomography era. Leuk Lymphoma. 2012 Mar;53(3):381–5. PMID:21877882
2478. Ricordel C, Friboulet L, Facchinetti F, et al. Molecular mechanisms of acquired resistance to third-generation EGFR-TKIs in EGFR T790M-mutant lung cancer. Ann Oncol. 2018 Jan 1;29(suppl_1):i28–37. PMID:29462256
2479. Rieger M, Österborg A, Pettengell R, et al. Primary mediastinal B-cell lymphoma treated with CHOP-like chemotherapy with or without rituximab: results of the Mabthera International Trial Group study. Ann Oncol. 2011 Mar;22(3):664–70. PMID:20724576
2480. Rieker RJ, Aulmann S, Penzel R, et al. Chromosomal imbalances in sporadic neuroendocrine tumours of the thymus. Cancer Lett. 2005 Jun 1;223(1):169–74. PMID:15890250
2481. Rieker RJ, Quentmeier A, Weiss C, et al. Cystic lymphangioma of the small-bowel mesentery: case report and a review of the literature. Pathol Oncol Res. 2000;6(2):146–8. PMID:10936792
2482. Rieker RJ, Schirmacher P, Schnabel PA, et al. Thymolipoma. A report of nine cases, with emphasis on its association with myasthenia gravis. Surg Today. 2010;40(2):132–6. PMID:20107952
2483. Righi L, Graziano P, Fornari A, et al. Immunohistochemical subtyping of nonsmall cell lung cancer not otherwise specified in fine-needle aspiration cytology: a retrospective study of 103 cases with surgical correlation. Cancer. 2011 Aug 1;117(15):3416–23. PMID:21246522
2484. Righi L, Vavalà T, Rapa I, et al. Impact of non-small-cell lung cancer-not otherwise specified immunophenotyping on treatment outcome. J Thorac Oncol. 2014 Oct;9(10):1540–6. PMID:25521399
2485. Righi L, Volante M, Rapa I, et al. Therapeutic biomarkers in lung neuroendocrine neoplasia. Endocr Pathol. 2014 Dec;25(4):371–7. PMID:25252622
2486. Riihimäki M, Thomsen H, Sundquist K, et al. Clinical landscape of cancer metastases. Cancer Med. 2018 Nov;7(11):5534–42. PMID:30328287
2487. Rikova K, Guo A, Zeng Q, et al. Global survey of phosphotyrosine signaling identifies oncogenic kinases in lung cancer. Cell. 2007 Dec 14;131(6):1190–203. PMID:18083107
2488. Rimner A, Yao X, Huang J, et al. Postoperative radiation therapy is associated with longer overall survival in completely resected stage II and III thymoma-an analysis of the International Thymic Malignancies Interest Group retrospective database. J Thorac Oncol. 2016 Oct;11(10):1785–92. PMID:27346413
2489. Rindi G, Klersy C, Inzani F, et al. Grading the neuroendocrine tumors of the lung: an evidence-based proposal. Endocr Relat Cancer. 2013 Dec 16;21(1):1–16. PMID:24344249
2490. Rindi G, Klimstra DS, Abedi-Ardekani B, et al. A common classification framework for neuroendocrine neoplasms: an International Agency for Research on Cancer (IARC) and World Health Organization (WHO) expert consensus proposal. Mod Pathol. 2018 Dec;31(12):1770–86. PMID:30140036
2491. Ríos JC, Chávarri F, Morales G, et al. Cardiac myxoma with prenatal diagnosis. World J Pediatr Congenit Heart Surg. 2013 Apr;4(2):210–2. PMID:23799738
2492. Ripamonti D, Marini B, Rambaldi A, et al. Treatment of primary effusion lymphoma with highly active antiviral therapy in the setting of HIV infection. AIDS. 2008 Jun 19;22(10):1236–7. PMID:18525275
2493. Ritter JH, Wick MR. Primary carcinomas of the thymus gland. Semin Diagn Pathol. 1999 Feb;16(1):18–31. PMID:10355651
2494. Ritterhouse LL, Vivero M, Mino-Kenudson M, et al. GNAS mutations in primary mucinous and non-mucinous lung adenocarcinomas. Mod Pathol. 2017 Dec;30(12):1720–7. PMID:28776576
2495. Ritterhouse LL, Wu EY, Kim WG, et al. Loss of SMAD4 protein expression in gastrointestinal and extra-gastrointestinal carcinomas. Histopathology. 2019 Oct;75(4):546–51. PMID:31054158
2496. Rittmeyer A, Barlesi F, Waterkamp D, et al. Atezolizumab versus docetaxel in patients with previously treated non-small-cell lung cancer (OAK): a phase 3, open-label, multicentre randomised controlled trial. Lancet. 2017 Jan 21;389(10066):255–65. PMID:27979383
2497. Rivera GA, Wakelee H. Lung cancer in never smokers. Adv Exp Med Biol. 2016;893:43–57. PMID:26667338
2498. Rizvi SM, Goodwill J, Lim E, et al. The frequency of neuroendocrine cell hyperplasia in patients with pulmonary neuroendocrine tumours and non-neuroendocrine cell carcinomas. Histopathology. 2009 Sep;55(3):332–7. PMID:19723148
2499. Rizzardi G, Marulli G, Calabrese F, et al. Bronchial carcinoid tumours in children: surgical treatment and outcome in a single institution. Eur J Pediatr Surg. 2009 Aug;19(4):228–31. PMID:19513967
2500. Robelin P, Hadoux J, Forestier J, et al. Characterization, prognosis, and treatment of patients with metastatic lung carcinoid tumors. J Thorac Oncol. 2019 Jun;14(6):993–1002. PMID:30771520
2501. Robinson DR, Wu YM, Kalyana-Sundaram S, et al. Identification of recurrent NAB2-STAT6 gene fusions in solitary fibrous tumor by integrative sequencing. Nat Genet. 2013 Feb;45(2):180–5. PMID:23313952
2502. Rocha RV, Butany J, Cusimano RJ. Adipose tumors of the heart. J Card Surg. 2018 Aug;33(8):432–7. PMID:29992619
2503. Rod J, Orbach D, Verité C, et al. Surgical management of thymic epithelial tumors in children: lessons from the French Society of Pediatric Oncology and review of the literature. Pediatr Blood Cancer. 2014 Nov;61(11):1910–5. PMID:25130986
2504. Roden AC, Erickson-Johnson MR, Yi ES, et al. Analysis of MAML2 rearrangement in mucoepidermoid carcinoma of the thymus. Hum Pathol. 2013 Dec;44(12):2799–805. PMID:24134933
2505. Roden AC, Fang W, Shen Y, et al. Distribution of mediastinal lesions across multi-institutional, international, radiology databases. J Thorac Oncol. 2020 Apr;15(4):568–79. PMID:31870881
2506. Roden AC, García JJ, Wehrs RN, et al. Histopathologic, immunophenotypic and cytogenetic features of pulmonary mucoepidermoid carcinoma. Mod Pathol. 2014 Nov;27(11):1479–88. PMID:24743219
2507. Roden AC, Greipp PT, Knutson DL, et al. Histopathologic and cytogenetic features of pulmonary adenoid cystic carcinoma. J Thorac Oncol. 2015 Nov;10(11):1570–5. PMID:26309189
2508. Roden AC, Hu X, Kip S, et al. BRAF V600E expression in Langerhans cell histiocytosis: clinical and immunohistochemical study on 25 pulmonary and 54 extrapulmonary cases. Am J Surg Pathol. 2014 Apr;38(4):548–51. PMID:24625419
2509. Rodney AJ, Tannir NM, Siefker-Radtke AO, et al. Survival outcomes for men with mediastinal germ-cell tumors: the University of Texas M. D. Anderson Cancer Center experience. Urol Oncol. 2012 Nov-Dec;30(6):879–85. PMID:20933444
2510. Rodriguez E, Reuter VE, Mies C, et al.

Abnormalities of 2q: a common genetic link between rhabdomyosarcoma and hepatoblastoma? Genes Chromosomes Cancer. 1991 Mar;3(2):122–7. PMID:1676906

2511. Rodriguez EF, Dacic S, Pantanowitz L, et al. Cytopathology of pulmonary adenocarcinoma with a single histological pattern using the proposed International Association for the Study of Lung Cancer/American Thoracic Society/European Respiratory Society (IASLC/ATS/ERS) classification. Cancer Cytopathol. 2015 May;123(5):306–17. PMID:25788465

2512. Rodriguez FJ, Aubry MC, Tazelaar HD, et al. Pulmonary chondroma: a tumor associated with Carney triad and different from pulmonary hamartoma. Am J Surg Pathol. 2007 Dec;31(12):1844–53. PMID:18043038

2512A. Rodríguez M, Mallidi HR, da Silva A, et al. Recurrence of pericardial mesothelioma affecting the myocardium after pericardial resection. Ann Thorac Surg. 2018 Nov;106(5):e243–5. PMID:29792828

2513. Roemer MG, Advani RH, Ligon AH, et al. PD-L1 and PD-L2 genetic alterations define classical Hodgkin lymphoma and predict outcome. J Clin Oncol. 2016 Aug 10;34(23):2690–7. PMID:27069084

2514. Roeser A, Cohen-Aubart F, Breillat P, et al. Autoimmunity associated with Erdheim-Chester disease improves with BRAF/MEK inhibitors. Haematologica. 2019 Nov;104(11):e502–5. PMID:30923093

2515. Rogalla P, Lemke I, Kazmierczak B, et al. An identical HMGIC-LPP fusion transcript is consistently expressed in pulmonary chondroid hamartomas with t(3;12)(q27-28;q14-15). Genes Chromosomes Cancer. 2000 Dec;29(4):363–6. PMID:11066083

2516. Roggli VL. Pericardial mesothelioma after exposure to asbestos. N Engl J Med. 1981 Apr 23;304(17):1045. PMID:7207561

2517. Roh MH. The utilization of cytologic fine-needle aspirates of lung cancer for molecular diagnostic testing. J Pathol Transl Med. 2015 Jul;49(4):300–9. PMID:26076721

2518. Rohani A, Akbari V. A colossal atrial myxoma. J Cardiovasc Dis Res. 2010 Jul;1(3):158–60. PMID:21187871

2519. Roller MB, Manoharan A, Lvoff R. Primary cardiac lymphoma. Acta Haematol. 1991;85(1):47–8. PMID:2011932

2520. Roma A, Varsegi M, Magi-Galluzzi C, et al. The distinction of bronchogenic cyst from metastatic testicular teratoma: a light microscopic and immunohistochemical study. Am J Clin Pathol. 2008 Aug;130(2):265–73. PMID:18628097

2521. Ronchi A, Cozzolino I, Montella M, et al. Extragonadal germ cell tumors: not just a matter of location. A review about clinical, molecular and pathological features. Cancer Med. 2019 Nov;8(16):6832–40. PMID:31568647

2522. Rooper LM, Bishop JA, Westra WH. INSM1 is a sensitive and specific marker of neuroendocrine differentiation in head and neck tumors. Am J Surg Pathol. 2018 May;42(5):665–71. PMID:29438167

2523. Rooper LM, Sharma R, Li QK, et al. INSM1 demonstrates superior performance to the individual and combined use of synaptophysin, chromogranin and CD56 for diagnosing neuroendocrine tumors of the thoracic cavity. Am J Surg Pathol. 2017 Nov;41(11):1561–9. PMID:28719469

2524. Roper N, Gao S, Maity TK, et al. APOBEC mutagenesis and copy-number alterations are drivers of proteogenomic tumor evolution and heterogeneity in metastatic thoracic tumors. Cell Rep. 2019 Mar 5;26(10):2651–2666.e6. PMID:30840888

2525. Roque L, Oliveira P, Martins C, et al. A non-balanced translocation (10;16) demonstrated

by FISH analysis in a case of alveolar adenoma of the lung. Cancer Genet Cytogenet. 1996 Jul 1;89(1):34–7. PMID:8689607

2526. Rosado-de-Christenson ML, Pugatch RD, Moran CA, et al. Thymolipoma: analysis of 27 cases. Radiology. 1994 Oct;193(1):121–6. PMID:8090879

2527. Rosado-de-Christenson ML, Strollo DC, Marom EM. Imaging of thymic epithelial neoplasms. Hematol Oncol Clin North Am. 2008 Jun;22(3):409–31. PMID:18514124

2528. Rosado-de-Christenson ML, Templeton PA, Moran CA. From the archives of the AFIP. Mediastinal germ cell tumors: radiologic and pathologic correlation. Radiographics. 1992 Sep;12(5):1013–30. PMID:1326777

2529. Rosai J, Levine GD. Tumors of the thymus. Washington, DC: Armed Forces Institute of Pathology; 1976. (AFIP atlas of tumor pathology, series 2; fascicle 13).

2530. Rosell R, Carcereny E, Gervais R, et al. Erlotinib versus standard chemotherapy as first-line treatment for European patients with advanced EGFR mutation-positive non-small-cell lung cancer (EURTAC): a multicentre, open-label, randomised phase 3 trial. Lancet Oncol. 2012 Mar;13(3):239–46. PMID:22285168

2531. Rosen EY, Goldman DA, Hechtman JF, et al. TRK fusions are enriched in cancers with uncommon histologies and the absence of canonical driver mutations. Clin Cancer Res. 2020 Apr 1;26(7):1624–32. PMID:31871300

2532. Rosen LE, Karrison T, Ananthanarayanan V, et al. Nuclear grade and necrosis predict prognosis in malignant epithelioid pleural mesothelioma: a multi-institutional study. Mod Pathol. 2018 Apr;31(4):598–606. PMID:29327706

2533. Rosenbaum DG, Teruya-Feldstein J, Price AP, et al. Radiologic features of NUT midline carcinoma in an adolescent. Pediatr Radiol. 2012 Feb;42(2):249–52. PMID:22057302

2534. Rosenthal R, Cadieux EL, Salgado R, et al. Neoantigen-directed immune escape in lung cancer evolution. Nature. 2019 Mar;567(7749):479–85. PMID:30894752

2535. Rosenwald A, Wright G, Leroy K, et al. Molecular diagnosis of primary mediastinal B cell lymphoma identifies a clinically favorable subgroup of diffuse large B cell lymphoma related to Hodgkin lymphoma. J Exp Med. 2003 Sep 15;198(6):851–62. PMID:12975453

2536. Roslyn JJ, Gordon HE, Mulder DG. Mediastinal parathyroid adenomas. A cause of persistent hyperparathyroidism. Am Surg. 1983 Oct;49(10):523–7. PMID:6678542

2537. Rossi G, Bertero L, Marchiò C, et al. Molecular alterations of neuroendocrine tumours of the lung. Histopathology. 2018 Jan;72(1):142–52. PMID:29239031

2538. Rossi G, Cadioli A, Mengoli MC, et al. Napsin A expression in pulmonary sclerosing haemangioma. Histopathology. 2012 Jan;60(2):361–3. PMID:22074388

2539. Rossi G, Cavazza A, Marchioni A, et al. Role of chemotherapy and the receptor tyrosine kinases KIT, PDGFRalpha, PDGFRbeta, and Met in large-cell neuroendocrine carcinoma of the lung. J Clin Oncol. 2005 Dec 1;23(34):8774–85. PMID:16314638

2540. Rossi G, Cavazza A, Righi L, et al. Napsin-A, TTF-1, EGFR, and ALK status determination in lung primary and metastatic mucin-producing adenocarcinomas. Int J Surg Pathol. 2014 Aug;22(5):401–7. PMID:24651909

2541. Rossi G, Cavazza A, Spagnolo P, et al. Diffuse idiopathic pulmonary neuroendocrine cell hyperplasia syndrome. Eur Respir J. 2016 Jun;47(6):1829–41. PMID:27076588

2542. Rossi G, Cavazza A, Sturm N, et al. Pulmonary carcinomas with pleomorphic, sarcomatoid, or sarcomatous elements: a

clinicopathologic and immunohistochemical study of 75 cases. Am J Surg Pathol. 2003 Mar;27(3):311–24. PMID:12604887

2543. Rossi G, Marchioni A, Milani M, et al. TTF-1, cytokeratin 7, 34betaE12, and CD56/NCAM immunostaining in the subclassification of large cell carcinomas of the lung. Am J Clin Pathol. 2004 Dec;122(6):884–93. PMID:15595193

2544. Rossi G, Mengoli MC, Cavazza A, et al. Large cell carcinoma of the lung: clinically oriented classification integrating immunohistochemistry and molecular biology. Virchows Arch. 2014 Jan;464(1):61–8. PMID:24221342

2545. Rossi G, Murer B, Cavazza A, et al. Primary mucinous (so-called colloid) carcinomas of the lung: a clinicopathologic and immunohistochemical study with special reference to CDX-2 homeobox gene and MUC2 expression. Am J Surg Pathol. 2004 Apr;28(4):442–52. PMID:15087663

2546. Rossi G, Pelosi G, Barbareschi M, et al. Subtyping non-small cell lung cancer: relevant issues and operative recommendations for the best pathology practice. Int J Surg Pathol. 2013 Aug;21(4):326–36. PMID:23740564

2547. Rossi S, Fletcher CD. Angiosarcoma arising in hemangioma/vascular malformation: report of four cases and review of the literature. Am J Surg Pathol. 2002 Oct;26(10):1319–29. PMID:12360047

2548. Rossi S, Orvieto E, Furlanetto A, et al. Utility of the immunohistochemical detection of FLI-1 expression in round cell and vascular neoplasm using a monoclonal antibody. Mod Pathol. 2004 May;17(5):547–52. PMID:15001993

2549. Rossi V, Donini M, Sergio P, et al. When a thymic carcinoma "becomes" a GIST. Lung Cancer. 2013 Apr;80(1):106–8. PMID:23375402

2550. Rosti G, Secondino S, Necchi A, et al. Primary mediastinal germ cell tumors. Semin Oncol. 2019 Apr;46(2):107–11. PMID:31076171

2551. Roszik J, Khan A, Conley AP, et al. Unique aberrations in intimal sarcoma identified by next-generation sequencing as potential therapy targets. Cancers (Basel). 2019 Aug 31;11(9):E1283. PMID:31480474

2552. Rothstein DH, Voss SD, Isakoff M, et al. Thymoma in a child: case report and review of the literature. Pediatr Surg Int. 2005 Jul;21(7):548–51. PMID:15926048

2553. Rotstein DL, Bril V. A family with myasthenia gravis with and without thymoma. Can J Neurol Sci. 2012 Jul;39(4):539–40. PMID:22728868

2554. Rouquette I, Taranchon-Clermont E, Gilhodes J, et al. Immune biomarkers in thymic epithelial tumors: expression patterns, prognostic value and comparison of diagnostic tests for PD-L1. Biomark Res. 2019 Dec 4;7:28. PMID:31827799

2555. Roux FJ, Lantuéjoul S, Brambilla E, et al. Mucinous cystadenoma of the lung. Cancer. 1995 Nov 1;76(9):1540–4. PMID:8635055

2556. Roviaro G, Montorsi M, Varoli F, et al. Primary pulmonary tumours of neurogenic origin. Thorax. 1983 Dec;38(12):942–5. PMID:6665754

2557. Rowsell C, Sirbovan J, Rosenblum MK, et al. Primary chordoid meningioma of lung. Virchows Arch. 2005 Mar;446(3):333–7. PMID:15714337

2558. Roxas RBS, Bernardo MCF, Jacoba AP, et al. Primary thymic signet ring cell adenocarcinoma: a currently unrecognized variant. Int J Surg Pathol. 2019 May;27(3):315–21. PMID:30259765

2559. Ruan SY, Chen KY, Yang PC. Recurrent respiratory papillomatosis with pulmonary involvement: a case report and review of the literature. Respirology. 2009 Jan;14(1):137–40.

PMID:19144058

2560. Ruano R, Takashi E, Schultz R, et al. Prenatal diagnosis of posterior mediastinal lymphangioma by two- and three-dimensional ultrasonography. Ultrasound Obstet Gynecol. 2008 Jun;31(6):697–700. PMID:18435512

2561. Rubin MA, Snell JA, Tazelaar HD, et al. Cardiac papillary fibroelastoma: an immunohistochemical investigation and unusual clinical manifestations. Mod Pathol. 1995 May;8(4):402–7. PMID:7567939

2562. Rudin CM, Avila-Tang E, Harris CC, et al. Lung cancer in never smokers: molecular profiles and therapeutic implications. Clin Cancer Res. 2009 Sep 15;15(18):5646–61. PMID:19755392

2563. Rudin CM, Durinck S, Stawiski EW, et al. Comprehensive genomic analysis identifies SOX2 as a frequently amplified gene in small-cell lung cancer. Nat Genet. 2012 Oct;44(10):1111–6. PMID:22941189

2564. Rudin CM, Poirier JT, Byers LA, et al. Molecular subtypes of small cell lung cancer: a synthesis of human and mouse model data. Nat Rev Cancer. 2019 May;19(5):289–97. PMID:30926931

2565. Rudzinski ER, Anderson JR, Chi YY, et al. Histology, fusion status, and outcome in metastatic rhabdomyosarcoma: a report from the Children's Oncology Group. Pediatr Blood Cancer. 2017 Dec;64(12):10.1002/pbc.26645. PMID:28521080

2566. Ruffini E, Detterbeck F, Van Raemdonck D, et al. Thymic carcinoma: a cohort study of patients from the European Society of Thoracic Surgeons database. J Thorac Oncol. 2014 Apr;9(4):541–8. PMID:24736078

2567. Ruffini E, Fang W, Guerrera F, et al. The International Association for the Study of Lung Cancer Thymic Tumors Staging Project: the impact of the eighth edition of the Union for International Cancer Control and American Joint Committee on Cancer TNM stage classification of thymic tumors. J Thorac Oncol. 2020 Mar;15(3):436–47. PMID:31783179

2568. Rusch A, Ziltener G, Nackaerts K, et al. Prevalence of BRCA-1 associated protein 1 germline mutation in sporadic malignant pleural mesothelioma cases. Lung Cancer. 2015 Jan;87(1):77–9. PMID:25468148

2569. Rusch VW. Extrapleural pneumonectomy and extended pleurectomy/decortication for malignant pleural mesothelioma: the Memorial Sloan-Kettering Cancer Center approach. Ann Cardiothorac Surg. 2012 Nov;1(4):523–31. PMID:23977547

2570. Rusch VW, Chansky K, Kindler HL, et al. The IASLC Mesothelioma Staging Project: proposals for the M descriptors and for revision of the TNM stage groupings in the forthcoming (eighth) edition of the TNM classification for mesothelioma. J Thorac Oncol. 2016 Dec;11(12):2112–9. PMID:27687962

2571. Rusch VW, Gill R, Mitchell A, et al. A multicenter study of volumetric computed tomography for staging malignant pleural mesothelioma. Ann Thorac Surg. 2016 Oct;102(4):1059–66. PMID:27596916

2572. Rusch VW, Giroux D. Do we need a revised staging system for malignant pleural mesothelioma? Analysis of the IASLC database. Ann Cardiothorac Surg. 2012 Nov;1(4):438–48. PMID:23977534

2573. Rusch VW, Giroux D, Kennedy C, et al. Initial analysis of the International Association for the Study of Lung Cancer mesothelioma database. J Thorac Oncol. 2012 Nov;7(11):1631–9. PMID:23070243

2574. Rusch VW, Rimner A, Krug LM. The challenge of malignant pleural mesothelioma: new directions. J Thorac Oncol. 2014 Mar;9(3):271–2. PMID:24518084

2575. Rusner C, Trabert B, Katalinic A, et al. Incidence patterns and trends of malignant gonadal and extragonadal germ cell tumors in Germany, 1998-2008. Cancer Epidemiol. 2013 Aug;37(4):370–3. PMID:23683844
2576. Russell CF, Edis AJ, Scholz DA, et al. Mediastinal parathyroid tumors: experience with 38 tumors requiring mediastinotomy for removal. Ann Surg. 1981 Jun;193(6):805–9. PMID:7247524
2577. Russell PA, Barnett SA, Walkiewicz M, et al. Correlation of mutation status and survival with predominant histologic subtype according to the new IASLC/ATS/ERS lung adenocarcinoma classification in stage III (N2) patients. J Thorac Oncol. 2013 Apr;8(4):461–8. PMID:23486266
2578. Russell PA, Rogers TM, Solomon B, et al. Correlation between molecular analysis, diagnosis according to the 2015 WHO classification of unresected lung tumours and TTF1 expression in small biopsies and cytology specimens from 344 non-small cell lung carcinoma patients. Pathology. 2017 Oct;49(6):604–10. PMID:28811082
2579. Russell PA, Wainer Z, Wright GM, et al. Does lung adenocarcinoma subtype predict patient survival?: A clinicopathologic study based on the new International Association for the Study of Lung Cancer/American Thoracic Society/European Respiratory Society international multidisciplinary lung adenocarcinoma classification. J Thorac Oncol. 2011 Sep;6(9):1496–504. PMID:21642859
2580. Rychik J, Khalek N, Gaynor JW, et al. Fetal intrapericardial teratoma: natural history and management including successful in utero surgery. Am J Obstet Gynecol. 2016 Dec;215(6):780.e1–7. PMID:27530489
2581. Ryu HS, Koh JS, Park S, et al. Classification of thymoma by fine needle aspiration biopsy according to WHO classification: a cytological algorithm for stepwise analysis in the classification of thymoma. Acta Cytol. 2012;56(5):487–94. PMID:23075888
2581A. Ryu JH, Moss J, Beck GJ, et al. The NHLBI lymphangioleiomyomatosis registry: characteristics of 230 patients at enrollment. Am J Respir Crit Care Med. 2006 Jan 1;173(1):105–11. PMID:16210669
2582. Ryu YJ, Yoo SH, Jung MJ, et al. Embryonal rhabdomyosarcoma arising from a mediastinal teratoma: an unusual case report. J Korean Med Sci. 2013 Mar;28(3):476–9. PMID:23487585
2583. Saad ED, Paoletti X, Burzykowski T, et al. Precision medicine needs randomized clinical trials. Nat Rev Clin Oncol. 2017 May;14(5):317–23. PMID:28169302
2584. Saad RS, Silverman JF. Respiratory cytology: differential diagnosis and pitfalls. Diagn Cytopathol. 2010 Apr;38(4):297–307. PMID:19856422
2585. Saarinen S, Kaasinen E, Karjalainen-Lindsberg ML, et al. Primary mediastinal large B-cell lymphoma segregating in a family: exome sequencing identifies MLL as a candidate predisposition gene. Blood. 2013 Apr 25;121(17):3428–30. PMID:23457195
2586. Saccomanno G, Archer VE, Auerbach O, et al. Development of carcinoma of the lung as reflected in exfoliated cells. Cancer. 1974 Jan;33(1):256–70. PMID:4810100
2587. Saccomanno G, Saunders RP, Archer VE, et al. Cancer of the lung: the cytology of sputum prior to the development of carcinoma. Acta Cytol. 1965 Nov-Dec;9(6):413–23. PMID:5218351
2588. Sadler DW, Coghill SB. Histopathologists, malignancies, and undefined high-power fields. Lancet. 1989 Apr 8;1(8641):785–6. PMID:2564592
2589. Saglietti C, Volante M, La Rosa S, et al. Cytology of primary salivary gland-type tumors of the lower respiratory tract: report of 15 cases and review of the literature. Front Med (Lausanne). 2017 Apr 24;4:43. PMID:28484699
2590. Saha K, Sit NK, Jash D, et al. Diagnosis of sclerosing hemangioma of lung: don't rely on fine-needle aspiration cytology diagnosis alone. J Cancer Res Ther. 2013 Oct-Dec;9(4):748–50. PMID:24518736
2591. Sahn SA. Pleural diseases related to metastatic malignancies. Eur Respir J. 1997 Aug;10(8):1907–13. PMID:9272937
2592. Said JW, Shintaku IP, Asou H, et al. Herpesvirus 8 inclusions in primary effusion lymphoma: report of a unique case with T-cell phenotype. Arch Pathol Lab Med. 1999 Mar;123(3):257–60. PMID:10086517
2593. Saito A, Watanabe K, Kusakabe T, et al. Mediastinal mature teratoma with coexistence of angiosarcoma, granulocytic sarcoma and a hematopoietic region in the tumor: a rare case of association between hematological malignancy and mediastinal germ cell tumor. Pathol Int. 1998 Sep;48(9):749–53. PMID:9778115
2594. Saito T, Kimoto M, Nakai S, et al. Ectopic ACTH syndrome associated with large cell neuroendocrine carcinoma of the thymus. Intern Med. 2011;50(14):1471–5. PMID:21757832
2595. Sak SD, Koseoglu RD, Demirag F, et al. Alveolar adenoma of the lung. Immunohistochemical and flow cytometric characteristics of two new cases and a review of the literature. APMIS. 2007 Dec;115(12):1443–9. PMID:18184418
2596. Sakakibara A, Inagaki Y, Imaoka E, et al. Divergence and heterogeneity of neoplastic PD-L1 expression: two autopsy case reports of intravascular large B-cell lymphoma. Pathol Int. 2019 Mar;69(3):148–54. PMID:30688388
2597. Sakakibara A, Kohno K, Iwakoshi A, et al. Diagnostic utility of programmed cell death ligand 1 (clone SP142) in mediastinal composite lymphoma: a report of two cases. Pathol Int. 2020 Feb;70(2):116–22. PMID:31894883
2598. Sakakura N, Tateyama H, Nakamura S, et al. Diagnostic reproducibility of thymic epithelial tumors using the World Health Organization classification: note for thoracic clinicians. Gen Thorac Cardiovasc Surg. 2013 Feb;61(2):89–95. PMID:23229995
2599. Sakakura N, Tateyama H, Usami N, et al. Thymic basaloid carcinoma with pleural dissemination that developed after a curative resection: report of a case. Surg Today. 2010 Nov;40(11):1073–8. PMID:21046508
2600. Sakamoto H, Sakamaki T, Sumino H, et al. Production of endothelin-1 and big endothelin-1 by human cardiac myxoma cells–implications of the origin of myxomas–. Circ J. 2004 Dec;68(12):1230–2. PMID:15564714
2601. Sakamoto H, Shimizu J, Horio Y, et al. Disproportionate representation of KRAS gene mutation in atypical adenomatous hyperplasia, but even distribution of EGFR gene mutation from preinvasive to invasive adenocarcinomas. J Pathol. 2007 Jul;212(3):287–94. PMID:17534846
2602. Sakamoto I, Tomiyama N, Sugita A, et al. A case of sclerosing hemangioma surrounded by emphysematous change. Radiat Med. 2004 Mar-Apr;22(2):123–5. PMID:15176609
2603. Sakane T, Murase T, Okuda K, et al. A comparative study of PD-L1 immunohistochemical assays with four reliable antibodies in thymic carcinoma. Oncotarget. 2018 Jan 8;9(6):6993–7009. PMID:29467945
2604. Sakane T, Murase T, Okuda K, et al. A mutation analysis of the EGFR pathway genes, RAS, EGFR, PIK3CA, AKT1 and BRAF, and TP53 gene in thymic carcinoma and thymoma type A/B3. Histopathology. 2019 Nov;75(5):755–66. PMID:31179560
2605. Sakane T, Okuda K, Hattori H, et al. Blastomatoid pulmonary carcinosarcoma: a rare case report and review of the literature. Thorac Cancer. 2018 Oct;9(10):1323–6. PMID:30106243
2606. Sakanoue I, Hamakawa H, Fujimoto D, et al. KRAS mutation-positive mucinous adenocarcinoma originating in the thymus. J Thorac Dis. 2017 Aug;9(8):E694–7. PMID:28932588
2607. Sakharpe A, Lahat G, Gulamhusein T, et al. Epithelioid sarcoma and unclassified sarcoma with epithelioid features: clinicopathological variables, molecular markers, and a new experimental model. Oncologist. 2011;16(4):512–22. PMID:21357725
2608. Sakuma F, Tsuchida K, Minaguchi T, et al. A rare case of pulmonary lepidic metastasis in patient with branch-type intraductal papillary mucinous carcinoma of the pancreas. Clin J Gastroenterol. 2019 Dec;12(6):621–5. PMID:31123981
2609. Sakurai A, Imai T, Kikumori T, et al. Thymic neuroendocrine tumour in multiple endocrine neoplasia type 1: female patients are not rare exceptions. Clin Endocrinol (Oxf). 2013 Feb;78(2):248–54. PMID:22690831
2610. Sakurai H, Hasegawa T, Watanabe Si, et al. Inflammatory myofibroblastic tumor of the lung. Eur J Cardiothorac Surg. 2004 Feb;25(2):155–9. PMID:14747105
2611. Sakurai H, Kaji M, Yamazaki K, et al. Intrathoracic lipomas: their clinicopathological behaviors are not as straightforward as expected. Ann Thorac Surg. 2008 Jul;86(1):261–5. PMID:18573434
2612. Sakurai H, Miyashita Y, Oyama T. Adenocarcinoma arising in anterior mediastinal mature cystic teratoma: report of a case. Surg Today. 2008;38(4):348–51. PMID:18368326
2613. Salazar MC, Rosen JE, Arnold BN, et al. Adjuvant chemotherapy for T3 non-small cell lung cancer with additional tumor nodules in the same lobe. J Thorac Oncol. 2016 Jul;11(7):1090–100. PMID:27013407
2614. Salem A, Bell D, Sepesi B, et al. Clinicopathologic and genetic features of primary bronchopulmonary mucoepidermoid carcinoma: the MD Anderson Cancer Center experience and comprehensive review of the literature. Virchows Arch. 2017 Jun;470(6):619–26. PMID:28343305
2615. Sales LM, Vontz FK. Teratoma and Di Guglielmo syndrome. South Med J. 1970 Apr;63(4):448–50. PMID:5265820
2616. Salpea P, Horvath A, London E, et al. Deletions of the PRKAR1A locus at 17q24.2-q24.3 in Carney complex: genotype-phenotype correlations and implications for genetic testing. J Clin Endocrinol Metab. 2014 Jan;99(1):E183–8. PMID:24170103
2617. Salvador-Coloma C, Saigí M, Díaz-Beveridge R, et al. Identification of actionable genetic targets in primary cardiac sarcomas. Onco Targets Ther. 2019 Nov 7;12:9265–75. PMID:31807008
2618. Samaniego F, Rodriguez E, Houldsworth J, et al. Cytogenetic and molecular analysis of human male germ cell tumors: chromosome 12 abnormalities and gene amplification. Genes Chromosomes Cancer. 1990 Mar;1(4):289–300. PMID:2177638
2619. Sammassimo S, Pruneri G, Andreola G, et al. A retrospective international study on primary extranodal marginal zone lymphoma of the lung (BALT lymphoma) on behalf of International Extranodal Lymphoma Study Group (IELSG). Hematol Oncol. 2016 Dec;34(4):177–83. PMID:26152851
2620. Sands JM, Nguyen T, Shivdasani P, et al. Next-generation sequencing informs diagnosis and identifies unexpected therapeutic targets in lung squamous cell carcinomas. Lung Cancer. 2020 Feb;140:35–41. PMID:31855703
2621. Sane AC, Roggli VL. Curative resection of a well-differentiated papillary mesothelioma of the pericardium. Arch Pathol Lab Med. 1995 Mar;119(3):266–7. PMID:7887781
2622. Sanfilippo R, Miceli R, Grosso F, et al. Myxofibrosarcoma: prognostic factors and survival in a series of patients treated at a single institution. Ann Surg Oncol. 2011 Mar;18(3):720–5. PMID:20878245
2623. Sangoi AR, McKenney JK, Schwartz EJ, et al. Adenomatoid tumors of the female and male genital tracts: a clinicopathological and immunohistochemical study of 44 cases. Mod Pathol. 2009 Sep;22(9):1228–35. PMID:19543245
2624. Santagata S, Ligon KL, Hornick JL. Embryonic stem cell transcription factor signatures in the diagnosis of primary and metastatic germ cell tumors. Am J Surg Pathol. 2007 Jun;31(6):836–45. PMID:17527070
2625. Santangeli P, Pieroni M, Marzo F, et al. Cardiac myxoma presenting with sensory neuropathy. Int J Cardiol. 2010 Aug 6;143(1):e14–6. PMID:19162348
2626. Santillan A, Knopman J, Patsalides A, et al. Delayed intracranial aneurysm formation after cardiac myxoma resection: report of two cases and review of the literature. Interv Neuroradiol. 2019 Apr;25(2):177–81. PMID:30394840
2627. Santos C, Montesinos J, Castañer E, et al. Primary pericardial mesothelioma. Lung Cancer. 2008 May;60(2):291–3. PMID:17936406
2628. Saqi A, Shaham D, Scognamiglio T, et al. Incidence and cytological features of pulmonary hamartomas indeterminate on CT scan. Cytopathology. 2008 Jun;19(3):185–91. PMID:17388933
2629. Saraya T, Fujiwara M, Kimura H, et al. A 17-year-old woman with a solitary, mixed squamous cell and glandular papilloma of the bronchus. Respirol Case Rep. 2018 Nov 30;7(2):e00393. PMID:30519472
2630. Sarkaria IS, Bains MS, Sood S, et al. Resection of primary mediastinal non-seminomatous germ cell tumors: a 28-year experience at memorial sloan-kettering cancer center. J Thorac Oncol. 2011 Jul;6(7):1236–41. PMID:21610519
2631. Sarkaria IS, Iyoda A, Roh MS, et al. Neoadjuvant and adjuvant chemotherapy in resected pulmonary large cell neuroendocrine carcinomas: a single institution experience. Ann Thorac Surg. 2011 Oct;92(4):1180–6, discussion 1186–7. PMID:21867986
2632. Sarkozy C, Copie-Bergman C, Damotte D, et al. Gray-zone lymphoma between cHL and large B-cell lymphoma: a histopathologic series from the LYSA. Am J Surg Pathol. 2019 Mar;43(3):341–51. PMID:30540571
2633. Sarkozy C, Molina T, Ghesquières H, et al. Mediastinal gray zone lymphoma: clinico-pathological characteristics and outcomes of 99 patients from the Lymphoma Study Association. Haematologica. 2017 Jan;102(1):150–9. PMID:27758822
2634. Saruwatari K, Ikemura S, Sekihara K, et al. Aggressive tumor microenvironment of solid predominant lung adenocarcinoma subtype harboring with epidermal growth factor receptor mutations. Lung Cancer. 2016 Jan;91:7–14. PMID:26711928
2635. Sasajima Y, Yamabe H, Kobashi Y, et al. High expression of the Epstein-Barr virus latent protein EB nuclear antigen-2 on pyothorax-associated lymphomas. Am J Pathol. 1993 Nov;143(5):1280–5. PMID:8238246
2636. Sasaki Y, Minamiya Y, Okuyama M, et al. [A case of lung cancer with skin metastases responding to erlotinib]. Gan To Kagaku

Ryoho. 2011 Feb;38(2):271–4. Japanese. PMID:21368493

2637. Satish OS, Aditya MS, Rao MA, et al. Sporadic cardiac myxoma involving all the cardiac chambers. Circulation. 2013 Jan 29;127(4):e360–1. PMID:23357665

2638. Sato S, Koike T, Yamato Y, et al. Resected well-differentiated fetal pulmonary adenocarcinoma and summary of 25 cases reported in Japan. Jpn J Thorac Cardiovasc Surg. 2006 Dec;54(12):539–42. PMID:17236658

2639. Satoh H, Takayashiki N, Shiozawa T, et al. Recurrent pulmonary synovial sarcoma effectively treated with amrubicin: a case report. Exp Ther Med. 2015 May;9(5):1947–9. PMID:26136920

2640. Satoh Y, Tsuchiya E, Weng SY, et al. Pulmonary sclerosing hemangioma of the lung. A type II pneumocytoma by immunohistochemical and immunoelectron microscopic studies. Cancer. 1989 Sep 15;64(6):1310–7. PMID:2548701

2641. Sattar N, Durrance R, Khan A, et al. Malignant mesothelioma presenting as recurrent hydro-pneumothorax: an atypical case presentation and literature review. Respir Med Case Rep. 2018 Feb 24;23:152–5. PMID:29719805

2642. Satturwar S, Malenie R, Sutton A, et al. Validation of immunohistochemical tests performed on cytology cell block material: practical application of the College of American Pathologists' guidelines. Cytojournal. 2019 Mar 15;16:6. PMID:31031816

2643. Sauter JL, Graham RP, Larsen BT, et al. SMARCA4-deficient thoracic sarcoma: a distinctive clinicopathological entity with undifferentiated rhabdoid morphology and aggressive behavior. Mod Pathol. 2017 Oct;30(10):1422–32. PMID:28643792

2643A. Sauter JL, Grogg KL, Vrana JA, et al. Young investigator challenge: validation and optimization of immunohistochemistry protocols for use on cellient cell block specimens. Cancer Cytopathol. 2016 Feb;124(2):89–100. PMID:26882197

2644. Savage KJ, Monti S, Kutok JL, et al. The molecular signature of mediastinal large B-cell lymphoma differs from that of other diffuse large B-cell lymphomas and shares features with classical Hodgkin lymphoma. Blood. 2003 Dec 1;102(12):3871–9. PMID:12933571

2645. Sawabata N, Miyaoka E, Asamura H, et al. Japanese lung cancer registry study of 11,663 surgical cases in 2004: demographic and prognosis changes over decade. J Thorac Oncol. 2011 Jul;6(7):1229–35. PMID:21610521

2646. Sawai T, Inoue Y, Doi S, et al. Tubular adenocarcinoma of the thymus: case report and review of the literature. Int J Surg Pathol. 2006 Jul;14(3):243–6. PMID:16959713

2647. Saygin C, Uzunaslan D, Ozguroglu M, et al. Dendritic cell sarcoma: a pooled analysis including 462 cases with presentation of our case series. Crit Rev Oncol Hematol. 2013 Nov;88(2):253–71. PMID:23755890

2648. Sbrana F, Mannucci F, Airò E, et al. Cardiac tamponade due to apixaban therapy in patient with unknown pericardial hemangioma. Intern Emerg Med. 2018 Mar;13(2):297–9. PMID:28803417

2648A. Scagliotti G, Brodowicz T, Shepherd FA, et al. Treatment-by-histology interaction analyses in three phase III trials show superiority of pemetrexed in nonsquamous non-small cell lung cancer. J Thorac Oncol. 2011 Jan;6(1):64–70. PMID:21119545

2649. Schaefer IM, Dong F, Garcia EP, et al. Recurrent SMARCB1 inactivation in epithelioid malignant peripheral nerve sheath tumors. Am J Surg Pathol. 2019 Jun;43(6):835–43. PMID:30864974

2650. Schaefer IM, Fletcher CD. Myxoid variant of so-called angiomatoid "malignant fibrous histiocytoma": clinicopathologic characterization in a series of 21 cases. Am J Surg Pathol. 2014 Jun;38(6):816–23. PMID:24503754

2651. Schaefer IM, Fletcher CD, Hornick JL. Loss of H3K27 trimethylation distinguishes malignant peripheral nerve sheath tumors from histologic mimics. Mod Pathol. 2016 Jan;29(1):4–13. PMID:26585554

2652. Schaefer IM, Sahlmann CO, Overbeck T, et al. Blastomatoid pulmonary carcinosarcoma: report of a case with a review of the literature. BMC Cancer. 2012 Sep 25;12:424. PMID:23006472

2653. Schaefer IM, Zardo P, Freermann S, et al. Neuroendocrine carcinoma in a mediastinal teratoma as a rare variant of somatic-type malignancy. Virchows Arch. 2013 Nov;463(5):731–5. PMID:23979407

2654. Schaffer BE, Park KS, Yiu G, et al. Loss of p130 accelerates tumor development in a mouse model for human small-cell lung carcinoma. Cancer Res. 2010 May 15;70(10):3877–83. PMID:20406986

2655. Schalper KA, Brown J, Carvajal-Hausdorf D, et al. Objective measurement and clinical significance of TILs in non-small cell lung cancer. J Natl Cancer Inst. 2015 Feb 3;107(3):dju435. PMID:25650315

2656. Scherpereel A, Astoul P, Baas P, et al. [Guidelines of the European Respiratory Society and the European Society of Thoracic Surgeons for the management of malignant pleural mesothelioma]. Zhongguo Fei Ai Za Zhi. 2010 Oct;13(10):C23–45. Chinese. PMID:20976998

2657. Schiavetti A, Indolfi P, Hill DA, et al. Primary pulmonary rhabdomyosarcoma in childhood: clinico-biologic features in two cases with review of the literature–erratum. Pediatr Blood Cancer. 2009 Jan;52(1):146. PMID:18802940

2658. Schimke RN, Madigan CM, Silver BJ, et al. Choriocarcinoma, thyrotoxicosis, and the Klinefelter syndrome. Cancer Genet Cytogenet. 1983 May;9(1):1–7. PMID:6682351

2659. Schirosi L, Nannini N, Nicoli D, et al. Activating c-KIT mutations in a subset of thymic carcinoma and response to different c-KIT inhibitors. Ann Oncol. 2012 Sep;23(9):2409–14. PMID:22357254

2660. Schirosi L, Nannini N, Nicoli D, et al. Activating c-KIT mutations in a subset of thymic carcinoma and response to different c-KIT inhibitors. Ann Oncol. 2012 Sep;23(9):2409–14. PMID:22357254

2661. Schleiermacher G, Mosseri V, London WB, et al. Segmental chromosomal alterations have prognostic impact in neuroblastoma: a report from the INRG project. Br J Cancer. 2012 Oct 9;107(8):1418–22. PMID:22976801

2662. Schmaltz AA, Apitz J. Primary rhabdomyosarcoma of the heart. Pediatr Cardiol. 1982;2(1):73–5. PMID:7063430

2663. Schmidt LA, Myers JL, McHugh JB. Napsin A is differentially expressed in sclerosing hemangiomas of the lung. Arch Pathol Lab Med. 2012 Dec;136(12):1580–4. PMID:23194051

2664. Schmidt RL, Witt BL, Lopez-Calderon LE, et al. The influence of rapid onsite evaluation on the adequacy rate of fine-needle aspiration cytology: a systematic review and meta-analysis. Am J Clin Pathol. 2013 Mar;139(3):300–8. PMID:23429365

2665. Schmitz R, Hansmann ML, Bohle V, et al. TNFAIP3 (A20) is a tumor suppressor gene in Hodgkin lymphoma and primary mediastinal B cell lymphoma. J Exp Med. 2009 May 11;206(5):981–9. PMID:19380639

2666. Schmitz R, Wright GW, Huang DW, et al. Genetics and pathogenesis of diffuse large B-cell lymphoma. N Engl J Med. 2018 Apr 12;378(15):1396–407. PMID:29641966

2667. Schneider BJ, Saxena A, Downey RJ. Surgery for early-stage small cell lung cancer. J Natl Compr Canc Netw. 2011 Oct;9(10):1132–9. PMID:21975913

2668. Schneider DT, Calaminus G, Koch S, et al. Epidemiologic analysis of 1,442 children and adolescents registered in the German germ cell tumor protocols. Pediatr Blood Cancer. 2004 Feb;42(2):169–75. PMID:14752882

2669. Schneider DT, Calaminus G, Reinhard H, et al. Primary mediastinal germ cell tumors in children and adolescents: results of the German cooperative protocols MAKEI 83/86, 89, and 96. J Clin Oncol. 2000 Feb;18(4):832–9. PMID:10673525

2670. Schneider DT, Schuster AE, Fritsch MK, et al. Genetic analysis of childhood germ cell tumors with comparative genomic hybridization. Klin Padiatr. 2001 Jul-Aug;213(4):204–11. PMID:11528555

2671. Schneider DT, Schuster AE, Fritsch MK, et al. Genetic analysis of mediastinal nonseminomatous germ cell tumors in children and adolescents. Genes Chromosomes Cancer. 2002 May;34(1):115–25. PMID:11921289

2672. Schneider DT, Schuster AE, Fritsch MK, et al. Multipoint imprinting analysis indicates a common precursor cell for gonadal and nongonadal pediatric germ cell tumors. Cancer Res. 2001 Oct 1;61(19):7268–76. PMID:11585765

2673. Schneider F, Derrick V, Davison JM, et al. Morphological and molecular approach to synchronous non-small cell lung carcinomas: impact on staging. Mod Pathol. 2016 Jul;29(7):735–42. PMID:27080983

2674. Schoenmakers EF, Wanschura S, Mols R, et al. Recurrent rearrangements in the high mobility group protein gene, HMGI-C, in benign mesenchymal tumours. Nat Genet. 1995 Aug;10(4):436–44. PMID:7670494

2675. Scholten ET, Kreel L. Distribution of lung metastases in the axial plane. A combined radiological-pathological study. Radiol Clin (Basel). 1977;46(4):248–65. PMID:195302

2676. Schrader AMR, Jansen PM, Willemze R, et al. High prevalence of MYD88 and CD79B mutations in intravascular large B-cell lymphoma. Blood. 2018 May 3;131(18):2086–9. PMID:29514783

2677. Schrader KA, Nelson TN, De Luca A, et al. Multiple granular cell tumors are an associated feature of LEOPARD syndrome caused by mutation in PTPN11. Clin Genet. 2009 Feb;75(2):185–9. PMID:19054014

2678. Schrock AB, Frampton GM, Suh J, et al. Characterization of 298 patients with lung cancer harboring MET exon 14 skipping alterations. J Thorac Oncol. 2016 Sep;11(9):1493–502. PMID:27343443

2679. Schrock AB, Li SD, Frampton GM, et al. Pulmonary sarcomatoid carcinomas commonly harbor either potentially targetable genomic alterations or high tumor mutational burden as observed by comprehensive genomic profiling. J Thorac Oncol. 2017 Jun;12(6):932–42. PMID:28315738

2680. Schulte MA, Ramzy I, Greenberg SD. Immunocytochemical characterization of large-cell carcinomas of the lung. Role, limitations and technical considerations. Acta Cytol. 1991 Mar-Apr;35(2):175–80. PMID:1709321

2681. Schwaederle M, Elkin SK, Tomson BN, et al. Squamousness: next-generation sequencing reveals shared molecular features across squamous tumor types. Cell Cycle. 2015;14(14):2355–61. PMID:26030731

2682. Schwartz AM, Henson DE. Analysis of Surveillance, Epidemiology, and End Results database for carcinoid tumors. Chest. 2015 Sep;148(3):e104–5. PMID:26324138

2683. Schwartz BE, Hofer MD, Lemieux ME, et al. Differentiation of NUT midline carcinoma by epigenomic reprogramming. Cancer Res. 2011 Apr 1;71(7):2686–96. PMID:21447744

2684. Schwartz EJ, Longacre TA. Adenomatoid tumors of the female and male genital tracts express WT1. Int J Gynecol Pathol. 2004 Apr;23(2):123–8. PMID:15084840

2685. Schweiger T, Lang G, Klepetko W, et al. Prognostic factors in pulmonary metastasectomy: spotlight on molecular and radiological markers. Eur J Cardiothorac Surg. 2014 Mar;45(3):408–16. PMID:23729747

2686. Schweigert M, Kaiser J, Fuchs T, et al. Thymoma within a giant congenital thymic cyst. Interact Cardiovasc Thorac Surg. 2011 Oct;13(4):442–3. PMID:21788299

2687. Schweizer L, Koelsche C, Sahm F, et al. Meningeal hemangiopericytoma and solitary fibrous tumors carry the NAB2-STAT6 fusion and can be diagnosed by nuclear expression of STAT6 protein. Acta Neuropathol. 2013 May;125(5):651–8. PMID:23575898

2688. Schwering I, Bräuninger A, Klein U, et al. Loss of the B-lineage-specific gene expression program in Hodgkin and Reed-Sternberg cells of Hodgkin lymphoma. Blood. 2003 Feb 15;101(4):1505–12. PMID:12393731

2689. Sclafani LM, Woodruff JM, Brennan MF. Extraadrenal retroperitoneal paragangliomas: natural history and response to treatment. Surgery. 1990 Dec;108(6):1124–9, discussion 1129–30. PMID:2174194

2690. Scott DW, Wright GW, Williams PM, et al. Determining cell-of-origin subtypes of diffuse large B-cell lymphoma using gene expression in formalin-fixed paraffin-embedded tissue. Blood. 2014 Feb 20;123(8):1214–7. PMID:24398326

2691. Sears D, Hajdu SI. The cytologic diagnosis of malignant neoplasms in pleural and peritoneal effusions. Acta Cytol. 1987 Mar-Apr;31(2):85–97. PMID:3469856

2692. Sebenik M, Ricci A Jr, DiPasquale B, et al. Undifferentiated intimal sarcoma of large systemic blood vessels: report of 14 cases with immunohistochemical profile and review of the literature. Am J Surg Pathol. 2005 Sep;29(9):1184–93. PMID:16096408

2693. Secondino S, Grazioli V, Valentino F, et al. Multimodal approach of pulmonary artery intimal sarcoma: a single-institution experience. Sarcoma. 2017;2017:7941432. PMID:28912665

2694. Seeger RC, Brodeur GM, Sather H, et al. Association of multiple copies of the N-myc oncogene with rapid progression of neuroblastomas. N Engl J Med. 1985 Oct 31;313(18):1111–6. PMID:4047115

2695. Segletes LA, Steffee CH, Geisinger KR. Cytology of primary pulmonary mucoepidermoid and adenoid cystic carcinoma. A report of four cases. Acta Cytol. 1999 Nov-Dec;43(6):1091–7. PMID:10578983

2696. Sehested M, Hirsch FR, Osterlind K, et al. Morphologic variations of small cell lung cancer. A histopathologic study of pretreatment and posttreatment specimens in 104 patients. Cancer. 1986 Feb 15;57(4):804–7. PMID:3002587

2697. Sehn LH, Berry B, Chhanabhai M, et al. The revised International Prognostic Index (R-IPI) is a better predictor of outcome than the standard IPI for patients with diffuse large B-cell lymphoma treated with R-CHOP. Blood. 2007 Mar 1;109(5):1857–61. PMID:17105812

2698. Seki M, Yoshida K, Shiraishi Y, et al. Biallelic DICER1 mutations in sporadic pleuropulmonary blastoma. Cancer Res. 2014 May 15;74(10):2742–9. PMID:24675358

2699. Sekimizu M, Sunami S, Nakazawa A, et al. Chromosome abnormalities in advanced stage T-cell lymphoblastic lymphoma of children and adolescents: a report from Japanese Paediatric Leukaemia/Lymphoma Study Group (JPLSG) and review of the literature. Br J Haematol.

2011 Sep;154(5):612–7. PMID:21689091
2700. Sekimizu M, Yoshida A, Mitani S, et al. Frequent mutations of genes encoding vacuolar H+ -ATPase components in granular cell tumors. Genes Chromosomes Cancer. 2019 Jun;58(6):373–80. PMID:30597645
2701. Sekine I, Kodama T, Yokose T, et al. Rare pulmonary tumors - a review of 32 cases. Oncology. 1998 Sep-Oct;55(5):431–4. PMID:9732221
2702. Sekine S, Shibata T, Matsuno Y, et al. Beta-catenin mutations in pulmonary blastomas: association with morule formation. J Pathol. 2003 Jun;200(2):214–21. PMID:12754743
2703. Selby DM, Stocker JT, Ishak KG. Angiosarcoma of the liver in childhood: a clinicopathologic and follow-up study of 10 cases. Pediatr Pathol. 1992 Jul-Aug;12(4):485–98. PMID:1409148
2703A. Selvaggi G, Scagliotti GV. Histologic subtype in NSCLC: Does it matter? Oncology (Williston Park). 2009 Nov 30;23(13):1133–40. PMID:20043461
2704. Sen S, Dişcigil B, Badak I, et al. Lipoma of the diaphragm: a rare presentation. Ann Thorac Surg. 2007 Jun;83(6):2203–5. PMID:17532428
2705. Seo JB, Im JG, Goo JM, et al. Atypical pulmonary metastases: spectrum of radiologic findings. Radiographics. 2001 Mar-Apr;21(2):403–17. PMID:11259704
2706. Seo JS, Lee JW, Kim A, et al. Whole exome and transcriptome analyses integrated with microenvironmental immune signatures of lung squamous cell carcinoma. Cancer Immunol Res. 2018 Jul;6(7):848–59. PMID:29720381
2707. Seol SH, Kim DI, Jang JS, et al. Left atrial myxoma presenting as paroxysmal supraventricular tachycardia. Heart Lung Circ. 2014 Feb;23(2):e65–6. PMID:23891308
2708. Sequist LV, Waltman BA, Dias-Santagata D, et al. Genotypic and histological evolution of lung cancers acquiring resistance to EGFR inhibitors. Sci Transl Med. 2011 Mar 23;3(75):75ra26. PMID:21430269
2709. Sequist LV, Yang JC, Yamamoto N, et al. Phase III study of afatinib or cisplatin plus pemetrexed in patients with metastatic lung adenocarcinoma with EGFR mutations. J Clin Oncol. 2013 Sep 20;31(27):3327–34. PMID:23816960
2709A. Sereno M, He Z, Smith CR, et al. Inclusion of multiple high-risk histopathological criteria improves the prediction of adjuvant chemotherapy efficacy in lung adenocarcinoma. Histopathology. 2020 Nov 6 [Epub ahead of print]. PMID:33155719
2710. Settas N, Faucz FR, Stratakis CA. Succinate dehydrogenase (SDH) deficiency, Carney triad and the epigenome. Mol Cell Endocrinol. 2018 Jul 5;469:107–11. PMID:28739378
2711. Shah AA, Mehrad M, Kelting SM, et al. An uncommon primary lung tumour: hyalinizing clear cell carcinoma, salivary gland-type. Histopathology. 2015 Aug;67(2):274–6. PMID:25545688
2712. Shah MH, Goldner WS, Halfdanarson TR, et al. NCCN Guidelines Insights: Neuroendocrine and Adrenal Tumors, Version 2.2018. J Natl Compr Canc Netw. 2018 Jun;16(6):693–702. PMID:29891520
2713. Shaher RM, Mintzer J, Farina M, et al. Clinical presentation of rhabdomyoma of the heart in infancy and childhood. Am J Cardiol. 1972 Jul 11;30(1):95–103. PMID:4260837
2714. Shahi M, Dolan M, Murugan P. Hyalinizing clear cell carcinoma of the bronchus. Head Neck Pathol. 2017 Dec;11(4):575–9. PMID:28508996
2715. Shanbhag S, Ambinder RF. Hodgkin lymphoma: a review and update on recent progress. CA Cancer J Clin. 2018 Mar;68(2):116–32. PMID:29194581
2716. Shanks JH, Harris M, Banerjee SS, et al. Mesotheliomas with deciduoid morphology: a morphologic spectrum and a variant not confined to young females. Am J Surg Pathol. 2000 Feb;24(2):285–94. PMID:10680897
2717. Shao D, Wang SX. Pericardial solitary fibrous tumor on FDG PET/CT. Clin Nucl Med. 2019 Jan;44(1):85–7. PMID:30371588
2718. Sharma A, DeValeria PA, Scherber RM, et al. Angiosarcoma causing cardiac constriction late after radiation therapy for breast carcinoma. Tex Heart Inst J. 2016 Feb 1;43(1):81–3. PMID:27047293
2719. Sharma P, Jha V, Kumar N, et al. Clinicopathological analysis of mediastinal masses: a mixed bag of non-neoplastic and neoplastic etiologies. Turk Patoloji Derg. 2017;33(1):37–46. PMID:28044305
2720. Sharma S, Gupta N, Rajwanshi A, et al. Inflammatory myofibroblastic tumour: a diagnostic challenge on fine needle aspiration cytology. Cytopathology. 2016 Dec;27(6):512–6. PMID:27087029
2721. Shaw AT, Ou SH, Bang YJ, et al. Crizotinib in ROS1-rearranged non-small-cell lung cancer. N Engl J Med. 2014 Nov 20;371(21):1963–71. PMID:25264305
2722. Shehata BM, Cundiff CA, Lee K, et al. Exome sequencing of patients with histiocytoid cardiomyopathy reveals a de novo NDUFB11 mutation that plays a role in the pathogenesis of histiocytoid cardiomyopathy. Am J Med Genet A. 2015 Sep;167A(9):2114–21. PMID:25921236
2723. Shehata BM, Patterson K, Thomas JE, et al. Histiocytoid cardiomyopathy: three new cases and a review of the literature. Pediatr Dev Pathol. 1998 Jan-Feb;1(1):56–69. PMID:10463272
2724. Shehata BM, Steelman CK, Abramowsky CR, et al. NUT midline carcinoma in a newborn with multiorgan disseminated tumor and a 2-year-old with a pancreatic/hepatic primary. Pediatr Dev Pathol. 2010 Nov-Dec;13(6):481–5. PMID:20017639
2725. Shen C, Wang X, Che G. A rare case of primary peripheral epithelial myoepithelial carcinoma of lung: case report and literature review. Medicine (Baltimore). 2016 Aug;95(35):e4371. PMID:27583848
2726. Shen J, Fang Z, Zhang Y, et al. Primary cardiac dedifferentiated liposarcoma in a middle-aged female: a case report. J Cardiothorac Surg. 2019 Aug 30;14(1):156. PMID:31470882
2727. Sheppard MN, Burke L, Kennedy M. TTF-1 is useful in the diagnosis of pulmonary papillary adenoma. Histopathology. 2003 Oct;43(4):404–5. PMID:14511264
2728. Shern JF, Chen L, Chmielecki J, et al. Comprehensive genomic analysis of rhabdomyosarcoma reveals a landscape of alterations affecting a common genetic axis in fusion-positive and fusion-negative tumors. Cancer Discov. 2014 Feb;4(2):216–31. PMID:24436047
2729. Shern JF, Yohe ME, Khan J. Pediatric rhabdomyosarcoma. Crit Rev Oncog. 2015;20(3-4):227–43. PMID:26349418
2730. Shetty Roy AN, Radin M, Sarabi D, et al. Familial recurrent atrial myxoma: Carney's complex. Clin Cardiol. 2011 Feb;34(2):83–6. PMID:21298650
2731. Shewale JB, Mitchell KG, Nelson DB, et al. Predictors of survival after resection of primary sarcomas of the chest wall-A large, single-institution series. J Surg Oncol. 2018 Sep;118(3):518–24. PMID:30109699
2732. Shi J, Bai ZX, Zhang BG, et al. Papillary fibroelastoma of the aortic valve in association with rheumatic heart disease: a case report. J Cardiothorac Surg. 2016 Jan 16;11:6. PMID:26772603
2733. Shi Y, Bing Z, Xu X, et al. Primary pulmonary malignant melanoma: case report and literature review. Thorac Cancer. 2018 Sep;9(9):1185–9. PMID:30062692
2734. Shia J, Qin J, Erlandson RA, et al. Malignant mesothelioma with a pronounced myxoid stroma: a clinical and pathological evaluation of 19 cases. Virchows Arch. 2005 Nov;447(5):828–34. PMID:16021506
2735. Shiba S, Imaoka H, Shioji K, et al. Clinical characteristics of Japanese patients with epithelioid hemangioendothelioma: a multicenter retrospective study. BMC Cancer. 2018 Oct 19;18(1):993. PMID:30340559
2736. Shibusa T, Shijubo N, Abe S. Tumor angiogenesis and vascular endothelial growth factor expression in stage I lung adenocarcinoma. Clin Cancer Res. 1998 Jun;4(6):1483–7. PMID:9626466
2737. Shibuya K, Hoshino H, Chiyo M, et al. High magnification bronchovideoscopy combined with narrow band imaging could detect capillary loops of angiogenic squamous dysplasia in heavy smokers at high risk for lung cancer. Thorax. 2003 Nov;58(11):989–95. PMID:14586056
2738. Shibuya K, Nakajima T, Fujiwara T, et al. Narrow band imaging with high-resolution bronchovideoscopy: a new approach for visualizing angiogenesis in squamous cell carcinoma of the lung. Lung Cancer. 2010 Aug;69(2):194–202. PMID:20541831
2739. Shields TW. Surgical technics in the diagnosis of intrathoracic disease. SD J Med Pharm. 1961 Oct;14:379–84. PMID:14039213
2740. Shields WE. Lesions masquerading as primary mediastinal tumors or cysts. In: Shields TW, LoCicero J, Reed CE, et al., editors. General thoracic surgery. Volume 2. 7th ed. Philadelphia (PA): Lippincott Williams & Wilkins; 2009. pp. 2201–23.
2741. Shih AR, Uruga H, Bozkurtlar E, et al. Problems in the reproducibility of classification of small lung adenocarcinoma: an international interobserver study. Histopathology. 2019 Nov;75(5):649–59. PMID:31107973
2742. Shilo K, Foss RD, Franks TJ, et al. Pulmonary mucoepidermoid carcinoma with prominent tumor-associated lymphoid proliferation. Am J Surg Pathol. 2005 Mar;29(3):407–11. PMID:15725811
2743. Shim HS, Kenudson M, Zheng Z, et al. Unique genetic and survival characteristics of invasive mucinous adenocarcinoma of the lung. J Thorac Oncol. 2015 Aug;10(8):1156–62. PMID:26200269
2744. Shimada H, Ambros IM, Dehner LP, et al. Terminology and morphologic criteria of neuroblastic tumors: recommendations by the International Neuroblastoma Pathology Committee. Cancer. 1999 Jul 15;86(2):349–63. PMID:10421272
2745. Shimada H, Ambros IM, Dehner LP, et al. The International Neuroblastoma Pathology Classification (the Shimada system). Cancer. 1999 Jul 15;86(2):364–72. PMID:10421273
2746. Shimada K, Kinoshita T, Naoe T, et al. Presentation and management of intravascular large B-cell lymphoma. Lancet Oncol. 2009 Sep;10(9):895–902. PMID:19717091
2747. Shimada K, Matsue K, Yamamoto K, et al. Retrospective analysis of intravascular large B-cell lymphoma treated with rituximab-containing chemotherapy as reported by the IVL Study Group in Japan. J Clin Oncol. 2008 Jul 1;26(19):3189–95. PMID:18506023
2748. Shimazaki H, Aida S, Sato M, et al. Lung carcinoma with rhabdoid cells: a clinicopathological study and survival analysis of 14 cases. Histopathology. 2001 May;38(5):425–34. PMID:11422479
2749. Shimizu J, Arano Y, Murata T, et al. A case of intrathoracic giant malignant peripheral nerve sheath tumor in neurofibromatosis type I (von Recklinghausen's disease). Ann Thorac Cardiovasc Surg. 2008 Feb;14(1):42–7. PMID:18292741
2750. Shin BK, Kim MK, Park SH, et al. Fine-needle aspiration cytology of pleuropulmonary blastoma: a case report with unusual features. Diagn Cytopathol. 2001 Dec;25(6):397–402. PMID:11747237
2751. Shin J, Vincent JG, Cuda JD, et al. Sox10 is expressed in primary melanocytic neoplasms of various histologies but not in fibrohistiocytic proliferations and histiocytoses. J Am Acad Dermatol. 2012 Oct;67(4):717–26. PMID:22325460
2752. Shin SJ, Dodd-Eaton EB, Peng G, et al. Penetrance of different cancer types in families with Li-Fraumeni syndrome: a validation study using multicenter cohorts. Cancer Res. 2020 Jan 15;80(2):354–60. PMID:31719101
2753. Shin SY, Kim MY, Oh SY, et al. Pulmonary sclerosing pneumocytoma of the lung: CT characteristics in a large series of a tertiary referral center. Medicine (Baltimore). 2015 Jan;94(4):e498. PMID:25634202
2753A. Shinozaki-Ushiku A, Ushiku T, Morita S, et al. Diagnostic utility of BAP1 and EZH2 expression in malignant mesothelioma. Histopathology. 2017 Apr;70(5):722–33. PMID:27859460
2754. Shiono S, Ishii G, Nagai K, et al. Histopathologic prognostic factors in resected colorectal lung metastases. Ann Thorac Surg. 2005 Jan;79(1):278–82, discussion 283. PMID:15620957
2755. Shiono S, Matsutani N, Okumura S, et al. The prognostic impact of lymph-node dissection on lobectomy for pulmonary metastasis. Eur J Cardiothorac Surg. 2015 Oct;48(4):616–21, discussion 621. PMID:25605827
2756. Shiota H, Elya JE, Alekseyenko AA, et al. "Z4" complex member fusions in NUT carcinoma: implications for a novel oncogenic mechanism. Mol Cancer Res. 2018 Dec;16(12):1826–33. PMID:30139738
2756A. Shirsat H, Zhou F, Chang JC, et al. Bronchiolar adenoma/pulmonary ciliated muconodular papillary tumor. Am J Clin Pathol. 2020 Dec 14 [Epub ahead of print]. PMID:33313677
2757. Shlien A, Tabori U, Marshall CR, et al. Excessive genomic DNA copy number variation in the Li-Fraumeni cancer predisposition syndrome. Proc Natl Acad Sci U S A. 2008 Aug 12;105(32):11264–9. PMID:18685109
2758. Sholl LM. Large-cell carcinoma of the lung: a diagnostic category redefined by immunohistochemistry and genomics. Curr Opin Pulm Med. 2014 Jul;20(4):324–31. PMID:24811836
2759. Sholl LM, Aisner DL, Varella-Garcia M, et al. Multi-institutional oncogenic driver mutation analysis in lung adenocarcinoma: the Lung Cancer Mutation Consortium experience. J Thorac Oncol. 2015 May;10(5):768–77. PMID:25738220
2760. Sholl LM, Do K, Shivdasani P, et al. Institutional implementation of clinical tumor profiling on an unselected cancer population. JCI Insight. 2016 Nov 17;1(19):e87062. PMID:27882345
2760A. Sholl LM, Long KB, Hornick JL. Sox2 expression in pulmonary non-small cell and neuroendocrine carcinomas. Appl Immunohistochem Mol Morphol. 2010 Jan;18(1):55–61. PMID:19661786
2761. Sholl LM, Nishino M, Pokharel S, et al. Primary pulmonary NUT midline carcinoma: clinical, radiographic, and pathologic characterizations. J Thorac Oncol. 2015 Jun;10(6):951–9. PMID:26001144
2762. Sholl LM, Yeap BY, Iafrate AJ, et al. Lung adenocarcinoma with EGFR amplification has

distinct clinicopathologic and molecular features in never-smokers. Cancer Res. 2009 Nov 1;69(21):8341–8. PMID:19826035
2763. Shrestha R, Nabavi N, Lin YY, et al. BAP1 haploinsufficiency predicts a distinct immunogenic class of malignant peritoneal mesothelioma. Genome Med. 2019 Feb 18;11(1):8. PMID:30777124
2764. Sica G, Wagner PL, Altorki N, et al. Immunohistochemical expression of estrogen and progesterone receptors in primary pulmonary neuroendocrine tumors. Arch Pathol Lab Med. 2008 Dec;132(12):1889–95. PMID:19061285
2765. Sickles EA, Belliveau RE, Wiernik PH. Primary mediastinal choriocarcinoma in the male. Cancer. 1974 Apr;33(4):1196–203. PMID:4856444
2766. Siddiqui S, Connelly T, Keita L, et al. Thymic carcinoma presenting as atypical chest pain. BMJ Case Rep. 2015 Nov 25;2015:bcr2015211374. PMID:26607199
2767. Sidwell RU, Rouse P, Owen RA, et al. Granular cell tumor of the scrotum in a child with Noonan syndrome. Pediatr Dermatol. 2008 May-Jun;25(3):341–3. PMID:18577039
2768. Siegal GP, Dehner LP, Rosai J. Histiocytosis X (Langerhans' cell granulomatosis) of the thymus. A clinicopathologic study of four childhood cases. Am J Surg Pathol. 1985 Feb;9(2):117–24. PMID:3883820
2769. Siegel RJ, Bueso-Ramos C, Cohen C, et al. Pulmonary blastoma with germ cell (yolk sac) differentiation: report of two cases. Mod Pathol. 1991 Sep;4(5):566–70. PMID:1722041
2770. Siegel RL, Miller KD, Jemal A. Cancer statistics, 2020. CA Cancer J Clin. 2020 Jan;70(1):7–30. PMID:31912902
2771. Sievers S, Alemazkour K, Zahn S, et al. IGF2/H19 imprinting analysis of human germ cell tumors (GCTs) using the methylation-sensitive single-nucleotide primer extension method reflects the origin of GCTs in different stages of primordial germ cell development. Genes Chromosomes Cancer. 2005 Nov;44(3):256–64. PMID:16001432
2772. Sigel CS, Moreira AL, Travis WD, et al. Subtyping of non-small cell lung carcinoma: a comparison of small biopsy and cytology specimens. J Thorac Oncol. 2011 Nov;6(11):1849–56. PMID:21841504
2773. Sim JK, Chung SM, Choi JH, et al. Clinical and molecular characteristics of pulmonary sarcomatoid carcinoma. Korean J Intern Med. 2018 Jul;33(4):737–44. PMID:29458244
2774. Simbolo M, Barbi S, Fassan M, et al. Gene expression profiling of lung atypical carcinoids and large cell neuroendocrine carcinomas identifies three transcriptomic subtypes with specific genomic alterations. J Thorac Oncol. 2019 Sep;14(9):1651–61. PMID:31085341
2775. Simbolo M, Mafficini A, Sikora KO, et al. Lung neuroendocrine tumours: deep sequencing of the four World Health Organization histotypes reveals chromatin-remodelling genes as major players and a prognostic role for TERT, RB1, MEN1 and KMT2D. J Pathol. 2017 Mar;241(4):488–500. PMID:27873319
2776. Simonato L, Agudo A, Ahrens W, et al. Lung cancer and cigarette smoking in Europe: an update of risk estimates and an assessment of inter-country heterogeneity. Int J Cancer. 2001 Mar 15;91(6):876–87. PMID:11275995
2777. Simpson L, Kumar SK, Okuno SH, et al. Malignant primary cardiac tumors: review of a single institution experience. Cancer. 2008 Jun;112(11):2440–6. PMID:18428209
2778. Singh Ospina N, Thompson GB, C Nichols F 3rd, et al. Thymic and bronchial carcinoid tumors in multiple endocrine neoplasia type 1: the Mayo Clinic experience from 1977 to 2013. Horm Cancer. 2015 Dec;6(5-6):247–53. PMID:26070346
2779. Sioletic S, Dal Cin P, Fletcher CD, et al. Well-differentiated and dedifferentiated liposarcomas with prominent myxoid stroma: analysis of 56 cases. Histopathology. 2013 Jan;62(2):287–93. PMID:23020289
2780. Siontis BL, Leja M, Chugh R. Current clinical management of primary cardiac sarcoma. Expert Rev Anticancer Ther. 2020 Jan;20(1):45–51. PMID:31914831
2781. Siontis BL, Zhao L, Leja M, et al. Primary cardiac sarcoma: a rare, aggressive malignancy with a high propensity for brain metastases. Sarcoma. 2019 Mar 10;2019:1960593. PMID:30962762
2782. Sirajuddin A, Raparia K, Lewis VA, et al. Primary pulmonary lymphoid lesions: radiologic and pathologic findings. Radiographics. 2016 Jan-Feb;36(1):53–70. PMID:26761531
2783. Sirvent N, Coindre JM, Maire G, et al. Detection of MDM2-CDK4 amplification by fluorescence in situ hybridization in 200 paraffin-embedded tumor samples: utility in diagnosing adipocytic lesions and comparison with immunohistochemistry and real-time PCR. Am J Surg Pathol. 2007 Oct;31(10):1476–89. PMID:17895748
2784. Sivakumar S, Lucas FAS, McDowell TL, et al. Genomic landscape of atypical adenomatous hyperplasia reveals divergent modes to lung adenocarcinoma. Cancer Res. 2017 Nov 15;77(22):6119–30. PMID:28951454
2785. Sivakumar S, San Lucas FA, Jakubek YA, et al. Genomic landscape of allelic imbalance in premalignant atypical adenomatous hyperplasias of the lung. EBioMedicine. 2019 Apr;42:296–303. PMID:30905849
2786. Skalidis EI, Parthenakis FI, Zacharis EA, et al. Pulmonary tumor embolism from primary cardiac B-cell lymphoma. Chest. 1999 Nov;116(5):1489–90. PMID:10559123
2787. Skapek SX, Ferrari A, Gupta AA, et al. Rhabdomyosarcoma. Nat Rev Dis Primers. 2019 Jan 7;5(1):1. PMID:30617281
2788. Sklair-Levy M, Polliack A, Shaham D, et al. CT-guided core-needle biopsy in the diagnosis of mediastinal lymphoma. Eur Radiol. 2000;10(5):714–8. PMID:10823620
2789. Skov BG, Clementsen P, Larsen KR, et al. The prevalence of ALK rearrangement in pulmonary adenocarcinomas in an unselected Caucasian population from a defined catchment area: impact of smoking. Histopathology. 2017 May;70(6):889–95. PMID:27943404
2790. Smadhi H, Boudaya MS, Abdannadher M, et al. Pulmonary sarcomatoid carcinoma: a surgical diagnosis and prognostic factors. Tunis Med. 2019 Jan;97(1):128–32. PMID:31535704
2791. Smith CJ, Perfetti TA, Garg R, et al. IARC carcinogens reported in cigarette mainstream smoke and their calculated log P values. Food Chem Toxicol. 2003 Jun;41(6):807–17. PMID:12738186
2792. Smith M, Chaudhry MA, Lozano P, et al. Cardiac myxoma induced paraneoplastic syndromes: a review of the literature. Eur J Intern Med. 2012 Dec;23(8):669–73. PMID:23122392
2793. Smith SC, Palanisamy N, Betz BL, et al. At the intersection of primary pulmonary myxoid sarcoma and pulmonary angiomatoid fibrous histiocytoma: observations from three new cases. Histopathology. 2014 Jul;65(1):144–6. PMID:24372335
2794. Smith SC, Poznanski AA, Fullen DR, et al. CD34-positive superficial myxofibrosarcoma: a potential diagnostic pitfall. J Cutan Pathol. 2013 Jul;40(7):639–45. PMID:23600956
2795. Sneddon S, Leon JS, Dick IM, et al. Absence of germline mutations in BAP1 in sporadic cases of malignant mesothelioma. Gene. 2015 May 25;563(1):103–5. PMID:25796603
2796. Snover DC, Levine GD, Rosai J. Thymic carcinoma. Five distinctive histological variants. Am J Surg Pathol. 1982 Jul;6(5):451–70. PMID:7125053
2797. Soda M, Choi YL, Enomoto M, et al. Identification of the transforming EML4-ALK fusion gene in non-small-cell lung cancer. Nature. 2007 Aug 2;448(7153):561–6. PMID:17625570
2798. Soeberg MJ, Leigh J, van Zandwijk N. Malignant mesothelioma in Australia 2015: current incidence and asbestos exposure trends. J Toxicol Environ Health B Crit Rev. 2016;19(5-6):173–89. PMID:27705544
2799. Soerensen TR, Raedkjaer M, Jørgensen PH, et al. Soft tissue sarcomas of the thoracic wall: more prone to higher mortality, and local recurrence-A single institution long-term follow-up study. Int J Surg Oncol. 2019 Mar 4;2019:2350157. PMID:30956820
2800. Soga J, Yakuwa Y. Bronchopulmonary carcinoids: an analysis of 1,875 reported cases with special reference to a comparison between typical carcinoids and atypical varieties. Ann Thorac Cardiovasc Surg. 1999 Aug;5(4):211–9. PMID:10508944
2801. Soga J, Yakuwa Y, Osaka M. Evaluation of 342 cases of mediastinal/thymic carcinoids collected from literature: a comparative study between typical carcinoids and atypical varieties. Ann Thorac Cardiovasc Surg. 1999 Oct;5(5):285–92. PMID:10550713
2802. Sogge MR, McDonald SD, Cofold PB. The malignant potential of the dysgenetic germ cell in Klinefelter's syndrome. Am J Med. 1979 Mar;66(3):515–8. PMID:571203
2803. Soh J, Toyooka S, Ichihara S, et al. Sequential molecular changes during multistage pathogenesis of small peripheral adenocarcinomas of the lung. J Thorac Oncol. 2008 Apr;3(4):340–7. PMID:18379350
2804. Sökücü SN, Kocatürk C, Urer N, et al. Evaluation of six patients with pulmonary carcinosarcoma with a literature review. ScientificWorldJournal. 2012;2012:167317. PMID:22619609
2805. Sokullu O, Sanioglu S, Deniz H, et al. Primary cardiac rhabdomyosarcoma of the right atrium: case report. Heart Surg Forum. 2008;11(2):E117–9. PMID:18430653
2806. Solé F, Bosch F, Woessner S, et al. Refractory anemia with excess of blasts and isochromosome 12p in a patient with primary mediastinal germ-cell tumor. Cancer Genet Cytogenet. 1994 Oct 15;77(2):111–3. PMID:7954319
2807. Soler-Soler J, Romero-González R. Calcified intramural fibroma of the left ventricle. Eur J Cardiol. 1975 Jun;3(1):71–3. PMID:1132411
2808. Solomon BJ, Mok T, Kim DW, et al. First-line crizotinib versus chemotherapy in ALK-positive lung cancer. N Engl J Med. 2014 Dec 4;371(23):2167–77. PMID:25470694
2809. Sommeling C, Santens P. Anti-N-methyl-D-aspartate (anti-NMDA) receptor antibody encephalitis in a male adolescent with a large mediastinal teratoma. J Child Neurol. 2014 May;29(5):688–90. PMID:24563471
2810. Song DH, Choi IH, Ha SY, et al. Epithelial-myoepthelial carcinoma of the tracheobronchial tree: the prognostic role of myoepithelial cells. Lung Cancer. 2014 Mar;83(3):416–9. PMID:24485468
2811. Song HJ, Qiu ZL, Shen CT, et al. Pulmonary metastases in differentiated thyroid cancer: efficacy of radioiodine therapy and prognostic factors. Eur J Endocrinol. 2015 Sep;173(3):399–408. PMID:26104753
2812. Song JS, Kim D, Kwon JH, et al. Clinicopathologic significance and immunogenomic analysis of programmed death-ligand 1 (PD-L1) and programmed death 1 (PD-1) expression in thymic epithelial tumors. Front Oncol. 2019 Oct 15;9:1055. PMID:31681591
2813. Song JY, Pittaluga S, Dunleavy K, et al. Lymphomatoid granulomatosis–a single institute experience: pathologic findings and clinical correlations. Am J Surg Pathol. 2015 Feb;39(2):141–56. PMID:25321327
2814. Sonobe H, Ohtsuki Y, Nakayama H, et al. A thymic squamous cell carcinoma with complex chromosome abnormalities. Cancer Genet Cytogenet. 1998 May;103(1):83–5. PMID:9595055
2815. Sonobe H, Takeuchi T, Ohtsuki Y, et al. A thymoma with clonal complex chromosome abnormalities. Cancer Genet Cytogenet. 1999 Apr;110(1):72–4. PMID:10198628
2816. Sonzogni A, Bianchi F, Fabbri A, et al. Pulmonary adenocarcinoma with mucin production modulates phenotype according to common genetic traits: a reappraisal of mucinous adenocarcinoma and colloid adenocarcinoma. J Pathol Clin Res. 2017 Mar 22;3(2):139–52. PMID:28451462
2817. Soo RA, Stone ECA, Cummings KM, et al. Scientific advances in thoracic oncology 2016. J Thorac Oncol. 2017 Aug;12(8):1183–209. PMID:28579481
2818. Sordillo PP, Epremian B, Koziner B, et al. Lymphomatoid granulomatosis: an analysis of clinical and immunologic characteristics. Cancer. 1982 May 15;49(10):2070–6. PMID:6978760
2819. Sorrell AD, Espenschied CR, Culver JO, et al. Tumor protein p53 (TP53) testing and Li-Fraumeni syndrome : current status of clinical applications and future directions. Mol Diagn Ther. 2013 Feb;17(1):31–47. PMID:23355100
2820. Souhami RL, Bradbury I, Geddes DM, et al. Prognostic significance of laboratory parameters measured at diagnosis in small cell carcinoma of the lung. Cancer Res. 1985 Jun;45(6):2878–82. PMID:2985256
2820A. Soura E, Eliades PJ, Shannon K, et al. Hereditary melanoma: update on syndromes and management: emerging melanoma cancer complexes and genetic counseling. J Am Acad Dermatol. 2016 Mar;74(3):411–20. PMID:26892651
2821. Sousa V, Espírito Santo J, Silva M, et al. EGFR/erB-1, HER2/erB-2, CK7, LP34, Ki67 and P53 expression in preneoplastic lesions of bronchial epithelium: an immunohistochemical and genetic study. Virchows Arch. 2011 May;458(5):571–81. PMID:21424799
2822. Souza FF, Fennessy FM, Yang Q, et al. Case report. PET/CT appearance of desmoid tumour of the chest wall. Br J Radiol. 2010 Feb;83(986):e39–42. PMID:20139256
2823. Sowithayasakul P, Sinlapamongkolkul P, Treetipsatit J, et al. Hematologic malignancies associated with mediastinal germ cell tumors: 10 years' experience at Thailand's National Pediatric Tertiary Referral Center. J Pediatr Hematol Oncol. 2018 Aug;40(6):450–5. PMID:29864110
2824. Sozzi G, Pastorino U, Moiraghi L, et al. Loss of FHIT function in lung cancer and preinvasive bronchial lesions. Cancer Res. 1998 Nov 15;58(22):5032–7. PMID:9823304
2825. Spartalis M, Tzatzaki E, Spartalis E, et al. Primary cardiac intimal sarcoma masquerading as mitral stenosis. Clin Case Rep. 2017 Jul 14;5(8):1422–3. PMID:28781875
2826. Specht K, Sung YS, Zhang L, et al. Distinct transcriptional signature and immunoprofile of CIC-DUX4 fusion-positive round cell tumors compared to EWSR1-rearranged Ewing sarcomas: further evidence toward distinct pathologic entities. Genes Chromosomes Cancer. 2014 Jul;53(7):622–33. PMID:24723486
2827. Specht K, Zhang L, Sung YS, et al. Novel BCOR-MAML3 and ZC3H7B-BCOR gene fusions in undifferentiated small blue round cell sarcomas. Am J Surg Pathol. 2016 Apr;40(4):433–42. PMID:26752546

2828. Speights VO Jr, Dobin SM, Truss LM. A cytogenetic study of a cardiac papillary fibroelastoma. Cancer Genet Cytogenet. 1998 Jun;103(2):167–9. PMID:9614918
2829. Spencer H. The pulmonary plasma cell/histiocytoma complex. Histopathology. 1984 Nov;8(6):903–16. PMID:6098549
2830. Spencer H, Dail DH, Arneaud J. Non-invasive bronchial epithelial papillary tumors. Cancer. 1980 Mar 15;45(6):1486–97. PMID:7357529
2831. Spillane AJ, Thomas JM, Fisher C. Epithelioid sarcoma: the clinicopathological complexities of this rare soft tissue sarcoma. Ann Surg Oncol. 2000 Apr;7(3):218–25. PMID:10791853
2832. Spinelli M, Khorshad J, Viola P. When tumor doesn't read textbook. Third case of TTF1 and p40 co-expression in the same tumour cells in a non-small cell carcinoma. A potential new entity to consider? Pathologica. 2019 Jun;111(2):58–61. PMID:31388196
2833. Sponholz S, Schirren M, Baldes N, et al. Repeat resection for recurrent pulmonary metastasis of colorectal cancer. Langenbecks Arch Surg. 2017 Feb;402(1):77–85. PMID:28058514
2834. Srivali N, Yi ES, Ryu JH. Pulmonary artery sarcoma mimicking pulmonary embolism: a case series. QJM. 2017 May 1;110(5):283–6. PMID:28040708
2835. Srivastava A, Hornick JL. Immunohistochemical staining for CDX-2, PDX-1, NESP-55, and TTF-1 can help distinguish gastrointestinal carcinoid tumors from pancreatic endocrine and pulmonary carcinoid tumors. Am J Surg Pathol. 2009 Apr;33(4):626–32. PMID:19065104
2836. Staats P, Tavora F, Burke AP. Intimal sarcomas of the aorta and iliofemoral arteries: a clinicopathological study of 26 cases. Pathology. 2014 Dec;46(7):596–603. PMID:25393249
2837. Stachowicz-Stencel T, Orbach D, Brecht I, et al. Thymoma and thymic carcinoma in children and adolescents: a report from the European Cooperative Study Group for Pediatric Rare Tumors (EXPeRT). Eur J Cancer. 2015 Nov;51(16):2444–52. PMID:26259494
2838. Stankovic B, Bjørhovde HAK, Skarshaug R, et al. Immune cell composition in human non-small cell lung cancer. Front Immunol. 2019 Feb 1;9:3101. PMID:30774636
2839. Star P, Goodwin A, Kapoor R, et al. Germline BAP1-positive patients: the dilemmas of cancer surveillance and a proposed interdisciplinary consensus monitoring strategy. Eur J Cancer. 2018 Mar;92:48–53. PMID:29413689
2840. Starrett GJ, Luengas EM, McCann JL, et al. The DNA cytosine deaminase APOBEC3H haplotype I likely contributes to breast and lung cancer mutagenesis. Nat Commun. 2016 Sep 21;7:12918. PMID:27650891
2841. Stathis A, Zucca E, Bekradda M, et al. Clinical response of carcinomas harboring the BRD4-NUT oncoprotein to the targeted bromodomain inhibitor OTX015/MK-8628. Cancer Discov. 2016 May;6(5):492–500. PMID:26976114
2842. Stathopoulos GT, Sherrill TP, Karabela SP, et al. Host-derived interleukin-5 promotes adenocarcinoma-induced malignant pleural effusion. Am J Respir Crit Care Med. 2010 Nov 15;182(10):1273–81. PMID:20595227
2843. Staudt LM. The molecular and cellular origins of Hodgkin's disease. J Exp Med. 2000 Jan 17;191(2):207–12. PMID:10637266
2844. Stayner L, Bena J, Sasco AJ, et al. Lung cancer risk and workplace exposure to environmental tobacco smoke. Am J Public Health. 2007 Mar;97(3):545–51. PMID:17267733
2845. Steele KE, Brown C. Multiplex immunohistochemistry for image analysis of tertiary lymphoid structures in cancer. Methods Mol Biol. 2018;1845:87–98. PMID:30141009
2845A. Steelman C, Katzenstein H, Parham D, et al. Unusual presentation of congenital infantile fibrosarcoma in seven infants with molecular-genetic analysis. Fetal Pediatr Pathol. 2011;30(5):329–37. PMID:21843073
2846. Stefanovic A, Morgensztern D, Fong T, et al. Pulmonary marginal zone lymphoma: a single centre experience and review of the SEER database. Leuk Lymphoma. 2008 Jul;49(7):1311–20. PMID:18604720
2847. Steger C, Steiner HJ, Moser K, et al. A typical thymic carcinoid tumour within a thymolipoma: report of a case and review of combined tumours of the thymus. BMJ Case Rep. 2010 Nov 2;2010:bcr0420102958. PMID:22791779
2848. Steidl C, Connors JM, Gascoyne RD. Molecular pathogenesis of Hodgkin's lymphoma: increasing evidence of the importance of the microenvironment. J Clin Oncol. 2011 May 10;29(14):1812–26. PMID:21483001
2849. Steidl C, Gascoyne RD. The molecular pathogenesis of primary mediastinal large B-cell lymphoma. Blood. 2011 Sep 8;118(10):2659–69. PMID:21700770
2850. Steidl C, Shah SP, Woolcock BW, et al. MHC class II transactivator CIITA is a recurrent gene fusion partner in lymphoid cancers. Nature. 2011 Mar 17;471(7338):377–81. PMID:21368758
2851. Stein MG, Mayo J, Müller N, et al. Pulmonary lymphangitic spread of carcinoma: appearance on CT scans. Radiology. 1987 Feb;162(2):371–5. PMID:3797649
2852. Steiropoulos P, Kouliatsis G, Karpathiou G, et al. Rare cases of primary pleural Hodgkin and non-Hodgkin lymphomas. Respiration. 2009;77(4):459–63. PMID:18503251
2853. Stelow EB, Bellizzi AM, Taneja K, et al. NUT rearrangement in undifferentiated carcinomas of the upper aerodigestive tract. Am J Surg Pathol. 2008 Jun;32(6):828–34. PMID:18391746
2854. Stelow EB, French CA. Carcinomas of the upper aerodigestive tract with rearrangement of the nuclear protein of the testis (NUT) gene (NUT midline carcinomas). Adv Anat Pathol. 2009 Mar;16(2):92–6. PMID:19550370
2854A. Stemberger-Papić S, Vrdoljak-Mozetic D, Ostojić DV, et al. Expression of CD133 and CD117 in 64 serous ovarian cancer cases. Coll Antropol. 2015 Sep;39(3):745–53. PMID:26898076
2855. Stéphan JL, Galambrun C, Boucheron S, et al. Epstein-Barr virus–positive undifferentiated thymic carcinoma in a 12-year-old white girl. J Pediatr Hematol Oncol. 2000 Mar-Apr;22(2):162–6. PMID:10779032
2856. Stephens P, Hunter C, Bignell G, et al. Lung cancer: intragenic ERBB2 kinase mutations in tumours. Nature. 2004 Sep 30;431(7008):525–6. PMID:15457249
2857. Stephens PJ, Davies HR, Mitani Y, et al. Whole exome sequencing of adenoid cystic carcinoma. J Clin Invest. 2013 Jul;123(7):2965–8. PMID:23778141
2858. Stephenson TJ, Mills PM. Adenomatoid tumours: an immunohistochemical and ultrastructural appraisal of their histogenesis. J Pathol. 1986 Apr;148(4):327–35. PMID:3517266
2859. Sterlacci W, Fiegl M, Hilbe W, et al. Clinical relevance of neuroendocrine differentiation in non-small cell lung cancer assessed by immunohistochemistry: a retrospective study on 405 surgically resected cases. Virchows Arch. 2009 Aug;455(2):125–32. PMID:19652998
2860. Sterner DJ, Mori M, Roggli VL, et al. Prevalence of pulmonary atypical alveolar cell hyperplasia in an autopsy population: a study of 100 cases. Mod Pathol. 1997 May;10(5):469–73. PMID:9160312
2861. Stevens TM, Morlote D, Xiu J, et al. NUTM1-rearranged neoplasia: a multi-institution experience yields novel fusion partners and expands the histologic spectrum. Mod Pathol. 2019 Jun;32(6):764–73. PMID:30723300
2862. Stewart DR, Best AF, Williams GM, et al. Neoplasm risk among individuals with a pathogenic germline variant in DICER1. J Clin Oncol. 2019 Mar 10;37(8):668–76. PMID:30715996
2863. Stewart PA, Welsh EA, Slebos RJC, et al. Proteogenomic landscape of squamous cell lung cancer. Nat Commun. 2019 Aug 8;10(1):3578. PMID:31395880
2864. Stoll LM, Johnson MW, Gabrielson E, et al. The utility of napsin-A in the identification of primary and metastatic lung adenocarcinoma among cytologically poorly differentiated carcinomas. Cancer Cytopathol. 2010 Dec 25;118(6):441–9. PMID:20830690
2865. Stolz A, Harustiak T, Simonek J, et al. Long-term outcomes and prognostic factors of patients with pulmonary carcinoid tumors. Neoplasma. 2015;62(3):478–83. PMID:25866229
2866. Storck S, Kennedy AL, Marcus KJ, et al. Pediatric NUT-midline carcinoma: therapeutic success employing a sarcoma based multimodal approach. Pediatr Hematol Oncol. 2017 May;34(4):231–7. PMID:29040054
2867. Storm PB, Fallon B, Bunge RG. Mediastinal choriocarcinoma in a chromatin-positive boy. J Urol. 1976 Dec;116(6):838–40. PMID:1034031
2868. Stransky N, Egloff AM, Tward AD, et al. The mutational landscape of head and neck squamous cell carcinoma. Science. 2011 Aug 26;333(6046):1157–60. PMID:21798893
2869. Stratakis CA, Carney JA. The triad of paragangliomas, gastric stromal tumours and pulmonary chondromas (Carney triad), and the dyad of paragangliomas and gastric stromal sarcomas (Carney-Stratakis syndrome): molecular genetics and clinical implications. J Intern Med. 2009 Jul;266(1):43–52. PMID:19522824
2870. Stratakis CA, Kirschner LS, Carney JA. Clinical and molecular features of the Carney complex: diagnostic criteria and recommendations for patient evaluation. J Clin Endocrinol Metab. 2001 Sep;86(9):4041–6. PMID:11549623
2871. Strauchen JA. Indolent T-lymphoblastic proliferation: report of a case with an 11-year history and association with myasthenia gravis. Am J Surg Pathol. 2001 Mar;25(3):411–5. PMID:11224614
2872. Ströbel P, Bargou R, Wolff A, et al. Sunitinib in metastatic thymic carcinomas: laboratory findings and initial clinical experience. Br J Cancer. 2010 Jul 13;103(2):196–200. PMID:20571495
2873. Ströbel P, Bauer A, Puppe B, et al. Tumor recurrence and survival in patients treated for thymomas and thymic squamous cell carcinomas: a retrospective analysis. J Clin Oncol. 2004 Apr 15;22(8):1501–9. PMID:15084623
2874. Ströbel P, Hartmann E, Rosenwald A, et al. Corticomedullary differentiation and maturational arrest in thymomas. Histopathology. 2014 Mar;64(4):557–66. PMID:24236644
2875. Ströbel P, Hartmann M, Jakob A, et al. Thymic carcinoma with overexpression of mutated KIT and the response to imatinib. N Engl J Med. 2004 Jun 17;350(25):2625–6. PMID:15201427
2876. Ströbel P, Helmreich M, Menioudakis G, et al. Paraneoplastic myasthenia gravis correlates with generation of mature naive CD4(+) T cells in thymomas. Blood. 2002 Jul 1;100(1):159–66. PMID:12070022
2877. Ströbel P, Hohenberger P, Marx A. Thymoma and thymic carcinoma: molecular pathology and targeted therapy. J Thorac Oncol. 2010 Oct;5(10 Suppl 4):S286–90. PMID:20859121
2878. Ströbel P, Marino M, Feuchtenberger M, et al. Micronodular thymoma: an epithelial tumour with abnormal chemokine expression setting the stage for lymphoma development. J Pathol. 2005 Sep;207(1):72–82. PMID:15965907
2879. Ströbel P, Rosenwald A, Beyersdorf N, et al. Selective loss of regulatory T cells in thymomas. Ann Neurol. 2004 Dec;56(6):901–4. PMID:15562414
2880. Ströbel P, Zettl A, Shilo K, et al. Tumor genetics and survival of thymic neuroendocrine neoplasms: a multi-institutional clinicopathologic study. Genes Chromosomes Cancer. 2014 Sep;53(9):738–49. PMID:24764238
2881. Strollo DC, Rosado-de-Christenson ML. Primary mediastinal malignant germ cell neoplasms: imaging features. Chest Surg Clin N Am. 2002 Nov;12(4):645–58. PMID:12471868
2882. Strollo DC, Rosado de Christenson ML, Jett JR. Primary mediastinal tumors. Part 1: tumors of the anterior mediastinum. Chest. 1997 Aug;112(2):511–22. PMID:9266892
2883. Stubbins RJ, Alami Laroussi N, Peters AC, et al. Epstein-Barr virus associated smooth muscle tumors in solid organ transplant recipients: incidence over 31 years at a single institution and review of the literature. Transpl Infect Dis. 2019 Feb;21(1):e13010. PMID:30298678
2884. Sturm N, Lantuéjoul S, Laverrière MH, et al. Thyroid transcription factor 1 and cytokeratins 1, 5, 10, 14 (34betaE12) expression in basaloid and large-cell neuroendocrine carcinomas of the lung. Hum Pathol. 2001 Sep;32(9):918–25. PMID:11567220
2885. Sturm N, Rossi G, Lantuéjoul S, et al. 34BetaE12 expression along the whole spectrum of neuroendocrine proliferations of the lung, from neuroendocrine cell hyperplasia to small cell carcinoma. Histopathology. 2003 Feb;42(2):156–66. PMID:12558748
2886. Su PH, Luh SP, Yieh DM, et al. Anterior mediastinal immature teratoma with precocious puberty in a child with Klinefelter syndrome. J Formos Med Assoc. 2005 Aug;104(8):601–4. PMID:16193184
2887. Su XY, Wang WY, Li JN, et al. Immunohistochemical differentiation between type B3 thymomas and thymic squamous cell carcinomas. Int J Clin Exp Pathol. 2015 May 1;8(5):5354–62. PMID:26191237
2888. Subitha K, Thambi R, Sheeja S, et al. Role of imprint cytology in intra-operative diagnosis of an unusual variant of teratoma. J Cytol. 2013 Apr;30(2):148–9. PMID:23833409
2889. Sudour-Bonnange H, Faure-Conter C, Martelli H, et al. Primary mediastinal and retroperitoneal malignant germ cell tumors in children and adolescents: results of the TGM95 trial, a study of the French Society of Pediatric Oncology (Société Française des Cancers de l'Enfant). Pediatr Blood Cancer. 2017 Sep;64(9). PMID:28306215
2890. Suehara Y, Sakata-Yanagimoto M, Hattori K, et al. Liquid biopsy for the identification of intravascular large B-cell lymphoma. Haematologica. 2018 Jun;103(6):e241–4. PMID:29472348
2891. Suemitsu R, Takeo S, Momosaki S, et al. Thymic basaloid carcinoma with aggressive invasion of the lung and pericardium: report of a case. Surg Today. 2011 Jul;41(7):986–8. PMID:21748617
2892. Sugano M, Nagasaka T, Sasaki E, et al. HNF4α as a marker for invasive mucinous adenocarcinoma of the lung. Am J Surg Pathol. 2013 Feb;37(2):211–8. PMID:23108025
2893. Sugio K, Osaki T, Oyama T, et al. Genetic alteration in carcinoid tumors of the lung. Ann Thorac Cardiovasc Surg. 2003 Jun;9(3):149–54. PMID:12875635
2894. Suh JH, Shin OR, Kim YH. Multiple

calcifying fibrous pseudotumor of the pleura. J Thorac Oncol. 2008 Nov;3(11):1356–8. PMID:18978573

2895. Suh YJ, Park CM, Han K, et al. Utility of FDG PET/CT for preoperative staging of non-small cell lung cancers manifesting as subsolid nodules with a solid portion of 3 cm or smaller. AJR Am J Roentgenol. 2020 Mar;214(3):514–23. PMID:31846374

2896. Sumegi J, Streblow R, Frayer RW, et al. Recurrent t(2;2) and t(2;8) translocations in rhabdomyosarcoma without the canonical PAX-FOXO1 fuse PAX3 to members of the nuclear receptor transcriptional coactivator family. Genes Chromosomes Cancer. 2010 Mar;49(3):224–36. PMID:19953635

2897. Sumerauer D, Vicha A, Zuntova A, et al. Teratoma in an adolescent with malignant transformation into embryonal rhabdomyosarcoma: case report. J Pediatr Hematol Oncol. 2006 Oct;28(10):688–92. PMID:17023832

2898. Sun D, Wu Y, Liu Y, et al. Primary cardiac myxofibrosarcoma: case report, literature review and pooled analysis. BMC Cancer. 2018 May 2;18(1):512. PMID:29720127

2899. Sun J, Garfield DH, Lam B, et al. The value of autofluorescence bronchoscopy combined with white light bronchoscopy compared with white light alone in the diagnosis of intraepithelial neoplasia and invasive lung cancer: a meta-analysis. J Thorac Oncol. 2011 Aug;6(8):1336–44. PMID:21642863

2900. Sun JM, Ahn MJ, Ahn JS, et al. Chemotherapy for pulmonary large cell neuroendocrine carcinoma: similar to that for small cell lung cancer or non-small cell lung cancer? Lung Cancer. 2012 Aug;77(2):365–70. PMID:22579297

2901. Sun M, Zhao L, Weng Lao I, et al. Well-differentiated papillary mesothelioma: a 17-year single institution experience with a series of 75 cases. Ann Diagn Pathol. 2019 Feb;38:43–50. PMID:30419426

2902. Sun W, Feng L, Yang X, et al. Clonality assessment of multifocal lung adenocarcinoma by pathology evaluation and molecular analysis. Hum Pathol. 2018 Nov;81:261–71. PMID:30420048

2903. Sun Y, Li J, Zheng C, et al. Study on polymorphisms in CHRNA5/CHRNA3/CHRNB4 gene cluster and the associated with the risk of non-small cell lung cancer. Oncotarget. 2017 Dec 20;9(2):2435–44. PMID:29416783

2904. Sunami S, Sekimizu M, Takimoto T, et al. Prognostic impact of intensified maintenance therapy on children with advanced lymphoblastic lymphoma: a report from the Japanese Pediatric Leukemia/Lymphoma Study Group ALB-NHL03 study. Pediatr Blood Cancer. 2016 Mar;63(3):451–7. PMID:26585702

2905. Sundaram M, McGuire MH, Herbold DR, et al. High signal intensity soft tissue masses on T1 weighted pulsing sequences. Skeletal Radiol. 1987;16(1):30–6. PMID:3823958

2906. Sundling KE, Cibas ES. Ancillary studies in pleural, pericardial, and peritoneal effusion cytology. Cancer Cytopathol. 2018 Aug;126 Suppl 8:590–8. PMID:30156768

2907. Sung MT, Maclennan GT, Lopez-Beltran A, et al. Primary mediastinal seminoma: a comprehensive assessment integrated with histology, immunohistochemistry, and fluorescence in situ hybridization for chromosome 12p abnormalities in 23 cases. Am J Surg Pathol. 2008 Jan;32(1):146–55. PMID:18162782

2908. Sur A, Manraj H, Lavoie PM, et al. Multiple successful angioembolizations for refractory cardiac failure in a preterm with rapidly involuting congenital hemangioma. AJP Rep. 2016 Mar;6(1):e99–103. PMID:26929881

2909. Surabhi VR, Chua S, Patel RP, et al. Inflammatory myofibroblastic tumors:

current update. Radiol Clin North Am. 2016 May;54(3):553–63. PMID:27153788

2910. Surveillance, Epidemiology, and End Results (SEER) Program [Internet]. Bethesda (MD): National Cancer Institute; 2020. Available from: https://seer.cancer.gov/.

2911. Surveillance, Epidemiology, and End Results (SEER) Program [Internet]. Bethesda (MD): National Cancer Institute; 2020. Cancer Stat Facts: lung and bronchus cancer. Available from: https://seer.cancer.gov/statfacts/html/lungb.html.

2912. Sussman W, Stasney J. Congenital glycogenic tumor of the heart. Am Heart J. 1950 Aug;40(2):312–5. PMID:15432292

2913. Suster D, Pihan G, Mackinnon AC, et al. Expression of PD-L1/PD-1 in lymphoepithelioma-like carcinoma of the thymus. Mod Pathol. 2018 Dec;31(12):1801–6. PMID:29973653

2914. Suster D, Pihan G, Mackinnon AC, et al. Poorly differentiated nonkeratinizing squamous cell carcinoma of the thymus: clinicopathologic and molecular genetic study of 25 cases. Am J Surg Pathol. 2018 Sep;42(9):1224–36. PMID:29975245

2915. Suster S. Thymic carcinoma: update of current diagnostic criteria and histologic types. Semin Diagn Pathol. 2005 Aug;22(3):198–212. PMID:16711401

2916. Suster S, Moran CA. Diffuse pulmonary meningotheliomatosis. Am J Surg Pathol. 2007 Apr;31(4):624–31. PMID:17414111

2917. Suster S, Moran CA. Micronodular thymoma with lymphoid B-cell hyperplasia: clinicopathologic and immunohistochemical study of eighteen cases of a distinctive morphologic variant of thymic epithelial neoplasm. Am J Surg Pathol. 1999 Aug;23(8):955–62. PMID:10435566

2918. Suster S, Moran CA. Neuroendocrine neoplasms of the mediastinum. Am J Clin Pathol. 2001 Jun;115 Suppl:S17–27. PMID:11993687

2919. Suster S, Moran CA. Primary thymic epithelial neoplasms showing combined features of thymoma and thymic carcinoma. A clinicopathologic study of 22 cases. Am J Surg Pathol. 1996 Dec;20(12):1469–80. PMID:8944040

2920. Suster S, Moran CA. Problem areas and inconsistencies in the WHO classification of thymoma. Semin Diagn Pathol. 2005 Aug;22(3):188–97. PMID:16711400

2921. Suster S, Moran CA. Spindle cell thymic carcinoma: clinicopathologic and immunohistochemical study of a distinctive variant of primary thymic epithelial neoplasm. Am J Surg Pathol. 1999 Jun;23(6):691–700. PMID:10366152

2922. Suster S, Moran CA. Thymic carcinoid with prominent mucinous stroma. Report of a distinctive morphologic variant of thymic neuroendocrine neoplasm. Am J Surg Pathol. 1995 Nov;19(11):1277–85. PMID:7573690

2923. Suster S, Moran CA, Chan JK. Thymoma with pseudosarcomatous stroma: report of an unusual histologic variant of thymic epithelial neoplasm that may simulate carcinosarcoma. Am J Surg Pathol. 1997 Nov;21(11):1316–23. PMID:9351569

2924. Suster S, Moran CA, Dominguez-Malagon H, et al. Germ cell tumors of the mediastinum and testis: a comparative immunohistochemical study of 120 cases. Hum Pathol. 1998 Jul;29(7):737–42. PMID:9670832

2925. Suster S, Moran CA, Koss MN. Epithelioid hemangioendothelioma of the anterior mediastinum. Clinicopathologic, immunohistochemical, and ultrastructural analysis of 12 cases. Am J Surg Pathol. 1994 Sep;18(9):871–81. PMID:8067508

2926. Suster S, Rosai J. Cystic thymomas. A clinicopathologic study of ten cases. Cancer. 1992 Jan 1;69(1):92–7. PMID:1727679

2927. Suster S, Rosai J. Thymic carcinoma. A clinicopathologic study of 60 cases. Cancer. 1991 Feb 15;67(4):1025–32. PMID:1991250

2928. Suurmeijer AJ, Dickson BC, Swanson D, et al. The histologic spectrum of soft tissue spindle cell tumors with NTRK3 gene rearrangements. Genes Chromosomes Cancer. 2019 Nov;58(11):739–46. PMID:31112350

2929. Suzuki A, Hirokawa M, Takada N, et al. Utility of monoclonal PAX8 antibody for distinguishing intrathyroid thymic carcinoma from follicular cell-derived thyroid carcinoma. Endocr J. 2018 Dec 28;65(12):1171–5. PMID:30210064

2930. Suzuki E, Sasaki H, Kawano O, et al. Expression and mutation statuses of epidermal growth factor receptor in thymic epithelial tumors. Jpn J Clin Oncol. 2006 Jun;36(6):351–6. PMID:16762968

2931. Suzuki K, Nagai K, Yoshida J, et al. The prognosis of resected lung carcinoma associated with atypical adenomatous hyperplasia: a comparison of the prognosis of well-differentiated adenocarcinoma associated with atypical adenomatous hyperplasia and intrapulmonary metastasis. Cancer. 1997 Apr 15;79(8):1521–6. PMID:9118033

2932. Suzuki K, Saji H, Aokage K, et al. Comparison of pulmonary segmentectomy and lobectomy: safety results of a randomized trial. J Thorac Cardiovasc Surg. 2019 Sep;158(3):895–907. PMID:31078312

2933. Suzuki K, Takahashi K, Yoshida J, et al. Synchronous double primary lung carcinomas associated with multiple atypical adenomatous hyperplasia. Lung Cancer. 1998 Feb;19(2):131–9. PMID:9567250

2934. Suzuki M, Nakatani Y, Ito H, et al. Pulmonary adenocarcinoma with high-grade fetal adenocarcinoma component has a poor prognosis, comparable to that of micropapillary adenocarcinoma. Mod Pathol. 2018 Sep;31(9):1404–17. PMID:29785018

2935. Suzuki M, Yazawa T, Ota S, et al. High-grade fetal adenocarcinoma of the lung is a tumour with a fetal phenotype that shows diverse differentiation, including high-grade neuroendocrine carcinoma: a clinicopathological, immunohistochemical and mutational study of 20 cases. Histopathology. 2015 Dec;67(6):806–16. PMID:25851923

2936. Svec A, Rangaiah M, Giles M, et al. EBV+ diffuse large B-cell lymphoma arising within atrial myxoma. An example of a distinct primary cardiac EBV+ DLBCL of immunocompetent patients. Pathol Res Pract. 2012 Mar 15;208(3):172–6. PMID:22326256

2937. Swarts DR, Henfling ME, Van Neste L, et al. CD44 and OTP are strong prognostic markers for pulmonary carcinoids. Clin Cancer Res. 2013 Apr 15;19(8):2197–207. PMID:23444222

2938. Swarts DR, Rudelius M, Claessen SM, et al. Limited additive value of the Ki-67 proliferative index on patient survival in World Health Organization-classified pulmonary carcinoids. Histopathology. 2017 Feb;70(3):412–22. PMID:27701763

2939. Swarts DR, Scarpa A, Corbo V, et al. MEN1 gene mutation and reduced expression are associated with poor prognosis in pulmonary carcinoids. J Clin Endocrinol Metab. 2014 Feb;99(2):E374–8. PMID:24276465

2940. Swartz MF, Lutz CJ, Chandan VS, et al. Atrial myxomas: pathologic types, tumor location, and presenting symptoms. J Card Surg. 2006 Jul-Aug;21(4):435–40. PMID:16846432

2941. Swerdlow SH, Campo E, Harris NL, et al., editors. WHO classification of tumours of haematopoietic and lymphoid tissues. Lyon (France): International Agency for Research on Cancer; 2017. (WHO classification of tumours series, 4th rev. ed.; vol. 2). https://publications.iarc.fr/556.

2942. Szczepański T, Langerak AW, Willemse MJ, et al. T cell receptor gamma (TCRG) gene rearrangements in T cell acute lymphoblastic leukemia refelct 'end-stage' recombinations: implications for minimal residual disease monitoring. Leukemia. 2000 Jul;14(7):1208–14. PMID:10914544

2943. Szczepański T, Pongers-Willemse MJ, Langerak AW, et al. Ig heavy chain gene rearrangements in T-cell acute lymphoblastic leukemia exhibit predominant DH6-19 and DH7-27 gene usage, can result in complete V-D-J rearrangements, and are rare in T-cell receptor alpha beta lineage. Blood. 1999 Jun 15;93(12):4079–85. PMID:10361104

2944. Szuhai K, de Jong D, Leung WY, et al. Transactivating mutation of the MYOD1 gene is a frequent event in adult spindle cell rhabdomyosarcoma. J Pathol. 2014 Feb;232(3):300–7. PMID:24272621

2945. Tachibana M, Saito M, Kobayashi J, et al. Distal-type bronchiolar adenoma of the lung expressing p16INK4a - morphologic, immunohistochemical, ultrastructural and genomic analysis - report of a case and review of the literature. Pathol Int. 2020 Mar;70(3):179–85. PMID:32030846

2946. Tagawa T, Ohta M, Kuwata T, et al. S-1 plus cisplatin chemotherapy with concurrent radiation for thymic basaloid carcinoma. J Thorac Oncol. 2010 Apr;5(4):572–3. PMID:20357624

2947. Taguchi R, Higuchi K, Sudo M, et al. A case of anaplastic lymphoma kinase (ALK)-positive ciliated muconodular papillary tumor (CMPT) of the lung. Pathol Int. 2017 Feb;67(2):99–104. PMID:28093881

2948. Tajima S, Aki M, Yajima K, et al. Primary epithelial-myoepithelial carcinoma of the lung: a case report demonstrating high-grade transformation-like changes. Oncol Lett. 2015 Jul;10(1):175–81. PMID:26170995

2949. Tajima S, Takanashi Y, Koda K. Enlarging cystic lymphangioma of the mediastinum in an adult: Is this a neoplastic lesion related to the recently discovered PIK3CA mutation? Int J Clin Exp Pathol. 2015 May 1;8(5):5924–8. PMID:26191320

2950. Tajima S, Yanagiya M, Sato M, et al. Metaplastic thymoma with myasthenia gravis presumably caused by an accumulation of intratumoral immature T cells: a case report. Int J Clin Exp Pathol. 2015 Nov 1;8(11):15375–80. PMID:26823897

2951. Takahashi F, Tsuta K, Matsuno Y, et al. Adenocarcinoma of the thymus: mucinous subtype. Hum Pathol. 2005 Feb;36(2):219–23. PMID:15754301

2952. Takahashi M, Kanamori Y, Takahashi M, et al. Detection of a metastatic lesion and tiny yolk sac tumors in two teenage patients by FDG-PET: report of two cases. Surg Today. 2014 Oct;44(10):1962–5. PMID:23801057

2953. Takahashi Y, Eguchi T, Kameda K, et al. Histologic subtyping in pathologic stage I-IIA lung adenocarcinoma provides risk-based stratification for surveillance. Oncotarget. 2018 Nov 6;9(87):35742–51. PMID:30515266

2954. Takakuwa T, Ham MF, Luo WJ, et al. Loss of expression of Epstein-Barr virus nuclear antigen-2 correlates with a poor prognosis in cases of pyothorax-associated lymphoma. Int J Cancer. 2006 Jun 1;118(11):2782–9. PMID:16385574

2955. Takakuwa T, Luo WJ, Ham MF, et al. Establishment and characterization of unique cell lines derived from pyothorax-associated lymphoma which develops in long-standing pyothorax and is strongly associated with Epstein-Barr virus infection. Cancer Sci. 2003 Oct;94(10):858–63. PMID:14556658

2956. Takakuwa T, Tresnasari K, Rahadiani N,

et al. Cell origin of pyothorax-associated lymphoma: a lymphoma strongly associated with Epstein-Barr virus infection. Leukemia. 2008 Mar;22(3):620–7. PMID:18079737
2957. Takamatsu M, Sato Y, Muto M, et al. Hyalinizing clear cell carcinoma of the bronchial glands: presentation of three cases and pathological comparisons with salivary gland counterparts and bronchial mucoepidermoid carcinomas. Mod Pathol. 2018 Jun;31(6):923–33. PMID:29434341
2958. Takamochi K, Ogura T, Suzuki K, et al. Loss of heterozygosity on chromosomes 9q and 16p in atypical adenomatous hyperplasia concomitant with adenocarcinoma of the lung. Am J Pathol. 2001 Nov;159(5):1941–8. PMID:11696455
2959. Takamori S, Noguchi M, Morinaga S, et al. Clinicopathologic characteristics of adenosquamous carcinoma of the lung. Cancer. 1991 Feb 1;67(3):649–54. PMID:1985759
2960. Takanami I, Takeuchi K, Giga M. The prognostic value of natural killer cell infiltration in resected pulmonary adenocarcinoma. J Thorac Cardiovasc Surg. 2001 Jun;121(6):1058–63. PMID:11385371
2961. Takao M, Takagi T, Suzuki H, et al. Resection of mucinous lung adenocarcinoma presenting with intractable bronchorrhea. J Thorac Oncol. 2010 Apr;5(4):576–8. PMID:20357626
2962. Takeda M, Kasai T, Enomoto Y, et al. 9p21 deletion in the diagnosis of malignant mesothelioma, using fluorescence in situ hybridization analysis. Pathol Int. 2010 May;60(5):395–9. PMID:20518890
2963. Takeda M, Tani Y, Saijo N, et al. Cytopathological features of SMARCA4-deficient thoracic sarcoma: report of 2 cases and review of the literature. Int J Surg Pathol. 2020 Feb;28(1):109–14. PMID:31448657
2964. Takeda S, Miyoshi S, Akashi A, et al. Clinical spectrum of primary mediastinal tumors: a comparison of adult and pediatric populations at a single Japanese institution. J Surg Oncol. 2003 May;83(1):24–30. PMID:12722093
2965. Takeda S, Miyoshi S, Ohta M, et al. Primary germ cell tumors in the mediastinum: a 50-year experience at a single Japanese institution. Cancer. 2003 Jan 15;97(2):367–76. PMID:12518361
2966. Takenaka S, Hashimoto N, Araki N, et al. Eleven cases of cardiac metastases from soft-tissue sarcomas. Jpn J Clin Oncol. 2011 Apr;41(4):514–8. PMID:21247968
2967. Takeshima Y, Amatya VJ, Kushitani K, et al. Value of immunohistochemistry in the differential diagnosis of pleural sarcomatoid mesothelioma from lung sarcomatoid carcinoma. Histopathology. 2009 May;54(6):667–76. PMID:19438742
2968. Takeshima Y, Nakayori F, Nakano T, et al. Extra-abdominal desmoid tumor presenting as an intrathoracic tumor: case report and literature review. Pathol Int. 2001 Oct;51(10):824–8. PMID:11881738
2969. Takeuchi E, Shimizu E, Sano N, et al. A case of pleomorphic adenoma of the lung with multiple distant metastases–observations on its oncogene and tumor suppressor gene expression. Anticancer Res. 1998 May-Jun;18(3B):2015–20. PMID:9677459
2970. Takeuchi K, Soda M, Togashi Y, et al. Pulmonary inflammatory myofibroblastic tumor expressing a novel fusion, PPFIBP1-ALK: reappraisal of anti-ALK immunohistochemistry as a tool for novel ALK fusion identification. Clin Cancer Res. 2011 May 15;17(10):3341–8. PMID:21430068
2971. Takeuchi K, Soda M, Togashi Y, et al. RET, ROS1 and ALK fusions in lung cancer. Nat Med. 2012 Feb 12;18(3):378–81. PMID:22327623
2972. Taki M, Inada S, Ariyasu R, et al. Anaplastic large cell lymphoma mimicking fibrosing mediastinitis. Intern Med. 2013;52(23):2645–51. PMID:24292756
2973. Takiff H, Calabria R, Yin L, et al. Mesenteric cysts and intra-abdominal cystic lymphangiomas. Arch Surg. 1985 Nov;120(11):1266–9. PMID:4051731
2974. Takikita M, Altekruse S, Lynch CF, et al. Associations between selected biomarkers and prognosis in a population-based pancreatic cancer tissue microarray. Cancer Res. 2009 Apr 1;69(7):2950–5. PMID:19276352
2975. Takino H, Li C, Yamada S, et al. Thymic extranodal marginal zone lymphoma of mucosa-associated lymphoid tissue: a gene methylation study. Leuk Lymphoma. 2013 Aug;54(8):1742–6. PMID:23320886
2976. Tam CG, Broome DR, Shannon RL. Desmoid tumor of the anterior mediastinum: CT and radiologic features. J Comput Assist Tomogr. 1994 May-Jun;18(3):499–501. PMID:8188925
2977. Tamai M, Ishida M, Ebisu Y, et al. Thymic enteric type adenocarcinoma: a case report with cytological features. Diagn Cytopathol. 2018 Jan;46(1):92–7. PMID:28888068
2978. Tamboli P, Toprani TH, Amin MB, et al. Carcinoma of lung with rhabdoid features. Hum Pathol. 2004 Jan;35(1):8–13. PMID:14745719
2979. Tamborini E, Casieri P, Miselli F, et al. Analysis of potential receptor tyrosine kinase targets in intimal and mural sarcomas. J Pathol. 2007 Jun;212(2):227–35. PMID:17471466
2980. Tamin SS, Maleszewski JJ, Scott CG, et al. Prognostic and bioepidemiologic implications of papillary fibroelastomas. J Am Coll Cardiol. 2015 Jun 9;65(22):2420–9. PMID:26046736
2981. Tan MH, Morrison C, Wang P, et al. Loss of parafibromin immunoreactivity is a distinguishing feature of parathyroid carcinoma. Clin Cancer Res. 2004 Oct 1;10(19):6629–37. PMID:15475453
2982. Tanaka H, Akiyama Y, Kitamura A, et al. Malignant mesothelioma with squamous differentiation. Histopathology. 2018 Jun;72(7):1216–20. PMID:29430704
2983. Tanaka M, Kato K, Gomi K, et al. NUT midline carcinoma: report of 2 cases suggestive of pulmonary origin. Am J Surg Pathol. 2012 Mar;36(3):381–8. PMID:22301500
2984. Tanaka M, Kato K, Gomi K, et al. Perivascular epithelioid cell tumor with SFPQ/PSF-TFE3 gene fusion in a patient with advanced neuroblastoma. Am J Surg Pathol. 2009 Sep;33(9):1416–20. PMID:19606011
2984A. Tanaka M, Kohashi K, Kushitani K, et al. Inflammatory myofibroblastic tumors of the lung carrying a chimeric A2M-ALK gene: report of 2 infantile cases and review of the differential diagnosis of infantile pulmonary lesions. Hum Pathol. 2017 Aug;66:177–82. PMID:28705706
2985. Tanaka R, Emerson LL, Karwande SV, et al. Growing pulmonary nodule with increased 18-fluorodeoxyglucose uptake in a former smoker. Chest. 2005 May;127(5):1848–51. PMID:15888868
2986. Tanas MR, Ma S, Jadaan FO, et al. Mechanism of action of a WWTR1(TAZ)-CAMTA1 fusion oncoprotein. Oncogene. 2016 Feb 18;35(7):929–38. PMID:25961935
2987. Tanas MR, Sboner A, Oliveira AM, et al. Identification of a disease-defining gene fusion in epithelioid hemangioendothelioma. Sci Transl Med. 2011 Aug 31;3(98):98ra82. PMID:21885404
2988. Tang TT, Segura AD, Oechler HW, et al. Inflammatory myofibrohistiocytic proliferation simulating sarcoma in children. Cancer. 1990 Apr 1;65(7):1626–34. PMID:2311072
2989. Tang VK, Vijhani P, Cherian SV, et al. Primary pulmonary lymphoproliferative neoplasms. Lung India. 2018 May-Jun;35(3):220–30. PMID:29697079
2990. Tani E, Wejde J, Åström K, et al. FNA cytology of solitary fibrous tumors and the diagnostic value of STAT6 immunocytochemistry. Cancer Cytopathol. 2018 Jan;126(1):36–43. PMID:28914981
2991. Taniguchi A, Hashida Y, Nemoto Y, et al. Epstein-Barr virus-positive pyothorax-associated lymphoma arising from a posttraumatic empyema. Acta Haematol. 2015;134(3):155–60. PMID:25968626
2992. Tanimura S, Tomoyasu H, Kohno T, et al. [Basaloid carcinoma originated from the wall of thymic cyst presenting as pericardial and thoracic effusion; report of a case]. Kyobu Geka. 2002 Jul;55(7):571–5. Japanese. PMID:12136587
2993. Tao TY, Yahyavi-Firouz-Abadi N, Singh GK, et al. Pediatric cardiac tumors: clinical and imaging features. Radiographics. 2014 Jul-Aug;34(4):1031–46. PMID:25019440
2994. Tapias LF, Mercier O, Ghigna MR, et al. Validation of a scoring system to predict recurrence of resected solitary fibrous tumors of the pleura. Chest. 2015 Jan;147(1):216–23. PMID:25103552
2995. Tapias LF, Mino-Kenudson M, Lee H, et al. Risk factor analysis for the recurrence of resected solitary fibrous tumours of the pleura: a 33-year experience and proposal for a scoring system. Eur J Cardiothorac Surg. 2013 Jul;44(1):111–7. PMID:23233072
2996. Tateishi U, Müller NL, Johkoh T, et al. Primary mediastinal lymphoma: characteristic features of the various histological subtypes on CT. J Comput Assist Tomogr. 2004 Nov-Dec;28(6):782–9. PMID:15538151
2997. Tateyama H, Eimoto T, Tada T, et al. Immunoreactivity of a new CD5 antibody with normal epithelium and malignant tumors including thymic carcinoma. Am J Clin Pathol. 1999 Feb;111(2):235–40. PMID:9930146
2998. Tateyama H, Eimoto T, Tada T, et al. p53 protein expression and p53 gene mutation in thymic epithelial tumors. An immunohistochemical and DNA sequencing study. Am J Clin Pathol. 1995 Oct;104(4):375–81. PMID:7572785
2999. Tateyama H, Saito Y, Fujii Y, et al. The spectrum of micronodular thymic epithelial tumours with lymphoid B-cell hyperplasia. Histopathology. 2001 Jun;38(6):519–27. PMID:11422495
3000. Tavora F, Miettinen M, Fanburg-Smith J, et al. Pulmonary artery sarcoma: a histologic and follow-up study with emphasis on a subset of low-grade myofibroblastic sarcomas with a good long-term follow-up. Am J Surg Pathol. 2008 Dec;32(12):1751–61. PMID:18779732
3001. Taylor MS, Chougule A, MacLeay AR, et al. Morphologic overlap between inflammatory myofibroblastic tumor and IgG4-related disease: lessons from next-generation sequencing. Am J Surg Pathol. 2019 Mar;43(3):314–24. PMID:30451733
3002. Tazelaar HD, Kerr D, Yousem SA, et al. Diffuse pulmonary lymphangiomatosis. Hum Pathol. 1993 Dec;24(12):1313–22. PMID:8276379
3003. Tazelaar HD, Locke TJ, McGregor CG. Pathology of surgically excised primary cardiac tumors. Mayo Clin Proc. 1992 Oct;67(10):957–65. PMID:1434856
3004. Tazi A, de Margerie C, Naccache JM, et al. The natural history of adult pulmonary Langerhans cell histiocytosis: a prospective multicentre study. Orphanet J Rare Dis. 2015 Mar 14;10:30. PMID:25887097
3005. Tazi A, Marc K, Dominique S, et al. Serial computed tomography and lung function testing in pulmonary Langerhans' cell histiocytosis. Eur Respir J. 2012 Oct;40(4):905–12. PMID:22441752
3006. Teh BT. Thymic carcinoids in multiple endocrine neoplasia type 1. J Intern Med. 1998 Jun;243(6):501–4. PMID:9681849
3007. Teh BT, Hayward NK, Walters MK, et al. Genetic studies of thymic carcinoids in multiple endocrine neoplasia type 1. J Med Genet. 1994 Mar;31(3):261–2. PMID:7912288
3008. Teh BT, McArdle J, Chan SP, et al. Clinicopathologic studies of thymic carcinoids in multiple endocrine neoplasia type 1. Medicine (Baltimore). 1997 Jan;76(1):21–9. PMID:9064485
3009. Teh BT, Zedenius J, Kytölä S, et al. Thymic carcinoids in multiple endocrine neoplasia type 1. Ann Surg. 1998 Jul;228(1):99–105. PMID:9671073
3010. Tehrani OS, Chen EQ, Schaebler DL, et al. Thymoma associated with malignancies may herald a hereditary cancer syndrome. Fam Cancer. 2010 Dec;9(4):655–7. PMID:20734236
3011. Teilum G. Endodermal sinus tumors of the ovary and testis. Comparative morphogenesis of the so-called mesoephroma ovarii (Schiller) and extraembryonic (yolk sac-allantoic) structures of the rat's placenta. Cancer. 1959 Nov-Dec;12:1092–105. PMID:13837288
3012. Teixeira VH, Pipinikas CP, Pennycuick A, et al. Deciphering the genomic, epigenomic, and transcriptomic landscapes of pre-invasive lung cancer lesions. Nat Med. 2019 Mar;25(3):517–25. PMID:30664780
3013. Templeton AK, Miyamoto S, Babu A, et al. Cancer stem cells: progress and challenges in lung cancer. Stem Cell Investig. 2014 Apr 15;1:9. PMID:27358855
3014. ten Heuvel SE, Hoekstra HJ, Bastiaannet E, et al. The classic prognostic factors tumor stage, tumor size, and tumor grade are the strongest predictors of outcome in synovial sarcoma: no role for SSX fusion type or ezrin expression. Appl Immunohistochem Mol Morphol. 2009 May;17(3):189–95. PMID:18997619
3015. Teo M, Crotty P, O'Sullivan M, et al. NUT midline carcinoma in a young woman. J Clin Oncol. 2011 Apr 20;29(12):e336–9. PMID:21263084
3016. Terada T. CD5-positive marginal zone B-cell lymphoma of the mucosa-associated lymphoid tissue (MALT) of the lung. Diagn Pathol. 2012 Feb 14;7:16. PMID:22333190
3017. Terada T. Mediastinal seminoma with multiple KIT gene mutations. Pathology. 2009;41(7):695–7. PMID:20001354
3018. Terada T. Primary sarcomatoid malignant mesothelioma of the pericardium. Med Oncol. 2012 Jun;29(2):1345–6. PMID:21328086
3019. Teramoto K, Kawaguchi Y, Hori T, et al. Thymic papillo-tubular adenocarcinoma containing a cyst: report of a case. Surg Today. 2012 Oct;42(10):988–91. PMID:22407350
3020. Terasaki Y, Okumura H, Saito K, et al. HHV-8/KSHV-negative and CD20-positive primary effusion lymphoma successfully treated by pleural drainage followed by chemotherapy containing rituximab. Intern Med. 2008;47(24):2175–8. PMID:19075546
3021. Terenziani M, D'Angelo P, Inserra A, et al. Mature and immature teratoma: a report from the second Italian pediatric study. Pediatr Blood Cancer. 2015 Jul;62(7):1202–8. PMID:25631333
3022. Terra SB, Jang JS, Bi L, et al. Molecular characterization of pulmonary sarcomatoid carcinoma: analysis of 33 cases. Mod Pathol. 2016 Aug;29(8):824–31. PMID:27174587
3023. Terra SBSP, Aesif SW, Maleszewski JJ, et al. Mediastinal synovial sarcoma: clinicopathologic analysis of 21 cases with molecular confirmation. Am J Surg Pathol. 2018 Jun;42(6):761–6. PMID:29543673

3024. Terry J, Saito T, Subramanian S, et al. TLE1 as a diagnostic immunohistochemical marker for synovial sarcoma emerging from gene expression profiling studies. Am J Surg Pathol. 2007 Feb;31(2):240–6. PMID:17255769

3025. Teruya-Feldstein J, Jaffe ES, Burd PR, et al. The role of Mig, the monokine induced by interferon-gamma, and IP-10, the interferon-gamma-inducible protein-10, in tissue necrosis and vascular damage associated with Epstein-Barr virus-positive lymphoproliferative disease. Blood. 1997 Nov 15;90(10):4099–105. PMID:9354680

3026. Testa JR, Cheung M, Pei J, et al. Germline BAP1 mutations predispose to malignant mesothelioma. Nat Genet. 2011 Aug 28;43(10):1022–5. PMID:21874000

3027. The Non-Hodgkin's Lymphoma Classification Project. A clinical evaluation of the International Lymphoma Study Group classification of non-Hodgkin's lymphoma. Blood. 1997 Jun 1;89(11):3909–18. PMID:9166827

3028. Thomas de Montpréville V, Ghigna MR, Lacroix L, et al. Thymic carcinomas: clinicopathologic study of 37 cases from a single institution. Virchows Arch. 2013 Mar;462(3):307–13. PMID:23319214

3029. Thomas de Montpréville V, Quilhot P, Chalabreysse L, et al. Glut-1 intensity and pattern of expression in thymic epithelial tumors are predictive of WHO subtypes. Pathol Res Pract. 2015 Dec;211(12):996–1002. PMID:26534878

3030. Thomas JM, Musani AI. Malignant pleural effusions: a review. Clin Chest Med. 2013 Sep;34(3):459–71. PMID:23993817

3031. Thomas RK, Re D, Zander T, et al. Epidemiology and etiology of Hodgkin's lymphoma. Ann Oncol. 2002;13 Suppl 4:147–52. PMID:12401681

3032. Thomas-de-Montpréville V, Nottin R, Dulmet E, et al. Heart tumors in children and adults: clinicopathological study of 59 patients from a surgical center. Cardiovasc Pathol. 2007 Jan-Feb;16(1):22–8. PMID:17218211

3033. Thomas De Montpréville V, Zemoura L, Dulmet E. [Thymoma with epithelial micronodules and lymphoid hyperplasia: six cases of a rare and equivocal subtype]. Ann Pathol. 2002 Jun;22(3):177–82. French. PMID:12410100

3034. Thomason R, Schlegel W, Lucca M, et al. Primary malignant mesothelioma of the pericardium. Case report and literature review. Tex Heart Inst J. 1994;21(2):170–4. PMID:8061543

3035. Thun MJ, Hannan LM, Adams-Campbell LL, et al. Lung cancer occurrence in never-smokers: an analysis of 13 cohorts and 22 cancer registry studies. PLoS Med. 2008 Sep 30;5(9):e185. PMID:18788891

3036. Thunnissen E, Beasley MB, Borczuk AC, et al. Reproducibility of histopathological subtypes and invasion in pulmonary adenocarcinoma. An international interobserver study. Mod Pathol. 2012 Dec;25(12):1574–83. PMID:22814311

3037. Thunnissen E, Beliën JA, Kerr KM, et al. In compressed lung tissue microscopic sections of adenocarcinoma in situ may mimic papillary adenocarcinoma. Arch Pathol Lab Med. 2013 Dec;137(12):1792–7. PMID:24283861

3038. Thunnissen E, Borczuk AC, Flieder DB, et al. The use of immunohistochemistry improves the diagnosis of small cell lung cancer and its differential diagnosis. An international reproducibility study in a demanding set of cases. J Thorac Oncol. 2017 Feb;12(2):334–46. PMID:27998793

3039. Thunnissen E, Noguchi M, Aisner S, et al. Reproducibility of histopathological diagnosis in poorly differentiated NSCLC: an international multiobserver study. J Thorac Oncol. 2014 Sep;9(9):1354–62. PMID:25122431

3040. Thunnissen FB, Arends JW, Buchholtz RT, et al. Fine needle aspiration cytology of inflammatory pseudotumor of the lung (plasma cell granuloma). Report of four cases. Acta Cytol. 1989 Nov-Dec;33(6):917–21. PMID:2588924

3041. Thway K, Nicholson AG, Lawson K, et al. Primary pulmonary myxoid sarcoma with EWSR1-CREB1 fusion: a new tumor entity. Am J Surg Pathol. 2011 Nov;35(11):1722–32. PMID:21997693

3042. Thway K, Nicholson AG, Wallace WA, et al. Endobronchial pulmonary angiomatoid fibrous histiocytoma: two cases with EWSR1-CREB1 and EWSR1-ATF1 fusions. Am J Surg Pathol. 2012 Jun;36(6):883–8. PMID:22588066

3043. Tiffet O, Nicholson AG, Ladas G, et al. A clinicopathologic study of 12 neuroendocrine tumors arising in the thymus. Chest. 2003 Jul;124(1):141–6. PMID:12853516

3044. Tinat J, Bougeard G, Baert-Desurmont S, et al. 2009 version of the Chompret criteria for Li Fraumeni syndrome. J Clin Oncol. 2009 Sep 10;27(26):e108–9, author reply e110. PMID:19652052

3045. Tokarek T, Szpor J, Pankowski J, et al. Desmoid tumor of lung with pleural involvement - the case of unique location of aggressive fibromatosis. Folia Med Cracov. 2015;55(1):53–9. PMID:26774632

3046. Tolstrup K, Shiota T, Gurudevan S, et al. Left atrial myxomas: correlation of two-dimensional and live three-dimensional transesophageal echocardiography with the clinical and pathologic findings. J Am Soc Echocardiogr. 2011 Jun;24(6):618–24. PMID:21367578

3047. Tomita S, Mori KL, Sakajiri S, et al. B-cell marker negative (CD7+, CD19-) Epstein-Barr virus-related pyothorax-associated lymphoma with rearrangement in the JH gene. Leuk Lymphoma. 2003 Apr;44(4):727–30. PMID:12769353

3048. Tomiyama N, Johkoh T, Mihara N, et al. Using the World Health Organization classification of thymic epithelial neoplasms to describe CT findings. AJR Am J Roentgenol. 2002 Oct;179(4):881–6. PMID:12239030

3049. Tomizawa K, Suda K, Onozato R, et al. Prognostic and predictive implications of HER2/ERBB2/neu gene mutations in lung cancers. Lung Cancer. 2011 Oct;74(1):139–44. PMID:21353324

3050. Tonon G, Modi S, Wu L, et al. t(11;19) (q21;p13) translocation in mucoepidermoid carcinoma creates a novel fusion product that disrupts a Notch signaling pathway. Nat Genet. 2003 Feb;33(2):208–13. PMID:12539049

3051. Tonon G, Wong KK, Maulik G, et al. High-resolution genomic profiles of human lung cancer. Proc Natl Acad Sci U S A. 2005 Jul 5;102(27):9625–30. PMID:15983384

3052. Toomes H, Delphendahl A, Manke HG, et al. The coin lesion of the lung. A review of 955 resected coin lesions. Cancer. 1983 Feb 1;51(3):534–7. PMID:6821831

3053. Toprani TH, Tamboli P, Amin MB, et al. Thymic carcinoma with rhabdoid features. Ann Diagn Pathol. 2003 Apr;7(2):106–11. PMID:12715336

3054. Torii I, Tateishi U, Terauchi T, et al. Prognostic implications of diffusion-weighted magnetic resonance imaging in patients with superior sulcus tumors receiving induction chemoradiation therapy. Jpn J Clin Oncol. 2016 Mar;46(3):264–9. PMID:26848076

3055. Toriyama A, Mori T, Sekine S, et al. Utility of PAX8 mouse monoclonal antibody in the diagnosis of thyroid, thymic, pleural and lung tumours: a comparison with polyclonal PAX8 antibody. Histopathology. 2014 Oct;65(4):465–72. PMID:24592933

3056. Torniai M, Scortichini L, Tronconi F, et al. Systemic treatment for lung carcinoids: from bench to bedside. Clin Transl Med. 2019 Jul 4;8(1):22. PMID:31273555

3057. Toufan M, Jodati A, Safaei N, et al. Myxomas in all cardiac chambers. Echocardiography. 2012 Nov;29(10):E270–2. PMID:22957665

3058. Toyokawa G, Takenoyama M, Taguchi K, et al. The first case of lung carcinosarcoma harboring in-frame deletions at exon19 in the EGFR gene. Lung Cancer. 2013 Sep;81(3):491–4. PMID:23891513

3059. Tozbikian GH, Zynger DL. A combination of GATA3 and SOX10 is useful for the diagnosis of metastatic triple-negative breast cancer. Hum Pathol. 2019 Mar;85:221–7. PMID:30468800

3060. Tran TA, Fabre M, Pariente D, et al. Erdheim-Chester disease in childhood: a challenging diagnosis and treatment. J Pediatr Hematol Oncol. 2009 Oct;31(10):782–6. PMID:19755920

3061. Tranchant R, Quetel L, Tallet A, et al. Co-occurring mutations of tumor suppressor genes, LATS2 and NF2, in malignant pleural mesothelioma. Clin Cancer Res. 2017 Jun 15;23(12):3191–202. PMID:28003305

3062. Traub B. Mucinous cystadenoma of the lung. Arch Pathol Lab Med. 1991 Aug;115(8):740–1. PMID:1863181

3063. Traverse-Glehen A, Pittaluga S, Gaulard P, et al. Mediastinal gray zone lymphoma: the missing link between classic Hodgkin's lymphoma and mediastinal large B-cell lymphoma. Am J Surg Pathol. 2005 Nov;29(11):1411–21. PMID:16224207

3064. Travis WD. Lung cancer pathology: current concepts. Clin Chest Med. 2020 Mar;41(1):67–85. PMID:32008630

3065. Travis WD. Pathology and diagnosis of neuroendocrine tumors: lung neuroendocrine. Thorac Surg Clin. 2014 Aug;24(3):257–66. PMID:25065926

3065A. Travis WD. Sarcomatoid neoplasms of the lung and pleura. Arch Pathol Lab Med. 2010 Nov;134(11):1645–58. PMID:21043818

3066. Travis WD. Update on small cell carcinoma and its differentiation from squamous cell carcinoma and other non-small cell carcinomas. Mod Pathol. 2012 Jan;25 Suppl 1:S18–30. PMID:22214967

3067. Travis WD, Asamura H, Bankier AA, et al. The IASLC Lung Cancer Staging Project: proposals for coding T categories for subsolid nodules and assessment of tumor size in part-solid tumors in the forthcoming eighth edition of the TNM classification of lung cancer. J Thorac Oncol. 2016 Aug;11(8):1204–23. PMID:27107787

3068. Travis WD, Brambilla E, Burke AP, et al., editors. WHO classification of tumours of the lung, pleura, thymus and heart. Lyon (France): International Agency for Research on Cancer; 2015. (WHO classification of tumours series, 4th ed.; vol. 7). https://publications.iarc.fr/17.

3069. Travis WD, Brambilla E, Müller-Hermelink HK, et al., editors. Pathology and genetics of tumours of the lung, pleura, thymus and heart. Lyon (France): International Agency for Research on Cancer; 2004. (WHO classification of tumours series, 3rd ed.; vol. 10). https://publications.iarc.fr/10.

3070. Travis WD, Brambilla E, Nicholson AG. Testing for neuroendocrine immunohistochemical markers should not be performed in poorly differentiated NSCCs in the absence of neuroendocrine morphologic features according to the 2015 WHO classification. J Thorac Oncol. 2016 Feb;11(2):e26–7. PMID:26811228

3071. Travis WD, Brambilla E, Nicholson AG, et al. The 2015 World Health Organization classification of lung tumors: impact of genetic, clinical and radiologic advances since the 2004 classification. J Thorac Oncol. 2015 Sep;10(9):1243–60. PMID:26291008

3072. Travis WD, Brambilla E, Noguchi M, et al. Diagnosis of lung adenocarcinoma in resected specimens: implications of the 2011 International Association for the Study of Lung Cancer/American Thoracic Society/European Respiratory Society classification. Arch Pathol Lab Med. 2013 May;137(5):685–705. PMID:22913371

3073. Travis WD, Brambilla E, Noguchi M, et al. Diagnosis of lung cancer in small biopsies and cytology: implications of the 2011 International Association for the Study of Lung Cancer/American Thoracic Society/European Respiratory Society classification. Arch Pathol Lab Med. 2013 May;137(5):668–84. PMID:22970842

3074. Travis WD, Brambilla E, Noguchi M, et al. International Association for the Study of Lung Cancer/American Thoracic Society/European Respiratory Society international multidisciplinary classification of lung adenocarcinoma. J Thorac Oncol. 2011 Feb;6(2):244–85. PMID:21252716

3075. Travis WD, Brambilla E, Noguchi M, et al. International Association for the Study of Lung Cancer/American Thoracic Society/European Respiratory Society: international multidisciplinary classification of lung adenocarcinoma: executive summary. Proc Am Thorac Soc. 2011 Sep;8(5):381–5. PMID:21926387

3076. Travis WD, Colby TV, Corrin B, et al., editors. Histological typing of lung and pleural tumors. Berlin (Germany): Springer; 1999.

3077. Travis WD, Dacic S, Wistuba I, et al. IASLC multidisciplinary recommendations for pathologic assessment of lung cancer resection specimens after neoadjuvant therapy. J Thorac Oncol. 2020 May;15(5):709–40. PMID:32004713

3077A. Travis WD, Gal AA, Colby TV, et al. Reproducibility of neuroendocrine lung tumor classification. Hum Pathol. 1998 Mar;29(3):272–9. PMID:9496831

3078. Travis WD, Giroux DJ, Chansky K, et al. The IASLC Lung Cancer Staging Project: proposals for the inclusion of broncho-pulmonary carcinoid tumors in the forthcoming (seventh) edition of the TNM classification for lung cancer. J Thorac Oncol. 2008 Nov;3(11):1213–23. PMID:18978555

3079. Travis WD, Linnoila RI, Tsokos MG, et al. Neuroendocrine tumors of the lung with proposed criteria for large-cell neuroendocrine carcinoma. An ultrastructural, immunohistochemical, and flow cytometric study of 35 cases. Am J Surg Pathol. 1991 Jun;15(6):529–53. PMID:1709558

3080. Travis WD, Lubin J, Ries L, et al. United States lung carcinoma incidence trends: declining for most histologic types among males, increasing among females. Cancer. 1996 Jun 15;77(12):2464–70. PMID:8640694

3081. Travis WD, Nicholson AG, Geisinger KR, et al. Tumors of the lower respiratory tract. Washington, DC: American Registry of Pathology; 2019. (AFIP atlas of tumor pathology, series 4; fascicle 29).

3082. Travis WD, Rekhtman N. Pathological diagnosis and classification of lung cancer in small biopsies and cytology: strategic management of tissue for molecular testing. Semin Respir Crit Care Med. 2011 Feb;32(1):22–31. PMID:21500121

3083. Travis WD, Rekhtman N, Riley GJ, et al. Pathologic diagnosis of advanced lung cancer based on small biopsies and cytology: a paradigm shift. J Thorac Oncol. 2010 Apr;5(4):411–4. PMID:20357614

3084. Travis WD, Rush W, Flieder DB, et al. Survival analysis of 200 pulmonary neuroendocrine tumors with clarification of criteria for atypical carcinoid and its separation from

typical carcinoid. Am J Surg Pathol. 1998 Aug;22(8):934–44. PMID:9706973
3085. Tremblay A, Taghizadeh N, McWilliams AM, et al. Low prevalence of high-grade lesions detected with autofluorescence bronchoscopy in the setting of lung cancer screening in the Pan-Canadian Lung Cancer Screening Study. Chest. 2016 Nov;150(5):1015–22. PMID:27142184
3086. Trinquand A, Tanguy-Schmidt A, Ben Abdelali R, et al. Toward a NOTCH1/FBXW7/RAS/PTEN-based oncogenetic risk classification of adult T-cell acute lymphoblastic leukemia: a Group for Research in Adult Acute Lymphoblastic Leukemia study. J Clin Oncol. 2013 Dec 1;31(34):4333–42. PMID:24166518
3087. Trivedi M, Chandar R, Nair M, et al. Primary mediastinal large B-cell lymphoma in a child presenting with superior mediastinal syndrome and chylous pleural and pericardial effusion. J Pediatr Hematol Oncol. 2020 Jul;42(5):e369–72. PMID:30951026
3088. Truong LD, Mody DR, Cagle PT, et al. Thymic carcinoma. A clinicopathologic study of 13 cases. Am J Surg Pathol. 1990 Feb;14(2):151–66. PMID:1689123
3089. Truong T, Hung RJ, Amos CI, et al. Replication of lung cancer susceptibility loci at chromosomes 15q25, 5p15, and 6p21: a pooled analysis from the International Lung Cancer Consortium. J Natl Cancer Inst. 2010 Jul 7;102(13):959–71. PMID:20548021
3090. Tryfon S, Dramba V, Zoglopitis F, et al. Solitary papillomas of the lower airways: epidemiological, clinical, and therapeutic data during a 22-year period and review of the literature. J Thorac Oncol. 2012 Apr;7(4):643–8. PMID:22425912
3091. Tsang P, Cesarman E, Chadburn A, et al. Molecular characterization of primary mediastinal B cell lymphoma. Am J Pathol. 1996 Jun;148(6):2017–25. PMID:8669486
3092. Tsao MS, Marguet S, Le Teuff G, et al. Subtype classification of lung adenocarcinoma predicts benefit from adjuvant chemotherapy in patients undergoing complete resection. J Clin Oncol. 2015 Oct 20;33(30):3439–46. PMID:25918286
3093. Tsim S, Kelly C, Alexander L, et al. Diagnostic and Prognostic Biomarkers in the Rational Assessment of Mesothelioma (DIAPHRAGM) study: protocol of a prospective, multicentre, observational study. BMJ Open. 2016 Nov 24;6(11):e013324. PMID:27884852
3094. Tsubokawa N, Mimae T, Sasada S, et al. Negative prognostic influence of micropapillary pattern in stage IA lung adenocarcinoma. Eur J Cardiothorac Surg. 2016 Jan;49(1):293–9. PMID:25762400
3095. Tsuchida M, Umezu H, Hashimoto T, et al. Absence of gene mutations in KIT-positive thymic epithelial tumors. Lung Cancer. 2008 Dec;62(3):321–5. PMID:18486988
3096. Tsuchida M, Yamato Y, Hashimoto T, et al. Recurrent thymic carcinoid tumor in the pleural cavity. 2 cases of long-term survivors. Jpn J Thorac Cardiovasc Surg. 2001 Nov;49(11):666–8. PMID:11757339
3097. Tsui DWY, Murtaza M, Wong ASC, et al. Dynamics of multiple resistance mechanisms in plasma DNA during EGFR-targeted therapies in non-small cell lung cancer. EMBO Mol Med. 2018 Jun;10(6):e7945. PMID:29848757
3098. Tsukioka T, Inoue K, Iwata T, et al. Thymolipoma associated with myasthenia gravis. Gen Thorac Cardiovasc Surg. 2007 Jan;55(1):26–8. PMID:17444169
3099. Tsunoda Y, Tanaka K, Okada K, et al. [Thymic basaloid carcinoma]. Kyobu Geka. 2010 Sep;63(10):857–61. Japanese. PMID:20845693
3100. Tsuruoka K, Horinouchi H, Goto Y, et al. PD-L1 expression in neuroendocrine tumors of the lung. Lung Cancer. 2017 Jun;108:115–20. PMID:28625622
3101. Tsuta K, Ishii G, Nitadori J, et al. Comparison of the immunophenotypes of signet-ring cell carcinoma, solid adenocarcinoma with mucin production, and mucinous bronchioloalveolar carcinoma of the lung characterized by the presence of cytoplasmic mucin. J Pathol. 2006 May;209(1):78–87. PMID:16463270
3102. Tsuta K, Kawago M, Inoue E, et al. The utility of the proposed IASLC/ATS/ERS lung adenocarcinoma subtypes for disease prognosis and correlation of driver gene alterations. Lung Cancer. 2013 Sep;81(3):371–6. PMID:23891509
3103. Tsuta K, Kawago M, Yoshida A, et al. Primary lung adenocarcinoma with morule-like components: a unique histologic hallmark of aggressive behavior and EGFR mutation. Lung Cancer. 2014 Jul;85(1):12–8. PMID:24768118
3104. Tsutani Y, Miyata Y, Mimae T, et al. The prognostic role of pathologic invasive component size, excluding lepidic growth, in stage I lung adenocarcinoma. J Thorac Cardiovasc Surg. 2013 Sep;146(3):580–5. PMID:23778085
3105. Tsutani Y, Miyata Y, Yamanaka T, et al. Solid tumors versus mixed tumors with a ground-glass opacity component in patients with clinical stage IA lung adenocarcinoma: prognostic comparison using high-resolution computed tomography findings. J Thorac Cardiovasc Surg. 2013 Jul;146(1):17–23. PMID:23246051
3106. Tsyganov MM, Pevzner AM, Ibragimova MK, et al. Human papillomavirus and lung cancer: an overview and a meta-analysis. J Cancer Res Clin Oncol. 2019 Aug;145(8):1919–37. PMID:31236668
3107. Tuna IC, Julsrud PR, Click RL, et al. Tissue characterization of an unusual right atrial mass by magnetic resonance imaging. Mayo Clin Proc. 1991 May;66(5):498–501. PMID:2030616
3108. Turner AR, MacDonald RN, Gilbert JA, et al. Mediastinal germ cell cancers in Klinefelter's syndrome. Ann Intern Med. 1981 Feb;94(2):279. PMID:7469226
3109. Turner SR, Buonocore D, Desmeules P, et al. Feasibility of endobronchial ultrasound transbronchial needle aspiration for massively parallel next-generation sequencing in thoracic cancer patients. Lung Cancer. 2018 May;119:85–90. PMID:29656758
3110. Turunen JA, Markkinen S, Wilska R, et al. BAP1 germline mutations in Finnish patients with uveal melanoma. Ophthalmology. 2016 May;123(5):1112–7. PMID:26876698
3111. Tutak E, Satar M, Ozbarlas N, et al. A newborn infant with intrapericardial rhabdomyosarcoma: a case report. Turk J Pediatr. 2008 Mar-Apr;50(2):179–81. PMID:18664085
3112. Twa DD, Chan FC, Ben-Neriah S, et al. Genomic rearrangements involving programmed death ligands are recurrent in primary mediastinal large B-cell lymphoma. Blood. 2014 Mar 27;123(13):2062–5. PMID:24497532
3113. Tzouvelekis A, Karampitsakos T, Gomatou G, et al. Lung cancer in patients with idiopathic pulmonary fibrosis. A retrospective multicenter study in Greece. Pulm Pharmacol Ther. 2020 Feb;60:101880. PMID:31874284
3114. U.S. Department of Health and Human Services. The health consequences of smoking: 50 years of progress. A report of the Surgeon General. Atlanta (GA): U.S. Department of Health and Human Services, Centers for Disease Control and Prevention, National Center for Chronic Disease Prevention and Health Promotion, Office on Smoking and Health; 2014 [printed with corrections 2014 Jan]. Available from: https://www.cdc.gov/tobacco/data_statistics/sgr/50th-anniversary/index.htm.
3115. Uchida N, Fujita K, Okamura M, et al. The clinical benefits of immune checkpoint inhibitor for thymic carcinomas ~experience of single public hospital in Japan~. Respir Med Case Rep. 2018 Nov 13;26:39–41. PMID:30505679
3116. Udo E, Furusato B, Sakai K, et al. Ciliated muconodular papillary tumors of the lung with KRAS/BRAF/AKT1 mutation. Diagn Pathol. 2017 Aug 22;12(1):62. PMID:28830562
3117. Ueda Y, Omasa M, Taki T, et al. Thymic neuroblastoma within a thymic cyst in an adult. Case Rep Oncol. 2012 May;5(2):459–63. PMID:23109922
3117A. Ueno M, Fujiyama J, Yamazaki I, et al. Cytology of primary pulmonary meningioma. Report of the first multiple case. Acta Cytol. 1998 Nov-Dec;42(6):1424–30. PMID:9850654
3118. UICC [Internet]. Geneva (Switzerland): Union for International Cancer Control; 2020. TNM Publications and Resources; updated 2020 Oct 6. Available from: https://www.uicc.org/resources/tnm/publications-resources.
3119. Ulbright TM, Loehrer PJ, Roth LM, et al. The development of non-germ cell malignancies within germ cell tumors. A clinicopathologic study of 11 cases. Cancer. 1984 Nov 1;54(9):1824–33. PMID:6090001
3120. Ulbright TM, Roth LM, Brodhecker CA. Yolk sac differentiation in germ cell tumors. A morphologic study of 50 cases with emphasis on hepatic, enteric, and parietal yolk sac features. Am J Surg Pathol. 1986 Mar;10(3):151–64. PMID:2420222
3121. Ulbright TM, Tickoo SK, Berney DM, et al. Best practices recommendations in the application of immunohistochemistry in testicular tumors: report from the International Society of Urological Pathology consensus conference. Am J Surg Pathol. 2014 Aug;38(8):e50–9. PMID:24832161
3122. Uner A, Dogan M, Sal E, et al. Stroke and recurrent peripheral embolism in left atrial myxoma. Acta Cardiol. 2010 Feb;65(1):101–3. PMID:20306900
3123. Urban C, Lackner H, Schwinger W, et al. Fatal hemophagocytic syndrome as initial manifestation of a mediastinal germ cell tumor. Med Pediatr Oncol. 2003 Apr;40(4):247–9. PMID:12555254
3124. Ushiku T, Shinozaki A, Shibahara J, et al. SALL4 represents fetal gut differentiation of gastric cancer, and is diagnostically useful in distinguishing hepatoid gastric carcinoma from hepatocellular carcinoma. Am J Surg Pathol. 2010 Apr;34(4):533–40. PMID:20182341
3125. Usuda K, Saito Y, Nagamoto N, et al. Relation between bronchoscopic findings and tumor size of roentgenographically occult bronchogenic squamous cell carcinoma. J Thorac Cardiovasc Surg. 1993 Dec;106(6):1098–103. PMID:8246545
3126. Uzun O, Wilson DG, Vujanic GM, et al. Cardiac tumours in children. Orphanet J Rare Dis. 2007 Mar 1;2:11. PMID:17331235
3127. Vaideeswar P, Gupta R, Mishra P, et al. Atypical cardiac myxomas: a clinicopathologic analysis and their comparison to 64 typical myxomas. Cardiovasc Pathol. 2012 May-Jun;21(3):180–7. PMID:21839650
3128. Vaishnavi A, Capelletti M, Le AT, et al. Oncogenic and drug-sensitive NTRK1 rearrangements in lung cancer. Nat Med. 2013 Nov;19(11):1469–72. PMID:24162815
3129. Vallés-Torres J, Izquierdo-Villarroya MB, Vallejo-Gil JM, et al. Cardiac undifferentiated pleomorphic sarcoma mimicking left atrial myxoma. J Cardiothorac Vasc Anesth. 2019 Feb;33(2):493–6. PMID:29551281
3130. Valli M, Fabris GA, Dewar A, et al. Atypical carcinoid tumour of the lung: a study of 33 cases with prognostic features. Histopathology. 1994 Apr;24(4):363–9. PMID:8045525
3131. Valli M, Fabris GA, Dewar A, et al. Atypical carcinoid tumour of the thymus: a study of eight cases. Histopathology. 1994 Apr;24(4):371–5. PMID:8045526
3132. van Boerdonk RA, Daniels JM, Bloemena E, et al. High-risk human papillomavirus-positive lung cancer: molecular evidence for a pattern of pulmonary metastasis. J Thorac Oncol. 2013 Jun;8(6):711–8. PMID:23571474
3133. van Boerdonk RA, Daniels JM, Snijders PJ, et al. DNA copy number aberrations in endobronchial lesions: a validated predictor for cancer. Thorax. 2014 May;69(5):451–7. PMID:24227199
3134. van Boerdonk RA, Smesseim I, Heideman DA, et al. Close surveillance with long-term follow-up of subjects with preinvasive endobronchial lesions. Am J Respir Crit Care Med. 2015 Dec 15;192(12):1483–9. PMID:26275031
3135. van Boerdonk RA, Sutedja TG, Snijders PJ, et al. DNA copy number alterations in endobronchial squamous metaplastic lesions predict lung cancer. Am J Respir Crit Care Med. 2011 Oct 15;184(8):948–56. PMID:21799074
3136. van de Rijn M, Barr FG, Xiong QB, et al. Poorly differentiated synovial sarcoma: an analysis of clinical, pathologic, and molecular genetic features. Am J Surg Pathol. 1999 Jan;23(1):106–12. PMID:9888710
3137. Van den Berghe I, Debiec-Rychter M, Proot L, et al. Ring chromosome 6 may represent a cytogenetic subgroup in benign thymoma. Cancer Genet Cytogenet. 2002 Aug;137(1):75–7. PMID:12377419
3138. van den Bosch JM, Wagenaar SS, Corrin B, et al. Mesenchymoma of the lung (so called hamartoma): a review of 154 parenchymal and endobronchial cases. Thorax. 1987 Oct;42(10):790–3. PMID:3321538
3139. Van Dievel J, Sciot R, Delcroix M, et al. Single-center experience with intimal sarcoma, an ultra-orphan, commonly fatal mesenchymal malignancy. Oncol Res Treat. 2017;40(6):353–9. PMID:28501860
3140. van Echten J, de Jong B, Sinke RJ, et al. Definition of a new entity of malignant extragonadal germ cell tumors. Genes Chromosomes Cancer. 1995 Jan;12(1):8–15. PMID:7534118
3141. van Meerbeeck JP, Gaafar R, Manegold C, et al. Randomized phase III study of cisplatin with or without raltitrexed in patients with malignant pleural mesothelioma: an intergroup study of the European Organisation for Research and Treatment of Cancer Lung Cancer Group and the National Cancer Institute of Canada. J Clin Oncol. 2005 Oct 1;23(28):6881–9. PMID:16192580
3142. van Noesel J, van der Ven WH, van Os TA, et al. Activating germline R776H mutation in the epidermal growth factor receptor associated with lung cancer with squamous differentiation. J Clin Oncol. 2013 Apr 1;31(10):e161–4. PMID:23358982
3143. Van Schil PE, Asamura H, Rusch VW, et al. Surgical implications of the new IASLC/ATS/ERS adenocarcinoma classification. Eur Respir J. 2012 Feb;39(2):478–86. PMID:21828029
3144. Van Schil PE, Opitz I, Weder W, et al. Multimodal management of malignant pleural mesothelioma: Where are we today? Eur Respir J. 2014 Sep;44(3):754–64. PMID:24525443
3145. van Spronsen DJ, Vrints LW, Hofstra G, et al. Disappearance of prognostic significance of histopathological grading of nodular sclerosing Hodgkin's disease for unselected patients, 1972-92. Br J Haematol. 1997 Feb;96(2):322–7. PMID:9029020
3146. van Velthuysen ML, Groen EJ, van der Noort V, et al. Grading of neuroendocrine neoplasms: mitoses and Ki-67 are both essential. Neuroendocrinology. 2014;100(2-3):221–7.

PMID:25358267
3147. Van Vlierberghe P, Pieters R, Beverloo HB, et al. Molecular-genetic insights in paediatric T-cell acute lymphoblastic leukaemia. Br J Haematol. 2008 Oct;143(2):153–68. PMID:18691165
3148. Vandevenne JE, De Schepper AM, De Beuckeleer L, et al. New concepts in understanding evolution of desmoid tumors: MR imaging of 30 lesions. Eur Radiol. 1997;7(7):1013–9. PMID:9265665
3149. Vanhentenrijk V, Vanden Bempt I, Dierickx D, et al. Relationship between classic Hodgkin lymphoma and overlapping large cell lymphoma investigated by comparative expressed sequence hybridization expression profiling. J Pathol. 2006 Oct;210(2):155–62. PMID:16874743
3150. van Meerbeeck JP, Fennell DA, De Ruysscher DK. Small-cell lung cancer. Lancet. 2011 Nov 12;378(9804):1741–55. PMID:21565397
3151. Van Vlierberghe P, Ferrando A. The molecular basis of T cell acute lymphoblastic leukemia. J Clin Invest. 2012 Oct;122(10):3398–406. PMID:23023710
3152. Vargas SO, French CA, Faul PN, et al. Upper respiratory tract carcinoma with chromosomal translocation 15;19: evidence for a distinct disease entity of young patients with a rapidly fatal course. Cancer. 2001 Sep 1;92(5):1195–203. PMID:11571733
3153. Varghese AM, Zakowski MF, Yu HA, et al. Small-cell lung cancers in patients who never smoked cigarettes. J Thorac Oncol. 2014 Jun;9(6):892–6. PMID:24828667
3154. Vasey PA, Dunlop DJ, Kaye SB. Primary mediastinal germ cell tumour and acute monocytic leukaemia occurring concurrently in a 15-year-old boy. Ann Oncol. 1994 Sep;5(7):649–52. PMID:7993843
3155. Vassallo R, Harari S, Tazi A. Current understanding and management of pulmonary Langerhans cell histiocytosis. Thorax. 2017 Oct;72(10):937–45. PMID:28689173
3156. Vassallo R, Jensen EA, Colby TV, et al. The overlap between respiratory bronchiolitis and desquamative interstitial pneumonia in pulmonary Langerhans cell histiocytosis: high-resolution CT, histologic, and functional correlations. Chest. 2003 Oct;124(4):1199–205. PMID:14555547
3157. Vassallo R, Ryu JH, Schroeder DR, et al. Clinical outcomes of pulmonary Langerhans'-cell histiocytosis in adults. N Engl J Med. 2002 Feb 14;346(7):484–90. PMID:11844849
3158. Vassella E, Langsch S, Dettmer MS, et al. Molecular profiling of lung adenosquamous carcinoma: hybrid or genuine type? Oncotarget. 2015 Sep 15;6(27):23905–16. PMID:26068980
3159. Vaughan CJ, Veugelers M, Basson CT. Tumors and the heart: molecular genetic advances. Curr Opin Cardiol. 2001 May;16(3):195–200. PMID:11357016
3160. Vaughan CJ, Weremowicz S, Goldstein MM, et al. A t(2;19)(p13;p13.2) in a giant invasive cardiac lipoma from a patient with multiple lipomatosis. Genes Chromosomes Cancer. 2000 Jun;28(2):133–7. PMID:10824997
3161. Vaziri M, Rad K. Progressive dyspnea in a 40-year-old man caused by giant mediastinal thymolipoma. Case Rep Surg. 2016;2016:3469395. PMID:27293949
3162. Vazquez MF, Koizumi JH, Henschke CI, et al. Reliability of cytologic diagnosis of early lung cancer. Cancer. 2007 Aug 25;111(4):252–8. PMID:17614298
3163. Vega F, Padula A, Valbuena JR, et al. Lymphomas involving the pleura: a clinicopathologic study of 34 cases diagnosed by pleural biopsy. Arch Pathol Lab Med. 2006 Oct;130(10):1497–502. PMID:17090191
3164. Veinot JP. Cardiac tumors of adipocytes and cystic tumor of the atrioventricular node. Semin Diagn Pathol. 2008 Feb;25(1):29–38. PMID:18350920
3165. Velankar MM, Nathwani BN, Schlutz MJ, et al. Indolent T-lymphoblastic proliferation: report of a case with a 16-year course without cytotoxic therapy. Am J Surg Pathol. 1999 Aug;23(8):977–81. PMID:10435569
3166. Verbeke SL, de Jong D, Bertoni F, et al. Array CGH analysis identifies two distinct subgroups of primary angiosarcoma of bone. Genes Chromosomes Cancer. 2015 Feb;54(2):72–81. PMID:25231439
3167. Verkkala K, Kupari M, Maamies T, et al. Primary cardiac tumours–operative treatment of 20 patients. Thorac Cardiovasc Surg. 1989 Dec;37(6):361–4. PMID:2617502
3168. Vermi W, Lonardi S, Bosisio D, et al. Identification of CXCL13 as a new marker for follicular dendritic cell sarcoma. J Pathol. 2008 Nov;216(3):356–64. PMID:18792075
3169. Veugelers M, Wilkes D, Burton K, et al. Comparative PRKAR1A genotype-phenotype analyses in humans with Carney complex and prkar1a haploinsufficient mice. Proc Natl Acad Sci U S A. 2004 Sep 28;101(39):14222–7. PMID:15371594
3169A. Vidarsdottir H, Tran L, Nodin B, et al. Immunohistochemical profiles in primary lung cancers and epithelial pulmonary metastases. Hum Pathol. 2019 Feb;84:221–30. PMID:30389437
3170. Viganò S, Papini GD, Cotticelli B, et al. Prevalence of cerebral aneurysms in patients treated for left cardiac myxoma: a prospective study. Clin Radiol. 2013 Nov;68(11):e624–8. PMID:23937828
3170A. Villa JK, Amador P, Janovsky J, et al. A genome-wide search for ionizing-radiation-responsive elements in Deinococcus radiodurans reveals a regulatory role for the DNA gyrase subunit A gene's 5' untranslated region in the radiation and desiccation response. Appl Environ Microbiol. 2017 May 31;83(12):e00039–17. PMID:28411225
3171. Villacampa VM, Villarreal M, Ros LH, et al. Cardiac rhabdomyosarcoma: diagnosis by MR imaging. Eur Radiol. 1999;9(4):634–7. PMID:10354875
3172. Villani A, Shore A, Wasserman JD, et al. Biochemical and imaging surveillance in germline TP53 mutation carriers with Li-Fraumeni syndrome: 11 year follow-up of a prospective observational study. Lancet Oncol. 2016 Sep;17(9):1295–305. PMID:27501770
3173. Vincenten JPL, van Essen HF, Lissenberg-Witte BI, et al. Clonality analysis of pulmonary tumors by genome-wide copy number profiling. PLoS One. 2019 Oct 16;14(10):e0223827. PMID:31618260
3174. Viola P, Vroobel KM, Devaraj A, et al. Follicular dendritic cell tumour/sarcoma: a commonly misdiagnosed tumour in the thorax. Histopathology. 2016 Nov;69(5):752–61. PMID:27206572
3175. Viswanathan K, Borczuk AC, Siddiqui MT. Orthopedia homeobox protein (OTP) is a sensitive and specific marker for primary pulmonary carcinoid tumors in cytologic and surgical specimens. J Am Soc Cytopathol. 2019 Jan-Feb;8(1):39–46. PMID:30929758
3176. Vivero M, Davineni P, Nardi V, et al. Metaplastic thymoma: a distinctive thymic neoplasm characterized by YAP1-MAML2 gene fusions. Mod Pathol. 2020 Apr;33(4):560–5. PMID:31641231
3177. Vladislav IT, Gökmen-Polar Y, Kesler KA, et al. The role of histology in predicting recurrence of type A thymomas: a clinicopathologic correlation of 23 cases. Mod Pathol. 2013 Aug;26(8):1059–64. PMID:23579619
3178. Vlasveld LT, Splinter TA, Hagemeijer A, et al. Acute myeloid leukaemia with +i(12p) shortly after treatment of mediastinal germ cell tumour. Br J Haematol. 1994 Sep;88(1):196–8. PMID:7803244
3179. Völkl TM, Langer T, Aigner T, et al. Klinefelter syndrome and mediastinal germ cell tumors. Am J Med Genet A. 2006 Mar 1;140(5):471–81. PMID:16470792
3179A. Vollmer RT, Ogden L, Crissman JD. Separation of small-cell from non-small-cell lung cancer. The Southeastern Cancer Study Group pathologists' experience. Arch Pathol Lab Med. 1984 Oct;108(10):792–4. PMID:6089696
3180. von Ahsen I, Rogalla P, Bullerdiek J. Expression patterns of the LPP-HMGA2 fusion transcript in pulmonary chondroid hamartomas with t(3;12)(q27 approximately 28;q14 approximately 15). Cancer Genet Cytogenet. 2005 Nov;163(1):68–70. PMID:16271958
3180A. Voutsadakis IA, Mozarowski P. Expression of TTF-1 in breast cancer independently of ER expression: a case report and pathogenic implications. Breast Dis. 2017;37(1):1–6. PMID:27983521
3181. Vuong HG, Ho ATN, Altibi AMA, et al. Clinicopathological implications of MET exon 14 mutations in non-small cell lung cancer - a systematic review and meta-analysis. Lung Cancer. 2018 Sep;123:76–82. PMID:30089599
3182. Waddell N, Pajic M, Patch AM, et al. Whole genomes redefine the mutational landscape of pancreatic cancer. Nature. 2015 Feb 26;518(7540):495–501. PMID:25719666
3183. Wadt KA, Aoude LG, Johansson P, et al. A recurrent germline BAP1 mutation and extension of the BAP1 tumor predisposition spectrum to include basal cell carcinoma. Clin Genet. 2015 Sep;88(3):267–72. PMID:25225168
3184. Wakelee HA, Chang ET, Gomez SL, et al. Lung cancer incidence in never smokers. J Clin Oncol. 2007 Feb 10;25(5):472–8. PMID:17290054
3185. Wakely PE Jr. Cytopathology-histopathology of the mediastinum: epithelial, lymphoproliferative, and germ cell neoplasms. Ann Diagn Pathol. 2002 Feb;6(1):30–43. PMID:11842377
3186. Wakely PE Jr. Fine needle aspiration in the diagnosis of thymic epithelial neoplasms. Hematol Oncol Clin North Am. 2008 Jun;22(3):433–42. PMID:18514125
3187. Walch AK, Zitzelsberger HF, Aubele MM, et al. Typical and atypical carcinoid tumors of the lung are characterized by 11q deletions as detected by comparative genomic hybridization. Am J Pathol. 1998 Oct;153(4):1089–98. PMID:9777940
3188. Walpole S, Pritchard AL, Cebulla CM, et al. Comprehensive study of the clinical phenotype of germline BAP1 variant-carrying families worldwide. J Natl Cancer Inst. 2018 Dec 1;110(12):1328–41. PMID:30517737
3189. Walters M, Pittelkow MR, Hasserjian RP, et al. Follicular dendritic cell sarcoma with indolent T-lymphoblastic proliferation is associated with paraneoplastic autoimmune multiorgan syndrome. Am J Surg Pathol. 2018 Dec;42(12):1647–52. PMID:30222603
3190. Walts AE, Hiroshima K, Marchevsky AM. Desmoglein 3 and p40 immunoreactivity in neoplastic and nonneoplastic thymus: a potential adjunct to help resolve selected diagnostic and staging problems. Ann Diagn Pathol. 2015 Aug;19(4):216–20. PMID:25979154
3191. Walts AE, Hiroshima K, McGregor SM, et al. BAP1 immunostain and CDKN2A (p16) FISH analysis: clinical applicability for the diagnosis of malignant mesothelioma in effusions. Diagn Cytopathol. 2016 Jul;44(7):599–606. PMID:27121152
3192. Walts AE, Ines D, Marchevsky AM. Limited role of Ki-67 proliferative index in predicting overall short-term survival in patients with typical and atypical pulmonary carcinoid tumors. Mod Pathol. 2012 Sep;25(9):1258–64. PMID:22575865
3193. Wanebo HJ, Rao B, Miyazawa N, et al. Immune reactivity in primary carcinoma of the lung and its relation to prognosis. J Thorac Cardiovasc Surg. 1976 Sep;72(3):339–50. PMID:183063
3194. Wang C, Gaz RD, Moncure AC. Mediastinal parathyroid exploration: a clinical and pathologic study of 47 cases. World J Surg. 1986 Aug;10(4):687–95. PMID:3751094
3195. Wang CP, Chang YL, Ko JY, et al. Lymphoepithelial carcinoma versus large cell undifferentiated carcinoma of the major salivary glands. Cancer. 2004 Nov 1;101(9):2020–7. PMID:15389474
3196. Wang CX, Liu B, Wang YF, et al. Pulmonary enteric adenocarcinoma: a study of the clinicopathologic and molecular status of nine cases. Int J Clin Exp Pathol. 2014 Feb 15;7(3):1266–74. PMID:24696747
3197. Wang DY, Kuo SH, Chang DB, et al. Fine needle aspiration cytology of thymic carcinoid tumor. Acta Cytol. 1995 May-Jun;39(3):423–7. PMID:7762327
3198. Wang E, Lin D, Wang Y, et al. Immunohistochemical and ultrastructural markers suggest different origins for cuboidal and polygonal cells in pulmonary sclerosing hemangioma. Hum Pathol. 2004 Apr;35(4):503–8. PMID:15116333
3199. Wang EH, Dai SD, Qi FJ, et al. Gene expression and clonality analysis of the androgen receptor and phosphoglycerate kinase genes in polygonal cells and cuboidal cells in so-called pulmonary sclerosing hemangioma. Mod Pathol. 2007 Nov;20(11):1208–15. PMID:17873892
3200. Wang F, Lan H. A case report on the effect of rituximab on pyothorax-associated lymphoma. Medicine (Baltimore). 2019 Dec;98(50):e18393. PMID:31852157
3201. Wang F, Liu A, Peng Y, et al. Diagnostic utility of SALL4 in extragonadal yolk sac tumors: an immunohistochemical study of 59 cases with comparison to placental-like alkaline phosphatase, alpha-fetoprotein, and glypican-3. Am J Surg Pathol. 2009 Oct;33(10):1529–39. PMID:19574883
3202. Wang GY, Thomas DG, Davis JL, et al. EWSR1-NFATC2 translocation-associated sarcoma clinicopathologic findings in a rare aggressive primary bone or soft tissue tumor. Am J Surg Pathol. 2019 Aug;43(8):1112–22. PMID:30994538
3203. Wang H, Sun L, Sang Y, et al. A study of ALK-positive pulmonary squamous-cell carcinoma: from diagnostic methodologies to clinical efficacy. Lung Cancer. 2019 Apr;130:135–42. PMID:30885334
3204. Wang HW, Balakrishna JP, Pittaluga S, et al. Diagnosis of Hodgkin lymphoma in the modern era. Br J Haematol. 2019 Jan;184(1):45–59. PMID:30407610
3205. Wang J, Kragel AH, Friedlander ER, et al. Granular cell tumor of the sinus node. Am J Cardiol. 1993 Feb 15;71(5):490–2. PMID:8430653
3206. Wang J, Lian B, Ye L, et al. Clinicopathological characteristics and survival outcomes in adenosquamous carcinoma of the lung: a population-based study from the SEER database. Oncotarget. 2017 Dec 21;9(8):8133–46. PMID:29487721
3207. Wang J, Ye L, Cai H, et al. Comparative study of large cell neuroendocrine carcinoma and small cell lung carcinoma in high-grade neuroendocrine tumors of the lung: a large population-based study. J Cancer. 2019 Jul 10;10(18):4226–36. PMID:31413741
3208. Wang JG, Cui L, Jiang T, et al. Primary

cardiac leiomyosarcoma: an analysis of clinical characteristics and outcome patterns. Asian Cardiovasc Thorac Ann. 2015 Jun;23(5):623–30. PMID:25740020
3209. Wang JG, Han J, Jiang T, et al. Cardiac paragangliomas. J Card Surg. 2015 Jan;30(1):55–60. PMID:25331372
3210. Wang JG, Li NN. Primary cardiac synovial sarcoma. Ann Thorac Surg. 2013 Jun;95(6):2202–9. PMID:23647858
3211. Wang JG, Wang B, Hu Y, et al. Clinicopathologic features and outcomes of primary cardiac tumors: a 16-year-experience with 212 patients at a Chinese medical center. Cardiovasc Pathol. 2018 Mar-Apr;33:45–54. PMID:29414432
3212. Wang LL, Teshiba R, Ikegaki N, et al. Augmented expression of MYC and/or MYCN protein defines highly aggressive MYC-driven neuroblastoma: a Children's Oncology Group study. Br J Cancer. 2015 Jun 30;113(1):57–63. PMID:26035700
3213. Wang QB, Chen YQ, Shen JJ, et al. Sixteen cases of pulmonary sclerosing haemangioma: CT findings are not definitive for preoperative diagnosis. Clin Radiol. 2011 Aug;66(8):708–14. PMID:21529795
3214. Wang R, Hu H, Pan Y, et al. RET fusions define a unique molecular and clinicopathologic subtype of non-small-cell lung cancer. J Clin Oncol. 2012 Dec 10;30(35):4352–9. PMID:23150706
3215. Wang R, Pan Y, Li C, et al. Analysis of major known driver mutations and prognosis in resected adenosquamous lung carcinomas. J Thorac Oncol. 2014 Jun;9(6):760–8. PMID:24481316
3216. Wang S, Yang DM, Rong R, et al. Artificial intelligence in lung cancer pathology image analysis. Cancers (Basel). 2019 Oct 28;11(11):E1673. PMID:31661863
3217. Wang VE, Urisman A, Albacker L, et al. Checkpoint inhibitor is active against large cell neuroendocrine carcinoma with high tumor mutation burden. J Immunother Cancer. 2017 Sep 19;5(1):75. PMID:28923100
3218. Wang XL, Jiang GJ, Zhang XZ, et al. Pulmonary papillary adenoma: report of two cases. J Coll Physicians Surg Pak. 2017 Sep;27(9):582–3. PMID:29017679
3219. Wang XL, Mu YM, Dou JT, et al. Medullar thyroid carcinoma in mediastinum initially presenting as ectopic ACTH syndrome. A case report. Neuro Endocrinol Lett. 2011;32(4):421–4. PMID:21876495
3220. Wang Y, Ma C, Yang J, et al. Incomplete excision or postoperative hematoma: primary right ventricular intramyocardial lipoma involving the right ventricular outflow tract. J Med Ultrason (2001). 2015 Oct;42(4):541–5. PMID:26576979
3221. Wang Y, Thomas A, Lau C, et al. Mutations of epigenetic regulatory genes are common in thymic carcinomas. Sci Rep. 2014 Dec 8;4:7336. PMID:25482724
3222. Wang Y, Wenzl K, Manske MK, et al. Amplification of 9p24.1 in diffuse large B-cell lymphoma identifies a unique subset of cases that resemble primary mediastinal large B-cell lymphoma. Blood Cancer J. 2019 Aug 30;9(9):73. PMID:31471540
3222A. Wang YF, Liu B, Fan XS, et al. Thyroid carcinoma showing thymus-like elements: a clinicopathologic, immunohistochemical, ultrastructural, and molecular analysis. Am J Clin Pathol. 2015 Feb;143(2):223–33. PMID:25596248
3223. Wang YL, Yi XH, Chen G, et al. [Thymoma associated with an lipofibroadenoma: report of a case]. Zhonghua Bing Li Xue Za Zhi. 2009 Aug;38(8):556–7. Chinese. PMID:20021971
3224. Wang Z, Yang MQ, Huang WJ, et al. Sclerosing pneumocytoma mixed with a typical carcinoid tumor: a case report and review of literature. Medicine (Baltimore). 2019 Feb;98(5):e14315. PMID:30702609
3225. Warth A, Cortis J, Fink L, et al. Training increases concordance in classifying pulmonary adenocarcinomas according to the novel IASLC/ATS/ERS classification. Virchows Arch. 2012 Aug;461(2):185–93. PMID:22729141
3226. Warth A, Muley T, Harms A, et al. Clinical relevance of different papillary growth patterns of pulmonary adenocarcinoma. Am J Surg Pathol. 2016 Jun;40(6):818–26. PMID:26927890
3227. Warth A, Muley T, Herpel E, et al. Large-scale comparative analyses of immunomarkers for diagnostic subtyping of non-small-cell lung cancer biopsies. Histopathology. 2012 Dec;61(6):1017–25. PMID:22882703
3228. Warth A, Muley T, Kossakowski C, et al. Prognostic impact and clinicopathological correlations of the cribriform pattern in pulmonary adenocarcinoma. J Thorac Oncol. 2015 Apr;10(4):638–44. PMID:25634008
3229. Warth A, Muley T, Kossakowski CA, et al. Prognostic impact of intra-alveolar tumor spread in pulmonary adenocarcinoma. Am J Surg Pathol. 2015 Jun;39(6):793–801. PMID:25723114
3230. Warth A, Muley T, Meister M, et al. The novel histologic International Association for the Study of Lung Cancer/American Thoracic Society/European Respiratory Society classification system of lung adenocarcinoma is a stage-independent predictor of survival. J Clin Oncol. 2012 May 1;30(13):1438–46. PMID:22393100
3231. Wassef M, Blei F, Adams D, et al. Vascular anomalies classification: recommendations from the International Society for the Study of Vascular Anomalies. Pediatrics. 2015 Jul;136(1):e203–14. PMID:26055853
3232. Watanabe H, Saito H, Yokose T, et al. Relation between thin-section computed tomography and clinical findings of mucinous adenocarcinoma. Ann Thorac Surg. 2015 Mar;99(3):975–81. PMID:25624054
3233. Watanabe J, Togo S, Sumiyoshi I, et al. Clinical features of squamous cell lung cancer with anaplastic lymphoma kinase (ALK)-rearrangement: a retrospective analysis and review. Oncotarget. 2018 May 8;9(35):24000–13. PMID:29844868
3234. Watanabe M, Yamamoto H, Hashida S, et al. Primary pulmonary melanoma: a report of two cases. World J Surg Oncol. 2015 Sep 17;13:274. PMID:26376781
3235. Watanabe R, Ito I, Kenmotsu H, et al. Large cell neuroendocrine carcinoma of the lung: Is it possible to diagnose from biopsy specimens? Jpn J Clin Oncol. 2013 Mar;43(3):294–304. PMID:23381206
3236. Watanabe Y, Tsuta K, Kusumoto M, et al. Clinicopathologic features and computed tomographic findings of 52 surgically resected adenosquamous carcinomas of the lung. Ann Thorac Surg. 2014 Jan;97(1):245–51. PMID:24206962
3237. Watchell M, Heritage DW, Pastore L, et al. Cytogenetic study of cardiac papillary fibroelastoma. Cancer Genet Cytogenet. 2000 Jul 15;120(2):174–5. PMID:10991617
3238. Waters R, Horvai A, Greipp P, et al. Atypical lipomatous tumour/well-differentiated liposarcoma and de-differentiated liposarcoma in patients aged ≤ 40 years: a study of 116 patients. Histopathology. 2019 Dec;75(6):833–42. PMID:31471922
3239. Watson GH. Cardiac rhabdomyomas in tuberous sclerosis. Ann N Y Acad Sci. 1991;615:50–7. PMID:2039167
3240. Watson R, Frye J, Trieu M, et al. Primary undifferentiated pleomorphic cardiac sarcoma with MDM2 amplification presenting as acute left-sided heart failure. BMJ Case Rep. 2018 Sep 30;2018:bcr-2018-226073. PMID:30275026
3241. Watson S, Perrin V, Guillemot D, et al. Transcriptomic definition of molecular subgroups of small round cell sarcomas. J Pathol. 2018 May;245(1):29–40. PMID:29431183
3242. Wayman CP, Wilson JF. Long-term potentiation of hypothalamic alpha-MSH release by NMDA. Ann N Y Acad Sci. 1993 May 31;680:646–8. PMID:8390208
3243. Weaver J, Downs-Kelly E, Goldblum JR, et al. Fluorescence in situ hybridization for MDM2 gene amplification as a diagnostic tool in lipomatous neoplasms. Mod Pathol. 2008 Aug;21(8):943–9. PMID:18500263
3244. Weber C, Pautex S, Zulian GB, et al. Primary pulmonary malignant meningioma with lymph node and liver metastasis in a centenary woman, an autopsy case. Virchows Arch. 2013 Apr;462(4):481–5. PMID:23443940
3245. Weber TR, Connors RH, Tracy TF Jr, et al. Complex hemangiomas of infants and children. Individualized management in 22 cases. Arch Surg. 1990 Aug;125(8):1017–20, discussion 1020–1. PMID:2198856
3246. Webster P, Wujanto L, Fisher C, et al. Malignancies confined to disused arteriovenous fistulae in renal transplant patients: an important differential diagnosis. Am J Nephrol. 2011;34(1):42–8. PMID:21659738
3247. Weidle UH, Birzele F, Kollmorgen G, et al. Molecular basis of lung tropism of metastasis. Cancer Genomics Proteomics. 2016 Mar-Apr;13(2):129–39. PMID:26912803
3248. Weidle UH, Birzele F, Kollmorgen G, et al. The multiple roles of exosomes in metastasis. Cancer Genomics Proteomics. 2017 Jan 2;14(1):1–15. PMID:28031234
3249. Weidner N. Germ-cell tumors of the mediastinum. Semin Diagn Pathol. 1999 Feb;16(1):42–50. PMID:10355653
3250. Weinbreck N, Vignaud JM, Begueret H, et al. SYT-SSX fusion is absent in sarcomatoid mesothelioma allowing its distinction from synovial sarcoma of the pleura. Mod Pathol. 2007 Jun;20(6):617–21. PMID:17507990
3251. Weirich G, Schneider P, Fellbaum C, et al. p53 alterations in thymic epithelial tumours. Virchows Arch. 1997 Jul;431(1):17–23. PMID:9247629
3252. Weis CA, Yao X, Deng Y, et al. The impact of thymoma histotype on prognosis in a worldwide database. J Thorac Oncol. 2015 Feb;10(2):367–72. PMID:25616178
3253. Weiss LM, Bindl JM, Picozzi VJ, et al. Lymphoblastic lymphoma: an immunophenotype study of 26 cases with comparison to T cell acute lymphoblastic leukemia. Blood. 1986 Feb;67(2):474–8. PMID:3080041
3254. Weiss LM, Movahed LA, Warnke RA, et al. Detection of Epstein-Barr viral genomes in Reed-Sternberg cells of Hodgkin's disease. N Engl J Med. 1989 Feb 23;320(8):502–6. PMID:2536894
3255. Weiss SW, Ishak KG, Dail DH, et al. Epithelioid hemangioendothelioma and related lesions. Semin Diagn Pathol. 1986 Nov;3(4):259–87. PMID:3303234
3256. Weissferdt A. Large cell carcinoma of lung: on the verge of extinction? Semin Diagn Pathol. 2014 Jul;31(4):278–88. PMID:25023633
3257. Weissferdt A, Fujimoto J, Kalhor N, et al. Expression of PD-1 and PD-L1 in thymic epithelial neoplasms. Mod Pathol. 2017 Jun;30(6):826–33. PMID:28281549
3258. Weissferdt A, Hernandez JC, Kalhor N, et al. Spindle cell thymomas: an immunohistochemical study of 30 cases. Appl Immunohistochem Mol Morphol. 2011 Jul;19(4):329–35. PMID:21386704
3259. Weissferdt A, Kalhor N, Correa AM, et al. "Sarcomatoid" carcinomas of the lung: a clinicopathological study of 86 cases with a new perspective on tumor classification. Hum Pathol. 2017 May;63:14–26. PMID:27993578
3260. Weissferdt A, Kalhor N, Moran CA. Combined thymoma-thymic seminoma. Report of 2 cases of a heretofore unreported association. Hum Pathol. 2014 Oct;45(10):2168–72. PMID:25090916
3261. Weissferdt A, Kalhor N, Moran CA. Cystic well-differentiated squamous cell carcinoma of the thymus: a clinicopathological and immunohistochemical study of six cases. Histopathology. 2016 Feb;68(3):333–8. PMID:26031186
3262. Weissferdt A, Kalhor N, Rodriguez Canales J, et al. Primary mediastinal yolk sac tumors: an immunohistochemical analysis of 14 cases. Appl Immunohistochem Mol Morphol. 2019 Feb;27(2):125–33. PMID:27643524
3263. Weissferdt A, Kalhor N, Suster S, et al. Primary angiosarcomas of the anterior mediastinum: a clinicopathologic and immunohistochemical study of 9 cases. Hum Pathol. 2010 Dec;41(12):1711–7. PMID:20709359
3264. Weissferdt A, Moran CA. Anaplastic thymic carcinoma: a clinicopathologic and immunohistochemical study of 6 cases. Hum Pathol. 2012 Jun;43(6):874–7. PMID:22055398
3265. Weissferdt A, Moran CA. Lipomatous tumors of the anterior mediastinum with muscle differentiation: a clinicopathological and immunohistochemical study of three cases. Virchows Arch. 2014 Apr;464(4):489–93. PMID:24558031
3266. Weissferdt A, Moran CA. Malignant biphasic tumors of the lungs. Adv Anat Pathol. 2011 May;18(3):179–89. PMID:21490435
3267. Weissferdt A, Moran CA. Mediastinal seminoma with florid follicular lymphoid hyperplasia: a clinicopathological and immunohistochemical study of six cases. Virchows Arch. 2015 Feb;466(2):209–15. PMID:25425477
3268. Weissferdt A, Moran CA. Micronodular thymic carcinoma with lymphoid hyperplasia: a clinicopathological and immunohistochemical study of five cases. Mod Pathol. 2012 Jul;25(7):993–9. PMID:22388764
3269. Weissferdt A, Moran CA. Neuroendocrine differentiation in thymic carcinomas: a diagnostic pitfall: an immunohistochemical analysis of 27 cases. Am J Clin Pathol. 2016 Mar;145(3):393–400. PMID:27124922
3270. Weissferdt A, Moran CA. Pax8 expression in thymic epithelial neoplasms: an immunohistochemical analysis. Am J Surg Pathol. 2011 Sep;35(9):1305–10. PMID:21836478
3271. Weissferdt A, Moran CA. Primary pulmonary primitive neuroectodermal tumor (PNET): a clinicopathological and immunohistochemical study of six cases. Lung. 2012 Dec;190(6):677–83. PMID:22802134
3272. Weissferdt A, Moran CA. Pulmonary salivary gland-type tumors with features of malignant mixed tumor (carcinoma ex pleomorphic adenoma): a clinicopathologic study of five cases. Am J Clin Pathol. 2011 Nov;136(5):793–8. PMID:22031319
3273. Weissferdt A, Moran CA. Spindle cell thymomas with neuroendocrine morphology: a clinicopathological and immunohistochemical study of 18 cases. Histopathology. 2014 Jul;65(1):111–8. PMID:24702597
3274. Weissferdt A, Moran CA. The spectrum of ectopic thymomas. Virchows Arch. 2016 Sep;469(3):245–54. PMID:27255665
3275. Weissferdt A, Moran CA. Thymic carcinoma associated with multilocular thymic cyst: a clinicopathologic study of 7 cases. Am J Surg Pathol. 2011 Jul;35(7):1074–9. PMID:21677542

3276. Weissferdt A, Moran CA. Thymic carcinoma, part 1: a clinicopathologic and immunohistochemical study of 65 cases. Am J Clin Pathol. 2012 Jul;138(1):103–14. PMID:22706865
3277. Weissferdt A, Moran CA. Thymic carcinoma, part 2: a clinicopathologic correlation of 33 cases with a proposed staging system. Am J Clin Pathol. 2012 Jul;138(1):115–21. PMID:22706866
3278. Weissferdt A, Rodriguez-Canales J, Liu H, et al. Primary mediastinal seminomas: a comprehensive immunohistochemical study with a focus on novel markers. Hum Pathol. 2015 Mar;46(3):376–83. PMID:25576290
3279. Weissferdt A, Suster S, Moran CA. Primary mediastinal "thymic" seminomas. Adv Anat Pathol. 2012 Mar;19(2):75–80. PMID:22313835
3280. Weissferdt A, Tang X, Wistuba II, et al. Comparative immunohistochemical analysis of pulmonary and thymic neuroendocrine carcinomas using PAX8 and TTF-1. Mod Pathol. 2013 Dec;26(12):1554–60. PMID:23787439
3281. Weissferdt A, Wistuba II, Moran CA. Molecular aspects of thymic carcinoma. Lung Cancer. 2012 Nov;78(2):127–32. PMID:22921473
3282. Weitzel JN, Chao EC, Nehoray B, et al. Somatic TP53 variants frequently confound germ-line testing results. Genet Med. 2018 Aug;20(8):809–16. PMID:29189820
3283. Weksler B, Dhupar R, Parikh V, et al. Thymic carcinoma: a multivariate analysis of factors predictive of survival in 290 patients. Ann Thorac Surg. 2013 Jan;95(1):299–303. PMID:23141529
3284. Welsh TJ, Green RH, Richardson D, et al. Macrophage and mast-cell invasion of tumor cell islets confers a marked survival advantage in non-small-cell lung cancer. J Clin Oncol. 2005 Dec 10;23(35):8959–67. PMID:16219934
3285. Wen J, Chen J, Chen D, et al. Evaluation of the prognostic value of surgery and postoperative radiotherapy for patients with thymic neuroendocrine tumors: a propensity-matched study based on the SEER database. Thorac Cancer. 2018 Dec;9(12):1603–13. PMID:30276969
3286. Wen J, Li HZ, Ji ZG, et al. A decade of clinical experience with extra-adrenal paragangliomas of retroperitoneum: report of 67 cases and a literature review. Urol Ann. 2010 Jan;2(1):12–6. PMID:20842251
3287. Wendroth SM, Mentrikoski MJ, Wick MR. GATA3 expression in morphologic subtypes of breast carcinoma: a comparison with gross cystic disease fluid protein 15 and mammaglobin. Ann Diagn Pathol. 2015 Feb;19(1):6–9. PMID:25544392
3288. Wessendorf S, Barth TF, Viardot A, et al. Further delineation of chromosomal consensus regions in primary mediastinal B-cell lymphomas: an analysis of 37 tumor samples using high-resolution genomic profiling (array-CGH). Leukemia. 2007 Dec;21(12):2463–9. PMID:17728785
3289. West JA, Viswanathan SR, Yabuuchi A, et al. A role for Lin28 in primordial germ-cell development and germ-cell malignancy. Nature. 2009 Aug 13;460(7257):909–13. PMID:19578360
3290. Westra WH, Baas IO, Hruban RH, et al. K-ras oncogene activation in atypical alveolar hyperplasias of the human lung. Cancer Res. 1996 May 1;56(9):2224–8. PMID:8616876
3291. Wetterskog D, Wilkerson PM, Rodrigues DN, et al. Mutation profiling of adenoid cystic carcinomas from multiple anatomical sites identifies mutations in the RAS pathway, but no KIT mutations. Histopathology. 2013 Mar;62(4):543–50. PMID:23398044
3292. Wheler J, Hong D, Swisher SG, et al. Thymoma patients treated in a phase I clinic at MD Anderson Cancer Center: responses to mTOR inhibitors and molecular analyses. Oncotarget. 2013 Jun;4(6):890–8. PMID:23765114
3293. Wheler JJ, Falchook GS, Tsimberidou AM, et al. Aberrations in the epidermal growth factor receptor gene in 958 patients with diverse advanced tumors: implications for therapy. Ann Oncol. 2013 Mar;24(3):838–42. PMID:23139256
3294. Whitaker D, Henderson DW, Shilkin KB. The concept of mesothelioma in situ: implications for diagnosis and histogenesis. Semin Diagn Pathol. 1992 May;9(2):151–61. PMID:1609157
3295. White JE, Fincher RM, D'Cruz IA. Pericardial metastasis from testicular seminoma: appearance and disappearance by echocardiography. Am J Med Sci. 1991 Mar;301(3):182–5. PMID:2000890
3296. White W, Shiu MH, Rosenblum MK, et al. Cellular schwannoma. A clinicopathologic study of 57 patients and 58 tumors. Cancer. 1990 Sep 15;66(6):1266–75. PMID:2400975
3297. WHO Classification of Tumours Editorial Board. Digestive system tumours. Lyon (France): International Agency for Research on Cancer; 2019. (WHO classification of tumours series, 5th ed.; vol. 1). https://publications.iarc.fr/579.
3298. WHO Classification of Tumours Editorial Board. Soft tissue and bone tumours. Lyon (France): International Agency for Research on Cancer; 2020. (WHO classification of tumours series, 5th ed.; vol. 3). https://publications.iarc.fr/588.
3299. Wiatrowska BA, Krol J, Zakowski MF. Large-cell neuroendocrine carcinoma of the lung: proposed criteria for cytologic diagnosis. Diagn Cytopathol. 2001 Jan;24(1):58–64. PMID:11135471
3300. Wick MR. Mediastinal cysts and intrathoracic thyroid tumors. Semin Diagn Pathol. 1990 Nov;7(4):285–94. PMID:2284514
3301. Wick MR. Primary lesions that may imitate metastatic tumors histologically: a selective review. Semin Diagn Pathol. 2018 Mar;35(2):123–42. PMID:29174934
3302. Wick MR, Carney JA, Bernatz PE, et al. Primary mediastinal carcinoid tumors. Am J Surg Pathol. 1982 Apr;6(3):195–205. PMID:6285747
3303. Wick MR, Ritter JH, Nappi O. Inflammatory sarcomatoid carcinoma of the lung: report of three cases and clinicopathologic comparison with inflammatory pseudotumors in adult patients. Hum Pathol. 1995 Sep;26(9):1014–21. PMID:7672783
3304. Wick MR, Rosai J. Neuroendocrine neoplasms of the mediastinum. Semin Diagn Pathol. 1991 Feb;8(1):35–51. PMID:1646476
3305. Wick MR, Scheithauer BW. Oat-cell carcinoma of the thymus. Cancer. 1982 Apr 15;49(8):1652–7. PMID:6279270
3306. Wick MR, Scheithauer BW, Weiland LH, et al. Primary thymic carcinomas. Am J Surg Pathol. 1982 Oct;6(7):613–30. PMID:6295194
3307. Wiegand S, Eivazi B, Barth PJ, et al. Pathogenesis of lymphangiomas. Virchows Arch. 2008 Jul;453(1):1–8. PMID:18500536
3308. Wiesner T, Obenauf AC, Murali R, et al. Germline mutations in BAP1 predispose to melanocytic tumors. Nat Genet. 2011 Aug 28;43(10):1018–21. PMID:21874003
3309. Wijesuriya S, Chandratreya L, Medford AR. Chronic pulmonary emboli and radiologic mimics on CT pulmonary angiography: a diagnostic challenge. Chest. 2013 May;143(5):1460–71. PMID:23648910
3310. Wilkerson MD, Yin X, Hoadley KA, et al. Lung squamous cell carcinoma mRNA expression subtypes are reproducible, clinically important, and correspond to normal cell types. Clin Cancer Res. 2010 Oct 1;16(19):4864–75. PMID:20643781
3311. Willems SM, Debiec-Rychter M, Szuhai K, et al. Local recurrence of myxofibrosarcoma is associated with increase in tumour grade and cytogenetic aberrations, suggesting a multistep tumour progression model. Mod Pathol. 2006 Mar;19(3):407–16. PMID:16415793
3312. Willén H, Akerman M, Dal Cin P, et al. Comparison of chromosomal patterns with clinical features in 165 lipomas: a report of the CHAMP study group. Cancer Genet Cytogenet. 1998 Apr 1;102(1):46–9. PMID:9530339
3313. William J, Variakojis D, Yeldandi A, et al. Lymphoproliferative neoplasms of the lung: a review. Arch Pathol Lab Med. 2013 Mar;137(3):382–91. PMID:23451749
3314. Williams LA, Pankratz N, Lane J, et al. Klinefelter syndrome in males with germ cell tumors: a report from the Children's Oncology Group. Cancer. 2018 Oct 1;124(19):3900–8. PMID:30291793
3315. Williams WT, Parsons WH. Intrathoracic lipomas. J Thorac Surg. 1957 Jun;33(6):785–90. PMID:13429696
3316. Willis RA. The borderland of embryology and pathology. Bull N Y Acad Med. 1950 Jul;26(7):440–60. PMID:15426876
3317. Wilson CI, Inchausti BC, Griffith KM, et al. Cardiac myxoma with chondroid features. Ann Diagn Pathol. 1999 Oct;3(5):309–14. PMID:10556479
3318. Wilson KS, McKenna RW, Kroft SH, et al. Primary effusion lymphomas exhibit complex and recurrent cytogenetic abnormalities. Br J Haematol. 2002 Jan;116(1):113–21. PMID:11841403
3319. Wilson RW, Gallateau-Salle F, Moran CA. Desmoid tumors of the pleura: a clinicopathologic mimic of localized fibrous tumor. Mod Pathol. 1999 Jan;12(1):9–14. PMID:9950156
3320. Wilson RW, Moran CA. Primary melanoma of the lung: a clinicopathologic and immunohistochemical study of eight cases. Am J Surg Pathol. 1997 Oct;21(10):1196–202. PMID:9331292
3321. Wilson WH, Kingma DW, Raffeld M, et al. Association of lymphomatoid granulomatosis with Epstein-Barr viral infection of B lymphocytes and response to interferon-alpha 2b. Blood. 1996 Jun 1;87(11):4531–7. PMID:8639820
3322. Wilson WH, Pittaluga S, Nicolae A, et al. A prospective study of mediastinal gray-zone lymphoma. Blood. 2014 Sep 4;124(10):1563–9. PMID:25024303
3323. Winter L, Langrehr J, Hänninen EL. Primary angiosarcoma of the abdominal aorta: multi-row computed tomography. Abdom Imaging. 2010 Aug;35(4):485–7. PMID:19462198
3324. Wirtschafter E, Walts AE, Liu ST, et al. Diffuse idiopathic pulmonary neuroendocrine cell hyperplasia of the lung (DIPNECH): current best evidence. Lung. 2015 Oct;193(5):659–67. PMID:26104490
3325. Wislez M, Antoine M, Baudrin L, et al. Non-mucinous and mucinous subtypes of adenocarcinoma with bronchioloalveolar carcinoma features differ by biomarker expression and in the response to gefitinib. Lung Cancer. 2010 May;68(2):185–91. PMID:19581016
3326. Wistuba II, Behrens C, Milchgrub S, et al. Sequential molecular abnormalities are involved in the multistage development of squamous cell lung carcinoma. Oncogene. 1999 Jan 21;18(3):643–50. PMID:9989814
3327. Wistuba II, Behrens C, Virmani AK, et al. Allelic losses at chromosome 8p21-23 are early and frequent events in the pathogenesis of lung cancer. Cancer Res. 1999 Apr 15;59(8):1973–9. PMID:10213509
3328. Wistuba II, Gazdar AF. Lung cancer preneoplasia. Annu Rev Pathol. 2006;1:331–48. PMID:18039118
3329. Wistuba II, Lam S, Behrens C, et al. Molecular damage in the bronchial epithelium of current and former smokers. J Natl Cancer Inst. 1997 Sep 17;89(18):1366–73. PMID:9308707
3330. Witkin GB, Rosai J. Solitary fibrous tumor of the mediastinum. A report of 14 cases. Am J Surg Pathol. 1989 Jul;13(7):547–57. PMID:2735490
3331. Wittekind C, Compton CC, Brierley JD, et al., editors. TNM supplement: a commentary on uniform use. 4th ed. Oxford (UK): Wiley-Blackwell; 2012.
3332. Wittenberg KH, Swensen SJ, Myers JL. Pulmonary involvement with Erdheim-Chester disease: radiographic and CT findings. AJR Am J Roentgenol. 2000 May;174(5):1327–31. PMID:10789787
3333. Wittersheim M, Heydt C, Hoffmann F, et al. KRAS mutation in papillary fibroelastoma: a true cardiac neoplasm? J Pathol Clin Res. 2017 Mar 7;3(2):100–4. PMID:28451458
3333A. Wolf J, Seto T, Han JY, et al. Capmatinib in MET exon 14-mutated or MET-amplified non-small-cell lung cancer. N Engl J Med. 2020 Sep 3;383(10):944–57. PMID:32877583
3334. Wolfe JT 3rd, Wick MR, Banks PM, et al. Clear cell carcinoma of the thymus. Mayo Clin Proc. 1983 Jun;58(6):365–70. PMID:6855274
3335. Wolff AC, Hammond ME, Hicks DG, et al. Recommendations for human epidermal growth factor receptor 2 testing in breast cancer: American Society of Clinical Oncology/College of American Pathologists clinical practice guideline update. Arch Pathol Lab Med. 2014 Feb;138(2):241–56. PMID:24099077
3336. Woo WL, Panagiotopoulos N, Gvinianidze L, et al. Primary mucoepidermoid carcinoma of the thymus presenting with myasthenia gravis. J Thorac Dis. 2014 Oct;6(10):E223–5. PMID:25364536
3337. Wood B, Swarbrick N, Frost F. Diagnosis of pulmonary hamartoma by fine needle biopsy. Acta Cytol. 2008 Jul-Aug;52(4):412–7. PMID:18702357
3338. Wood DE. Mediastinal germ cell tumors. Semin Thorac Cardiovasc Surg. 2000 Oct;12(4):278–89. PMID:11154723
3338A. Wu B, Sun T, Gu Y, et al. CT and MR imaging of thyroid carcinoma showing thymus-like differentiation (CASTLE): a report of ten cases. Br J Radiol. 2016;89(1060):20150726. PMID:26954328
3339. Wu CY, Wang J, Chang NY. A comparative study of intraoperative cytology and frozen sections of sclerosing pneumocytoma. Int J Surg Pathol. 2016 Oct;24(7):600–6. PMID:27160435
3340. Wu G, Jones J, Sequeira IB, et al. Congenital pericardial hemangioma responding to high-dose corticosteroid therapy. Can J Cardiol. 2009 Apr;25(4):e139–40. PMID:19340361
3341. Wu J, Chu PG, Jiang Z, et al. Napsin A expression in primary mucin-producing adenocarcinomas of the lung: an immunohistochemical study. Am J Clin Pathol. 2013 Feb;139(2):160–6. PMID:23355200
3341A. Wu M, Krishnamurthy K. Peutz-Jeghers syndrome. 2020 Jul 22. In: StatPearls. Treasure Island (FL): StatPearls Publishing; 2020 Jan–. PMID:30570978
3342. Wu M, Sun K, Gil J, et al. Immunohistochemical detection of p63 and XIAP in thymic hyperplasia and thymomas. Am J Clin Pathol. 2009 May;131(5):689–93. PMID:19369629
3343. Wu SC, Lin ZQ, Xu CW, et al. Multiple primary lung cancers. Chest. 1987 Nov;92(5):892–6. PMID:3665605
3344. Wu SG, Li Y, Li B, et al. Unusual

combined thymic mucoepidermoid carcinoma and thymoma: a case report and review of literature. Diagn Pathol. 2014 Jan 20;9:8. PMID:24444077
3345. Wu TC, Kuo TT. Study of Epstein-Barr virus early RNA 1 (EBER1) expression by in situ hybridization in thymic epithelial tumors of Chinese patients in Taiwan. Hum Pathol. 1993 Mar;24(3):235–8. PMID:8454269
3346. Wu W, Youm W, Rezk SA, et al. Human herpesvirus 8-unrelated primary effusion lymphoma-like lymphoma: report of a rare case and review of 54 cases in the literature. Am J Clin Pathol. 2013 Aug;140(2):258–73. PMID:23897264
3347. Wu X, Huang Y, Li Y, et al. 18F-FDG PET/CT imaging in pulmonary sarcomatoid carcinoma and correlation with clinical and genetic findings. Ann Nucl Med. 2019 Sep;33(9):647–56. PMID:31165974
3348. Wychulis AR, Payne WS, Clagett OT, et al. Surgical treatment of mediastinal tumors: a 40 year experience. J Thorac Cardiovasc Surg. 1971 Sep;62(3):379–92. PMID:4331304
3349. Xia H, Nakayama T, Sakuma H, et al. Analysis of API2-MALT1 fusion, trisomies, and immunoglobulin VH genes in pulmonary mucosa-associated lymphoid tissue lymphoma. Hum Pathol. 2011 Sep;42(9):1297–304. PMID:21396678
3350. Xie M, Wu X, Wang F, et al. Clinical significance of plasma Epstein-Barr virus DNA in pulmonary lymphoepithelioma-like carcinoma (LELC) patients. J Thorac Oncol. 2018 Feb;13(2):218–27. PMID:29191777
3351. Xie Y, Xie K, Gou Q, et al. Recurrent desmoid tumor of the mediastinum: a case report. Oncol Lett. 2014 Nov;8(5):2276–8. PMID:25295113
3352. Xu J, Zhao J, Geng S, et al. Primary seminoma arising in the middle mediastinum: a case report. Oncol Lett. 2016 Jul;12(1):348–50. PMID:27347149
3353. Xu S, Zhao Q, Wei S, et al. Next generation sequencing uncovers potential genetic driver mutations of malignant pulmonary granular cell tumor. J Thorac Oncol. 2015 Oct;10(10):e106–9. PMID:26398830
3353A. Xu XY, Yang GY, Yang JH, et al. Analysis of clinical characteristics and differential diagnosis of the lung biopsy specimens in 99 adenocarcinoma cases and 111 squamous cell carcinoma cases: utility of an immunohistochemical panel containing CK5/6, CK34βE12, p63, CK7 and TTF-1. Pathol Res Pract. 2014 Oct;210(10):680–5. PMID:25063315
3354. Yabuki H, Kuwana K, Minowa M. Resection of primary malignant lung melanoma: a case report. Asian Cardiovasc Thorac Ann. 2018 Nov;26(9):710–2. PMID:30360631
3355. Yahata S, Endo T, Honma H, et al. Sunray appearance on enhanced magnetic resonance image of cardiac angiosarcoma with pericardial obliteration. Am Heart J. 1994 Feb;127(2):468–71. PMID:8296726
3356. Yalçın B, Demir HA, Tanyel FC, et al. Mediastinal germ cell tumors in childhood. Pediatr Hematol Oncol. 2012 Oct;29(7):633–42. PMID:22877235
3357. Yamada T, Chiba W, Hitomi S. [Thymic basaloid carcinoma]. Kyobu Geka. 2006 Dec;59(13):1154–8. Japanese. PMID:17163206
3358. Yamada Y, Tomaru U, Ishizu A, et al. Expression of proteasome subunit β5t in thymic epithelial tumors. Am J Surg Pathol. 2011 Sep;35(9):1296–304. PMID:21836487
3359. Yamaguchi H, Soda H, Kitazaki T, et al. Thymic carcinoma with epidermal growth factor receptor gene mutations. Lung Cancer. 2006 May;52(2):261–2. PMID:16545487
3360. Yamaji I, Iimura O, Mito T, et al. An ectopic, ACTH producing, oncocytic carcinoid tumor of the thymus: report of a case. Jpn J Med. 1984 Feb;23(1):62–6. PMID:6748352
3361. Yamamoto H, Higasa K, Sakaguchi M, et al. Novel germline mutation in the transmembrane domain of HER2 in familial lung adenocarcinomas. J Natl Cancer Inst. 2014 Jan;106(1):djt338. PMID:24317180
3362. Yamamoto H, Yoshida A, Taguchi K, et al. ALK, ROS1 and NTRK3 gene rearrangements in inflammatory myofibroblastic tumours. Histopathology. 2016 Jul;69(1):72–83. PMID:26647767
3363. Yamamoto T, Horiguchi H, Shibagaki T, et al. Encapsulated type II pneumocyte adenoma: a case report and review of the literature. Respiration. 1993;60(6):373–7. PMID:8290804
3363A. Yamamoto Y, Kodama K, Maniwa T, et al. Anaplastic lymphoma kinase-positive squamous cell carcinoma of the lung: a case report. Mol Clin Oncol. 2016 Jul;5(1):61–3. PMID:27330767
3364. Yamamoto Y, Kodama K, Maniwa T, et al. Primary malignant melanoma of the lung: a case report. Mol Clin Oncol. 2017 Jul;7(1):39–41. PMID:28685072
3365. Yamani F, Chen W. Cytokeratin-positive primary effusion lymphoma: a diagnostic challenge. Br J Haematol. 2018 Jan;180(1):9. PMID:28880367
3366. Yamaoka O, Matsui T, Nishiyama K, et al. Indolent primary effusion lymphoma-like lymphoma in the pericardium: a case report and review of the literature. J Cardiol Cases. 2019 Jan 23;19(5):148–52. PMID:31073346
3367. Yamatani C, Abe M, Shimoji M, et al. Pulmonary adenosquamous carcinoma with mucoepidermoid carcinoma-like component with characteristic p63 staining pattern: either a novel subtype originating from bronchial epithelium or variant mucoepidermoid carcinoma. Lung Cancer. 2014 Apr;84(1):45–50. PMID:24513264
3368. Yamato H, Ohshima K, Suzumiya J, et al. Evidence for local immunosuppression and demonstration of c-myc amplification in pyothorax-associated lymphoma. Histopathology. 2001 Aug;39(2):163–71. PMID:11493333
3369. Yamauchi K, Yasuda M. Comparison in treatments of nonleukemic granulocytic sarcoma: report of two cases and a review of 72 cases in the literature. Cancer. 2002 Mar 15;94(6):1739–46. PMID:11920536
3370. Yamazaki K. Type-II pneumocyte differentiation in pulmonary sclerosing hemangioma: ultrastructural differentiation and immunohistochemical distribution of lineage-specific transcription factors (TTF-1, HNF-3 alpha, and HNF-3 beta) and surfactant proteins. Virchows Arch. 2004 Jul;445(1):45–53. PMID:15138814
3371. Yamazaki K, Abe S, Takekawa H, et al. Tumor angiogenesis in human lung adenocarcinoma. Cancer. 1994 Oct 15;74(8):2245–50. PMID:7522947
3372. Yan J, Luo D, Zhang F, et al. Diffuse large B cell lymphoma associated with chronic inflammation arising within atrial myxoma: aggressive histological features but indolent clinical behaviour. Histopathology. 2017 Dec;71(6):951–9. PMID:28782131
3373. Yanagawa N, Shiono S, Abiko M, et al. The clinical impact of solid and micropapillary patterns in resected lung adenocarcinoma. J Thorac Oncol. 2016 Nov;11(11):1976–83. PMID:27374456
3374. Yanagawa N, Wang A, Kohler D, et al. Human papilloma virus genome is rare in North American non-small cell lung carcinoma patients. Lung Cancer. 2013 Mar;79(3):215–20. PMID:23254264
3375. Yandrapalli S, Mehta B, Mondal P, et al. Cardiac papillary fibroelastoma: the need for a timely diagnosis. World J Clin Cases. 2017 Jan 16;5(1):9–13. PMID:28138441
3376. Yang C, Sanchez-Vega F, Chang JC, et al. Lung-only melanoma: UV mutational signature supports origin from occult cutaneous primaries and argues against the concept of primary pulmonary melanoma. Mod Pathol. 2020 Nov;33(11):2244–55. PMID:32581366
3377. Yang CF, Chan DY, Speicher PJ, et al. Role of adjuvant therapy in a population-based cohort of patients with early-stage small-cell lung cancer. J Clin Oncol. 2016 Apr 1;34(10):1057–64. PMID:26786925
3378. Yang CH, Lee LY. Pulmonary sclerosing pneumocytoma remains a diagnostic challenge using frozen sections: a clinicopathological analysis of 59 cases. Histopathology. 2018 Feb;72(3):500–8. PMID:28881050
3379. Yang GC, Hwang SJ, Yee HT. Fine-needle aspiration cytology of unusual germ cell tumors of the mediastinum: atypical seminoma and parietal yolk sac tumor. Diagn Cytopathol. 2002 Aug;27(2):69–74. PMID:12203871
3380. Yang L, Wang N, Yuan Y, et al. Secular trends in incidence of lung cancer by histological type in Beijing, China, 2000-2016. Chin J Cancer Res. 2019 Apr;31(2):306–15. PMID:31156301
3381. Yang Q, Xu Z, Chen X, et al. Clinicopathological characteristics and prognostic factors of pulmonary large cell neuroendocrine carcinoma: a large population-based analysis. Thorac Cancer. 2019 Apr;10(4):751–60. PMID:30734490
3382. Yang S, Gao Y, Zhao H, et al. Cardiac embryonal rhabdomyosarcoma in an adult. Eur J Cardiothorac Surg. 2014 Jun;45(6):e233. PMID:24634480
3383. Yang YJ, Steele CT, Ou XL, et al. Diagnosis of high-grade pulmonary neuroendocrine carcinoma by fine-needle aspiration biopsy: nonsmall-cell or small-cell type? Diagn Cytopathol. 2001 Nov;25(5):292–300. PMID:11747218
3384. Yano M, Sasaki H, Yokoyama T, et al. Thymic carcinoma: 30 cases at a single institution. J Thorac Oncol. 2008 Mar;3(3):265–9. PMID:18317069
3385. Yano S, Shinohara H, Herbst RS, et al. Production of experimental malignant pleural effusions is dependent on invasion of the pleura and expression of vascular endothelial growth factor/vascular permeability factor by human lung cancer cells. Am J Pathol. 2000 Dec;157(6):1893–903. PMID:11106562
3386. Yao DX, Shia J, Erlandson RA, et al. Lymphohistiocytoid mesothelioma: a clinical, immunohistochemical and ultrastructural study of four cases and literature review. Ultrastruct Pathol. 2004 Jul-Aug;28(4):213–28. PMID:15693633
3387. Yao JC, Hassan M, Phan A, et al. One hundred years after "carcinoid": epidemiology of and prognostic factors for neuroendocrine tumors in 35,825 cases in the United States. J Clin Oncol. 2008 Jun 20;26(18):3063–72. PMID:18565894
3388. Yao W, Yang H, Huang G, et al. Massive localized malignant pleural mesothelioma (LMPM): manifestations on computed tomography in 6 cases. Int J Clin Exp Med. 2015 Oct 15;8(10):18367–74. PMID:26770440
3389. Yaris N, Nas Y, Cobanoglu U, et al. Thymic carcinoma in children. Pediatr Blood Cancer. 2006 Aug;47(2):224–7. PMID:16007580
3390. Yatabe Y, Dacic S, Borczuk AC, et al. Best practices recommendations for diagnostic immunohistochemistry in lung cancer. J Thorac Oncol. 2019 Mar;14(3):377–407. PMID:30572031
3391. Yatabe Y, Koga T, Mitsudomi T, et al. CK20 expression, CDX2 expression, K-ras mutation, and goblet cell morphology in a subset of lung adenocarcinomas. J Pathol. 2004 Jun;203(2):645–52. PMID:15141379
3392. Yatabe Y, Kosaka T, Takahashi T, et al. EGFR mutation is specific for terminal respiratory unit type adenocarcinoma. Am J Surg Pathol. 2005 May;29(5):633–9. PMID:15832087
3393. Yatabe Y, Takahashi T, Mitsudomi T. Epidermal growth factor receptor gene amplification is acquired in association with tumor progression of EGFR-mutated lung cancer. Cancer Res. 2008 Apr 1;68(7):2106–11. PMID:18381415
3394. Yates DH, Corrin B, Stidolph PN, et al. Malignant mesothelioma in south east England: clinicopathological experience of 272 cases. Thorax. 1997 Jun;52(6):507–12. PMID:9227715
3395. Yaziji H, Battifora H, Barry TS, et al. Evaluation of 12 antibodies for distinguishing epithelioid mesothelioma from adenocarcinoma: identification of a three-antibody immunohistochemical panel with maximal sensitivity and specificity. Mod Pathol. 2006 Apr;19(4):514–23. PMID:16554731
3396. Ye B, Cappel J, Findeis-Hosey J, et al. hASH1 is a specific immunohistochemical marker for lung neuroendocrine tumors. Hum Pathol. 2016 Feb;48:142–7. PMID:26596584
3397. Yeh YC, Ho HL, Wu YC, et al. AKT1 internal tandem duplications and point mutations are the genetic hallmarks of sclerosing pneumocytoma. Mod Pathol. 2020 Mar;33(3):391–403. PMID:31527710
3398. Yeh YC, Kao HL, Lee KL, et al. Epstein-Barr virus-associated pulmonary carcinoma: proposing an alternative term and expanding the histologic spectrum of lymphoepithelioma-like carcinoma of the lung. Am J Surg Pathol. 2019 Feb;43(2):211–9. PMID:30334830
3399. Yi ES, Lee GK. Updates on selected topics in lung cancers: air space invasion in adenocarcinoma and Ki-67 staining in carcinoid tumors. Arch Pathol Lab Med. 2018 Aug;142(8):947–51. PMID:29869902
3400. Yim J, Zhu LC, Chiriboga L, et al. Histologic features are important prognostic indicators in early stages lung adenocarcinomas. Mod Pathol. 2007 Feb;20(2):233–41. PMID:17192789
3401. Yin J, Yang Y, Ma K, et al. Clinicopathological characteristics and prognosis of pulmonary pleomorphic carcinoma: a population-based retrospective study using SEER data. J Thorac Dis. 2018 Jul;10(7):4262–73. PMID:30174872
3402. Yin Z, Kirschner LS. The Carney complex gene PRKAR1A plays an essential role in cardiac development and myxomagenesis. Trends Cardiovasc Med. 2009 Feb;19(2):44–9. PMID:19577711
3403. Yip PY, Yu B, Cooper WA, et al. Patterns of DNA mutations and ALK rearrangement in resected node negative lung adenocarcinoma. J Thorac Oncol. 2013 Apr;8(4):408–14. PMID:23392229
3404. Yoh K, Nishiwaki Y, Ishii G, et al. Mutational status of EGFR and KIT in thymoma and thymic carcinoma. Lung Cancer. 2008 Dec;62(3):316–20. PMID:18448188
3405. Yokoi K, Kondo K, Fujimoto K, et al. JLCS medical practice guidelines for thymic tumors: summary of recommendations. Jpn J Clin Oncol. 2017 Dec 1;47(12):1119–22. PMID:29036455
3406. Yokose T, Ito Y, Ochiai A. High prevalence of atypical adenomatous hyperplasia of the lung in autopsy specimens from elderly patients with malignant neoplasms. Lung Cancer. 2000 Aug;29(2):125–30. PMID:10963842
3407. Yokota K, Sasaki H, Okuda K, et al.

KIF5B/RET fusion gene in surgically-treated adenocarcinoma of the lung. Oncol Rep. 2012 Oct;28(4):1187–92. PMID:22797671
3408. Yokoyama S, Hayashida R, Yoshiyama K, et al. Ectopic cervical thymoma excised through a transcervical approach combined with video-assisted thoracoscopic surgery: a case report. Ann Thorac Cardiovasc Surg. 2015;21(3):293–7. PMID:25740445
3409. Yokoyama S, Miyoshi H, Nishi T, et al. Clinicopathologic and prognostic implications of programmed death ligand 1 expression in thymoma. Ann Thorac Surg. 2016 Apr;101(4):1361–9. PMID:26794891
3410. Yokoyama S, Murakami T, Tao H, et al. Tumor spread through air spaces identifies a distinct subgroup with poor prognosis in surgically resected lung pleomorphic carcinoma. Chest. 2018 Oct;154(4):838–47. PMID:29932891
3411. Yoneda S, Marx A, Heimann S, et al. Low-grade metaplastic carcinoma of the thymus. Histopathology. 1999 Jul;35(1):19–30. PMID:10383710
3412. Yoneda S, Marx A, Müller-Hermelink HK. Low-grade metaplastic carcinomas of the thymus: biphasic thymic epithelial tumors with mesenchymal metaplasia–an update. Pathol Res Pract. 1999;195(8):555–63. PMID:10483586
3413. Yoo H, Jeong BH, Chung MJ, et al. Risk factors and clinical characteristics of lung cancer in idiopathic pulmonary fibrosis: a retrospective cohort study. BMC Pulm Med. 2019 Aug 14;19(1):149. PMID:31412851
3414. Yoon DH, Roberts W. Sex distribution in cardiac myxomas. Am J Cardiol. 2002 Sep 1;90(5):563–5. PMID:12208428
3415. Yoon JH, Nouraie M, Chen X, et al. Characteristics of lung cancer among patients with idiopathic pulmonary fibrosis and interstitial lung disease - analysis of institutional and population data. Respir Res. 2018 Oct 3;19(1):195. PMID:30285867
3416. Yoon JY, Pal P, Ko HM. Primary pulmonary lymphoepithelioma-like carcinoma: a potential source of misdiagnosis on radial probe endobronchial ultrasound-guided transbronchial aspiration cytology. Cytopathology. 2019 Nov;30(6):653–6. PMID:31423666
3417. Yoon JY, Sigel K, Martin J, et al. Evaluation of the prognostic significance of TNM staging guidelines in lung carcinoid tumors. J Thorac Oncol. 2019 Feb;14(2):184–92. PMID:30414942
3418. Yoon RG, Kim MY, Song JW, et al. Primary endobronchial marginal zone B-cell lymphoma of bronchus-associated lymphoid tissue: CT findings in 7 patients. Korean J Radiol. 2013 Mar-Apr;14(2):366–74. PMID:23483549
3419. Yoshida A, Arai Y, Hama N, et al. Expanding the clinicopathologic and molecular spectrum of BCOR-associated sarcomas in adults. Histopathology. 2020 Mar;76(4):509–20. PMID:31647130
3420. Yoshida A, Goto K, Kodaira M, et al. CIC-rearranged sarcomas: a study of 20 cases and comparisons with Ewing sarcomas. Am J Surg Pathol. 2016 Mar;40(3):313–23. PMID:26685084
3421. Yoshida A, Kobayashi E, Kubo T, et al. Clinicopathological and molecular characterization of SMARCA4-deficient thoracic sarcomas with comparison to potentially related entities. Mod Pathol. 2017 Jun;30(6):797–809. PMID:28256572
3422. Yoshida A, Kohno T, Tsuta K, et al. ROS1-rearranged lung cancer: a clinicopathologic and molecular study of 15 surgical cases. Am J Surg Pathol. 2013 Apr;37(4):554–62. PMID:23426121
3423. Yoshida A, Sekine S, Tsuta K, et al. NKX2.2 is a useful immunohistochemical marker for Ewing sarcoma. Am J Surg Pathol. 2012 Jul;36(7):993–9. PMID:22446943
3424. Yoshida A, Tsuta K, Watanabe S, et al. Frequent ALK rearrangement and TTF-1/p63 co-expression in lung adenocarcinoma with signet-ring cell component. Lung Cancer. 2011 Jun;72(3):309–15. PMID:21036415
3425. Yoshida A, Wakai S, Ryo E, et al. Expanding the phenotypic spectrum of mesenchymal tumors harboring the EWSR1-CREM fusion. Am J Surg Pathol. 2019 Dec;43(12):1622–30. PMID:31305268
3426. Yoshida M, Okabe M, Eimoto T, et al. Immunoglobulin VH genes in thymic MALT lymphoma are biased toward a restricted repertoire and are frequently unmutated. J Pathol. 2006 Feb;208(3):415–22. PMID:16353132
3427. Yoshida Y, Shibata T, Kokubu A, et al. Mutations of the epidermal growth factor receptor gene in atypical adenomatous hyperplasia and bronchioloalveolar carcinoma of the lung. Lung Cancer. 2005 Oct;50(1):1–8. PMID:15950315
3428. Yoshikai M, Kamohara K, Fumoto H, et al. Left ventricular myxoma originating from the papillary muscle. J Heart Valve Dis. 2003 Mar;12(2):177–9. PMID:12701789
3429. Yoshikawa T, Noguchi Y, Matsukawa H, et al. Thymus carcinoid producing parathyroid hormone (PTH)-related protein: report of a case. Surg Today. 1994;24(6):544–7. PMID:7919739
3430. Yoshimoto T, Matsubara D, Nakano T, et al. Frequent loss of the expression of multiple subunits of the SWI/SNF complex in large cell carcinoma and pleomorphic carcinoma of the lung. Pathol Int. 2015 Nov;65(11):595–602. PMID:26345631
3431. Yoshimura M, Kinoshita Y, Hamasaki M, et al. Highly expressed EZH2 in combination with BAP1 and MTAP loss, as detected by immunohistochemistry, is useful for differentiating malignant pleural mesothelioma from reactive mesothelial hyperplasia. Lung Cancer. 2019 Apr;130:187–93. PMID:30885343
3432. Yoshino M, Hiroshima K, Motohashi S, et al. Papillary carcinoma of the thymus gland. Ann Thorac Surg. 2005 Aug;80(2):741–2. PMID:16039252
3433. Yoshizawa A, Motoi N, Riely GJ, et al. Impact of proposed IASLC/ATS/ERS classification of lung adenocarcinoma: prognostic subgroups and implications for further revision of staging based on analysis of 514 stage I cases. Mod Pathol. 2011 May;24(5):653–64. PMID:21252858
3434. Yoshizawa A, Sumiyoshi S, Sonobe M, et al. Validation of the IASLC/ATS/ERS lung adenocarcinoma classification for prognosis and association with EGFR and KRAS gene mutations: analysis of 440 Japanese patients. J Thorac Oncol. 2013 Jan;8(1):52–61. PMID:23242438
3435. You MJ, Medeiros LJ, Hsi ED. T-lymphoblastic leukemia/lymphoma. Am J Clin Pathol. 2015 Sep;144(3):411–22. PMID:26276771
3436. Young L, Lee HS, Inoue Y, et al. Serum VEGF-D a concentration as a biomarker of lymphangioleiomyomatosis severity and treatment response: a prospective analysis of the Multicenter International Lymphangioleiomyomatosis Efficacy of Sirolimus (MILES) trial. Lancet Respir Med. 2013 Aug;1(6):445–52. PMID:24159565
3437. Young LR, Brody AS, Inge TH, et al. Neuroendocrine cell distribution and frequency distinguish neuroendocrine cell hyperplasia of infancy from other pulmonary disorders. Chest. 2011 May;139(5):1060–71. PMID:20884725
3438. Young LR, Deutsch GH, Bokulic RE, et al. A mutation in TTF1/NKX2.1 is associated with familial neuroendocrine cell hyperplasia of infancy. Chest. 2013 Oct;144(4):1199–206. PMID:23787483
3439. Yousefi M, Nosrati R, Salmaninejad A, et al. Organ-specific metastasis of breast cancer: molecular and cellular mechanisms underlying lung metastasis. Cell Oncol (Dordr). 2018 Apr;41(2):123–40. PMID:29568985
3440. Yousem SA. Peripheral squamous cell carcinoma of lung: patterns of growth with particular focus on airspace filling. Hum Pathol. 2009 Jun;40(6):861–7. PMID:19269005
3441. Yousem SA. Pulmonary intestinal-type adenocarcinoma does not show enteric differentiation by immunohistochemical study. Mod Pathol. 2005 Jun;18(6):816–21. PMID:15605076
3442. Yousem SA, Hochholzer L. Alveolar adenoma. Hum Pathol. 1986 Oct;17(10):1066–71. PMID:3759064
3443. Yousem SA, Hochholzer L. Mucoepidermoid tumors of the lung. Cancer. 1987 Sep 15;60(6):1346–52. PMID:3040215
3444. Yousem SA, Weiss LM, Colby TV. Primary pulmonary Hodgkin's disease. A clinicopathologic study of 15 cases. Cancer. 1986 Mar 15;57(6):1217–24. PMID:3943043
3445. Yousem SA, Weiss LM, Warnke RA. Primary mediastinal non-Hodgkin's lymphomas: a morphologic and immunologic study of 19 cases. Am J Clin Pathol. 1985 Jun;83(6):676–80. PMID:3923821
3446. Yousem SA, Wick MR, Randhawa P, et al. Pulmonary blastoma. An immunohistochemical analysis with comparison with fetal lung in its pseudoglandular stage. Am J Clin Pathol. 1990 Feb;93(2):167–75. PMID:2301281
3447. Yu DC, Grabowski MJ, Kozakewich HP, et al. Primary lung tumors in children and adolescents: a 90-year experience. J Pediatr Surg. 2010 Jun;45(6):1090–5. PMID:20620301
3448. Yu GH, Kussmaul WG, DiSesa VJ, et al. Adult intracardiac rhabdomyoma resembling the extracardiac variant. Hum Pathol. 1993 Apr;24(4):448–51. PMID:8491485
3449. Yu HA, Arcila ME, Rekhtman N, et al. Analysis of tumor specimens at the time of acquired resistance to EGFR-TKI therapy in 155 patients with EGFR-mutant lung cancers. Clin Cancer Res. 2013 Apr 15;19(8):2240–7. PMID:23470965
3450. Yu J, Astrinidis A, Henske EP. Chromosome 16 loss of heterozygosity in tuberous sclerosis and sporadic lymphangiomyomatosis. Am J Respir Crit Care Med. 2001 Oct 15;164(8 Pt 1):1537–40. PMID:11704609
3451. Yu JF, Cui H, Ji GM, et al. Clinical and imaging manifestations of primary cardiac angiosarcoma. BMC Med Imaging. 2019 Feb 14;19(1):16. PMID:30764784
3452. Yu JQ, Yang ZG, Austin JH, et al. Adenosquamous carcinoma of the lung: CT-pathological correlation. Clin Radiol. 2005 Mar;60(3):364–9. PMID:15710140
3453. Yu K, Liu Y, Wang H, et al. Epidemiological and pathological characteristics of cardiac tumors: a clinical study of 242 cases. Interact Cardiovasc Thorac Surg. 2007 Oct;6(5):636–9. PMID:17670730
3454. Yu M, Meng Y, Xu B, et al. Ectopic micronodular thymoma with lymphoid stroma in the cervical region: a rare case associated with Langerhans cells proliferation. Onco Targets Ther. 2016 Jul 18;9:4317–22. PMID:27486334
3455. Yu N, Kim HR, Cha YJ, et al. Development of acute megakaryoblastic leukemia with isochromosome (12p) after a primary mediastinal germ cell tumor in Korea. J Korean Med Sci. 2011 Aug;26(8):1099–102. PMID:21860563
3456. Yu W, Mi L, Cong J, et al. Diffuse pulmonary lymphangiomatosis: a rare case report in an adult. Medicine (Baltimore). 2019 Oct;98(43):e17349. PMID:31651839
3457. Yu XY, Zhang XW, Wang F, et al. Correlation and prognostic significance of PD-L1 and P53 expression in resected primary pulmonary lymphoepithelioma-like carcinoma. J Thorac Dis. 2018 Mar;10(3):1891–902. PMID:29707344
3458. Yuan L, Katabi N, Antonescu CR, et al. Pulmonary myoepithelial tumors with exuberant reactive pneumocytes: proposed reclassification of so-called pneumocytic adenomyoepithelioma. Am J Surg Pathol. 2020 Jan;44(1):140–7. PMID:31567188
3459. Yuan Y, Lu C, Xue L, et al. Association between TERT rs2736100 polymorphism and lung cancer susceptibility: evidence from 22 case-control studies. Tumour Biol. 2014 May;35(5):4435–42. PMID:24390616
3460. Yurick BS, Ottoman RE. Primary mediastinal choriocarcinoma. Radiology. 1960 Dec;75:901–7. PMID:13787562
3461. Yusuf SW, Bathina JD, Qureshi S, et al. Cardiac tumors in a tertiary care cancer hospital: clinical features, echocardiographic findings, treatment and outcomes. Heart Int. 2012 Feb 3;7(1):e4. PMID:22690297
3462. Yvorel V, Forest F, Parietti E, et al. B3 thymoma arising within thymolipoma. Pathology. 2015 Dec;47(7):702–5. PMID:26517631
3463. Zacharias J, Nicholson AG, Ladas GP, et al. Large cell neuroendocrine carcinoma and large cell carcinomas with neuroendocrine morphology of the lung: prognosis after complete resection and systematic nodal dissection. Ann Thorac Surg. 2003 Feb;75(2):348–52. PMID:12607637
3464. Zaghloul TI, Embaby AM, Elmahdy AR. Biodegradation of chicken feathers waste directed by Bacillus subtilis recombinant cells: scaling up in a laboratory scale fermentor. Bioresour Technol. 2011 Feb;102(3):2387–93. PMID:21094599
3465. Zakowski MF, Huang J, Bramlage MP. The role of fine needle aspiration cytology in the diagnosis and management of thymic neoplasia. J Thorac Oncol. 2010 Oct;5(10 Suppl 4):S281–5. PMID:20859120
3466. Zakowski MF, Rekhtman N, Auger M, et al. Morphologic accuracy in differentiating primary lung adenocarcinoma from squamous cell carcinoma in cytology specimens. Arch Pathol Lab Med. 2016 Oct;140(10):1116–20. PMID:27552093
3467. Zaman M, Huissoon A, Buckland M, et al. Clinical and laboratory features of seventy-eight UK patients with Good's syndrome (thymoma and hypogammaglobulinaemia). Clin Exp Immunol. 2019 Jab;195(1):132–8. PMID:30216434
3468. Zaman SS, van Hoeven KH, Slott S, et al. Distinction between bronchioloalveolar carcinoma and hyperplastic pulmonary proliferations: a cytologic and morphometric analysis. Diagn Cytopathol. 1997 May;16(5):396–401. PMID:9143840
3469. Zamboni MM, da Silva CT Jr, Baretta R, et al. Important prognostic factors for survival in patients with malignant pleural effusion. BMC Pulm Med. 2015 Mar 28;15:29. PMID:25887349
3470. Zanelli M, Zizzo M, Montanaro M, et al. Fibrin-associated large B-cell lymphoma: first case report within a cerebral artery aneurysm and literature review. BMC Cancer. 2019 Sep 13;19(1):916. PMID:31519155
3471. Zangwill SD, Trost BA, Zlotocha J, et al. Orthotopic heart transplantation in a child with histiocytoid cardiomyopathy. J Heart Lung Transplant. 2004 Jul;23(7):902–4. PMID:15261188
3472. Zanini G, Gorga E, Pasini F, et al. Seaweed floating in the pericardium: a rare case of primary dedifferentiated liposarcoma.

Cardiovasc Pathol. 2016 Jul-Aug;25(4):333–5. PMID:26525285
3473. Zaric B, Perin B, Stojsic V, et al. Relation between vascular patterns visualized by narrow band imaging (NBI) videobronchoscopy and histological type of lung cancer. Med Oncol. 2013 Mar;30(1):374. PMID:23275117
3474. Zauderer MG, Jayakumaran G, DuBoff M, et al. Prevalence and preliminary validation of screening criteria to identify carriers of germline BAP1 mutations. J Thorac Oncol. 2019 Nov;14(11):1989–94. PMID:31323388
3475. Zebrowski BK, Yano S, Liu W, et al. Vascular endothelial growth factor levels and induction of permeability in malignant pleural effusions. Clin Cancer Res. 1999 Nov;5(11):3364–8. PMID:10589746
3476. Zenali MJ, Weissferdt A, Solis LM, et al. An update on clinicopathological, immunohistochemical, and molecular profiles of colloid carcinoma of the lung. Hum Pathol. 2015 Jun;46(6):836–42. PMID:25776025
3477. Zeng Q, Vogtmann E, Jia MM, et al. Tobacco smoking and trends in histological subtypes of female lung cancer at the Cancer Hospital of the Chinese Academy of Medical Sciences over 13 years. Thorac Cancer. 2019 Aug;10(8):1717–24. PMID:31293059
3478. Zeng Z, Ding W, Luo F, et al. Lung cavity accompanied by hemoptysis: lymphoepithelioma-like carcinoma. QJM. 2018 Sep 1;111(9):643–4. PMID:29722879
3479. Zettl A, Ströbel P, Wagner K, et al. Recurrent genetic aberrations in thymoma and thymic carcinoma. Am J Pathol. 2000 Jul;157(1):257–66. PMID:10880395
3480. Zhan Y, Peng X, Shan F, et al. Attenuation and morphologic characteristics distinguishing a ground-glass nodule measuring 5-10 mm in diameter as invasive lung adenocarcinoma on thin-slice CT. AJR Am J Roentgenol. 2019 Oct;213(4):W162–70. PMID:31216199
3481. Zhang C, Huang C, Zhang X, et al. Clinical characteristics associated with primary cardiac angiosarcoma outcomes: a Surveillance, Epidemiology and End Result analysis. Eur J Med Res. 2019 Aug 19;24(1):29. PMID:31426842
3482. Zhang C, Schmidt LA, Hatanaka K, et al. Evaluation of napsin A, TTF-1, p63, p40, and CK5/6 immunohistochemical stains in pulmonary neuroendocrine tumors. Am J Clin Pathol. 2014 Sep;142(3):320–4. PMID:25125621
3483. Zhang C, Yang H, Lang B, et al. Surgical significance and efficacy of epidermal growth factor receptor tyrosine kinase inhibitors in patients with primary lung adenosquamous carcinoma. Cancer Manag Res. 2018 Aug 2;10:2401–7. PMID:30122989
3484. Zhang C, Zhang J, Xu FP, et al. Genomic landscape and immune microenvironment features of preinvasive and early invasive lung adenocarcinoma. J Thorac Oncol. 2019 Nov;14(11):1912–23. PMID:31446140
3485. Zhang G, Yu Z, Shen G, et al. Association between Epstein-Barr virus and thymic epithelial tumors: a systematic review. Infect Agent Cancer. 2019 Nov 6;14:32. PMID:31709004
3486. Zhang H, Yu Y, Zhou L, et al. Circulating tumor microparticles promote lung metastasis by reprogramming inflammatory and mechanical niches via a macrophage-dependent pathway. Cancer Immunol Res. 2018 Sep;6(9):1046–56. PMID:30002156
3487. Zhang J, Sun J, Liang XL, et al. Differences between low and high grade fetal adenocarcinoma of the lung: a clinicopathological and molecular study. J Thorac Dis. 2017 Jul;9(7):2071–8. PMID:28840008
3488. Zhang J, Xiang C, Han Y, et al. Differential diagnosis of pulmonary enteric adenocarcinoma and metastatic colorectal carcinoma with the assistance of next-generation sequencing and immunohistochemistry. J Cancer Res Clin Oncol. 2019 Jan;145(1):269–79. PMID:30415301
3489. Zhang M, Ding L, Liu Y, et al. Cardiac myxoma with glandular elements: a clinicopathological and immunohistochemical study of five new cases with an emphasis on differential diagnosis. Pathol Res Pract. 2014 Jan;210(1):55–8. PMID:24238992
3490. Zhang M, Wang Y, Jones S, et al. Somatic mutations of SUZ12 in malignant peripheral nerve sheath tumors. Nat Genet. 2014 Nov;46(11):1170–2. PMID:25305755
3491. Zhang M, Wu QC. Giant cardiac myxoma involving the left atrium, left ventricle, right atrium and superior vena cava. J Card Surg. 2013 Nov;28(6):704. PMID:23837537
3492. Zhang PJ, Brooks JS, Goldblum JR, et al. Primary cardiac sarcomas: a clinicopathologic analysis of a series with follow-up information in 17 patients and emphasis on long-term survival. Hum Pathol. 2008 Sep;39(9):1385–95. PMID:18602663
3493. Zhang PJ, Livolsi VA, Brooks JJ. Malignant epithelioid vascular tumors of the pleura: report of a series and literature review. Hum Pathol. 2000 Jan;31(1):29–34. PMID:10665909
3494. Zhang T, Pu XH, Yuan M, et al. Histogram analysis combined with morphological characteristics to discriminate adenocarcinoma in situ or minimally invasive adenocarcinoma from invasive adenocarcinoma appearing as pure ground-glass nodule. Eur J Radiol. 2019 Apr;113:238–44. PMID:30927953
3495. Zhang TM, Lu BH, Cai YR, et al. Well-differentiated fetal adenocarcinoma of the lung: clinicopathologic features of 45 cases in China. Int J Clin Exp Pathol. 2018 Mar 1;11(3):1587–98. PMID:31938258
3496. Zhang X, Wang T, Wang W, et al. Does familial breast cancer and thymoma suggest a cancer syndrome? A family perspective. Gene. 2015 Dec 1;573(2):333–7. PMID:26344711
3497. Zhang XC, Wang J, Shao GG, et al. Comprehensive genomic and immunological characterization of Chinese non-small cell lung cancer patients. Nat Commun. 2019 Apr 16;10(1):1772. PMID:30992440
3498. Zhang Y, Bi L, Qiu Y, et al. Primary pulmonary intravascular large B-cell lymphoma: a report of three cases and literature review. Oncol Lett. 2018 Mar;15(3):3610–3. PMID:29467882
3498A. Zhang YL, Yuan JQ, Wang KF, et al. The prevalence of EGFR mutation in patients with non-small cell lung cancer: a systematic review and meta-analysis. Oncotarget. 2016 Nov 29;7(48):78985–93. PMID:27738317
3499. Zhang YZ, Brambilla C, Molyneaux PL, et al. Utility of nuclear grading system in epithelioid malignant pleural mesothelioma in biopsy-heavy setting: an external validation study of 563 cases. Am J Surg Pathol. 2020 Mar;44(3):347–56. PMID:32045387
3500. Zhao C, Rajan A. Immune checkpoint inhibitors for treatment of thymic epithelial tumors: how to maximize benefit and optimize risk? Mediastinum. 2019 Sep;3:35. PMID:31608320
3501. Zhao GQ, Dowell JE. Hematologic malignancies associated with germ cell tumors. Expert Rev Hematol. 2012 Aug;5(4):427–37. PMID:22992236
3502. Zhao J, Bhatnagar V, Ding L, et al. A systematic review of paraneoplastic syndromes associated with thymoma: treatment modalities, recurrence, and outcomes in resected cases. J Thorac Cardiovasc Surg. 2020 Jul;160(1):306–314.e14. PMID:31982129
3503. Zhao J, Shao J, Zhao R, et al. Histological evolution from primary lung adenocarcinoma harboring EGFR mutation to high-grade neuroendocrine carcinoma. Thorac Cancer. 2018 Jan;9(1):129–35. PMID:29120087
3504. Zhao J, Zuo T, Zheng R, et al. Epidemiology and trend analysis on malignant mesothelioma in China. Chin J Cancer Res. 2017 Aug;29(4):361–8. PMID:28947868
3505. Zhao L, Huang S, Liu J, et al. Clinicopathological, radiographic, and oncogenic features of primary pulmonary enteric adenocarcinoma in comparison with invasive adenocarcinoma in resection specimens. Medicine (Baltimore). 2017 Sep;96(39):e8153. PMID:28953659
3506. Zhao W, Chen T, Yang Y. Primary extragenital choriocarcinoma in posterior mediastinum in a male adult: a case report. Ann Transl Med. 2019 Nov;7(22):703. PMID:31930104
3507. Zhao XG, Wang H, Wang YL, et al. Malignant solitary fibrous tumor of the right atrium. Am J Med Sci. 2012 Nov;344(5):422–5. PMID:22986609
3508. Zhao Y, Zhao H, Hu D, et al. Surgical treatment and prognosis of thymic squamous cell carcinoma: a retrospective analysis of 105 cases. Ann Thorac Surg. 2013 Sep;96(3):1019–24. PMID:23866799
3509. Zhao ZR, To KF, Mok TS, et al. Is there significance in identification of non-predominant micropapillary or solid components in early-stage lung adenocarcinoma? Interact Cardiovasc Thorac Surg. 2017 Jan;24(1):121–5. PMID:27600912
3510. Zheng Q, Luo R, Jin Y, et al. So-called "non-classic" ciliated muconodular papillary tumors: a comprehensive comparison of the clinicopathological and molecular features with classic ciliated muconodular papillary tumors. Hum Pathol. 2018 Dec;82:193–201. PMID:30092236
3511. Zheng Q, Zheng M, Jin Y, et al. ALK-rearrangement neuroendocrine carcinoma of the lung: a comprehensive study of a rare case series and review of literature. Onco Targets Ther. 2018 Aug 17;11:4991–8. PMID:30154667
3512. Zhi Q, Wang Y, Wang X, et al. Predictive and prognostic value of preoperative serum tumor markers in resectable adenosqamous lung carcinoma. Oncotarget. 2016 Oct 4;7(40):64798–809. PMID:27623437
3513. Zhou F, Hou L, Ding T, et al. Distinct clinicopathologic features, genomic characteristics and survival of central and peripheral pulmonary large cell neuroendocrine carcinoma: from different origin cells? Lung Cancer. 2018 Feb;116:30–7. PMID:29413048
3514. Zhou J, Zhao J, Zheng J, et al. A prediction model for ROS1-rearranged lung adenocarcinomas based on histologic features. PLoS One. 2016 Sep 20;11(9):e0161861. PMID:27648828
3515. Zhou Q, Han L, Ke X, et al. Ectopic thymoma: retrospective analysis of eight cases with clinical features and computed tomography findings. Clin Imaging. 2020 Apr;60(2):153–9. PMID:31927170
3516. Zhou X, Zhou Y, Zhaoshun Y, et al. Hamartoma of mature cardiomyocytes in right atrium: a case report and literature review. Medicine (Baltimore). 2019 Aug;98(31):e16640. PMID:31374034
3517. Zhou Z, Sehn LH, Rademaker AW, et al. An enhanced International Prognostic Index (NCCN-IPI) for patients with diffuse large B-cell lymphoma treated in the rituximab era. Blood. 2014 Feb 6;123(6):837–42. PMID:24264230
3518. Zhrebker L, Cherni I, Gross LM, et al. Case report: whole exome sequencing of primary cardiac angiosarcoma highlights potential for targeted therapies. BMC Cancer. 2017 Jan 5;17(1):17. PMID:28056866
3519. Zhu B, Laskin W, Chen Y, et al. NUT midline carcinoma: a neoplasm with diagnostic challenges in cytology. Cytopathology. 2011 Dec;22(6):414–7. PMID:21210877
3519A. Zhu E, Xie H, Gu C, et al. Recognition of filigree pattern expands the concept of micropapillary subtype in patients with surgically resected lung adenocarcinoma. Mod Pathol. 2020 Nov 16 [Epub ahead of print]. PMID:33199840
3520. Zhu F, Liu Z, Hou Y, et al. Primary salivary gland-type lung cancer: clinicopathological analysis of 88 cases from China. J Thorac Oncol. 2013 Dec;8(12):1578–84. PMID:24389442
3521. Zhu P, Yan F, Ao Q. Langerhans cells proliferation in ectopic micronodular thymoma with lymphoid stroma: a case report. Int J Clin Exp Pathol. 2014 Sep 15;7(10):7262–7. PMID:25400824
3522. Zhuo M, Guan Y, Yang X, et al. The prognostic and therapeutic role of genomic subtyping by sequencing tumor or cell-free DNA in pulmonary large-cell neuroendocrine carcinoma. Clin Cancer Res. 2020 Feb 15;26(4):892–901. PMID:31694833
3523. Zinzani PL, Martelli M, Poletti V, et al. Practice guidelines for the management of extranodal non-Hodgkin's lymphomas of adult non-immunodeficient patients. Part I: primary lung and mediastinal lymphomas. A project of the Italian Society of Hematology, the Italian Society of Experimental Hematology and the Italian Group for Bone Marrow Transplantation. Haematologica. 2008 Sep;93(9):1364–71. PMID:18603558
3524. Zlotchenko G, Futuri S, Dillon E, et al. A rare case of lymphoma involving the tricuspid valve. J Cardiovasc Comput Tomogr. 2013 May-Jun;7(3):207–9. PMID:23849494
3525. Zon R, Orazi A, Neiman RS, et al. Benign hematologic neoplasm associated with mediastinal mature teratoma in a patient with Klinefelter's syndrome: a case report. Med Pediatr Oncol. 1994;23(4):376–9. PMID:8058011
3526. Zoppo F, Rizzo S, Corrado A, et al. Morphology of right atrial appendage for permanent atrial pacing and risk of iatrogenic perforation of the aorta by active fixation lead. Heart Rhythm. 2015 Apr;12(4):744–50. PMID:25533584
3527. Zu Y, Perle MA, Yan Z, et al. Chromosomal abnormalities and p53 gene mutation in a cardiac angiosarcoma. Appl Immunohistochem Mol Morphol. 2001 Mar;9(1):24–8. PMID:11277410
3528. Zwiebel BR, Austin JH, Grimes MM. Bronchial carcinoid tumors: assessment with CT of location and intratumoral calcification in 31 patients. Radiology. 1991 May;179(2):483–6. PMID:2014296
3529. Zynger DL, Dimov ND, Luan C, et al. Glypican 3: a novel marker in testicular germ cell tumors. Am J Surg Pathol. 2006 Dec;30(12):1570–5. PMID:17122513
3530. Zynger DL, Everton MJ, Dimov ND, et al. Expression of glypican 3 in ovarian and extragonadal germ cell tumors. Am J Clin Pathol. 2008 Aug;130(2):224–30. PMID:18628091

Subject index

Bold page numbers indicate the main discussion(s) of the topic.

inflammatory myofibroblastic tumour   6, 104, 166, 274–275, 286, 288
INI1   *See* SMARCB1
INSM1   135–136, 138, 141, 146, 304, 397
interferon-α   225
interferon-γ   233
International Agency for Research on Cancer (IARC)   3–4, 6, 20, 24, 127, 133, 475
International Association for the Study of Lung Cancer (IASLC)   11–14, 27, 31, 71, 73–74, 218
International Thymic Malignancy Interest Group (ITMIG)   14, 328, 331–332, 335–336, 339–341, 344, 358–360, 363, 372, 379, 383, 385, 387
interstitial pneumonitis   321
intimal sarcoma   2, 164–165, 262–263, 265
intravascular large B-cell lymphoma   3, 174, 184
intravascular lymphoma   174
invasive mucinous adenocarcinoma   2, 30, 32, 58–59, 62–63, 67, **75–78,** 80
invasive non-mucinous adenocarcinoma   2, 27, 55, 59–62, **64,** 68, 75, 100
involucrin   324
IRF4   179, 225, 270, 428, 436, 439
IRS2   140
Isaacs syndrome   321
isochromosome 12p   403, 408, 410, 412, 420, 422–423

J

JAK2   428, 439
Japan Lung Cancer Society (JLCS)   322
juvenile xanthogranuloma   306

K

kaposins   222
Kaposi sarcoma   15, 159, 221, 274
Kaposi sarcoma–associated herpesvirus   *See* HHV8
kappa   176, 183
KDR   258, 300
KEAP1   90–91, 112, 129, 145
keratinizing squamous cell carcinoma   35, 90–93, 100
Kerner–Morrison syndrome   311
Ki-67   36, 46, 67, 87, 91, 127–129, 131, 134–138, 141–142, 145, 147–149, 176, 242, 248, 259, 271, 324, 328, 330, 348, 366, 384, 390, 392–396, 398, 434, 442
KIAA1211   *See* CRACD
KIF5B   67
KIT   92, 117–118, 131, 151, 165, 263, 323–325, 327, 336, 338, 342–343, 348,

351, 355–358, 360, 363, 369, 371, 373, 375–377, 381–382, 384, 386–387, 398, 401, 403–404, 406, 409–410, 423, 433, 444, 455, 464
KL1   211
KLC1   67
KLF17   125
Klinefelter syndrome   400, 408, 412, 415, 418, 422
Klippel–Trénaunay syndrome   252
KMT2   90, 258
KMT2A   427, 433
KMT2D   91, 258
KRAS   26–27, 48, 55, 58, 61, 65–66, 72–73, 75, 77–78, 80, 82, 84, 95, 97, 102, 105, 109, 112, 129, 131, 145, 151, 228, 231, 258, 323, 336, 355, 377, 401–402, 456
Ks20.8   324
KSR1   325

L

L1CAM   197
L26   324
lambda   176, 183
Lambert–Eaton myasthenic syndrome   25, 139
Lambl excrescence   230, 232
laminin   118
LANA1   222
LANA2   222
Langerhans cell histiocytosis   3, 174, 186–187, 189–190, 426
Langerhans cells   186–188, 345–346
langerin   187–188, 190, 346
large cell carcinoma   2, 20–21, 29–31, 35, 91, **97–98,** 103, 109–110, 113, 127, 139, 147–148, 388
large cell neuroendocrine carcinoma   2, 7, 27, 31, 36, 72, 92, 98, 105, 109, 127–128, 134, 136–137, 139, **144–149,** 352, 358, 389–390, 392–393, **397–398**
latency-associated nuclear antigen   221–222, 271
LATS1   208, 308
LATS2   208, 218, 308
LCA   *See* CD45
LCK   433
LDH   224, 226, 401, 404–405, 434–435
leiomyosarcoma   5, 166, 260–261, 264–265, 275, 421
LEOPARD syndrome   305
lepidic   2, 12, 27, 29–30, 32, 35, 49, 51, 57–64, 66–69, 72–73, 76, 78, 234–235, 455, 457
lepidic adenocarcinoma   2, 62–64, 67–69

let-7   161
leukaemia   8, 366, 405, 423, 426, 432–434, 443–444, 468, 474
LewisY   460
lichen planus   321
Li–Fraumeni–like   228, 258
Li–Fraumeni syndrome   65, 274, 472–474
limbic encephalopathy   139, 321
LIN28   409–410
lipofibroadenoma   7, 349
lipoleiomyosarcoma   281
lipoma   5–6, 155, 243–244, 246, 250, 274, **276**
lipomatous hamartoma of the atrioventricular valve   229, 245
lipomatous hypertrophy of the atrial septum   228, 243–244
liposarcoma   6, 109, 214, 244, 265, 276, **280–281,** 291
LKB1   *See* STK11
LMNA   289
LMO   433
LMP1   95, 179–180, 183, 222, 225–226, 271, 435–436
LN3   254
localized mesothelioma   4, 194, 202–203
long QT syndrome   254
loss of heterozygosity   55, 62, 66, 86, 112, 114, 117, 170, 172, 206–207, 301
low-grade papillary adenocarcinoma   7, 352–353, **370–371,** 379
low-molecular-weight cytokeratin   143
LPP   154
Lugano classification   17, 180, 268, 271, 431, 437, 440
LYL1   433
lymphangiectasis   159
lymphangioleiomyomatosis   2, 56, 159, 170–172, 274, 473
lymphangioma   6, 45, 158, 197, 294
lymphangitic carcinomatosis   452–453
lymphoblastic lymphoma   325, 403, 444
lymphocytic interstitial pneumonia   176
lymphoepithelial carcinoma   2, 7, 26, 92, 94–96, 209, 353, 358, 361–363
lymphoepithelial lesions   175–177, 431
lymphomatoid granulomatosis   3, 174, 180–183
Lynch syndrome   320
lysozyme   423, 442, 444
LZTR1   308, 473

M

MAC387   254
Maffucci syndrome   300

The World Health Organization Classification of Tumours

Urinary system and male genital organs
Moch H, Humphrey PA, Ulbright TM, et al., editors. WHO classification of tumours of the urinary system and male genital organs. Lyon (France): International Agency for Research on Cancer; 2016. (WHO classification of tumours series, 4th ed.; vol. 8). https://publications.iarc.fr/540.

Central nervous system
Louis DN, Ohgaki H, Wiestler OD, et al., editors. WHO classification of tumours of the central nervous system. Lyon (France): International Agency for Research on Cancer; 2016. (WHO classification of tumours series, 4th rev. ed.; vol. 1). https://publications.iarc.fr/543.

Head and neck
El-Naggar AK, Chan JKC, Grandis JR, et al., editors. WHO classification of head and neck tumours. Lyon (France): International Agency for Research on Cancer; 2017. (WHO classification of tumours series, 4th ed.; vol. 9). https://publications.iarc.fr/548.

Endocrine organs
Lloyd RV, Osamura RY, Klöppel G, et al., editors. WHO classification of tumours of endocrine organs. Lyon (France): International Agency for Research on Cancer; 2017. (WHO classification of tumours series, 4th ed.; vol. 10). https://publications.iarc.fr/554.

Haematopoietic and lymphoid tissues
Swerdlow SH, Campo E, Harris NL, et al., editors. WHO classification of tumours of haematopoietic and lymphoid tissues. Lyon (France): International Agency for Research on Cancer; 2017. (WHO classification of tumours series, 4th rev. ed.; vol. 2). https://publications.iarc.fr/556.

Skin
Elder DE, Massi D, Scolyer RA, et al., editors. WHO classification of skin tumours. Lyon (France): International Agency for Research on Cancer; 2018. (WHO classification of tumours series, 4th ed.; vol. 11). https://publications.iarc.fr/560.

Eye
Grossniklaus HE, Eberhart CG, Kivelä TT, editors. WHO classification of tumours of the eye. Lyon (France): International Agency for Research on Cancer; 2018. (WHO classification of tumours series, 4th ed.; vol. 12). https://publications.iarc.fr/561.

Digestive system
WHO Classification of Tumours Editorial Board. Digestive system tumours. Lyon (France): International Agency for Research on Cancer; 2019. (WHO classification of tumours series, 5th ed.; vol. 1). https://publications.iarc.fr/579.

Breast
WHO Classification of Tumours Editorial Board. Breast tumours. Lyon (France): International Agency for Research on Cancer; 2019. (WHO classification of tumours series, 5th ed.; vol. 2). https://publications.iarc.fr/581.

Soft tissue and bone
WHO Classification of Tumours Editorial Board. Soft tissue and bone tumours. Lyon (France): International Agency for Research on Cancer; 2020. (WHO classification of tumours series, 5th ed.; vol. 3). https://publications.iarc.fr/588.

Female genital tract
WHO Classification of Tumours Editorial Board. Female genital tumours. Lyon (France): International Agency for Research on Cancer; 2020. (WHO classification of tumours series, 5th ed.; vol. 4). https://publications.iarc.fr/592.

Thorax
WHO Classification of Tumours Editorial Board. Thoracic tumours. Lyon (France): International Agency for Research on Cancer; 2021. (WHO classification of tumours series, 5th ed.; vol. 5). https://publications.iarc.fr/595.

WHO Classification of Tumours Online
The content of this renowned classification series is now also available in a convenient digital format:
https://tumourclassification.iarc.who.int